American Medical Association
Physicians dedicated to the health of America

Health Professions Education Directory

1997-1998

Comments or Inquiries

Fred Donini-Lenhoff
Medical Education Products
American Medical Association
515 N State St
Chicago, IL 60610
312 464-4635
312 464-5830 Fax
E-mail: Fred_Lenhoff@ama-assn.org

Order Information

The *Health Professions Education Directory* is available
for $54.95 ($44.95 AMA members) from
American Medical Association
Order Department OP417597
PO Box 7046
Dover, DE 19903-7046
800 621-8335
312 464-5600 Fax

ISBN 0-89970-834-X
BP19:96-889:5M:5/97

Table of Contents

351 Section III—Institutions Sponsoring Accredited Programs

447 Section IV—Health Professions Education Data

Preface

New This Year

The *1997-1998 Health Professions Education Directory* has been expanded to include program listings, occupational descriptions, and educational program information for six additional professions accredited by five agencies (238 programs total)—the American Art Therapy Association, Commission on Opticianry Accreditation, Commission on Standards and Accreditation of the Council on Rehabilitation Education, Council on Accreditation of the National Recreation and Park Association, and National Association for Schools of Music.

The *Directory* now encompasses

- Nearly 5,000 programs enrolling approximately 150,000 students
- 2,094 sponsoring institutions
- 40 occupations
- 13 accrediting agencies
- Aggregate enrollment, graduate, and attrition data for 3,557 programs, nationally and by state

Organization of the *Directory*

The *Health Professions Education Directory* contains information on accredited educational programs in 40 health professions.

Section I: Health Professions Accreditation provides information on the accreditation of nearly 5,000 health professions education programs accredited by 13 agencies: the Accreditation Council for Occupational Therapy Education, American Art Therapy Association, Commission on Accreditation of Allied Health Education Programs, Commission on Accreditation/Approval for Dietetics Education of The American Dietetic Association, Commission on Dental Accreditation of the American Dental Association, Commission on Opticianry Accreditation, Commission on Standards and Accreditation of the Council on Rehabilitation Education, Council on Academic Accreditation in Audiology and Speech-Language Pathology, Council on Accreditation of the National Recreation and Park Association, Joint Review Committee on Educational Programs in Nuclear Medicine Technology, Joint Review Committee on Education in Radiologic Technology, National Accrediting Agency for Clinical Laboratory Sciences, and National Association for Schools of Music.

Section II: Occupational Descriptions and Educational Programs summarizes the historical development for the majority of the 40 occupations listed and includes occupational descriptions, job descriptions, employment characteristics, and information about educational programs, such as length, curriculum, and educational standards. Section II also provides sources for information on accreditation, program evaluation, careers, certification, licensure, and registration. This information is followed by a complete list of accredited educational programs in alphabetical order by state, for each occupation. The majority of the program listings include the name and address of each educational program, program director's name and telephone/fax numbers, medical director name (if applicable), evening/weekend course availability, class capacity, month(s) classes begin, yearly tuition cost, and academic award(s) granted.

Section III: Institutions Sponsoring Accredited Programs lists 2,094 institutions sponsoring nearly 5,000 health professions education programs. Sponsoring institutions are listed by state and city in alphabetical order. The majority of entries for each institution include the name, address, and telephone number of the chief executive officer and a list of the accredited health education programs for which the institution is a sponsor.

Section IV: Health Professions Education Data summarizes data collected on the Annual Survey of Accredited Health Education Programs conducted by the AMA, with cooperation from accredited programs and 10 of the 13 agencies that accredit health professions education programs.

Mailing Labels

Mailing labels of deans, CEOs, and program directors of professional health educational programs are available from the AMA. Contact Sylvia Etzel at 312 464-4693 for pricing and availability.

Disclaimer

The AMA does not certify or register health personnel and does not recognize or approve certifying agencies. The certifying agencies listed in Section II do not represent an inclusive listing. For more information on certifying agencies, contact the National Organization for Competency Assurance, 1200 19th St NW/Ste 300, Washington, DC 20036; 202 857-1165.

Nondiscriminatory Language

Language used in the *Directory* is intended to promote equal treatment of the sexes. Gender-related words that refer to a group of which women may be a part are intended to refer to both sexes.

Corrections and Suggestions for Improvement

Corrections to the listings of accredited programs or sponsoring institutions in Sections II and III should be made through the 13 accrediting agencies. Information may also be provided to the AMA, Medical Education Products, 515 N State St, Chicago IL 60640; 312 464-4635 or 312 464-5830 (fax).

Acknowledgments

The AMA gratefully acknowledges the cooperative relationships with the 13 health professions accrediting agencies; these relationships and the hard work of accrediting agency staff throughout the year are essential for establishing the survey population and for providing information about accredited programs. The AMA also expresses its deep appreciation for the continued cooperation of program directors, nearly all of whom respond to the Annual Survey of Accredited Health Education Programs.

Acknowledgments are also due to Enza Messineo for survey and data assistance; J.D. Kinney and Suzanne Fraker for assistance in disseminating this product to the various professional, counseling, and health information organizations; Rod Hill for production support; and customer service staff for handling the questions generated by the complexities of this cooperative product.

Fred Donini-Lenhoff, Editor
Maria Gudewicz, Publications Coordinator
Hannah Hedrick, PhD, Director, Medical Education Products

Figure 1. Thirteen accrediting agencies and the 40 occupations for which they accredit programs

Accrediting Agency	Occupations
Accreditation Council for Occupational Therapy Education (ACOTE)	Occupational Therapist Occupational Therapy Assistant
American Art Therapy Association (AATA)	Art Therapist
Commission on Accreditation of Allied Health Education Programs (CAAHEP)	Anesthesiologist Assistant Athletic Trainer Cardiovascular Technologist Cytotechnologist Diagnostic Medical Sonographer Electroneurodiagnostic Technologist Emergency Medical Technician-Paramedic Health Information Administrator Health Information Technician Medical Assistant Medical Illustrator Ophthalmic Medical Technician/Technologist Orthotist/Prosthetist Perfusionist Physician Assistant Respiratory Therapist Respiratory Therapy Technician Specialist in Blood Bank Technology Surgical Technologist
Commission on Accreditation/Approval for Dietetics Education (CAADE) of the American Dietetic Association	Dietetic Technician Dietitian/Nutritionist
Commission on Dental Accreditation (CDA) of the American Dental Association	Dental Assistant Dental Hygienist Dental Laboratory Technician
Commission of Opticianry Accreditation	Ophthalmic Dispensing Optician Ophthalmic Laboratory Technician
Commission on Standards and Accreditation of the Council on Rehabilitation Education	Rehabilitation Counselor
Council on Academic Accreditation in Audiology and Speech-Language Pathology	Audiologist Speech-language Pathologist
Council on Accreditation of the National Recreation and Park Association	Therapeutic Recreation Specialist
Joint Review Committee on Education in Radiologic Technology (JRCERT)	Radiation Therapist Radiographer
Joint Review Committee on Educational Programs in Nuclear Medicine Technology (JRCNMT)	Nuclear Medicine Technologist
National Accrediting Agency for Clinical Laboratory Sciences (NAACLS)	Clinical Laboratory Technician/Medical Laboratory Technician-Associate Degree Clinical Laboratory Technician/Medical Laboratory Technician-Certificate Clinical Laboratory Scientist/Medical Technologist Histologic Technician/Technologist Pathologists' Assistant
National Association for Schools of Music (NASM)	Music Therapist

Section I

Health Professions Accreditation

Section I: Health Professions Accreditation provides a summary description of the following accrediting agencies, as well as descriptions of the occupations for which they accredit programs:

- Accreditation Council for Occupational Therapy Education (ACOTE)
- American Art Therapy Association (AATA)
- Commission on Accreditation of Allied Health Education Programs (CAAHEP)
- Commission on Accreditation/Approval for Dietetics Education of The American Dietetic Association (CAADE)
- Commission on Dental Accreditation of the American Dental Association (CDA)
- Commission on Opticianry Accreditation (COA)
- Commission on Standards and Accreditation of the Council on Rehabilitation Education (CORE)
- Council on Academic Accreditation in Audiology and Speech-Language Pathology (CAA)
- Council on Accreditation of the National Recreation and Park Association (NRPA)
- Joint Review Committee on Educational Programs in Nuclear Medicine Technology (JRCNMT)
- Joint Review Committee on Education in Radiologic Technology (JRCERT)
- National Accrediting Agency for Clinical Laboratory Sciences (NAACLS)
- National Association for Schools of Music (NASM)

Occupational information and program/institution data for five occupations—art therapist, ophtlalmic dispensing optician, ophthalmic laobratory technician, rehabilitation counselor, and therapeutic recreation specialist—appear for the first time in this edition of the *Health Professions Education Directory*. Refer to Figure 1 at left for a complete list of the occupations accredited by the above 13 agencies.

Participating in the *Directory*

Accrediting agencies meeting the criteria described below may participate in the process that results in the publication of educational programs in the *Directory.*

Accrediting agencies, including those that use the term "approve" instead of "accredit," may either

1. participate in the annual Survey of Health Professions Education Programs and agree to subsequent publication of program information in the *Directory* or
2. provide program information for publication in the *Directory.*

To be included in the *Directory*, professions are generally required to meet the following criteria.

Educational programs and credential(s): The profession requires formal postsecondary education through a program in an art, science, or therapy related to health care that meets national standards and that culminates in a certificate, diploma, associate degree, baccalaureate degree, masters degree, doctorate, or post-degree certificate. (Not included are degrees of doctor of medicine, osteopathy, dentistry, veterinary medicine, optometry, podiatry, chiropractic, or clinical psychology; any level of nursing education; any level of pharmacy education; or graduate degrees in public health or health administration.)

Educational programs for the professions in this *Directory* are sponsored by a variety of institutions, including 4-year colleges, universities, academic health centers, and health care institutions. Programs are also sponsored by junior and community colleges, vocational and technical schools, proprietary schools, medical schools, blood banks, consortia, and US government institutions.

Professional responsibility: Members of the profession participate in the delivery of health care, diagnostic and rehabilitation services, therapeutic treatments, or related services, such as

- identifying, evaluating, treating, or preventing diseases or disorders
- providing dietetic and nutrition counseling and services
- promoting healthy behaviors
- providing health maintenance, rehabilitative, or therapeutic services
- managing health or information services
- addressing psychosocial and cognitive needs (music and art therapy)

Recognition of accreditation or approval process: The agency evaluating the educational programs in accordance with national standards developed by the profession must be recognized for that purpose by the US Department of Education, the Council on Recognition of Postsecondary Accreditation, or an equivalent agency.

Educational Standards

To become accredited, programs are assessed for their compliance with national educational standards, which generally state the responsibilities and qualifications of a program director, a medical director, and other program officials and faculty, along with requirements related to curriculum, physical resources, financing, and records. Standards are usually flexible enough to allow educational programs to respond to continuous technological changes.

Definition and Benefits of Accreditation

Accreditation is a process of external peer review in which a private, nongovernment agency or association grants public recognition to an institution or specialized program of study that meets established qualifications and educational standards, as determined through initial and subsequent periodic evaluations. The process encourages educational institutions and programs to continuously evaluate and improve their processes and outcomes. Accreditation helps prospective students identify institutions with programs that meet standards established by and for the field(s) in which they are interested and assists those who wish to transfer from one institution to another. For institutions, accreditation protects against internal and external pressures to modify programs for reasons that are not educationally sound, involves faculty and staff in comprehensive program and institutional evaluation and planning, and stimulates self-improvement by providing national standards against which the institution can evaluate the program it sponsors.

Accreditation also benefits society by providing reasonable assurance of quality educational preparation for professional certification, registration, or licensure. It may be used, along with other considerations, as a basis for determining eligibility for some types of federal assistance and for identifying institutions and programs for the investment of public and private funds.

Collaborative Data Collection and Dissemination Continue

This *Directory* continues to reflect nearly 60 years of cooperation in the complex processes related to allied health and rehabilitation professions' education and accreditation and in efforts to disseminate information about accredited programs to as wide an audience as possible. The current edition comprises 13 agencies accrediting nearly 5,000 educational programs in 41 professions.

For nearly 20 years (1976 to 1994), the American Medical Association (AMA), in collaboration with more than 50 national allied health and rehabilitation professional organizations and medical specialty societies, cooperated with as many as 22 review committees to accredit more than 3,000 programs in 27 professions. That process today is conducted by the accrediting agencies described below, including CAAHEP, which retains 19 of the professions and 17 of the review committees formerly in CAAHEP's predecessor, the CAHEA system (Commission on Allied Health Education and Accreditation). ACOTE, JRCERT, JRCNMT, and NAACLS were formerly a part of that system.

All former members of the CAHEA system participate in the annual survey of accredited programs conducted by the AMA, which requests correct program and institution names, addresses, and personnel; availability of evening/weekend classes; changes in tuition, class capacity, starting date, and credential awarded; and statistics on enrollments, graduates, and attrition by gender. Accrediting agency and AMA staff cooperate in updating the program and institution population in the database, verifying the accuracy of the data, and designing the survey instrument.

Beginning with the 1996-1997 *Directory*, basic program and institution information was also provided for more than 1,300 programs in seven professions accredited by the Commission on Accreditation/Approval for Dietetics Education of The American Dietetic Association, the Commission on Dental Accreditation of the American Dental Association, and the Council on Academic Accreditation in Audiology and Speech-Language Pathology.

For the current edition, five additional agencies agreed to participate in the annual survey and to list the 238 programs they accredit in the *Directory*—the American Art Therapy Association, Commission on Opticianry Accreditation, Commission on Standards and Accreditation of the Council on Rehabilitation Education, Council on Accreditation of the National Recreation and Park Association, and National Association for Schools of Music.

Accreditation Council for Occupational Therapy Education

Structure and Functions

The American Occupational Therapy Association (AOTA) Accreditation Council for Occupational Therapy Education (ACOTE), recognized by the Commission on Recognition of Postsecondary Accreditation (CORPA) and the US Department of Education (ED), is a standing committee of the AOTA Executive Board. ACOTE evaluates professional and technical curricula, reviews and revises the *Essentials and Guidelines for an Accredited Educational Program for the Occupational Therapist* and *Essentials and Guidelines for an Accredited Educational Program for the Occupational Therapy Assistant*, and accredits occupational therapist and occupational therapy assistant programs.

Purpose and Responsibilities

The purposes of the ACOTE accreditation process are to

1. Encourage continuous self-analysis and improvement of the occupational therapy program by representatives of the institution's administrative staff, teaching faculty, students, governing body, and other appropriate constituencies, with the ultimate aim of assuring students of quality education and assuring recipients of services appropriate occupational therapy care.
2. Accredit entry-level occupational therapy educational programs, evaluate other occupational therapy programs as appropriate, and review and revise the *Essentials and Guidelines for an Accredited Educational Program for the Occupational Therapist*

and *Essentials and Guidelines for an Accredited Educational Program for the Occupational Therapy Assistant.*

3. Determine whether the occupational therapy educational program meets the appropriate approved educational standards.
4. Provide counsel and assistance during the accreditation process to the faculty and administrative personnel of the occupational therapy program and the institution in which it is located and to aid them in recognizing the program's strengths and limitations.
5. Encourage faculty to anticipate and accommodate new trends and developments in the practice of occupational therapy that should be incorporated into the educational process.
6. Assure the educational community, general public, and other agencies or organizations that the program has both clearly defined and appropriate objectives, maintains conditions under which these objectives can reasonably be expected to be achieved, appears to be accomplishing them substantially, and can be expected to continue to do so.

Composition

ACOTE consists of 17 members selected from its Roster of Accreditation Evaluators, which includes the chair of ACOTE, and two public members. The AOTA staff liaison serves as member without voting privileges. The 17 members represent professional and technical levels of education and practice (fieldwork experience). To provide for continuity within the agency, not more than one-third of the membership may rotate off the ACOTE in a single year.

The ACOTE Roster of Accreditation Evaluators consists of 95 trained evaluators who do not serve on ACOTE. The Roster includes registered occupational therapists (OTR) and certified occupational therapy assistants (COTA) with expertise in either professional or technical levels of education or practice, three members at large, and six members with administrative experience or special expertise. The Roster is maintained on a 3-year staggered rotational basis. New members are recommended for the Roster by ACOTE. Individuals may self-nominate directly to the Director, Accreditation Department.

ACOTE Members

Ben Atchison, PhD, OTR, FAOTA
Anne K Brown, MS, OTR
Marianne F Christiansen, MA, OTR
Melissa J Dill, MS, OTR
Florence Hannes, MS, OTR
Artice W Harmon, MPH, OTR/L
Stephen L Heater, EdD, OTR/L, FAOTA
Christine L Hischmann, MS, OTR/L
Karla Keller, COTA
Paula Kramer, PhD, OTR, FAOTA
Ronna Linroth, OTR, ROH
Sister Carolita Mauer, MA, OTR/L
Barbara J Natell, MSEd, OTR/L
Karin J Opacich, MHPE, OTR/L, FAOTA
Collins E "Hugh" Smith, Jr, FACHE
Barbara B Sussenberger, MS, OTR
Carol B Traxler, PhD

ACOTE Information

Doris Gordon, MS, MPH, OTR, FAOTA, Director
  Accreditation Department
American Occupational Therapy Association
4270 Montgomery Lane/PO Box 31220
Bethesda, MD 20824-1220
301 652-2682
301 652-7711 Fax

American Art Therapy Association

Structure and Functions

The American Art Therapy Association (AATA) establishes and publishes educational, professional, and ethical standards for art therapy education and practice. It is governed and directed by a nine-member board elected by the membership. AATA committees actively work on governmental affairs, clinical issues, and professional development. The AATA's committment to continuing education and research in art therapy is demonstrated by its annual national conferences and regional symposia, publications, videos, and awards.

The Art Therapy Credentials Board (ATCB), an independent, nonprofit organization, grants postgraduate registration (ATR) after reviewing documentation of completion of graduate education and supervised postgraduate experience. The Registered Art Therapist who successfully completes the written examination administered by the ATCB is qualified as board-certified (ATR-BC). Recertification is required every 5 years by examination or documentation of continuing education credits.

Purpose and Responsibilities

The AATA's mission is to serve its members and the public by providing standards of professional competence and developing and promoting knowledge in, and of, art therapy. The AATA's Education Committee
1. establishes and promotes education standards;
2. supports the development of educational programs and encourages diversity among these programs;
3. fosters communication among educators; and
4. provides information to the public regarding educational standards and opportunities.

AATA Information

Virgina Minar, ATR-BC, President
American Art Therapy Association
1202 Allanson Rd
Mundelein, IL 60060
847 949-6064
847 566-4580 Fax

Commission on Accreditation of Allied Health Education Programs

Structure and Functions

The Commission on Accreditation of Allied Health Education Programs (CAAHEP) is the largest allied health accreditation system in the country, accrediting educational programs in 17 allied health disciplines. CAAHEP is a diverse organization consisting of 85 commissioners from 49 professional allied health organizations and related medical specialty groups, including 17 Committees on Accreditation (CoA). The Commission, creating a system of checks and balances, carries out its chief accreditation and leadership functions through a seven-member Executive Board, a seven-member Council on Accreditation and Recognition (CAR), and leadership from the 17 CoAs.

CAAHEP is incorporated in the State of Illinois as a 501(3)(c) nonprofit agency. From July 1994 through December 1996, the American Medical Association provided modified financial support and management services under contract for CAAHEP. In January 1997, CAAHEP became an independent agency. It is recognized nationally by the Council for Higher Education Accreditation and the US Department of Education (ED) for seven CoAs that perform a federal gatekeeper role: the Accreditation Committee for Perfusion Education, Accreditation Review Committee on Education for the Physician Assistant, Cytotechnology Programs Review Committee, Joint Review Committee on Education in Cardiovascular Technology, Joint Review Committee on Education in Diagnostic Medical Sonography, Joint Review Committee on Education in Electroneurodiagnostic Technology, and Joint Review Committee on Educational Programs for the Emergency Medical Technician-Paramedic. The ED is a federal agency authorized to publish a list of accrediting agencies and associations recognized as reliable authorities on educational quality.

Purposes and Responsibilities

The purposes of CAAHEP are to
1. Promote and support the education of competent and caring allied health professionals and the continued improvement of allied health education programs.
2. Protect, document, and inform the public of the integrity of allied health education programs.
3. Establish standards of accreditation based on professional standards, programmatic self-study, and peer review.
4. Maintain the integrity and ensure the credibility of the process of accrediting allied health education programs.
5. Enhance and promote dialogue among all parties and accrediting agencies in the allied health professions regarding the issues that affect the accreditation of allied health education programs and take a leadership role in coordinating a collective approach to addressing the resolution of problems in the allied health professions.
6. Provide accreditation and related coordination services for allied health education and recognize any bodies offering allied health education programs that meet or exceed established minimum criteria.
7. Compile, analyze, and disseminate information and data on allied health education and accreditation within the allied health educational system.
8. Promote the study of critical issues in allied health education and accreditation and respond to the changing health care needs of society by assisting bodies offering allied health education programs that seek to respond creatively and appropriately to public policy initiatives.

CAAHEP commissioners are responsible for approving CAAHEP bylaws, policies, mission, and vision statements; determining whether a profession is to be recognized as an allied health profession; monitoring CAR's activities related to the development of accreditation standards and accreditation activities to ensure the quality and equity of its accreditation practices; monitoring the application of CAAHEP accreditation standards; maintaining national recognition as an accrediting agency; and securing liability insurance coverage and retaining legal counsel for CAAHEP, its appointed and elected committees, CAR, and all Committees on Accreditation.

CAR is responsible for awarding or denying accreditation in the name of CAAHEP, after reviewing and reaching agreement with the recommendations submitted by a CoA; participating in the establishment of accreditation standards, criteria, policies, and procedures; establishing the criteria for recognizing CoAs and recommending that CAAHEP should recognize a given CoA; establishing quality assurance and improvement criteria for CoAs and monitoring the activities of CoAs; establishing policy, procedures, and practices for standardized, equitable programmatic evaluation; and maintaining confidentiality of information collected during the accreditation review process.

Composition

Figure 2, on page 6, summarizes the three classifications of CAAHEP membership.

CAAHEP Executive Board Members

Kirby H Cox, MNS, President
William W Goding, MEd, RRT
William Horgan, CCP, Secretary
Thomas R Lunsford, MSE, CO
Jerome M Sullivan, MS, RRT, Treasurer
William J Teutsch
Jack Trufant, EdD, Vice President

Council on Accreditation and Recognition

W Chuck Philip, EdD, Chair
David Gale, PhD
Janet Ghigo, R EEG/EP T, Secretary
John E McCarty, PA-C
Maria Piantanida, PhD
Diana Yankowitz, Vice Chair

Commissioners—CoAs and Organizations

Accreditation Committee for Perfusion Education
William J Horgan, CCP

Accreditation Review Committee for the Medical Illustrator
Alice Katz, MS

Accreditation Review Committee on Anesthesiologist's Assistant
Richard Brouillard, MMSc

Accreditation Review Committee on Education for the Physician Assistant
John E McCarty, PA-C

Accreditation Review Committee on Education in Surgical Technology
Margrethe May, MS, CST

American Academy of Anesthesiologists' Assistants
Theresa Green, MS, AA-C, AAAA

American Academy of Cardiovascular Perfusion
Jeri Dobbs

American Academy of Family Physicians
Jerry P Rogers, MD, FAAFP

American Academy of Pediatrics
Leslie C Ellwood, MD, FAAP

American Academy of Physician Assistants
Laura J Stuetzer, MS, PA-C

American Academy of Physical Medicine & Rehabilitation
Jay V S Subbarao, MD, MS

Committee on Accreditation of Specialist in Blood Bank Technology Schools
Jane Mesnard, MS, MT (ASCP) SBB

American Association for Respiratory Care
Jerome M Sullivan, MS, RRT

American Association for Thoracic Surgery
Stanton P Nolan, MD, FACS

American Association of Blood Banks
Carol J Grant, MS, MT (ASCP) SBBB

American Association of Medical Assistants
Nancy L Walters, MT(ASCP), CMA

American Board of Cardiovascular Perfusion
David Ogella, CCP

American Clinical Neurophysiology Society
Lawrence Green, MD

American College of Cardiology
John P Parker, MD

American College of Chest Physicians
A Wallace Conerly, MD, FCCP

American College of Emergency Physicians
David R Johnson, MD, FACEP

American College of Physicians
Raymond Murray, MD

American College of Radiology
Samuel L Hissong, MD, FACR

American College of Surgeons
Fred Luchette, MD

American Health Information Management Association (AHIMA)
Patricia Thierry, MBA, RRA

American Hospital Association
Helen F Heidelbaugh, RN, MS

American Institute of Ultrasound in Medicine
Kenneth J W Taylor, MD, PhD

American Kinesiotherapy Association
Bridget Collins, MS, RKT

American Medical Association
Thomas S Harle, MD

American Orthopaedic Society for Sports Medicine
Robert E Hunter, MD

American Society of Anesthesiologists
Ronald W Dunbar, MD, FASA

American Society of Cytopathology
Barbara Guidos, SCT(ASCP)

American Society of Echocardiography
Keith Comess, MD

American Society of Electroneurodiagnostic Technologists
Janet Ghigo, R EEG/EP T

American Society of Extra-Corporeal Technology
Bruce Bartel, CCP

American Society of Radiologic Technologists
Greg Morrison

American Thoracic Society
Michael Altman, MD, FACS

Association for Anesthesiologists' Assistants Education
James Redford, MD

Association of Medical Illustrators
Mark Pederson, MS

Association of Physician Assistant Programs
Sherry Stolberg

Association of Schools of Allied Health Professions
David D Gale, PhD
Marilyn S Harrington, RDH, PhD
Frances L Horvath, MD
Lindsay L Rettie, EdD
John E Trufant, EdD

Association of Surgical Technologists
William J Teutsch

Association of Technical Personnel in Ophthalmology
Norma Garber, CO, COMT

Committee on Accreditation for Ophthalmic Medical Personnel
Jeanne Kapeller

Council on Accreditation (AHIMA)
Margaret A Skurka, MS, RRA

Curriculum Review Board of the American Association of Medical
    Assistants' Endowment
Julianna S Drumheller, CMA

Cytotechnology Programs Review Committee
Fritz Lin, MD

Hospitals
Jeanne M Clerc, EdD
Carol A Hamer, PhD
Jack Lylis, PhD
Mark H Mattes, JD

Joint Commission on Allied Health Personnel in Ophthalmology
Melvin I Freeman, MD

Joint Review Committee for Respiratory Therapy Education
William W Goding, MEd, RRT

Joint Review Committee on Education in Cardiovascular Technology
Randy Christian, RCPT

Joint Review Committee on Education in Diagnostic Medical
    Sonography
Diana Kawai Yankowitz, RDMS

Joint Review Committee on Education in Electroneurodiagnostic
    Technology
Wendi Nugent, R EEG T, RPSGT

Joint Review Committe on Educational Programs for the
    Emergency Medical Technician-Paramedic
Debra Cason, RN, MS

Joint Review Committee on Educational Programs in Athletic
    Training
Robert S Benke, HSD, ATC

National Athletic Trainers' Association
Larry J Leverenz, PhD

National Commission on Orthotic and Prosthetic Education
Ira Schoenwald, PhD

National Council on State Emergency Medication Services Training
    Coordinators
Liza K Burril

National Network of Health Career Programs in Two-Year Colleges
Kirby H Cox, MNS
John Cromer, PhD
Sondra Flemming, MS
Judy Kilmer, MS, MT
Frederick Law, MD

Orthotists and Prothetists National Office
Thomas R Lunsford, MSE, CO

National Registry of Emergency Medical Technicians
William E Brown, Jr, MS, NREMT-P

Perfusion Program Directors' Council
Patrick F Plunkett, EdD

Society of Cardiovascular Anesthesiologists
Frederick A Hensley, Jr, MD, FAAA

Society of Diagnostic Medical Sonographers
Beth Anderhub, MEd, RT, CNMT, RDMS

Society of Thoracic Surgeons
Walter H Merrill, MD, FACS

Society of Vascular Technology
Robert S McGrath, RN, BSN, RVT

US Department of Defense
Mortimer W Lockett, EdD

US Department of Veterans Affairs
Linda Johnson, PhD

Vocational Technical Education
Jolene K Miller
Carole Stacy

Public Representative
Maria Piantanida, PhD

Public Representative (alternate)
Mary K Garrett, EdD

Student Representative
Susan D Keithley

CAAHEP Information

Commission on Accreditation of Allied Health Education Programs
35 E Wacker Dr/Ste 1970
Chicago, IL 60601-2208
312 553-9355
312 553-9616 Fax
E-mail: 75767,1444@CompuServe.com

CAAHEP Staff

Lawrence M Detmer, MHA, Executive Director
Wendi Williams, MS, Publications Assistant
Anne Wood, Secretary

Membership Classification	Number of Commissioners
Class I	
sponsoring organizations	one
committees on accreditation	one
communities of interest	one
Class II	
educational program sponsors	
4-year institutions (appointed by the Association of Schools of Allied Health Professions)	five
2-year institutions (appointed or elected by the National Network of Health Career Programs in Two-Year Colleges)	five
Class III	
hospitals	four
proprietary institutions; Department of Veterans' Affairs; Department of Defense; and vocational and technical institutions	four
at-large members: one representative each from 4-year and 2-year institutions who are not members of ASAHP or the National Network public representative	three

Fig. 2 Three classifications of CAAHEP membership and the number of commissioners in each classification.

Commission on Accreditation/Approval for Dietetics Education of The American Dietetic Association

Current Accreditation and Approval Activities

The Commission on Accreditation/Approval for Dietetics Education (CAADE) is The American Dietetic Association (ADA) accrediting body for Dietetic Internships, Coordinated Programs, and Dietetic Technician Programs. CAADE also approves Didactic Programs in Dietetics and Preprofessional Practice Programs. Preprofessional Practice Programs (AP4s) will be phased into the accreditation process by 2004.

As stated in the ADA Bylaws, the purpose of CAADE is to protect the public by encouraging high standards for the educational preparation of dietetics professionals and by establishing a quality management process for recognition of dietetics education programs.

Overview of Accreditation and Approval of Dietetics Education Programs

CAADE accredits and approves programs by evaluating their compliance with the Standards of Education. The difference between the accreditation and approval processes for dietetics education programs is that accreditation requires a site visit. Professional peer review is used throughout both processes.

The purpose of both accreditation and approval is to evaluate how effectively an educational program meets stated minimum criteria for educational quality and to encourage program improvements. Programs voluntarily seek accreditation or approval by demonstrating compliance with the stated criteria. Accreditation and approval criteria ensure that the institution or program fulfills responsibilities to students and the profession within the framework of traditions basic to higher education, such as protecting academic and intellectual freedom and encouraging flexibility in program development.

Members of the public are included on the accreditation decision-making body; persons not associated with the profession of dietetics or a dietetics program play an active role in the accreditation decision-making process. Public disclosure of accreditation decisions also is required.

CAADE has chosen to be recognized as an accrediting body by two agencies, the Commission on Recognition of Postsecondary Accreditation (CORPA) and the US Department of Education (ED). CORPA is the nongovernmental body and ED is the governmental body that recognize the authority of CAADE as the accrediting body for dietetics education programs. Recognition by both agencies provides opportunity for interaction with other accrediting bodies and review of CAADE accrediting procedures. Recognition by ED allows students enrolled in CAADE-accredited dietetic internships to qualify for federal funding.

Composition

CAADE consists of the chair, chair-elect, six review panel chairs, and two public members (see list below). In addition, five review panels, composed of educators and practitioners, are responsible for reviewing programs based on policies and procedures developed by the commission. The Review Panel/Site Visitors for Accreditation of Coordinated Programs in Dietetics has one chair and 25 additional members. The Review Panel/Site Visitors for Accreditation of Dietetic Internship Programs has two co-chairs and 52 additional members. The Review Panel/Site Visitors for Accreditation of Dietetic Technician Programs has one chair and 10 additional members. There are two Review Panels for Approval of Didactic Programs in Dietetics, each with one chair and 12 additional members, for a total of 24.

The commission functions as the governing unit and grants final accreditation and approval awards. Its 1997-1998 members are

Chair
Joyce Mooty, EdM, MPH, RD, Renal Dietitian, Mercy Renal Center and Veterans Affairs Medical Center, Detroit, Michigan

Chair-Elect
Kara Caldwell-Freeman, DrPH, RD, Professor, California State Polytechnic University, Pomona, California

Public members
Sharon M McPherron, Executive Director, Craft Alliance, St Louis, Missouri
Glenda Price, PhD, Provost, Spelman College, Atlanta, Georgia

Co-Chair (Review Panel/Site Visitors for Accreditation of Dietetic Internship Programs)
Denise M. Brown, PhD, RD, LD, Assistant Professor, William Carey College, Golf Port, Mississippi

Co-Chair (Review Panel/Site Visitors for Accreditation of Dietetic Internship Programs)
Lt Col Esther F Myers, PhD, RD, Associate Chief, Biomedical Science Corp, US Air Force, Andrews AFB, Maryland

Chair (Review Panel/Site Visitors for Accreditation of Coordinated Programs in Dietetics)
Katherine Y Southworth, MS, RD, LD, CHE, Specialist and Assistant Director, Coordinated Program in Dietetics, University of Texas at Austin, Austin, Texas

Chair (Review Panel/Site Visitors for Accreditation of Dietetic Technician Programs)
Vidya K Kudva, MS, RD, CDE, CNSD, Chief Clinical Dietitian, San Antonio Community Hospital, Alta Loma, California

Chair (Review Panel for Approval of Didactic Programs in Dietetics-A)
Jane K Ross, PhD, RD, Associate Professor, University of Vermont, Burlington, Vermont

Chair (Review Panel for Approval of Didactic Programs in Dietetics-B)
Charlette R Gallagher, PhD, RD, LD, Manager, Geriatrics and Long Term Care Service, Ross Products Division, Columbus, Ohio

CAADE Information
Beverly E Mitchell, MBA, RD
Education and Accreditation Team
Commission on Accreditation/Approval for Dietetics Education
The American Dietetic Association
216 W Jackson Blvd
Chicago, IL 60606-6995
312 899-0040, ext 4872
312 899-4817 Fax
E-mail: bmitche@eatright.org

Commission on Dental Accreditation of the American Dental Association

History

From the early 1940s until 1975, the American Dental Association's Council on Dental Education was the agency recognized as the national accrediting organization for dentistry and dental-related educational programs. On January 1, 1975, the Council on Dental Education's accreditation authority was transferred to the Commission on Accreditation and Dental Auxiliary Educational Programs, an expanded agency established to provide representation of all groups affected by its accrediting activities. In 1979, the name of the Commission was changed to the Commission on Dental Accreditation.

Structure and Functions

Maintaining and improving the quality of dental-related educational programs is a primary aim of the Commission. In meeting its responsibilities as a specialized accrediting agency accepted by the dental profession, the Commission on Recognition of Postsecondary Accreditation, and the US Department of Education, the Commission on Dental Accreditation

- evaluates dental assisting, dental hygiene, and dental laboratory technology education programs based on the extent to which program goals, institutional objectives, and approved accreditation standards are met;

- supports continuing evaluation of and improvements in dental-related educational programs through institutional self-evaluation;
- encourages innovations in program design based on sound educational principles; and
- provides consultation in initial and ongoing program development.

The programs listed in this *Directory* for the occupations of dental assistant, dental hygienist, and dental laboratory technician are conducted in accordance with published accreditation standards. A student who enrolls in and completes any of these programs will be considered a graduate of an accredited program.

If an institution in this *Directory* offers more than one version of its dental assisting or dental laboratory technology program, only the program identified in the directory is accredited by the Commission. All listed programs are conducted at the post-secondary level.

Although other programs may be either under development or in operation, this *Directory* lists only those programs accredited by the Commission as of July 1996.

Composition

The Commission on Dental Accreditation has 20 members:
- four from the American Dental Association (ADA)
- four from the American Association of Dental Schools (AADS)
- four from the American Association of Dental Examiners (AADE)
- two from among the eight dental specialty organizations representing dental public health, periodontics, pediatric dentistry, oral and maxillofacial surgery, endodontics, orthodontics and dentofacial orthopedics, oral pathology, and prosthodontics
- two public members
- one dental student member
- one from the American Dental Hygienists' Association (ADHA)
- one from the American Dental Assistants Association (ADAA)
- one from the National Association of Dental Laboratories (NADL)

Commission Members

The members of the 1996-97 Commission on Dental Accreditation:

David R Myers, DDS (AADAS), chairman
Dennis J Brandstetter, DDS (ADA), vice chairman
Christopher C Babcock (student)
Arnold Baker, DDS (ADA)
Phyllis L Beemsterboer, RDH, EdD (ADHA)
Jack S Broussard, Jr, DDS (ADA)
Donald E Demkee, DDS (AADE)
Patrick J Ferrillo, Jr, DDS, (AADS)
Henry W Fields, Jr, DDS (AADS)
George E Goodboe, CDT (NADL)
Rowland A Hutchinson, DDS (AADS)
Robert W Koch, DDS (ADA)
Ronald J Peterson, DDS (AADE)
Joseph W Rossa, DDS (AADE)
R Gary Rozier, DDS (Dental Public Health)
Thomas J Savage, PhD (Public)
Charles E Tomich, DDS (Oral and Maxillofacial Pathology)
Rose Walls, CDA, MS (ADAA)
James D Watkins, DDS (AADE)

Information

Commission on Dental Accreditation, American Dental Association
211 E Chicago Ave
Chicago, IL 60611-2678
312 440-2718
312 440-2915 Fax
Internet: http://www.ada.org

Commission on Opticianry Accreditation

The Commission on Opticianry Accreditation (COA) was formed in 1979 with the sole purpose of accrediting ophthalmic dispensing optician and ophthalmic laboratory technician educational programs, formerly a function of the National Academy of Opticianry. In 1985, the US Department of Education recognized the commission as the accrediting body for 2-year ophthalmic dispensing and 1-year ophthalmic laboratory technology programs.

Purpose and Responsibilities

The COA develops and maintains standards for ophthalmic dispensing and laboratory technician programs that meet the changing needs of programs, students, and the public. The commission strives to ensure the competence of opticianry professionals and the provision of quality professional care to the public.

The COA's accreditation process certifies that a program has voluntarily undergone a comprehensive study indicating that the program has set appropriate educational objectives for students; that the school performs the functions it claims; and that the school furnishes materials and services to enable students to meet those stated objectives.

Accreditation assures the public that program graduates are skilled practitioners and makes programs eligible for many grants and other funding. In addition, many of the states that license opticians specify graduation from an accredited program as a licensure requirement.

COA Information

Floyd H Holmgrain, Jr, EdD, Executive Director
Commission on Opticianry Accreditation
10111 Martin Luther King Jr Hwy/Ste 100
Bowie, MD 20720-4200
301 459-8075
301 577-3880 Fax

Council on Academic Accreditation in Audiology and Speech-Language Pathology

Accreditation from the Council on Academic Accreditation in Audiology and Speech-Language Pathology is sought voluntarily by educational programs that offer graduate degrees in speech-language pathology, audiology, or both. For more information on the council, contact

Tess Kirsch
Accreditation Program Coordinator
American Speech-Language-Hearing Association (ASHA)
10801 Rockville Pike
Rockville, MD 20852
301 897-5700
301 571-0457 Fax

Council on Accreditation of the National Recreation and Park Association

Structure and Functions

The Council on Accreditation of the National Recreation and Park Association (NRPA), in cooperation with the American Association for Leisure and Recreation (AALR), is authorized by the NRPA Board of Trustees to accredit programs at the baccalaureate level in recreation, therapeutic recreation, park resources, and leisure services. Established in 1974, the Council is recognized by the Commission on Recognition of Postsecondary Accreditation (CORPA). The Council on Accreditation publishes the *Handbook of the NRPA/AALR Accreditation Process*, *Procedural Guidelines for the Accreditation Process*, and *Standards and Evaluative Criteria for Baccalaureate Programs in Recreation, Park Resources and Leisure Services*.

Purpose and Responsibilities

The Council believes that accreditation serves the public by promoting and maintaining standards of professional preparation; assists the academic unit and the institution's administration in establishing and attaining appropriate goals for therapeutic recreation programs; ensures continual self-study for development and improvement of professional preparation programs; and encourages innovation and experimentation within acceptable academic and professional standards.

Accredited programs have undergone a rigorous process of self-assessment and peer review and have met standards established by the profession itself as essential to prepare graduates for competence in entry-level positions in the profession. Programs are reviewed every 5 years to ensure continued compliance with the standards.

Composition

The Council on Accreditation meets twice annually to review accredited programs, revise and update accreditation standards and procedures, and conduct business. The Council consists of 10 members, who are appointed by the two sponsoring organizations—five educators, three practitioners, one college/university administrator, and one public representative. Each member serves a 3-year term.

Information

Jeanne Houghton, Accreditation Coordinator
Council on Accreditation
2775 S Quincy St/Ste 300
Arlington, VA 22206-2236
703 578-5570
703 671-6772 Fax

Council on Rehabilitation Education

Structure and Functions

In 1969, a group of rehabilitation professionals met to discuss the need for accreditation of rehabilitation counselor education (RCE) programs. After 2 years of planning, the Council on Rehabilitation Education (CORE) was formed in 1971 and incorporated in 1972. Five professional rehabilitation organizations were represented by CORE:

- American Rehabilitation Association (ARA), formerly the International Association of Rehabilitation Facilities
- American Rehabilitation Counseling Association (ARCA)
- Council of State Administrators of Vocational Rehabilitation (CSAVR)
- National Council on Rehabilitation Education (NCRE), formerly the Council on Rehabilitation Educators
- National Rehabilitation Counseling Association (NRCA).

Today, these five organizations—except ARA, which has been replaced by the National Council of State Agencies of the Blind (NCSAB)—compose CORE and as such represent the professional and organizational constituencies concerned with the training, evaluation, and employment of rehabilitation counselors.

Purpose and Responsibilities

Each new rehabilitation counseling education program is assessed in accordance with the *Standards for Rehabilitation Counselor Education Programs*, published by CORE, and accredited programs are periodically reviewed to ensure that they remain in substantial compliance. The *Standards* are not intended to limit program creativity or limit variability; programs may adopt innovative procedures or experiences that meet the standards in a different manner.

As stated in the CORE bylaws, the accreditation process serves the following purposes:

- To promote the effective delivery of rehabiltation services by stimulating and fostering continual review and improvement of master's degree rehabilitation counselor educational programs.
- To promote a high standard of professional education in rehabilitation couseling and to foster program development based on a vocationally oriented, service-to-people attitude.
- To encourage sound educational experimentation and innovations and to stimulate continuous self-study and improvement.
- To reassess, redefine, and reevaluate program criteria as the needs of the profession and the public change.
- To evolve a consultative model for developing programs.
- To review admissions and other requirements of RCE programs to ensure that all qualified applicants may participate.
- To foster mutual respect and cooperation between RCE programs and the programs of other helping professions.
- To emphasize the vocational aspect of services in the broader context of human development and thereby help reduce dependency among all vulnerable consumer groups, especially individuals with the most severe and multiple disabilities.
- To meet the personnel needs of public and private rehabilitation agencies.
- To publish periodically a roster of recognized programs for members of the profession, the public, government agencies, and prospective students.
- To enhance the position of mutual respect and acceptance of RCE programs in the academic community and on campus.
- To develop an accreditation system based on the objective assessment of outcomes of the educational program.

Composition

CORE is composed of representatives, appointed to 4-year terms, from each of the five national professional organizations concerned with rehabilitation counseling: ARCA, CSAVR, NCRE, NRCA, and the NCSAB. CORE also has two public members, one who represents the consumer public and one the public at large.

CORE Information

Jeanne Patterson, Executive Director
Council on Rehabilitation Education (CORE)
1835 Rohlwing Rd/Ste E
Rolling Meadows, IL 60008
847 394-1785
847 394-2108 Fax
E-mail: patters@polaris.net

Joint Review Committee on Educational Programs in Nuclear Medicine Technology

Structure and Functions

The Joint Review Committee on Educational Programs in Nuclear Medicine Technology (JRCNMT) was established in 1970 to provide accreditation recognition for educational programs in nuclear medicine technology in collaboration with the American Medical Association. In 1994, the JRCNMT was recognized by the US Department of Education (ED) and the Commission on Recognition of Postsecondary Accreditation (CORPA) as an independent accrediting agency responsible for accrediting nuclear medicine technology programs. The JRCNMT is sponsored by the American College of Radiology, American Society of Radiologic Technologists, Society of Nuclear Medicine, and Society of Nuclear Medicine-Technologist Section.

The JRCNMT reviews and revises the *Essentials and Guidelines for an Accredited Educational Program for the Nuclear Medicine Technologist*, evaluates nuclear medicine technology programs, grants accreditation status to qualified programs, maintains a directory of accredited nuclear medicine technology programs, and publishes accreditation actions to provide information to prospective students, employers, and the public.

Purpose and Responsibilities

The JRCNMT establishes, maintains, and promotes standards of quality for educational programs in nuclear medicine technology to ensure the preparation of skilled professionals, and provides recognition for educational programs that meet or exceed the minimum standards outlined in the *Essentials*. The JRCNMT

1. Establishes appropriate standards through comprehensive review and revision of the *Essentials and Guidelines for an Accredited Educational Program for the Nuclear Medicine Technologist* every 5 years. The JRCNMT conducts formal workshops, invites written comments, and disseminates proposed revisions of the *Essentials* to the community of interest and the public. At the conclusion of the review process, the *Essentials* are submitted to each of the sponsoring organizations for adoption.
2. Provides accreditation recognition for nuclear medicine technology programs that meet or exceed the minimum educational standards. The JRCNMT and its staff provide consultative services to programs seeking initial or continuing reaccreditation. The accreditation process is enhanced by the use of program self-analysis and volunteer peer on-site evaluation. Accreditation actions are reached after consideration of the self-analysis, the onsite evaluation report, and follow-up communication. The JRCNMT disseminates information on accreditation actions to ED, CORPA, and the public. Information on approved educational programs in nuclear medicine technology is also provided to the AMA for publication in this *Directory*.
3. Monitors the outcomes of the educational process on a regular basis. These outcomes are measured by a variety of means including graduates' success in career placement, job satisfaction, employer satisfaction, certification results, and patient satisfaction. The final product of quality educational programs is a graduate qualified to provide skilled professional services to patients.

Composition

The JRCNMT is composed of 14 members—12 professional members representing nuclear medicine and two public members. The selection of members is based on ED requirements and includes practitioners, educators, and public interests.

JRCNMT Members

William L Ashburn, MD
Robert E Henkin, MD (Secretary-Treasurer)
Jack A Ziffer, MD
Barbara Hente, BA, RT-N(ARRT), CNMT (Vice Chair)
Elaine M Markon MS, RT(N), CNMT
Johnny W Scott, MD (Chair)
Patricia Bynum, MEd, RT(R)(N), CNMT
Michael J Blend, PhD, DO
Susan C Weiss, CNMT
Louis N Morgan, PhD
Paul Christian, CNMT
Peter T Kirchner, MD
Sterling R Provost, PhD, Public Member
G Kirk Olsen, Public Member

JRCNMT Information

Elaine Cuklanz, MT(ASCP)NM, Executive Director
Joint Review Committee on Educational Programs in Nuclear Medicine Technology
350 South 400 East/Ste 200
Salt Lake City, UT 84111-2938
801 364-4310
801 364-9234 Fax
E-mail: jrcnmt@lgcy.com

Joint Review Committee on Education in Radiologic Technology

Structure and Functions

The Joint Review Committee on Education in Radiologic Technology (JRCERT) was established in 1969 by the American Society of Radiologic Technologists and the American College of Radiology within the structure for allied health education accreditation provided by the AMA. In 1994, the US Department of Education (ED) recognized the JRCERT as the independent accrediting agency for radiography and radiation therapy education programs. The JRCERT board of directors awards accreditation to programs that are in compliance with federal law and ED regulations, as well as with the *Standards for an Accredited Educational Program in Radiologic Sciences*.

The Value of JRCERT Accreditation

The most significant benefit of JRCERT accreditation is to assure the public that professionals providing radiologic technology services have appropriate knowledge and skills to perform quality diagnostic and therapeutic procedures on patients.

In the broadest sense, accreditation assures acceptable educational quality. The process of accreditation involves an assessment of program quality, and contributes to a continuing enhancement of program operation. The provision of peer review based on national educational standards established by radiologic science professionals and the communities of interest is of utmost importance in this process. Accreditation offers assurance to the public that a program accepts and fulfills its commitment to educational quality.

Accreditation assures prospective students that the programs to which they apply meet educational standards established by radiological science professionals. Accreditation assists students in transferring from one accredited program to another by ensuring a comparable curriculum among programs. Student eligibility for federal financial assistance as well as financial support from states and the private sector can be met through JRCERT program accreditation. Accreditation supports the efforts of national and state certification/licensing agencies in assuring program reliability and validity for professional certification, registration, or licensure activities. Also, graduates of accredited programs are more marketable, as employers can be assured that these graduates possess the necessary knowledge, skills, attributes, and values to competently perform professional tasks.

Business and industry look to programmatic accreditation for quality assurance when financing employee tuition reimbursement, scholarship, and grant programs. Accreditation also identifies institutions and programs for investment of public and private funds.

JRCERT Purpose and Responsibilities

The JRCERT is dedicated to excellence in education and to quality and safety of patient care through the accreditation of educational programs in radiation and imaging sciences. With this objective, the JRCERT joins other organizations in the radiologic sciences to assure the public of quality care as recipients of radiological services.

The JRCERT awards accreditation to educational programs through a peer review process that includes documentation and an on-site visit substantiating compliance with the Educational Standards. The site visitors identified by the JRCERT to evaluate programs are an integral part of the accreditation process. The JRCERT provides training for these volunteer peer evaluators and monitors their performance. The JRCERT board of directors meets periodically to evaluate the documents submitted by the program in pursuit of initial or continuing accreditation, as well as the report of the site visit team. The directors award accreditation to those programs that have demonstrated substantial compliance with accreditation requirements. Once accredited, each program must periodically provide reports, pay fees, and submit to the continuing accreditation process to maintain accreditation.

Composition

The JRCERT is composed of directors meeting the requirements of the US Department of Higher Education Act. The JRCERT maintains majority technologist representation and includes appropriately credentialed professionals in diagnostic radiology, radiography, radiation oncology, and radiation therapy, as well as public representation.

JRCERT Board of Directors

Sarah S Baker, MEd, RT(R), FASRT
Nadia Bugg, PhD, RT(R), FAERS
Donna Dunn, MS, RT(R)
D Gay Lancaster, MS
Paul A Larson, MD

Jordan B Renner, MD
V Amod Saxena, MD, FRCR, FACR
Leroy R Sparks, EdD, RT(R)
Janis Stiewing, MS, RT(R)

JRCERT Information

Marilyn Fay, MA, RT(R), Executive Director
Joint Review Committee on Education in Radiologic Technology
20 N Wacker Dr/Ste 900
Chicago, IL 60606-2901
312 704-5300
312 704-5304 Fax
E-mail: jrcert@mail.idt.net

National Accrediting Agency for Clinical Laboratory Sciences

Structure and Functions

The National Accrediting Agency for Clinical Laboratory Sciences (NAACLS), recognized by the US Department of Education, is a nonprofit organization that independently accredits clinical laboratory science/medical technology, clinical laboratory technician/medical laboratory technician (associate degree and certificate), histologic technician/histotechnologist, and pathologists' assistant programs. NAACLS approves phlebotomy and cytogenetic technology educational programs. NAACLS was established in 1973 as the successor to the American Society of Clinical Pathologists' (ASCP) Board of Schools. ASCP and the American Society for Clinical Laboratory Science (ASCLS) are sponsoring organizations of NAACLS. The National Society for Histotechnology and the Association of Genetic Technologists are participating organizations. The American Association of Pathologists' Assistants is an affiliating organization.

Purpose and Responsibilities

Program Accreditation

Primary aspects of NAACLS' programmatic accreditation process include the self-study and site visit processes, evaluation by a review committee, and evaluation by the NAACLS Board of Directors. Evaluation is based on the *Essentials*, which are the minimum criteria NAACLS uses when awarding programmatic accreditation.

NAACLS conducts various functions of programmatic accreditation, which include:
1. Drafting and reviewing *Essentials* for the operation of educational programs.
2. Selecting knowledgeable volunteers to review Self-Study Reports and to serve as site visitors.
3. Selecting representatives to serve on the review committees and the Board of Directors.
4. Granting accreditation awards based on a program's self-study and site visit processes.

Program Approval

NAACLS' program approval process identifies phlebotomy and cytogenetic technology educational programs that are structured to assure that graduates possess stated career entry-level competencies. Program approval provides this measure of assurance to potential students, prospective employers, and the public. Primary aspects of the NAACLS program approval process are the self-study process, evaluation by the Programs Approval Review Committee (PARC), and evaluation by the Board of Directors. Evaluation is based on *Standards*, which are the minimum criteria NAACLS uses when awarding program approval.

The NAACLS program approval functions include:

1. Drafting and reviewing *Standards* and *Competencies* for the operation of specialized programs.
2. Developing *Guidelines* that explain and interpret the *Standards*.
3. Selecting representatives to serve on the Programs Approval Review Committee and the Board of Directors.
4. Granting approval awards based on a program's self-study process.

Composition

The composition of NAACLS includes three review committees, the Board of Directors, and the executive office staff. The Clinical Laboratory Sciences Programs Review Committee (CLSPRC) reviews clinical laboratory science/medical technology, clinical laboratory technician/medical laboratory technician (associate degree and certificate), and histologic technician/histotechnologist programs for accreditation. The Affiliated Professions Review Committee (APRC) reviews pathologists' assistant programs for accreditation. The Programs Approval Review Committee (PARC) reviews phlebotomy and cytogenetic technology programs for approval. The Board of Directors functions as the governing unit and grants final accreditation and approval awards. The executive office staff facilitates both the accreditation and approval processes.

The CLSPRC is composed of educators and practitioners from the clinical laboratory science disciplines. The APRC has representatives from review committees and members selected by the affiliated profession. The PARC is composed of educators and practitioners representing the disciplines of phlebotomy and cytogenetic technology. All three review committees are represented by a Board of Directors liaison. Members are appointed by the Board of Directors for staggered terms to assure continuity on each committee. The chairman and vice chairman are selected annually by committee members at the summer meeting. Each review committee meets annually, in the winter and summer.

The Board of Directors has 13 members, each serving a term of 4 years or until a successor is chosen. Officers are elected every year at the Board of Directors' fall meeting. The Board of Directors, which meets annually in the spring and fall, includes three clinical laboratory scientists who are active members of and selected by the ASCLS (two clinical laboratory science/medical technology educators and one laboratory administrator); three clinical pathologists, selected by the ASCP, who are fellows or associate members of that organization (two clinical pathologist educators and one laboratory director); two educators, who are neither clinical laboratory scientists nor physicians, one of whom is employed by a community or junior college and one by a senior college, elected by the board; two public representatives, whose primary livelihoods are not derived from the laboratory industry, elected by the board; one representative practitioner, who is a clinical laboratory science technician (associate degree or certificate), elected by the board; and one member selected by each participating organization from among its active members.

Board of Directors

Cynthia Wells, EdD, CLS(NCA), MT(ASCP), President
Joeline D Davidson, MBA, CLS(NCA), Vice President
Dorryl L Buck, Jr, MD
Constance L Churchill, PhD
Richard J De Luca, MPH, MA
Barbara Douglas, MLT(ASCP)
H Elise Galloway, PhD, MS, MT(ASCP)
Edwin B Herring, MD
David Anderson Hooker, MA, MPA, MPH, JD

Michael Laposata, MD, PhD
Frederick W Pairent, PhD
John Ryan, MBA, HT/HTL(ASCP)
Peggy Stupca, MS, CLSp(CG), CLSup

Clinical Laboratory Sciences Programs Review Committee (CLSPRC)

Lucille Contois, MA, MT(ASCP), Chairman
Katherine Nisi Zell, EdS, MT(ASCP)SH, Vice Chairman
Shauna Anderson, PhD, MT(ASCP)C, CLS
Sue G Barr, EdD, MT(ASCP)
Betty Craft, EdD, MT(ASCP), CLS(NCA)
Norton I German, MD
Jean Holter, EdD
Rhoda P Levin, MS
Sergey Lyubsky, MD, PhD
Phyllis Ann Muellenberg, MA, MT(ASCP)
Susan M Reynolds, MA, HTL(ASCP)
Shirley Richmond, EdD, MT(ASCP)
Mary Jean Rutherford, MEd, MT(ASCP)SC
Cecile Sanders, MEd, MT(ASCP)
Mary Christine Steuterman, MD
Peggy A Wenk, BS, HTL(ASCP)

Programs Approval Review Committee (PARC)

Halcyon St Hill, EdD, MS, MT(ASCP), CLS(NCA), Chairman
Betty Dunn, MS, CLSp(CG), Vice Chairman
Benna Boutty, MA, MT(ASCP)
Helen M Jenks, MT(ASCP), CLSp(CG)
Virginia Narlock, PhD, CLS(NCA), MT(ASCP)
Susan E Phelan, MHS, MT(ASCP)
Irene Roeckel, MD
Kathryn L Smith, CLPlb(NCA), PBT(ASCP)

Affiliated Professions Review Committee (APRC)

Jerry Phipps, Path Asst, Chairman
Charles W Ford, PhD
Irene E Roeckel, MD
Steven Suvalsky, BSMT, MHS

NAACLS Information

Olive M Kimball, EdD, Executive Director
National Accrediting Agency for Clinical Laboratory Sciences
8410 W Bryn Mawr Ave/Ste 670
Chicago, IL 60631-3415
773 714-8880 Phone
773 714-8886 Fax
E-mail: NAACLS@mcs.net
Internet: http://www.mcs.net/~naacls

National Association of Schools of Music

Structure and Functions

The National Association of Schools of Music (NASM) was founded in 1924 to secure a better understanding among institutions of higher education engaged in work in music (including music therapy); to establish a more uniform method of granting credit; and to set minimum standards for granting degrees and other credentials. In 1975, representatives of member institutions agreed to create a category of membership for nondegree-granting institutions. The services of NASM are available to all types of degree-granting institutions in higher education and to nondegree-granting institutions offering preprofessional programs or general music training programs. Membership in NASM is voluntary.

NASM is recognized by the US Department of Education (ED) as the agency responsible for accrediting all music curricula.

Purpose and Responsibilites

NASM works to

- provide a national forum for the discusson and consideration of concerns relevant to the preservation and advancement of standards in the field of music in higher education;
- develop a national unity and strength to maintain the position of music study in the family of fine arts and humanities in universities, colleges, and schools of music;
- maintain professional leadership in music training and develop a national context for the artist's professional growth;
- establish minimum achievement standards in music curricula without restricting an administration or school in its freedom to develop new ideas, to experiment, or to expand its program;
- recognize that inspired teaching may rightly reject a status quo philosophy; and
- establish that the prime objective of all educational programs in music is to provide the opportunity for every music student to develop individual potential to the utmost.

Composition

NASM is composed of three commissions, the board of directors, and the executive office staff. The NASM board of directors is composed of the officers (president, vice president, treasurer, secretary, executive director [ex officio], and nine regional chairs) as well as the immediate past president, the chair and the associate chair of the Commission on Accreditation, the chairs of the Commission on Community/Junior College Accreditation and Non-Degree-Granting Accreditation, and three public members.

NASM Board of Directors

President
Harold Best, Wheaton College

Vice President
William Hipp, University of Miami

Treasurer
Karen L Wolff, Oberlin College Conservatory of Music

Secretary
Dorothy Payne, University of South Carolina

Immediate Past President
Robert J Werner, University of Cincinnati

Chair, Commission on Non-Degree-Granting Accreditation
Deborah Berman, San Francisco Conservatory of Music

Chair, Commission on Community/Junior College Accreditation
Lynn Asper, Grand Rapids Community College

Chair, Commission on Accreditation
Joyce J Bolden, Alcorn State University

Associate Chair, Commission on Accreditation
Daniel Sher, University of Colorado at Boulder

Regional Chairs
Donald Para, California State University, Long Beach
Erich Lear, Washington State University
Jim Cargill, Black Hills State University
Judith Kritzmire, University of Minnesota, Duluth
Edwin L Williams, Ohio Northern University

Ronald Lee, University of Rhode Island
Charlotte Collins, Shenandoah University
Peter Ciurczak, University of Southern Mississippi
Annette Hall, University of Arkansas at Monticello

Public Members
Leandra G Armour, Nashville, Tennessee
Christie K Bohner, Alexandria, Virginia
Cindy Boyd, Dallas, Texas

Ex Officio
Samuel Hope, NASM Executive Director

NASM Information

Karen P Moynahan, Associate Director
National Association of Schools of Music
11250 Roger Bacon Dr/Ste 21
Reston, VA 22090
703 437-0700
703 437-6312 Fax
E-mail: kpmnasm@aol.com

Section II

Occupational Descriptions and Educational Programs

Section II—Occupational Descriptions and Educational Program Information—summarizes the historical development of each of the allied health occupations for which programs are accredited. Occupational descriptions, job descriptions, employment characteristics, and information about educational programs, including length, curriculum, and educational standards, are provided for the majority of professions listed.

Section II also includes a brief list of information sources for accreditation, program evaluation, careers, certification, licensure, and registration. This information is followed by a list of accredited educational programs in alphabetical order, by state, then city, for each occupation. Each of the program listings includes the name and address of the educational program; name and telephone number of the program director, as well as fax number and e-mail address, where available; name of the medical director; class capacity; month(s) classes begin; yearly tuition cost; academic award(s) granted; availability of evening/weekend courses; and clinical affiliates, where applicable.

Inquiries regarding information about a specific educational program should be made directly to program officials.

Anesthesiologist Assistant

History

Anesthesiologist assistant (AA) educational programs began in 1969 at Case Western University in Cleveland, Ohio, and at Emory University in Atlanta, Georgia. The impetus for these new programs was task analysis studies showing the increased need for anesthetists with technical backgrounds. Although the Case Western curriculum was originally designed toward a baccalaureate degree, both programs currently award a master's degree for successful completion of their program.

In 1975, the American Society of Anesthesiologists (ASA) took action in support of this new emerging profession, on the basis of its review of the educational and clinical objectives. In 1976, the ASA petitioned the American Medical Association (AMA) Council on Medical Education (CME) for recognition of the anesthesiologist assistant as an emerging health profession. The CME's recognition followed in 1978. This authorized the initiation of a collaborative activity between the AMA's Division of Allied Health Education and Accreditation and the ASA on the development of a body of educational Standards.

In 1981, ASA withdrew from this collaborative activity with the CME owing to internal differences of opinion and the ASA's desire not to appear preferential to AAs over other members of the anesthesia care team. This action prompted members of the ASA who strongly supported the AA programs to establish a new physician-sponsoring group called the Association for Anesthesiologists' Assistants Education (AAAE).

In 1983, the AAAE and the American Academy of Anesthesiologists' Assistants (AAAA) petitioned the CME to recognize them as collaborative sponsors for the programs designed to educate the anesthesiologist assistant. In 1984, the CME reinstated AMA's recognition of anesthesiologist assistants, and in 1987, *Standards* for the education of the AA were adopted by the AMA, the AAAE, and the AAAA. The Emory and Case Western programs were evaluated and initially accredited by the Committee on Allied Health Education and Accreditation (CAHEA) in 1988, and continue to be fully accredited by the Commission on Accreditation of Allied Health Education Programs, CAHEA's successor organization.

Occupational Description

Anesthesiologist assistants function under the direction of a licensed and qualified anesthesiologist, principally in medical centers. The AA assists the anesthesiologist in developing and implementing the anesthesia care plan. This may include collecting preoperative data, such as taking an appropriate health history; performing various preoperative tasks, such as the insertion of intravenous and arterial catheters and special catheters for central venous pressure monitoring, if necessary; performing airway management and drug administration for induction and maintenance of anesthesia; assisting in the administering and monitoring of regional and peripheral nerve blockade; administering supportive therapy, for example, with intravenous fluids and cardiovascular drugs; adjusting anesthetic levels on a minute-to-minute basis; performing intraoperative monitoring; providing recovery room care; or functioning in the intensive care unit. The anesthesiologist assistant may also be used in pain clinics or may participate in administrative and educational activities.

Job Description

In addition to the duties described in the occupational description above, anesthesiologist assistants provide other support according to established protocols. Such activities may include pretesting anesthesia delivery systems and patient monitors and operating special monitors and support devices for critical cardiac, pulmonary, and neurological systems. Anesthesiologist assistants may be involved in the operation of bedside electronic computer-based monitors and have supervisory responsibilities for laboratory functions associated with anesthesia and operating room care. They provide cardiopulmonary resuscitation in association with other anesthesia care team members and in accordance with approved emergency protocols.

Employment Characteristics

Anesthesiologist assistants work as members of the anesthesia care team in any locale where they may be appropriately directed by legally responsible anesthesiologists. AA anesthetists most often work within organizations that also employ nurse anesthetists, and their responsibilities are usually identical. Experience has shown that AAs are most commonly employed in larger facilities that perform procedures such as cardiac surgery, neurosurgery, transplant surgery, and trauma care, given the training in extensive patient monitoring devices and complex patients and procedures emphasized in AA educational programs. However, anesthesiologist assistants are used in hospitals of all sizes and assist anesthesiologists in a variety of settings and for a wide range of procedures. Starting salaries are in the $60,000 to $70,000 range for the 40-hour work week plus benefits and consideration of on-call activity.

Educational Programs

Length. These postbaccalaureate programs are essentially 2 years.
Prerequisites. The programs require an undergraduate premedical background (premedical courses in biology, chemistry, physics, and math) and a baccalaureate degree. Although any baccalaureate major is acceptable (if premedical requirements are met), majors typically are biology, chemistry, physics, mathematics, computer science, or one of the allied health professions, including respiratory therapy, medical technology, or nursing.
Standards. *Standards* are minimum educational standards adopted by the collaborating organizations. Each applicant program is assessed for its relative compliance with the *Standards*. Once accredited, programs are reviewed periodically to determine whether they continue to meet the *Standards*. The *Standards* are available

on written request from the Accreditation Review Committee for the Anesthesiologist Assistant, in care of Theresa Green.

Inquiries

Accreditation

Requests for information on program accreditation, including the *Standards*, preparing the self-study report, and arranging a site visit, should be submitted to

Theresa Green, AA-C (ARC-AA)
Department of Anesthesiology
University Hospitals
11000 Euclid Ave
Cleveland, OH 44106

Careers

Curriculum inquiries should be directed to the individual programs. Inquiries regarding anesthesiologist assistant careers should be directed to

American Academy of Anesthesiologists' Assistants
PO Box 33876
Decatur, GA 30033-0876
800 757-5858

Certification

Inquiries on certification should be directed to

National Commission for Certification of Anesthesiologist Assistants
PO Box 15519
Atlanta, GA 30333-0519

Anesthesiologist Assistant

Georgia

Emory University

Anesthesiologist Asst Prgm
School of Medicine
475 Woodruff Memorial Bldg
Atlanta, GA 30322
Prgm Dir: Wesley T Frazier, MD
Tel: 404 727-5910
Class Cap: 60   *Begins:* Jun
Length: 27 mos   *Award:* Dipl, MMSc
Tuition per yr: $12,600

Ohio

Case-Western Reserve University

Anesthesiologist Asst Prgm
11100 Euclid Ave
Cleveland, OH 44106
Prgm Dir: James E Redford, MD
Tel: 216 844-8077   *Fax:* 216 844-3781
Class Cap: 10   *Begins:* Jun
Length: 24 mos   *Award:* MS
Tuition per yr: $18,000

Art Therapist

History

Although visual expressions have been basic to humanity throughout history, art therapy did not emerge as a distinct profession until the 1930s. At the beginning of the 20th century, psychiatrists became interested in and began studying artwork done by patients to see if there might be a link between a patient's art and his/her illness. At this same time, art educators were discovering that the free and spontaneous art expression of children represented both emotional and symbolic communications.

Educator and psychotherapist Margaret Naumburg is considered the founder of art therapy as a separate profession in the United States. The profession's first journal, the *Bulletin of Art Therapy* (today the *American Journal of Art Therapy*), was published in 1961. The American Art Therapy Association (AATA) was founded in 1969. The AATA sponsors annual conferences and regional symposia, approves educational programs, and publishes *ART THERAPY: Journal of the American Art Therapy Association* (first published in 1983). In the 1970s, the first graduate degrees in art therapy were awarded; today, college curricula across the country include undergraduate introductory courses and preparatory programs in art therapy, as well as 27 master's degree programs approved by the AATA.

The AATA establishes and publishes standards for art therapy education, ethics, and practice. AATA committees actively work on governmental affairs, clinical issues, and professional development. The AATA's committment to continuing education and research in art therapy is demonstrated by its annual national conferences and regional symposia, publications, videos, and awards.

Occupational Description

Art therapy is a human service profession that uses art media, images, the creative art process, and patient/client responses to the artwork as reflections of an individual's development, abilities, personality, interests, concerns, and conflicts. Art therapy, through the nonverbal qualities of art media, can help individuals access and express memories, trauma, and intrapsychic conflict often not easily reached with words. Art therapy helps individuals reconcile their emotions, foster self-awareness, increase self-esteem, develop their social skills, manage behavior, solve problems, and reduce anxiety.

Job Description

Art therapists use drawings and other art/media forms to assess, treat, and rehabilitate patients with mental, emotional, physical, and/or developmental disorders. Art therapists use and facilitate the art process, providing materials, instruction, and structuring of tasks tailored either to individuals or groups. Using their skills of assessment and interpretation, they understand and plan the appropriateness of materials applicable to the client's therapeutic needs.

With the growing acceptance of alternative therapies and increased scientific understanding of the link between mind, body, and spirit, art therapy is becoming more prevalent as a parallel and supportive therapy for almost any medical condition. For example, art therapists work with cancer, burn, pain, HIV-positive, asthma, and substance abuse patients, among others, in pediatric, geriatric, and other settings.

Art therapists also maintain appropriate charts, records, and periodic reports on patient progress as required by agency guidelines and professional standards; participate in professional staff meetings and conferences; and provide information and consultation regarding the client's clinical progress. They also may function as supervisors, administrators, consultants, and expert witnesses.

Programs

An art therapist must be sensitive to human needs and expressions and possess emotional stability, patience, a capacity for insight into psychological processes, and an understanding of art media. An art therapist also must be an attentive listener and keen observer and be able to develop a rapport with people. Flexibility and a sense of humor are important in adapting to changing circumstances, frustration, and disappointment.

Employment Characteristics

Art therapists work in private offices, art rooms, or meeting rooms in facilities such as medical and psychiatric hospitals, outpatient facilities, clinics, residential treatment centers, day treatment centers, rehabilitation centers, halfway houses, shelters, schools and universities, correctional facilities, elder-care facilities, pain clinics, and art studios.

The art therapist may work as part of a team that includes physicians, psychologists, nurses, rehabilitation counselors, social workers, and teachers. Together, they determine and implement a client's therapeutic, school, or mental health program. Art therapists also work as primary therapists in private practice.

Earnings for art therapists vary depending on type of practice, job responsibilities, and practice location. Entry-level income is approximately $25,000, median income between $28,000 and $38,000, and top earning potential for salaried administrators between $40,000 and $60,000. Art therapists who possess doctoral degrees or state licensure or who qualify in their state to conduct a private practice can earn $75 to $90 per hour in private practice.

Registration and Certification

The Art Therapy Credentials Board (ATCB), an independent, nonprofit organization, grants postgraduate registration (ATR) after reviewing documentation of completion of graduate education and supervised postgraduate experience. The Registered Art Therapist who successfully completes the written examination administered by the ATCB is qualified as board certified (ATR-BC). Recertification is required every 5 years by examination or by documentation of continuing education credits.

Educational Programs

Length. Art therapy masters' degree programs are no less than 2 years and must include a minimum of 21 graduate credit hours in the art therapy core curriculum.

Prerequisites. Applicants must hold a baccalaureate degree from an accredited US institution or have equivalent academic preparation from an institution outside the United States. In addition, prospective students must submit a portfolio of original artwork and must document 15 semester hours in studio art and 12 semester hours in psychology.

Curriculum. The core curriculum for art therapy includes history, theory, and practice techniques of art therapy; psychopathology; assessment of patients and diagnostic categories; and practice standards, ethical and legal issues, and matters of cultural diversity related to art therapy.

Standards. The *Education Standards* published by the AATA describe the standards by which graduate-level art therapy programs may apply to the AATA Education Program Approval Board (EPAB) for approval. Each new art therapy education program is assessed in accordance with the *Education Standards*, and approved programs are periodically reviewed to ensure that they remain in substantial compliance.

Inquiries

Education, Program Approval, Careers, Resources

Requests for information on education, program approval, careers, and resources should be directed to

American Art Therapy Association
1202 Allanson Rd
Mundelein, IL 60060
847 949-6064
847 566-4580 Fax
E-mail: estygariii@aol.com
Internet: http://www.arttherapy.org

Registration/Certification

Requests for information on registration/certification should be directed to

Art Therapy Credentials Board
401 N Michigan Ave
Chicago, IL 60611
312 527-6764
312 644-1815 Fax

Art Therapist

Canada

Concordia University

Art Therapist Prgm
1455 de Maisonneuve Blvd
West Montreal, QU H3G 1M8
Prgm Dir: Leland Peterson, MA ATR
Tel: 514 848-4643
Award: MA

California

College of Notre Dame

Art Therapist Prgm
1500 Ralston Ave
Belmont, CA 94002
Prgm Dir: Doris Arrington, EdD ATR-BC
Tel: 415 508-3556   *Fax:* 415 508-3736
E-mail: daarin@cnd.edu
Class Cap: 35   *Begins:* Sep Jan May
Length: 36 mos   *Award:* MAT , MFT
Evening or weekend classes available

Loyola Marymount University

Art Therapist Prgm
Grad Dept of Marital and Family Therapy
7900 Loyola Blvd
Los Angeles, CA 90045-8215
Prgm Dir: Debra Lineach, ATR-BC
Tel: 310 338-4562
Class Cap: 20   *Begins:* Aug
Length: 24 mos, 36 mos   *Award:* MA
Tuition per yr: $12,000 res, $12,000 non-res

District of Columbia

George Washington University

Art Therapist Prgm
2129 G St NW
Bldg L
Washington, DC 20052
Prgm Dir: Katherine J Williams, ATR-BC
Tel: 202 994-6285   *Fax:* 202 994-1404
E-mail: kathwagw1s2.circ.gwu.edu
Class Cap: 25   *Begins:* Sep
Length: 24 mos, 48 mos   *Award:* Dipl, MA
Tuition per yr: $12,889 res, $12,889 non-res
Evening or weekend classes available

Illinois

School of the Art Institute of Chicago

Art Therapist Prgm
Dept of Art Educ and Art Therapy
112 S Michigan Ave
Chicago, IL 60603
Prgm Dir: Randy M Vick, ATR-BC
Tel: 312 345-3516   *Fax:* 312 541-8063
E-mail: rvick@artic.edu
Class Cap: 30   *Begins:* Sep
Length: 20 mos   *Award:* MA
Tuition per yr: $17,760 res, $17,760 non-res
Evening or weekend classes available

Univ of Illinois at Chicago

Art Therapist Prgm
929 W Harrison St
M/C 036
Chicago, IL 60607
Prgm Dir: Harriet Wadeson, PhD ATR-BC HLM
Tel: 312 996-5728   *Fax:* 312 413-2333
Class Cap: 16   *Begins:* Sep
Length: 24 mos   *Award:* MA
Tuition per yr: $4,748 res, $11,002 non-res

Southern Illinois Univ at Edwardsville

Art Therapist Prgm
Box 1764
Dept of Art and Design
Edwardsville, IL 62026-1764
Prgm Dir: P Gussie Klorer, PhD ATR-BC, LCPC
Tel: 618 692-3183   *Fax:* 618 692-3106
Class Cap: 10   *Begins:* Aug
Length: 24 mos   *Award:* MA
Tuition per yr: $2,160 res, $6,480 non-res
Evening or weekend classes available

Kansas

Emporia State University

Art Therapist Prgm
1200 Commercial
Emporia, KS 66801
Prgm Dir: Nancy Knapp, ATR-BC
Tel: 316 343-5807   *Fax:* 316 341-5785
Class Cap: 20   *Begins:* Sep
Length: 24 mos   *Award:* MS
Tuition per yr: $1,840 res, $4,740 non-res
Evening or weekend classes available

Kentucky

University of Louisville

Art Therapist Prgm
Expressive Therapies Program
Gardiner Hall 331
Louisville, KY 40292
Prgm Dir: Abby Calisch, PsyD ATR-BC
Tel: 502 852-5265   *Fax:* 502 852-4598
E-mail: accali01@ulkyum.louisville.edu
Class Cap: 18   *Begins:* Aug
Length: 17 mos   *Award:* MA
Tuition per yr: $3,430 res, $9,738 non-res
Evening or weekend classes available

Massachusetts

Lesley College

Art Therapist Prgm
Expressive Therapies
29 Everett St
Cambridge, MA 02138
Prgm Dir: Julia Byers, ATR
Tel: 617 349-8436   *Fax:* 617 349-8431
E-mail: jbyers@mail.lesley.edu
Class Cap: 70   *Begins:* Aug
Length: 24 mos, 36 mos   *Award:* MA
Tuition per yr: $7,900

Michigan

Wayne State University

Art Therapist Prgm
163 Community Arts Bldg
Detroit, MI 48202
Prgm Dir: Holly Feen-Calligan, ATR-BC
Tel: 313 577-0490   Fax: 313 577-4091
Class Cap: 25   *Begins:* Sep
Length: 28 mos, 32 mos   *Award:* MEd
Tuition per yr: $2,700

Missouri

St Louis Institute of Art Psychotherapy

Art Therapist Prgm
308A N Euclid
St Louis, MO 63108
Prgm Dir: Mary N St Clair, ATR-BC
Tel: 314 367-8550   *Fax:* 314 367-4998
Class Cap: 12   *Begins:* Sep Jan Jun
Length: 16 mos   *Award:* Cert
Tuition per yr: $8,100
Evening or weekend classes available

New Mexico

University of New Mexico

Art Therapist Prgm
Art Education/Art Therapy
Albuquerque, NM 87131-1236
Prgm Dir: Linney Wix, ATR
Tel: 505 277-4112   *Fax:* 505 277-8362
Class Cap: 15   *Begins:* Aug
Length: 30 mos   *Award:* MA
Tuition per yr: $1,710 res, $6,000 non-res
Evening or weekend classes available

New York

Pratt Institute

Art Therapist Prgm
200 Willoughby Ave
East 3
Brooklyn, NY 11205
Prgm Dir: Laurel Thompson, MPS,ADTR,ATR-BC
Tel: 718 636-3428   *Fax:* 718 636-3597
Class Cap: 24   *Begins:* Aug
Length: 24 mos   *Award:* MPS
Tuition per yr: $14,898 res, $14,898 non-res

Long Island Univ - C W Post Campus

Art Therapist Prgm
720 Northern Blvd
Brookville, NY 11548
Prgm Dir: David R Henley, ATR
Tel: 516 299-2464   *Fax:* 516 299-2858
Class Cap: 10   *Begins:* Sep Jan
Length: 24 mos   *Award:* MA
Tuition per yr: $11,480 res, $11,480 non-res
Evening or weekend classes available

Programs

Hofstra University

Art Therapist Prgm
Counseling, Research, Spec Ed and Rehab
212 Mason Hall/124 Hofstra University
Hempstead, NY 11550-1090
Prgm Dir: Beth Gonzalez-Dolginko, ATR-BC
Tel: 516 463-5755   *Fax:* 516 754-2278
E-mail: cprbgd@vaxc.hofstra.edu
Class Cap: 25   *Begins:* Sep Jan
Length: 24 mos   *Award:* MA, MS
Tuition per yr: $10,000
Evening or weekend classes available

College of New Rochelle

Art Therapist Prgm
29 Castle Pl
New Rochelle, NY 10805
Prgm Dir: Patricia St John, ATR-BC
Tel: 914 654-5280   *Fax:* 914 654-5593
Class Cap: 30   *Begins:* Sep Jan May Jul
Length: 24 mos   *Award:* MS
Tuition per yr: $7,296 res, $7,296 non-res
Evening or weekend classes available

New York University

Art Therapist Prgm
34 Stuyvesant St
New York, NY 10003
Prgm Dir: Laurie Wilson, PhD ATR-BC
Tel: 212 998-5727   *Fax:* 212 995-4320
Class Cap: 22   *Begins:* Sep
Length: 24 mos   *Award:* MAT
Tuition per yr: $13,650 res, $13,650 non-res
Evening or weekend classes available

Nazareth College of Rochester

Art Therapist Prgm
4245 East Ave
Rochester, NY 14618-3790
Prgm Dir: Ellen G Horovitz, ATR MA
Tel: 716 389-2815   *Fax:* 716 586-2452
E-mail: eghorovi@naz.edu
Class Cap: 14   *Begins:* Sep
Length: 24 mos   *Award:* MS
Tuition per yr: $8,910 res, $8,910 non-res
Evening or weekend classes available

Ohio

Ursuline College

Art Therapist Prgm
2550 Lander Rd
Pepper Pike, OH 44124
Prgm Dir: S Kathleen Burke, OSU PhD ATR LPC
Tel: 216 646-8139   *Fax:* 216 449-3180
Class Cap: 20   *Begins:* Aug Jan Jun
Length: 24 mos   *Award:* MAT
Tuition per yr: $10,192 res, $10,192 non-res
Evening or weekend classes available

Oregon

Marylhurst College

Art Therapist Prgm
Marylhurst, OR 97036
Prgm Dir: Christine Turner, ATR-BC
Tel: 503 699-6244   *Fax:* 503 636-1957
Class Cap: 16   *Begins:* Sep
Length: 21 mos   *Award:* Cert, MAT
Evening or weekend classes available

Pennsylvania

Allegheny University of the Health Sciences

Art Therapist Prgm
Broad and Vine Sts
Mail Stop 905
Philadelphia, PA 19102-1192
Prgm Dir: Nancy Gerber, MS ATR-BC
Tel: 215 762-6925   *Fax:* 215 762-6933
E-mail: gerber@allegheny.edu
Begins: Aug
Length: 24 mos, 48 mos   *Award:* Dipl, MA
Tuition per yr: $5,800 res, $5,800 non-res

Marywood College

Art Therapist Prgm
Art Dept
2300 Adams Ave
Scranton, PA 18509
Prgm Dir: Bruce Moon, ATR
Tel: 717 348-6278
Class Cap: 15   *Begins:* Sep Jan Jun
Length: 24 mos   *Award:* Cert, MA
Tuition per yr: $9,600
Evening or weekend classes available

Vermont

Vermont College of Norwich University

Art Therapist Prgm
Montpelier, VT 05602
Prgm Dir: Gladys Agell, PhD ATR-BC HLM
Tel: 802 828-8810   *Fax:* 802 828-8585
E-mail: gagell@norwich.edu
Class Cap: 20   *Begins:* Jun
Length: 15 mos   *Award:* MAAT
Tuition per yr: $5,550

Virginia

Eastern Virginia Medical School

Art Therapist Prgm
PO Box 1980
Norfolk, VA 23501
Prgm Dir: Trudy Manning Rauch, ATR-BC
Tel: 757 446-5895   *Fax:* 757 446-5918
E-mail: art@picar.evms.edu
Class Cap: 15   *Begins:* Aug
Length: 24 mos   *Award:* MS
Tuition per yr: $13,500 res, $13,500 non-res

Wisconsin

Mt Mary College

Art Therapist Prgm
2900 N Menomonee River Pkwy
Milwaukee, WI 53222
Prgm Dir: Lynn Kapitan, ATR
Tel: 414 256-1215   *Fax:* 414 245-1205
Class Cap: 18   *Begins:* June
Length: 24 mos   *Award:* MS
Tuition per yr: $15,075
Evening or weekend classes available

Athletic Trainer

History

Work on establishing standards for athletic training educational programs was initiated in 1959 by the National Athletic Trainers' Association (NATA). In 1969, the NATA Committee on Curriculum Development approved the first two programs. By 1979, there were 23 undergraduate programs and two graduate programs approved by NATA. In 1982, the NATA Certification Committee completed a role delineation study that led to the NATA Professional Education Committee's development of an entry-level list of competencies. Another role-delineation study was conducted in 1990, resulting in a 1990 revision of the athletic training entry-level competencies. A third role-delineation study was completed in 1994. By 1996, NATA had approved 84 entry-level and 14 graduate athletic training educational programs.

During 1989, the NATA, through its Professional Education Committee, applied to the American Medical Association (AMA) Council on Medical Education (CME) for recognition of athletic training as an allied health occupation. Recognition was granted on June 22, 1990.

In October 1990, an initial meeting was conducted for the development of the *Standards (Essentials)* for accreditation of educational programs for athletic trainers. Individuals attending that meeting represented the AMA's Division of Allied Health Education and Accreditation (DAHEA), the American Academy of Pediatrics (AAP), the American Academy of Family Physicians (AAFP), the American Orthopaedic Society for Sports Medicine (AOSSM), and the NATA.

In late 1991, the *Standards* were adopted by the AMA CME and the sponsors of the Joint Review Committee on Educational Programs in Athletic Training (JRC-AT), including the AAFP, AAP, and NATA. In January 1995, the AOSSM also became a cosponsor of the JRC-AT. As of January 1997, all *Standards* are adopted by the Commission on Accreditation of Allied Health Education Programs (CAAHEP) in conjunction with CAAHEP Committees on Accreditation and sponsoring organizations.

Occupational Description

The athletic trainer, with the consultation and supervision of attending and/or consulting physicians, is an integral part of the health-care system associated with physical activity and sports. Through preparation in both academic and practical experience, the athletic trainer provides a variety of services, including injury prevention, recognition, immediate care, treatment, and rehabilitation after physical trauma.

Job Description

Role delineation studies conducted by the profession in 1982, 1990, and 1994 concluded that the role of an athletic trainer includes, but may not be limited to, six major domains: prevention, recognition and evaluation, management and treatment, rehabilitation, organization and administration, and education and counseling.

Employment Characteristics

Athletic trainers typically provide their services in one or more of the following settings: secondary schools, colleges and universities, professional athletic organizations, industry, and private or hospital-based clinics.

According to the NATA, entry-level salaries in 1994 averaged $22,750.

Educational Programs

Length. Baccalaurcate degree programs require 4 years of study. Postbaccalaureate programs are generally 1 to 2 years.

Prerequisites. Applicants for the 4-year baccalaureate degree programs should have a high school diploma or equivalent and meet institutional entrance requirements. Applicants for postbaccalaureate programs should have a baccalaureate degree that includes appropriate course work and clinical experience, as specified by the institution.

Curriculum. The professional curriculum includes formal instruction in prevention and evaluation of athletic injuries and illnesses, first aid and emergency care, therapeutic exercise, administration of athletic training programs, human anatomy, human physiology, exercise physiology, kinesiology and biomechanics, nutrition, psychology, and personal and community health. The curriculum also includes a series of structured laboratory and clinical experiences.

Standards. *Standards* are minimum educational standards developed by the NATA, AAP, AAFP, AOSSM, and AMA. Each new program is assessed in accordance with the *Standards and Guidelines of an Accredited Educational Program for the Athletic Trainer*, and accredited programs are reviewed periodically to determine whether they remain in compliance. The *Standards and Guidelines* are available on written request from the Joint Review Committee on Educational Programs in Athletic Training.

Inquiries

Accreditation

Requests for information on program accreditation, including *Standards*, preparing the self-study report, and arranging a site visit, should be submitted to

Joint Review Committee on Educational Programs in
Athletic Training (JRC-AT)
School of Health and Human Performance
Rm C-33 Arena
Indiana State University
Terre Haute, IN 47809
812 237-3026
812 237-4338 Fax

Careers

Inquiries regarding careers should be addressed to

National Athletic Trainers' Association, Inc
2952 Stemmons Frwy/Ste 200
Dallas, TX 75247
214 637-6282 (1-800-TRY-NATA)
214 637-2206 Fax

Certification

Inquiries regarding certification may be addressed to

NATA Board of Certification
3725 National Dr/Ste 213
Raleigh, NC 27612
919 787-5321
919 781-3186 Fax

Athletic Trainer

Alabama

University of Alabama
Athletic Trainer Prgm
Area of Professional Studies
PO Box 870312
Tuscaloosa, AL 35487-0312
Prgm Dir: Kenneth E Wright, DA ATC
Tel: 205 348-8683 *Fax:* 205 348-4707
Med Dir: James B Robinson, MD
Class Cap: 45 *Begins:* Aug
Length: 36 mos *Award:* BS
Tuition per yr: $3,263 res, $4,954 non-res

California

California State University - Northridge
Athletic Trainer Prgm
18111 Nordhoff St
Northridge, CA 91330-8287
Prgm Dir: Alice J McLaine, MS ATC
Tel: 818 677-3205 *Fax:* 818 677-3207
E-mail: alice.mclaine@email.esun.edu
Med Dir: Eric Sletten, MD
Class Cap: 14 *Begins:* Sep Jan
Length: 36 mos *Award:* BA
Tuition per yr: $958 res, $1,204 non-res

California State University - Sacramento
Athletic Trainer Prgm
CSUS 6000 J St
Sacramento, CA 95819
Prgm Dir: Doris E Fennessy Flores, MS
Tel: 916 278-6401 *Fax:* 916 278-7664
Class Cap: 40 *Begins:* Aug
Length: 36 mos *Award:* BS
Tuition per yr: $1,860

Colorado

University of Northern Colorado
Athletic Trainer Prgm
Sch of Kinesiology and Phys Ed
Butler-Hancock 124
Greeley, CO 80639
Prgm Dir: Dan Libera, ATC
Tel: 970 351-2822 Fax: 970 351-1762
Med Dir: Aaron Parkhurst, MD
Class Cap: 16 *Begins:* Aug
Length: 40 mos *Award:* BA
Tuition per yr: $2,920 res, $8,606 non-res

Connecticut

Southern Connecticut State University
Athletic Trainer Prgm
501 Crescent St
New Haven, CT 06515
Prgm Dir: Sharon P Misasi, MS NATAC
Tel: 203 392-6091 *Fax:* 203 392-6093
E-mail: misasi@scsud.ctstateu.edu
Med Dir: William Lewis, MD
Class Cap: 40 *Begins:* Aug
Length: 36 mos *Award:* BS
Tuition per yr: $3,128 res, $8,220 non-res
Evening or weekend classes available

Delaware

University of Delaware
Athletic Trainer Prgm
Bob Carpenter Center
Newark, DE 19716
Prgm Dir: Keith A Handling, MS ATC PT
Tel: 302 831-2287 *Fax:* 302 831-8653
Med Dir: Kevin N Waninger, MD
Class Cap: 32 *Begins:* Sep
Length: 27 mos *Award:* BS
Tuition per yr: $3,690 res, $10,220 non-res

Florida

Barry University
Athletic Trainer Prgm
11300 NE 2nd Ave
Miami Shores, FL 33161-6695
Prgm Dir: Carl R Cramer, EdD RKT ATC
Tel: 305 899-3497 *Fax:* 305 899-3556
E-mail: cramer@dominic.barry.edu
Med Dir: Philip R Lozman
Class Cap: 15 *Begins:* Jan May Jun Sep
Length: 48 mos *Award:* BS
Tuition per yr: $12,790 res, $12,790 non-res
Evening or weekend classes available

Georgia

Valdosta State University
Athletic Trainer Prgm
Dept of HPEA
Valdosta, GA 31698
Prgm Dir: James A Madaleno, MS
Tel: 912 333-7161 *Fax:* 912 333-5972
E-mail: jmadalen@grits.valdosta.peachnet.edu
Class Cap: 16 *Begins:* Sep
Length: 18 mos *Award:* BS
Tuition per yr: $1,887 res, $5,097 non-res
Evening or weekend classes available

Idaho

Boise State University
Athletic Trainer Prgm
Dept of HPER/G-209
1910 University Dr
Boise, ID 83725
Prgm Dir: John McChesney, MS ATC
Tel: 208 385-1570 *Fax:* 208 385-1894
Class Cap: 28 *Begins:* Sep
Length: 48 mos *Award:* BS
Tuition per yr: $1,876 res, $6,062 non-res

Illinois

Southern Illinois Univ at Carbondale
Athletic Trainer Prgm
Southern Illinois University
Dept of Physical Education
Carbondale, IL 62901-4310
Prgm Dir: Sally A Perkins, ATC/L
Tel: 618 453-5482 *Fax:* 618 453-5152
E-mail: sallyatc@siu.edu
Med Dir: Rollin Perkins, MD
Class Cap: 13 *Begins:* Aug
Length: 18 mos, 36 mos *Award:* Dipl, BS
Tuition per yr: $2,400 res, $7,200 non-res

Eastern Illinois University
Athletic Trainer Prgm
Lantz Training Rm
Charleston, IL 61920
Prgm Dir: Rob Doyle, PhD AT C/R
Tel: 217 581-3811 *Fax:* 217 581-6434
E-mail: cfrd@eiu.edu
Med Dir: Joseph D Wall, MD
Class Cap: 35 *Begins:* Aug
Length: 31 mos *Award:* Dipl, BS
Tuition per yr: $2,905 res, $7,009 non-res

Univ of Illinois at Urbana - Champaign
Athletic Trainer Prgm
Dept of Kinesiology/209 Freer Hall
906 S Goodwin Ave
Urbana, IL 61801-3895
Prgm Dir: Gerald W Bell, EdD PT ATC/L
Tel: 217 333-7699 *Fax:* 217 244-7322
E-mail: g-bell@uiuc.edu
Med Dir: Pam Kulinna, MA
Class Cap: 12 *Begins:* Aug
Length: 33 mos *Award:* BS
Tuition per yr: $4,168 res, $10,468 non-res

Indiana

Anderson University
Athletic Trainer Prgm
1100 E 5th St
Anderson, IN 46012-1362
Prgm Dir: Steven D Risinger, BA MA ATC
Tel: 317 641-4491 *Fax:* 317 641-4491
Med Dir: Stephen Hampton, MD
Class Cap: 28 *Begins:* Sep
Length: 27 mos *Award:* Dipl, BA
Tuition per yr: $11,040 res, $11,040 non-res
Evening or weekend classes available

Ball State University

Athletic Trainer Prgm
HP 222
Muncie, IN 47306
Prgm Dir: Michael S Ferrara, PhD
Tel: 317 285-5128   *Fax:* 317 285-8254
E-mail: mferrara@wa.bsu.edu
Begins: Aug
Length: 24 mos, 36 mos   *Award:* BS
Tuition per yr: $2,864 res, $4,380 non-res

Purdue University

Athletic Trainer Prgm
Dept of HKLS
1362 Lambert
West Lafayette, IN 47907
Prgm Dir: Larry J Leverenz, PhD
Tel: 317 494-3167   *Fax:* 317 496-1239
E-mail: llevere@purdue.edu
Med Dir: Stephen F Badylak, MD PhD
Class Cap: 10   *Begins:* Aug
Length: 27 mos   *Award:* BA
Tuition per yr: $1,604 res, $5,318 non-res

Iowa

University of Iowa

Athletic Trainer Prgm
110 CHA
Iowa City, IA 52242-1020
Prgm Dir: Danny T Foster, PhD ATC
Tel: 319 335-9393   *Fax:* 319 335-9398
E-mail: danny-foster@uiowa.edu
Med Dir: John P Albright, MD
Class Cap: 16   *Begins:* Aug Jan Jun
Length: 29 mos   *Award:* BS
Tuition per yr: $2,470 res, $9,068 non-res
Evening or weekend classes available

Kansas

Kansas State University

Athletic Trainer Prgm
364 Bluemont Hall
Manhattan, KS 66506-0302
Prgm Dir: Jeffrey P Rudy, BS MS ATC
Tel: 913 532-6991   *Fax:* 913 532-7358
Begins: Aug Jan
Length: 28 mos   *Award:* BS
Tuition per yr: $1,210 res, $4,272 non-res

Kentucky

Eastern Kentucky University

Athletic Trainer Prgm
Alumni Coliseum 128
Richmond, KY 40475
Prgm Dir: Eva Clifton, MA
Tel: 606 622-2134   *Fax:* 606 622-1230
E-mail: phecliftehcs.eku.edu
Med Dir: Mary Lloyd Ireland, MD
Class Cap: 14   *Begins:* Aug
Length: 48 mos   *Award:* Dipl, BS
Tuition per yr: $1,980 res, $5,450 non-res

Massachusetts

Bridgewater State College

Athletic Trainer Prgm
School of Education
Allied Studies
Bridgewater, MA 02325
Prgm Dir: Marcia Anderson, PhD ATC
Tel: 508 697-1215   *Fax:* 508 697-1717
E-mail: mkandrerson@bridgew.edu
Med Dir: Joseph F Zabilski, MD
Class Cap: 14   *Begins:* Sep
Length: 36 mos   *Award:* BS
Tuition per yr: $704 res, $2,771 non-res
Evening or weekend classes available

Springfield College

Athletic Trainer Prgm
Allied Health Science Center
Springfield, MA 01109
Prgm Dir: Charles J Redmond, MEd MSPT
Tel: 413 748-3231   *Fax:* 413 748-3371
Class Cap: 120   *Begins:* Sep
Length: 48 mos   *Award:* BS
Tuition per yr: $10,368 res, $10,368 non-res

Michigan

Grand Valley State University

Athletic Trainer Prgm
One Campus Dr
Allendale, MI 49401
Prgm Dir: Deborah J Springer, MA BS
Tel: 616 895-3140   *Fax:* 616 895-3838
E-mail: springed@gvsu.edu
Class Cap: 10   *Begins:* Sep Jan
Length: 36 mos   *Award:* Cert
Tuition per yr: $2,700 res, $6,200 non-res
Evening or weekend classes available

Central Michigan University

Athletic Trainer Prgm
Sports Medicine Curriculum
Rose 145
Mt Pleasant, MI 48859
Prgm Dir: David A Kaiser, EdD ATC
Tel: 517 774-6687   *Fax:* 517 774-5391
E-mail: david.kaiser@cmich.edu
Class Cap: 26   *Begins:* Aug Jan
Length: 36 mos   *Award:* Dipl, BS
Tuition per yr: $2,302 res, $5,977 non-res
Evening or weekend classes available

Minnesota

Mankato State University

Athletic Trainer Prgm
MSU Box 28
PO Box 8400
Mankato, MN 56002-8400
Prgm Dir: Kent K Kalm, EdD ATC/R
Tel: 507 389-6715   *Fax:* 507 389-6447
Class Cap: 32   *Begins:* Sep
Length: 24 mos   *Award:* BS
Tuition per yr: $2,242 res, $4,867 non-res

Gustavus Adolphus College

Athletic Trainer Prgm
800 W College Ave
St Peter, MN 56082
Prgm Dir: Gary D Reinholtz, MA ATC
Tel: 507 933-7612   *Fax:* 507 933-8412
E-mail: gdratcr.gac.edu
Med Dir: Alan Markman, MD
Class Cap: 16   *Begins:* Sep
Length: 36 mos   *Award:* BA
Tuition per yr: $15,350 res, $15,350 non-res

Mississippi

University of Southern Mississippi

Athletic Trainer Prgm
Sch of Human Performance and Recreation
Hattiesburg, MS 39406-5142
Prgm Dir: James B Gallaspy, MEd
Tel: 601 266-5577   *Fax:* 601 266-4668
Class Cap: 60   *Begins:* Aug
Length: 36 mos   *Award:* BS
Tuition per yr: $1,196 res, $2,426 non-res

Missouri

Southwest Missouri State University

Athletic Trainer Prgm
Sports Med & Athletic Train Curriculum
Springfield, MO 65804
Prgm Dir: Karen R Toburen, EdD ATC
Tel: 417 836-8553   *Fax:* 417 836-6905
E-mail: krt858f@wpgate.smsu.edu
Med Dir: Richard A Seagrave, MD
Class Cap: 30   *Begins:* Aug
Length: 32 mos   *Award:* BS
Tuition per yr: $2,888 res, $5,558 non-res
Evening or weekend classes available

New Hampshire

University of New Hampshire

Ahtletic Trainer Prgm
Dept of Physical Education
145 Main St/Field House
Durham, NH 03824
Prgm Dir: Daniel R Sedory, MS ATC
Tel: 603 862-1831   *Fax:* 603 862-0154
Med Dir: Gary Kish, MD
Class Cap: 50   *Begins:* Sep
Length: 6 mos   *Award:* BS
Tuition per yr: $4,880

New Jersey

William Paterson College

Athletic Trainer Prgm
300 Pompton Rd
Wayne, NJ 07470
Prgm Dir: David Middlemas, MA ATC
Tel: 201 595-2267   *Fax:* 201 595-2034
Med Dir: Alan E Schultz, MD
Class Cap: 24   *Begins:* Sep
Length: 48 mos   *Award:* BS
Tuition per yr: $1,500 res, $1,976 non-res

Programs

New Mexico

New Mexico State University
Athletic Trainer Prgm
Box 30001/Dept 3SMC
Las Cruces, NM 88003-0001
Prgm Dir: Leah Putnam, MS ATC
Tel: 505 646-5038   *Fax:* 505 646-4065
Class Cap: 40   *Begins:* Aug
Length: 32 mos   *Award:* BS
Tuition per yr: $2,188 res, $6,798 non-res

New York

Canisius College
Athletic Trainer Prgm
2001 Main St
Buffalo, NY 14208-1098
Prgm Dir: Peter Koehneke, MS ATC
Tel: 716 888-2954   *Fax:* 716 888-3219
E-mail: koehneke@canisius.edu
Med Dir: Joseph Cervi, MD
Class Cap: 15   *Begins:* Aug
Length: 45 mos   *Award:* BS
Tuition per yr: $12,600 res, $12,600 non-res

SUNY College at Cortland
Athletic Trainer Prgm
Box 2000
Cortland, NY 13045
Prgm Dir: John Cottone, EdD ATC
Tel: 607 753-4962   *Fax:* 607 753-4929
E-mail: cottoneJ@syncorva.edu
Class Cap: 30   *Begins:* Sep
Length: 30 mos   *Award:* Cert
Tuition per yr: $3,400 res, $8,300 non-res

North Carolina

Appalachian State University
Athletic Trainer Prgm
Hlth Leisure and Exercise Sci
Boone, NC 28608
Prgm Dir: Jamie Moul, EdD ATC
Tel: 704 262-3140   *Fax:* 704 262-3138
E-mail: mouljl@apstate.edu
Class Cap: 12   *Begins:* Aug Jan
Length: 32 mos   *Award:* BS
Tuition per yr: $802 res, $4,044 non-res

East Carolina University
Athletic Trainer Prgm
ECU-Sports Medicine Div
245 Ward Sports Medicine Bldg
Greenville, NC 27858
Prgm Dir: Katie W Walsh, EdD ATC
Tel: 919 328-4560   *Fax:* 919 328-4537
Med Dir: John Siegel, MD
Class Cap: 40   *Begins:* Aug
Length: 18 mos   *Award:* BS
Tuition per yr: $1,620 res, $8,515 non-res

High Point University
Athletic Trainer Prgm
University Station
Montlieu Ave
High Point, NC 27262
Prgm Dir: Rick Proctor, BS MAT ATC
Tel: 910 841-9267   *Fax:* 910 841-9182
E-mail: rproctor@acme.highpoint.edu
Class Cap: 15   *Begins:* Aug Jan
Length: 18 mos   *Award:* Dipl, BS
Tuition per yr: $8,230

North Dakota

University of Mary
Athletic Trainer Prgm
7500 University Dr
Bismarck, ND 58504-9652
Prgm Dir: T Mic McCrory, MEd LATC
Tel: 701 255-2500   *Fax:* 701 255-7687
Med Dir: Jeffrey Smith, MD
Class Cap: 36   *Begins:* Aug
Length: 36 mos   *Award:* Dipl, BS
Tuition per yr: $7,230 non-res
Evening or weekend classes available

North Dakota State University
Athletic Trainer Prgm
Bison Sports Arena
Fargo, ND 58105-5600
Prgm Dir: Elise L Erickson, MS L/ATC
Tel: 701 231-8093   *Fax:* 701 231-8022
Med Dir: Lee A Christoferson Jr, MD
Class Cap: 39   *Begins:* Aug
Length: 38 mos   *Award:* BS
Tuition per yr: $1,947 res, $5,198 non-res

Univ of N Dakota Sch of Med and Hlth Sci
Athletic Trainer Prgm
Div of Sports Medicine
Box 9013
Grand Forks, ND 58202-9013
Prgm Dir: James D Rudd, MS ATC
Tel: 701 777-3102   *Fax:* 701 777-4352
Med Dir: William Mann, MD
Class Cap: 45   *Begins:* Aug
Length: 36 mos   *Award:* BS
Tuition per yr: $2,428 res, $5,952 non-res

Ohio

Capital University
Athletic Trainer Prgm
Troutman Hall
2199 E Main St
Columbus, OH 43209
Prgm Dir: Russ Hoff, MS ATC
Tel: 614 236-6569   *Fax:* 614 236-6178
E-mail: rhoff@capital.edu
Class Cap: 10   *Begins:* Aug
Length: 14 mos, 21 mos   *Award:* BA
Tuition per yr: $14,200 res, $14,200 non-res

Marietta College
Athletic Trainer Prgm
215 Fifth St
Marietta, OH 45750
Prgm Dir: Paul Spear, RN BS MS
Tel: 614 376-4772   *Fax:* 614 376-4896
Med Dir: David Lacey, MD
Class Cap: 40   *Begins:* Aug
Length: 16 mos   *Award:* BS
Tuition per yr: $14,450
Evening or weekend classes available

University of Toledo
Athletic Trainer Prgm
2801 W Bancroft St
Toledo, OH 43606
Prgm Dir: James M Rankin, PhD ATC
Tel: 419 530-2752   *Fax:* 419 530-4759
Med Dir: Roger J Kruse, MD
Class Cap: 30   *Begins:* Sep
Length: 27 mos   *Award:* BS, BE
Tuition per yr: $3,398 res, $8,147 non-res

Oregon

Oregon State University
Athletic Trainer Prgm
Langton Hall 226
Corvallis, OR 97331-3302
Prgm Dir: Rod A Harter, PhD ATC
Tel: 541 737-6801   *Fax:* 541 737-2788
E-mail: harterr@ccmail.orst.edu
Med Dir: Richard V Cronk, MD
Class Cap: 18   *Begins:* Sep
Length: 18 mos   *Award:* Dipl, BS
Tuition per yr: $3,347 res, $11,085 non-res

Pennsylvania

East Stroudsburg University
Athletic Trainer Prgm
200 Prospect St
East Stroudsburg, PA 18301
Prgm Dir: John R Thatcher, MEd ATC
Tel: 717 422-3065   Fax: 717 424-3306
Class Cap: 40   *Begins:* Sep
Length: 48 mos   *Award:* BS
Tuition per yr: $3,224 res, $8,198 non-res

Messiah College
Athletic Trainer Prgm
Grantham, PA 17027
Prgm Dir: Edwin A Bush, MS ATC
Tel: 717 691-2511   *Fax:* 717 691-6044
Med Dir: Thomas Yucha, MD
Class Cap: 10   *Begins:* Aug
Length: 9 mos   *Award:* BA
Tuition per yr: $5,435

Lock Haven University
Athletic Trainer Prgm
Himes 116
Lock Haven, PA 17745
Prgm Dir: David J Tomasi, ATC
Tel: 717 893-2214   *Fax:* 717 893-2650
Med Dir: John H Bailey, MD
Class Cap: 15   *Begins:* Aug
Length: 18 mos   *Award:* Dipl, BS
Tuition per yr: $3,368 res, $8,566 non-res
Evening or weekend classes available

Temple University
Athletic Trainer Prgm
Philadelphia, PA 19122
Prgm Dir: Michael R Sitler, EdD ATC
Tel: 215 204-1950 *Fax:* 215 204-8705
Class Cap: 24 *Begins:* Sep
Length: 48 mos *Award:* BS
Tuition per yr: $5,086 res, $9,662 non-res

Duquesne University
Athletic Trainer Prgm
123 Health Sciences Bldg
Pittsburgh, PA 15282
Prgm Dir: Paula S Turocy, EdD ATC
Tel: 412 396-5695 *Fax:* 412 396-5554
E-mail: sammaron@dug2.cc.dug.edu
Class Cap: 30 *Begins:* Sep
Length: 36 mos *Award:* Dipl, BS
Tuition per yr: $14,486
Evening or weekend classes available

Slippery Rock University
Athletic Trainer Prgm
Allied Health Dept
Slippery Rock, PA 16057
Prgm Dir: Bonnie Jo Siple, MS ATC
Tel: 412 738-2930
Med Dir: R Kreider, MD
Class Cap: 40 *Begins:* Aug
Length: 36 mos *Award:* BS
Tuition per yr: $3,224 res, $8,198 non-res

West Chester University
Athletic Trainer Prgm
Department of Sports Medicine
West Chester, PA 19383
Prgm Dir: Neil Curtis, EdD ATC
Tel: 610 436-2969 *Fax:* 610 436-2803
E-mail: ncurtis@wcupa.edu
Class Cap: 24 *Begins:* Aug
Length: 45 mos *Award:* BS
Tuition per yr: $3,368 res, $8,566 non-res

South Carolina

University of South Carolina
Athletic Trainer Prgm
Blatt Physical Education Center
Columbia, SC 29208
Prgm Dir: Malissa Martin, EdD ATC
Tel: 803 777-7301 *Fax:* 803 777-6250
Med Dir: Robert Peele, MD
Class Cap: 40 *Begins:* Aug *Award:* BS
Evening or weekend classes available

Texas

Texas Christian University
Athletic Trainer Prgm
PO 32909
Ft Worth, TX 76129
Prgm Dir: T Ross Bailey, BS MEd LAT CAT
Tel: 817 921-7984 *Fax:* 817 921-7323
E-mail: r.bailey@tcu.edu
Med Dir: Bert Franks, MD
Class Cap: 5 *Begins:* Aug
Length: 10 mos *Award:* BS
Tuition per yr: $7,000

Utah

Brigham Young University
Athletic Trainer Prgm
212 Richards Bldg
Provo, UT 84602
Prgm Dir: Gaye Merrill, MS ATC
Tel: 801 378-4670 *Fax:* 801 378-3665
E-mail: gaye_merrill@byu.edu
Med Dir: Darrell Stacey, MD
Class Cap: 40 *Begins:* Sep Jan
Length: 32 mos *Award:* BS
Tuition per yr: $2,520 res, $3,800 non-res
Evening or weekend classes available

Vermont

University of Vermont
Athletic Trainer Prgm
Sports Therapy
Patrick Gymnasium
Burlington, VT 05405
Prgm Dir: Denise M Alosa, ATC
Tel: 802 656-7678 *Fax:* 802 656-0949
E-mail: dalosa@zoo.uvm.edu
Med Dir: Michael E Sargent, MD
Class Cap: 10 *Begins:* Aug
Length: 27 mos *Award:* Dipl,Cert, BS, BA
Tuition per yr: $6,800 res, $16,800 non-res

Washington

Washington State University
Athletic Trainer Prgm
Kinesiology & Leisure Studies
PEB 104
Pullman, WA 99164-1410
Prgm Dir: Carol Zweifel, MS PE
Tel: 509 335-0307 *Fax:* 509 335-4729
E-mail: carolz@wsu.edu
Med Dir: Lloyd Perino, MD
Class Cap: 30 *Begins:* Sep
Length: 23 mos *Award:* BS
Tuition per yr: $3,142 res, $8,866 non-res

West Virginia

West Virginia University
Athletic Trainer Prgm
PO Box 6116 Coliseum
Morgantown, WV 26506
Prgm Dir: Vincent Stilger, HSD ATC
Tel: 304 293-3295, Ext 148 *Fax:* 304 293-4641
E-mail: stilger@wvnvm.wvnet.edu
Med Dir: Dana Brooks
Class Cap: 15 *Begins:* Oct
Length: 27 mos *Award:* Cert
Tuition per yr: $2,128 res, $6,370 non-res

Wisconsin

University of Wisconsin - LaCrosse
Athletic Trainer Prgm
134 Mitchell Hall
LaCrosse, WI 54601
Prgm Dir: Mark H Gibson, MS ATC PT
Tel: 608 785-8190 *Fax:* 608 785-6520
E-mail: gibso_mh@mail.uwlac.edu
Class Cap: 30 *Begins:* Sep
Length: 33 mos *Award:* BS
Tuition per yr: $2,633 res, $7,157 non-res

Audiologist

Speech Language Pathologist

Accreditation

The following list of institutions of higher learning provides information on graduate degree programs in speech-language pathology and/or audiology accredited by the Council on Academic Accreditation (CAA) in Audiology and Speech-Language Pathology. Accreditation by the CAA is sought voluntarily by educational programs that offer graduate degrees in speech-language pathology, audiology, or both. The CAA accreditation program is recognized by the Commission on Recognition of Postsecondary Accreditation (CORPA) and the US Department of Education.

Accreditation is awarded initially for a 5-year period and then for an 8-year period for reaccreditation. Programs seeking reaccreditation for the first time are reviewed by the CAA on the fourth anniversary of their accreditation period; those seeking reaccreditation for the second or subsequent times are reviewed on the seventh anniversary of their accreditation period.

Accreditation by the CAA offers a graduate the assurance that the academic and clinical practicum experience obtained in an accredited program meets nationally established standards. Accreditation means that a program has

- engaged in extensive self-study, often over a period of years;
- prepared and submitted a complex application, often 100 pages long;
- undergone an on-site visit by a team of specially trained peers;
- received, and responded to, a digest of the report submitted by the site visitors;
- had its application, the site visit report, and its response studied by the CAA;
- undergone final evaluation and approval by the CAA; and
- submitted annual reports during the period of its accreditation.

Information

For information about a specific educational program, write to the director of the speech-language pathology and/or audiology program in care of the institution listed.

For additional information about the professions, contact

The American Speech-Language-Hearing Association (ASHA)
10801 Rockville Pike
Rockville, MD 20852
301 897-5700
301 571-0457 Fax

Audiologist

Alabama

University of South Alabama
Audiologist Prgm
Speech and Hearing Ctr
2000 University Commons
Mobile, AL 36688
Tel: 334 380-2600

University of Montevallo
Audiologist Prgm
Comm Science and Disorders
Station 6720
Montevallo, AL 35115-6720
Tel: 205 665-6720

University of Alabama
Audiologist Prgm
Dept of Comm Disorders
PO Box 870242
Tuscaloosa, AL 35487-0242
Tel: 205 348-7131

Auburn University
Audiologist Prgm
Dept of Comm Disorders
1199 Haley Ctr
University, AL 36849-5232
Tel: 334 844-9600

Arizona

Arizona State University
Audiologist Prgm
Speech and Hearing Science
Tempe, AZ 85287-0102
Tel: 602 965-2374

University of Arizona
Audiologist Prgm
Speech and Hearing Sciences
Bldg 71 Rm 214
Tucson, AZ 85721
Tel: 602 621-1644

Arkansas

University of Arkansas at Little Rock
Audiologist Prgm
Communicative Disorders
2601 S University
Little Rock, AR 72204
Tel: 501 569-3155

California

California State University - Long Beach
Audiologist Prgm
Communicative Disorders
1250 Bellflower Blvd
Long Beach, CA 90840
Tel: 310 985-5370

California State University - Los Angeles
Audiologist Prgm
Communication Disorders
5151 State University Dr
Los Angeles, CA 90032
Tel: 213 343-4690

California State University - Northridge
Audiologist Prgm
Communicative Disorders
18111 Nordhoff St
Northridge, CA 91330
Tel: 818 885-2852

California State University - Sacramento
Audiologist Prgm
Speech Pathology & Audiology
6000 J St
Sacramento, CA 95819
Tel: 916 278-6601

San Diego State University
Audiologist Prgm
Communicative Disorders
San Diego, CA 92182
Tel: 619 594-7746

San Francisco State University
Audiologist Prgm
1600 Holloway Ave
Burk Hall Rm 104
San Francisco, CA 94132
Tel: 415 338-1001

San Jose State University
Audiologist Prgm
Speech and Hearing Ctr
Washington Sq
San Jose, CA 95192
Tel: 408 277-2651

Colorado

University of Colorado
Audiologist Prgm
Campus Box 409
Boulder, CO 80309-0409
Tel: 303 492-6445

University of Northern Colorado
Audiologist Prgm
Communication Disorders
Greeley, CO 80639
Tel: 970 351-1726

Connecticut

Southern Connecticut State University
Audiologist Prgm
Communication Disorders
501 Crescent St
New Haven, CT 06515
Tel: 203 392-5954

University of Connecticut
Audiologist Prgm
Communication Sciences
U-85
Storrs, CT 06268
Tel: 203 486-2817

District of Columbia

Gallaudet University
Audiologist Prgm
Audiology & Speech-Lang Path
800 Florida Ave NE
Washington, DC 20002
Tel: 202 651-5329

George Washington University
Audiologist Prgm
Dept of Speech and Hearing
2201 G St NW
Washington, DC 20052
Tel: 202 994-7364

Howard University
Audiologist Prgm
Comm Sciences and Disorders
2400 6th St NW
Washington, DC 20059
Tel: 202 806-6990

Florida

University of Florida
Audiologist Prgm
Comm Processes and Disorders
335 Dauer Hall
Gainesville, FL 32611
Tel: 352 392-2035

University of South Florida
Audiologist Prgm
Comm Sciences and Disorders
BEH 255
Tampa, FL 33620-8150
Tel: 813 974-2006

Georgia

University of Georgia
Audiologist Prgm
Comm Sciences and Disorders
576 Aderhold Hall
Athens, GA 30602
Tel: 706 542-4561

Hawaii

University of Hawaii at Manoa
Audiologist Prgm
John A Burns School of Med
1410 Lower Campus Dr
Honolulu, HI 96822
Tel: 808 956-8279

Idaho

Idaho State University
Audiologist Prgm
Speech Pathology & Audiology
Box 8116
Pocatello, ID 83209-0009
Tel: 208 236-2196

Illinois

Univ of Illinois at Urbana - Champaign
Audiologist Prgm
220 Speech & Hearing Sci Bldg
901 S 6th St
Champaign, IL 61820
Tel: 217 333-2230

Rush University
Audiologist Prgm
Comm Disorders and Sciences
1653 W Harrison St
Chicago, IL 60612
Tel: 312 942-5332

Northern Illinois University
Audiologist Prgm
Communicative Disorders
DeKalb, IL 60115-2899
Tel: 815 753-1486

Northwestern University
Audiologist Prgm
Comm Sciences and Disorders
2299 Sheridan Rd
Evanston, IL 60201
Tel: 847 491-3066

Western Illinois University
Audiologist Prgm
Dept of Communication
1 University Circle
Macomb, IL 61455
Tel: 309 298-1955

Illinois State University
Audiologist Prgm
Speech Pathology & Audiology
Fairchild Hall #204
Normal, IL 61761
Tel: 309 438-8643

Indiana

Indiana University - Bloomington
Audiologist Prgm
Speech and Hearing Sciences
Bloomington, IN 47405
Tel: 812 855-0285

Ball State University
Audiologist Prgm
Speech Pathology & Audiology
2000 University Ave
Muncie, IN 47306-0555
Tel: 317 285-8162

Purdue University
Audiologist Prgm
Audiology and Speech Sciences
West Lafayette, IN 47907
Tel: 317 494-3788

Iowa

University of Northern Iowa
Audiologist Prgm
Communicative Disorders
Cedar Falls, IA 50614
Tel: 319 273-2560

Programs

University of Iowa
Audiologist Prgm
Speech Pathology & Audiology
Iowa City, IA 52242
Tel: 319 335-8718

Kansas

University of Kansas
Audiologist Prgm
Intercampus Prgm
3031 Dole Ctr
Lawrence, KS 66045
Tel: 913 864-0630

Wichita State University
Audiologist Prgm
Comm Disorders and Sciences
1845 Fairmont
Wichita, KS 67260-0075
Tel: 316 689-3240

Kentucky

University of Louisville
Audiologist Prgm
Communicative Disorders
Meyers Hall 129 E Broadway
Louisville, KY 40292
Tel: 502 588-5274

Louisiana

Louisiana State Univ and A & M College
Audiologist Prgm
Communication Disorders
Music/Dramatic Arts Bldg #163
Baton Rouge, LA 70803-2606
Tel: 504 388-2545

University of Southwestern Louisiana
Audiologist Prgm
Communicative Disorders
104 University Circle
Lafayette, LA 70504-3170
Tel: 318 482-6721

Louisiana State Univ Med Ctr - New Orleans
Audiologist Prgm
Communication Disorders
1900 Gravier St
New Orleans, LA 70112-2262
Tel: 504 568-4348

Louisiana Tech University
Audiologist Prgm
Dept of Speech
PO Box 3165
Ruston, LA 71272
Tel: 318 257-4764

Maryland

Univ of Maryland at College Park
Audiologist Prgm
Hearing and Speech Science
College Park, MD 20742
Tel: 301 405-4213

Towson State University
Audiologist Prgm
Comm Sciences and Disorders
Towson, MD 21204-7097
Tel: 410 830-3099

Massachusetts

University of Massachusetts - Amherst
Audiologist Prgm
Communication Disorders
Arnold House Rm 6
Amherst, MA 01003
Tel: 413 545-0131

Boston University
Audiologist Prgm
Communication Disorders
635 Commonwealth Ave
Boston, MA 02215
Tel: 617 353-3252

Northeastern University
Audiologist Prgm
Speech-Lang Path & Audiology
133 Forsyth Ave
Boston, MA 02115
Tel: 617 373-3698

Michigan

Wayne State University
Audiologist Prgm
Comm Disorders and Sciences
555 Manoogian Hall
Detroit, MI 48202
Tel: 313 577-3339

Michigan State University
Audiologist Prgm
Audiology and Speech Sciences
378 Comm Arts & Sciences Bldg
East Lansing, MI 48824-1212
Tel: 517 353-8788

Western Michigan University
Audiologist Prgm
Speech Pathology & Audiology
Kalamazoo, MI 49008
Tel: 616 383-0963

Central Michigan University
Audiologist Prgm
Communication Disorders
Mt Pleasant, MI 48859
Tel: 517 774-7288

Minnesota

University of Minnesota - Twin Cities
Audiologist Prgm
115 Shevlin Hall
164 Pillsbury Dr SE
Minneapolis, MN 55455
Tel: 612 624-3322

Mississippi

University of Southern Mississippi
Audiologist Prgm
Speech and Hearing Sciences
PO Box 5092 Southern Station
Hattiesburg, MS 39406-5092
Tel: 601 266-5216

University of Mississippi
Audiologist Prgm
Communicative Disorders
University, MS 38677
Tel: 601 232-7652

Missouri

Southwest Missouri State University
Audiologist Prgm
Communication Disorders
901 S National
Springfield, MO 65804-0095
Tel: 417 836-5368

Central Institute for the Deaf
Audiologist Prgm
Washington University
818 S Euclid Ave
St Louis, MO 63110-1594
Tel: 314 652-3200

Central Missouri State University
Audiologist Prgm
Speech Pathology & Audiology
Warrensburg, MO 64093
Tel: 816 543-4606

Nebraska

University of Nebraska - Lincoln
Audiologist Prgm
Speech Pathology & Audiology
301 Barkley Memorial Ctr
Lincoln, NE 68583-0738
Tel: 402 472-5496

New Jersey

Trenton State College
Audiologist Prgm
Speech Pathology & Audiology
Hillwood Lakes CN 4700
Trenton, NJ 08650-4700
Tel: 609 771-2322

New Mexico

University of New Mexico
Audiologist Prgm
Communicative Disorders
901 Vassar NE
Albuquerque, NM 87131-1191
Tel: 505 277-4453

New York

CUNY Herbert H Lehman College
Audiologist Prgm
Speech and Hearing Sciences
Bedford Park Blvd W
Bronx, NY 10468
Tel: 718 960-8138

CUNY Brooklyn College
Audiologist Prgm
Speech and Hearing Center
Bedford Ave and Ave H
Brooklyn, NY 11210
Tel: 718 951-5186

SUNY at Buffalo
Audiologist Prgm
Comm Disorders and Sciences
109 Park Hall
Buffalo, NY 14260
Tel: 716 636-3400

CUNY Queens College
Audiologist Prgm
Comm Sciences and Disorders
65-30 Kissena Blvd
Flushing, NY 11367
Tel: 718 520-7358

SUNY College at Fredonia
Audiologist Prgm
Speech Pathology & Audiology
W121 Thompson Hall
Fredonia, NY 14063
Tel: 716 673-3202

Adelphi University
Audiologist Prgm
Speech Arts & Comm Disorders
Hy Weinberg Ctr/Cambridge Ave
Garden City, NY 11530
Tel: 516 877-4770

Hofstra University
Audiologist Prgm
Speech-Lang-Hearing Sciences
Rm 106 Davison Hall
Hempstead, NY 11550
Tel: 516 463-5508

Ithaca College
Audiologist Prgm
Speech Pathology & Audiology
Ithaca, NY 14850
Tel: 607 274-3248

St John's University
Audiologist Prgm
Speech and Hearing Ctr
Grand Central Pkwy
Jamaica, NY 11439
Tel: 718 990-6480

SUNY College at New Paltz
Audiologist Prgm
Communication Disorders
New Paltz, NY 12561
Tel: 914 257-3464

CUNY Hunter College
Audiologist Prgm
School of Health Sciences
425 E 25th St
New York, NY 10010
Tel: 212 481-4467

SUNY College at Plattsburgh
Audiologist Prgm
Hearing and Speech Science
226 Sibley Hall
Plattsburgh, NY 12901
Tel: 518 564-2170

Syracuse University Main Campus
Audiologist Prgm
Comm Sciences and Disorders
805 S Crouse Ave
Syracuse, NY 13244
Tel: 315 443-9648

North Carolina

Univ of North Carolina at Chapel Hill
Audiologist Prgm
Speech and Hearing Sciences
CB 7180 Wing D Medical School
Chapel Hill, NC 27599
Tel: 919 966-1006

Univ of North Carolina at Greensboro
Audiologist Prgm
Comm Sciences and Disorders
FERG 300 UNCG
Greensboro, NC 27412-5001
Tel: 910 334-5939

East Carolina University
Audiologist Prgm
Speech-Lang & Auditory Path
Greenville, NC 27858
Tel: 919 757-4405

North Dakota

Minot State University
Audiologist Prgm
Communication Disorders
500 Ninth Ave NW
Minot, ND 58701
Tel: 701 857-3030

Ohio

University of Akron
Audiologist Prgm
Communicative Disorders
302 E Buchtel Ave
Akron, OH 44325-3001
Tel: 330 972-6803

Ohio University Main Campus
Audiologist Prgm
Hearing and Speech Sciences
Lindley Hall
Athens, OH 45701
Tel: 614 593-1407

Bowling Green State University
Audiologist Prgm
Communication Disorders
Bowling Green, OH 43403
Tel: 419 372-2515

Univ of Cincinnati
Audiologist Prgm
Communication Disorders
Mail Station 379
Cincinnati, OH 45221-0379
Tel: 513 556-4480

Cleveland State University
Audiologist Prgm
Dept of Speech and Hearing
1899 E 22nd St
Cleveland, OH 44115
Tel: 216 687-3804

Ohio State University
Audiologist Prgm
110 Pressey Hall
1070 Carmack Rd
Columbus, OH 43210-1372
Tel: 614 292-8207

Kent State University
Audiologist Prgm
Speech Pathology & Audiology
A104 Music and Speech Ctr
Kent, OH 44242
Tel: 216 672-2672

Miami University
Audiologist Prgm
Speech Pathology & Audiology
2 Bachelor Hall
Oxford, OH 45056
Tel: 513 529-2500

Oklahoma

Univ of Oklahoma Health Sciences Center
Audiologist Prgm
Communication Disorders
825 NE 14th/PO Box 26901
Oklahoma City, OK 73190
Tel: 405 271-4214

Oregon

Portland State University
Audiologist Prgm
Speech and Hearing Sciences
Box 751
Portland, OR 97207-0751
Tel: 503 725-3143

Pennsylvania

Bloomsburg University
Audiologist Prgm
Comm Disorders & Spec Educ
Bloomsburg, PA 17815
Tel: 717 389-4436

Clarion University of Pennsylvania
Audiologist Prgm
Speech Pathology & Audiology
Clarion, PA 16214
Tel: 814 226-2581

Programs

Temple University
Audiologist Prgm
Speech-Lang-Hearing Sciences
Dept of Speech
Philadelphia, PA 19122
Tel: 215 204-8537

University of Pittsburgh
Audiologist Prgm
1117 Cathedral of Learning
5th Ave & Bigelow Blvd
Pittsburgh, PA 15260
Tel: 412 624-6807

Penn State University - Main Campus
Audiologist Prgm
Communication Disorders
110 Moore Bldg
University Park, PA 16802
Tel: 814 865-3177

Rhode Island

University of Rhode Island
Audiologist Prgm
Communicative Disorders
Adams Hall
Kingston, RI 02881
Tel: 401 792-5969

South Dakota

University of South Dakota
Audiologist Prgm
Communication Disorders
414 E Clark St
Vermillion, SD 57069-2390
Tel: 605 677-5474

Tennessee

East Tennessee State University
Audiologist Prgm
Public & Allied Health
Comm Disorders Box 70,643
Johnson City, TN 37614-0643
Tel: 615 929-4272

University of Tennessee - Knoxville
Audiologist Prgm
Audiology & Speech Pathology
457 S Stadium Hall
Knoxville, TN 37996-0740
Tel: 615 974-5019

University of Memphis
Audiologist Prgm
Audiology & Speech Pathology
807 Jefferson Ave
Memphis, TN 38105
Tel: 901 678-5800

Vanderbilt University Medical Center
Audiologist Prgm
Hearing and Speech Sciences
1114 19th Ave S
Nashville, TN 37212
Tel: 615 320-5353

Texas

University of Texas at Austin
Audiologist Prgm
Communication Disorders
Austin, TX 78712
Tel: 512 471-4119

Lamar Univ Institute of Tech - Beaumont
Audiologist Prgm
Dept of Communication
Box 10076 - Lamar Station
Beaumont, TX 77710
Tel: 409 880-8170

University of Texas at Dallas
Audiologist Prgm
Communication Disorders
1966 Inwood Rd
Dallas, TX 75235
Tel: 214 883-3060

University of North Texas
Audiologist Prgm
Communication Disorders
Denton, TX 76203-5008
Tel: 817 565-2481

Baylor College of Medicine
Audiologist Prgm
Audiology & Speech Pathology
One Baylor Plaza
Houston, TX 77030-3498
Tel: 713 798-5916

Texas Tech Univ Hlth Sci Ctr
Audiologist Prgm
Communication Disorders
MS 2073
Lubbock, TX 79409-2073
Tel: 806 742-3908

Utah

Utah State University
Audiologist Prgm
Comm Disorders & Deaf Educ
Logan, UT 84322-1000
Tel: 801 797-1375

Brigham Young University
Audiologist Prgm
Comm Sciences and Disorders
136 John Taylor Bldg
Provo, UT 84602
Tel: 801 378-5117

Univ of Utah Health Sciences Center
Audiologist Prgm
Communication Disorders
1201 Behavioral Science Bldg
Salt Lake City, UT 84112
Tel: 801 581-6726

Virginia

Univ of Virginia Health Sciences Center
Audiologist Prgm
Communication Disorders
PO Box 9022
Charlottesville, VA 22906-9022
Tel: 804 924-7107

James Madison University
Audiologist Prgm
Speech Pathology & Audiology
Harrisonburg, VA 22807
Tel: 540 568-6630

Radford University
Audiologist Prgm
Comm Sciences and Disorders
Radford, VA 24142
Tel: 540 831-5453

Washington

Western Washington University
Audiologist Prgm
Speech Pathology & Audiology
Bellingham, WA 98225
Tel: 206 650-3199

Washington State University
Audiologist Prgm
Speech and Hearing Sciences
Pullman, WA 99164-2420
Tel: 509 335-4525

University of Washington
Audiologist Prgm
Speech and Hearing Sciences
Seattle, WA 98195
Tel: 206 543-7966

West Virginia

West Virginia University
Audiologist Prgm
Speech Pathology & Audiology
PO Box 6122/805 Allen Hall
Morgantown, WV 26506-6122
Tel: 304 293-4241

Wisconsin

University of Wisconsin - Madison
Audiologist Prgm
Communicative Disorders
1975 Willow Dr
Madison, WI 53706
Tel: 608 262-3951

University of Wisconsin - Oshkosh
Audiologist Prgm
Communicative Disorders
Oshkosh, WI 54901
Tel: 414 424-2421

University of Wisconsin - Stevens Point
Audiologist Prgm
Communicative Disorders
2100 Main St
Stevens Point, WI 54481
Tel: 715 346-4511

Wyoming

University of Wyoming
Audiologist Prgm
Speech-Lang Path & Audiology
PO Box 3311/Univ Station
Laramie, WY 82071
Tel: 307 766-5710

Speech Language Pathologist

Alabama

University of South Alabama
Speech Language Pathologist Prgm
Speech and Hearing Ctr
2000 University Commons
Mobile, AL 36688
Tel: 334 380-2600

University of Montevallo
Speech Language Pathologist Prgm
Comm Science and Disorders
Station 6720
Montevallo, AL 35115-6720
Tel: 205 665-6720

Alabama A & M University
Speech Language Pathologist Prgm
Dept of Special Education
PO Box 580
Normal, AL 35762
Tel: 205 851-5533

University of Alabama
Speech Language Pathologist Prgm
Communicative Disorders
PO Box 870242
Tuscaloosa, AL 35487-0242
Tel: 205 348-7131

Auburn University
Speech Language Pathologist Prgm
Communication Disorders
1199 Haley Ctr
University, AL 36849-5232
Tel: 334 844-9600

Arizona

Northern Arizona University
Speech Language Pathologist Prgm
Speech Pathology & Audiology
NAU Box 15045
Flagstaff, AZ 86011
Tel: 602 523-2969

Arizona State University
Speech Language Pathologist Prgm
Speech and Hearing Science
Tempe, AZ 85287-0102
Tel: 602 965-2374

University of Arizona
Speech Language Pathologist Prgm
Speech & Hearing Sciences
Bldg 71 Rm 214
Tucson, AZ 85721
Tel: 520 621-1644

Arkansas

University of Central Arkansas
Speech Language Pathologist Prgm
Box 4985
Conway, AR 72032
Tel: 501 450-3176

University of Arkansas Main Campus
Speech Language Pathologist Prgm
Prgm in Comm Disorders
410 Arkansas Ave
Fayetteville, AR 72701
Tel: 501 575-4509

University of Arkansas at Little Rock
Speech Language Pathologist Prgm
Communicative Disorders
2601 S University
Little Rock, AR 72204
Tel: 501 569-3155

Arkansas State University
Speech Language Pathologist Prgm
Spec Educ & Comm Disorders
PO Box 940
State University, AR 72467
Tel: 501 972-3061

California

California State University - Chico
Speech Language Pathologist Prgm
Speech Pathology & Audiology
Dept of Education
Chico, CA 95929-0222
Tel: 916 898-5871

California State University - Fresno
Speech Language Pathologist Prgm
Laboratory School Rm 125
5048 N Jackson
Fresno, CA 93740-0080
Tel: 209 278-2423

California State University - Fullerton
Speech Language Pathologist Prgm
Dept of Speech Communication
800 N State College Blvd
Fullerton, CA 92634
Tel: 714 773-3617

California State University - Hayward
Speech Language Pathologist Prgm
Comm Sciences and Disorders
25800 Carlos Bee Blvd
Hayward, CA 94542
Tel: 510 881-3086

Loma Linda University
Speech Language Pathologist Prgm
Speech-Lang Path/Audiology
Nichol Hall Rm A506
Loma Linda, CA 92350
Tel: 909 824-4998

California State University - Long Beach
Speech Language Pathologist Prgm
Communicative Disorders
1250 Bellflower Blvd
Long Beach, CA 90840
Tel: 310 985-5370

California State University - Los Angeles
Speech Language Pathologist Prgm
Communication Disorders
5151 State University Dr
Los Angeles, CA 90032
Tel: 213 343-4690

California State University - Northridge
Speech Language Pathologist Prgm
Communicative Disorders
18111 Nordhoff St
Northridge, CA 91330
Tel: 818 885-2852

University of Redlands
Speech Language Pathologist Prgm
Communicative Disorders
PO Box 3080/1200 E Colton Ave
Redlands, CA 92373-0999
Tel: 714 335-4061

California State University - Sacramento
Speech Language Pathologist Prgm
Speech Pathology & Audiology
6000 J St
Sacramento, CA 95819
Tel: 916 278-6601

San Diego State University
Speech Language Pathologist Prgm
Communicative Disorders
San Diego, CA 92182
Tel: 619 594-7746

San Francisco State University
Speech Language Pathologist Prgm
1600 Holloway Ave
Burk Hall Rm 104
San Francisco, CA 94132
Tel: 415 338-1001

San Jose State University
Speech Language Pathologist Prgm
Speech and Hearing Ctr
Washington Square
San Jose, CA 95192
Tel: 408 277-2651

University of the Pacific
Speech Language Pathologist Prgm
Communicative Disorders
3601 Pacific Ave
Stockton, CA 95211
Tel: 209 946-2381

Colorado

University of Colorado
Speech Language Pathologist Prgm
Campus Box 409
Boulder, CO 80309-0409
Tel: 303 492-6445

University of Northern Colorado
Speech Language Pathologist Prgm
Communication Disorders
Greeley, CO 80639
Tel: 970 351-1726

Connecticut

Southern Connecticut State University
Speech Language Pathologist Prgm
Communication Disorders
501 Crescent St
New Haven, CT 06515
Tel: 203 392-5954

University of Connecticut
Speech Language Pathologist Prgm
Communication Sciences
U-85
Storrs, CT 06268
Tel: 203 486-2817

District of Columbia

Gallaudet University
Speech Language Pathologist Prgm
Audiology & Speech-Lang Path
800 Florida Ave NE
Washington, DC 20002
Tel: 202 651-5329

George Washington University
Speech Language Pathologist Prgm
Dept of Speech and Hearing
2201 G St NW
Washington, DC 20052
Tel: 202 994-7364

Howard University
Speech Language Pathologist Prgm
Comm Sciences and Disorders
2400 6th St NW
Washington, DC 20059
Tel: 202 806-6990

University of the District of Columbia
Speech Language Pathologist Prgm
Communication Sciences
4200 Connecticut Ave NW
Washington, DC 20001
Tel: 202 727-2318

Florida

Florida Atlantic University
Speech Language Pathologist Prgm
Communication Disorders
PO Box 3091
Boca Raton, FL 33431
Tel: 561 367-2258

Nova Southeastern University
Speech Language Pathologist Prgm
Comm Sciences and Disorders
3375 SW 75th Ave
Ft Lauderdale, FL 33324
Tel: 305 475-7075

University of Florida
Speech Language Pathologist Prgm
Comm Processes and Disorders
335 Dauer Hall
Gainesville, FL 32611
Tel: 352 392-2035

University of Central Florida
Speech Language Pathologist Prgm
Communicative Disorders
4000 Central Florida Blvd
Orlando, FL 32816
Tel: 407 249-4798

Florida State University
Speech Language Pathologist Prgm
Communication Disorders
107 RRC (R-89)
Tallahassee, FL 32306-2007
Tel: 904 644-8456

University of South Florida
Speech Language Pathologist Prgm
Comm Sciences and Disorders
BEH 255
Tampa, FL 33620-8150
Tel: 813 974-2006

Georgia

University of Georgia
Speech Language Pathologist Prgm
Comm Sciences and Disorders
576 Aderhold Hall
Athens, GA 30602
Tel: 706 542-4561

Georgia State University
Speech Language Pathologist Prgm
Communication Disorders
University Plaza
Atlanta, GA 30303
Tel: 404 651-2310

Valdosta State University
Speech Language Pathologist Prgm
Dept of Special Education
Valdosta, GA 31698
Tel: 912 333-5931

Hawaii

University of Hawaii at Manoa
Speech Language Pathologist Prgm
John A Burns School of Med
1410 Lower Campus Dr
Honolulu, HI 96822
Tel: 808 956-8279

Idaho

Idaho State University
Speech Language Pathologist Prgm
Speech Pathology & Audiology
Box 8116
Pocatello, ID 83209-0009
Tel: 208 236-2196

Illinois

Southern Illinois Univ at Carbondale
Speech Language Pathologist Prgm
Comm Disorders and Sciences
Carbondale, IL 62901
Tel: 618 453-4301

Univ of Illinois at Urbana - Champaign
Speech Language Pathologist Prgm
220 Speech & Hearing Sci Bldg
901 S 6th St
Champaign, IL 61820
Tel: 217 333-2230

Eastern Illinois University
Speech Language Pathologist Prgm
Comm Disorders and Sciences
Charleston, IL 61920
Tel: 217 581-2712

Rush University
Speech Language Pathologist Prgm
Comm Disorders and Sciences
1653 W Harrison St
Chicago, IL 60612
Tel: 312 942-5332

Saint Xavier University
Speech Language Pathologist Prgm
Comm Disorders and Sciences
3700 W 103rd St
Chicago, IL 60655
Tel: 773 298-3561

Northern Illinois University
Speech Language Pathologist Prgm
Communicative Disorders
DeKalb, IL 60115-2899
Tel: 815 753-1486

Southern Illinois Univ at Edwardsville
Speech Language Pathologist Prgm
Speech Pathology & Audiology
Box 1776
Edwardsville, IL 62026-1776
Tel: 618 692-3662

Northwestern University
Speech Language Pathologist Prgm
Comm Sciences and Disorders
2299 Sheridan Rd
Evanston, IL 60201
Tel: 847 491-3066

Western Illinois University
Speech Language Pathologist Prgm
Dept of Communication
1 University Circle
Macomb, IL 61455
Tel: 309 298-1955

Illinois State University
Speech Language Pathologist Prgm
Speech Pathology & Audiology
Fairchild Hall #204
Normal, IL 61761
Tel: 309 438-8643

Governors State University
Speech Language Pathologist Prgm
Communication Disorders
University Park, IL 60466
Tel: 708 534-5000, Ext 2370

Indiana

Indiana University - Bloomington
Speech Language Pathologist Prgm
Speech and Hearing Sciences
Bloomington, IN 47405
Tel: 812 855-0285

Ball State University
Speech Language Pathologist Prgm
Speech Pathology & Audiology
2000 University Ave
Muncie, IN 47306-0555
Tel: 317 285-8162

Indiana State University
Speech Language Pathologist Prgm
Communication Disorders
8th and Sycamore Sts
Terre Haute, IN 47809
Tel: 812 237-2804

Purdue University
Speech Language Pathologist Prgm
Audiology and Speech Sciences
West Lafayette, IN 47907
Tel: 317 494-3788

Iowa

University of Northern Iowa
Speech Language Pathologist Prgm
Communicative Disorders
Cedar Falls, IA 50614
Tel: 319 273-2560

University of Iowa
Speech Language Pathologist Prgm
Speech Pathology & Audiology
Iowa City, IA 52242
Tel: 319 335-8718

Kansas

Ft Hays State University
Speech Language Pathologist Prgm
Communication Disorders
600 Park St
Hays, KS 67601
Tel: 913 628-5366

University of Kansas
Speech Language Pathologist Prgm
Intercampus Program
3031 Dole Ctr
Lawrence, KS 66045
Tel: 913 864-0630

Kansas State University
Speech Language Pathologist Prgm
Comm Sciences and Disorders
Justin Hall 303
Manhattan, KS 66506
Tel: 913 532-5510

Wichita State University
Speech Language Pathologist Prgm
Comm Disorders and Sciences
1845 Fairmont
Wichita, KS 67260-0075
Tel: 316 689-3240

Kentucky

Western Kentucky University
Speech Language Pathologist Prgm
Communication Disorders
Tate Page Hall Rm 111
Bowling Green, KY 42101
Tel: 502 745-4303

University of Kentucky
Speech Language Pathologist Prgm
Communication Disorders
1028 S Broadway Ste 3
Lexington, KY 40504-2605
Tel: 606 257-7918

University of Louisville
Speech Language Pathologist Prgm
Communicative Disorders
Meyers Hall/129 E Broadway
Louisville, KY 40292
Tel: 502 588-5274

Murray State University
Speech Language Pathologist Prgm
Communication Disorders
16th and Main Sts
Murray, KY 42071
Tel: 502 762-6810

Eastern Kentucky University
Speech Language Pathologist Prgm
Communication Disorders
Richmond, KY 40475
Tel: 606 622-4442

Louisiana

Louisiana State Univ and A & M College
Speech Language Pathologist Prgm
Communication Disorders
Music/Dramatic Arts Bldg #163
Baton Rouge, LA 70803-2606
Tel: 504 388-2545

Southern Univ and A & M College
Speech Language Pathologist Prgm
Speech Pathology & Audiology
PO Box 9888
Baton Rouge, LA 70813
Tel: 504 771-3950

Southeastern Louisiana University
Speech Language Pathologist Prgm
Dept of Special Education
PO Box 879
Hammond, LA 70402
Tel: 504 549-2214

University of Southwestern Louisiana
Speech Language Pathologist Prgm
Communicative Disorders
104 University Circle
Lafayette, LA 70504-3170
Tel: 318 482-6721

Northeast Louisiana University
Speech Language Pathologist Prgm
School of Communication
700 University Ave
Monroe, LA 71209-0321
Tel: 318 342-1395

Louisiana State Univ Med Ctr - New Orleans
Speech Language Pathologist Prgm
Communication Disorders
1900 Gravier St
New Orleans, LA 70112-2262
Tel: 504 568-4348

Louisiana Tech University
Speech Language Pathologist Prgm
Dept of Speech
PO Box 3165
Ruston, LA 71272
Tel: 318 257-4764

Maine

University of Maine - Orono
Speech Language Pathologist Prgm
Communication Disorders
N Stevens Hall
Orono, ME 04469
Tel: 207 581-2006

Maryland

Loyola College of Maryland
Speech Language Pathologist Prgm
Speech-Lang Path & Audiology
4501 N Charles St
Baltimore, MD 21210
Tel: 301 323-1010, Ext 2241

Univ of Maryland at College Park
Speech Language Pathologist Prgm
Hearing and Speech Science
College Park, MD 20742
Tel: 301 405-4213

Towson State University
Speech Language Pathologist Prgm
Comm Sciences and Disorders
Towson, MD 21204-7097
Tel: 410 830-3099

Massachusetts

University of Massachusetts - Amherst
Speech Language Pathologist Prgm
Communication Disorders
Arnold House Rm 6
Amherst, MA 01003
Tel: 413 545-0131

Boston University
Speech Language Pathologist Prgm
Communication Disorders
635 Commonwealth Ave
Boston, MA 02215
Tel: 617 353-3252

Emerson College
Speech Language Pathologist Prgm
Communication Disorders
100 Beacon St
Boston, MA 02116
Tel: 617 578-8732

MGH Institute of Health Professions
Speech Language Pathologist Prgm
Comm Sciences and Disorders
101 Merrimac St
Boston, MA 02114
Tel: 617 726-8019

Northeastern University
Speech Language Pathologist Prgm
Speech-Lang Path & Audiology
133 Forsyth Ave
Boston, MA 02115
Tel: 617 373-3698

Worcester State College
Speech Language Pathologist Prgm
Communication Disorders
486 Chandler St
Worcester, MA 01602-2597
Tel: 508 793-8055

Michigan

Wayne State University
Speech Language Pathologist Prgm
Comm Disorders and Sciences
555 Manoogian Hall
Detroit, MI 48202
Tel: 313 577-3339

Michigan State University
Speech Language Pathologist Prgm
Audiology and Speech Sciences
378 Comm Arts & Sciences Bldg
East Lansing, MI 48824-1212
Tel: 517 353-8788

Western Michigan University
Speech Language Pathologist Prgm
Speech Pathology & Audiology
Kalamazoo, MI 49008
Tel: 616 383-0963

Northern Michigan University
Speech Language Pathologist Prgm
Communication Disorders
1401 Presque Isle Ave
Marquette, MI 49855-5337
Tel: 906 227-2125

Central Michigan University
Speech Language Pathologist Prgm
Communication Disorders
Mt Pleasant, MI 48859
Tel: 517 774-7288

Eastern Michigan University
Speech Language Pathologist Prgm
Ypsilanti, MI 48197
Tel: 313 487-4412

Minnesota

University of Minnesota - Duluth
Speech Language Pathologist Prgm
Communicative Disorders
10 Univ Dr/252 Montague Hall
Duluth, MN 55812
Tel: 218 726-7974

Mankato State University
Speech Language Pathologist Prgm
Communication Disorders
Ellis and Stadium Rds
Mankato, MN 56002-8400
Tel: 507 389-1415

University of Minnesota - Twin Cities
Speech Language Pathologist Prgm
115 Shevlin Hall
164 Pillsbury Dr SE
Minneapolis, MN 55455
Tel: 612 624-3322

Moorhead State University
Speech Language Pathologist Prgm
Speech-Lang-Hearing Sciences
1104 7th Ave S
Moorhead, MN 56563
Tel: 218 236-2286

St Cloud State University
Speech Language Pathologist Prgm
A216 Education Bldg
720 4th Ave S
St Cloud, MN 56301
Tel: 320 255-2092

Mississippi

Mississippi University for Women
Speech Language Pathologist Prgm
Speech Pathology & Audiology
PO Box W-1340
Columbus, MS 39701
Tel: 601 329-7270

University of Southern Mississippi
Speech Language Pathologist Prgm
Speech and Hearing Sciences
PO Box 5092/Southern Station
Hattiesburg, MS 39406-5092
Tel: 601 266-5216

University of Mississippi
Speech Language Pathologist Prgm
Communicative Disorders
University, MS 38677
Tel: 601 232-7652

Missouri

Southeast Missouri State University
Speech Language Pathologist Prgm
Communication Disorders
Cape Girardeau, MO 63701
Tel: 573 651-2488

University of Missouri - Columbia
Speech Language Pathologist Prgm
Communicative Disorders
303 Lewis Hall
Columbia, MO 65211
Tel: 573 882-3873

Truman State University
Speech Language Pathologist Prgm
Human Potential & Performance
Violette Hall 164
Kirksville, MO 63501
Tel: 816 785-4669

Southwest Missouri State University
Speech Language Pathologist Prgm
Communication Disorders
901 S National
Springfield, MO 65804-0095
Tel: 417 836-5368

Fontbonne College
Speech Language Pathologist Prgm
Communication Disorders
6800 Wydown Blvd
St Louis, MO 63105
Tel: 314 862-3456

St Louis University Health Sciences Ctr
Speech Language Pathologist Prgm
Communication Disorders
3733 W Pine Blvd
St Louis, MO 63108
Tel: 314 658-2939

Central Missouri State University
Speech Language Pathologist Prgm
Speech Pathology & Audiology
Warrensburg, MO 64093
Tel: 816 543-4606

Nebraska

University of Nebraska at Kearney
Speech Language Pathologist Prgm
Communication Disorders
Kearney, NE 68849
Tel: 308 234-8300

University of Nebraska - Lincoln
Speech Language Pathologist Prgm
Speech Pathology & Audiology
301 Barkley Memorial Ctr
Lincoln, NE 68583-0738
Tel: 404 472-5496

University of Nebraska at Omaha
Speech Language Pathologist Prgm
Spec Educ and Comm Disorders
Omaha, NE 68182-0167
Tel: 402 554-3336

Nevada

University of Nevada - Reno
Speech Language Pathologist Prgm
Speech Pathology & Audiology
108 Redfield Bldg/152
Reno, NV 89557
Tel: 702 784-4887

New Hampshire

University of New Hampshire
Speech Language Pathologist Prgm
Communication Disorders
4 Library Way/Hewitt Hall
Durham, NH 03824
Tel: 603 862-2538

New Jersey

Trenton State College
Speech Language Pathologist Prgm
Speech Pathology & Audiology
Hillwood Lakes CN 4700
Trenton, NJ 08650-4700
Tel: 609 771-2322

Kean College of New Jersey
Speech Language Pathologist Prgm
Morris Ave
Union, NJ 07083
Tel: 908 527-2218

Montclair State University
Speech Language Pathologist Prgm
Comm Sciences and Disorders
Speech Bldg K-119 Normal Ave
Upper Montclair, NJ 07043
Tel: 201 655-4232

William Paterson College
Speech Language Pathologist Prgm
Communication Disorders
300 Pompton Rd
Wayne, NJ 07470
Tel: 201 595-2209

New Mexico

University of New Mexico
Speech Language Pathologist Prgm
Communicative Disorders
901 Vassar NE
Albuquerque, NM 87131-1191
Tel: 505 277-4453

New Mexico State University
Speech Language Pathologist Prgm
Communication Disorders
Box 3001-3 SPE
Las Cruces, NM 88003
Tel: 505 646-4121

Eastern New Mexico University
Speech Language Pathologist Prgm
Communicative Arts & Sciences
Station #3
Portales, NM 88130
Tel: 505 562-2157

New York

College of St Rose
Speech Language Pathologist Prgm
Communication Disorders
432 Western Ave
Albany, NY 12203
Tel: 518 454-5122

CUNY Herbert H Lehman College
Speech Language Pathologist Prgm
Speech and Hearing Sciences
Bedford Park Blvd W
Bronx, NY 10468
Tel: 718 960-8138

CUNY Brooklyn College
Speech Language Pathologist Prgm
Speech and Hearing Ctr
Bedford Ave and Ave H
Brooklyn, NY 11210
Tel: 718 951-5186

Long Island University - Brooklyn Campus
Speech Language Pathologist Prgm
Speech Comm Sci & Theater
One University Plaza
Brooklyn, NY 11201
Tel: 718 488-1252

Long Island Univ - C W Post Campus
Speech Language Pathologist Prgm
Northern Blvd
Brookville, NY 11548
Tel: 516 299-2436

SUNY at Buffalo
Speech Language Pathologist Prgm
Comm Disorders and Sciences
109 Park Hall
Buffalo, NY 14260
Tel: 716 636-3400

SUNY College at Buffalo
Speech Language Pathologist Prgm
Communication Disorders
1300 Elmwood Ave
Buffalo, NY 14222
Tel: 716 878-5502

CUNY Queens College
Speech Language Pathologist Prgm
Comm Sciences and Disorders
65-30 Kissena Blvd
Flushing, NY 11367
Tel: 718 520-7358

SUNY College at Fredonia
Speech Language Pathologist Prgm
Speech Pathology & Audiology
W121 Thompson Hall
Fredonia, NY 14063
Tel: 716 673-3202

Adelphi University
Speech Language Pathologist Prgm
Speech Arts & Comm Disorders
Hy Wienberg Ctr/Cambridge Ave
Garden City, NY 11530
Tel: 516 877-4770

SUNY College at Geneseo
Speech Language Pathologist Prgm
Comm Disorders and Sciences
1 College Circle
Geneseo, NY 14454
Tel: 716 245-5328

Hofstra University
Speech Language Pathologist Prgm
Speech-Lang-Hearing Sciences
Rm 106 Davison Hall
Hempstead, NY 11550
Tel: 516 463-5508

Ithaca College
Speech Language Pathologist Prgm
Speech Pathology & Audiology
Ithaca, NY 14850
Tel: 607 274-3248

Programs

St John's University
Speech Language Pathologist Prgm
Speech and Hearing Ctr
Grand Central Pkwy
Jamaica, NY 11439
Tel: 718 990-6480

SUNY College at New Paltz
Speech Language Pathologist Prgm
Communication Disorders
New Paltz, NY 12561
Tel: 914 257-3464

CUNY Hunter College
Speech Language Pathologist Prgm
School of Health Sciences
425 E 25th St
New York, NY 10010
Tel: 212 481-4467

New York University
Speech Language Pathologist Prgm
Speech-Lang Path & Audiology
719 Broadway 2nd Fl
New York, NY 10003
Tel: 212 998-5265

Teachers College Columbia University
Speech Language Pathologist Prgm
Speech-Lang Path & Audiology
525 W 120th St
New York, NY 10027
Tel: 212 678-3892

SUNY College at Plattsburgh
Speech Language Pathologist Prgm
Hearing and Speech Science
226 Sibley Hall
Plattsburgh, NY 12901
Tel: 518 564-2170

Nazareth College of Rochester
Speech Language Pathologist Prgm
4245 East Ave
Rochester, NY 14618-2790
Tel: 716 586-2525, Ext 314

Syracuse University Main Campus
Speech Language Pathologist Prgm
Comm Sciences and Disorders
805 S Crouse Ave
Syracuse, NY 13244
Tel: 315 443-9648

North Carolina

Appalachian State University
Speech Language Pathologist Prgm
Communication Disorders
Boone, NC 28608
Tel: 704 262-2182

Univ of North Carolina at Chapel Hill
Speech Language Pathologist Prgm
Speech and Hearing Sciences
CB 7180 Wing D Medical School
Chapel Hill, NC 27599
Tel: 919 966-1006

Western Carolina University
Speech Language Pathologist Prgm
Dept of Human Services
School of Educ and Psych
Cullowhee, NC 28723-9043
Tel: 704 227-7310

North Carolina Central University
Speech Language Pathologist Prgm
Speech Hearing Lang & Reading
School of Education
Durham, NC 27707
Tel: 919 560-6470

Univ of North Carolina at Greensboro
Speech Language Pathologist Prgm
Comm Sciences and Disorders
FERG 300 UNCG
Greensboro, NC 27412-5001
Tel: 910 334-5939

East Carolina University
Speech Language Pathologist Prgm
Speech-Lang & Auditory Path
Greenville, NC 27858
Tel: 919 757-4405

North Dakota

Univ of N Dakota Sch of Med and Hlth Sci
Speech Language Pathologist Prgm
Communication Disorders
PO Box 8040/Univ Station
Grand Forks, ND 58202-8040
Tel: 701 777-3232

Minot State University
Speech Language Pathologist Prgm
Communication Disorders
500 Ninth Ave NW
Minot, ND 58701
Tel: 701 857-3030

Ohio

University of Akron
Speech Language Pathologist Prgm
Communicative Disorders
302 E Buchtel Ave
Akron, OH 44325-3001
Tel: 330 972-6803

Ohio University Main Campus
Speech Language Pathologist Prgm
Hearing and Speech Sciences
Lindley Hall
Athens, OH 45701
Tel: 614 593-1407

Bowling Green State University
Speech Language Pathologist Prgm
Communication Disorders
Bowling Green, OH 43403
Tel: 419 372-2515

Univ of Cincinnati
Speech Language Pathologist Prgm
Communication Disorders
Mail Station 379
Cincinnati, OH 45221-0379
Tel: 513 556-4480

Case-Western Reserve University
Speech Language Pathologist Prgm
Communication Sciences
10900 Euclid Ave
Cleveland, OH 44106
Tel: 216 368-2470

Cleveland State University
Speech Language Pathologist Prgm
Dept of Speech and Hearing
1899 E 22nd St
Cleveland, OH 44115
Tel: 216 687-3804

Ohio State University
Speech Language Pathologist Prgm
110 Pressey Hall
1070 Carmack Rd
Columbus, OH 43210-1372
Tel: 614 292-8207

Kent State University
Speech Language Pathologist Prgm
Speech Pathology & Audiology
A104 Music and Speech Center
Kent, OH 44242
Tel: 216 672-2672

Miami University
Speech Language Pathologist Prgm
Speech Pathology & Audiology
2 Bachelor Hall
Oxford, OH 45056
Tel: 513 529-2500

University of Toledo
Speech Language Pathologist Prgm
Special Education Services
2801 W Bancroft St
Toledo, OH 43606
Tel: 419 530-7733

Oklahoma

University of Central Oklahoma
Speech Language Pathologist Prgm
Curriculum & Instruction
100 N University Dr
Edmond, OK 73034
Tel: 405 341-2980

Univ of Oklahoma Health Sciences Center
Speech Language Pathologist Prgm
Communication Disorders
825 NE 14th/PO Box 26901
Oklahoma City, OK 73190
Tel: 405 271-4214

Oklahoma State University Main Campus
Speech Language Pathologist Prgm
Speech-Lang Path & Audiology
120 Hanner Hall
Stillwater, OK 74078
Tel: 405 744-6021

Northeastern State University
Speech Language Pathologist Prgm
Special Services Bldg
Tahlequah, OK 74464
Tel: 918 456-5511, Ext 3778

University of Tulsa
Speech Language Pathologist Prgm
Comm Disorders and Sciences
600 S College Ave
Tulsa, OK 74104
Tel: 918 631-2903

Oregon

University of Oregon
Speech Language Pathologist Prgm
354 Clinical Services Bldg
Eugene, OR 97403
Tel: 503 346-3593

Portland State University
Speech Language Pathologist Prgm
Speech and Hearing Sciences
Box 751
Portland, OR 97207-0751
Tel: 503 725-3143

Pennsylvania

Bloomsburg University
Speech Language Pathologist Prgm
Comm Disorders & Spec Educ
Bloomsburg, PA 17815
Tel: 717 389-4436

California University of Pennsylvania
Speech Language Pathologist Prgm
Speech Pathology & Audiology
Learning Research Ctr
California, PA 15419
Tel: 412 938-4175

Clarion University of Pennsylvania
Speech Language Pathologist Prgm
Speech Pathology & Audiology
Clarion, PA 16214
Tel: 814 226-2581

Edinboro University of Pennsylvania
Speech Language Pathologist Prgm
Speech and Comm Studies
Campton Hall
Edinboro, PA 16444
Tel: 814 732-2730

Indiana University of Pennsylvania
Speech Language Pathologist Prgm
Spec Educ & Clinical Services
203 Davis Hall
Indiana, PA 15701
Tel: 412 357-2450

Temple University
Speech Language Pathologist Prgm
Speech-Lang-Hearing Sciences
Dept of Speech
Philadelphia, PA 19122
Tel: 215 204-8537

University of Pittsburgh
Speech Language Pathologist Prgm
1117 Cathedral of Learning
5th Ave and Bigelow Blvd
Pittsburgh, PA 15260
Tel: 412 624-6807

Penn State University - Main Campus
Speech Language Pathologist Prgm
Communication Disorders
110 Moore Bldg
University Park, PA 16802
Tel: 814 865-3177

West Chester University
Speech Language Pathologist Prgm
Communication Disorders
West Chester, PA 19383
Tel: 610 436-3447

Rhode Island

University of Rhode Island
Speech Language Pathologist Prgm
Communicative Disorders
Adams Hall
Kingston, RI 02881
Tel: 401 792-5969

South Carolina

University of South Carolina
Speech Language Pathologist Prgm
Speech-Lang Path-Audiology
Columbia, SC 29208
Tel: 803 777-4813

South Carolina State University
Speech Language Pathologist Prgm
Speech Pathology & Audiology
300 College St NE
Orangeburg, SC 29117
Tel: 803 536-8074

South Dakota

University of South Dakota
Speech Language Pathologist Prgm
Communication Disorders
414 E Clark St
Vermillion, SD 57069-2390
Tel: 605 677-5474

Tennessee

East Tennessee State University
Speech Language Pathologist Prgm
Public & Allied Health
Comm Disorders Box 70,643
Johnson City, TN 37614-0643
Tel: 615 929-4272

University of Tennessee - Knoxville
Speech Language Pathologist Prgm
Audiology & Speech Pathology
457 S Stadium Hall
Knoxville, TN 37996-0740
Tel: 615 974-5019

University of Memphis
Speech Language Pathologist Prgm
Audiology & Speech Pathology
807 Jefferson Ave
Memphis, TN 38105
Tel: 901 678-5800

Tennessee State University
Speech Language Pathologist Prgm
Speech Pathology & Audiology
3500 John Merritt Blvd
Nashville, TN 37209-1561
Tel: 615 963-7081

Vanderbilt University Medical Center
Speech Language Pathologist Prgm
Hearing and Speech Sciences
1114 19th Ave S
Nashville, TN 37212
Tel: 615 320-5353

Texas

University of Texas at Austin
Speech Language Pathologist Prgm
Communication Disorders
Austin, TX 78712
Tel: 512 471-4119

Lamar Univ Institute of Tech - Beaumont
Speech Language Pathologist Prgm
Dept of Communication
Box 10076 - Lamar Station
Beaumont, TX 77710
Tel: 409 880-8170

University of Texas at Dallas
Speech Language Pathologist Prgm
Communication Disorders
1966 Inwood Rd
Dallas, TX 75235
Tel: 214 883-3060

Texas Woman's University
Speech Language Pathologist Prgm
Comm Sciences and Disorders
Box 425737/TWU Station
Denton, TX 76204-3737
Tel: 817 898-2033

University of North Texas
Speech Language Pathologist Prgm
Communication Disorders
Denton, TX 76203-5008
Tel: 817 565-2481

Univ of Texas - Pan American
Speech Language Pathologist Prgm
Hlth Sci & Human Svcs 2.140
1201 W University Dr
Edinburg, TX 78539-2999
Tel: 210 316-7040

University of Texas at El Paso
Speech Language Pathologist Prgm
Speech Hearing & Lang Devel
El Paso, TX 79968-0639
Tel: 915 747-5250

Texas Christian University
Speech Language Pathologist Prgm
Speech Communication
2800 S University Dr
Ft Worth, TX 76129
Tel: 817 921-7621

Programs

University of Houston
Speech Language Pathologist Prgm
Communication Disorders
Rm 146-D SOA Bldg
Houston, TX 77204
Tel: 713 743-2896

Texas Tech Univ Hlth Sci Ctr
Speech Language Pathologist Prgm
Communication Disorders
MS 2073
Lubbock, TX 79409-2073
Tel: 806 742-3908

Stephen F Austin State University
Speech Language Pathologist Prgm
Counseling & Spec Education
SFA Box 13019
Nacogdoches, TX 75962
Tel: 409 468-1252

Our Lady of the Lake University
Speech Language Pathologist Prgm
Comm and Learning Disorders
411 S 24th St
San Antonio, TX 78207
Tel: 210 434-6711

Southwest Texas State University
Speech Language Pathologist Prgm
Speech Hearing & Lang Clinic
Communication Disorders
San Marcos, TX 78666-4616
Tel: 512 245-2330

Baylor University
Speech Language Pathologist Prgm
Communication Disorders
PO Box 97332
Waco, TX 76798-7332
Tel: 817 755-2567

Utah

Utah State University
Speech Language Pathologist Prgm
Comm Disorders & Deaf Educ
Logan, UT 84322-1000
Tel: 801 797-1375

Brigham Young University
Speech Language Pathologist Prgm
Comm Sciences and Disorders
136 John Taylor Bldg
Provo, UT 84602
Tel: 801 378-5117

Univ of Utah Health Sciences Center
Speech Language Pathologist Prgm
Communication Disorders
1201 Behavioral Science Bldg
Salt Lake City, UT 84112
Tel: 801 581-6726

Vermont

University of Vermont
Speech Language Pathologist Prgm
Comm Science and Disorders
Allen House
Burlington, VT 05405-0350
Tel: 802 656-3861

Virginia

Univ of Virginia Health Sciences Center
Speech Language Pathologist Prgm
Communication Disorders
PO Box 9022
Charlottesville, VA 22906-9022
Tel: 804 924-7107

Hampton University
Speech Language Pathologist Prgm
Communication Disorders
Hampton, VA 23668
Tel: 804 727-5435

James Madison University
Speech Language Pathologist Prgm
Speech Pathology & Audiology
Harrisonburg, VA 22807
Tel: 540 568-6630

Old Dominion University
Speech Language Pathologist Prgm
Speech Pathology & Audiology
Child Study Ctr
Norfolk, VA 23529-0136
Tel: 757 440-4117

Radford University
Speech Language Pathologist Prgm
Comm Sciences and Disorders
Radford, VA 24142
Tel: 540 831-5453

Washington

Western Washington University
Speech Language Pathologist Prgm
Speech Pathology & Audiology
Bellingham, WA 98225
Tel: 206 650-3199

Eastern Washington University
Speech Language Pathologist Prgm
Comm Disorders MS 106
526 Fifth St
Cheney, WA 99004-2431
Tel: 509 359-6622

Washington State University
Speech Language Pathologist Prgm
Speech and Hearing Sciences
Pullman, WA 99164-2420
Tel: 509 335-4525

University of Washington
Speech Language Pathologist Prgm
Speech and Hearing Sciences
Seattle, WA 98195
Tel: 206 543-7966

West Virginia

Marshall University
Speech Language Pathologist Prgm
Communication Disorders
400 Hall Greer Blvd
Huntington, WV 25705
Tel: 304 696-3640

West Virginia University
Speech Language Pathologist Prgm
Speech Pathology & Audiology
PO Box 6122/805 Allen Hall
Morgantown, WV 26506-6122
Tel: 304 293-4241

Wisconsin

University of Wisconsin - Eau Claire
Speech Language Pathologist Prgm
Communication Disorders
Eau Claire, WI 54702-4004
Tel: 715 836-4919

University of Wisconsin - Madison
Speech Language Pathologist Prgm
Communicative Disorders
1975 Willow Dr
Madison, WI 53706
Tel: 608 262-3951

Marquette University
Speech Language Pathologist Prgm
Speech Pathology & Audiology
619 N 16th St
Milwaukee, WI 53233
Tel: 414 288-3428

University of Wisconsin - Milwaukee
Speech Language Pathologist Prgm
Comm Sciences and Disorders
PO Box 413
Milwaukee, WI 53201
Tel: 414 229-5076

University of Wisconsin - Oshkosh
Speech Language Pathologist Prgm
Communicative Disorders
Oshkosh, WI 54901
Tel: 414 424-2421

University of Wisconsin - River Falls
Speech Language Pathologist Prgm
Communicative Disorders
235 Kleinpell Fine Arts Bldg
River Falls, WI 54022
Tel: 715 425-3830

University of Wisconsin - Stevens Point
Speech Language Pathologist Prgm
Communicative Disorders
2100 Main St
Stevens Point, WI 54481
Tel: 715 346-4511

University of Wisconsin - Whitewater
Speech Language Pathologist Prgm
Communicative Disorders
Whitewater, WI 53190-1790
Tel: 414 472-5201

Wyoming

University of Wyoming
Speech Language Pathologist Prgm
Speech-Lang Path & Audiology
PO Box 3311/Univ Station
Laramie, WY 82071
Tel: 307 766-5710

Specialist in Blood Bank Technology

History

In 1954, the first examination for blood bank technologists was administered by the American Society of Clinical Pathologists' Board of Registry. It is significant that both the examination and the process for approving blood bank schools were the result of a cooperative effort between the Board of Registry and the American Association of Blood Banks (AABB). Technologists working for 5 years in blood banking were eligible to take the examination.

After 1960, individuals could attend a 12-month educational program at an accredited school in lieu of the 5-year experience route. Levels of competency were established, and the scope of knowledge pertinent to the field was prescribed to ensure that the institutions would maintain acceptable standards of practice; would follow a curriculum that included all phases of blood bank technology, laboratory management, and transfusion services; and would support a faculty adequate to assume teaching responsibilities. To date, more than 4,000 individuals have been certified as specialists in blood bank technology.

Because the number of programs had increased by 1969, *Standards (Essentials)* were prepared by the Committee on Education of the AABB and were adopted by the House of Delegates of the American Medical Association (AMA) in 1971. Subsequently, the *Standards* underwent major revisions in 1977, 1983, and 1991 and were adopted by the AMA Council on Medical Education and the AABB.

Occupational Description

Specialists in blood bank technology perform both routine and specialized tests in blood bank immunohematology in technical areas of the modern blood bank and perform transfusion services, using methodology that conforms to the Standards for Blood Banks and Transfusion Services of the AABB.

Job Description

Specialists in blood bank technology demonstrate a superior level of technical proficiency and problem-solving ability in such areas as (1) testing for blood group antigens, compatibility, and antibody identification; (2) investigating abnormalities such as hemolytic diseases of the newborn, hemolytic anemias, and adverse responses to transfusion; (3) supporting physicians in transfusion therapy, including for patients with coagulopathies or candidates for organ transplant; and (4) performing blood collection and processing, including selecting donors, drawing and typing blood, and performing pretransfusion tests to ensure the safety of the patient. Supervision, management, and/or teaching make up a considerable part of the responsibilities of the specialist in blood bank technology.

Employment Characteristics

Specialists in blood banking work in many types of facilities, including community blood centers, private hospital blood banks, university-affiliated blood banks, transfusion services, and independent laboratories; they also may be part of a university faculty. Specialists may work some weekend and night duty, including emergency calls. Qualified specialists may advance to supervisory or administrative positions or move into teaching or research activities. The criteria for advancement in this field are experience, technical expertise, and completion of advanced education courses.

Entry-level salaries for specialists in blood banking average between $32,000 and $42,000, depending on previous experience.

Educational Programs

Length. Most of the educational programs are approximately 12 months. Some programs offer a master's degree and take longer to complete.

Prerequisites. Applicants must be certified in medical technology by the Board of Registry and possess a baccalaureate degree from a regionally accredited college or university. If applicants are not certified in medical technology by the Board of Registry, they must possess both a baccalaureate degree from a regionally accredited college or university with a major in any of the biological or physical sciences and have work experience in a blood bank.

Curriculum. Each specific educational program defines its own criteria for measurement of student achievement, and the sequence of instruction is at the discretion of the medical director and the program director and/or educational coordinator of the program. The clinical material available in the educational program provides the student with a full range of experiences. The educational design and environment are conducive to the development of competence in all technical areas of the modern blood bank and transfusion services. The didactic experience covers all theoretical concepts of blood bank immunohematology.

Standards. *Standards* are minimum educational standards adopted by the AABB in collaboration with the Commission on Accreditation of Allied Health Education Programs. Each new program is assessed in accordance with the *Standards*, and accredited programs are reviewed periodically to determine whether they continue to meet the standards. The *Standards* are available on written request from the AABB Committee on Accreditation of Specialist in Blood Bank Technology (SBB) Schools.

Inquiries

Accreditation

Requests for information on program accreditation, including *Standards*, preparing the self-study report, and arranging a site visit, should be submitted to

AABB Committee on Accreditation of SBB Schools
American Association of Blood Banks
8101 Glenbrook Rd
Bethesda, MD 20814-2749
301 215-6482
E-mail: education@aabb.org
Internet: http://www.aabb.org

Careers

Inquiries regarding careers and curriculum should be addressed to

American Association of Blood Banks
8101 Glenbrook Rd
Bethesda, MD 20814-2749
301 907-6977
E-mail: education@aabb.org
Internet: http://www.aabb.org

Certification/Registration

Inquiries regarding certification may be addressed to

Board of Registry
PO Box 12270
Chicago, IL 60612-0270

Specialist in Blood Bank Technology

Alabama

Univ of Alabama at Birmingham Hospital
Specialist in BB Tech Prgm
Rm 381, SHRB Building
1714 9th Ave S
Birmingham, AL 35294-1270
Prgm Dir: Margaret G Fritsma, MA
  MT(ASCP)SBB
Tel: 205 934-5987 *Fax:* 205 975-7302
Med Dir: Shu T Huang, MD
Class Cap: 2 *Begins:* Jun
Length: 12 mos, 24 mos *Award:* Dipl,Cert,
  MSCLS
Tuition per yr: $3,162 res, $6,240 non-res

California

Sacramento Medical Foundation Blood Ctr
Specialist in BB Tech Prgm
1625 Stockton Blvd
Sacramento, CA 95816
Prgm Dir: Valerie E Webber, MT SBB(ASCP)
Tel: 916 456-1500 *Fax:* 916 452-9232
Med Dir: Paul V Holland, MD
Class Cap: 3 *Begins:* Jan
Length: 12 mos *Award:* Cert

District of Columbia

Walter Reed Army Medical Center
Specialist in BB Tech Prgm
US Army Blood Bank Fellowship
Dept of Pathology, ALS
6825 16th St NW
Washington, DC 20307-5001
Prgm Dir: LTC Michael Fitzpatrick, PhD
Tel: 202 782-6210 *Fax:* 202 782-4985
Med Dir: Maj D Joe Chaffin, MD
Class Cap: 8 *Begins:* Feb
Length: 12 mos, 18 mos *Award:* Dipl,Cert, MS
Tuition per yr: $7,200

Florida

Central Florida Blood Bank
Specialist in BB Tech Prgm
32 W Gore St
Orlando, FL 32806
Prgm Dir: Michael L Pratt, MS MT(ASCP) SBB
Tel: 407 849-6100 *Fax:* 407 649-8517
Med Dir: Neil Newburg, MD
Class Cap: 5 *Begins:* Sep
Length: 12 mos *Award:* Cert, SBB

Transfusion Med Acad Ctr FL Blood Svcs
Specialist in BB Tech Prgm
445 31st St N
St Petersburg, FL 33713
Prgm Dir: Alice Putman, MT(ASCP) SBB
Tel: 813 327-0168 *Fax:* 813 327-4602
Med Dir: German F Leparc, MD
Class Cap: 4 *Begins:* Feb
Length: 12 mos, 24 mos *Award:* Cert
Tuition per yr: $1,200

Georgia

American Red Cross Blood Services Southern Region
Specialist in BB Tech Prgm
1925 Monroe Dr NE
Atlanta, GA 30324
Prgm Dir: Lisbeth Fabiny, MHS MT(ASCP)
Tel: 404 881-0668 *Fax:* 404 876-6984
Med Dir: Alfred J Grindon, MD
Class Cap: 6 *Begins:* Feb
Length: 12 mos *Award:* Cert

Illinois

Univ of Illinois at Chicago
Specialist in BB Tech Prgm
Dept of Medical Laboratory Sciences
808 S Wood St Rm 690
Chicago, IL 60612-7305
Prgm Dir: Veronica N Lewis, MS MT(ASCP)SB
Tel: 312 996-7767 *Fax:* 312 996-9296
E-mail: veronica@uic.edu
Med Dir: Glenn Ramsey, MD
Class Cap: 10 *Begins:* Sep
Length: 12 mos, 31 mos *Award:* Cert, MS
Tuition per yr: $5,365 res, $15,160 non-res

Louisiana

Medical Center of LA - Charity Campus
Specialist in BB Tech Prgm
1532 Tulane Ave
New Orleans, LA 70112-2860
Prgm Dir: Cynthia A Eicher, MHS MT(ASCP)SBB
Tel: 504 568-2466 *Fax:* 504 568-2635
Med Dir: Yuan S Kao, MD
Class Cap: 4 *Begins:* Jan
Length: 12 mos, 24 mos *Award:* Cert

Maryland

Johns Hopkins Hospital
Specialist in BB Tech Prgm
Carnegie Bldg, Rm 667
600 N Wolfe St
Baltimore, MD 21287-6667
Prgm Dir: Michael Baldwin, MBA MT(ASCP)SBB
Tel: 410 955-6580 Fax: 410 955-0618
Med Dir: Paul M Ness, MD
Class Cap: 3 *Begins:* Feb
Length: 12 mos *Award:* Cert

NIH Clinical Center Blood Bank
Specialist in BB Tech Prgm
NIH/CC/DTM
Bldg 10 Rm 1C-711
10 Center Dr, MSC 1184
Bethesda, MD 20892
Prgm Dir: Sherry Sheldon, MT(ASCP)SBB
Tel: 301 496-8335 *Fax:* 301 402-1360
Med Dir: Cathy Conry-Cantilena, MD
Class Cap: 3 *Begins:* Jan
Length: 12 mos *Award:* Cert

Massachusetts

Deaconess Hospital
Specialist in BB Tech Prgm
One Deaconess Rd
Boston, MA 02215
Prgm Dir: Maruditsa Mitsiu, MS MT(ASCP)SBB
Tel: 617 632-0433 *Fax:* 617 632-0432
Med Dir: Walter H Dzik, MD
Class Cap: 3 *Begins:* Jan Sep
Length: 12 mos *Award:* Cert

Ohio

Hoxworth Blood Center
Specialist in BB Tech Prgm
3130 Highland Ave/PO Box 670055
Cincinnati, OH 45267-0055
Prgm Dir: Susan L Wilkinson, EdD
  MT(ASCP)SBB
Tel: 513 558-1271 *Fax:* 513 558-1279
E-mail: susan.wilkinson@uc.edu
Med Dir: Thomas Zuck, MD
Class Cap: 7 *Begins:* Sep
Length: 12 mos, 24 mos *Award:* Dipl,Cert, MS

Amer Red Cross Blood Services - Northern Ohio Reg
Specialist in BB Tech Prgm
3747 Euclid Ave
Cleveland, OH 44115-2501
Prgm Dir: Jane Mesnard, PhD MS MT(ASCP)SBB
Tel: 216 431-3288 *Fax:* 216 431-3246
Med Dir: John P Miller, MD, PhD
Class Cap: 4 *Begins:* Sep
Length: 12 mos, 24 mos *Award:* Cert
Tuition per yr: $250

Ohio State University Medical Center Blood Bank and American Red Cross Blood Services - Central Ohio Reg
Specialist in BB Tech Prgm
995 E Broad St
Columbus, OH 43205
Prgm Dir: Mary E Wissel, MD
Tel: 614 253-2740, Ext 270 *Fax:* 614 253-2945
Class Cap: 8 *Begins:* Jan
Length: 24 mos *Award:* Cert

Texas

Univ of Tx Southwestern Med Ctr

Specialist in BB Tech Prgm
5323 Harry Hines Blvd
Dallas, TX 75235-8878
Prgm Dir: Lynn M Little, PhD MT(ASCP)
Tel: 214 648-1780   *Fax:* 214 648-1565
E-mail: llittl@mednet.swmed.edu
Med Dir: Harold Kaplan, MD
Class Cap: 4   *Begins:* Aug
Length: 12 mos, 24 mos   *Award:* Cert
Tuition per yr: $1,110 res, $6,512 non-res

**University of Texas Medical Branch Blood
  Bank**

Specialist in BB Tech Prgm
301 University Blvd
Galveston, TX 77555-0717
Prgm Dir: Janet Vincent, MS SBB(ASCP)
Tel: 409 772-4866   *Fax:* 409 772-3193
E-mail: jvincent@mspo6.med.utmb.edu
Med Dir: Gerald Shulman, MD
Class Cap: 4   *Begins:* Feb
Length: 12 mos   *Award:* Cert

Gulf Coast Regional Blood Center

Specialist in BB Tech Prgm
1400 La Concha Ln
Houston, TX 77054-1802
Prgm Dir: Lee Ann Prihoda, MT(ASCP)SBB
Tel: 713 791-6201   *Fax:* 713 790-1007
Med Dir: Arthur Bracey, MD
Class Cap: 6   *Begins:* Jan
Length: 12 mos   *Award:* Cert

University Health System

Specialist in BB Tech Prgm
4502 Medical Dr, MS 75
San Antonio, TX 78229-4495
Prgm Dir: Milka M Montiel, MD
Tel: 210 616-2807   Fax: 210 616-3992
Med Dir: Chantal R Harrison, MD
Class Cap: 2   *Begins:* Sep
Length: 12 mos   *Award:* Cert

Wisconsin

Blood Center of Southeast Wisconsin

Specialist in BB Tech Prgm
638 N 18th St/PO Box 2178
Milwaukee, WI 53201-2178
Prgm Dir: Susan Johnson, MT(ASCP)SBB
Tel: 414 933-5000   *Fax:* 414 937-6332
E-mail: sue_j@smtp.gate.bcsew.edu
Med Dir: Janice G McFarland, MD
Class Cap: 4   *Begins:* Aug Feb
Length: 12 mos   *Award:* Cert

Cardiovascular Technologist

History

In December 1981, the American Medical Association (AMA) Council on Medical Education (CME) officially recognized cardiovascular technology as an allied health profession. Subsequently, organizations that had indicated an interest in sponsoring accreditation activities for the cardiovascular technologist were invited to appoint a representative to an ad hoc committee to develop *Standards (Essentials)*. Interested individuals were also invited to join the committee.

The ad hoc committee on development of *Standards* for the cardiovascular technologist held its first meeting on April 29, 1982, in Atlanta, Georgia. Twenty-one individuals attended the first meeting representing the following organizations: American College of Cardiology; AMA; American Society of Echocardiography; American College of Radiology; American Registry of Diagnostic Medical Sonographers; Grossmont College, El Cajon, California; American Society of Radiologic Technologists; Society of Diagnostic Medical Sonographers; National Alliance of Cardiovascular Technologists; Society of Non-Invasive Vascular Technology; American College of Chest Physicians; American Cardiology Technologists Association; Santa Fe Community College, Gainesville, Florida; and National Society for Cardiopulmonary Technology.

An initial draft of the proposed *Standards and Guidelines of an Accredited Educational Program in Cardiovascular Technology* was developed as a result of this meeting. Subsequent meetings were held to refine and polish the *Standards*. In September 1983, the committee members reached agreement on the *Standards*. The Joint Review Committee on Education in Cardiovascular Technology (JRC-CVT) held its first meeting in November 1985 in preparation for its ongoing review of programs seeking accreditation in cardiovascular technology.

The *Standards* are adopted by the Commission on Accreditation of Alllied Health Education Programs and the following sponsor organizations of the JRC-CVT: the American College of Cardiology, American College of Chest Physicians, American College of Radiology, American Society of Echocardiography, American Society of Cardiovascular Professionals, and Society of Vascular Technology (formerly the Society of Non-Invasive Vascular Technology).

Occupational Description

The cardiovascular technologist performs diagnostic examinations at the request or direction of a physician in one or more of the following three areas: (1) invasive cardiology, (2) noninvasive cardiology, and (3) noninvasive peripheral vascular study. Through subjective sampling and/or recording, the technologist creates an easily definable foundation of data from which a correct anatomic and physiologic diagnosis may be established for each patient.

Job Description

The cardiovascular technologist is qualified by specific technological education to perform various cardiovascular/peripheral vascular diagnostic procedures. The role of the cardiovascular technologist may include but is not limited to (1) reviewing and/or recording pertinent patient history and supporting clinical data; (2) performing appropriate procedures and obtaining a record of anatomical, pathological, and/or physiological data for interpretation by a physician; and (3) exercising discretion and judgment in the performance of cardiovascular diagnostic services.

Employment Characteristics

Cardiovascular technologists may provide their services to patients in any medical setting, under the supervision of a doctor of medicine or osteopathy. The procedures performed by the cardiovascular technologist may be found in, but are not limited to, one of the following general settings: (1) invasive cardiovascular laboratories, including cardiac catheterization, blood gas, and electrophysiology laboratories; (2) noninvasive cardiovascular laboratories, including echocardiography, exercise stress test, and electrocardiography laboratories; and (3) noninvasive peripheral vascular studies laboratories, including Doppler ultrasound, thermography, and plethysmography laboratories.

According to the 1992 CAHEA Annual Supplemental Survey, entry-level salaries average $28,490.

Educational Programs

Length. Programs may be from 1 to 4 years, depending on student qualifications and number of areas of diagnostic evaluation selected: invasive cardiology, noninvasive cardiology, or noninvasive peripheral vascular study.

Prerequisites. High school diploma or equivalent or qualifications in a clinically related allied health profession.

Curriculum. Curricula of accredited programs include both didactic instruction and formal laboratory experiences. Suggested areas of instruction in the core curriculum include an introduction to the field of cardiovascular technology, general and/or applied sciences, human anatomy and physiology, basic pharmacology, and basic medical electronics and medical instrumentation. Emphasis, following the core curriculum, is given in the area(s) of diagnostic evaluation selected: invasive cardiology, noninvasive cardiology, and noninvasive peripheral vascular study. Both didactic instruction and clinical experiences are provided in these areas.

Standards. *Standards* are minimum educational standards adopted by the several collaborating organizations and the AMA CME. Each new program is assessed in accordance with the *Standards,* and accredited programs are periodically reviewed to determine continuing substantial compliance. The *Standards and Guidelines* are available on written request from the JRC-CVT.

Inquiries

Accreditation

Requests for information on program accreditation, including the *Standards,* preparing the self-study report, and arranging a site visit, should be submitted to:

Joint Review Committee on Education in Cardiovascular Technology
3525 Ellicott Mills Dr/Ste N
Ellicott City, MD 21043-4547
410 418-4800
410 418-4805 Fax
E-mail: assnhdqtrs@aol.com

Careers

Inquiries regarding careers and curriculum should be addressed to

Society of Vascular Technology
4601 Presidents Dr/Ste 260
Lanham, MD 20706-4365
301 459-7550
800 SVT-VEIN
301 459-5651 Fax

American Society of Echocardiography
4101 Lake Boone Trail/Ste 201
Raleigh, NC 27607
919 787-5181
919 787-4916 Fax

American Society of Cardiovascular Professionals/Society of Cardiovascular Managers (ASCP/SCM)
910 Charles St
Fredericksburg, VA 22401
540 370-0102
540 370-0015 Fax

Certification/Registration

Inquiries regarding registration should be addressed to

Cardiovascular Credentialing International
4456 Corporation Ln/Ste 120
Virginia Beach, VA 23462
800 326-0268
804 628-3259 Fax

American Registry of Diagnostic Medical Sonographers
600 Jefferson Plaza/Ste 360
Rockville, MD 20852-1150
301 738-8401
301 738-0312 Fax

Cardiovascular Technologist

California

Grossmont College

Cardiovascular Technologist Prgm
8800 Grossmont College Dr
El Cajon, CA 92020-1799
Prgm Dir: Rickey D Kirby, MA
Tel: 619 465-1700   *Fax:* 619 461-3396
E-mail: rick_kirby@gcccd.cc.ca.us
Med Dir: William Ceretto, MD
Class Cap: 54   *Begins:* Aug
Length: 22 mos   *Award:* Cert, AS
Tuition per yr: $377 res, $3,596 non-res
Evening or weekend classes available

Florida

Edison Community College

Cardiovascular Technologist Prgm
9909 College Prkwy
Ft Myers, FL 33906
Prgm Dir: Robert J Davis, RRT RCVT
Tel: 941 489-9430   *Fax:* 941 489-9037
Med Dir: Steven R West, MD
Class Cap: 25   *Begins:* Aug
Length: 20 mos   *Award:* AS
Tuition per yr: $1,474 res, $5,482 non-res

Georgia

Augusta Technical Inst/University Hosp

Ga Heart Inst Sch Cardiovascular Tech
Invasive & Noninvasive Tracks
1350 Walton Way
Augusta, GA 30901-2629
Prgm Dir: Patricia L Thomas, MBA RCVT BSRT
Tel: 706 774-5044   *Fax:* 706 774-8644
Med Dir: John W Kelly, MD
Class Cap: 20   *Begins:* Jul
Length: 24 mos   *Award:* AAT
Tuition per yr: $2,516 res, $2,516 non-res
Evening or weekend classes available

Maryland

Naval School of Health Sciences - MD

Cardiovascular Technologist Prgm
Naval Sch of Hlth Sciences
Bethesda, MD 20889-5611
Prgm Dir: Kenneth D Horton, HMC
Tel: 301 295-0124   *Fax:* 301 295-0621
E-mail: khorton@nsh20.navy
Med Dir: David Ferguson, MD
Class Cap: 15   *Begins:* Mar Jul
Length: 12 mos   *Award:* Cert

Minnesota

Northwest Technical Coll - E Grand Forks

Cardiovascular Technologist Prgm
Hwy 220 N
PO Box 111
East Grand Forks, MN 56721
Prgm Dir: Susan Rick, RN RCVT
Tel: 218 773-3441
Med Dir: Noah Chelliah, MD
Class Cap: 10   *Begins:* Aug
Length: 24 mos   *Award:* AD
Tuition per yr: $3,735 res, $4,665 non-res

New Jersey

Morristown Memorial Hospital

Cardiovascular Technologist Prgm
100 Madison Ave
Morristown, NJ 07962-1956
Prgm Dir: Kathleen Sauter
Tel: 201 971-5096   *Fax:* 201 540-0336
Med Dir: John Banas, MD
Class Cap: 12   *Begins:* Sep
Length: 18 mos   *Award:* Cert
Tuition per yr: $2,700 res, $2,700 non-res

Ohio

Cuyahoga Community College

Cardiovascular Technologist Prgm
11000 Pleasant Valley Rd
Parma, OH 44130
Prgm Dir: B Edward Stacey, MA ACSM
Tel: 216 987-5574   *Fax:* 216 987-5066
E-mail: ed.stacey@tri-c.cc.oh.us
Class Cap: 20   *Begins:* Sep
Length: 22 mos   *Award:* AAS
Tuition per yr: $2,068 res, $2,567 non-res
Evening or weekend classes available

University of Toledo

Cardiovascular Technologist Prgm
2801 W Bancroft St
Toledo, OH 43606-3390
Prgm Dir: Suzanne Wambold, RN MEd RDGS
Tel: 419 530-3193   *Fax:* 419 530-3096
Med Dir: Wilson Felix, MD
Class Cap: 10   *Begins:* Sep
Length: 21 mos   *Award:* AS
Tuition per yr: $4,302 res, $10,321 non-res
Evening or weekend classes available

Pennsylvania

Eastern College

Cardiovascular Technologist Prgm
130 S Bryn Mawr Ave
Bryn Mawr, PA 19010
Prgm Dir: Melissa Mabry, MBA RCVT
Tel: 610 526-3388
Med Dir: Harold J Robinson, MD
Class Cap: 20   *Begins:* Sep
Length: 24 mos   *Award:* Cert, AS
Tuition per yr: $15,850 res, $10,620 non-res
Evening or weekend classes available

Geisinger Medical Center

Cardiovascular Technologist Prgm
100 N Academy Ave
Danville, PA 17822-2011
Prgm Dir: William L Fisher, RCVT
Tel: 717 271-8002
Med Dir: William Kimber, MD
Class Cap: 5   *Begins:* Jan
Length: 12 mos   *Award:* Dipl
Tuition per yr: $4,000

Gwynedd-Mercy College

Cardiovascular Technologist Prgm
Sumneytown Pike
Gwynedd Valley, PA 19437
Prgm Dir: Andrea Reiley-Helzner, MS RCVT
Tel: 610 646-7300   *Fax:* 610 646-7300
Med Dir: Otto F Muller, MD
Class Cap: 16   *Begins:* Sept
Length: 24 mos, 12 mos   *Award:* Cert, AS
Tuition per yr: $18,370 res, $12,670 non-res

Lancaster Institute for Health Education

Cardiovascular Technologist Prgm
PO Box 3555
555 N Duke St
Lancaster, PA 17604-3555
Prgm Dir: William L Fisher, RCVT
Tel: 717 290-5511   *Fax:* 717 290-5970
Med Dir: John P Slovak, MD
Class Cap: 8   *Begins:* Jul
Length: 12 mos   *Award:* Dipl
Tuition per yr: $4,000

South Dakota

Southeast Technical Institute

Cardiovascular Technologist Prgm
2301 Career Pl
Sioux Falls, SD 57107
Prgm Dir: Randall Lee Townley, RDCS CCT MS
Tel: 605 367-8459   *Fax:* 605 367-8305
E-mail: seti.tec.jd.us
Med Dir: Greg Schultz, MD
Class Cap: 60   *Begins:* Jun
Length: 24 mos   *Award:* AAS
Tuition per yr: $3,202 res, $3,202 non-res

Texas

El Centro College

Cardiovascular Technologist Prgm
Main & Lamar Sts
Dallas, TX 75202-3604
Prgm Dir: Leland R Christian, BA RCPT
Tel: 214 860-2314   *Fax:* 214 860-2268
E-mail: lrc5527@dcccd.edu
Med Dir: Jack Schwade, MD
Class Cap: 20   *Begins:* Sep
Length: 24 mos   *Award:* AAS
Tuition per yr: $539 res, $1,055 non-res

Virginia

Sentara Norfolk General Hospital
Cardiovascular Technologist Prgm
600 Gresham Dr
Norfolk, VA 23507
Prgm Dir: Kathy Butterbaugh
Tel: 757 628-2827   *Fax:* 757 668-2905
Med Dir: John P Parker, MD
Class Cap: 10   *Begins:* Aug
Length: 18 mos   *Award:* Cert
Tuition per yr: $5,287

Washington

Spokane Community College
Cardiovascular Technologist Prgm
Invasive & Noninvasive Tracks
N 1810 Greene St MS 2090
Spokane, WA 99207-5499
Prgm Dir: Dennis K Carney, AS RCVT
Tel: 509 533-7309   *Fax:* 509 533-8621
E-mail: dcarney@ctc.ctc.edu
Med Dir: Pierre Leimgruber, MD
Class Cap: 30   *Begins:* Sep
Length: 20 mos   *Award:* AAS
Tuition per yr: $1,401 res, $5,511 non-res
Evening or weekend classes available

Clinical Laboratory Science/ Medical Technology

History

The American Society of Clinical Pathologists (ASCP) began program accreditation review as one of the functions of its Board of Registry of Medical Technologists in 1933, working with the American Medical Association (AMA) Council on Medical Education (CME). The first set of *Essentials of an Acceptable School for Clinical Laboratory Technicians* was prepared by the ASCP Board of Registry and subsequently adopted by the AMA House of Delegates in 1937. The first list of 211 accredited programs was issued by the ASCP Board of Registry in 1933. The program title was changed to medical technology in 1947 with that year's revised *Essentials*.

The American Society for Clinical Laboratory Sciences (ASCLS) was organized in 1932. ASCLS joined ASCP in periodically revising the *Essentials* and was represented on the ASCP Board of Registry and the ASCP Board of Schools (established in 1949). ASCLS was recognized by the CME as one of the organizations collaborating with the AMA in accrediting educational programs.

In 1972, representatives of ASCLS and ASCP began talks that culminated in the incorporation of the National Accrediting Agency for Clinical Laboratory Sciences (NAACLS), in October 1973, as an organization independent of the professional organizations to which the authority to approve *Essentials* was delegated. NAACLS is the first agency of its kind to conduct the processes of detailed program review and recommendations through which the Committee on Allied Health Education and Accreditation (CAHEA) accredited programs. NAACLS is now an independent agency recognized by the US Department of Education.

Units within NAACLS include the Board of Directors, the Clinical Laboratory Sciences Programs Review Committee, and the executive office staff. The Board of Directors is the governing unit. The Bylaws provide for sponsoring and participating organization representation on the board. ASCP and ASCLS are sponsoring organizations. Current participating organizations are the National Society for Histotechnology and the Association of Genetic Technologists. In addition to representatives from these professional organizations, the membership of the board includes two college educators, two public members, and a technician practitioner. The programs review committee includes technologist and pathologist program officials and educators/practitioners.

The American Association of Pathologists' Assistants is an affiliating organization and cooperates in the accreditation of training programs for pathologists' assistants.

In addition to the work associated with conducting program reviews, NAACLS provides workshops and publishes a periodic newsletter, as well as publications related to clinical laboratory scientist/medical technologist, clinical laboratory technician/medical laboratory technician, histologic technician/technologist, pathologists' assistant, phlebotomy, and cytogenetic technology programs.

Clinical Laboratory Scientist/ Medical Technologist

Occupational Description

Laboratory tests play an important role in the detection, diagnosis, and treatment of many diseases. Clinical laboratory scientists/medical technologists perform these tests in conjunction with pathologists (physicians who diagnose the causes and nature of disease) and other physicians or scientists who specialize in clinical chemistry, microbiology, or the other biological sciences. Clinical laboratory scientists/medical technologists develop data on the blood, tissues, and fluids of the human body by using a variety of precision instruments.

Job Description

In addition to possessing the skills of clinical laboratory technicians/medical laboratory technicians, clinical laboratory scientists/medical technologists perform complex analyses, fine-line discrimination, and error correction. They are able to recognize interdependency of tests and have knowledge of physiological conditions affecting test results so that they can confirm these results and develop data that may be used by a physician in determining the presence, extent, and, as far as possible, cause of disease.

Clinical laboratory scientists/medical technologists assume responsibility and are held accountable for accurate results. They establish and monitor quality control and quality assurance programs and design or modify procedures as necessary. Tests and procedures performed or supervised by clinical laboratory scientists/medical technologists in the clinical laboratory focus on major areas of hematology, microbiology, immunohematology, immunology, clinical chemistry, and urinalysis.

Employment Characteristics

Most clinical laboratory scientists/medical technologists are employed in hospital laboratories. The remainder are employed chiefly in physicians' private laboratories and clinics; by the armed forces; by city, state, and federal health agencies; in industrial medical laboratories; in pharmaceutical houses; in numerous public and private research programs dedicated to the study of specific diseases; and as faculty of accredited programs preparing medical laboratory personnel. Salaries vary depending on the employer and geographic location.

Based on a 1994 survey by the American Society of Clinical Pathologists' Board of Registry, the median entry-level salary was $25,126 and the supervisor entry-level salary was $30,680.

Educational Programs

Length. At least 1 year of professional/clinical education.
Prerequisites. College courses and numbers of required credits are those necessary to ensure admission of a student who is prepared for the educational program. Content areas should include general chemistry, general biological sciences, organic and/or biochemistry, microbiology, immunology, and mathematics. Survey courses do not qualify as fulfillment of chemistry and biological science prerequisites, and remedial mathematics courses will not satisfy the mathematics requirement.

College/university programs that integrate preprofessional and professional coursework are structured with professional courses in the junior and senior years.
Curriculum. There must be a structured laboratory program, including instruction pertaining to theory and practice in hematology, clinical chemistry, microbiology, immunology, and immunohematology. The program must culminate in a baccalaureate degree for those students not already possessing the degree.
Standards. *Essentials* are minimum educational standards adopted by NAACLS. Each new program is assessed in accordance with the *Essentials*, and accredited programs are periodically reviewed to determine whether they remain in substantial compliance.

Clinical Laboratory Technician/ Medical Laboratory Technician- Associate Degree

Occupational Description

Laboratory tests play an important role in the detection, diagnosis, and treatment of many diseases and in the promotion of health. Clinical laboratory technicians/medical laboratory technicians perform these tests under the supervision or direction of pathologists (physicians who diagnose the causes and nature of disease) and other physicians, clinical laboratory scientists/medical technologists, or other scientists who specialize in clinical chemistry, microbiology, or the other biological sciences. Clinical laboratory technicians/medical laboratory technicians (associate degree) develop data on the blood, tissues, and fluids of the human body by using a variety of precision instruments.

Job Description

Clinical laboratory technicians/medical laboratory technicians (associate degree) perform all the routine tests in an up-to-date medical laboratory and can demonstrate discrimination between closely similar items and correction of errors by use of preset strategies. The technician has knowledge of specific techniques and instruments and is able to recognize factors that directly affect procedures and results. The technician also monitors quality control programs within predetermined parameters.

Employment Characteristics

Most clinical laboratory technicians/medical laboratory technicians (associate degree) work in hospital laboratories, averaging a 40-hour week. Salaries vary, depending upon the employer and geographic location. Based upon a 1994 survey by the American Society of Clinical Pathologists' Board of Registry, the median entry-level salary was $20,176, and the average salary was $24,544.

Educational Programs

Length. The period of education is usually 2 academic years, with graduates receiving an associate degree.
Prerequisites. High school diploma or equivalent. The applicant also must meet the admission requirements of the sponsoring educational institution.
Curriculum. Clinical laboratory technician/medical laboratory technician (associate degree) programs are conducted in junior or community colleges, in 2-year divisions of universities and colleges, or in other recognized institutions granting associate degrees. Courses are taught on campus and usually in affiliated hospitals. Classroom and laboratory classes focus on general knowledge and basic skills; understanding principles and mastering procedures of laboratory testing; and basic laboratory mathematics, computer technology, communication skills, and interpersonal relationships and responsibilities. The clinical courses include application of basic principles commonly used in the diagnostic laboratory. Technical instruction includes procedures in hematology, microbiology, immunohematology, immunology, clinical chemistry, and urinalysis.
Standards. *Essentials* are minimum educational standards adopted by NAACLS. Each new program is assessed in accordance with the *Essentials*, and accredited programs are periodically reviewed to determine whether they remain in substantial compliance.

Clinical Laboratory Technician/ Medical Laboratory Technician- Certificate

Occupational Description

Laboratory tests play an important role in the detection, diagnosis, and treatment of many diseases and in the promotion of health. Clinical laboratory technicians/medical laboratory technicians perform these tests under the supervision or direction of pathologists (physicians who diagnose the causes and nature of disease) and other physicians, clinical laboratory scientists/medical technologists, or other scientists who specialize in clinical chemistry, microbiology, or biological sciences. Clinical laboratory technicians/ medical laboratory technicians (certificate) perform many routine procedures in the clinical laboratory under the direction of a qualified physician and/or clinical laboratory scientist/medical technologist.

Job Description

Clinical laboratory technicians/medical laboratory technicians (certificate) perform routine, uncomplicated procedures in the medical laboratory. These procedures involve the use of common laboratory instruments in processes where discrimination is clear, errors are few and easily corrected, and results of the procedures can be confirmed with a reference test or source within the working area.

Employment Characteristics

Most clinical laboratory technicians/medical laboratory technicians (certificate) work in hospital laboratories, averaging a 40-hour week. Based on a 1994 survey by the American Society of Clinical Pathologists' Board of Registry, the median entry-level salary was $20,176, and the average salary was $24,544.

Educational Programs

Length. The period of clinical education is usually 12 months, with graduates receiving a certificate.
Prerequisites. High school diploma or equivalent.
Curriculum. Clinical laboratory technician/medical laboratory technician (certificate) programs are conducted in junior and community colleges or in other recognized instructional institutions. The curriculum focuses on knowledge and basic skills and on understanding principles and mastering procedures of laboratory testing, as well as on basic laboratory mathematics, computer technology, communication skills and interpersonal relationships, and social responsibilities. Technical instruction includes procedures in hematology, microbiology, immunohematology, immunology, clinical chemistry, and urinalysis.
Standards. *Essentials* are minimum educational standards adopted by NAACLS. Each new program is assessed in accordance with the *Essentials*, and accredited programs are periodically reviewed to determine whether they remain in substantial compliance.

Histologic Technician/ Histotechnologist

Occupational Description

Physicians (usually pathologists) and other scientists specializing in biological sciences or related clinical areas such as chemistry work in partnership with medical laboratory workers to analyze blood, tissues, and fluids from humans (and sometimes animals), using a variety of precision instruments. The results of these tests are used to detect and diagnose disease and other abnormalities.

The main responsibility of the histologic technician/histotechnologist in the clinical laboratory is preparing sections of body tissue for examination by a pathologist. This includes the preparation of tissue specimens of human and animal origin for diagnostic, research, or teaching purposes. Tissue sections prepared by the histologic technician/technologist for a variety of disease entities enable the pathologist to diagnose body dysfunction and malignancy.

Job Description

Histologic technicians process sections of body tissue by fixation, dehydration, embedding, sectioning, decalcification, microincineration, mounting, and routine and special staining. Histotechnologists perform all functions of the histotechnician, as well as the more complex procedures for processing tissues. They identify tissue structures, cell components, and their staining characteristics and relate them to physiological functions; implement and test new techniques and procedures; make judgments concerning the results of quality control measures; and institute proper procedures to maintain accuracy and precision. Histotechnologists apply the principles of management and supervision when they function as section supervisors and of educational methodology when they teach students. (Histotechnologist programs are designated in the program listings with an asterisk.)

Employment Characteristics

Most histologic technicians/histotechnologists work in hospital laboratories, averaging a 40-hour week.

Based on a 1994 survey by the American Society of Clinical Pathologists' Board of Registry, the median entry-level salary for histologic technicians was $20,800, the median entry-level salary for histotechnologists was $24,752, and the supervisor entry-level salary was $29,099.

Educational Programs

Length. Twelve months for the histotechnician, unless the curriculum is an integral part of a college program; for the histotechnologist, a baccalaureate degree program of 4 years.
Prerequisites. High school diploma or equivalent.
Curriculum. The curriculum includes both didactic instruction and practical demonstration in the areas of medical ethics, medical terminology, chemistry, laboratory mathematics, computer technology, organic and/or biochemistry, immunology, electron microscopy, management, anatomy, histology, histochemistry, quality control, instrumentation, microscopy, processing techniques, preparation of museum specimens, and record and administration procedures. It is recommended that the curriculum be an integral part of a junior or community college program culminating in an associate degree and that the course of study include chemistry, biology, and mathematics. The baccalaureate-level program includes coursework designed to provide supervisors and teachers with advanced capabilities.

Standards. *Essentials* are minimum educational standards adopted by NAACLS. Each new program is assessed in accordance with the *Essentials*, and accredited programs are periodically reviewed to determine whether they remain in substantial compliance.

Pathologists' Assistant

Occupational Description

Anatomic pathologists are physicians who examine tissue specimens from patients and perform autopsies to diagnose the disease processes involved. Pathologists' assistants participate in autopsies and in the examination, dissection, and processing of tissue specimens. They function as physician extenders.

Job Description

The following services are provided under the direct supervision of a licensed and board-certified pathologist and should include, but are not limited to:

Surgical Pathology. Assisting in the preparation and performance of surgical specimen dissection by assuring appropriate specimen accessioning, obtaining pertinent clinical information and studies, describing gross anatomic features, dissecting surgical specimens, preparing and submitting tissue for histologic processing, obtaining and submitting specimens for additional analytic procedures (immunostaining, flow cytometry, image analysis, bacterial and viral cultures, toxicology, etc), and assisting in photographing gross and microscopic specimens.

Autopsy Pathology. Assisting in the performance of postmortem examination by ascertaining proper legal authorization; obtaining and reviewing the patient's chart and other pertinent clinical data and studies; notifying involved personnel of all special procedures and techniques required; coordinating special requests for specimens; notifying involved clinicians and appropriate authorities and individuals; assisting in the postmortem examination; selecting and preparing tissue for histologic processing and special studies; obtaining specimens for biological and toxicologic analysis; assisting in photographing gross and microscopic specimens and photomicrography; and participating in the completion of the autopsy report.

Additional duties. Assuming duties as may be assigned relative to teaching, administrative, supervisory, and budgetary functions in anatomic pathology.

Employment Characteristics

Pathologists' assistants are employed in a variety of settings, including community and regional hospitals, university medical centers, private pathology laboratories, and medical examiners/coroners offices. Most work 40-55 hours per week. Salaries vary with geographic location and type of employing institution. Entry-level salaries are between $45,000 and $50,000.

Educational Programs

Length. Minimum 22 months.
Degree. Baccalaureate and master's level programs.
Prerequisites. Variable among programs and dependent on the degree offered. Baccalaureate programs require a minimum of 60 hours of acceptable credits, with variable specific requirements.
Curriculum. Curricula include both didactic and practical training to provide a sound background in the basic medical sciences and the necessary skills to work in an anatomic pathology laboratory. Course work includes anatomy, physiology, and medical terminology, as well as general, systemic, pediatric, and forensic pathology.

Practical training includes autopsy pathology, surgical pathology, forensic pathology, and medical photography.
Standards. *Essentials* are minimum educational standards adopted by NAACLS and the American Association of Pathologists' Assistants (AAPA). Each new training program is assessed in accordance with the *Essentials*, and accredited programs are periodically reviewed to determine whether they remain in substantial compliance.

Inquiries

Accreditation

Requests for information on program accreditation, including *Essentials*, preparing the self-study report, and arranging a site visit, should be submitted to NAACLS.

Approval

Requests for information on program approval, including *Standards* and *Competencies*, and preparing the Self-Study Report, should be submitted to NAACLS.

National Accrediting Agency for Clinical Laboratory Sciences
8410 W Bryn Mawr Ave/Ste 670
Chicago, IL 60631-3415
773 714-8880
773 714-8886 Fax
E-mail: NAACLS@mcs.net
http://www.mcs.net/~naacls

Careers

Inquiries regarding careers and curriculum should be addressed to

American Society for Clinical Laboratory Science
7910 Woodmont Ave/Ste 1301
Bethesda, MD 20814
301 657-2768

American Society of Clinical Pathologists
2100 W Harrison St
Chicago, IL 60612
312 738-1336
E-mail: info@asco.org *or* info@ascp.org
http://www.ascp.org

Association of Genetic Technologists (AGT)
Executive Office
PO Box 15945-288
Lenexa, KS 66285
913 541-9077

National Society for Histotechnology
4201 Northview Dr/Ste 502
Bowie, MD 20716-2604
301 262-6221

American Association of Pathologists' Assistants
8030 Old Cedar Ave S/#225
Bloomington, MN 55425-1215
800 532-AAPA

Certification/Registration

Inquiries regarding certification may be addressed to

Board of Registry
PO Box 12270
Chicago, IL 60612
312 738-1336, Ext 341

National Certification Agency for
Medical Laboratory Personnel
PO Box 15945-289
Lenexa, KS 66285
913 438-5110

Clinical Laboratory Scientist/Medical Technologist

Alabama

Baptist Health System Inc

Clin Lab Scientist/Med Tech Prgm
800 Montclair Rd
Birmingham, AL 35213
Prgm Dir: Pamela Crider, MBA MT(ASCP)
Tel: 205 592-5413 *Fax:* 205 592-1228
E-mail: pam.crider@bhsala.com
Med Dir: George V Eisenhart, MD
Class Cap: 4 *Begins:* Jan Jul
Length: 12 mos *Award:* Cert, BS

University of Alabama at Birmingham

Clin Lab Scientist/Med Tech Prgm
Sch of Hlth Related Professions
1714 9th Ave S Rm 381
Birmingham, AL 35294-1270
Prgm Dir: Virginia R Randolph, MA MT(ASCP)
Tel: 205 934-4683 *Fax:* 205 975-7302
E-mail: randolpv@admin.shrp.uab.edu
Med Dir: John A Smith, MD PhD
Class Cap: 25 *Begins:* Aug
Length: 15 mos *Award:* Cert, BS
Tuition per yr: $4,800 res, $9,600 non-res
Evening or weekend classes available

University of South Alabama

Clin Lab Scientist/Med Tech Prgm
Dept of Medical Technology
1504 Springhill Ave Rm 2309
Mobile, AL 36604
Prgm Dir: William J Korzun, PhD MT(ASCP)
Tel: 334 434-3461 *Fax:* 334 434-3403
Med Dir: William Gardner, Jr, MD
Class Cap: 14 *Begins:* Sep
Length: 21 mos *Award:* BSMT
Tuition per yr: $2,198 res, $2,798 non-res

Alabama Reference Laboratories, Inc

Clin Lab Scientist/Med Tech Prgm
543 S Hull St
PO Box 4600
Montgomery, AL 36103-4600
Prgm Dir: Kathy W Young, MT(ASCP)
Tel: 334 263-5745 *Fax:* 334 241-0513
Med Dir: Robert B Adams, MD
Class Cap: 7 *Begins:* Jun Jul
Length: 12 mos *Award:* Cert

Auburn University at Montgomery

Clin Lab Scientist/Med Tech Prgm
School of Science
Dept of Biology
Montgomery, AL 36193
Prgm Dir: Richard Hebert, PhD MT(ASCP)
Tel: 334 244-3302 *Fax:* 334 244-3826
Med Dir: Richard W Miller, MD
Class Cap: 12 *Begins:* Mar
Length: 24 mos *Award:* Dipl,Cert, BS
Tuition per yr: $2,840 res, $8,520 non-res

Baptist Medical Center
Clin Lab Scientist/Med Tech Prgm
2105 E South Blvd
Montgomery, AL 36116
Prgm Dir: Denise Z Jackson, MT(ASCP)
Tel: 205 286-2899
Med Dir: William M Bridger, MD
Class Cap: 8 *Begins:* Jan Jul
Length: 12 mos *Award:* Cert, BS

Tuskegee University
Clin Lab Scientist/Med Tech Prgm
Basil O'Connor Hall
Tuskegee, AL 36088
Prgm Dir: Mary Edith Powell, EdD MPA
  MT(ASCP)
Tel: 334 727-8696 *Fax:* 334 727-5461
Med Dir: Madhuri Singh, MD
Class Cap: 10 *Begins:* Sep
Length: 24 mos *Award:* BS
Tuition per yr: $9,876 res, $9,876 non-res

Arizona

Arizona State University
Clin Lab Scientist/Med Tech Prgm
Clinical Lab Sciences
Dept of Microbiology
Tempe, AZ 85287
Prgm Dir: Diana Mass, MA MT(ASCP)CLS
Tel: 602 965-7090 *Fax:* 602 965-0098
E-mail: atdim@asuvm.inre.asu.edu
Med Dir: Joseph Spataro, MD
Class Cap: 14 *Begins:* Jan
Length: 16 mos *Award:* BS
Tuition per yr: $1,940 res, $8,308 non-res

University of Arizona
Clin Lab Scientist/Med Tech Prgm
Sch of Hlth Related Professions
1435 N Fremont
Tucson, AZ 85719
Prgm Dir: Harold L Potter Jr, PhD MT(ASCP)
Tel: 520 626-4084 *Fax:* 520 622-4656
Med Dir: Kenneth J Ryan, MD
Class Cap: 22 *Begins:* Aug Jan
Length: 18 mos *Award:* Dipl,Cert, BS
Tuition per yr: $2,010 res, $8,378 non-res

Arkansas

Baptist Medical System
Clin Lab Scientist/Med Tech Prgm
11900 Colonel Glenn Rd
Ste 1000
Little Rock, AR 72210-2820
Prgm Dir: Sandra G Ackerman, MT(ASCP)SH
Tel: 501 223-7409 *Fax:* 501 223-7406
Med Dir: John Edward Slaven, MD
Class Cap: 12 *Begins:* Jul
Length: 12 mos *Award:* Cert, BS, MT
Tuition per yr: $2,500

Univ of Arkansas for Medical Sciences
Clin Lab Scientist/Med Tech Prgm
4301 W Markham
Slot 597
Little Rock, AR 72205
Prgm Dir: Martha J Lake, MT(ASCP)
Tel: 501 686-5776 *Fax:* 501 686-6513
E-mail: mlake@chrp.uams.edu
Med Dir: Alexandros A Pappas, MD
Class Cap: 23 *Begins:* Aug
Length: 18 mos, 27 mos *Award:* Dipl, BSMT
Tuition per yr: $2,100 res, $5,250 non-res

Arkansas State University
Clin Lab Scientist/Med Tech Prgm
PO Box 69
State University, AR 72467
Prgm Dir: Mary Jean Rutherford, MEd
  MT(ASCP)SC
Tel: 501 972-3073 *Fax:* 501 972-2040
E-mail: mjruth@crow.astate.edu
Med Dir: Don B Vollman, Jr, MD
Class Cap: 24 *Begins:* Jan
Length: 18 mos *Award:* BS
Tuition per yr: $2,400 res, $4,200 non-res
Evening or weekend classes available

California

California State University - Bakersfield
Clin Lab Scientist/Med Tech Prgm
9001 Stockdale Hwy
Bakersfield, CA 93311
Prgm Dir: Landy J McBride, PhD MT(ASCP)
Tel: 805 664-2228
Med Dir: William R Schmalhorst, MD
Begins: Sep Jan
Length: 9 mos *Award:* Cert, BS
Tuition per yr: $1,440 res, $8,492 non-res

California State Univ-Dominguez Hills
Clin Lab Scientist/Med Tech Prgm
1000 E Victoria St
Carson, CA 90747
Prgm Dir: Cheryl Jackson-Harris, MS
  MT(ASCP)SH
Tel: 310 243-3748 *Fax:* 310 516-3865
E-mail: charris@dnox20.csudn.edu
Med Dir: Karen Cove, MD
Class Cap: 12 *Begins:* Jan Jul
Length: 12 mos *Award:* Cert, BS, MS
Tuition per yr: $1,791 res, $6,888 non-res

Fresno Community Hospital & Medical Ctr
Clin Lab Scientist/Med Tech Prgm
PO Box 1232
Fresno, CA 93715
Prgm Dir: Sue M McGowen, MT(ASCP)
Tel: 209 442-3982 *Fax:* 209 442-6542
Class Cap: 10 *Begins:* Jul
Length: 12 mos *Award:* Cert

Valley Children's Hospital
Clin Lab Scientist/Med Tech Prgm
3151 N Millbrook Ave
Fresno, CA 93703
Prgm Dir: Percy F Lee, MS MT(ASCP)
Tel: 209 225-3000
Med Dir: Stephen Kassel, MD
Class Cap: 4 *Begins:* Jan Jul
Length: 12 mos *Award:* Cert, BS

Scripps Memorial Hospitals
Clin Lab Scientist/Med Tech Prgm
Pathology Med Lab/Dept 8970
9888 Genesee Ave
La Jolla, CA 92037
Prgm Dir: Gerald S Rea, MT(ASCP)
Tel: 619 453-3141 *Fax:* 619 550-3289
Med Dir: Phillips L Gausewitz, MD
Class Cap: 8 *Begins:* Feb Aug
Length: 12 mos *Award:* Cert

Loma Linda University
Clin Lab Scientist/Med Tech Prgm
11234 Anderson Ave
Loma Linda, CA 92350
Prgm Dir: Samuel L Chafin, MS MT(ASCP)
Tel: 909 824-4966 *Fax:* 909 824-4832
E-mail: chabay@prmenet.com
Med Dir: James M Pappas, MD
Class Cap: 16 *Begins:* Sep
Length: 18 mos *Award:* BS
Tuition per yr: $11,026

St Mary Medical Center
Clin Lab Scientist/Med Tech Prgm
1050 Linden Ave
Long Beach, CA 90813
Prgm Dir: Linda C Kovac, MT(ASCP)CLS(NCA)
Tel: 310 491-9694
Med Dir: Andrew Burg, MD
Begins: Feb Jul
Length: 12 mos *Award:* Cert, BS

Veterans Affairs Medical Center
Clin Lab Scientist/Med Tech Prgm
5901 E Seventh St (113ED)
Long Beach, CA 90822
Prgm Dir: Leila Bradford, MT(ASCP)
Tel: 310 494-2611
Med Dir: Galli S Ascher, MD
Class Cap: 12 *Begins:* Jan Jul
Length: 12 mos *Award:* Cert

Cedars Sinai Medical Center
Clin Lab Scientist/Med Tech Prgm
8700 Beverly Blvd
Rm 3722B
Los Angeles, CA 90048
Prgm Dir: Sharron E Kelly
Tel: 310 855-5334
Med Dir: Stephen Lee, MD
Class Cap: 10 *Begins:* Jul
Length: 12 mos *Award:* Cert

Charles R Drew Univ of Med & Science
Clin Lab Scientist/Med Tech Prgm
King/Drew Medical Ctr
12021 S Wilmington Ave
Los Angeles, CA 90059
Prgm Dir: Mary Ann Bradley, MS MT(ASCP)
Tel: 310 668-4477 *Fax:* 310 608-2420
Med Dir: Elias Amador, MD
Class Cap: 3 *Begins:* Jul
Length: 12 mos *Award:* Cert

Programs

Los Angeles County - USC Medical Center

Clin Lab Scientist/Med Tech Prgm
1200 N State St
GH2636
Los Angeles, CA 90033
Prgm Dir: Susan Wilcox, MHA MT(ASCP)SH
    DLM CLS(NCA)
Tel: 213 226-7050   *Fax:* 213 226-4582
Med Dir: Edward T Wong, MD
Class Cap: 20   *Begins:* Varies
Length: 12 mos   *Award:* Cert

Veterans Affairs Med Ctr W Los Angeles

Clin Lab Scientist/Med Tech Prgm
11301 Wilshire Blvd (113)
Los Angeles, CA 90073
Prgm Dir: Elizabeth Kaupp, MT(ASCP)CT
Tel: 310 478-3711, Ext 44628   *Fax:* 310 268-4983
Med Dir: Joan H Howanitz, MD
Class Cap: 6   *Begins:* Jul
Length: 12 mos   *Award:* Cert

St Joseph Hospital

Clin Lab Scientist/Med Tech Prgm
1100 Stewart Dr
PO Box 5600
Orange, CA 92268
Prgm Dir: Mary Ann Kovach, MT(ASCP)
Tel: 714 771-8155   *Fax:* 714 744-8522
Med Dir: Thomas R Heinz, MD
Class Cap: 8   *Begins:* Aug
Length: 12 mos   *Award:* Cert

Univ of California Irvine Med Ctr

Clin Lab Scientist/Med Tech Prgm
101 City Dr S
Orange, CA 92868-3298
Prgm Dir: Marie Pezzlo, MA MT(ASCP)
Tel: 714 456-5037   *Fax:* 714 456-8272
E-mail: mtpezzlo@uci.edu
Med Dir: Luis M de la Maza, MD PhD
Class Cap: 4   *Begins:* Aug
Length: 12 mos   *Award:* Cert

Huntington Memorial Hospital

Clin Lab Scientist/Med Tech Prgm
100 W California Blvd
PO Box 7013
Pasadena, CA 91109-7013
Prgm Dir: Cheryl Ward, MS MT(ASCP)
Tel: 818 397-5229   *Fax:* 818 397-3800
Med Dir: Charles E Marshall, MD
Begins: Jan Jul
Length: 12 mos   *Award:* Cert

Eisenhower Memorial Hospital

Clin Lab Scientist/Med Tech Prgm
39000 Bob Hope Dr
Rancho Mirage, CA 92270
Prgm Dir: Joan M Steiner, MA MS MT(ASCP)
Tel: 619 773-4525   *Fax:* 619 773-1577
Med Dir: William M Burleigh, MD
Class Cap: 4   *Begins:* Jul
Length: 12 mos   *Award:* Cert

Univ of California Davis Med Ctr

Clin Lab Scientist/Med Tech Prgm
Clinical Laboratory Bldg
4625 2nd Ave
Sacramento, CA 95817
Prgm Dir: Claramae H Miller, PhD
Tel: 916 734-0231   *Fax:* 916 734-0320
Med Dir: Robert D Cardiff, MD PhD
Class Cap: 12   *Begins:* Aug
Length: 12 mos   *Award:* Cert

San Bernardino County Medical Center

Clin Lab Scientist/Med Tech Prgm
780 E Gilbert St
San Bernardino, CA 92415-0935
Prgm Dir: Susan E Liddle, MT(ASCP)
Tel: 909 387-7975   *Fax:* 909 387-7877
Med Dir: Theodore A Friedman, MD
Class Cap: 3   *Begins:* Jul Feb
Length: 12 mos   *Award:* Cert

San Francisco State University

Clin Lab Scientist/Med Tech Prgm
Ctr for Advanced Med Tech
San Francisco, CA 94132
Prgm Dir: Jerrold Haas, MT(ASCP)
Tel: 415 338-1696   *Fax:* 415 338-7747
E-mail: jbh@sfsu.edu
Med Dir: Paul Ortega, MD
Class Cap: 32   *Begins:* Jan Jul
Length: 12 mos   *Award:* Cert
Tuition per yr: $2,332 res, $9,712 non-res

Columbia San Jose Medical Center

Clin Lab Scientist/Med Tech Prgm
675 E Santa Clara St
San Jose, CA 95112
Prgm Dir: Arlene T Susbilla, MT(ASCP)
Tel: 408 977-7330   *Fax:* 408 993-7160
Med Dir: Gerald A Weiss, MD
Class Cap: 4   *Begins:* Feb Jul
Length: 12 mos   *Award:* Cert

Santa Barbara Cottage Hospital

Clin Lab Scientist/Med Tech Prgm
Pueblo at Bath Sts
PO Box 689
Santa Barbara, CA 93102
Prgm Dir: Lynette Hansen, MHA MT(ASCP)
Tel: 805 569-7378   *Fax:* 805 569-8223
Med Dir: Peter Lorenz Morris, MD
Class Cap: 4   *Begins:* Aug
Length: 12 mos   *Award:* Cert

LA County Harbor UCLA Medical Center

Clin Lab Scientist/Med Tech Prgm
1000 W Carson St
PO Box 12
Torrance, CA 90509-2910
Prgm Dir: Michael Coover, MS MT(ASCP)
Tel: 310 222-3014   *Fax:* 310 618-0249
Med Dir: Robert J Morin, MD
Class Cap: 4   *Begins:* Jan Jul
Length: 12 mos   *Award:* Cert

Colorado

Penrose-St Francis Health System

Clin Lab Scientist/Med Tech Prgm
2215 N Cascade Ave
PO Box 7021
Colorado Springs, CO 80933
Prgm Dir: Sr Rose V Brown, MEd MT(ASCP)
Tel: 719 776-5221   *Fax:* 719 776-5584
Med Dir: Cosimo G Sciotto, MD PhD
Class Cap: 6   *Begins:* Aug
Length: 12 mos   *Award:* Cert, BS
Tuition per yr: $1,000 res, $1,000 non-res

HealthONE Ctr for Health Sciences Educ

Clin Lab Scientist/Med Tech Prgm
1719 E 19th Ave
Denver, CO 80218
Prgm Dir: Karen E Myers, MA MT(ASCP)SC
Tel: 303 839-6485
Med Dir: Thomas A Merrick, MD
Class Cap: 14   *Begins:* Aug
Length: 12 mos   *Award:* Dipl,Cert, BS
Tuition per yr: $3,300

University of Colorado Hlth Science Ctr

Clin Lab Scientist/Med Tech Prgm
4200 E Ninth Ave
B-173
Denver, CO 80262
Prgm Dir: George A Harwell, EdD MT(ASCP)SC
Tel: 303 270-8178   *Fax:* 303 270-4792
Med Dir: Ronald Lepoff, MD
Class Cap: 20   *Begins:* Aug
Length: 12 mos   *Award:* Dipl, BS, MLS
Tuition per yr: $4,600 res, $22,579 non-res

Parkview Episcopal Medical Center

Clin Lab Scientist/Med Tech Prgm
400 W 16th St
Pueblo, CO 81003
Prgm Dir: Mary Chasteen, MT(ASCP)SBB
Tel: 719 584-4405   *Fax:* 719 584-4658
Med Dir: Domingo Baitlon, MD
Class Cap: 6   *Begins:* Jul
Length: 12 mos   *Award:* Cert, BS

Connecticut

Bridgeport Hospital

Clin Lab Scientist/Med Tech Prgm
267 Grant St
Bridgeport, CT 06602
Prgm Dir: Patricia A Clark, MS MT(ASCP)SM
Tel: 203 384-3108
Med Dir: Larry H Bernstein, MD
Class Cap: 6   *Begins:* Jun
Length: 12 mos   *Award:* Cert, BS

St Vincent's Medical Center

Clin Lab Scientist/Med Tech Prgm
2800 Main St
Bridgeport, CT 06606
Prgm Dir: Diana M Luca, MS MT(ASCP)SC SH
Tel: 203 576-5036   *Fax:* 203 579-5034
Med Dir: James A Spencer, MD
Class Cap: 6   *Begins:* Jun
Length: 11 mos   *Award:* Cert

Danbury Hospital

Clin Lab Scientist/Med Tech Prgm
24 Hospital Ave
Danbury, CT 06810
Prgm Dir: Rebecca Brewer, MT(ASCP)
Tel: 203 797-7522
Med Dir: Ramon N Kranwinkel, MD
Class Cap: 13   *Begins:* Aug
Length: 12 mos   *Award:* Cert, BS

Quinnipiac College

Clin Lab Scientist/Med Tech Prgm
275 Mt Carmel Ave
Hamden, CT 06518
Prgm Dir: Thomas C Brady, PhD MT(ASCP)
Tel: 203 281-8609   *Fax:* 203 281-8706
Med Dir: Romeo Vidone, MD
Class Cap: 24   *Begins:* Sep Jan
Length: 12 mos   *Award:* Dipl,Cert, BS
Tuition per yr: $12,800

Hartford Hospital

Clin Lab Scientist/Med Tech Prgm
School of Allied Health
80 Seymour St
Hartford, CT 06115
Prgm Dir: Wayne A Aguiar, MS MT(ASCP)
Tel: 860 545-2612   *Fax:* 860 545-5066
Med Dir: Herbert Silver, MD
Class Cap: 12   *Begins:* Jun
Length: 12 mos   *Award:* Dipl, BS
Tuition per yr: $1,000

St Mary's Hospital

Clin Lab Scientist/Med Tech Prgm
56 Franklin St
Waterbury, CT 06706
Prgm Dir: Joseph A Vaccarelli, MS MT(ASCP)
Tel: 203 597-3152   *Fax:* 203 597-3130
Med Dir: William C Frederick, PhD MD
Class Cap: 6   *Begins:* Aug
Length: 12 mos   *Award:* Cert, BS

University of Hartford

Clin Lab Scientist/Med Tech Prgm
Dana Hall/Rm 232
200 Bloomfield Ave
West Hartford, CT 06117-1599
Prgm Dir: Karen Barrett, MS MT(ASCP)
Tel: 860 768-4489   *Fax:* 860 768-5244
E-mail: bitnet:barrett@hartford.edu
Med Dir: George Barrows, MD
Class Cap: 16   *Begins:* Jan Jun Sep
Length: 12 mos, 48 mos   *Award:* Cert, BS
Tuition per yr: $7,800 res, $15,600 non-res
Evening or weekend classes available

Delaware

University of Delaware

Clin Lab Scientist/Med Tech Prgm
050 McKinly Laboratory
Dept of Medical Technology
Newark, DE 19716
Prgm Dir: Anna P Ciulla, MCC MT(ASCP)SC
Tel: 302 831-2849   *Fax:* 302 831-2281
E-mail: anna.ciulla@mvs.udel.edu
Med Dir: Robert Knowles, MD
Class Cap: 26   *Begins:* Sep
Length: 18 mos   *Award:* Dipl, BS
Tuition per yr: $3,990 res, $11,250 non-res
Evening or weekend classes available

District of Columbia

George Washington University

Clin Lab Scientist/Med Tech Prgm
2300 K St NW
Washington, DC 20037
Prgm Dir: Sylvia Silver, DA MT(ASCP)
Tel: 202 994-2945   *Fax:* 202 994-5056
E-mail: ssilver@qwis2.circ.gwu.edu
Med Dir: Donald S Karcher, MD
Class Cap: 12   *Begins:* Aug
Length: 12 mos   *Award:* Cert, BS
Tuition per yr: $11,400

Howard University

Clin Lab Scientist/Med Tech Prgm
Sixth & Bryant Sts NW
C/AHS
Washington, DC 20059
Prgm Dir: Hemant B Karnik, PhD MT(ASCP)
Tel: 202 806-7565   *Fax:* 202 806-7918
Med Dir: Josephine J Marshalleck, MD
Class Cap: 20   *Begins:* Aug
Length: 18 mos   *Award:* BSMT
Tuition per yr: $8,825

Walter Reed Army Medical Center

Clin Lab Scientist/Med Tech Prgm
Clinical Lab Officer Course
6825 16th St NW Rm 2B72
Washington, DC 20307-5001
Prgm Dir: Nancy P Johnson, PhD MT(ASCP)
Tel: 202 782-0733   *Fax:* 202 782-0692
Med Dir: Renata B Greenspan, Col MD
Class Cap: 6   *Begins:* Aug
Length: 12 mos   *Award:* Cert

Washington Hospital Center

Clin Lab Scientist/Med Tech Prgm
110 Irving St NW
Washington, DC 20010
Prgm Dir: Sue W Lawton, MA MT(ASCP) MS
Tel: 202 877-3346   *Fax:* 202 877-5263
E-mail: seli@mgh.edu
Med Dir: Mary E Kass, MD
Class Cap: 14   *Begins:* Aug
Length: 12 mos   *Award:* Cert, BS
Tuition per yr: $2,000 res, $2,000 non-res

Florida

Florida Atlantic University

Clin Lab Scientist/Med Tech Prgm
777 Glades Rd
Boca Raton, FL 33431
Prgm Dir: Cynthia Butler, EdD MT(ASCP)
Tel: 561 367-3394   *Fax:* 561 367-3613
E-mail: cbutler@acc.fau.edu
Med Dir: Fred W Reineke, MD
Class Cap: 18   *Begins:* Aug
Length: 12 mos   *Award:* BSMT
Tuition per yr: $933 res, $3,253 non-res
Evening or weekend classes available

Bethune-Cookman College

Clin Lab Scientist/Med Tech Prgm
640 Mary McLeod Bethune Blvd
Daytona Beach, FL 32114-3099
Prgm Dir: John B Kennedy, EdD MT(ASCP)
Tel: 904 255-1401   *Fax:* 904 253-7726
Med Dir: William Schildecker, MD
Class Cap: 10   *Begins:* Aug
Length: 24 mos   *Award:* Cert, BS
Tuition per yr: $7,611

St Vincent's Medical Center

Clin Lab Scientist/Med Tech Prgm
St. Vincent's Medical Center
1800 Barrs St
Jacksonville, FL 32203
Prgm Dir: Lynnette Chakkaphak, MS MT(ASCP)
Tel: 904 308-3817   *Fax:* 904 308-2970
Med Dir: Matthew C Patterson, MD
Class Cap: 10   *Begins:* Jan Jul
Length: 12 mos   *Award:* Cert, BS

University Medical Center

Clin Lab Scientist/Med Tech Prgm
655 W Eighth St
Jacksonville, FL 32209
Prgm Dir: James D Sigler, MT(ASCP)
Tel: 904 549-4660   *Fax:* 904 549-4629
Med Dir: Ned M Hardy, MD
Class Cap: 3   *Begins:* Jul Jan
Length: 12 mos   *Award:* Cert

Florida International University

Clin Lab Scientist/Med Tech Prgm
University Park Campus
Miami, FL 33199
Prgm Dir: Barbara V Anderson, MS
   MT(ASCP)SBB
Tel: 305 348-3186   *Fax:* 305 348-1997
Med Dir: William Riemer, MD
Class Cap: 20   *Begins:* Jul
Length: 24 mos   *Award:* BS
Tuition per yr: $2,439 res, $9,264 non-res
Evening or weekend classes available

Florida Hospital Medical Center

Clin Lab Scientist/Med Tech Prgm
601 E Rollins St
Orlando, FL 32803
Prgm Dir: Patricia L Rogers, MT(ASCP)SBB
Tel: 407 897-1855   *Fax:* 407 893-6943
Med Dir: Rodney F Holcomb, MD
Class Cap: 20   *Begins:* Aug
Length: 12 mos   *Award:* Dipl, BS
Tuition per yr: $1,000

Programs

University of Central Florida
Clin Lab Scientist/Med Tech Prgm
4000 Central Florida Blvd
B10 103
Orlando, FL 32816-2360
Prgm Dir: Dorilyn J Hitchcock, MS MT(ASCP)
Tel: 407 823-2968 *Fax:* 407 823-3095
E-mail: hitchcod@pegasus.cc.ucf.us
Med Dir: Raymond B Franklin Jr, MD PhD
Class Cap: 18 *Begins:* Aug
Length: 24 mos *Award:* BS
Tuition per yr: $1,770 res, $6,839 non-res

University of West Florida
Clin Lab Scientist/Med Tech Prgm
Dept of Biology Univ of W Florida
11000 University Pkwy
Pensacola, FL 32514-5751
Prgm Dir: Swarna Krothapalli, MS MT(ASCP)
Tel: 904 474-2988 *Fax:* 904 474-3130
E-mail: skrothap@nautilus.uwf.edu
Med Dir: James Potter, MD
Class Cap: 20 *Begins:* May
Length: 15 mos *Award:* BS
Tuition per yr: $1,819 res, $1,819 non-res

Bayfront Medical Center
Clin Lab Scientist/Med Tech Prgm
701 Sixth St S
St Petersburg, FL 33701
Prgm Dir: June P Schurig, MT(ASCP)
Tel: 813 893-6604 *Fax:* 813 893-6977
Med Dir: Larry Davis, MD
Class Cap: 8 *Begins:* Aug
Length: 12 mos *Award:* Cert, BS
Tuition per yr: $500 res, $500 non-res

Tallahassee Memorial Regional Med Center
Clin Lab Scientist/Med Tech Prgm
Magnolia and Miccosukee Rds
Tallahassee, FL 32308
Prgm Dir: Virginia Dell Craig, MT(ASCP)
Tel: 904 681-5809 *Fax:* 904 942-3336
Med Dir: Woodward Burgert, Jr, MD
Class Cap: 3 *Begins:* Feb Jul
Length: 12 mos *Award:* Cert, BS

Tampa General Hospital
Clin Lab Scientist/Med Tech Prgm
PO Box 1289
Tampa, FL 33601
Prgm Dir: Laura Ferguson, MT(ASCP)
Tel: 813 251-7246 *Fax:* 813 253-4073
Med Dir: Irwin L Browarsky, MD
Class Cap: 6 *Begins:* Aug
Length: 12 mos *Award:* Cert, BS
Tuition per yr: $800

Georgia

Emory University Hospital
Clin Lab Scientist/Med Tech Prgm
1364 Clifton Rd NE
Atlanta, GA 30322
Prgm Dir: Theressa Y Vincent, MT(ASCP)SBB
Tel: 404 712-7304
Med Dir: John A Bryan, MD
Class Cap: 12 *Begins:* Sep
Length: 15 mos, 25 mos *Award:* Dipl,Cert, BS
Tuition per yr: $3,560 res, $12,760 non-res

Emory University System of Health Care
Clin Lab Scientist/Med Tech Prgm
1364 Clifton Rd NE
Atlanta, GA 30322
Prgm Dir: Anne Roebuck, MS MT(ASCP)
Tel: 404 712-4376 *Fax:* 404 686-4980
Med Dir: John Bryan, MD
Class Cap: 12 *Begins:* Sep
Length: 15 mos *Award:* Dipl,Cert, BS
Tuition per yr: $4,134 res, $13,935 non-res

Georgia State University
Clin Lab Scientist/Med Tech Prgm
University Plaza
Atlanta, GA 30303-3090
Prgm Dir: Susan B Roman, MMSc MT(ASCP)SM
Tel: 404 651-3034 *Fax:* 404 651-2015
Med Dir: L David Stacy, MD
Class Cap: 30 *Begins:* Sep
Length: 15 mos *Award:* Dipl, BS
Tuition per yr: $4,134 res, $13,935 non-res

Grady Health System
Clin Lab Scientist/Med Tech Prgm
80 Butler St SE
PO Box 26095
Atlanta, GA 30335-3801
Prgm Dir: Marilea Grider, MS MT (ASCP)
Tel: 404 616-4806 *Fax:* 404 616-9913
Med Dir: Victor M Napoli, MD
Class Cap: 12 *Begins:* Sep
Length: 15 mos, 24 mos *Award:* Cert, BS
Tuition per yr: $4,134 res, $13,934 non-res

Medical College of Georgia
Clin Lab Scientist/Med Tech Prgm
AL-106
Augusta, GA 30912-0500
Prgm Dir: Julia R Crowley, EdD MT(ASCP)
Tel: 706 721-3046 *Fax:* 706 721-7631
E-mail: jcrowley@mail.mcg.edu
Med Dir: Charles Robert Baisden, MD
Class Cap: 20 *Begins:* Sep Jun
Length: 12 mos, 21 mos *Award:* Cert, BS
Tuition per yr: $1,722 res, $7,208 non-res

Columbus State University
Clin Lab Scientist/Med Tech Prgm
4225 University Ave
Columbus, GA 31907-5645
Prgm Dir: Mae E Allen, PhD MT(ASCP)
Tel: 706 568-2051 *Fax:* 706 568-2084
E-mail: allen.mae@colstate.edu
Med Dir: Hans J Peters, MD
Class Cap: 16 *Begins:* Jun
Length: 15 mos *Award:* BS
Tuition per yr: $3,075 res, $9,540 non-res
Evening or weekend classes available

Armstrong Atlantic State University
Clin Lab Scientist/Med Tech Prgm
11935 Abercorn St
Savannah, GA 31419-1997
Prgm Dir: Lester Hardegree Jr, MEd MT(ASCP)
Tel: 912 927-5204 *Fax:* 912 921-5505
E-mail:
  lester_hardegree@mailgate.armstrong.edu
Med Dir: John Ralph Edgar, MD
Class Cap: 12 *Begins:* Sep
Length: 15 mos *Award:* Cert, BSMT
Tuition per yr: $2,448 res, $7,620 non-res

Hawaii

University of Hawaii at Manoa
Clin Lab Scientist/Med Tech Prgm
1960 E-W Rd
Bio C206
Honolulu, HI 96822
Prgm Dir: Patricia L Taylor, MS MT(ASCP)CLS
Tel: 808 956-8557 *Fax:* 808 956-5506
E-mail: ptaylor@hawaii.edu
Med Dir: William Wong, PhD
Class Cap: 20 *Begins:* Aug
Length: 30 mos *Award:* Cert, BS
Tuition per yr: $2,832 res, $9,312 non-res
Evening or weekend classes available

Idaho

St Alphonsus Regl Medical Center
Clin Lab Scientist/Med Tech Prgm
1055 N Curtis Rd
Boise, ID 83706
Prgm Dir: Sandra K Perotto, MT(ASCP)
Tel: 208 378-2182 *Fax:* 208 378-2920
Med Dir: Steven H Wilson, MD
Begins: Jul
Length: 12 mos *Award:* Cert

Idaho State University
Clin Lab Scientist/Med Tech Prgm
Dept Biological Sciences
Box 8007
Pocatello, ID 83209
Prgm Dir: Kathleen Spiegel, PhD MT(ASCP)
Tel: 208 236-3765
Med Dir: Charles O Garrison, MD
Class Cap: 12 *Begins:* Sep July Jan
Length: 12 mos, 24 mos *Award:* Cert, BS
Tuition per yr: $750 res, $3,500 non-res
Evening or weekend classes available

Illinois

St Elizabeth Hospital
Clin Lab Scientist/Med Tech Prgm
211 S Third St
Belleville, IL 62222
Prgm Dir: JoAnn B Denaro, MT(ASCP)
Tel: 618 234-2120 *Fax:* 618 234-8713
Med Dir: Paul A Rusnack, MD
Class Cap: 4 *Begins:* Jul
Length: 12 mos *Award:* Cert
Tuition per yr: $1,000 res, $1,000 non-res

Rush University
Clin Lab Scientist/Med Tech Prgm
1653 W Harrison St
Chicago, IL 60612
Prgm Dir: Herbert J Miller, PhD MT(ASCP)
Tel: 312 942-7251 *Fax:* 312 942-6989
E-mail: hmiller@rush.edu
Med Dir: Meryl Haber, MD
Begins: Sep
Length: 18 mos, 9 mos *Award:* Dipl,Cert, BS
Tuition per yr: $10,254

Univ of Illinois at Chicago

Clin Lab Scientist/Med Tech Prgm
808 S Wood St Rm 690
M/C 518
Chicago, IL 60612-7305
Prgm Dir: Donna H Weaver, MEd MT(ASCP)SH
Tel: 312 996-7767   *Fax:* 312 996-9296
E-mail: dweaver@uic.edu
Med Dir: Phillip J DeChristopher, MD PhD
Class Cap: 24   *Begins:* Sept
Length: 12 mos, 21 mos   *Award:* BS
Tuition per yr: $5,069 res, $11,484 non-res

Decatur Memorial Hospital

Clin Lab Scientist/Med Tech Prgm
2300 N Edward St
Decatur, IL 62526
Prgm Dir: Connie Myers, MS MT(ASCP)
Tel: 217 876-5000   *Fax:* 217 876-5013
Med Dir: David M Johnson, MD
Class Cap: 10   *Begins:* Jun
Length: 12 mos   *Award:* Cert, BS

Northern Illinois University

Clin Lab Scientist/Med Tech Prgm
DeKalb, IL 60115
Prgm Dir: Dianne M Cearlock, PhD CLS(NCA)
Tel: 815 753-1382   *Fax:* 815 753-1653
E-mail: dcearlock@iu.edu
Med Dir: A R Tammes, MD
Class Cap: 24   *Begins:* Aug
Length: 18 mos   *Award:* BS
Tuition per yr: $4,128 res, $10,990 non-res

National-Louis University

Clin Lab Scientist/Med Tech Prgm
2840 Sheridan Rd
Evanston, IL 60201
Prgm Dir: Claudia Miller, PhD MT(ASCP)CLS
Tel: 847 256-5150   *Fax:* 847 256-1057
Med Dir: James Perkins, MD
Class Cap: 12   *Begins:* Sep
Length: 12 mos   *Award:* Cert, BA
Tuition per yr: $11,250
Evening or weekend classes available

Edward Hines Jr VA Hospital

Clin Lab Scientist/Med Tech Prgm
PO Box 5000/113/School
Hines, IL 60141-5113
Prgm Dir: Donna M Wray, MT(ASCP)
Tel: 708 216-2611   *Fax:* 708 216-2588
Med Dir: Myron E Rubnitz, MD
Class Cap: 10   *Begins:* Aug
Length: 12 mos   *Award:* Cert, BS

Foster G McGaw Hosp of Loyola University

Clin Lab Scientist/Med Tech Prgm
2160 S First Ave
Maywood, IL 60153
Prgm Dir: Jacqueline S Streid, MEd MT(ASCP)
Tel: 708 216-8939   *Fax:* 708 216-6676
E-mail: jstreid@luc.edu
Med Dir: Robert E Lee, MD
Class Cap: 8   *Begins:* Jun
Length: 12 mos   *Award:* Cert
Tuition per yr: $1,500

Finch U of Hlth Science/Chicago Med Sch

Clin Lab Scientist/Med Tech Prgm
3333 Green Bay Rd
North Chicago, IL 60064
Prgm Dir: Janet M DeRobertis, MS MT(ASCP)
Tel: 847 578-3303   *Fax:* 847 578-8651
Med Dir: Satinder K Singh, MD
Class Cap: 20   *Begins:* Sep Dec Mar
Length: 24 mos   *Award:* BS
Tuition per yr: $10,857

St Francis Medical Center

Clin Lab Scientist/Med Tech Prgm
530 NE Glen Oak Ave
Peoria, IL 61637
Prgm Dir: Cathy R Moewe, MT(ASCP)CLS
Tel: 309 655-2479   *Fax:* 309 655-7658
E-mail: camoewe@heartland.bradley.edu
Med Dir: Michael P Hayes, MD
Class Cap: 10   *Begins:* Aug
Length: 11 mos   *Award:* Cert, BS
Tuition per yr: $1,000 res, $1,000 non-res

Rockford Memorial Hospital

Clin Lab Scientist/Med Tech Prgm
2400 N Rockton Ave
Rockford, IL 61103
Prgm Dir: Nancy Knight, MT(ASCP)
Tel: 815 968-6861   *Fax:* 815 971-5797
Med Dir: A R Tammes, MD
Class Cap: 8   *Begins:* Aug
Length: 9 mos   *Award:* Cert, BS

St Anthony Medical Center

Clin Lab Scientist/Med Tech Prgm
5666 E State St
Rockford, IL 61108
Prgm Dir: James F Beam, MT(ASCP)
Tel: 815 395-5119   *Fax:* 815 395-5364
Med Dir: William C Lane, MD
Class Cap: 5   *Begins:* Aug
Length: 9 mos   *Award:* Cert, BS

Swedish American Hospital

Clin Lab Scientist/Med Tech Prgm
1400 Charles St
Rockford, IL 61104
Prgm Dir: Lorinda Schiller, MEd MT(ASCP)
Tel: 815 968-4400   *Fax:* 815 966-3967
Med Dir: Luis R Owano, MD
Class Cap: 7   *Begins:* Aug
Length: 9 mos   *Award:* Cert, BS
Tuition per yr: $800 res, $800 non-res

St John's Hospital

Clin Lab Scientist/Med Tech Prgm
800 E Carpenter
Springfield, IL 62769
Prgm Dir: Gilma Roncancio, MS MT(ASCP)
Tel: 217 757-6788   *Fax:* 217 535-3996
Med Dir: Donald Van Fossan, MD PhD
Class Cap: 6   *Begins:* Jun
Length: 12 mos   *Award:* Dipl, BS, BA
Tuition per yr: $800

University of Illinois at Springfield

Clin Lab Scientist/Med Tech Prgm
Shepherd Rd
Springfield, IL 62794
Prgm Dir: Paula Garrott, EdM
    MT(ASCP)CLS(NCA)
Tel: 217 786-6589   *Fax:* 217 786-7188
E-mail: garrott.paula@uis.edu
Med Dir: Joan Barenfanger, MD
Class Cap: 20   *Begins:* Aug Jan
Length: 21 mos   *Award:* BS
Tuition per yr: $2,720 res, $8,160 non-res

Indiana

St Francis Hospital and Health Centers

Clin Lab Scientist/Med Tech Prgm
1600 Albany St
Beech Grove, IN 46107
Prgm Dir: DeAnne S Maxwell, MT(ASCP)
Tel: 317 783-8195   *Fax:* 317 783-8801
Med Dir: F Donald McGovern, Jr, MD
Class Cap: 10   *Begins:* Jul
Length: 12 mos   *Award:* Cert, BA, BS
Tuition per yr: $1,500

Lutheran Hospital of Indiana, Inc

Clin Lab Scientist/Med Tech Prgm
7950 W Jefferson Blvd
Ft Wayne, IN 46804-1677
Prgm Dir: Karen D Johnson, MT(ASCP)
Tel: 219 435-7178   *Fax:* 219 435-7633
Med Dir: Jeffrey P Squires, MD
Class Cap: 12   *Begins:* Aug
Length: 12 mos   *Award:* Cert
Tuition per yr: $1,500

Parkview Memorial Hospital

Clin Lab Scientist/Med Tech Prgm
2200 Randallia
Ft Wayne, IN 46805
Prgm Dir: Frances M Williams, MS MT(ASCP)
Tel: 219 484-6636   *Fax:* 219 483-1373
Med Dir: Darryl R Smith, MD
Class Cap: 6   *Begins:* Jun Jan
Length: 12 mos   *Award:* Cert, BS
Tuition per yr: $1,500
Evening or weekend classes available

St Margaret Hospital & Health Centers

Clin Lab Scientist/Med Tech Prgm
5454 Hohman Ave
Hammond, IN 46320
Prgm Dir: Rosemary Ann Butkiewicz,
    MT/I(ASCP)
Tel: 312 891-9305   *Fax:* 219 933-2136
Med Dir: Lisbeth Gallagher, MD
Class Cap: 9   *Begins:* Aug
Length: 12 mos   *Award:* Cert, BS
Tuition per yr: $1,000

St Mary Medical Center

Clin Lab Scientist/Med Tech Prgm
1500 S Lake Park Ave
Hobart, IN 46342
Prgm Dir: Mary Sue Demitroulas, MT(ASCP)
Tel: 219 947-6271
Med Dir: Amarjit S Kochar, MD
Class Cap: 16   *Begins:* Jun
Length: 12 mos   *Award:* Cert, BS

Programs

Indiana University School of Medicine

Clin Lab Scientist/Med Tech Prgm
1120 S Dr Fesler Hall
Rm 409
Indianapolis, IN 46202-5113
Prgm Dir: Linda M Kasper, MS MT(ASCP)SC
Tel: 317 274-1265 *Fax:* 317 278-0643
E-mail: lmkasper@indyunix.iupui.edu
Med Dir: James W Smith, MD
Class Cap: 32 *Begins:* Aug
Length: 11 mos *Award:* Dipl, BS
Tuition per yr: $3,780 res, $11,673 non-res

Methodist Hospital of Indiana, Inc

Clin Lab Scientist/Med Tech Prgm
1701 N Senante Blvd
PO Box 1367
Indianapolis, IN 46206
Prgm Dir: Cheryl Oliver, MS MT(ASCP)
Tel: 317 929-8280 *Fax:* 317 929-2102
Med Dir: Charles Miraglia, MD
Class Cap: 24 *Begins:* Jun
Length: 12 mos *Award:* Cert, BS
Tuition per yr: $1,500

St Vincent Hosp & Health Care Ctr, Inc

Clin Lab Scientist/Med Tech Prgm
2001 W 86 St
Indianapolis, IN 46260
Prgm Dir: Anne Kornafel, MS MT(ASCP) SH
Tel: 317 338-2290 *Fax:* 317 338-3213
Med Dir: John Michael Irons, MD
Class Cap: 6 *Begins:* Jun
Length: 12 mos *Award:* Cert, BS
Tuition per yr: $1,500

Ball Memorial Hospital

Clin Lab Scientist/Med Tech Prgm
2401 University Ave
Muncie, IN 47303
Prgm Dir: Shirley A Replogle, MT(ASCP)
Tel: 317 747-3327 *Fax:* 317 747-3326
Med Dir: Richard W Pearson, MD
Class Cap: 8 *Begins:* Jul
Length: 12 mos *Award:* Cert, BS
Tuition per yr: $1,500

Good Samaritan Hospital

Clin Lab Scientist/Med Tech Prgm
520 S Seventh St
Vincennes, IN 47591
Prgm Dir: Philip H Bousley, MA MT(ASCP)
Tel: 812 885-3367 *Fax:* 812 885-3135
Med Dir: Mark C Mills, MD
Class Cap: 6 *Begins:* Aug Feb
Length: 12 mos *Award:* Cert, BS

Iowa

Mercy/St Luke's Hospitals

Clin Lab Scientist/Med Tech Prgm
1026 A Ave NE
Cedar Rapids, IA 52402
Prgm Dir: Nadine Sojka, MS MT(ASCP)SH
Tel: 319 369-7309
Med Dir: Dorryl Buck, MD
Class Cap: 6 *Begins:* Jul
Length: 12 mos *Award:* Cert, BS, BA
Tuition per yr: $2,000 res, $2,000 non-res

Iowa Methodist Medical Center

Clin Lab Scientist/Med Tech Prgm
1200 Pleasant St
Des Moines, IA 50309-1453
Prgm Dir: Linda L Blair, MS MT(ASCP)
   CLS(NCA)
Tel: 515 241-4470 *Fax:* 515 241-8535
Med Dir: Richard Kent Schupham, MD
Class Cap: 8 *Begins:* Jun
Length: 12 mos *Award:* Cert
Tuition per yr: $2,000 res, $2,000 non-res

Mercy Hospital Medical Center

Clin Lab Scientist/Med Tech Prgm
400 University
Des Moines, IA 51314
Prgm Dir: Marianne Samorey, MS BS MT(ASCP)
   CLS(NCA)
Tel: 515 247-4469 *Fax:* 515 248-8810
Med Dir: Vijaya Dhannavada, MD
Begins: Aug
Length: 12 mos *Award:* Dipl,Cert, BS
Tuition per yr: $2,000

University of Iowa

Clin Lab Scientist/Med Tech Prgm
U IA Hosps & Clins-Pathology
150A Medical Laboratories
Iowa City, IA 52242
Prgm Dir: Marian Schwabbauer, PhD MT(ASCP)
Tel: 319 335-8248 *Fax:* 319 335-8348
E-mail: marian_schwabbauer@uiowa.edu
Med Dir: Robert Tucker, MD
Class Cap: 16 *Begins:* Jun
Length: 12 mos *Award:* Cert, BS
Tuition per yr: $3,191 res, $11,714 non-res
Evening or weekend classes available

Marian Health Center

Clin Lab Scientist/Med Tech Prgm
801 5th St
Sioux City, IA 51101
Prgm Dir: Marvin L Pansegrau, MT(ASCP)M
Tel: 712 279-2095 *Fax:* 712 279-2371
Med Dir: Askar A Qalbani, MD
Class Cap: 10 *Begins:* Aug
Length: 12 mos *Award:* Cert, BS
Tuition per yr: $2,000

St Luke's Regional Medical Center

Clin Lab Scientist/Med Tech Prgm
2720 Stone Park Blvd
Sioux City, IA 51104
Prgm Dir: Sharon K Collier, MT(ASCP)
Tel: 712 279-3967 *Fax:* 712 279-7983
Med Dir: Gene Herbek, MD
Class Cap: 10 *Begins:* Aug
Length: 12 mos *Award:* Cert, BS
Tuition per yr: $2,000 res, $2,000 non-res

Kansas

Hays Pathology Laboratories

Clin Lab Scientist/Med Tech Prgm
1300 E 13th St
Hays, KS 67601
Prgm Dir: Janet Hudzicki, MA MT(ASCP)SM
Tel: 913 625-5646 *Fax:* 913 625-0013
Med Dir: Ward M Newcomb, MD
Class Cap: 4 *Begins:* Jan Jul
Length: 12 mos *Award:* Cert
Tuition per yr: $6,300 res, $6,300 non-res

University of Kansas Medical Center

Clin Lab Scientist/Med Tech Prgm
3901 Rainbow Blvd
1014 Kansas Univ Hospital
Kansas City, KS 66160-7608
Prgm Dir: Venus J Ward, PhD MT(ASCP)
Tel: 913 588-5220 *Fax:* 913 588-5222
E-mail: vward@kumc.edu
Med Dir: Masahiro Chiga, MD
Class Cap: 24 *Begins:* Jun
Length: 12 mos *Award:* BS
Tuition per yr: $2,898 res, $12,180 non-res

Wichita State University

Clin Lab Scientist/Med Tech Prgm
Campus Box 43
Wichita, KS 67208
Prgm Dir: Mary E Conrad, PhD MT(ASCP)
Tel: 316 689-3146 *Fax:* 316 978-3025
E-mail: conrad@1wsu.chp.edu
Med Dir: William Reals, MD
Class Cap: 50 *Begins:* Jan Aug Jun
Length: 18 mos, 24 mos *Award:* Dipl,Cert, BSMT
Tuition per yr: $4,956 res, $17,448 non-res
Evening or weekend classes available

Kentucky

St Elizabeth Medical Center

Clin Lab Scientist/Med Tech Prgm
One Medical Village Dr
Edgewood, KY 41017
Prgm Dir: Christopher M Barczak, MT(ASCP)
Tel: 606 344-2170 *Fax:* 606 344-5560
Med Dir: Jackson Pemberton, MD
Class Cap: 5 *Begins:* Jun Jan
Length: 12 mos *Award:* Cert
Tuition per yr: $2,000

Univ of Kentucky Chandler Med Ctr

Clin Lab Scientist/Med Tech Prgm
Div of Chemical Lab Sci
1 Medical Ctr Annex 2
Lexington, KY 40536-0080
Prgm Dir: Anne Stiene-Martin, PhD MT(ASCP)
Tel: 606 257-5402 *Fax:* 606 257-1816
E-mail: asmart00@pop.uky.edu
Med Dir: Diane Davey, MD
Class Cap: 25 *Begins:* May Aug
Length: 27 mos *Award:* Cert, BHS
Tuition per yr: $2,594 res, $7,114 non-res
Evening or weekend classes available

University of Louisville

Clin Lab Scientist/Med Tech Prgm
Health Sciences Ctr
Louisville, KY 40292
Prgm Dir: Susan A Miller, DA MT(ASCP)
Tel: 502 852-5345 *Fax:* 502 852-4597
E-mail: samillo1@ulkyvm.louisville.edu
Class Cap: 20 *Begins:* Jul Aug Jan
Length: 13 mos, 17 mos *Award:* Cert, BS, BHS
Tuition per yr: $4,494 res, $12,684 non-res

Owensboro Mercy Health System

Clin Lab Scientist/Med Tech Prgm
811 E Parrish Ave
Owensboro, KY 42303
Prgm Dir: Lisa Sellars Cecil, MT(ASCP)
Tel: 502 688-2934 *Fax:* 502 688-2938
Med Dir: Ritchie L Clark, MD
Class Cap: 10 *Begins:* Jul
Length: 12 mos *Award:* Dipl, BS
Tuition per yr: $700

Lourdes Hospital

Clin Lab Scientist/Med Tech Prgm
1530 Lone Oak Rd
Paducah, KY 42001
Prgm Dir: Kathy Kelley, MT(ASCP)
Tel: 502 444-2342 *Fax:* 502 444-2936
Med Dir: James R Roush, MD
Class Cap: 4 *Begins:* Jan Jul
Length: 12 mos *Award:* Cert, BS
Tuition per yr: $2,000

Pikeville Methodist Hospital

Clin Lab Scientist/Med Tech Prgm
911 S Bypass Rd
Pikeville, KY 41501
Prgm Dir: Betty S Martin, MT(ASCP)
Tel: 606 437-3967 *Fax:* 606 437-2339
Med Dir: James Dennis, MD
Class Cap: 6 *Begins:* Aug
Length: 12 mos *Award:* Cert, BS
Tuition per yr: $1,000 res, $1,000 non-res

Eastern Kentucky University

Clin Lab Scientist/Med Tech Prgm
Dizney 220
Richmond, KY 40475-3135
Prgm Dir: David C Hufford, PhD MT(ASCP)
Tel: 606 622-3078 *Fax:* 606 622-1140
E-mail: clshuffo@acs.eku.edu
Med Dir: Irene Roeckel, MD
Class Cap: 24 *Begins:* Jan Aug
Length: 17 mos *Award:* Dipl, BS
Tuition per yr: $1,970 res, $5,450 non-res

Louisiana

Rapides Regional Medical Center

Clin Lab Scientist/Med Tech Prgm
211 Fourth St
PO Box 30101
Alexandria, LA 71301
Prgm Dir: Laine O Poe, MT(ASCP)
Tel: 318 473-3175 *Fax:* 318 473-3079
Med Dir: James G Hair, MD
Class Cap: 8 *Begins:* Aug Feb
Length: 12 mos *Award:* Cert, BS

Our Lady of the Lake College

Clin Lab Scientist/Med Tech Prgm
General Studies Bldg
5120 Dijon
Baton Rouge, LA 70808
Prgm Dir: Beverly A Farrell, MS MT(ASCP)
Tel: 504 768-1706 *Fax:* 504 768-1703
E-mail: bfarrell@ololcollege.cc.la.us
Med Dir: Jack D Holden, MD
Class Cap: 12 *Begins:* Jan
Length: 12 mos *Award:* Cert, BS
Tuition per yr: $3,000

Lake Charles Mem Hosp Sch of Med Tech

Clin Lab Scientist/Med Tech Prgm
1701 Oak Park Blvd
Lake Charles, LA 70601
Prgm Dir: Dianne D Malveaux, MT(ASCP)
Tel: 318 494-2481 *Fax:* 318 494-2464
Med Dir: Carl G Bowling, MD
Class Cap: 8 *Begins:* Jan Aug
Length: 12 mos *Award:* Cert, BS
Tuition per yr: $50

St Patrick Hospital

Clin Lab Scientist/Med Tech Prgm
524 S Ryan St
PO Box 3401
Lake Charles, LA 70602-3401
Prgm Dir: Sheryl W Handy, MT(ASCP)
Tel: 318 491-7708 *Fax:* 318 494-0995
Med Dir: Lehrue Stevens, MD
Class Cap: 8 *Begins:* Dec May
Length: 12 mos *Award:* Cert, BS

St Francis Medical Center

Clin Lab Scientist/Med Tech Prgm
PO Box 1901
Monroe, LA 71201-1901
Prgm Dir: Charles Robert Starr Jr, MT(ASCP)
Tel: 318 327-4359 *Fax:* 318 327-4857
Med Dir: Richard J Blanchard Jr, MD
Class Cap: 12 *Begins:* Jul Jan
Length: 12 mos *Award:* Cert, BS

Alton Ochsner Medical Foundation

Clin Lab Scientist/Med Tech Prgm
1516 Jefferson Hwy
New Orleans, LA 70121
Prgm Dir: Susan L Kuemmel, MT(ASCP)SC
Tel: 504 842-3517 *Fax:* 504 842-3264
Med Dir: Willard T Dalton, MD
Class Cap: 10 *Begins:* Jul Jan
Length: 12 mos *Award:* Cert

Louisiana State Univ Med Ctr - New Orleans

Clin Lab Scientist/Med Tech Prgm
1900 Gravier St
New Orleans, LA 70112
Prgm Dir: Louann Lawrence, DrPH MT(ASCP)SH
Tel: 504 568-4271 *Fax:* 504 568-6761
E-mail: llawre@isumc.edu
Med Dir: Jack P Strong, MD
Class Cap: 45 *Begins:* May
Length: 14 mos *Award:* Dipl, BS
Tuition per yr: $3,359 res, $6,484 non-res

Touro Infirmary School of Med Tech

Clin Lab Scientist/Med Tech Prgm
1401 Foucher St
New Orleans, LA 70115
Tel: 504 897-8834
Med Dir: Jaeun M Kwon, MD
Class Cap: 12 *Begins:* Jul
Length: 12 mos *Award:* Cert, BS

Overton Brooks VA Medical Center

Clin Lab Scientist/Med Tech Prgm
510 E Stoner Ave
Shreveport, LA 71101-4295
Prgm Dir: Mary R McCole, MT(ASCP)SC
Tel: 318 221-8411 *Fax:* 318 424-6093
Med Dir: Aubrey A Lurie, MD
Class Cap: 10 *Begins:* Jan Jul
Length: 12 mos *Award:* Cert, BS

Maine

Eastern Maine Medical Center

Clin Lab Scientist/Med Tech Prgm
489 State St
Bangor, ME 04401
Prgm Dir: Ellen M Libby, MS MT(ASCP)
Tel: 207 973-7616 *Fax:* 207 973-7609
E-mail: emlibby@maine.maine.edu
Med Dir: Irwin Gross, MD
Class Cap: 6 *Begins:* Aug
Length: 11 mos *Award:* Cert
Tuition per yr: $3,808

Maine Medical Center

Clin Lab Scientist/Med Tech Prgm
22 Bramhall St
Portland, ME 04102-3175
Prgm Dir: Barry Corriveau, MEd MT(ASCP)
Tel: 207 871-2440 *Fax:* 207 871-6176
Med Dir: Allen L Pusch, MD
Class Cap: 5 *Begins:* Aug
Length: 11 mos *Award:* Dipl
Tuition per yr: $2,500 res, $2,500 non-res

Maryland

Malcolm Grow USAF Medical Center

Clin Lab Scientist/Med Tech Prgm
89th Medical Grp/SGAL
1050 W Perimeter Rd/Ste G1-15
Andrews AFB, MD 20762-6600
Prgm Dir: Maj Robert Zajac, MA MT(ASCP) SH
Tel: 301 981-3041 *Fax:* 301 981-3121
Med Dir: Kimberly D Schlack, MD
Class Cap: 8 *Begins:* Aug
Length: 12 mos *Award:* Dipl

Morgan State University

Clin Lab Scientist/Med Tech Prgm
Cold Spring Ln & Hillen Rd
Baltimore, MD 21239
Prgm Dir: Karim Mehrazar, PhD MT(ASCP)
Tel: 410 319-3611 *Fax:* 410 426-4732
Med Dir: Robert Jeffrey Johnson, MD
Class Cap: 14 *Begins:* Jun
Length: 12 mos *Award:* BS
Tuition per yr: $2,364 res, $7,288 non-res
Evening or weekend classes available

University of Maryland
Clin Lab Scientist/Med Tech Prgm
100 S Penn St
Baltimore, MD 21201
Prgm Dir: Denise M Harmening, PhD MT(ASCP)
Tel: 410 706-7729
Med Dir: Sanford A Stass, MD
Class Cap: 120 *Begins:* Sep
Length: 18 mos *Award:* Dipl,Cert, BS, MS
Tuition per yr: $3,390 res, $8,290 non-res

Salisbury State University
Clin Lab Scientist/Med Tech Prgm
Camden Ave
Salisbury, MD 21801
Prgm Dir: Johanna W Laird, MS MT(ASCP)
Tel: 410 543-6364 *Fax:* 410 548-3313
E-mail: jwlaird@ssu.edu
Med Dir: Stephen W Moore, MD
Begins: Sep
Length: 18 mos *Award:* Cert, BS
Tuition per yr: $2,566 res, $5,876 non-res

Columbia Union College
Clin Lab Scientist/Med Tech Prgm
7600 Flower Ave
Takoma Park, MD 20912
Prgm Dir: Juanita L Gurubatham, MA
    MT(ASCP)HT
Tel: 301 891-4184 *Fax:* 301 891-4191
E-mail: juanitag@cuc.edu
Med Dir: J D Mashburn, MD
Class Cap: 15 *Begins:* Sep
Length: 42 mos *Award:* BS
Tuition per yr: $10,940

Massachusetts

New England Deaconess Hospital
Clin Lab Scientist/Med Tech Prgm
One Deaconess Rd
Meissner G-21
Boston, MA 02215
Prgm Dir: Debra St George, MS MT(ASCP)
Tel: 617 632-9093 *Fax:* 617 632-0167
E-mail: dstgeorg@nedhmail.nedh.harvard.edu
Med Dir: Agnes Kim, MD
Class Cap: 8 *Begins:* Sep
Length: 12 mos *Award:* Cert
Tuition per yr: $1,000

Northeastern University
Clin Lab Scientist/Med Tech Prgm
360 Huntington Ave
Boston, MA 02215
Prgm Dir: Barbara E Martin, MHP MT(ASCP)CLS
Tel: 617 373-3664 *Fax:* 617 373-3030
Med Dir: Sanford Kurtz, MD
Class Cap: 32 *Begins:* Sep
Length: 57 mos, 18 mos *Award:* Cert, BS
Tuition per yr: $15,045

Veterans Administration Medical Center
Clin Lab Scientist/Med Tech Prgm
150 S Huntington Ave
Boston, MA 02130
Prgm Dir: Edward Hanchay, MT(ASCP)CLS
Tel: 617 232-9500 *Fax:* 617 278-4476
E-mail: hanchay.edward@boston.va.gov
Med Dir: John A Hayes, MD
Class Cap: 7 *Begins:* Jul
Length: 12 mos *Award:* Cert, BS

Fitchburg State College
Clin Lab Scientist/Med Tech Prgm
160 Pearl St
Fitchburg, MA 01420
Prgm Dir: Dorothy M Boisvert, EdD MT(ASCP)
Tel: 508 665-3080 *Fax:* 508 665-3578
E-mail: dboisvert@fsc.edu
Med Dir: Dieter Keller, MD
Class Cap: 40 *Begins:* Sep
Length: 48 mos *Award:* BS
Tuition per yr: $1,408 res, $5,542 non-res

Lawrence General Hospital
Clin Lab Scientist/Med Tech Prgm
One General St
Lawrence, MA 01842
Prgm Dir: Cynthia A Freyberger, MEd MT(ASCP)
Tel: 508 683-4000
Med Dir: Shashikala Dwarakanath, MD

University of Massachusetts - Lowell
Clin Lab Scientist/Med Tech Prgm
One University Ave
Weed Hall
Lowell, MA 01854
Prgm Dir: Kathleen Doyle, PhD MT(ASCP)
Tel: 508 934-4520 *Fax:* 508 934-3006
Med Dir: David McGoldrick, MD
Begins: Sep
Length: 36 mos *Award:* BS
Tuition per yr: $1,790 res, $7,253 non-res
Evening or weekend classes available

Newton Wellesley Hospital
Clin Lab Scientist/Med Tech Prgm
2014 Washington St
Newton Lower Falls, MA 02162
Prgm Dir: Anne M Pollock, MT(ASCP)
Tel: 617 243-6140 *Fax:* 617 342-6588
Med Dir: Richard J Sampson, MD
Class Cap: 12 *Begins:* Aug
Length: 12 mos *Award:* Cert, BS
Tuition per yr: $1,500

University of Massachusetts Dartmouth
Clin Lab Scientist/Med Tech Prgm
Dept of Med Lab Science
Old Westport Rd
North Dartmouth, MA 02747
Prgm Dir: Dorothy A Bergeron, MS CLS(NCA)
Tel: 508 999-8584 *Fax:* 508 999-8418
E-mail: dbergeron@umassd.edu
Med Dir: Gordon Bruce Robbins, MD
Begins: Sep
Length: 48 mos *Award:* Dipl, BS
Tuition per yr: $4,151 res, $10,733 non-res

Berkshire Medical Center
Clin Lab Scientist/Med Tech Prgm
725 North St
Pittsfield, MA 01201
Prgm Dir: Linda Billings, MT(ASCP)
Tel: 413 447-2580 *Fax:* 413 447-2097
Med Dir: Rebecca L Johnson, MD
Class Cap: 10 *Begins:* Jul
Length: 12 mos *Award:* Cert, BS

Life Laboratories
Clin Lab Scientist/Med Tech Prgm
299 Carew St
Springfield, MA 01104
Prgm Dir: Dorothy Lakoma, MST MS(ASCP) SC
Tel: 413 748-9562 *Fax:* 413 732-3349
Med Dir: Lewis Lefer, MD
Class Cap: 8 *Begins:* Sep
Length: 11 mos *Award:* Cert
Tuition per yr: $1,200

Michigan

Andrews University
Clin Lab Scientist/Med Tech Prgm
Berrien Springs, MI 49104
Prgm Dir: Marcia Kilsby, MS CLS(NCA)
    MT(ASCP)
Tel: 616 471-3336 *Fax:* 616 471-6218
E-mail: kilsby@andrews.edu
Med Dir: E Arthur Robertson, MD
Class Cap: 24 *Begins:* Sep
Length: 11 mos *Award:* Cert, BSMT
Tuition per yr: $10,476

Ferris State University
Clin Lab Scientist/Med Tech Prgm
200 Ferris Dr
VFS 404
Big Rapids, MI 49307-2740
Prgm Dir: Janice M Webster, PhD MT(ASCP)
Tel: 616 592-2314 *Fax:* 616 592-3788
E-mail: yes8@brusk.ferris.edu
Med Dir: Nicholas J Hruby, MD
Class Cap: 20 *Begins:* Aug
Length: 39 mos *Award:* BS
Tuition per yr: $3,630 res, $7,364 non-res

DMC University Laboratories
Clin Lab Scientist/Med Tech Prgm
4201 St Antoine
Detroit, MI 48201
Prgm Dir: Joyce Salancy, MS MT(ASCP)
Tel: 313 993-0482
Med Dir: Barbara J Anderson, MD
Class Cap: 15 *Begins:* Aug
Length: 11 mos *Award:* Cert

St John Hospital and Medical Center
Clin Lab Scientist/Med Tech Prgm
22101 Moross Rd
Detroit, MI 48236
Prgm Dir: Margaret Kluka, MS MT(ASCP)
Tel: 313 343-3508 *Fax:* 313 881-4727
Med Dir: Noel S Lawson, MD
Class Cap: 8 *Begins:* Jul
Length: 12 mos *Award:* Cert

Wayne State University
Clin Lab Scientist/Med Tech Prgm
233 Shapero Hall
Detroit, MI 48202
Prgm Dir: Carol A Watkins, MT(ASCP)MBA
Tel: 313 577-5524 *Fax:* 313 577-5497
Med Dir: Gilbert E Herman, PhD MD
Class Cap: 37 *Begins:* Sep
Length: 19 mos *Award:* BS
Tuition per yr: $4,680 res, $9,360 non-res

Michigan State University

Clin Lab Scientist/Med Tech Prgm
322 N Kedzie Lab
East Lansing, MI 48824-1031
Prgm Dir: Douglas W Estry, PhD MT(ASCP)CLS
Tel: 517 353-7800 *Fax:* 517 432-2006
E-mail: estry@pilot.msu.edu
Med Dir: Harold Bowman, MD
Begins: Aug
Length: 30 mos *Award:* BS
Tuition per yr: $5,006 res, $11,801 non-res

Hurley Medical Center

Clin Lab Scientist/Med Tech Prgm
1 Hurley Plaza
Flint, MI 48503
Prgm Dir: Debra S Liebler-Rogers, MHSA BS
  MT(ASCP)
Tel: 810 257-9131 *Fax:* 810 762-7082
Med Dir: Willys F Mueller, Jr, MD
Class Cap: 11 *Begins:* Aug
Length: 11 mos *Award:* Cert, BS

Garden City Hospital, Osteopathic

Clin Lab Scientist/Med Tech Prgm
6245 N Inkster Rd
Garden City, MI 48135
Prgm Dir: Barbara Cahalan Potts, MS MT(ASCP)
Tel: 313 458-4451
Med Dir: Nicholas S Sellas, DO
Class Cap: 8 *Begins:* Sep
Length: 9 mos *Award:* Cert

Butterworth Hospital

Clin Lab Scientist/Med Tech Prgm
100 Michigan St NE
Grand Rapids, MI 49503
Prgm Dir: Suzanne M Tomlinson, MS MT(ASCP)
Tel: 616 391-1840 *Fax:* 616 391-1986
E-mail: stomlinson@bw.brhn.org
Med Dir: Harold Hommerson, MD
Class Cap: 10 *Begins:* Aug
Length: 11 mos *Award:* Cert, BS

Northern Michigan University

Clin Lab Scientist/Med Tech Prgm
Learning Resources Bldg
Marquette, MI 49855-5346
Prgm Dir: Lucille A Contois, MA MT(ASCP)
Tel: 906 227-1660 *Fax:* 906 227-1658
E-mail: lcontois@nmu.edu
Med Dir: John Weiss, MD
Begins: Aug Jan
Length: 36 mos *Award:* BS
Tuition per yr: $3,690 res, $6,824 non-res

William Beaumont Hospital

Clin Lab Scientist/Med Tech Prgm
3601 W 13 Mile Rd
Royal Oak, MI 48073-6769
Prgm Dir: Deanna D Klosinski, PhD
  MT(ASCP)DLM
Tel: 810 551-8023 *Fax:* 810 551-3694
E-mail: dklosins@beaumont.edu
Med Dir: Joan C Mattson, MD
Class Cap: 12 *Begins:* Jul
Length: 10 mos *Award:* Cert

St Mary's Medical Center

Clin Lab Scientist/Med Tech Prgm
830 S Jefferson Ave
Saginaw, MI 48601
Prgm Dir: Nancy J Lier, MSA MT(ASCP)
Tel: 517 776-8145
Med Dir: George K Tong, MD
Class Cap: 4 *Begins:* Jun
Length: 12 mos *Award:* Cert, BS

Munson Medical Center

Clin Lab Scientist/Med Tech Prgm
1105 Sixth St
Traverse City, MI 49684
Prgm Dir: Mary Ann Urban, MT(ASCP)
Tel: 616 935-6100 *Fax:* 616 935-7389
Med Dir: John C Keep, MD
Class Cap: 6 *Begins:* Sep
Length: 10 mos *Award:* Cert, BS

Eastern Michigan University

Clin Lab Scientist/Med Tech Prgm
327 King Hall
Ypsilanti, MI 48197
Prgm Dir: Sandra L Drake, PhD MT (ASCP)
Tel: 313 487-0154 *Fax:* 313 427-4095
E-mail: sandra.drake@emich.edu
Med Dir: Jeffrey Warren, MD
Class Cap: 100 *Begins:* Sep Jan
Length: 12 mos *Award:* BS
Tuition per yr: $2,300 res, $6,000 non-res
Evening or weekend classes available

Minnesota

College of St Scholastica

Clin Lab Scientist/Med Tech Prgm
1200 Kenwood Ave
Duluth, MN 55811
Prgm Dir: Larry Birnbaum, PhD MT(ASCP)
Tel: 218 723-6621 *Fax:* 218 723-6472
E-mail: ibirnbau@fac1.css.edu
Med Dir: Thomas Nelson, MD
Class Cap: 8 *Begins:* Sep
Length: 21 mos *Award:* BA
Tuition per yr: $13,056 res, $13,056 non-res

Hennepin County Medical Center

Clin Lab Scientist/Med Tech Prgm
701 Park Ave S
Lab #812
Minneapolis, MN 55415
Prgm Dir: Patricia Ellinger, MSEd MT(ASCP)SBB
Tel: 612 347-3009 *Fax:* 612 904-4229
E-mail: pat.ellinger@co.hennepin.mn.us
Med Dir: John T Crosson, MD
Class Cap: 12 *Begins:* Jun
Length: 12 mos *Award:* Cert, BS
Tuition per yr: $1,200

Univ of Minnesota Hosp and Clinic

Clin Lab Scientist/Med Tech Prgm
420 Delaware St SE
PO Box 609 Mayo
Minneapolis, MN 55455
Prgm Dir: Karen Karni, PhD CLS(NCA)
Tel: 612 625-5136 *Fax:* 612 625-5901
E-mail: karni@maroon.tc.umn.edu
Med Dir: Leo T Furcht, MD
Class Cap: 32 *Begins:* Sep
Length: 24 mos *Award:* Dipl, BS
Tuition per yr: $4,000 res, $12,000 non-res
Evening or weekend classes available

St Cloud Hospital

Clin Lab Scientist/Med Tech Prgm
1406 Sixth Ave N
St Cloud, MN 56303
Prgm Dir: Jane Ceynar, MA MT(ASCP)
Tel: 320 255-5632
Med Dir: Stephen Bologna, MD
Class Cap: 4 *Begins:* Sep
Length: 12 mos *Award:* Cert, BS
Tuition per yr: $720

St Paul Ramsey Medical Center

Clin Lab Scientist/Med Tech Prgm
640 Jackson St
St Paul, MN 55101
Prgm Dir: Consoline L Brugler, MT(ASCP) CLS
Tel: 612 221-8846 *Fax:* 612 221-2741
E-mail:
  cbrugler@mis4.sprmc.healthpartners.com
Med Dir: Bruce Ellyson Hyde, MD
Class Cap: 8 *Begins:* Jul
Length: 12 mos *Award:* Cert
Tuition per yr: $2,020

Mississippi

University of Southern Mississippi

Clin Lab Scientist/Med Tech Prgm
PO Box 5134
Medical Technology Program
Hattiesburg, MS 39406-5134
Prgm Dir: M Jane Hudson, PhD MT(ASCP)SM
Tel: 601 266-4908 *Fax:* 601 266-4913
Med Dir: James E Williams III, MD
Class Cap: 36 *Begins:* Jan Aug
Length: 15 mos *Award:* Dipl,Cert, BS
Tuition per yr: $2,468 res, $5,288 non-res
Evening or weekend classes available

Mississippi Baptist Medical Center

Clin Lab Scientist/Med Tech Prgm
1225 N State St
Jackson, MS 39202
Prgm Dir: Bettye Covington, MA MT(ASCP)
Tel: 601 968-3070 *Fax:* 601 974-6286
Med Dir: William B Wilson, MD
Class Cap: 12 *Begins:* Jul
Length: 12 mos *Award:* Cert
Tuition per yr: $500 res, $500 non-res

Programs

University of Mississippi Medical Center
Clin Lab Scientist/Med Tech Prgm
2500 N State St
Jackson, MS 39216
Prgm Dir: David G Fowler, PhD
Tel: 601 984-6309 *Fax:* 601 984-6344
E-mail: fowler@shrp.umsmed.edu
Med Dir: William A Rock, Jr, MD
Class Cap: 20 *Begins:* Aug
Length: 24 mos *Award:* BS
Tuition per yr: $2,235 res, $4,192 non-res

North Mississippi Medical Center
Clin Lab Scientist/Med Tech Prgm
830 S Gloster
Tupelo, MS 38801
Prgm Dir: Lee H Montgomery, MT(ASCP)
Tel: 601 841-3082 *Fax:* 601 841-3337
Med Dir: Ishak L Enggano, MD
Class Cap: 14 *Begins:* Aug
Length: 12 mos *Award:* Cert, BS

Missouri

St John's Regional Medical Center
Clin Lab Scientist/Med Tech Prgm
2727 McClelland Blvd
Joplin, MO 64804-7170
Prgm Dir: Debbie Lorimer, MA MT(ASCP)
Tel: 417 625-2135 *Fax:* 417 659-6429
Med Dir: John Esther, MD
Class Cap: 8 *Begins:* Jan Jun
Length: 12 mos *Award:* Cert, BS
Tuition per yr: $2,000 res, $2,000 non-res

Avila College
Clin Lab Scientist/Med Tech Prgm
11901 Wornall Rd
Kansas City, MO 64145
Prgm Dir: Elaine Hostetler, MEd MT(ASCP)
Tel: 816 942-4511 *Fax:* 816 943-4585
E-mail: hostetlerev@mail.avila.edu
Med Dir: Pierre W Keitges, MD
Class Cap: 6 *Begins:* Aug
Length: 10 mos *Award:* Dipl, BSMT
Tuition per yr: $10,010
Evening or weekend classes available

St Luke's Hospital of Kansas City
Clin Lab Scientist/Med Tech Prgm
4400 Wornall Rd
Kansas City, MO 64111
Prgm Dir: Kay C Bertrand, MA MT(ASCP)CLS
Tel: 816 932-2410 *Fax:* 816 932-2259
Med Dir: Marjorie L Zucker, MD
Class Cap: 8 *Begins:* Jun
Length: 12 mos *Award:* Cert
Tuition per yr: $2,000 res, $2,000 non-res

North Kansas City Hospital
Clin Lab Scientist/Med Tech Prgm
2800 Clay Edwards Dr
North Kansas City, MO 64116
Prgm Dir: Jean E Cooper, MPA MT(ASCP)CT
Tel: 816 691-1321 *Fax:* 816 691-1317
Med Dir: Mark Stivers, MD
Class Cap: 8 *Begins:* Jun
Length: 12 mos *Award:* Cert, BS
Tuition per yr: $1,000

Cox Medical Centers
Clin Lab Scientist/Med Tech Prgm
3801 S National Ave
Springfield, MO 65807
Prgm Dir: Douglas D Hubbard, MT(ASCP)
Tel: 417 269-6633 *Fax:* 417 269-4600
Med Dir: Ronald M Wachter, MD
Class Cap: 8 *Begins:* Jan Jun
Length: 12 mos *Award:* Cert, BS
Tuition per yr: $3,000

St John's Regional Health Center
Clin Lab Scientist/Med Tech Prgm
1235 E Cherokee
Springfield, MO 65804
Prgm Dir: Claudette Millstead, EdD MT(ASCP)
Tel: 417 885-2880
Med Dir: Robert Druet, MD
Class Cap: 8 *Begins:* Jun
Length: 12 mos *Award:* Cert, BS
Tuition per yr: $1,000

Jewish Hosp-Coll of Nursing/Allied Hlth
Clin Lab Scientist/Med Tech Prgm
306 S Kingshighway Blvd
St Louis, MO 63110
Prgm Dir: Claudette M Millstead, EdD
    MT(ASCP) CLS(NCA)
Tel: 314 454-8486 *Fax:* 314 454-5239
Med Dir: Steven Teitelbaum, MD
Class Cap: 12 *Begins:* May
Length: 12 mos, 48 mos *Award:* Cert, BSCLS
Tuition per yr: $9,400
Evening or weekend classes available

St John's Mercy Medical Center
Clin Lab Scientist/Med Tech Prgm
615 S New Ballas Rd
St Louis, MO 63141-8277
Prgm Dir: Teresa A Taff, MT(ASCP)SM
Tel: 314 569-6855 *Fax:* 314 569-6866
Med Dir: Beverly B Kraemer, MD
Class Cap: 5 *Begins:* Jun
Length: 12 mos *Award:* Cert, BS
Tuition per yr: $3,800 res, $3,800 non-res

St Louis University Health Sciences Ctr
Clin Lab Scientist/Med Tech Prgm
1504 S Grand Blvd
St Louis, MO 63104-1395
Prgm Dir: Peggy A Edwards, MA MT(ASCP)
Tel: 314 577-8518 *Fax:* 314 577-8503
E-mail: edwardsp@sluvca.slu.edu
Med Dir: Marilyn Johnston, MD
Class Cap: 25 *Begins:* Aug Jan
Length: 12 mos, 39 mos *Award:* Cert, BS
Tuition per yr: $13,900 res, $13,900 non-res

Montana

Benefits Health Care-West Campus
Clin Lab Scientist/Med Tech Prgm
500 15th Ave S
Great Falls, MT 59405
Prgm Dir: Lois A Breidenbach, BS MT(ASCP)
Tel: 406 771-5018 *Fax:* 406 771-5126
Med Dir: J R Henneford, MD
Class Cap: 4 *Begins:* July
Length: 12 mos *Award:* Cert

Nebraska

Bishop Clarkson Memorial Hospital
Clin Lab Scientist/Med Tech Prgm
4350 Dewey Ave
Omaha, NE 68105
Prgm Dir: Cynthia D Owen, MT(ASCP)
Tel: 402 552-3121 Fax: 402 552-3625
Med Dir: Marc R Hapke, MD
Class Cap: 6 *Begins:* Jun
Length: 12 mos *Award:* Dipl, BS
Tuition per yr: $2,546 res, $6,939 non-res
Evening or weekend classes available

Nebraska Methodist Hospital
Clin Lab Scientist/Med Tech Prgm
8303 Dodge St
Omaha, NE 68114
Prgm Dir: Julie Richards, MPA MT(ASCP) BB
Tel: 402 354-4563 *Fax:* 402 354-4535
Med Dir: Jerald R Schenken, MD
Class Cap: 10 *Begins:* Jun
Length: 12 mos *Award:* Dipl, BSMT
Tuition per yr: $2,625 res, $7,140 non-res

University of Nebraska Medical Center
Clin Lab Scientist/Med Tech Prgm
600 S 42nd St
Omaha, NE 68198-3135
Prgm Dir: Phyllis Muellenberg, MA MT(ASCP)
Tel: 402 559-7628 *Fax:* 402 559-9044
E-mail: pmellen@mail.unmc.edu
Med Dir: James R Newland, MD
Class Cap: 24 *Begins:* Jun
Length: 12 mos *Award:* Dipl, BS
Tuition per yr: $2,625 res, $7,140 non-res

Nevada

University of Nevada Las Vegas
Clin Lab Scientist/Med Tech Prgm
4505 Maryland Pkwy
Las Vegas, NV 89154-3021
Prgm Dir: J Edgar Wakayama, PhD MT(ASCP)
Tel: 702 739-0973 *Fax:* 702 895-3872
E-mail: wakayama@nevada.edu
Med Dir: Henry Soloway, MD
Class Cap: 14 *Begins:* Sep
Length: 24 mos *Award:* BS
Tuition per yr: $1,536 res, $2,550 non-res

University of Nevada - Reno
Clin Lab Scientist/Med Tech Prgm
300 MacKay Science Bldg
Reno, NV 89557
Prgm Dir: Abraham Furmana, PhD MT(ASCP)
Tel: 702 784-4846
Med Dir: Dennis A Mackey, MD
Class Cap: 12 *Begins:* Jan Aug
Length: 22 mos *Award:* BS
Tuition per yr: $1,200 res, $2,700 non-res

New Hampshire

University of New Hampshire
Clin Lab Scientist/Med Tech Prgm
Hewitt Hall
4 Library Way
Durham, NH 03824
Prgm Dir: Jae O Kang, PhD MT(ASCP)
Tel: 603 862-1376 *Fax:* 603 862-3310
Med Dir: Walter Noll, MD
Class Cap: 25 *Begins:* Sep
Length: 38 mos *Award:* BS
Tuition per yr: $5,261 res, $14,221 non-res
Evening or weekend classes available

New Jersey

Cooper Hospital/University Medical Ctr
Clin Lab Scientist/Med Tech Prgm
One Cooper Plaza
Camden, NJ 08103
Prgm Dir: Diana M Hullihen, BS MT(ASCP)
Tel: 609 342-2456 *Fax:* 609 342-9718
Med Dir: Catalano Edison, MD
Class Cap: 8 *Begins:* Sep
Length: 12 mos *Award:* Cert, BS
Tuition per yr: $2,000

Monmouth Medical Center
Clin Lab Scientist/Med Tech Prgm
One Centennial Way
Long Branch, NJ 07740
Prgm Dir: John A Mihok, MT SM(ASCP) CLS
Tel: 908 870-5040 *Fax:* 908 870-5675
Med Dir: Louis J Zinterhofer, MD
Class Cap: 11 *Begins:* Sep
Length: 11.5 mos *Award:* Cert, BS
Tuition per yr: $800 res, $800 non-res

Morristown Memorial Hospital
Clin Lab Scientist/Med Tech Prgm
100 Madison Ave
Morristown, NJ 07960
Prgm Dir: Phyllis R Vail, EdM MT(ASCP)
Tel: 201 971-5282 *Fax:* 201 292-0401
Med Dir: Craig Dise, MD PhD
Class Cap: 8 *Begins:* Sep
Length: 12 mos *Award:* Cert, BS
Tuition per yr: $2,000 res, $2,000 non-res

Jersey Shore Medical Center
Clin Lab Scientist/Med Tech Prgm
1945 Corlies Ave
Neptune, NJ 07753
Prgm Dir: Perla L Simmons, MPA MT(ASCP)SH
  NCA CLSp(H)
Tel: 908 775-5500, Ext 4140 *Fax:* 908 776-4591
Med Dir: Martin Krumerman, MD
Class Cap: 8 *Begins:* Sep
Length: 12 mos *Award:* Cert
Tuition per yr: $1,000 res, $1,000 non-res

Univ of Med & Dent of New Jersey
Clin Lab Scientist/Med Tech Prgm
Schl Hlth Related Profs
65 Bergen St
Newark, NJ 07107-3006
Prgm Dir: Elaine M Keohane, PhD
Tel: 201 982-5510 *Fax:* 207 982-7028
E-mail: keohanem@umdnj.edu
Med Dir: Gabriel Mulcahy, MD
Class Cap: 24 *Begins:* Jun
Length: 15 mos *Award:* Cert, BS
Tuition per yr: $4,676 res, $7,014 non-res

The Valley Hospital
Clin Lab Scientist/Med Tech Prgm
223 N Van Dien Ave
Ridgewood, NJ 07450
Prgm Dir: Jacqueline M Opera, MT(ASCP)BB
Tel: 201 447-8234 *Fax:* 201 447-8657
Med Dir: Arthur Christiano, MD
Class Cap: 6 *Begins:* Jun
Length: 12 mos *Award:* Cert
Tuition per yr: $1,650

New Mexico

Univ of New Mexico School of Medicine
Clin Lab Scientist/Med Tech Prgm
Health Sciences & Service Bldg
Albuquerque, NM 87131
Prgm Dir: Barbara Fricke, MS MT(ASCP)CLS
Tel: 505 277-5434 *Fax:* 505 277-7011
E-mail: bfricke@unm.edu
Med Dir: Mary Lipscomb, MD
Class Cap: 16 *Begins:* Jan Jun
Length: 18 mos *Award:* Cert, BSMLS
Tuition per yr: $2,757 res, $7,698 non-res
Evening or weekend classes available

New York

Albany Medical Center Hospital
Clin Lab Scientist/Med Tech Prgm
47 New Scotland Ave
Albany, NY 12208
Prgm Dir: Jean Maatta, MS MT(ASCP) CLS
Tel: 518 262-4291 *Fax:* 518 262-4337
E-mail: jmaatta@cc.gateway.amc.edu
Med Dir: Jeffrey S Ross, MD
Class Cap: 8 *Begins:* Sep
Length: 12 mos *Award:* Cert
Tuition per yr: $4,950

Daemen College
Clin Lab Scientist/Med Tech Prgm
4380 Main St
Amherst, NY 14226-3592
Prgm Dir: Virginia Kotlarz, PhD MT(ASCP)
Tel: 716 839-8425 *Fax:* 716 834-8516
E-mail: vkortlarz@daemen.edu
Med Dir: Peter Vasilion, MD
Class Cap: 12 *Begins:* May
Length: 48 mos, 12 mos *Award:* Cert, BS
Tuition per yr: $9,950

New York Methodist Hospital
Clin Lab Scientist/Med Tech Prgm
506 Sixth St
Brooklyn, NY 11215
Prgm Dir: Lynda J Dines, MS MT(ASCP)
Tel: 718 780-3706 *Fax:* 718 780-3673
Med Dir: Pedro D Penha, MD
Class Cap: 10 *Begins:* Aug
Length: 12 mos *Award:* Cert, BS
Tuition per yr: $4,000

SUNY at Buffalo
Clin Lab Scientist/Med Tech Prgm
26 Cary Hall
3435 Main St
Buffalo, NY 14215
Prgm Dir: Robert Klick, MS MT(ASCP)
Tel: 716 829-3630 *Fax:* 716 829-3601
E-mail: klick@acsu.buffalo.edu
Med Dir: Edwin Jenis, MD
Class Cap: 36 *Begins:* Aug
Length: 24 mos *Award:* BS
Tuition per yr: $3,400 res, $8,300 non-res

Long Island Univ - C W Post Campus
Clin Lab Scientist/Med Tech Prgm
Northern Blvd
Clinical Lavoratory Sciences Program
Greenvale, NY 11548
Prgm Dir: Elizabeth O'Hara, MPA MT(ASCP)SH
Tel: 516 299-2485
Med Dir: Virginia Donavan, MD
Class Cap: 20 *Begins:* Sep Jan
Length: 18 mos *Award:* Cert, BS
Tuition per yr: $12,430 res, $12,430 non-res
Evening or weekend classes available

Woman's Christian Association Hospital
Clin Lab Scientist/Med Tech Prgm
207 Foote Ave
Jamestown, NY 14701-7077
Prgm Dir: Mary Kathryn C Kutschke, MA
  MT(ASCP)
Tel: 716 664-8258 *Fax:* 716 664-8306
Med Dir: Donald J Furman, MD
Class Cap: 10 *Begins:* Aug
Length: 11 mos *Award:* Cert, BS
Tuition per yr: $3,100 res, $3,100 non-res

St Vincent's Hosp & Med Ctr of New York
Clin Lab Scientist/Med Tech Prgm
153 W 11th St
New York, NY 10011
Prgm Dir: Sr Catherine Sherry, MS MT(ASCP)
Tel: 212 604-8385 *Fax:* 212 604-8426
Med Dir: John F Gillooley, MD
Class Cap: 10 *Begins:* Jun
Length: 12 mos *Award:* Cert, BS
Tuition per yr: $4,000

New York Institute of Technology
Clin Lab Scientist/Med Tech Prgm
Wheatley Rd
Old Westbury, NY 11568
Prgm Dir: Halina Diener, MS MT(ASCP)
Tel: 516 686-7607 *Fax:* 516 626-0673
E-mail: hdiener@admin.nyit.edu
Med Dir: Ahmed H Khapra, MD
Class Cap: 20 *Begins:* Sep Feb
Length: 36 mos *Award:* Dipl, BS
Tuition per yr: $10,180
Evening or weekend classes available

Marist College

Clin Lab Scientist/Med Tech Prgm
Medical Technology Dept
North Rd
Poughkeepsie, NY 12601
Prgm Dir: Catherine E Newkirk, MS MT(ASCP)
Tel: 914 575-3000 *Fax:* 914 471-6213
E-mail: jzmz@musicb.marist.edu
Med Dir: Phillip Lynch, MD
Class Cap: 20 *Begins:* Sep Jan
Length: 36 mos *Award:* BS
Tuition per yr: $12,070

Rochester General Hospital

Clin Lab Scientist/Med Tech Prgm
1425 Portland Ave
Rochester, NY 14621
Prgm Dir: Nancy C Mitchell, MS MT(ASCP)DLM
Tel: 716 338-4274 *Fax:* 716 338-4128
E-mail: nmitchell@rghnet.edu
Med Dir: Zygmunt M Tomkiewicz, MD
Class Cap: 18 *Begins:* Aug
Length: 12 mos *Award:* Cert
Tuition per yr: $2,600

St Mary's Hospital

Clin Lab Scientist/Med Tech Prgm
89 Genesee St
Rochester, NY 14611
Prgm Dir: Arlene Nikiel, MS MT(ASCP)SM
Tel: 716 464-3033 *Fax:* 716 464-3324
Med Dir: Pramod Carpenter, MD
Class Cap: 6 *Begins:* Aug
Length: 10 mos *Award:* Cert, BS
Tuition per yr: $2,650 res, $2,650 non-res

SUNY Health Science Ctr at Stony Brook

Clin Lab Scientist/Med Tech Prgm
Sch of Hlth Tech & Mgmt
Stony Brook, NY 11794-8205
Prgm Dir: Deborah T Firestone, MA
 MT(ASCP)SBB
Tel: 516 444-3221 *Fax:* 516 444-7621
E-mail: dfirestone@sunysb.hsc.edu
Med Dir: Marvin Kuschner, MD
Class Cap: 25 *Begins:* Sep
Length: 20 mos *Award:* Dipl, BS
Tuition per yr: $3,400 res, $8,300 non-res

SUNY Health Science Center at Syracuse

Clin Lab Scientist/Med Tech Prgm
750 Adams St
Syracuse, NY 13210
Prgm Dir: Harriet B Rolen-Mark, MA MT(ASCP)
Tel: 315 464-4608 *Fax:* 315 464-4609
E-mail: markh@vax.cs.hscsyr.edu
Med Dir: Robert E Hutchinson, MD
Class Cap: 20 *Begins:* Aug
Length: 21 mos *Award:* Dipl, BS
Tuition per yr: $5,477 res, $12,450 non-res

Catholic Medical Center

Clin Lab Scientist/Med Tech Prgm
89-15 Woodhaven Blvd
Woodhaven, NY 11421
Prgm Dir: Ann P Zero, MS MT(ASCP)
Tel: 718 805-4758 *Fax:* 718 805-7198
Med Dir: Usha C Ruder, MD
Class Cap: 18 *Begins:* Jun
Length: 12 mos *Award:* Cert, BS
Tuition per yr: $3,500

North Carolina

Univ of North Carolina at Chapel Hill

Clin Lab Scientist/Med Tech Prgm
Med Allied Hlth Professions
CB 7145 Medical School Wing E
Chapel Hill, NC 27599-7145
Prgm Dir: Susan J Beck, PhD MT(ASCP)
Tel: 919 966-3011 *Fax:* 919 966-3678
E-mail: sbeck@css.unc.edu
Med Dir: Lanier H Ayscue, MD
Class Cap: 20 *Begins:* Aug
Length: 20 mos *Award:* Dipl,Cert, BS
Tuition per yr: $2,161 res, $10,693 non-res

Carolinas College of Health Sciences

Clin Lab Scientist/Med Tech Prgm
PO Box 32861
Charlotte, NC 28232
Prgm Dir: Elizabeth T Anderson, MHDL
 MT(ASCP)
Tel: 704 355-4275 *Fax:* 704 355-3249
Med Dir: Edward H Lipford, MD
Class Cap: 9 *Begins:* Jul
Length: 12 mos *Award:* Cert
Tuition per yr: $500 res, $500 non-res

Western Carolina University

Clin Lab Scientist/Med Tech Prgm
134 Moore Hall
Cullowhee, NC 28723
Prgm Dir: Daniel K Southern, MS MT(ASCP)CLS
 p(H)NCA
Tel: 704 227-7114 *Fax:* 704 227-7446
E-mail: southern@wcu.edu
Med Dir: Joe P Hurt, MD PhD
Class Cap: 16 *Begins:* Aug
Length: 18 mos *Award:* BS
Tuition per yr: $762 res, $7,248 non-res
Evening or weekend classes available

Duke University Medical Center

Clin Lab Scientist/Med Tech Prgm
Education Service/Pathology
PO Box 2929
Durham, NC 27710
Prgm Dir: Margaret C Schmidt, EdD
 MT(ASCP)SH
Tel: 919 684-3872 *Fax:* 919 684-8671
E-mail: scmmibol@mc.duke.edu
Med Dir: Frances K Widmann, MD
Class Cap: 30 *Begins:* Jun
Length: 13 mos *Award:* Cert
Tuition per yr: $2,800 res, $2,800 non-res

Moses H Cone Memorial Hospital

Clin Lab Scientist/Med Tech Prgm
1200 N Elm St
Greensboro, NC 27401
Prgm Dir: Theresa W O'Laughlin, MCLT
 MT(ASCP)SH
Tel: 910 574-7485 *Fax:* 910 574-8270
Med Dir: Mary Christine Steuterman, MD
Begins: Jul
Length: 12 mos *Award:* Cert, BS

East Carolina University

Clin Lab Scientist/Med Tech Prgm
Dept Clinical Lab Science
Sch of Allied Hlth Sciences
Greenville, NC 27858
Prgm Dir: Susan T Smith, PhD MT(ASCP)
Tel: 919 328-4417 *Fax:* 919 328-4470
E-mail: cjsmith@ecuvm.cis.ecu.edu
Med Dir: H Thomas Norris, MD
Class Cap: 12 *Begins:* Aug
Length: 20 mos *Award:* BS
Tuition per yr: $2,371 res, $12,634 non-res
Evening or weekend classes available

New Hanover Regional Medical Center

Clin Lab Scientist/Med Tech Prgm
2131 S 17th St
PO Box 9000
Wilmington, NC 28402-7407
Prgm Dir: Clark Zervos, MHS MT(ASCP)SBB
Tel: 910 343-7072
Med Dir: Rebecca D McAfee, MD
Class Cap: 6 *Begins:* Aug
Length: 12 mos *Award:* Cert, BS

Bowman Gray School of Medicine

Clin Lab Scientist/Med Tech Prgm
Medical Ctr Blvd
Winston-Salem, NC 27157
Prgm Dir: Lenora W Flynn, MEd MT(ASCP)
Tel: 910 716-4727 *Fax:* 910 716-6359
E-mail: lflynn@bgsm.edu
Med Dir: Marbry B Hopkins III, MD
Class Cap: 12 *Begins:* July
Length: 12 mos *Award:* Cert
Tuition per yr: $2,000 res, $2,000 non-res

Forsyth Memorial Hospital

Clin Lab Scientist/Med Tech Prgm
3333 Silas Creek Pkwy
Winston-Salem, NC 27103
Prgm Dir: Donna G Basch, MT(ASCP)SC CLS
Tel: 910 718-2935 *Fax:* 910 718-9264
Med Dir: Joseph B Dudley, MD

Winston-Salem State University

Clin Lab Scientist/Med Tech Prgm
PO Box 13156
Winston-Salem, NC 27110
Prgm Dir: Simon O Ogamdi, PhD MT(ASCP)
Tel: 910 750-2510 *Fax:* 910 750-2517
Med Dir: William Karnes Poston, Jr, MD
Class Cap: 12 *Begins:* Aug
Length: 21 mos *Award:* BS
Tuition per yr: $3,926 res, $8,944 non-res

North Dakota

MeritCare

Clin Lab Scientist/Med Tech Prgm
737 Broadway
PO Box 2067
Fargo, ND 58123
Prgm Dir: Sandra Matthey, MS BS MT(ASCP)
Tel: 701 234-2489
Med Dir: James Coffey, MD
Class Cap: 15 *Begins:* Jun Aug
Length: 12 mos *Award:* Cert, BS
Tuition per yr: $2,110 res, $3,166 non-res

Univ of N Dakota Sch of Med and Hlth Sci

Clin Lab Scientist/Med Tech Prgm
Univ of North Dakota Sch of Medicine
Dept of Pathology PO Box 9037
Grand Forks, ND 582029037
Prgm Dir: A Wayne Bruce, PhD CLS(NCA)
Tel: 701 777-2636   *Fax:* 701 777-3108
E-mail: wbruce@mail.med.nodak.edu
Med Dir: Leslie Torgerson, MD
Class Cap: 45   *Begins:* May
Length: 24 mos, 24 mos   *Award:* Cert, BS
Tuition per yr: $2,528 res, $2,846 non-res
Evening or weekend classes available

Trinity Medical Center

Clin Lab Scientist/Med Tech Prgm
Main St & Burdick Expwy
Minot, ND 58701
Prgm Dir: Dolores Wood, MS MT(ASCP)
Tel: 701 857-5210   *Fax:* 701 857-5485
Med Dir: Robert W Cashmore, MD
Class Cap: 6   *Begins:* Jul
Length: 12 mos   *Award:* Cert, BS
Tuition per yr: $3,000

Ohio

Children's Hospital Medical Ctr of Akron

Clin Lab Scientist/Med Tech Prgm
One Perkins Square
Akron, OH 44308
Prgm Dir: Suzanne W Conner, MA CLS/CLDir
Tel: 330 379-8720
Med Dir: Robert Novak, MD
Class Cap: 12   *Begins:* Jul
Length: 12 mos   *Award:* Cert, BS
Tuition per yr: $1,500

Bowling Green State University

Clin Lab Scientist/Med Tech Prgm
504 Life Science Bldg
Bowling Green, OH 43403
Prgm Dir: Robert Harr, MS MT(ASCP)
Tel: 419 372-8109   *Fax:* 419 372-0332
E-mail: rharr@bgnet.bgsu.edu
Med Dir: Alcuin Bennett, MD
Class Cap: 16   *Begins:* June
Length: 14 mos   *Award:* Cert, BS
Tuition per yr: $6,285 res, $13,395 non-res

University of Cincinnati Medical Center

Clin Lab Scientist/Med Tech Prgm
231 Bethesda Ave
Cincinnati, OH 45267
Prgm Dir: Edward P Knepp, MEd MT(ASCP)
Tel: 513 558-2018   *Fax:* 513 558-2289
E-mail: kweppep@ucbeh.san.uc.edu
Med Dir: Colin R Macpherson, MD
Class Cap: 15   *Begins:* July
Length: 12 mos, 24 mos   *Award:* Cert, BS
Tuition per yr: $5,532 res, $13,952 non-res

Cleveland Clinic Foundation

Clin Lab Scientist/Med Tech Prgm
Cleveland Clinic Foundation
9500 Euclid Ave
Cleveland, OH 44195-5131
Prgm Dir: Sandra J Bodie, MT(ASCP)
Tel: 216 444-5155   *Fax:* 216 445-7253
Med Dir: Isobel Rutherford, MD
Begins: Jul
Length: 12 mos   *Award:* Cert, BS
Tuition per yr: $1,100 res, $1,100 non-res

University Hospitals of Cleveland

Clin Lab Scientist/Med Tech Prgm
2074 Abington Rd
Cleveland, OH 44106
Prgm Dir: Juanita R Wingenfeld, MS MT(ASCP)
Tel: 216 844-1812   *Fax:* 216 844-5601
Med Dir: Nancy S Rosenthal, MD
Class Cap: 12   *Begins:* Jul
Length: 12 mos   *Award:* Cert
Tuition per yr: $2,000

Ohio State University

Clin Lab Scientist/Med Tech Prgm
1583 Perry St
Columbus, OH 43210
Prgm Dir: Kory M Ward, PhD MT(ASCP)
Tel: 614 292-7303   *Fax:* 614 292-0210
E-mail: kward@postbox.acs.ohio-state.edu
Med Dir: Donald A Senhauser, MD
Class Cap: 27   *Begins:* Sep
Length: 23 mos   *Award:* Cert, BS
Tuition per yr: $3,424 res, $10,335 non-res

Wright State University

Clin Lab Scientist/Med Tech Prgm
Dept of Biological Sciences
208 Biological Sciences Bldg
Dayton, OH 45435
Prgm Dir: Kay R Zelenski-Low, PhD MT(ASCP)
Tel: 513 873-4229
Med Dir: James W Funkhouser, MD
Class Cap: 20   *Begins:* Jun
Length: 12 mos   *Award:* Dipl,Cert, BS
Tuition per yr: $3,600 res, $7,200 non-res
Evening or weekend classes available

Southwest General Health Center

Clin Lab Scientist/Med Tech Prgm
18697 Bagley Rd
Middleburg Hts, OH 44130
Prgm Dir: Carol J Miller, MA MT(ASCP)
Tel: 216 816-8859   *Fax:* 216 816-8690
Med Dir: Karen Gerken, MD
Class Cap: 6   *Begins:* Jul
Length: 12 mos   *Award:* Cert, BS
Tuition per yr: $1,500

St Charles Hospital

Clin Lab Scientist/Med Tech Prgm
2600 Navarre Ave
Oregon, OH 43616-3297
Prgm Dir: Peggy A Estes, MT(ASCP)
Tel: 419 698-7673   *Fax:* 419 698-7761
Med Dir: Lachman Chablani, MD
Begins: Jun
Length: 12 mos   *Award:* Cert

Trinity Medical Center East

Clin Lab Scientist/Med Tech Prgm
380 Summit Ave
Steubenville, OH 43952
Prgm Dir: Sheila C Hendricks, MEd MT(ASCP)
Tel: 614 283-7395   *Fax:* 614 283-7432
Med Dir: Chong-Sook Lee Sohn, MD
Class Cap: 8   *Begins:* Jul
Length: 12 mos   *Award:* Cert, BS
Tuition per yr: $1,000 res, $1,000 non-res

Riverside Hospital

Clin Lab Scientist/Med Tech Prgm
1600 N Superior St
Toledo, OH 43604
Prgm Dir: Karlyn J Lange, MT(ASCP)
Tel: 419 729-6015   *Fax:* 419 729-6298
Med Dir: Shaheda B Ahmed, MD
Class Cap: 4   *Begins:* Jul
Length: 12 mos   *Award:* Cert, BS
Tuition per yr: $150 res, $150 non-res

St Elizabeth Health Center

Clin Lab Scientist/Med Tech Prgm
1044 Belmont Ave
Youngstown, OH 44501-1790
Prgm Dir: Saeeda A Ghani, MS MT(ASCP)
Tel: 330 480-2808   *Fax:* 330 480-2913
Med Dir: Carl R Schaub, MD
Class Cap: 6   *Begins:* Jul
Length: 12 mos   *Award:* Cert, BS
Tuition per yr: $2,640

Western Reserve Care System

Clin Lab Scientist/Med Tech Prgm
500 Gypsy Ln
Youngstown, OH 44501
Prgm Dir: Sallie Lepore, MT(ASCP)
Tel: 330 740-3224   *Fax:* 330 740-3790
Med Dir: Tom E Campbell, MD
Class Cap: 4   *Begins:* Jan Jul
Length: 12 mos   *Award:* Cert
Tuition per yr: $1,400

Oklahoma

Valley View Regional Hospital

Clin Lab Scientist/Med Tech Prgm
430 N Monte Vista
Ada, OK 74820
Prgm Dir: Cheryl A Weems, MT(ASCP)C
Tel: 405 421-1550   *Fax:* 405 421-1525
Med Dir: Larry W Cartmell, MD
Class Cap: 6   *Begins:* Jul
Length: 12 mos   *Award:* Dipl, BS

St Mary's Hospital

Clin Lab Scientist/Med Tech Prgm
305 S Fifth St
Enid, OK 73702-0232
Prgm Dir: Christine Arnold, MT(ASCP)CLS
Tel: 405 249-3695   *Fax:* 405 249-3985
Med Dir: Ned M Austin, MD
Class Cap: 7   *Begins:* Aug
Length: 12 mos   *Award:* Cert, BS

Programs

Comanche County Memorial Hospital
Clin Lab Scientist/Med Tech Prgm
PO Box 129
Lawton, OK 73502
Prgm Dir: Gary Jackson, SH(ASCP)
Tel: 405 355-8620
Med Dir: Richard J Boatsman, MD
Begins: Aug
Length: 12 mos   *Award:* Cert, BS
Tuition per yr: $1,250

Muskogee Regional Medical Center
Clin Lab Scientist/Med Tech Prgm
300 Rockefeller Dr
Muskogee, OK 74401
Prgm Dir: Dorothy J Betts, MA MT(ASCP)
Tel: 918 684-2138   *Fax:* 918 684-2223
Med Dir: Harvey P Randall, MD
Class Cap: 8 *Begins:* Aug
Length: 12 mos   *Award:* Cert, BS
Tuition per yr: $1,284 res, $1,284 non-res

St Anthony Hospital
Clin Lab Scientist/Med Tech Prgm
1000 N Lee St
PO Box 205
Oklahoma City, OK 73101
Prgm Dir: Carolyn Novotny Anderson,
   MT(ASCP)SC
Tel: 405 272-7988   *Fax:* 405 272-6731
Med Dir: James M Brinkworth, MD
Class Cap: 8 *Begins:* Aug
Length: 12 mos   *Award:* Cert, BS

University Hospitals of Oklahoma City
Clin Lab Scientist/Med Tech Prgm
PO Box 26307/Rm EB400
Oklahoma City, OK 73126
Prgm Dir: Sandra K Johnson, MPH MT(ASCP)
Tel: 405 271-7732   *Fax:* 405 271-3133
Med Dir: John H Holliman, MD
Class Cap: 10 *Begins:* Aug
Length: 12 mos   *Award:* Cert

St Francis Hospital
Clin Lab Scientist/Med Tech Prgm
6161 S Yale Ave
Tulsa, OK 74136
Prgm Dir: Theresa D Foster, MPH MT(ASCP)SH
Tel: 918 494-6342   *Fax:* 918 494-1399
Med Dir: Robert S White, MD
Class Cap: 6 *Begins:* July
Length: 12 mos   *Award:* Cert, BS
Tuition per yr: $1,168

Oregon

Oregon Health Sciences University
Clin Lab Scientist/Med Tech Prgm
3181 SW Sam Jackson Pk
Portland, OR 97201
Prgm Dir: Marian Ewell, MT(ASCP)SBB
Tel: 503 494-8698   *Fax:* 503 494-2730
E-mail: ewellm@ohsu.edu
Med Dir: Victor C Marquardt, Jr, MD
Class Cap: 20 *Begins:* Aug
Length: 15 mos   *Award:* Dipl, BS
Tuition per yr: $10,000 res, $16,840 non-res
Evening or weekend classes available

Pennsylvania

Abington Memorial Hospital
Clin Lab Scientist/Med Tech Prgm
1200 Old York Rd
Abington, PA 19001
Prgm Dir: Barbara J Scheelje, MT(ASCP)
Tel: 215 576-2362   *Fax:* 215 576-4481
Med Dir: Paul J Cherney, MD
Class Cap: 6 *Begins:* Jul
Length: 12 mos   *Award:* Cert, BS
Tuition per yr: $3,500 res, $3,500 non-res

Sacred Heart Hospital
Clin Lab Scientist/Med Tech Prgm
421 Chew St
Allentown, PA 18102-3490
Prgm Dir: Deborah A Schwab, BS MT(ASCP)
Tel: 610 776-4745   *Fax:* 610 776-5159
Med Dir: James M Chiadis, MD
Class Cap: 4 *Begins:* Jul
Length: 12 mos   *Award:* Cert, BS
Tuition per yr: $1,000 res, $1,000 non-res

Altoona Hospital
Clin Lab Scientist/Med Tech Prgm
620 Howard Ave
Altoona, PA 16601-4899
Prgm Dir: Joseph R Noel, MT(ASCP)
Tel: 814 946-2835   *Fax:* 814 946-5279
Med Dir: Eugene M Sneff, MD
Begins: Jul
Length: 12 mos   *Award:* Cert, BS
Tuition per yr: $1,000 res, $1,000 non-res

Neumann College
Clin Lab Scientist/Med Tech Prgm
One Neumann Way
Aston, PA 19014
Prgm Dir: Sandra M Weiss, MA MT(ASCP)
Tel: 610 558-5607   *Fax:* 610 459-2370
E-mail: sweiss@smtpgate.neumann.edu
Med Dir: Harvey Spector, MD
Class Cap: 15 *Begins:* Sep
Length: 24 mos   *Award:* BS
Tuition per yr: $13,100
Evening or weekend classes available

Geisinger Medical Center
Clin Lab Scientist/Med Tech Prgm
100 N Academy Ave
Danville, PA 17822
Prgm Dir: Alvin Swartzentruber, MT(ASCP)
Tel: 717 271-6700   *Fax:* 717 271-6105
Med Dir: Peter J Cera, MD
Class Cap: 6 *Begins:* Jul
Length: 12 mos   *Award:* Dipl, BS
Tuition per yr: $1,920

Allegheny University Hospitals Elkins Park
Clin Lab Scientist/Med Tech Prgm
60 E Township Line Rd
Elkins Park, PA 19027
Prgm Dir: Phyllis Gotkin, PhD MT(ASCP)
Tel: 215 663-6101   *Fax:* 215 663-8842
Med Dir: Kathleen Sazama, MD JD
Class Cap: 8 *Begins:* Jun
Length: 12 mos   *Award:* Cert, BS
Tuition per yr: $3,000

St Vincent Health Center
Clin Lab Scientist/Med Tech Prgm
232 W 25th St
Erie, PA 16544
Prgm Dir: Stephen M Johnson, MS MT(ASCP)
Tel: 814 452-5365   *Fax:* 814 456-4784
E-mail: 104070.2643@campusarue.com
Med Dir: Kenneth H Jurgens, MD
Class Cap: 16 *Begins:* Aug
Length: 12 mos   *Award:* Cert, BS
Tuition per yr: $3,500

Health Hospitals/Polyclinic Hospital
Clin Lab Scientist/Med Tech Prgm
2601 N Third St
Harrisburg, PA 17110
Prgm Dir: Marcella I Anderson, MS MT(ASCP)
Tel: 717 782-2639   *Fax:* 717 782-4293
Med Dir: Frank J Rudy, MD
Class Cap: 6 *Begins:* Jul
Length: 12 mos   *Award:* Cert, BS
Tuition per yr: $2,000

Conemaugh Valley Memorial Hospital
Clin Lab Scientist/Med Tech Prgm
1086 Franklin St
Johnstown, PA 15905-4398
Prgm Dir: Patricia A Chappell, MT(ASCP)
Tel: 814 533-9831   *Fax:* 814 534-3253
Med Dir: Sidney A Goldblatt, MD
Class Cap: 12 *Begins:* July
Length: 12 mos   *Award:* Cert, BS
Tuition per yr: $2,500

Lancaster Institute for Health Education
Clin Lab Scientist/Med Tech Prgm
143 E Lemon St
Lancaster, PA 17602
Prgm Dir: Nadine E Gladfelter, MS MT(ASCP)
Tel: 717 290-5511   *Fax:* 717 290-5970
Med Dir: James T Eastman III, MD
Class Cap: 8 *Begins:* Jul
Length: 12 mos   *Award:* Cert
Tuition per yr: $4,000 res, $4,000 non-res

Latrobe Area Hospital
Clin Lab Scientist/Med Tech Prgm
121 W Second Ave
Latrobe, PA 15650
Prgm Dir: Joan A Grote, BS MT(ASCP)
Tel: 412 537-1577   *Fax:* 412 537-1818
Med Dir: Ronald S Bernardi, MD
Class Cap: 10 *Begins:* Jul
Length: 12 mos   *Award:* Dipl, BS
Tuition per yr: $1,850

Allegheny University of the Health Sciences
Clin Lab Scientist/Med Tech Prgm
Broad and Vines Sts MS 505
Philadelphia, PA 19102
Prgm Dir: Pamela Buccelli, EdD MT(ACSP)
Tel: 215 762-7176   *Fax:* 215 246-5397
E-mail: buccelli@allegheny.edu
Med Dir: Kathleen Sazama, MD JD
Class Cap: 30 *Begins:* Aug
Length: 21 mos, 33 mos   *Award:* BS
Tuition per yr: $9,840 res, $9,840 non-res
Evening or weekend classes available

Nazareth Hospital

Clin Lab Scientist/Med Tech Prgm
2601 Holme Ave
Philadelphia, PA 19152
Prgm Dir: Diane P Bejsiuk, MEd MT(ACSP)
Tel: 215 335-6248   *Fax:* 215 335-6155
Med Dir: William J Warren, MD
Begins: Jul
Length: 12 mos   *Award:* Cert, BS
Tuition per yr: $2,100

Pennsylvania Hospital

Clin Lab Scientist/Med Tech Prgm
800 Spruce St
Philadelphia, PA 19107
Prgm Dir: Caryn Lennon, MT(ASCP)SH
Tel: 215 829-5091   *Fax:* 215 829-7564
Med Dir: Michael J Warhol, MD
Class Cap: 6   *Begins:* Aug
Length: 12 mos   *Award:* Cert, BS
Tuition per yr: $2,500

Thomas Jefferson University

Clin Lab Scientist/Med Tech Prgm
130 S Ninth St
Edison Building
Philadelphia, PA 19107
Prgm Dir: Nancy M G Calder, MAEd MT(ASCP)
  CLS(NCA)
Tel: 215 503-8187   *Fax:* 215 503-2189
E-mail: calder@jeflin.tju.edu
Med Dir: Albert A Keshgegian, MD
Class Cap: 15   *Begins:* Sep
Length: 12 mos, 20 mos   *Award:* Cert, BS
Tuition per yr: $14,900 res, $14,900 non-res
Evening or weekend classes available

Allegheny General Hospital

Clin Lab Scientist/Med Tech Prgm
320 E North Ave
Pittsburgh, PA 15212-4772
Prgm Dir: Nancy J Brewer, PhD
Tel: 412 359-3530   *Fax:* 412 359-3598
Med Dir: Robert J Hartsock, MD
Class Cap: 15   *Begins:* Jun
Length: 12 mos   *Award:* Cert
Tuition per yr: $2,506

University of Pittsburgh

Clin Lab Scientist/Med Tech Prgm
209 Pennsylvania Hall
Pittsburgh, PA 15261
Prgm Dir: Ann C Albers, DrPH MT(ASCP)
Tel: 412 624-8951
Med Dir: Antonio J Amortegui, MD
Class Cap: 72   *Begins:* Sep
Length: 19 mos   *Award:* BS
Tuition per yr: $8,720 res, $18,711 non-res

Reading Hospital and Medical Center

Clin Lab Scientist/Med Tech Prgm
PO Box 16052
Reading, PA 19612-6052
Prgm Dir: Sharon K Strauss, MT(ASCP)
  CLS(NCA)
Tel: 610 378-5951   *Fax:* 610 208-5185
Med Dir: William K Natale, MD JD
Class Cap: 6   *Begins:* Jul
Length: 11 mos   *Award:* Cert

Robert Packer Hospital

Clin Lab Scientist/Med Tech Prgm
Guthrie Square
Sayre, PA 18840
Prgm Dir: Brian D Spezialetti, MS MT(ASCP)
Tel: 717 882-4736   *Fax:* 717 882-4413
E-mail: bspezial@inet.guthric.org
Med Dir: Joseph T King, MD
Class Cap: 10   *Begins:* Aug
Length: 12 mos   *Award:* Cert
Tuition per yr: $2,400

Scranton Medical Technology Consortium

Clin Lab Scientist/Med Tech Prgm
700 Quincy Ave
Scranton, PA 18510
Prgm Dir: Mary G Butler, MS MT(ASCP)
Tel: 717 961-5784
Med Dir: William Antognoli, MD
Class Cap: 20   *Begins:* Jul
Length: 12 mos   *Award:* Cert, BS
Tuition per yr: $3,500

Washington Hospital

Clin Lab Scientist/Med Tech Prgm
155 Wilson Ave
Washington, PA 15301
Prgm Dir: Cheryl D Asbury, MS MT(ASCP)
Tel: 412 223-3128   *Fax:* 412 229-2031
Med Dir: Richard S Pataki, MD
Class Cap: 4   *Begins:* Sep
Length: 12 mos   *Award:* Cert, BS, BA

Wilkes-Barre General Hospital

Clin Lab Scientist/Med Tech Prgm
N River and Auburn Sts
Wilkes-Barre, PA 18764
Prgm Dir: Maria E Nicoletti, CLS(NCA)
  MT(ASCP) SH
Tel: 717 552-1404   *Fax:* 717 552-1415
Med Dir: George A Grinaway, MD
Class Cap: 10   *Begins:* Jul
Length: 12 mos   *Award:* Cert
Tuition per yr: $1,200

Divine Providence Hospital

Clin Lab Scientist/Med Tech Prgm
1100 Grampian Blvd
Williamsport, PA 17701
Prgm Dir: Loretta A Moffatt, MT(ASCP)
Tel: 717 326-8854   *Fax:* 717 326-8929
Med Dir: Willem Lubbe, MD
Class Cap: 6   *Begins:* Aug
Length: 12 mos   *Award:* Cert
Tuition per yr: $1,000

York Hospital

Clin Lab Scientist/Med Tech Prgm
1001 S George St
York, PA 17405
Prgm Dir: Brenda L Kile, MA MT(ASCP)CLS
Tel: 717 851-2458   *Fax:* 717 851-2934
Med Dir: John P Whiteley, MD
Class Cap: 6   *Begins:* Jul
Length: 12 mos   *Award:* Cert, BS
Tuition per yr: $3,680 res, $3,680 non-res

Puerto Rico

Catholic University of Puerto Rico

Clin Lab Scientist/Med Tech Prgm
2250 Las Americas Ave Ste 588
Ponce, PR 00731-6382
Prgm Dir: Mara G de Santiago, MA MT(ASCP)
Tel: 787 841-2000   *Fax:* 787 840-4295
Med Dir: Adalberto Mendoza, MD
Class Cap: 24   *Begins:* Jul
Length: 12 mos   *Award:* Cert, BSMT
Tuition per yr: $4,750
Evening or weekend classes available

Interamerican University - San German

Clin Lab Scientist/Med Tech Prgm
Call Box 5100
San German, PR 00753
Prgm Dir: Ludai Rodriguez, MS MT (ASCP)
Tel: 809 834-6070
Med Dir: Jesus Vega, MD
Class Cap: 20   *Begins:* Aug Feb
Length: 12 mos   *Award:* Dipl,Cert, BS
Tuition per yr: $4,500

Interamerican University - Metro Campus

Clin Lab Scientist/Med Tech Prgm
PO Box 191293
San Juan, PR 00919-1293
Prgm Dir: Migdalia Texidor, MT(ASCP)
Tel: 787 767-5081   *Fax:* 787 250-8736
Med Dir: Jose Carrasco, MD
Class Cap: 25   *Begins:* Feb Aug
Length: 12 mos   *Award:* Dipl,Cert, BS
Tuition per yr: $4,500
Evening or weekend classes available

University of Puerto Rico

Clin Lab Scientist/Med Tech Prgm
PO Box 365067
San Juan, PR 00936-5067
Prgm Dir: Nelson Colon, MS MT(ASCP)CLS
Tel: 787 756-7220   *Fax:* 787 764-1760
Med Dir: German Lasala, MD
Class Cap: 45   *Begins:* Aug
Length: 15 mos   *Award:* Cert, BS
Tuition per yr: $1,260

University of the Sacred Heart

Clin Lab Scientist/Med Tech Prgm
PO Box 12383
Loiza Station
Santurce, PR 00914
Prgm Dir: Sara E A de Malave, MA MT(ASCP)
Tel: 787 728-1515   *Fax:* 787 727-7880
Med Dir: Eduardo de Leon, MD
Class Cap: 48   *Begins:* Feb Aug
Length: 12 mos, 60 mos   *Award:* Dipl,Cert, BS
Tuition per yr: $4,500 res, $4,500 non-res
Evening or weekend classes available

Programs

Rhode Island

Our Lady of Fatima Hospital
Clin Lab Scientist/Med Tech Prgm
School of Cytotechnology
200 High Service Ave
North Providence, RI 02904
Prgm Dir: Frances W Ingersoll, MS MT(ASCP)
Tel: 401 456-3215 *Fax:* 401 456-3156
Med Dir: Salvatore R Allegra, MD
Class Cap: 8 *Begins:* Jul
Length: 12 mos *Award:* Cert, BSMT
Tuition per yr: $3,500

Rhode Island Hospital
Clin Lab Scientist/Med Tech Prgm
593 Eddy St
Providence, RI 02903
Prgm Dir: David J Mello, MS MT(ASCP)CLS
Tel: 401 444-5724
Med Dir: Robert M Kenney, MD
Class Cap: 8 *Begins:* Aug
Length: 12 mos *Award:* Cert
Tuition per yr: $3,500

South Carolina

Anderson Area Medical Center
Clin Lab Scientist/Med Tech Prgm
800 N Fant St
Anderson, SC 29621
Prgm Dir: Georgia Lou Huff, MEd MT(ASCP)
Tel: 864 261-1390 *Fax:* 864 261-1649
Med Dir: E Eugene Baillie, MD
Class Cap: 8 *Begins:* Jul Jan
Length: 12 mos *Award:* Cert, BS
Tuition per yr: $2,600

Medical University of South Carolina
Clin Lab Scientist/Med Tech Prgm
Dept of Medical Lab Sciences
College of Health Professions
Charleston, SC 29425
Prgm Dir: Janice M Hundley, MS MT(ASCP)SH
Tel: 803 792-3169 *Fax:* 803 792-3383
E-mail: hundley@muse.edu
Med Dir: Elaine Jeter, MD
Class Cap: 25 *Begins:* Aug
Length: 12 mos *Award:* Dipl, BS
Tuition per yr: $4,401 res, $12,822 non-res

Baptist Medical Center at Columbia
Clin Lab Scientist/Med Tech Prgm
Taylor at Marion
Columbia, SC 29220
Prgm Dir: Joan M Savage, MT(ASCP) MA
Tel: 803 771-5014
Med Dir: Hoke F Henderson, MD
Class Cap: 3 *Begins:* Jan Jul
Length: 12 mos *Award:* Cert
Tuition per yr: $400 res, $400 non-res

McLeod Regional Medical Center
Clin Lab Scientist/Med Tech Prgm
555 E Cheves St
Florence, SC 29506-2617
Prgm Dir: Vicki T Anderson, MT(ASCP)
Tel: 803 667-2497 *Fax:* 803 667-2071
Med Dir: Vera C Hyman, MD
Class Cap: 8 *Begins:* Aug
Length: 12 mos *Award:* Cert, BS
Tuition per yr: $2,000

South Dakota

St Luke's-Midland Regional Medical Ctr
Clin Lab Scientist/Med Tech Prgm
305 S State St
Aberdeen, SD 57401
Prgm Dir: Etta Bassinger, MT(ASCP)
Tel: 605 622-5546
Med Dir: Roy G Burt, MD
Class Cap: 6 *Begins:* Aug
Length: 12 mos *Award:* Cert, BS
Tuition per yr: $2,300

Rapid City Regional Hospital
Clin Lab Scientist/Med Tech Prgm
353 Fairmont Blvd
Rapid City, SD 57701
Prgm Dir: Pam Kieffer, MS MT(ASCP) CLS
Tel: 605 341-8092 *Fax:* 605 399-2205
Med Dir: John F Barlow, MD
Class Cap: 8 *Begins:* Aug
Length: 12 mos *Award:* Cert, BS
Tuition per yr: $2,000

Sioux Valley Hospital
Clin Lab Scientist/Med Tech Prgm
1100 S Euclid Ave
Sioux Falls, SD 57117-5039
Prgm Dir: Marilyn J Barnett, MS MT(ASCP)CLS
Tel: 605 333-7104 *Fax:* 605 333-1532
Med Dir: David W Ohrt, MD PhD
Class Cap: 10 *Begins:* Jun
Length: 12 mos *Award:* Cert, BS
Tuition per yr: $2,600 res, $2,600 non-res

Tennessee

Austin Peay State University
Clin Lab Scientist/Med Tech Prgm
Clarksville, TN 37044
Prgm Dir: Robert T Crews, PhD MT(ASCP)
Tel: 615 648-7796 *Fax:* 615 648-5996
E-mail: crewsr@apsu02.apsu.edu
Med Dir: Randall R Haase, MD
Class Cap: 14 *Begins:* Jun
Length: 13 mos *Award:* Cert, BS
Tuition per yr: $882 res, $2,951 non-res
Evening or weekend classes available

Lincoln Memorial University
Clin Lab Scientist/Med Tech Prgm
Harrogate, TN 37752-0901
Prgm Dir: Patricia Ramsey, MS MT(ASCP)
Tel: 423 869-6232 *Fax:* 423 869-6244
Med Dir: Lynn F Blake, MD
Class Cap: 10 *Begins:* Aug
Length: 18 mos *Award:* BS
Tuition per yr: $6,800 res, $6,800 non-res
Evening or weekend classes available

Univ of Tennessee Med Ctr at Knoxville
Clin Lab Scientist/Med Tech Prgm
1924 Alcoa Hwy
Knoxville, TN 37920
Prgm Dir: Gail Maner, MS MT(ASCP)
Tel: 423 544-9087 *Fax:* 423 544-6866
Med Dir: John Carl Neff, MD
Class Cap: 14 *Begins:* Jan Jul
Length: 12 mos *Award:* Dipl,Cert, BS
Tuition per yr: $3,300 res, $9,844 non-res

University of Tennessee Memphis
Clin Lab Scientist/Med Tech Prgm
822 Beale Ave/Rm 321
Memphis, TN 38163
Prgm Dir: Brenta G Davis, EdD MT(ASCP)CLS
Tel: 901 448-6304 *Fax:* 901 448-7545
E-mail: bdavis@utmem1.utmem.edu
Med Dir: J T Francisco, MD
Class Cap: 30 *Begins:* Sep
Length: 21 mos *Award:* BS
Tuition per yr: $2,602 res, $6,532 non-res

St Thomas Hospital
Clin Lab Scientist/Med Tech Prgm
4220 Harding
PO Box 380
Nashville, TN 37202
Prgm Dir: Leigh Ann Hobbs, MT(ASCP)
Tel: 615 222-2044
Med Dir: Carla M Davis, MD
Class Cap: 8 *Begins:* Jul
Length: 12 mos *Award:* Cert, BS
Tuition per yr: $1,200

Tennessee State University
Clin Lab Scientist/Med Tech Prgm
Tennessee State University
3500 John A Merritt Blvd
Nashville, TN 37203
Prgm Dir: Theola Copeland, MS MT(ASCP)
Tel: 615 327-6459 *Fax:* 615 963-5926
E-mail: ddonovan@picard.tnstate.edu
Med Dir: Archie Powell, MD
Class Cap: 14 *Begins:* Aug
Length: 12 mos *Award:* BS
Tuition per yr: $2,925 res, $9,420 non-res

Vanderbilt University Medical Center
Clin Lab Scientist/Med Tech Prgm
4605D The Vanderbilt Clinic
1161 21st Ave S
Nashville, TN 37232-5310
Prgm Dir: Maralie Gaffron Exton, MT(ASCP)SH
Tel: 615 322-6940 *Fax:* 615 343-8420
Med Dir: John B Cousar Jr, MD
Begins: Jun
Length: 12 mos *Award:* Cert
Tuition per yr: $1,500 res, $1,500 non-res

Texas

Northwest Texas Healthcare System
Clin Lab Scientist/Med Tech Prgm
PO Box 1110
Amarillo, TX 79175
Prgm Dir: Barbara Jean Rogers, MT(ASCP)
Tel: 806 354-1946 *Fax:* 806 354-1059
Med Dir: James F Hamous, MD
Class Cap: 6 *Begins:* Jul
Length: 12 mos *Award:* Cert

Austin State Hospital
Clin Lab Scientist/Med Tech Prgm
4110 Guadalupe St
Austin, TX 78751
Prgm Dir: Judith D Larsen, MT(ASCP)SH
Tel: 512 419-2038
Med Dir: Dan G Hardy, MD
Class Cap: 7 *Begins:* Jul Aug
Length: 12 mos *Award:* Cert, BS
Tuition per yr: $275

St Elizabeth Hospital

Clin Lab Scientist/Med Tech Prgm
2830 Calder St
PO Box 5405
Beaumont, TX 77726-5405
Prgm Dir: Deborah R Zink, MT(ASCP) MBA
Tel: 409 899-7150 *Fax:* 409 899-7991
Med Dir: Terry W Bell, MD
Class Cap: 6 *Begins:* Aug
Length: 12 mos *Award:* Cert, BS

Corpus Christi State University

Clin Lab Scientist/Med Tech Prgm
College of Sci and Technology
6300 Ocean Dr
Corpus Christi, TX 78412
Prgm Dir: Christina Thompson, MT(ASCP)SBB
Tel: 512 994-2473 *Fax:* 512 994-2742
Med Dir: Joe Lewis, MD
Class Cap: 20 *Begins:* Sep
Length: 12 mos *Award:* Dipl,Cert, BS
Tuition per yr: $1,400 res, $7,800 non-res
Evening or weekend classes available

Univ of Tx Southwestern Med Ctr - Dallas

Clin Lab Scientist/Med Tech Prgm
5323 Harry Hines Blvd
Dallas, TX 75235-8878
Prgm Dir: Lynn M Little, PhD MT(ASCP)M
Tel: 214 648-2808
Med Dir: Robert W McKenna, MD
Class Cap: 24 *Begins:* Aug
Length: 12 mos *Award:* Dipl,Cert, BS
Tuition per yr: $1,696 res, $13,038 non-res

Univ of Texas - Pan American

Clin Lab Scientist/Med Tech Prgm
1201 W University Dr
Edinburg, TX 78539
Prgm Dir: Karen Chandler, MA MT(ASCP)
Tel: 210 381-2296 *Fax:* 210 384-5054
E-mail: kchandler@panam.edu
Med Dir: Domingo Useda, MD
Class Cap: 15 *Begins:* Sep
Length: 15 mos *Award:* Dipl,Cert, BS
Tuition per yr: $2,342 res, $9,049 non-res
Evening or weekend classes available

University of Texas at El Paso

Clin Lab Scientist/Med Tech Prgm
1101 N Campbell
Rm 615
El Paso, TX 79902
Prgm Dir: Richard C Mroz Jr, DA MT(ASCP) CLS
Tel: 915 747-7243 *Fax:* 915 747-7207
E-mail: rmroz@utep.edu
Med Dir: Arturo Vargas, MD
Class Cap: 24 *Begins:* Sep
Length: 20 mos *Award:* BS
Tuition per yr: $1,735 res, $6,298 non-res
Evening or weekend classes available

Harris Methodist Ft Worth

Clin Lab Scientist/Med Tech Prgm
1301 Pennsylvania
Harris Methodist Fort Worth
Ft Worth, TX 76104
Prgm Dir: Gail I Jones, PhD MT(ASCP)
Tel: 817 878-5621
E-mail: gail.jones@hmhs.com
Med Dir: John R Harbour, MD
Class Cap: 6 *Begins:* Jan Jul
Length: 12 mos *Award:* Cert, BS
Tuition per yr: $1,550 res, $1,550 non-res

Tarleton State University

Clin Lab Scientist/Med Tech Prgm
1625 W Myrtle St
Ft Worth, TX 76104
Prgm Dir: Karen R Murray, MBA MT(ASCP) SC
Tel: 817 926-1101 *Fax:* 817 922-8103
Med Dir: Richard C Schaffer, MD
Class Cap: 12 *Begins:* Jan Jul
Length: 13 mos *Award:* Dipl, BS
Tuition per yr: $3,000 res, $10,000 non-res

University of Texas Medical Branch

Clin Lab Scientist/Med Tech Prgm
Schl of Allied Hlth Sciences
J-28 Rm 4.442
Galveston, TX 77555-1028
Prgm Dir: Vicki S Freeman, PhD MT(ASCP)SC
Tel: 409 772-3055 *Fax:* 409 772-3014
E-mail: vfreeman@utmb.edu
Med Dir: Jack G Richmond, MD
Class Cap: 40 *Begins:* Jun
Length: 18 mos, 24 mos *Award:* Dipl, BSMT
Tuition per yr: $1,504 res, $11,562 non-res

Harris County Hosp Dist/Ben Taub Hosp

Clin Lab Scientist/Med Tech Prgm
1502 Taub Loop
Houston, TX 77030
Prgm Dir: Bettye H Riley, MT(ASCP)SBB
Tel: 713 793-3241
Med Dir: Jochewed Werch, MD
Class Cap: 10 *Begins:* Aug
Length: 12 mos *Award:* Cert, BS

Methodist Hospital

Clin Lab Scientist/Med Tech Prgm
6565 Fannin Mail St
STB1-20
Houston, TX 77030
Prgm Dir: Judy Jobe, MT(ASCP)
Tel: 713 790-2599 *Fax:* 713 703-7408
E-mail: jjobe@profsvcs.tmht.mc.edu
Med Dir: Abdus Saleem, MD
Class Cap: 8 *Begins:* Aug
Length: 12 mos *Award:* Cert, BS

Texas Southern University

Clin Lab Scientist/Med Tech Prgm
3100 Cleburne
Houston, TX 77004
Prgm Dir: Dorothy J Quiller, MEd MT(ASCP)
Tel: 713 527-7265 *Fax:* 713 313-1094
Med Dir: Sushma Mahajan, MD
Class Cap: 24 *Begins:* Sep Jan
Length: 48 mos, 48 mos *Award:* Cert, BS
Tuition per yr: $1,577 res, $5,128 non-res
Evening or weekend classes available

Univ of Texas Hlth Sci Ctr at Houston

Clin Lab Scientist/Med Tech Prgm
PO Box 20708
Houston, TX 77225
Prgm Dir: Carol T McCoy, PhD MT(ASCP)
Tel: 713 792-4466 *Fax:* 713 745-0772
E-mail: cmccoy@acad1.sahs.uth.tmc.edu
Med Dir: L Maximilian Buja, MD
Class Cap: 40 *Begins:* Aug
Length: 16 mos *Award:* BS
Tuition per yr: $1,040 res, $6,480 non-res

Univ of Texas M D Anderson Cancer Ctr

Clin Lab Scientist/Med Tech Prgm
1515 Holcombe Blvd
PO Box 73
Houston, TX 77030
Prgm Dir: Karen Rogge-McClure, MT(ASCP)SBB
Tel: 713 745-1688 *Fax:* 713 745-3337
E-mail: kmcclure@utmarc.uth.tmc.edu
Med Dir: Jeffrey J Tarrand, MD
Class Cap: 12 *Begins:* Aug
Length: 12 mos *Award:* Cert

Veterans Affairs Medical Center

Clin Lab Scientist/Med Tech Prgm
2002 Holcombe Blvd
Houston, TX 77030
Prgm Dir: Marion McNeal-Tresvant, MEd MT
ASCP
Tel: 713 794-7256 *Fax:* 713 794-7657
Med Dir: Alden W Dudley Jr, MD
Begins: Aug
Length: 12 mos *Award:* Cert

Texas Tech Univ Hlth Sci Ctr

Clin Lab Scientist/Med Tech Prgm
School of Allied Health
Lubbock, TX 79430
Prgm Dir: Hal S Larsen, PhD MT(ASCP)CLS
Tel: 806 743-3247 *Fax:* 806 743-3249
E-mail: alhhsl@ttuhsc.edu
Med Dir: David L Morgan, MD
Class Cap: 30 *Begins:* Aug
Length: 21 mos *Award:* BS
Tuition per yr: $2,100 res, $5,700 non-res

Memorial Hospital and Medical Center

Clin Lab Scientist/Med Tech Prgm
2200 W Illinois St
Midland, TX 79701
Prgm Dir: Peggy Jo Wheeler, MT(ASCP)
Tel: 915 685-1635 *Fax:* 915 685-6906
Med Dir: Sherri L Gillman, MD
Class Cap: 4 *Begins:* Jan Jul
Length: 12 mos *Award:* Cert, BS
Tuition per yr: $220

Shannon West Texas Memorial Hospital

Clin Lab Scientist/Med Tech Prgm
120 E Harris
PO Box 1879
San Angelo, TX 76902
Prgm Dir: Cleve Moore, MT(ASCP)
Tel: 915 653-6741 *Fax:* 915 657-5499
Med Dir: Martin Kulig, MD
Class Cap: 8 *Begins:* Jul Jan
Length: 12 mos *Award:* Cert, BS

Baptist Memorial Healthcare System

Clin Lab Scientist/Med Tech Prgm
111 Dallas St
San Antonio, TX 78286
Prgm Dir: Douglas Bearden, MA MT(ASCP)
Tel: 210 302-2386
Med Dir: Karen Magnon, MD
Class Cap: 12 *Begins:* Jul
Length: 12 mos *Award:* Cert
Tuition per yr: $1,550

Programs

Univ of Texas Hlth Sci Ctr at San Antonio

Clin Lab Scientist/Med Tech Prgm
7703 Floyd Curl Dr
San Antonio, TX 78284-7772
Prgm Dir: Shirlyn B McKenzie, PhD MS
Tel: 210 567-3081 *Fax:* 210 567-3089
E-mail: mckenzie@uthscsa.edu
Med Dir: Milka M Montiel, MD
Class Cap: 23 *Begins:* Aug Jan
Length: 24 mos, 39 mos *Award:* Cert, BS
Tuition per yr: $1,200 res, $8,048 non-res

Southwest Texas State University

Clin Lab Scientist/Med Tech Prgm
601 University Dr
San Marcos, TX 78666-4616
Prgm Dir: David M Falleur, MEd MT(ASCP)
Tel: 512 245-3500 *Fax:* 512 245-7860
E-mail: df03@admin.swt.edu
Med Dir: Margaret C Young, MD
Class Cap: 20 *Begins:* Jul
Length: 14 mos *Award:* Dipl, BCLS
Tuition per yr: $2,345 res, $8,810 non-res
Evening or weekend classes available

Scott & White Memorial Hosp and Clinic

Clin Lab Scientist/Med Tech Prgm
2401 S 31st St
Temple, TX 76508
Prgm Dir: Janet Duben-Engelkirk, EdD
 MT(ASCP)
Tel: 817 724-5177 *Fax:* 817 724-8396
E-mail: jengel@vvm.com
Med Dir: Daniel J Ladd, MD
Class Cap: 10 *Begins:* Aug
Length: 12 mos *Award:* Cert

Wadley Regional Medical Center

Clin Lab Scientist/Med Tech Prgm
1000 Pine St
Texarkana, TX 75501
Prgm Dir: Joyce Nantze, MT(ASCP)SBB
Tel: 903 798-7120 *Fax:* 903 798-7196
E-mail: jnantze@aol.com
Med Dir: J Keith Hairston, MD
Class Cap: 4 *Begins:* Aug
Length: 12 mos *Award:* Cert
Tuition per yr: $200 res, $200 non-res

University of Texas at Tyler

Clin Lab Scientist/Med Tech Prgm
3900 University Blvd
Tyler, TX 75701
Prgm Dir: James F Koukl, PhD MT(ASCP)
Tel: 903 566-7009 *Fax:* 903 566-7189
E-mail: jkoukl@mail.uttyl.edu
Med Dir: L R Hieger, MD
Class Cap: 12 *Begins:* Jun
Length: 12 mos *Award:* Cert, BS
Tuition per yr: $1,230 res, $9,102 non-res

Hillcrest Baptist Medical Center

Clin Lab Scientist/Med Tech Prgm
3000 Herring Ave
Waco, TX 76708
Prgm Dir: Alisa Petree, MT(ASCP)
Tel: 817 756-8653 *Fax:* 817 750-7922
E-mail: apetree@texnet.net
Med Dir: E B Morrison, MD
Class Cap: 4 *Begins:* Jan Jul
Length: 12 mos *Award:* Cert

Wichita General Hospital

Clin Lab Scientist/Med Tech Prgm
1600 Eighth St
Wichita Falls, TX 76301
Prgm Dir: Carolyn D Mass, MS MT(ASCP)
Tel: 817 723-1461 *Fax:* 817 761-8994
Med Dir: John H Scott, MD
Class Cap: 6 *Begins:* Jul
Length: 12 mos *Award:* Cert, BS
Tuition per yr: $2,000

Utah

Weber State University

Clin Lab Scientist/Med Tech Prgm
3750 Harrison Blvd
Ogden, UT 84408-3905
Prgm Dir: Roger C Nichols, MS MT(ASCP)SM
Tel: 801 626-6716 *Fax:* 801 626-7683
Med Dir: Dean Hammond, MD
Begins: Sep
Length: 36 mos *Award:* Dipl, BS
Tuition per yr: $2,324 res, $6,030 non-res
Evening or weekend classes available

Brigham Young University

Clin Lab Scientist/Med Tech Prgm
761 WIDB
Provo, UT 84602
Prgm Dir: Shauna C Anderson, PhD MT(ASCP)
Tel: 801 378-3132 *Fax:* 801 378-7499
E-mail: andersos@acd1.byu.edu
Med Dir: Robert G Lovell, MD
Begins: Aug Jan
Length: 12 mos *Award:* Dipl, BS
Tuition per yr: $2,530 res, $3,800 non-res

Univ of Utah Health Sciences Center

Clin Lab Scientist/Med Tech Prgm
Dept of Pathology
50 N Medical Dr
Salt Lake City, UT 84132
Prgm Dir: Larry Schoeff, MS MT(ASCP)
Tel: 801 581-7913 *Fax:* 801 581-4517
E-mail: lschoeff@hsc.utah.edu
Med Dir: Joseph A Knight, MD
Class Cap: 20 *Begins:* Mar
Length: 24 mos *Award:* Dipl, BS
Tuition per yr: $2,500 res, $7,700 non-res

Vermont

University of Vermont

Clin Lab Scientist/Med Tech Prgm
302 Rowell Bldg
Burlington, VT 05405
Prgm Dir: Anne E Huot, PhD
Tel: 802 656-3811 *Fax:* 802 656-2191
E-mail: ahuot@cosmos.uvm.edu
Med Dir: Edwin G Bovill, MD
Begins: Sep
Length: 48 mos *Award:* BS, MS
Tuition per yr: $6,732 res, $16,824 non-res

Virginia

Univ of Virginia Health Sciences Center

Clin Lab Scientist/Med Tech Prgm
Medical Ctr PO Box 168
Charlottesville, VA 22908
Prgm Dir: Cheryl V Leitch, MT(ASCP)SH
Tel: 804 924-5084 *Fax:* 804 982-1880
Med Dir: Michael R Wills, MD PhD
Class Cap: 16 *Begins:* Jun
Length: 12 mos *Award:* Cert
Tuition per yr: $2,202

Fairfax Hospital

Clin Lab Scientist/Med Tech Prgm
3300 Gallows Rd
Falls Church, VA 22046
Prgm Dir: Amy Shoemaker, MT(ASCP)
Tel: 703 698-2891 *Fax:* 703 698-2407
Med Dir: C Barrie Cook, MD
Begins: Jul
Length: 12 mos *Award:* Cert, BS
Tuition per yr: $2,000

Augusta Medical Center

Clin Lab Scientist/Med Tech Prgm
PO Box 1000
Fishersville, VA 22939
Prgm Dir: M Bernadette Bekken, MT(ASCP)BB
 CLS
Tel: 540 332-4539 *Fax:* 540 332-4543
Med Dir: Wayne P Jessee, MD
Class Cap: 5 *Begins:* Jul
Length: 12 mos *Award:* Cert, BS
Tuition per yr: $600

Rockingham Memorial Hospital

Clin Lab Scientist/Med Tech Prgm
235 Cantrell Ave
Harrisonburg, VA 22801
Prgm Dir: Randall G Vandevander, MT(ASCP)
Tel: 540 564-5407
Med Dir: Warren D Bannister, MD
Class Cap: 8 *Begins:* June
Length: 12 mos *Award:* Cert, BS

Norfolk State University

Clin Lab Scientist/Med Tech Prgm
2401 Corprew Ave
Norfolk, VA 23504
Prgm Dir: Mildred Fuller, PhD MT(ASCP)ClS
Tel: 757 683-2366 *Fax:* 757 683-2909
E-mail: mfuller@vger.nsu.edu
Med Dir: Anderson J Williams, MD
Class Cap: 11 *Begins:* Aug Jan
Length: 18 mos, 19 mos *Award:* BS
Tuition per yr: $2,865 res, $6,492 non-res
Evening or weekend classes available

Old Dominion University

Clin Lab Scientist/Med Tech Prgm
Schl of Med Lab Sciences
Health Sciences - 209
Norfolk, VA 23529
Prgm Dir: Faye E Coleman, MS MT(ASCP) CLS
Tel: 757 683-3588 *Fax:* 757 683-5028
E-mail: fecioou@cranium.hs.odu.edu
Med Dir: Richard P Moriarty, MD
Class Cap: 30 *Begins:* Aug
Length: 22 mos *Award:* BS
Tuition per yr: $4,690 res, $12,110 non-res
Evening or weekend classes available

Med Coll of VA/Virginia Commonwealth U
Clin Lab Scientist/Med Tech Prgm
PO Box 980583
MCV Campus
Richmond, VA 23298-0583
Prgm Dir: Barbara J Lindsey, MS CLSp(c)
Tel: 804 828-9469 *Fax:* 804 828-1911
E-mail: bjlindsey@gems.vcu.edu
Med Dir: Richard A McPherson, MD
Class Cap: 40 *Begins:* Aug Jan
Length: 20 mos *Award:* BS
Tuition per yr: $4,220 res, $12,476 non-res
Evening or weekend classes available

Carilion Health System/Carilion Roanoke Mem Hosp
Clin Lab Scientist/Med Tech Prgm
Roanoke Memorial Hospital
Belleview at Jefferson
Roanoke, VA 24033
Prgm Dir: Janet T Hiler, BS MT(ASCP)
Tel: 540 981-8032 *Fax:* 540 981-0156
Med Dir: Samuel F Vance, MD
Begins: Jul
Length: 12 mos *Award:* Cert, BS
Tuition per yr: $2,000 res, $2,000 non-res

Washington

University of Washington
Clin Lab Scientist/Med Tech Prgm
School of Medicine
Dept of Lab Medicine/Box 357110
Seattle, WA 98195-7110
Prgm Dir: Carol N LeCrone, MS MT(ASCP)
Tel: 206 548-6131 *Fax:* 206 548-6189
E-mail: lacrone@mail.labmed.washington.edu
Med Dir: James S Fine, MD
Class Cap: 30 *Begins:* Sep
Length: 24 mos *Award:* BS
Tuition per yr: $3,138 res, $9,753 non-res
Evening or weekend classes available

Sacred Heart Medical Center
Clin Lab Scientist/Med Tech Prgm
101 W Eighth Ave, PO Box 2555
TAF-C9
Spokane, WA 99220-2555
Prgm Dir: Cynthia Hamby, MEd MT(ASCP)
Tel: 509 455-3339 *Fax:* 509 455-2052
Med Dir: Mark E Williamson, MD
Class Cap: 8 *Begins:* Jul
Length: 12 mos *Award:* Cert

Central Washington University
Clin Lab Scientist/Med Tech Prgm
Center for Medical Technology
1120 W Spruce
Yakima, WA 98902
Prgm Dir: Claudia R Steen, MS MT(ASCP)
Tel: 509 248-7784
Med Dir: Stephen D Muehleck, MD
Class Cap: 8 *Begins:* Jul Dec
Length: 12 mos *Award:* Cert, BS
Tuition per yr: $2,430 res, $8,616 non-res

West Virginia

Marshall University
Clin Lab Scientist/Med Tech Prgm
400 Hall Greer Blvd
Huntington, WV 25701
Prgm Dir: Bruce J Brown, EdD MS MT(ASCP)
Tel: 304 696-3188 *Fax:* 304 696-3243
E-mail: brownbru@matshall.edu
Med Dir: John P Sheils, MD
Class Cap: 12 *Begins:* Aug
Length: 9 mos *Award:* BS
Tuition per yr: $2,316 res, $6,073 non-res
Evening or weekend classes available

West Virginia University
Clin Lab Scientist/Med Tech Prgm
PO Box 9211
2138 Health Sciences Ctr N
Morgantown, WV 26506-9211
Prgm Dir: Jean D Holter, EdD MT(ASCP)
Tel: 304 293-2069 *Fax:* 304 293-6249
Med Dir: Harry L Taylor, MD
Class Cap: 50 *Begins:* Aug
Length: 21 mos *Award:* BS
Tuition per yr: $2,706 res, $8,288 non-res

West Liberty State College
Clin Lab Scientist/Med Tech Prgm
Dept of Medical Technology
West Liberty, WV 26074
Prgm Dir: William C Wagener, PhD MT(ASCP)
Tel: 304 336-8177 *Fax:* 304 336-8266
Med Dir: Jaywant Philip Parmar, MD
Class Cap: 16 *Begins:* Aug
Length: 24 mos *Award:* BS
Tuition per yr: $1,800 res, $3,870 non-res

Wisconsin

St Elizabeth Hospital
Clin Lab Scientist/Med Tech Prgm
1506 S Oneida St
Appleton, WI 54915
Prgm Dir: Carla E Salmon, MT(ASCP)CLS
Tel: 414 738-2128 *Fax:* 414 730-5763
Med Dir: Peter V Podlusky, MD
Class Cap: 6 *Begins:* Aug
Length: 9 mos *Award:* Cert
Tuition per yr: $850

Sacred Heart Hospital
Clin Lab Scientist/Med Tech Prgm
900 W Clairemont Ave
Eau Claire, WI 54701
Prgm Dir: Jane Scheuermann, MS MT(ASCP)
Tel: 715 839-3973 *Fax:* 715 833-4941
Med Dir: Thomas W Hadley, MD
Class Cap: 5 *Begins:* Aug
Length: 10 mos *Award:* Cert
Tuition per yr: $850

St Vincent Hospital
Clin Lab Scientist/Med Tech Prgm
PO Box 13508
Green Bay, WI 54307
Prgm Dir: Harlan A Bloy, MT(ASCP)SM
Tel: 414 431-3050
Med Dir: Darrell P Skarphol, MD
Class Cap: 6 *Begins:* Aug
Length: 9 mos *Award:* Dipl, BS
Tuition per yr: $850

University of Wisconsin - Madison
Clin Lab Scientist/Med Tech Prgm
1300 University Ave
6175 MSC
Madison, WI 53706
Prgm Dir: Sharon Ehrmeyer, PhD MT(ASCP)
Tel: 608 262-2085 *Fax:* 608 262-9520
E-mail: ehrmeyer@facstaff.wisc.edu
Med Dir: Michael Hart, MD
Class Cap: 26 *Begins:* Jul
Length: 11 mos *Award:* BS
Tuition per yr: $2,549 res, $9,304 non-res
Evening or weekend classes available

St Joseph's Hospital
Clin Lab Scientist/Med Tech Prgm
611 St Joseph Ave
Marshfield, WI 54449
Prgm Dir: Virginia R Narlock, PhD MT(ASCP)CLS
Tel: 715 387-7202 *Fax:* 715 387-7121
Med Dir: Kurt Reed, MD
Class Cap: 12 *Begins:* Aug
Length: 9 mos *Award:* Cert, BS
Tuition per yr: $850 res, $850 non-res

Aurora Health Care
Clin Lab Scientist/Med Tech Prgm
Aurora Health Care
2900 W Oklahoma Ave Box 2901
Milwaukee, WI 53215
Prgm Dir: Christine M Schmus, MT(ASCP)MS
Tel: 414 649-7872 *Fax:* 414 649-7850
Med Dir: Reuben Eisenstein, MD
Class Cap: 12 *Begins:* May
Length: 12 mos *Award:* Cert, BS
Tuition per yr: $1,885

Clement J Zablocki VA Medical Center
Clin Lab Scientist/Med Tech Prgm
5000 W National Ave
Milwaukee, WI 53295
Prgm Dir: Mark J Maticek, MT(ASCP)
Tel: 414 384-2000 *Fax:* 414 384-2000
Med Dir: Bruce Edward Dunn, MD
Class Cap: 10 *Begins:* May
Length: 12 mos *Award:* BS

Froedtert Memorial Lutheran Hospital
Clin Lab Scientist/Med Tech Prgm
Dept of Pathology
PO Box 26509
Milwaukee, WI 53226
Prgm Dir: Ann H McDonald, PhD MT(ASCP)
Tel: 414 456-7615 *Fax:* 414 456-6305
E-mail: amedonah@post.its.mcw.edu
Med Dir: Carl G Becker, MD
Class Cap: 9 *Begins:* May
Length: 12 mos *Award:* Cert, BS
Tuition per yr: $1,000

University of Wisconsin - Milwaukee
Clin Lab Scientist/Med Tech Prgm
Sch of Allied Hlth Professions
PO Box 413
Milwaukee, WI 53201
Prgm Dir: Cindy Brown, MA MT(ASCP)
Tel: 414 229-5299 *Fax:* 414 229-2645
E-mail: cbrown@sahp2.uwm.edu
Med Dir: Jay F Schamberg, MD
Class Cap: 50 *Begins:* Sep
Length: 21 mos *Award:* Dipl, BS
Tuition per yr: $3,102 res, $9,965 non-res

Programs

Wausau Hospital
Clin Lab Scientist/Med Tech Prgm
333 Pine Ridge Blvd
Wausau, WI 54401
Prgm Dir: Susan Flaker-Johnson, MEd MT(ASCP)
Tel: 715 847-2136 *Fax:* 715 847-2930
Med Dir: Kathy P Belgea, MD
Class Cap: 5 *Begins:* Aug
Length: 9 mos *Award:* Cert, BS
Tuition per yr: $850

Wyoming

University of Wyoming
Clin Lab Scientist/Med Tech Prgm
Univ Station
PO Box 3837
Laramie, WY 82071
Prgm Dir: James E Thompson, MSA MT(ASCP)
Tel: 307 766-2180 *Fax:* 307 766-3445
E-mail: jthom@uwyo.edu
Med Dir: Gregory A Brondos, MD
Class Cap: 12 *Begins:* Jul
Length: 11 mos *Award:* BS
Tuition per yr: $2,652 res, $7,382 non-res
Evening or weekend classes available

Clinical Laboratory Technician/ Medical Laboratory Technician- AD

Alabama

Jefferson State Community College
Clin Lab Tech/Med Lab Tech-AD Prgm
2601 Carson Rd
Birmingham, AL 35215
Prgm Dir: Gail J Thomason, MA MT(ASCP) CIC
Tel: 205 856-6031 *Fax:* 205 856-7725
Med Dir: Donald R Cantley, MD
Class Cap: 12 *Begins:* Jun Jan
Length: 21 mos *Award:* Dipl, AAS
Tuition per yr: $1,800 res, $3,300 non-res
Evening or weekend classes available

George C Wallace State Comm College
Clin Lab Tech/Med Lab Tech-AD Prgm
Napier Rd
Dothan, AL 36303
Prgm Dir: Sylvia W Norton, EdD MT(ASCP)
Tel: 334 983-3521 *Fax:* 334 983-3600
Med Dir: Patrick Jones, MD
Class Cap: 9 *Begins:* Sep
Length: 24 mos *Award:* AAS
Tuition per yr: $2,898 res, $5,273 non-res
Evening or weekend classes available

Gadsden State Community College
Clin Lab Tech/Med Lab Tech-AD Prgm
PO Box 227
1001 George Wallace Dr
Gadsden, AL 35902-0227
Prgm Dir: Sunita M Graves, MS BS MT(ASCP)
Tel: 205 549-8470, Ext 328 *Fax:* 205 549-8465
Med Dir: E Max Sanders, MD
Class Cap: 34 *Begins:* Mar Sep
Length: 21 mos *Award:* AAS
Tuition per yr: $1,943 res, $3,618 non-res
Evening or weekend classes available

Wallace State College
Clin Lab Tech/Med Lab Tech-AD Prgm
PO Box 2000
Hanceville, AL 35077-2000
Prgm Dir: Marion A Slatsky, MT(ASCP)
Tel: 205 352-8330 *Fax:* 205 352-8228
Med Dir: James Lester Newsome, MD
Class Cap: 40 *Begins:* Sep Apr
Length: 21 mos *Award:* AAS
Tuition per yr: $1,332 res, $2,331 non-res
Evening or weekend classes available

Arizona

Phoenix College
Clin Lab Tech/Med Lab Tech-AD Prgm
1202 W Thomas Rd
Phoenix, AZ 85013
Prgm Dir: Marian Tadano, MA MT(ASCP)
Tel: 602 285-7114 *Fax:* 602 285-7700

Arkansas

Arkansas State University-Beebe
Clin Lab Tech/Med Lab Tech-AD Prgm
PO Drawer H
Beebe, AR 72012
Prgm Dir: Lynn W Baker Jr
Tel: 501 882-8214 *Fax:* 501 882-8387
Med Dir: John R Brineman, MD
Class Cap: 10 *Begins:* Aug
Length: 24 mos *Award:* AAS
Tuition per yr: $1,080 res, $1,824 non-res
Evening or weekend classes available

South Arkansas Community College
Clin Lab Tech/Med Lab Tech-AD Prgm
300 S West Ave
El Dorado, AR 71730
Prgm Dir: Paul C Smith, MT(ASCP)
Tel: 501 862-8131
Med Dir: Wayne Elliott, MD
Class Cap: 10 *Begins:* Aug
Length: 24 mos *Award:* Dipl, AAS
Tuition per yr: $1,120 res, $1,420 non-res
Evening or weekend classes available

Westark Community College
Clin Lab Tech/Med Lab Tech-AD Prgm
Grand at Waldron
PO Box 3649
Ft Smith, AR 72913
Prgm Dir: Ken Hamilton, DDS MT(ASCP)
Tel: 501 788-7852 *Fax:* 501 788-7869
Med Dir: Annette Landrum, MD
Class Cap: 10 *Begins:* Sep
Length: 19 mos *Award:* AS
Tuition per yr: $672 res, $1,560 non-res
Evening or weekend classes available

North Arkansas Comm and Tech Coll
Clin Lab Tech/Med Lab Tech-AD Prgm
420 Pioneer Ridge Dr
Harrison, AR 72601
Prgm Dir: Marion F Mosley, MHS MT(ASCP)
Tel: 501 743-3000, Ext 213
Med Dir: Robert L Miller, MD PhD
Class Cap: 8 *Begins:* Aug
Length: 22 mos *Award:* AAS
Tuition per yr: $816 res, $1,032 non-res

Phillips County Community College
Clin Lab Tech/Med Lab Tech-AD Prgm
PO Box 785
Helena, AR 72342
Prgm Dir: Maretta Locke, MEd MT(ASCP)
Tel: 501 338-6474 *Fax:* 501 338-7542
E-mail: mlocke@pccc.cc.ar.us
Med Dir: Francis Patton, MD
Class Cap: 14 *Begins:* Aug
Length: 22 mos *Award:* AAS
Tuition per yr: $840 res, $1,055 non-res

Garland County Community College
Clin Lab Tech/Med Lab Tech-AD Prgm
101 College Dr
Hot Springs, AR 71913-9174
Prgm Dir: Jay W Willborn, MEd BS MT(ASCP)
Tel: 501 767-9371, Ext 278 *Fax:* 501 767-6896
Med Dir: Vilasini Devi Jayaraman, MD
Class Cap: 10 *Begins:* Jan
Length: 18 mos *Award:* AS
Tuition per yr: $888 res, $1,104 non-res

Arkansas State University
Clin Lab Tech/Med Lab Tech-AD Prgm
PO Box 69
State University, AR 72467
Prgm Dir: Mary Jean Rutherford, MEd
MT(ASCP)SC
Tel: 501 972-3073   *Fax:* 501 972-2040
E-mail: mjruth@crow.astate.edu
Med Dir: Donald B Vollman, Jr, MD
Class Cap: 24   *Begins:* Aug
Length: 24 mos   *Award:* AS
Tuition per yr: $2,400 res, $4,200 non-res
Evening or weekend classes available

Colorado

Arapahoe Community College
Clin Lab Tech/Med Lab Tech-AD Prgm
2500 W College Dr
PO Box 9002
Littleton, CO 80160-9002
Prgm Dir: Linda Comeaux, MT(ASCP)
Tel: 303 797-5796   *Fax:* 303 797-5935
E-mail: lcomeaux@arapahoe.edu
Med Dir: Kenneth R Holloman, MD
Class Cap: 25   *Begins:* Aug
Length: 24 mos   *Award:* Dipl, AAS
Tuition per yr: $2,070 res, $8,115 non-res
Evening or weekend classes available

Connecticut

Housatonic Community Technical College
Clin Lab Tech/Med Lab Tech-AD Prgm
510 Barnum Ave
Bridgeport, CT 06608
Prgm Dir: Phyllis J Gutowski, MS MT(ASCP)
Tel: 203 579-6447   *Fax:* 203 579-6993
E-mail: ho_markos_25@comnet.edu
Med Dir: Uma Ayer, MD
Class Cap: 20   *Begins:* Sep
Length: 21 mos   *Award:* AS
Tuition per yr: $1,722 res, $4,842 non-res
Evening or weekend classes available

Manchester Community - Technical College
Clin Lab Tech/Med Lab Tech-AD Prgm
60 Bidwell St/PO Box 1046
Mail Station 19
Manchester, CT 06045-1046
Prgm Dir: Ellen P Digan, MA MT(ASCP)
Tel: 860 647-6190   *Fax:* 860 847-6238
E-mail: ma_digan@commnet.edu
Med Dir: Herbert Silver, MD
Class Cap: 14   *Begins:* Sep Aug
Length: 23 mos   *Award:* AS
Tuition per yr: $1,722 res, $4,842 non-res
Evening or weekend classes available

Delaware

Delaware Tech & Comm Coll - Owens Campus
Clin Lab Tech/Med Lab Tech-AD Prgm
PO Box 610
Georgetown, DE 19947
Prgm Dir: Rosanne B Arndt, MEd MT(ASCP)
Tel: 302 856-5400   *Fax:* 302 856-5758
E-mail: rarndt@outland.dtcc.edu
Med Dir: William A Diedrich Jr, MD
Class Cap: 42   *Begins:* Aug Jan Jun
Length: 24 mos   *Award:* AAS
Tuition per yr: $1,260 non-res
Evening or weekend classes available

Florida

Brevard Community College
Clin Lab Tech/Med Lab Tech-AD Prgm
1519 Clearlake Rd
Cocoa, FL 32922
Prgm Dir: Celine Marilyn Hulme, MEd MT(ASCP)
Tel: 407 632-1111   *Fax:* 407 634-3731
Med Dir: Carl Smedberg, MD
Class Cap: 16   *Begins:* Aug
Length: 22 mos   *Award:* AS
Tuition per yr: $1,406 res, $5,130 non-res
Evening or weekend classes available

Keiser College of Technology
Clin Lab Tech/Med Lab Tech-AD Prgm
1500 NW 49th St
Ft Lauderdale, FL 33309
Prgm Dir: Evelyn C Keiser, BS MT(ASCP)
Tel: 954 776-4456   *Fax:* 954 771-4894
Med Dir: Roshan Moraes, MD
Class Cap: 60   *Begins:* Aug Nov Feb May
Length: 13 mos, 24 mos   *Award:* AS, AA
Tuition per yr: $11,815
Evening or weekend classes available

Indian River Community College
Clin Lab Tech/Med Lab Tech-AD Prgm
3209 Virginia Ave
Ft Pierce, FL 34981-9003
Prgm Dir: Carol Daniels, MEd MT(ASCP)
Tel: 561 462-4405   *Fax:* 561 462-4796
E-mail: cdaniels@ircc.cc.fl.us
Med Dir: John L Rodgers, MD
Class Cap: 16   *Begins:* Aug
Length: 23 mos   *Award:* AS
Tuition per yr: $1,314 res, $4,860 non-res
Evening or weekend classes available

Florida Community College - Jacksonville
Clin Lab Tech/Med Lab Tech-AD Prgm
N Campus 4501 Capper Rd
Jacksonville, FL 32218
Prgm Dir: Peter P Mullen, MS MT(ASCP)
Tel: 904 766-6511   *Fax:* 904 766-6654
E-mail: pmullen@fccjvm.cc.fl.us
Med Dir: George Merrill Shore, MD
Class Cap: 40   *Begins:* Aug Jan May
Length: 24 mos   *Award:* AS
Tuition per yr: $2,903 res, $10,959 non-res
Evening or weekend classes available

Lake City Community College
Clin Lab Tech/Med Lab Tech-AD Prgm
Rte 19 PO Box 1030
Lake City, FL 32025
Prgm Dir: Gretchen L Miller, BS MT (ASCP)
Tel: 904 752-1822, Ext 1157   *Fax:* 904 758-9959
Med Dir: Francisco Ravelo, MD
Class Cap: 18   *Begins:* Aug
Length: 24 mos   *Award:* AS
Tuition per yr: $1,404 res, $5,441 non-res
Evening or weekend classes available

Miami-Dade Community College
Clin Lab Tech/Med Lab Tech-AD Prgm
Medical Ctr Campus
950 NW 20th St
Miami, FL 33127
Prgm Dir: Nilia Madan
Tel: 305 237-4041, Ext 30523
Med Dir: Susan R Baker, MD PhD
Class Cap: 44   *Begins:* Aug
Length: 20 mos, 35 mos   *Award:* AS
Tuition per yr: $1,898 res, $6,670 non-res
Evening or weekend classes available

St Petersburg Junior College
Clin Lab Tech/Med Lab Tech-AD Prgm
PO Box 13489
St Petersburg, FL 33733-3489
Prgm Dir: Valerie Polansky, MEd MT(ASCP)
Tel: 813 341-3670   *Fax:* 813 341-3744
E-mail: polanskyv@email.spjc.cc.fl.us
Med Dir: Rehana Nawab, MD
Class Cap: 40   *Begins:* Aug
Length: 24 mos   *Award:* AS
Tuition per yr: $1,551 res, $5,563 non-res

Georgia

Darton College
Clin Lab Tech/Med Lab Tech-AD Prgm
2400 Gillionville Rd
Albany, GA 31707
Prgm Dir: Nancy T York, MT(ASCP)
Tel: 912 430-6840   *Fax:* 912 430-6910
E-mail: nyork@dmail.dartnet.peachnet.edu
Med Dir: Frank Isele, MD
Class Cap: 12   *Begins:* Sep Jan Mar Jun
Length: 21 mos   *Award:* AS
Tuition per yr: $1,600 res, $5,472 non-res
Evening or weekend classes available

Augusta Technical Institute
Clin Lab Tech/Med Lab Tech-AD Prgm
3116 Deans Bridge Rd
Augusta, GA 30906
Prgm Dir: Jan Golden, MT(ASCP)SC
Tel: 706 771-4175
Med Dir: William Mullins, MD
Class Cap: 24   *Begins:* Jan
Length: 24 mos   *Award:* Dipl, AAT
Tuition per yr: $1,096

Programs

Coastal Georgia Community College
Clin Lab Tech/Med Lab Tech-AD Prgm
3700 Altama Ave
Brunswick, GA 31523
Prgm Dir: Katherine Nisi Zell, EdS MT(ASCP)SH
Tel: 912 264-7382 *Fax:* 912 262-3283
Med Dir: Milton J Arras, MD
Class Cap: 20 *Begins:* Sep Jan
Length: 21 mos *Award:* AS
Tuition per yr: $1,620 res, $5,492 non-res
Evening or weekend classes available

Dalton College
Clin Lab Tech/Med Lab Tech-AD Prgm
213 N College Dr
Dalton, GA 30720
Prgm Dir: Doris M Shoemaker, EdS MLN
  MT(ASCP)
Tel: 706 272-4512, Ext 257 *Fax:* 706 272-2517
E-mail:
  Dshoemaker@carpet.dalton.peachnet.edu
Med Dir: Floyd James, MD
Class Cap: 12 *Begins:* Sep Jan Mar Jun
Length: 24 mos *Award:* AS
Tuition per yr: $1,401 res, $3,204 non-res

Thomas Technical Institute
Clin Lab Tech/Med Lab Tech-AD Prgm
15689 US Hwy 19 N
Thomasville, GA 31792
Prgm Dir: Richard Miller, PhD MBA MT(ASCP)
  CLS(NCA)
Tel: 912 225-4078 *Fax:* 912 225-4030
E-mail: rmiller@ttin1.thomas.tec.ga.us
Med Dir: Jeff W Byrd, MD
Class Cap: 20 *Begins:* Sep
Length: 21 mos *Award:* AAT
Tuition per yr: $1,104 res, $2,112 non-res
Evening or weekend classes available

Hawaii

Kapiolani Community College
Clin Lab Tech/Med Lab Tech-AD Prgm
4303 Diamond Head Rd
Honolulu, HI 96816
Prgm Dir: Marcia A Armstrong, MS MT(ASCP)
Tel: 808 734-9231 *Fax:* 808 734-9126
E-mail: marmstro@leachie.kcc.hawaii.edu
Med Dir: L John Lockett, MD
Class Cap: 16 *Begins:* Aug
Length: 21 mos *Award:* AS
Tuition per yr: $788 res, $5,132 non-res

Illinois

Belleville Area College
Clin Lab Tech/Med Lab Tech-AD Prgm
2500 Carlyle Rd
Belleville, IL 62221
Prgm Dir: William E Meekins,
  MT(ASCP)SM(AAM)
Tel: 618 235-2700 *Fax:* 618 235-1578
Med Dir: Gregorio Sierra, MD
Class Cap: 16 *Begins:* Aug
Length: 20 mos *Award:* AAS
Tuition per yr: $1,573 res, $3,367 non-res
Evening or weekend classes available

Malcolm X College
Clin Lab Tech/Med Lab Tech-AD Prgm
1900 W Van Buren St
Chicago, IL 60612
Prgm Dir: Martha Garrett, MA BS MT(ASCP)
  CLS(NCA)
Tel: 312 850-7375 *Fax:* 312 850-7453
Med Dir: John L Kennedy, MD
Class Cap: 30 *Begins:* Sep
Length: 20 mos *Award:* AAS
Tuition per yr: $1,411 res, $3,407 non-res
Evening or weekend classes available

Oakton Community College
Clin Lab Tech/Med Lab Tech-AD Prgm
1600 E Golf Rd
Des Plaines, IL 60016
Prgm Dir: Lynne Lewis Steele, MMT MT(ASCP)
Tel: 847 635-1889 *Fax:* 847 635-1987
Med Dir: Ebrahim Amir-Mokri, MD
Class Cap: 20 *Begins:* Aug
Length: 21 mos *Award:* Dipl, AAS
Tuition per yr: $1,320 res, $4,720 non-res
Evening or weekend classes available

Sauk Valley Community College
Clin Lab Tech/Med Lab Tech-AD Prgm
173 Illinois Rt #2
Dixon, IL 61021-9110
Prgm Dir: Peggy White, MS MT(ASCP)
Tel: 815 288-5511 *Fax:* 815 288-5958
Med Dir: Tiem Lie, MD
Class Cap: 12 *Begins:* Aug
Length: 22 mos *Award:* Dipl, AAS
Tuition per yr: $2,345 res, $10,151 non-res

Elgin Community College
Clin Lab Tech/Med Lab Tech-AD Prgm
1700 Spartan Dr
Elgin, IL 60123-7193
Prgm Dir: Wendy L Miller, MS MT(ASCP)
Tel: 847 697-1000, Ext 7308 *Fax:* 847 622-0395
E-mail: wmiller@mail.elgin.cc.il.us
Med Dir: Patrick Garry, MD
Class Cap: 18 *Begins:* Aug
Length: 22 mos, 34 mos *Award:* AAS
Tuition per yr: $1,500 res, $6,784 non-res
Evening or weekend classes available

Lewis & Clark Community College
Clin Lab Tech/Med Lab Tech-AD Prgm
5800 Godfrey Rd
Godfrey, IL 62035-2466
Prgm Dir: Larry D Hostetler, BS MT(ASCP)
Tel: 618 466-3411, Ext 4421 *Fax:* 618 466-2798
Med Dir: Edward J Harrow, MD
Class Cap: 16 *Begins:* Aug
Length: 22 mos *Award:* Dipl, AAS
Tuition per yr: $1,600 res, $5,538 non-res
Evening or weekend classes available

College of Lake County
Clin Lab Tech/Med Lab Tech-AD Prgm
19351 W Washington St
Grayslake, IL 60030-1198
Prgm Dir: Remedios H Tesch, MS MSEd
  MT(ASCP)
Tel: 847 223-6601 *Fax:* 847 223-1357
E-mail: B10559@clc.cc.il.us
Med Dir: Fazia Batti, MD
Class Cap: 22 *Begins:* Aug
Length: 20 mos *Award:* AAS
Tuition per yr: $1,989 res, $7,587 non-res
Evening or weekend classes available

Kankakee Community College
Clin Lab Tech/Med Lab Tech-AD Prgm
River Rd
PO Box 888
Kankakee, IL 60901
Prgm Dir: Manuela Sawalha, MHS MT(ASCP)
Tel: 815 933-0296 *Fax:* 815 933-0217
Med Dir: Jesus Aquino, MD
Class Cap: 15 *Begins:* Aug
Length: 16 mos *Award:* AAS
Tuition per yr: $1,830 res, $2,332 non-res

Moraine Valley Community College
Clin Lab Tech/Med Lab Tech-AD Prgm
10900 S 88th Ave
Palos Hills, IL 60465
Prgm Dir: Janice L Swinarski, MT(ASCP)
Tel: 708 974-5223 *Fax:* 708 974-1184
E-mail: swinarsky@moraine.cc.il.us
Med Dir: Alvin M Ring, MD
Class Cap: 32 *Begins:* Aug
Length: 22 mos *Award:* AAS
Tuition per yr: $1,260 res, $4,830 non-res
Evening or weekend classes available

Illinois Central College
Clin Lab Tech/Med Lab Tech-AD Prgm
Health and Public Svcs Bldg
201 SW Adams
Peoria, IL 61635-0001
Prgm Dir: Janice M Kinsinger, MA MT(ASCP)CLS
Tel: 309 999-4661 *Fax:* 309 673-9626
Med Dir: Marvin Schmidt, MD
Class Cap: 16 *Begins:* Aug
Length: 20 mos *Award:* AAS
Tuition per yr: $1,470 res, $4,550 non-res
Evening or weekend classes available

Triton College
Clin Lab Tech/Med Lab Tech-AD Prgm
2000 Fifth Ave
River Grove, IL 60171
Prgm Dir: Carl Booker, MT(ASCP) MA
Tel: 708 456-0300
Med Dir: Marshall Short, MD
Class Cap: 25 *Begins:* Sep
Length: 22 mos *Award:* Dipl, AAS
Tuition per yr: $1,570 res, $4,886 non-res

Indiana

Indiana University Northwest
Clin Lab Tech/Med Lab Tech-AD Prgm
3400 Broadway
Gary, IN 46408
Prgm Dir: Janice G LaReau, MS MT(ASCP)SH
Tel: 219 980-6541 *Fax:* 219 980-6649
E-mail: jlareau@junhaw1.inu.indiana.edu
Med Dir: John A Griep, MD
Class Cap: 20 *Begins:* Jun
Length: 21 mos *Award:* AS
Tuition per yr: $3,395 res, $8,804 non-res
Evening or weekend classes available

Indiana Wesleyan University

Clin Lab Tech/Med Lab Tech-AD Prgm
4201 S Washington St
Marion, IN 46953
Prgm Dir: Jeanne Argot, PhD MT(ASCP)
Tel: 317 677-2296
Med Dir: Susan Rogers, MD
Begins: Sep Jan
Length: 21 mos   *Award:* Dipl, AS
Tuition per yr: $10,260 res, $10,260 non-res
Evening or weekend classes available

Ivy Tech State Coll NC - South Bend

Clin Lab Tech/Med Lab Tech-AD Prgm
1534 W Sample St
South Bend, IN 46619
Prgm Dir: Pamela B Primrose, MT(ASCP)
Tel: 219 289-7001   *Fax:* 219 236-7172
Med Dir: Robert J Tomec, MD
Class Cap: 18   *Begins:* Aug
Length: 22 mos   *Award:* AAS
Tuition per yr: $2,200 res, $4,440 non-res

Indiana State University

Clin Lab Tech/Med Lab Tech-AD Prgm
Dept of Life Sciences
Terre Haute, IN 47809
Prgm Dir: S Stevens
Tel: 812 237-2995
Med Dir: Roland M Kohr, MD
Class Cap: 24   *Begins:* Aug
Length: 24 mos   *Award:* Dipl, AS
Tuition per yr: $2,928 res, $7,224 non-res

Ivy Tech State Coll - Terre Haute

Clin Lab Tech/Med Lab Tech-AD Prgm
7999 US Hwy 41 S
Terre Haute, IN 47802-4894
Prgm Dir: Janee Gambill, MS MT(ASCP)
Tel: 812 299-1121   *Fax:* 812 299-1121
Med Dir: M Bashar Kashlar, MD
Class Cap: 24   *Begins:* Aug
Length: 21 mos   *Award:* AAS
Tuition per yr: $2,569 res, $4,678 non-res
Evening or weekend classes available

Vincennes University

Clin Lab Tech/Med Lab Tech-AD Prgm
1002 N First St
Vincennes, IN 47591
Prgm Dir: Joyce A Oglesby, MA MT(ASCP)
Tel: 812 888-5350   *Fax:* 812 888-4550
E-mail: joglesby@vunet.vina.edu
Med Dir: Mark C Mills, MD
Class Cap: 27   *Begins:* Aug
Length: 21 mos   *Award:* Dipl, AS
Tuition per yr: $2,758 res, $4,100 non-res
Evening or weekend classes available

Iowa

Des Moines Area Community College

Clin Lab Tech/Med Lab Tech-AD Prgm
2006 Ankeny Blvd
Ankeny, IA 50021
Prgm Dir: Jeannette Daehler, MT(ASCP)
Tel: 515 964-6296   *Fax:* 515 964-6440
E-mail: jdaehler@dmacc.cc.ia.us
Med Dir: David Baridon, MD
Class Cap: 24   *Begins:* Sep
Length: 21 mos   *Award:* AAS
Tuition per yr: $1,462 res, $2,927 non-res
Evening or weekend classes available

Scott Community College

Clin Lab Tech/Med Lab Tech-AD Prgm
500 Belmont Rd
Bettendorf, IA 52722
Prgm Dir: Pamela Bass, MS MT(ASCP)
Tel: 319 359-7531
E-mail: pbass@eiccd.cc.ia.us
Med Dir: Jack F Consamus, MD
Class Cap: 26   *Begins:* Aug
Length: 24 mos   *Award:* AAS
Tuition per yr: $3,900 res, $5,700 non-res
Evening or weekend classes available

Iowa Central Community College

Clin Lab Tech/Med Lab Tech-AD Prgm
330 Ave M
Fort Dodge, IA 50501
Prgm Dir: Diane C Edwards, BS MT(ASCP)
Tel: 515 576-7201, Ext 2393   *Fax:* 515 576-7206
E-mail: dedward@duke.icc.cc.ia.us
Med Dir: Doral E Colton, MD
Class Cap: 20   *Begins:* Aug
Length: 20 mos   *Award:* AAS
Tuition per yr: $2,393 res, $3,303 non-res

Hawkeye Community College

Clin Lab Tech/Med Lab Tech-AD Prgm
PO Box 8015
Waterloo, IA 50704
Prgm Dir: Joyce Timson, MT(ASCP)
Tel: 319 296-2320   *Fax:* 319 296-2874
Med Dir: Alan K Brown, MD
Class Cap: 18   *Begins:* Aug
Length: 22 mos   *Award:* AAS
Tuition per yr: $2,465 res, $4,930 non-res
Evening or weekend classes available

Kansas

Barton County Community College

Clin Lab Tech/Med Lab Tech-AD Prgm
Barton County Community College
RR 3 Box 136Z
Great Bend, KS 67530-9283
Prgm Dir: Leonard Bunselmeyer, MS MT(ASCP)
Tel: 316 792-2701   *Fax:* 316 792-3056
E-mail: bunselmeyer1@cougar.barton.cc.ks.us
Med Dir: Edward L Jones, MD
Class Cap: 18   *Begins:* Aug
Length: 24 mos   *Award:* Dipl, AAS
Tuition per yr: $1,554 res, $3,654 non-res
Evening or weekend classes available

Seward County Community College

Clin Lab Tech/Med Lab Tech-AD Prgm
PO Box 1137
Liberal, KS 67901
Prgm Dir: Suzanne Campbell, BS MT(ASCP)
Tel: 316 626-3077   *Fax:* 316 626-3026
E-mail: scampbel.sccc.sccc.cc.ks.us
Med Dir: Hubert C Peterson, MD
Class Cap: 11   *Begins:* Aug
Length: 24 mos   *Award:* Dipl, AAS
Tuition per yr: $1,782 res, $3,300 non-res
Evening or weekend classes available

Kentucky

Hazard Community College

Clin Lab Tech/Med Lab Tech-AD Prgm
One Community College Dr
Hwy 15 S
Hazard, KY 41701-2402
Prgm Dir: Deborah N Campbell, MHS BS MT(ASCP)
Tel: 606 436-5721   *Fax:* 606 439-1600
E-mail: dsulli01@ukcc.ury.edu
Med Dir: Rejeana K Mullins, MD
Class Cap: 15   *Begins:* Aug
Length: 24 mos   *Award:* Dipl, AAS
Tuition per yr: $980 res, $2,940 non-res
Evening or weekend classes available

Henderson Community College

Clin Lab Tech/Med Lab Tech-AD Prgm
2660 S Green St
Henderson, KY 42420
Prgm Dir: Randa Hawa, MT(ASCP) MS
Tel: 502 830-5318   *Fax:* 502 826-8391
Med Dir: Cathy L Freeman, MD
Class Cap: 14   *Begins:* Aug
Length: 22 mos   *Award:* AAS
Tuition per yr: $1,000 res, $1,000 non-res
Evening or weekend classes available

Eastern Kentucky University

Clin Lab Tech/Med Lab Tech-AD Prgm
Dizney 220
Richmond, KY 40475-3135
Prgm Dir: David C Hufford, PhD MT(ASCP)
Tel: 606 622-3078   *Fax:* 606 622-1140
E-mail: clshuffo@acs.eku.edu
Med Dir: Irene Roeckel, MD
Class Cap: 36   *Begins:* Aug Jan
Length: 22 mos   *Award:* Dipl, AS
Tuition per yr: $1,970 res, $5,450 non-res

Somerset Community College

Clin Lab Tech/Med Lab Tech-AD Prgm
Monticello Rd
Somerset, KY 42501
Prgm Dir: Nancy W Powell, MAEd MT(ASCP)
Tel: 606 679-8501   *Fax:* 606 679-5139
E-mail: nwpowel@ukcc.uky.edu
Med Dir: Marilyn McMillen, MD
Class Cap: 14   *Begins:* Aug
Length: 21 mos   *Award:* Dipl, AAS
Tuition per yr: $1,356 res, $3,818 non-res

Programs

Louisiana

Delgado Community College
Clin Lab Tech/Med Lab Tech-AD Prgm
501 City Park Ave
New Orleans, LA 70119
Prgm Dir: Sheila M Hickman, MEd
  MT(ASCP)SBB
Tel: 504 483-4198 *Fax:* 504 483-4609
Med Dir: Fred Brazda, MD
Class Cap: 12 *Begins:* Jan
Length: 24 mos *Award:* AS
Tuition per yr: $558 res, $1,428 non-res
Evening or weekend classes available

Southern Univ at Shreveport - Bossier City
Clin Lab Tech/Med Lab Tech-AD Prgm
3050 Martin Luther King Jr Dr
Shreveport, LA 71107
Prgm Dir: Regina S Robinson, MT(ASCP)
Tel: 318 674-3400
Med Dir: Warren D Grafton, MD
Class Cap: 15 *Begins:* Sep
Length: 24 mos *Award:* AS
Tuition per yr: $1,110 res, $2,240 non-res
Evening or weekend classes available

Maine

University of Maine at Augusta
Clin Lab Tech/Med Lab Tech-AD Prgm
46 University Dr
Augusta, ME 04330
Prgm Dir: Margaret Charette, MEd MT(ASCP)SC
Tel: 207 626-1407 *Fax:* 207 626-1143
Med Dir: James S Sweeney, MD
Class Cap: 10 *Begins:* Sep
Length: 21 mos *Award:* AS
Tuition per yr: $2,556 res, $6,228 non-res

Eastern Maine Technical College
Clin Lab Tech/Med Lab Tech-AD Prgm
354 Hogan Rd
Bangor, ME 04401
Prgm Dir: Anne D Merkel, MT(ASCP) MEd
Tel: 207 941-4645
Med Dir: John Chowning, MD
Class Cap: 12 *Begins:* Aug Jan
Length: 21 mos, 30 mos *Award:* AAS
Tuition per yr: $2,688 res, $5,922 non-res

University of Maine at Presque Isle
Clin Lab Tech/Med Lab Tech-AD Prgm
181 Main-317 South Hall
Presque Isle, ME 04769
Prgm Dir: Linda Graves, EdD MT(ASCP)
Tel: 207 768-9451 *Fax:* 207 768-9553
E-mail: graves@polaris.umpi.maine.edu
Med Dir: John Tewksbury, MD
Class Cap: 15 *Begins:* Sep
Length: 20 mos *Award:* Dipl, AS
Tuition per yr: $2,820 res, $6,870 non-res

Maryland

Essex Community College
Clin Lab Tech/Med Lab Tech-AD Prgm
7201 Rossville Blvd
Baltimore, MD 21237-3899
Prgm Dir: Lois Simmons, BS MT(ASCP)SH
Tel: 410 780-6406
Med Dir: Sandra L Butchart, MD
Class Cap: 20 *Begins:* Sep
Length: 18 mos, 24 mos *Award:* AAS
Tuition per yr: $2,580 res, $4,558 non-res

Allegany College of Maryland
Clin Lab Tech/Med Lab Tech-AD Prgm
12401 Willowbrook Rd SE
Cumberland, MD 21502-2596
Prgm Dir: Mary H Saunders, MEd MT(ASCP)
Tel: 301 724-7700 *Fax:* 301 777-8574
E-mail: molly@ac.cc.md.us
Med Dir: Giovanni Mastrangelo, MD
Class Cap: 18 *Begins:* Aug Sept
Length: 20 mos *Award:* AAS
Tuition per yr: $2,409 res, $3,069 non-res
Evening or weekend classes available

Villa Julie College
Clin Lab Tech/Med Lab Tech-AD Prgm
Green Spring Valley Rd
Stevenson, MD 21153
Prgm Dir: Vivi-Anne W Griffey, MS MT(ASCP)
Tel: 410 486-7000 *Fax:* 410 486-3552
E-mail: fac-grif@mail.vjc.edu
Med Dir: Alfred Paul Sanfilippo, MD PhD
Class Cap: 12 *Begins:* Sep
Length: 19 mos *Award:* AAS
Tuition per yr: $8,510
Evening or weekend classes available

Columbia Union College
Clin Lab Tech/Med Lab Tech-AD Prgm
7600 Flower Ave
Takoma Park, MD 20912
Prgm Dir: Juanita L Gurubatham, MA
  MT(ASCP)HT
Tel: 301 891-4184 *Fax:* 301 891-4191
E-mail: juanitag@cuc.edu
Med Dir: J D Mashburn, MD
Class Cap: 15 *Begins:* Sep
Length: 22 mos *Award:* AAS
Tuition per yr: $10,940

Massachusetts

Middlesex Community College - Bedford
Clin Lab Tech/Med Lab Tech-AD Prgm
Springs Rd
Bedford, MA 01730
Prgm Dir: Kenneth B Crowley Jr, MA MT(ASCP)
Tel: 617 280-3821 *Fax:* 617 275-2254
E-mail: crowleyK@admin.mcc.mass.edu
Med Dir: Constantine A Poppes, MD
Class Cap: 16 *Begins:* Sep Jan
Length: 18 mos *Award:* AAS
Tuition per yr: $3,630 res, $4,000 non-res
Evening or weekend classes available

Northeastern University
Clin Lab Tech/Med Lab Tech-AD Prgm
360 Huntington Ave
Boston, MA 02115
Prgm Dir: Barbara E Martin, MHP MT(ASCP)CLS
Tel: 617 373-3664 *Fax:* 617 373-3030
Med Dir: Jon Keller, MD
Class Cap: 20 *Begins:* Sep
Length: 36 mos *Award:* AS
Tuition per yr: $15,045

Massasoit Community College
Clin Lab Tech/Med Lab Tech-AD Prgm
Blue Hills Campus
900 Randolph St
Canton, MA 02021-1399
Prgm Dir: M Marie Waite, BS MT(ASCP)
Tel: 617 821-2222 *Fax:* 617 575-9428
Med Dir: Jon L Keller, MD
Class Cap: 30 *Begins:* Sep
Length: 16 mos *Award:* AAS
Tuition per yr: $2,923 res, $9,213 non-res

Bristol Community College
Clin Lab Tech/Med Lab Tech-AD Prgm
777 Elsbree St
Fall River, MA 02720
Prgm Dir: Sandra G Campos, MS CLS
Tel: 508 678-2811 *Fax:* 508 676-7146
E-mail: scampos@bristol.mass.educ
Med Dir: Gordon B Robbins, MD
Class Cap: 17 *Begins:* Sep Jan
Length: 18 mos *Award:* AS
Tuition per yr: $2,870 res, $8,050 non-res
Evening or weekend classes available

Mt Wachusett Community College
Clin Lab Tech/Med Lab Tech-AD Prgm
444 Green St
Gardner, MA 01440
Prgm Dir: Christine Kisiel, MA MT(ASCP)
Tel: 508 632-6600 *Fax:* 508 632-6155
Med Dir: Dieter H Keller, MD
Class Cap: 20 *Begins:* Sep
Length: 19 mos *Award:* AS
Tuition per yr: $1,400 res, $6,880 non-res
Evening or weekend classes available

Springfield Technical Community College
Clin Lab Tech/Med Lab Tech-AD Prgm
One Armory Square
Springfield, MA 01105-1204
Prgm Dir: Joanne U Cerrato, MA MT(ASCP)
Tel: 413 781-7822 *Fax:* 413 781-5805
Med Dir: John Sullivan, MD
Class Cap: 24 *Begins:* Sep
Length: 24 mos *Award:* AS
Tuition per yr: $1,681 res, $6,861 non-res
Evening or weekend classes available

Michigan

Kellogg Community College
Clin Lab Tech/Med Lab Tech-AD Prgm
450 North Ave
Battle Creek, MI 49016
Prgm Dir: Kathleen T Paff, MT(ASCP)
Tel: 616 965-3931
Med Dir: Jon L Neumann, MD
Class Cap: 16 *Begins:* Aug
Length: 20 mos *Award:* Dipl, AAS
Tuition per yr: $1,610 res, $2,604 non-res

Ferris State University

Clin Lab Tech/Med Lab Tech-AD Prgm
200 Ferris Dr
VFS 404
Big Rapids, MI 49307-2740
Prgm Dir: Janice M Webster, PhD MT(ASCP)
Tel: 616 592-2314   *Fax:* 616 592-3788
E-mail: ye58@music.ferris.edu
Med Dir: Nicholas J Hruby, MD
Class Cap: 25   *Begins:* Aug
Length: 21 mos   *Award:* AAS
Tuition per yr: $3,630 res, $7,364 non-res

Northern Michigan University

Clin Lab Tech/Med Lab Tech-AD Prgm
201 Magers Hall
Marquette, MI 49855
Prgm Dir: Lucille A Contois, MA MT(ASCP)
Tel: 906 227-1660   *Fax:* 906 227-1658
E-mail: lcontois@nmu.edu
Med Dir: John D Weiss, MD
Begins: Sep Jan
Length: 18 mos   *Award:* AAS
Tuition per yr: $2,952 res, $5,459 non-res

Baker College of Owosso

Clin Lab Tech/Med Lab Tech-AD Prgm
1020 S Washington St
Owosso, MI 48867
Prgm Dir: Diane Nelson, MA MT(ASCP)SH
Tel: 517 723-5251   *Fax:* 517 723-3355
Med Dir: Christopher Wiseman, MD
Begins: Sep
Length: 22 mos   *Award:* AS
Tuition per yr: $8,160 res, $8,160 non-res
Evening or weekend classes available

Minnesota

Alexandria Technical College

Clin Lab Tech/Med Lab Tech-AD Prgm
1601 Jefferson St
Alexandria, MN 56308
Prgm Dir: Judith A Hoffman, MS MT(ASCP)
Tel: 320 762-0221   *Fax:* 320 762-4501
E-mail: judyh@alx.tec.mn.us
Med Dir: Susan S Robey-Caffert, MD
Class Cap: 24   *Begins:* Sep
Length: 18 mos   *Award:* AAS
Tuition per yr: $2,760 res, $5,520 non-res

Medical Institute of Minnesota

Clin Lab Tech/Med Lab Tech-AD Prgm
5503 Green Valley Dr
Bloomington, MN 55437
Prgm Dir: Anna Franklin, MT(ASCP)
Tel: 612 844-0064   *Fax:* 612 844-0671
Med Dir: George Cembrowski, MD
Class Cap: 12   *Begins:* Oct Jan Apr Jul
Length: 20 mos   *Award:* AS
Tuition per yr: $7,275
Evening or weekend classes available

North Hennepin Community College

Clin Lab Tech/Med Lab Tech-AD Prgm
7411 85th Ave N
Brooklyn Park, MN 55445
Prgm Dir: Jane A Reinke, MS MT(ASCP)SH
Tel: 612 863-4674   *Fax:* 612 863-3089
E-mail: jreinke@nh.cc.mn.us
Med Dir: Cynthia J Lais, MD
Class Cap: 20   *Begins:* Sep
Length: 21 mos   *Award:* AS
Tuition per yr: $2,629 res, $5,085 non-res

Lake Superior College

Clin Lab Tech/Med Lab Tech-AD Prgm
2101 Trinity Rd
Duluth, MN 55811
Prgm Dir: JoAnn Wallgren, MA MT(ASCP)
Tel: 218 722-2801, Ext 329   *Fax:* 218 722-2899
Med Dir: Geoffrey A Witrak, MD
Class Cap: 25   *Begins:* Sep
Length: 20 mos   *Award:* AAS
Tuition per yr: $2,405 res, $4,875 non-res
Evening or weekend classes available

Northwest Technical Coll - E Grand Forks

Clin Lab Tech/Med Lab Tech-AD Prgm
2022 Central Ave NE
East Grand Forks, MN 56721
Prgm Dir: Gayle Melberg, MS MT(ASCP)
Tel: 218 773-3441
Med Dir: Albert Marvin Cooley, MD
Begins: Sep Dec Mar Jun
Length: 21 mos   *Award:* AD
Tuition per yr: $2,310 res, $2,310 non-res
Evening or weekend classes available

Minnesota Riverland Tech Coll-Faribault

Clin Lab Tech/Med Lab Tech-AD Prgm
1225 Third St SW
Faribault, MN 55021
Prgm Dir: Marlene J Vogelsang, BS MT(ASCP)
Tel: 507 334-3965   *Fax:* 507 332-5888
E-mail: mvogelsa@rtc.tec.mn.us
Med Dir: Dean T Clarke, MD
Class Cap: 16   *Begins:* Sep
Length: 22 mos   *Award:* AAS
Tuition per yr: $2,481 res, $4,961 non-res
Evening or weekend classes available

Fergus Falls Community College

Clin Lab Tech/Med Lab Tech-AD Prgm
1414 College Way
Fergus Falls, MN 56537
Prgm Dir: Eunice MacFarlane, MS MT(ASCP)
Tel: 218 739-7529   *Fax:* 218 739-7475
Med Dir: Gregory M Smith, MD
Class Cap: 15   *Begins:* Sep
Length: 18 mos   *Award:* AS
Tuition per yr: $2,800 res, $5,600 non-res
Evening or weekend classes available

Hibbing Community College

Clin Lab Tech/Med Lab Tech-AD Prgm
2900 E Beltline
Hibbing, MN 55746
Prgm Dir: Patricia Hinds
Tel: 218 262-7254   *Fax:* 218 262-7288
Med Dir: Tom Uncini, MD
Class Cap: 24   *Begins:* Sep
Length: 21 mos   *Award:* AAS
Tuition per yr: $2,390 res, $4,780 non-res

Lakeland Medical Dental Academy

Clin Lab Tech/Med Lab Tech-AD Prgm
1402 W Lake St
Minneapolis, MN 55408-2640
Prgm Dir: Lorrie Laurin, BA MT(ASCP)
Tel: 612 827-5656   *Fax:* 612 827-3833
Med Dir: Sherief A Mikhail, MD
Class Cap: 24   *Begins:* Mar Sep Jun Jan
Length: 24 mos   *Award:* AAS
Tuition per yr: $6,525 res, $6,525 non-res

St Paul Technical College

Clin Lab Tech/Med Lab Tech-AD Prgm
235 Marshall Ave
St Paul, MN 55102
Prgm Dir: Gladys E Westin, MT(ASCP) CLS
Tel: 612 221-1421   *Fax:* 612 221-1416
Med Dir: Virginia Dale, MD
Class Cap: 50   *Begins:* Sep
Length: 20 mos   *Award:* AAS
Tuition per yr: $2,740 res, $5,480 non-res
Evening or weekend classes available

Mississippi

Northeast Mississippi Community College

Clin Lab Tech/Med Lab Tech-AD Prgm
Cunningham Blvd
Booneville, MS 38829
Prgm Dir: Rilla K Jones, MT(ASCP) SM
Tel: 601 720-7388   *Fax:* 601 728-1165
Med Dir: Michael Todd, MD
Class Cap: 14   *Begins:* Aug
Length: 22 mos   *Award:* AD
Tuition per yr: $950 res, $2,050 non-res
Evening or weekend classes available

Mississippi Gulf Coast Community College

Clin Lab Tech/Med Lab Tech-AD Prgm
2300 Hwy 90 PO Box 100
Gautier, MS 39553
Prgm Dir: Gretahew Cunningham, MS MT(ASCP)
Tel: 601 497-9602   *Fax:* 601 497-7670
Med Dir: Lyman J Scripter
Begins: Aug Jan
Length: 24 mos   *Award:* Dipl, AAS
Tuition per yr: $1,335 res, $3,204 non-res
Evening or weekend classes available

Pearl River Community College

Clin Lab Tech/Med Lab Tech-AD Prgm
5448 US Hwy 49 S
Hattiesburg, MS 39401
Prgm Dir: Evelgn H Wallace, BA BS MT(ASCP)
Tel: 601 544-7722, Ext 123
Med Dir: James E Williams III, MD
Class Cap: 20   *Begins:* Aug
Length: 24 mos   *Award:* Dipl, AS
Tuition per yr: $425
Evening or weekend classes available

Hinds Community College District
Clin Lab Tech/Med Lab Tech-AD Prgm
Nursing/Allied Hlth Ctr
1750 Chadwick Dr
Jackson, MS 39204-3402
Prgm Dir: Nina Kerstine, MHS MT(ASCP)
Tel: 601 371-3515   *Fax:* 601 371-3529
Med Dir: Barbara Proctor, MD
Class Cap: 15   *Begins:* Aug Jan
Length: 24 mos   *Award:* AAS
Tuition per yr: $1,120
Evening or weekend classes available

Meridian Community College
Clin Lab Tech/Med Lab Tech-AD Prgm
910 Hwy 19 N
Meridian, MS 39307
Prgm Dir: Knox Poole, MA MT(ASCP)
Tel: 601 483-8241   *Fax:* 601 482-3936
Med Dir: Arthur Martin, MD
Class Cap: 16   *Begins:* Aug
Length: 24 mos   *Award:* AA
Tuition per yr: $1,440 res, $1,440 non-res
Evening or weekend classes available

Mississippi Delta Community College
Clin Lab Tech/Med Lab Tech-AD Prgm
PO Box 668
Moorhead, MS 38761
Prgm Dir: Jackie Brocato, MT(ASCP)SH
Tel: 601 246-6500   *Fax:* 601 246-6517
Med Dir: Donald Pierce, MD
Class Cap: 13   *Begins:* May
Length: 24 mos   *Award:* AAS
Tuition per yr: $11 res, $1,220 non-res
Evening or weekend classes available

Copiah - Lincoln Community College
Clin Lab Tech/Med Lab Tech-AD Prgm
PO Box 457
Wesson, MS 39191-0457
Prgm Dir: Mary E Shivers, MT(ASCP)
Tel: 601 643-5101   *Fax:* 601 446-1298
Med Dir: Robert B Britt, MD
Class Cap: 9   *Begins:* Aug Jan
Length: 24 mos   *Award:* AAS
Tuition per yr: $1,370 res, $1,970 non-res
Evening or weekend classes available

Missouri

Three Rivers Community College
Clin Lab Tech/Med Lab Tech-AD Prgm
2080 Three Rivers Blvd
Poplar Bluff, MO 63901
Prgm Dir: Denise Eubanks, MT(ASCP)
Tel: 314 840-9677
Med Dir: Robert J Cacchione, MD
Class Cap: 32   *Begins:* Aug
Length: 22 mos   *Award:* AAS
Tuition per yr: $1,598 res, $2,209 non-res

St Louis Comm College at Forest Park
Clin Lab Tech/Med Lab Tech-AD Prgm
5600 Oakland Ave
St Louis, MO 63110
Prgm Dir: Mary Ann Honti, MT(ASCP)
Tel: 314 644-9343   *Fax:* 314 644-9752
Med Dir: Gordon L Johnson, MD
Class Cap: 35   *Begins:* Aug
Length: 20 mos   *Award:* Dipl, AAS
Tuition per yr: $1,890 res, $2,385 non-res
Evening or weekend classes available

Nebraska

Southeast Community College
Clin Lab Tech/Med Lab Tech-AD Prgm
8800 O St
Lincoln, NE 68520
Prgm Dir: Janis K Bible, MT(ASCP)
Tel: 402 437-2760   *Fax:* 402 437-2404
Med Dir: George E Gammel, MD
Class Cap: 20   *Begins:* Jul
Length: 24 mos   *Award:* AAS
Tuition per yr: $1,773 res, $2,120 non-res
Evening or weekend classes available

Mid Plains Community College
Clin Lab Tech/Med Lab Tech-AD Prgm
601 W State Farm Rd
North Platte, NE 69101
Prgm Dir: Janice A Schulte, MT(ASCP)
Tel: 308 532-8980   *Fax:* 308 532-8980
Med Dir: Byron Barksdale, MD
Class Cap: 20   *Begins:* Aug
Length: 24 mos   *Award:* AA, AAS
Tuition per yr: $1,232 res, $1,430 non-res
Evening or weekend classes available

Nevada

Community College of Southern Nevada
Clin Lab Tech/Med Lab Tech-AD Prgm
6375 W Charleston Blvd
Las Vegas, NV 89102
Prgm Dir: Beth Pitonzo, PhD MT(ASCP)
CLS(NCA)
Tel: 702 651-5695   *Fax:* 702 651-5641
Med Dir: Robert Cranley, MD
Class Cap: 18   *Begins:* Sep
Length: 24 mos   *Award:* AAS
Tuition per yr: $1,132 res, $1,612 non-res
Evening or weekend classes available

New Hampshire

New Hampshire Community Technical College
Clin Lab Tech/Med Lab Tech-AD Prgm
Claremont, NH 03743
Prgm Dir: Andrea Gordon, MEd MT(ASCP)SH
Tel: 603 542-7744   *Fax:* 603 543-1844
E-mail: a_gordon@tec.nh.us
Med Dir: Charles C Cunningham, MD
Class Cap: 12   *Begins:* Aug
Length: 20 mos   *Award:* AAS
Tuition per yr: $4,100 res, $5,849 non-res
Evening or weekend classes available

New Jersey

Camden County College
Clin Lab Tech/Med Lab Tech-AD Prgm
PO Box 200
Blackwood, NJ 08012
Prgm Dir: Diane G Goldberg, MT(ASCP)
Tel: 609 227-7200   *Fax:* 609 374-4890
Med Dir: William Harrer, MD
Class Cap: 20   *Begins:* Sep
Length: 24 mos   *Award:* AAS
Tuition per yr: $2,293 res, $2,365 non-res
Evening or weekend classes available

Middlesex County College
Clin Lab Tech/Med Lab Tech-AD Prgm
155 Mill Rd
Edison, NJ 08818-3050
Prgm Dir: Stephen P Larkin III, MT(ASCP)SH
Tel: 908 906-2581
Med Dir: Henry G Schriever, MD
Class Cap: 38   *Begins:* Sep
Length: 21 mos   *Award:* Dipl, AAS
Tuition per yr: $1,800 res, $3,600 non-res
Evening or weekend classes available

Brookdale Community College
Clin Lab Tech/Med Lab Tech-AD Prgm
765 Newman Springs Rd
Lincroft, NJ 07738-1522
Prgm Dir: Andrew L Bryant, MS MT(ASCP)
Tel: 908 224-2853   *Fax:* 908 224-2772
Med Dir: Edwin Charles Leschhorn, MD
Class Cap: 12   *Begins:* Sep
Length: 20 mos   *Award:* AAS
Tuition per yr: $1,000 res, $2,000 non-res

Felician College
Clin Lab Tech/Med Lab Tech-AD Prgm
262 S Main St
Lodi, NJ 07644
Prgm Dir: Marilyn R Rubin, EdM MLT(ASCP)
Tel: 201 778-1190, Ext 6025   *Fax:* 201 778-4111
Med Dir: Arthur Christiano, MD
Class Cap: 18   *Begins:* Sep
Length: 20 mos   *Award:* Dipl, AAS
Tuition per yr: $12,000
Evening or weekend classes available

Atlantic Community College
Clin Lab Tech/Med Lab Tech-AD Prgm
Allied Health Division
5100 Black Horse Pike
Mays Landing, NJ 08330
Prgm Dir: Joseph Cofrancesco, MT(ASCP)
Tel: 609 343-5049   *Fax:* 609 343-4917
E-mail: lofaance@nsvm.atlantic.edu
Med Dir: Henry Seidel, MD
Begins: Sep
Length: 20 mos   *Award:* AAS
Tuition per yr: $1,584 res, $2,484 non-res
Evening or weekend classes available

Bergen Community College

Clin Lab Tech/Med Lab Tech-AD Prgm
400 Paramus Rd
Paramus, NJ 07652-1595
Prgm Dir: John F Lo Russo, MA MT(ASCP)
Tel: 201 447-7178 *Fax:* 201 612-8225
Med Dir: Rosalyn A Stahl, MD
Class Cap: 20 *Begins:* Sep
Length: 22 mos *Award:* AAS
Tuition per yr: $2,908 res, $5,816 non-res
Evening or weekend classes available

County College of Morris

Clin Lab Tech/Med Lab Tech-AD Prgm
Rte 10 and Ctr Grove Rd
Randolph, NJ 07869
Prgm Dir: Rita Alisauskas, PhD MT(ASCP)
Tel: 201 328-5370 *Fax:* 201 328-5379
E-mail: ralisauskas@ccm.edu
Med Dir: Mohammed Khan, MD
Class Cap: 20 *Begins:* Sep
Length: 23 mos *Award:* AAS
Tuition per yr: $1,386 res, $2,425 non-res
Evening or weekend classes available

Univ of Med & Dent of New Jersey

Clin Lab Tech/Med Lab Tech-AD Prgm
1776 Raritan Rd
Scotch Plains, NJ 07076
Prgm Dir: H Jesse Guiles, EdD MT(ASCP)
Tel: 201 982-5453 *Fax:* 908 889-2487
E-mail: guiles@umdnj.edu
Med Dir: Neena M Mirani, MD
Class Cap: 20 *Begins:* Sep
Length: 18 mos *Award:* AAS
Tuition per yr: $1,508 res, $3,016 non-res
Evening or weekend classes available

Mercer County Community College

Clin Lab Tech/Med Lab Tech-AD Prgm
1200 Old Trenton Rd
PO Box B
Trenton, NJ 08690
Prgm Dir: Jane O'Reilly, MEd MT(ASCP)
Tel: 609 586-4800 *Fax:* 609 586-2318
Med Dir: Todd Kolb, MD
Class Cap: 15 *Begins:* Aug
Length: 22 mos *Award:* Dipl, AAS
Tuition per yr: $2,571 res, $3,747 non-res
Evening or weekend classes available

New Mexico

New Mexico State U at Alamogordo

Clin Lab Tech/Med Lab Tech-AD Prgm
PO Box 477
Alamogordo, NM 88310
Prgm Dir: Jeanette H Ashwood, EdD MT(ASCP)
Tel: 505 439-3640 *Fax:* 505 439-3643
E-mail: ashwood@nmsua.nmsu.edu
Med Dir: William Gordon McGee, MD
Class Cap: 10 *Begins:* Aug
Length: 20 mos *Award:* AAS
Tuition per yr: $1,024 res, $2,288 non-res
Evening or weekend classes available

Albuquerque Tech Voc Institute

Clin Lab Tech/Med Lab Tech-AD Prgm
525 Buena Vista SE
Albuquerque, NM 87106
Prgm Dir: Monya Kmetz, MA MT(ASCP)
Tel: 505 224-4132 *Fax:* 505 224-4120
E-mail: monya@tvi.cc.nm.us
Med Dir: Mary Lipscomb, MD
Class Cap: 18 *Begins:* Jan
Length: 20 mos *Award:* AS
Tuition per yr: $773 res, $2,038 non-res
Evening or weekend classes available

Pima Medical Institute - Albuquerque

Clin Lab Tech/Med Lab Tech-AD Prgm
2201 San Pedro NE/Bldg 3
Albuquerque, NM 87110
Prgm Dir: Clare McCollough, MT(ASCP)
Tel: 505 881-1234 *Fax:* 505 884-8371
Med Dir: Scott Otteson, MD
Class Cap: 12 *Begins:* Varies
Length: 22 mos *Award:* AS
Tuition per yr: $6,684 res, $6,684 non-res

University of New Mexico - Gallup/IHS

Clin Lab Tech/Med Lab Tech-AD Prgm
Gallup Indian Med Ctr
200 College Rd
Gallup, NM 87301
Prgm Dir: Harry D Sheski, MA MT(ASCP)
Tel: 505 722-1721 *Fax:* 505 863-7513
E-mail: harrys@cigg.com
Med Dir: Wayne William Charland, MD
Class Cap: 10 *Begins:* Aug Jan
Length: 22 mos *Award:* AS
Tuition per yr: $720 res, $1,608 non-res
Evening or weekend classes available

New Mexico Junior College

Clin Lab Tech/Med Lab Tech-AD Prgm
5317 Lovington Hwy
Hobbs, NM 88240
Prgm Dir: Brenda Pierce, MT(ASCP)
Tel: 505 392-5304 *Fax:* 505 392-2527
E-mail: bpierce@nmjc.cc.nm.us
Med Dir: H V Beighley, MD
Class Cap: 20 *Begins:* Jul
Length: 24 mos *Award:* AAS
Tuition per yr: $500 res, $1,080 non-res
Evening or weekend classes available

New York

SUNY College of Technology at Alfred St

Clin Lab Tech/Med Lab Tech-AD Prgm
Alfred State College
Allied Hlth Bldg - Rm 206
Alfred, NY 14802
Prgm Dir: Victoria Bolton, MT(ASCP) MEd
Tel: 607 587-3617 *Fax:* 607 587-3684
E-mail: boltonvl@alfredtech.edu
Med Dir: Theodor K Mayer, MD PhD
Class Cap: 30 *Begins:* Aug
Length: 18 mos *Award:* AAS
Tuition per yr: $3,200 res, $8,300 non-res

Broome Community College

Clin Lab Tech/Med Lab Tech-AD Prgm
PO Box 1017
Binghamton, NY 13902
Prgm Dir: Julia E Peacock, MS M(ASCP)SI
Tel: 607 778-5211 *Fax:* 607 778-5345
E-mail: peacock-j@sunybroome.edu
Med Dir: Loren Wolsh, MD
Class Cap: 30 *Begins:* Aug Jan
Length: 22 mos *Award:* AAS
Tuition per yr: $2,168 res, $4,336 non-res
Evening or weekend classes available

CUNY New York City Technical College

Clin Lab Tech/Med Lab Tech-AD Prgm
300 Jay St
Brooklyn, NY 11201
Prgm Dir: Charles E Lavender, MS MT(ASCP)
Tel: 718 260-5671
Med Dir: Medghi Veseghi, MD
Begins: Sep Jan
Length: 24 mos *Award:* AAS
Tuition per yr: $725 res, $2,025 non-res

Trocaire College

Clin Lab Tech/Med Lab Tech-AD Prgm
110 Red Jacket Pkwy
Buffalo, NY 14220
Prgm Dir: Perka Kresic, MS MT(ASCP)CLS
Tel: 716 826-1200 *Fax:* 716 826-0059
Med Dir: David Scamurra, MD
Class Cap: 20 *Begins:* Aug
Length: 18 mos *Award:* AAS
Tuition per yr: $5,850

SUNY College of Technology at Canton

Clin Lab Tech/Med Lab Tech-AD Prgm
Cornell Dr
Canton, NY 13617
Prgm Dir: Linda D Pellett, MEd MT(ASCP)
Tel: 330 386-7400 *Fax:* 330 386-7959
E-mail: pellet@scnva.canto.edu
Med Dir: Phillip Bridgman
Class Cap: 20 *Begins:* Aug
Length: 18 mos *Award:* AAS
Tuition per yr: $3,200 res, $8,300 non-res

Programs

SUNY at Farmingdale
Clin Lab Tech/Med Lab Tech-AD Prgm
Rte 110/Gleeson Hall/Rm 304
Farmingdale, NY 11735
Prgm Dir: Karen M Escolas, MS MT (ASCP)
Tel: 516 420-2171 *Fax:* 516 420-2784
E-mail: escolakm@sunyfarva.cc.farmin6dale.edu
Med Dir: Paterno A Remigio, MD
Class Cap: 40 *Begins:* Sep
Length: 23 mos *Award:* AS
Tuition per yr: $3,200 res, $8,300 non-res
Evening or weekend classes available

Orange County Community College
Clin Lab Tech/Med Lab Tech-AD Prgm
115 South St
Middletown, NY 10940
Prgm Dir: Helen R Sherman, MS CLS(NCA)
Tel: 914 341-4273 *Fax:* 914 343-1228
E-mail: hsherman@mail.sunyorange.edu
Med Dir: Joseph B Naplitano, MD
Class Cap: 25 *Begins:* Sep
Length: 18 mos *Award:* AAS
Tuition per yr: $2,100 res, $4,200 non-res
Evening or weekend classes available

Clinton Community College
Clin Lab Tech/Med Lab Tech-AD Prgm
Lake Shore Rd Rt 9 S
136 Clinton Point Dr
Plattsburgh, NY 12901
Prgm Dir: Evelyn A Perry, MS MT(ASCP)
Tel: 518 562-4173 *Fax:* 518 561-8621
Med Dir: William J Strimel Jr, MD
Class Cap: 20 *Begins:* Sep
Length: 18 mos *Award:* AAS
Tuition per yr: $2,275 res, $4,550 non-res

Dutchess Community College
Clin Lab Tech/Med Lab Tech-AD Prgm
53 Pendell Rd
Poughkeepsie, NY 12601
Prgm Dir: Karen Ann Ingham, MT(ASCP)
Tel: 914 431-8321 *Fax:* 914 431-8991
E-mail: ingham@sunydutchess.edu
Med Dir: Neela Pushparaj, MD
Class Cap: 30 *Begins:* Sep
Length: 20 mos *Award:* AAS
Tuition per yr: $2,200 res, $2,200 non-res
Evening or weekend classes available

CUNY College of Staten Island
Clin Lab Tech/Med Lab Tech-AD Prgm
2800 Victory Blvd
Staten Island, NY 10314
Prgm Dir: Sharon D Bramson, PhD
Tel: 718 982-3690
Med Dir: Rudolph Howard, MD
Begins: Sep Feb Jun
Length: 24 mos *Award:* Dipl, AAS
Tuition per yr: $3,200 res, $6,800 non-res
Evening or weekend classes available

Hudson Valley Community College
Clin Lab Tech/Med Lab Tech-AD Prgm
80 Vanderburgh Ave
Troy, NY 12180
Prgm Dir: John M O'Leary, MS MT(ASCP)
Tel: 518 270-7407 *Fax:* 518 270-7594
E-mail: hylanpatelvcc.edu
Med Dir: An-Ya Wu, MD
Begins: Aug
Length: 18 mos *Award:* Dipl, AAS
Tuition per yr: $2,150 res, $5,000 non-res

Erie Community College - City Campus
Clin Lab Tech/Med Lab Tech-AD Prgm
6205 Main St
Williamsville, NY 14221-7095
Prgm Dir: Myrtle M Green, MS CMA MT(ASCP)
Tel: 716 851-1553
Med Dir: Adrian Vladutiu, MD PhD
Class Cap: 45 *Begins:* Sep
Length: 18 mos *Award:* AAS
Tuition per yr: $2,500 res, $5,000 non-res
Evening or weekend classes available

North Carolina

Asheville Buncombe Technical Comm Coll
Clin Lab Tech/Med Lab Tech-AD Prgm
340 Victoria Rd
Asheville, NC 28801
Prgm Dir: Laura S West, MT(ASCP)
Tel: 704 254-1921 *Fax:* 704 251-6355
Med Dir: Jane Lysko, MD
Class Cap: 16 *Begins:* Sep
Length: 21 mos *Award:* AAS
Tuition per yr: $770 res, $6,048 non-res

Alamance Community College
Clin Lab Tech/Med Lab Tech-AD Prgm
PO Box 8000
Graham, NC 27253-8000
Prgm Dir: Peggy Simpson, MT(ASCP)
Tel: 910 578-8727 *Fax:* 910 578-1987
Med Dir: Myra Lai-Goldman, MD
Class Cap: 40 *Begins:* Sep Mar
Length: 24 mos *Award:* AD
Tuition per yr: $742 res, $6,020 non-res
Evening or weekend classes available

Coastal Carolina Community College
Clin Lab Tech/Med Lab Tech-AD Prgm
444 Western Blvd
Jacksonville, NC 28546-6877
Prgm Dir: Christine N Weaver, MSAS MT(ASCP)
Tel: 910 938-6275 *Fax:* 910 455-7027
Med Dir: Charles L Garrett Jr, MD
Class Cap: 20 *Begins:* Sep
Length: 23 mos *Award:* AAS
Tuition per yr: $738 res, $5,828 non-res

Western Piedmont Community College
Clin Lab Tech/Med Lab Tech-AD Prgm
PO Box 680
Morganton, NC 28655-0680
Prgm Dir: Gary C Jennings, MS MT(ASCP)
Tel: 704 438-6126 *Fax:* 704 438-6015
Med Dir: James Parker, MD
Class Cap: 20 *Begins:* Sep
Length: 21 mos *Award:* AAS
Tuition per yr: $555 res, $4,515 non-res

Sandhills Community College
Clin Lab Tech/Med Lab Tech-AD Prgm
2200 Airport Rd
Pinehurst, NC 28374
Prgm Dir: D P Boswell, MA MT(ASCP)
Tel: 910 695-3839 *Fax:* 910 692-2756
Med Dir: James E Laningham, MD
Class Cap: 18 *Begins:* Sep
Length: 21 mos *Award:* AAS
Tuition per yr: $742 res, $6,020 non-res
Evening or weekend classes available

Wake Technical Community College
Clin Lab Tech/Med Lab Tech-AD Prgm
9101 Fayetteville Rd
Raleigh, NC 27603
Prgm Dir: Pamela Horton, BS MT(ASCP)
Tel: 919 231-4500 *Fax:* 919 779-3360
Med Dir: James R Edwards, MD
Class Cap: 24 *Begins:* Sep
Length: 21 mos *Award:* AS
Tuition per yr: $556 res, $4,515 non-res

Southwestern Community College
Clin Lab Tech/Med Lab Tech-AD Prgm
447 College Dr
PO Box 67
Sylva, NC 28779
Prgm Dir: Andrea Lambert, MT(ASCP)
Tel: 704 586-4091 *Fax:* 704 586-3129
Med Dir: Michael B Rohlfing, MD
Class Cap: 20 *Begins:* Sep
Length: 21 mos *Award:* AAS
Tuition per yr: $742 res, $6,020 non-res

Beaufort County Community College
Clin Lab Tech/Med Lab Tech-AD Prgm
PO Box 1069
Washington, NC 27889
Prgm Dir: Arthur S Keehnle, MS MT(ASCP)
Tel: 919 946-6194 *Fax:* 919 946-0271
Med Dir: Robert Hadley, MD
Class Cap: 13 *Begins:* Sep
Length: 21 mos *Award:* AD
Tuition per yr: $766 res, $6,044 non-res
Evening or weekend classes available

Halifax Community College
Clin Lab Tech/Med Lab Tech-AD Prgm
PO Box 809
Weldon, NC 27890
Prgm Dir: Sandra J Eisenmenger, MT(ASCP)
Tel: 919 536-2551 *Fax:* 919 536-4144
Med Dir: Gamlesh Gupta, MD
Class Cap: 10 *Begins:* Sep
Length: 21 mos *Award:* AAS
Tuition per yr: $742 res, $6,020 non-res
Evening or weekend classes available

North Dakota

Bismarck State College
Clin Lab Tech/Med Lab Tech-AD Prgm
1500 Edwards Ave
Bismarck, ND 58501
Prgm Dir: Mary Ann Durick, MS
Tel: 701 224-5469 *Fax:* 701 224-5550
E-mail: mdurick@badlands.nodak.edu
Med Dir: Dennis D Reinke, MD
Class Cap: 14 *Begins:* Aug
Length: 22 mos *Award:* AS
Tuition per yr: $1,809 res, $4,400 non-res

Ohio

Stark State College of Technology
Clin Lab Tech/Med Lab Tech-AD Prgm
6200 Frank Ave NW
Canton, OH 44720
Prgm Dir: Mel B Kallis, MT(ASCP)CLS
Tel: 330 494-6170 *Fax:* 330 966-6586
Med Dir: Artemio L Orlino, MD
Class Cap: 20 *Begins:* Aug
Length: 21 mos *Award:* Cert, AAS
Tuition per yr: $3,818 res, $4,933 non-res

Cincinnati State Tech and Comm College
Clin Lab Tech/Med Lab Tech-AD Prgm
3520 Central Pkwy
Cincinnati, OH 45223
Prgm Dir: Carolyn G Laemmle, EdD MT(ASCP)
Tel: 513 569-1689 *Fax:* 513 569-1659
Med Dir: Carl L Parrot, Jr, MD
Class Cap: 30 *Begins:* Sep
Length: 24 mos *Award:* Dipl, AAS
Tuition per yr: $4,000 res, $8,000 non-res
Evening or weekend classes available

Cuyahoga Community College
Clin Lab Tech/Med Lab Tech-AD Prgm
Metro Campus Sci & Tech 106
2900 Community College Ave
Cleveland, OH 44115-3196
Prgm Dir: Barbara Freeman, MT(ASCP)
Tel: 216 987-4438 *Fax:* 216 987-4438
Med Dir: Nancy S Rosenthal, MD
Begins: Sep
Length: 21 mos *Award:* Dipl, AAS
Tuition per yr: $1,326 res, $3,133 non-res
Evening or weekend classes available

Columbus State Community College
Clin Lab Tech/Med Lab Tech-AD Prgm
550 E Spring St
Columbus, OH 43215
Prgm Dir: Julie Dudas, MEd MT(ASCP)
Tel: 614 227-2518 *Fax:* 614 227-5144
E-mail: kkinzer%cscc@cougar.colstate.cc.oh.us
Med Dir: Rose Goodwin, MD
Class Cap: 20 *Begins:* Sep Mar
Length: 21 mos *Award:* Dipl, AAS
Tuition per yr: $2,736 res, $6,000 non-res

Lorain County Community College
Clin Lab Tech/Med Lab Tech-AD Prgm
1005 N Abbe Rd
Elyria, OH 44035
Prgm Dir: Roy B Anderson, MS MT(ASCP)
Tel: 216 365-4191 *Fax:* 216 366-4116
Med Dir: David A Dobrow, MD
Class Cap: 20 *Begins:* Sep
Length: 20 mos *Award:* AAS
Tuition per yr: $2,982 res, $3,582 non-res
Evening or weekend classes available

Lakeland Community College
Clin Lab Tech/Med Lab Tech-AD Prgm
7700 Clocktower Dr
Kirtland, OH 44094-5198
Prgm Dir: Donna C Pfeifer, MT(ASCP)SBB
Tel: 216 953-7257 *Fax:* 246 975-4733
Med Dir: Ronald Chapnick, MD
Class Cap: 24 *Begins:* Sep
Length: 22 mos *Award:* AAS
Tuition per yr: $2,711 res, $3,325 non-res
Evening or weekend classes available

Washington State Community College
Clin Lab Tech/Med Lab Tech-AD Prgm
710 Colegate Dr
Marietta, OH 45750
Prgm Dir: Dixie T Stone, PhD MT(ASCP)
Tel: 614 374-8716 *Fax:* 614 373-7496
Med Dir: F R Macatol, MD
Class Cap: 20 *Begins:* Sep
Length: 21 mos *Award:* Dipl, AAS
Tuition per yr: $2,900 res, $5,900 non-res
Evening or weekend classes available

Marion Technical College
Clin Lab Tech/Med Lab Tech-AD Prgm
1467 Mt Vernon Ave
Marion, OH 43302
Prgm Dir: Mary Ann Jenkins, MT(ASCP) CLS
Tel: 614 389-4636 *Fax:* 614 389-6136
Med Dir: Ted A Heckendorn, MD
Class Cap: 20 *Begins:* Sep
Length: 21 mos *Award:* AAS
Tuition per yr: $2,907 res, $5,253 non-res
Evening or weekend classes available

Shawnee State University
Clin Lab Tech/Med Lab Tech-AD Prgm
940 Second St
Portsmouth, OH 45662
Prgm Dir: Pamela J Staton, MS MT(ASCP)
Tel: 614 355-2250
E-mail: pstaton@shawnee.edu
Med Dir: Kathryn Skitarelic, MD
Class Cap: 21 *Begins:* Sep
Length: 21 mos *Award:* AAS
Tuition per yr: $3,968 res, $6,868 non-res
Evening or weekend classes available

University of Rio Grande
Clin Lab Tech/Med Lab Tech-AD Prgm
EE Davis Technical Career Ctr
Rio Grande, OH 45674
Prgm Dir: Russell F Cheadle, MS MT(ASCP)
Tel: 614 245-7319 *Fax:* 614 245-7440
E-mail: rcheadle@urgrgcc.edu
Med Dir: Frederic La Carbonara, MD
Class Cap: 20 *Begins:* Jun
Length: 24 mos, 36 mos *Award:* Dipl, AD
Tuition per yr: $3,119 res, $3,614 non-res
Evening or weekend classes available

Clark State Community College
Clin Lab Tech/Med Lab Tech-AD Prgm
570 E Leffel Ln
Springfield, OH 45505
Prgm Dir: Katherine D Kalinos, MA MT(ASCP)
Tel: 937 328-6112 *Fax:* 937 328-6138
Med Dir: G William Sickle, MD
Class Cap: 28 *Begins:* Sep
Length: 21 mos *Award:* Dipl, AD
Tuition per yr: $2,968 res, $2,968 non-res

Jefferson Community College
Clin Lab Tech/Med Lab Tech-AD Prgm
4000 Sunset Blvd
Steubenville, OH 43952
Prgm Dir: Barbara Smith, MEd MT(ASCP)
Tel: 614 264-5591
Med Dir: Chong Sook-Sohn, MD
Class Cap: 11 *Begins:* Aug
Length: 24 mos *Award:* AAS
Tuition per yr: $2,508 res, $2,728 non-res

Youngstown State University
Clin Lab Tech/Med Lab Tech-AD Prgm
Dept of Health Professions
1 University Plaza
Youngstown, OH 44555
Prgm Dir: Maria E Delost, MS MT(ASCP)
Tel: 330 742-1761 *Fax:* 330 742-2309
Med Dir: Norton German, MD
Class Cap: 20 *Begins:* Sep
Length: 24 mos *Award:* AAS
Tuition per yr: $4,488 res, $6,648 non-res
Evening or weekend classes available

Muskingum Area Technical College
Clin Lab Tech/Med Lab Tech-AD Prgm
1555 Newark Rd
Zanesville, OH 43701
Prgm Dir: Vicki Huntsman, BS MT(ASCP)
  CLS(NCA)
Tel: 614 454-2501, Ext 195 *Fax:* 614 454-0035
E-mail: vjhuntsman@sota-oh.com
Med Dir: Roger Little, MD
Class Cap: 24 *Begins:* Sep
Length: 23 mos *Award:* AAS
Tuition per yr: $2,577 res, $4,287 non-res
Evening or weekend classes available

Oklahoma

Northeastern Oklahoma A & M College
Clin Lab Tech/Med Lab Tech-AD Prgm
Second and I Sts NE
Miami, OK 74354
Prgm Dir: Rita Kay Harris, BA MT(ASCP)
Tel: 918 542-8441 *Fax:* 918 542-2680
Med Dir: Fred A Tweet, MD
Class Cap: 12 *Begins:* Aug
Length: 22 mos *Award:* Dipl,Cert, AD
Tuition per yr: $1,174 res, $3,252 non-res

Rose State College
Clin Lab Tech/Med Lab Tech-AD Prgm
6420 SE 15th St
Midwest City, OK 73110
Prgm Dir: Gail C Ingram, MT(ASCP)
Tel: 405 733-7577 *Fax:* 405 736-0338
Med Dir: Bill E Blevins, MD
Class Cap: 20 *Begins:* Aug
Length: 23 mos *Award:* AAS
Tuition per yr: $1,521 res, $3,861 non-res
Evening or weekend classes available

Seminole State College
Clin Lab Tech/Med Lab Tech-AD Prgm
PO Box 351
Seminole, OK 74818-0351
Prgm Dir: Perthena Latchaw, MS MT(ASCP)
Tel: 405 382-9950 *Fax:* 405 382-9950
E-mail: latchaw_p@ssc.cc.ok.us
Med Dir: Levi Jones, MD MT(ASCP)
Class Cap: 20 *Begins:* Aug
Length: 12 mos, 24 mos *Award:* AAS
Tuition per yr: $1,040 res, $2,700 non-res
Evening or weekend classes available

Programs

Tulsa Community College
Clin Lab Tech/Med Lab Tech-AD Prgm
909 S Boston Ave
Tulsa, OK 74119
Prgm Dir: Karen L Holmes, MA MT(ASCP)
Tel: 918 595-7008   *Fax:* 918 595-7298
E-mail: kholmes@tulsajc.tulsa.cc.ok.us
Med Dir: Melvin J VanBoven, DO
Class Cap: 16   *Begins:* Aug
Length: 24 mos   *Award:* Dipl, AA
Tuition per yr: $1,087 res, $3,033 non-res
Evening or weekend classes available

Oregon

Portland Community College
Clin Lab Tech/Med Lab Tech-AD Prgm
12000 SW 49th Ave
Portland, OR 97219
Prgm Dir: Terry L Emmons, MT(ASCP) CLS
Tel: 503 978-5671   *Fax:* 503 978-5257
E-mail: temmons@pcc.edu
Med Dir: Juan Millan, MD
Class Cap: 40   *Begins:* Sep
Length: 21 mos   *Award:* AAS
Tuition per yr: $1,610 res, $5,750 non-res
Evening or weekend classes available

Pennsylvania

Montgomery County Community College
Clin Lab Tech/Med Lab Tech-AD Prgm
340 DeKalb Pike
Blue Bell, PA 19422-1412
Prgm Dir: John C Flynn Jr, PhD MT(ASCP)SBB
Tel: 215 641-6486   *Fax:* 215 641-6434
Med Dir: Irwin J Hollander, MD
Class Cap: 20   *Begins:* Sep
Length: 21 mos   *Award:* Dipl, AAS
Tuition per yr: $2,240 res, $4,480 non-res
Evening or weekend classes available

Harcum College
Clin Lab Tech/Med Lab Tech-AD Prgm
Montgomery and Morris Aves
Bryn Mawr, PA 19010
Prgm Dir: Alexandra B Hilosky, MS (ASCP) EdD
Tel: 610 525-4100
Med Dir: Harry Schwamm, MD
Class Cap: 12   *Begins:* Sep
Length: 24 mos   *Award:* Dipl, AS
Tuition per yr: $6,500 res, $6,962 non-res

Mt Aloysius College
Clin Lab Tech/Med Lab Tech-AD Prgm
7373 Admiral Peary Hwy
Cresson, PA 16630-1999
Prgm Dir: Susan E Rozum, MEd MT(ASCP)
Tel: 814 886-6404   *Fax:* 814 886-2978
Med Dir: William Kirsch, MD
Class Cap: 25   *Begins:* Aug
Length: 20 mos   *Award:* AS
Tuition per yr: $10,760

Harrisburg Area Community College
Clin Lab Tech/Med Lab Tech-AD Prgm
One HACC Dr
Harrisburg, PA 17110-2999
Prgm Dir: Catherine A Lencioni, MS MT(ASCP)
Tel: 717 780-2311   *Fax:* 717 780-2551
Med Dir: Anthony E Maas, MD
Class Cap: 14   *Begins:* Jun
Length: 24 mos   *Award:* AA
Tuition per yr: $2,311 res, $4,583 non-res
Evening or weekend classes available

Penn State University - Hazleton
Clin Lab Tech/Med Lab Tech-AD Prgm
Hazleton, PA 18201
Prgm Dir: Patricia Ferry, MT(ASCP)
Tel: 717 450-3090   *Fax:* 717 450-3182
E-mail: pdf1@psu.edu
Med Dir: Johann Koenig, MD
Class Cap: 14   *Begins:* Aug
Length: 24 mos, 36 mos   *Award:* AD
Tuition per yr: $7,794 res, $10,224 non-res

Manor Junior College
Clin Lab Tech/Med Lab Tech-AD Prgm
Fox Chase Rd
Jenkintown, PA 19046
Prgm Dir: Nancy Ceranic, MT(ASCP)H(ASCP)
Tel: 215 885-2360   *Fax:* 215 576-6564
Med Dir: Christopher M Frauenhoffer, MD
Class Cap: 24   *Begins:* Sep Jan
Length: 20 mos   *Award:* Dipl, AS
Tuition per yr: $7,360
Evening or weekend classes available

Community College of Beaver County
Clin Lab Tech/Med Lab Tech-AD Prgm
College Dr
Monaca, PA 15061
Prgm Dir: Elizabeth A Valicenti, MS MT(ASCP)
Tel: 412 775-8561   *Fax:* 412 775-4055
Med Dir: Tae C Min, MD
Class Cap: 24   *Begins:* Sep
Length: 21 mos   *Award:* AAS
Tuition per yr: $2,870 res, $5,910 non-res
Evening or weekend classes available

Penn State Univ - New Kensington Campus
Clin Lab Tech/Med Lab Tech-AD Prgm
3550 Seventh St Rd
New Kensington, PA 15068
Prgm Dir: Julia R Young, MT(ASCP)
Tel: 412 339-6004   *Fax:* 412 339-5434
E-mail: try2@psu.edu
Med Dir: John Oehrle, MD
Class Cap: 40   *Begins:* Jun Aug Jan
Length: 24 mos   *Award:* Dipl, AD
Tuition per yr: $7,351 res, $11,437 non-res

Allegheny University of the Health Sciences
Clin Lab Tech/Med Lab Tech-AD Prgm
Broad and Vines Sts
Philadelphia, PA 19102
Prgm Dir: Pamela Buccelli, EdD MT(ASCP)
Tel: 215 762-7176   *Fax:* 215 246-5347
E-mail: buccelli@alleghney.edu
Med Dir: Kathleen Sazama, MD JD
Class Cap: 20   *Begins:* Aug
Length: 21 mos   *Award:* AAS
Tuition per yr: $8,120 res, $8,120 non-res

Community College of Philadelphia
Clin Lab Tech/Med Lab Tech-AD Prgm
1700 Spring Garden St
Philadelphia, PA 19130
Prgm Dir: Wendy M Blume, EdD MS MT(ASCP)
Tel: 215 751-8429   *Fax:* 215 751-8937
Med Dir: Stanley Burrows, MD
Class Cap: 36   *Begins:* Sep
Length: 21 mos   *Award:* AAS
Tuition per yr: $2,070 res, $4,180 non-res
Evening or weekend classes available

Reading Area Community College
Clin Lab Tech/Med Lab Tech-AD Prgm
10 S Second St
PO Box 1706
Reading, PA 19603
Prgm Dir: Sandra A Neiman, MA MT(ASCP)
Tel: 610 372-4721   *Fax:* 610 607-6254
Med Dir: James Welsh, MD
Class Cap: 24   *Begins:* Sep
Length: 20 mos   *Award:* AAS
Tuition per yr: $2,204 res, $4,408 non-res
Evening or weekend classes available

Comm Coll of Allegheny Cnty-South Campus
Clin Lab Tech/Med Lab Tech-AD Prgm
1750 Clairton Rd
Rte 885
West Mifflin, PA 15122
Prgm Dir: Jane Coughanour, MEd MT(ASCP)
Tel: 412 469-6280   *Fax:* 412 469-6371
Med Dir: Nirmal Kotwal, MD
Class Cap: 24   *Begins:* Aug
Length: 20 mos   *Award:* AS
Tuition per yr: $2,040 res, $4,080 non-res
Evening or weekend classes available

Rhode Island

Community College of Rhode Island
Clin Lab Tech/Med Lab Tech-AD Prgm
1762 Louisquisset Pike
Lincoln, RI 02865
Prgm Dir: Lela M Morgan, MA MT(ASCP)CLS
Tel: 401 333-7252   *Fax:* 401 333-7260
E-mail: lmorgan@ccri.cc.ri.us
Med Dir: Upendra Shah, MD
Class Cap: 20   *Begins:* Jun
Length: 18 mos   *Award:* AAS
Tuition per yr: $2,500 res, $6,900 non-res
Evening or weekend classes available

South Carolina

Trident Technical College
Clin Lab Tech/Med Lab Tech-AD Prgm
PO Box 118067
Charleston, SC 29423-8067
Prgm Dir: Ann H Smith, MA MT(ASCP)
Tel: 803 572-6067   *Fax:* 803 569-6585
E-mail: zsmitha@trident.tec.sc.us
Med Dir: John Columbus Cate IV, MD
Class Cap: 30   *Begins:* Aug
Length: 21 mos   *Award:* AHS
Tuition per yr: $1,536 res, $1,776 non-res
Evening or weekend classes available

Midlands Technical College

Clin Lab Tech/Med Lab Tech-AD Prgm
PO Box 2408
Columbia, SC 29202
Prgm Dir: Mary Breci-Swendrzynski, MAT
  MT(ASCP)
Tel: 803 822-3557   *Fax:* 803 822-3343
Med Dir: Ron G Burns, MD
Class Cap: 20   *Begins:* Sep
Length: 24 mos   *Award:* AS
Tuition per yr: $1,080 res, $1,344 non-res

Florence-Darlington Technical College

Clin Lab Tech/Med Lab Tech-AD Prgm
PO Box 100548
Florence, SC 29501-0548
Prgm Dir: John F Quinn, MEd MT(ASCP)
Tel: 803 661-8145, Ext 281   *Fax:* 803 661-8306
E-mail: quinnj@flo.tec.sc.us
Med Dir: Hans K Habermeier, MD
Class Cap: 30   *Begins:* Aug
Length: 24 mos   *Award:* AA
Tuition per yr: $1,650 res, $1,875 non-res
Evening or weekend classes available

Greenville Technical College

Clin Lab Tech/Med Lab Tech-AD Prgm
PO Box 5616/Station B
Greenville, SC 29606
Prgm Dir: Hugh B Batson, MA MT(ASCP)
Tel: 864 250-8292   *Fax:* 864 250-8462
E-mail: batsonhbb@gvltec.edu
Med Dir: Jackson H McCarter, MD
Class Cap: 22   *Begins:* Aug
Length: 21 mos   *Award:* AHS
Tuition per yr: $1,500 res, $2,400 non-res

Orangeburg Calhoun Technical College

Clin Lab Tech/Med Lab Tech-AD Prgm
3250 St Matthews Rd
Orangeburg, SC 29118
Prgm Dir: Bonnie D Fanning, MS MT(ASCP)
Tel: 803 536-0311   *Fax:* 803 535-1388
Med Dir: John E Shippey, Jr, MD
Class Cap: 18   *Begins:* Aug
Length: 21 mos   *Award:* AAS
Tuition per yr: $1,188 res, $1,452 non-res
Evening or weekend classes available

Tri-County Technical College

Clin Lab Tech/Med Lab Tech-AD Prgm
PO Box 587
Pendleton, SC 29670-0587
Prgm Dir: Dallas F Jones, MEd MT(ASCP)
Tel: 864 646-8361, Ext 251   *Fax:* 864 646-8256
E-mail: djones@tricty.tricounty.tec.sc.us
Med Dir: Albert A Hollingsworth, MD
Class Cap: 20   *Begins:* Aug
Length: 21 mos   *Award:* AAS
Tuition per yr: $1,350 res, $1,638 non-res
Evening or weekend classes available

York Technical College

Clin Lab Tech/Med Lab Tech-AD Prgm
452 S Anderson Rd
Rock Hill, SC 29730
Prgm Dir: Nancy G Westbrook, MS MT(ASCP)
  SBB
Tel: 803 981-7118   *Fax:* 803 327-8059
Med Dir: Earl Jenkins, Jr, MD
Class Cap: 20   *Begins:* Aug
Length: 21 mos   *Award:* AHS
Tuition per yr: $1,296 res, $1,548 non-res

Spartanburg Technical College

Clin Lab Tech/Med Lab Tech-AD Prgm
PO Drawer 4386
Spartanburg, SC 29305
Prgm Dir: Amelia Dickerson, MHS MT(ASCP)
Tel: 864 591-3866   *Fax:* 864 591-3708
E-mail: dickerson@spt.tec.sc.us
Med Dir: Michael Patton, MD
Class Cap: 23   *Begins:* Aug
Length: 21 mos   *Award:* AHS
Tuition per yr: $1,500 res, $1,875 non-res

South Dakota

Presentation College

Clin Lab Tech/Med Lab Tech-AD Prgm
1500 N Main St
Aberdeen, SD 57401
Prgm Dir: Roberta L Kervin, MAT MT(ASCP)
Tel: 605 229-8464   *Fax:* 605 229-8430
Med Dir: Roy Burt, MD
Class Cap: 10   *Begins:* Aug
Length: 21 mos   *Award:* AAS
Tuition per yr: $6,690
Evening or weekend classes available

Mitchell Technical Institute

Clin Lab Tech/Med Lab Tech-AD Prgm
821 N Capital
Mitchell, SD 57301
Prgm Dir: Barbara Feilmeier, BS MT(ASCP)
Tel: 605 995-3024   *Fax:* 605 996-3299
Med Dir: Kim Lorenzen, MD
Class Cap: 18   *Begins:* Aug
Length: 19 mos   *Award:* AAS
Tuition per yr: $1,850
Evening or weekend classes available

Lake Area Technical Institute

Clin Lab Tech/Med Lab Tech-AD Prgm
200 NE 9th St
Watertown, SD 57201
Prgm Dir: Mona Gleysteen, MS MT(ASCP)
Tel: 605 886-5872   *Fax:* 605 882-6347
E-mail: mgleyste@latiatec.sd.us
Med Dir: Melvin Gesink, MD
Class Cap: 20   *Begins:* Sep Jan
Length: 22 mos   *Award:* AAS
Tuition per yr: $2,225
Evening or weekend classes available

Tennessee

Cleveland State Community College

Clin Lab Tech/Med Lab Tech-AD Prgm
One Adkisson Rd
PO Box 3750
Cleveland, TN 37320
Prgm Dir: Joseph K Semak, EdD MT(ASCP)
Tel: 423 472-7141   *Fax:* 423 478-6255
E-mail: jsemak@clscc.cc.tn.us
Med Dir: W K Striker, MD
Begins: Aug
Length: 22 mos   *Award:* AAS
Tuition per yr: $1,300 res, $5,160 non-res

Columbia State Community College

Clin Lab Tech/Med Lab Tech-AD Prgm
Hwy 99 W
PO Box 1315
Columbia, TN 38401-1315
Prgm Dir: Nancy M Wells, MA MT(ASCP)
Tel: 615 540-2741   *Fax:* 615 540-2798
E-mail: wells@coscc.cc.tn.us
Med Dir: Harold Ferrell, MD
Class Cap: 20   *Begins:* Aug
Length: 21 mos   *Award:* AAS
Tuition per yr: $1,536 res, $4,614 non-res
Evening or weekend classes available

Cumberland School of Technology

Clin Lab Tech/Med Lab Tech-AD Prgm
1065 E 10th St
Cookeville, TN 38501
Prgm Dir: LaVerne Floyd, MA MT(ASCP)
Tel: 615 526-3660   *Fax:* 615 372-2603
Med Dir: Samuel Glasgow III, MD
Class Cap: 20   *Begins:* Jan May Jul Oct
Length: 18 mos   *Award:* AAS
Tuition per yr: $8,925 res, $8,925 non-res

East Tennessee State University

Clin Lab Tech/Med Lab Tech-AD Prgm
ETSU Nave Center
1000 West E St
Elizabethton, TN 37643
Prgm Dir: Linda S Lahr, MS MT(ASCP)
Tel: 423 547-4907   *Fax:* 423 547-4921
Med Dir: David Anthony Sibley, MD
Class Cap: 15   *Begins:* Aug
Length: 24 mos   *Award:* AAS
Tuition per yr: $2,892 res, $9,396 non-res
Evening or weekend classes available

Jackson State Community College

Clin Lab Tech/Med Lab Tech-AD Prgm
2046 N Parkway St
Jackson, TN 38301-3797
Prgm Dir: Glenda L Jones, MT(ASCP)
Tel: 901 425-2612   *Fax:* 901 425-2647
E-mail: GJONES@JSCC.CC.TN.US
Med Dir: Ben Sharpe, MD
Class Cap: 15   *Begins:* Sept
Length: 24 mos   *Award:* AAS
Tuition per yr: $1,491 res, $5,880 non-res
Evening or weekend classes available

Roane State Community College

Clin Lab Tech/Med Lab Tech-AD Prgm
8373 Kingston Pike
Knoxville, TN 37919
Prgm Dir: Evelyn H Bledsoe, MS MT(ASCP)
Tel: 423 539-6904   *Fax:* 423 539-6907
Med Dir: Bruce Bellomy, MD
Class Cap: 20   *Begins:* Aug
Length: 24 mos   *Award:* AAS
Tuition per yr: $1,482 res, $4,143 non-res
Evening or weekend classes available

Shelby State Community College

Clin Lab Tech/Med Lab Tech-AD Prgm
PO Box 40568
Memphis, TN 38174-0568
Prgm Dir: Darius Y Wilson, MAT MT(ASCP)
Tel: 901 544-5400   *Fax:* 901 544-5391
Med Dir: Michael F Bugg, MD
Class Cap: 30   *Begins:* Sep Jan
Length: 24 mos   *Award:* AAS
Tuition per yr: $1,536 res, $6,144 non-res
Evening or weekend classes available

Texas

Alvin Community College

Clin Lab Tech/Med Lab Tech-AD Prgm
3110 Mustang Rd
Alvin, TX 77511
Prgm Dir: Florence J Pipes, MS MT(ASCP)
Tel: 713 338-4696 *Fax:* 713 388-4736
Med Dir: Marion Rundel, MD
Begins: Aug
Length: 24 mos *Award:* AAS
Tuition per yr: $1,120 res, $3,080 non-res

Amarillo College

Clin Lab Tech/Med Lab Tech-AD Prgm
PO Box 447
Amarillo, TX 79178
Prgm Dir: Janet M Bohachef, BA MT(ASCP)
Tel: 806 354-6059 *Fax:* 806 354-6076
E-mail: jmsauer@actx.edu
Med Dir: Ralph Mennemeyer, MD
Class Cap: 20 *Begins:* Aug
Length: 24 mos *Award:* Dipl, AAS
Tuition per yr: $865 res, $1,265 non-res
Evening or weekend classes available

Austin Community College

Clin Lab Tech/Med Lab Tech-AD Prgm
1020 Grove Blvd
Austin, TX 78741
Prgm Dir: Carolyn Ragland, MS MT(ASCP) CLS
Tel: 512 223-6114 *Fax:* 512 369-6700
Med Dir: Paul LeBourgeosis, MD FCAP
Class Cap: 17 *Begins:* Aug
Length: 21 mos *Award:* AAS
Tuition per yr: $1,221 res, $4,884 non-res
Evening or weekend classes available

Univ TX at Brownsville/TX Southmost Coll

Clin Lab Tech/Med Lab Tech-AD Prgm
83 Ft Brown
Brownsville, TX 78520
Prgm Dir: Shamina Garcia Davis, MS MT(ASCP)
Tel: 210 544-8925 *Fax:* 210 544-8910
Med Dir: Luis M Garcia, MD
Begins: Sep
Length: 21 mos *Award:* Dipl, AAS
Tuition per yr: $1,158 res, $4,092 non-res

Del Mar College

Clin Lab Tech/Med Lab Tech-AD Prgm
Baldwin and Ayers
Corpus Christi, TX 78404
Prgm Dir: Duncan F Samo, MEd MT(ASCP)
Tel: 512 886-1107 *Fax:* 512 886-1598
Med Dir: James M Scherer, MD
Class Cap: 24 *Begins:* Sep
Length: 21 mos *Award:* Dipl, AAS
Tuition per yr: $1,000 res, $1,500 non-res
Evening or weekend classes available

El Centro College

Clin Lab Tech/Med Lab Tech-AD Prgm
Main and Lamar Sts
Dallas, TX 75202-3604
Prgm Dir: M La Cheeta McPherson, PhD MT(ASCP)
Tel: 214 860-2271 *Fax:* 214 860-2268
E-mail: mlm5544@dcccd.edu
Med Dir: Van E Telford, MD
Class Cap: 24 *Begins:* Aug
Length: 24 mos *Award:* AAS
Tuition per yr: $900 res, $2,000 non-res
Evening or weekend classes available

Grayson County College

Clin Lab Tech/Med Lab Tech-AD Prgm
6101 Grayson Dr
Denison, TX 75020
Prgm Dir: Shirley R Hagan, MS MT(ASCP)
Tel: 903 786-4468 *Fax:* 903 463-8779
Med Dir: Edgar G McKee, MD
Class Cap: 15 *Begins:* Jun Jul
Length: 23 mos *Award:* AAS
Tuition per yr: $1,050 res, $1,190 non-res
Evening or weekend classes available

El Paso Community College

Clin Lab Tech/Med Lab Tech-AD Prgm
PO Box 20500
El Paso, TX 79998
Prgm Dir: Arthur L Paul, MT(ASCP)
Tel: 915 534-4085 *Fax:* 915 534-4114
Med Dir: Joseph Lawrence, MD
Class Cap: 12 *Begins:* Jun
Length: 24 mos *Award:* AAS
Tuition per yr: $1,508 res, $3,238 non-res
Evening or weekend classes available

Houston Community College Central

Clin Lab Tech/Med Lab Tech-AD Prgm
5514 Clara
Houston, TX 77041
Prgm Dir: Mary Beth Murphy, MT(ASCP)
Tel: 713 718-5517 *Fax:* 713 849-4203
Med Dir: Oscar R Mangini, MD
Begins: Aug Jan
Length: 24 mos *Award:* AAS
Tuition per yr: $1,215 res, $1,741 non-res
Evening or weekend classes available

Kilgore College

Clin Lab Tech/Med Lab Tech-AD Prgm
1100 Broadway
Kilgore, TX 75662
Prgm Dir: Sarah Keith, MS MT(ASCP)NM
Tel: 903 983-8145 *Fax:* 903 983-8600
Med Dir: Kevin J McQuaid, MD
Class Cap: 12 *Begins:* Aug
Length: 21 mos *Award:* AAS
Tuition per yr: $950 non-res
Evening or weekend classes available

Central Texas College

Clin Lab Tech/Med Lab Tech-AD Prgm
US Hwy 190 W
PO Box 1800
Killeen, TX 76541-9990
Prgm Dir: Donna E Poteet, MA CLS(NCA)
Tel: 812 526-1187 *Fax:* 817 526-1765
Med Dir: Carlton E Hardin, MD
Class Cap: 40 *Begins:* Aug Jan
Length: 24 mos *Award:* AAS
Tuition per yr: $720
Evening or weekend classes available

Laredo Community College

Clin Lab Tech/Med Lab Tech-AD Prgm
W End Washington St
Laredo, TX 78040
Prgm Dir: David Hill, MS MT(ASCP)
Tel: 210 721-5264
Med Dir: Oscar Ramos, MD
Class Cap: 17 *Begins:* Aug
Length: 21 mos *Award:* Dipl, AAS
Tuition per yr: $500 res, $800 non-res

Odessa College

Clin Lab Tech/Med Lab Tech-AD Prgm
201 W University
Odessa, TX 79764-8299
Prgm Dir: Joel D Smith, MT(ASCP)
Tel: 915 335-6447 *Fax:* 915 335-6846
E-mail: cleach@odessa.edu
Med Dir: Kris Challapalli, MD
Class Cap: 16 *Begins:* Jul
Length: 22 mos *Award:* AAS
Tuition per yr: $532 res, $722 non-res
Evening or weekend classes available

San Jacinto College Central Campus

Clin Lab Tech/Med Lab Tech-AD Prgm
8060 Spencer Hwy
Pasadena, TX 77505
Prgm Dir: Charlyn Beth Goehring-Stahl, MS MT(ASCP) SBB
Tel: 713 478-2730 *Fax:* 713 478-2754
Med Dir: Dorothy Willis, MD
Class Cap: 25 *Begins:* Aug
Length: 23 mos *Award:* Dipl, AAS
Tuition per yr: $1,208 res, $1,872 non-res
Evening or weekend classes available

St Philip's College

Clin Lab Tech/Med Lab Tech-AD Prgm
1801 Martin Luther King Dr
San Antonio, TX 78203-2098
Prgm Dir: Rebecca E Sanchez, MS MT(ASCP)
Tel: 210 531-3553 *Fax:* 210 531-3459
E-mail: rsanchez@acc.d.edu
Med Dir: Desiree E D'Orsogna, MD
Class Cap: 18 *Begins:* Aug
Length: 24 mos *Award:* Dipl, AAS
Tuition per yr: $640 res, $1,320 non-res
Evening or weekend classes available

Temple College

Clin Lab Tech/Med Lab Tech-AD Prgm
2600 S 1st St
Temple, TX 76504
Prgm Dir: Billye Weaver, PhD MT(ASCP)CLS
Tel: 817 778-4811 *Fax:* 817 771-4528
Med Dir: Edwin H Johnson, MD
Class Cap: 25 *Begins:* Aug
Length: 24 mos *Award:* Dipl, AAS
Tuition per yr: $1,089 res, $1,540 non-res

Tyler Junior College

Clin Lab Tech/Med Lab Tech-AD Prgm
PO Box 9020
Tyler, TX 75711-9020
Prgm Dir: Patricia L Hobbs, MS MT(ASCP)
Tel: 903 510-2367 *Fax:* 903 510-2592
E-mail: lhob@tjc.tyler.cc.tx.us
Med Dir: Marian Fagan, MD
Class Cap: 23 *Begins:* Sep
Length: 22 mos *Award:* Dipl, AAS
Tuition per yr: $940 res, $1,461 non-res
Evening or weekend classes available

Victoria College

Clin Lab Tech/Med Lab Tech-AD Prgm
2200 E Red River
Victoria, TX 77901
Prgm Dir: Larry S Dunn, MS MT(ASCP)
Tel: 512 572-6455   *Fax:* 512 572-6441
E-mail: dunn@mailhost.vc.cc.tx.us
Med Dir: Joe David Ibanez, MD
Class Cap: 14   *Begins:* Aug
Length: 20 mos   *Award:* Dipl, AAS
Tuition per yr: $688 res, $1,032 non-res

McLennan Community College

Clin Lab Tech/Med Lab Tech-AD Prgm
1400 College Dr
Waco, TX 76708
Prgm Dir: Bridgit R Moore, MSHP MT(ASCP)
Tel: 817 299-8417
E-mail: brm@mcc.cc.tx.us
Med Dir: Daniel R Samples, MD PhD
Class Cap: 20   *Begins:* Aug
Length: 24 mos   *Award:* AAS
Tuition per yr: $1,266 res, $1,456 non-res
Evening or weekend classes available

Wharton County Junior College

Clin Lab Tech/Med Lab Tech-AD Prgm
911 Boling Hwy
Wharton, TX 77488
Prgm Dir: Janice Harbich, MA MT(ASCP)
Tel: 409 532-4560   *Fax:* 409 532-6489
Med Dir: Hector Perches, MD
Class Cap: 13   *Begins:* Aug Sep
Length: 24 mos   *Award:* AAS
Tuition per yr: $1,053 res, $1,794 non-res

Utah

Weber State University

Clin Lab Tech/Med Lab Tech-AD Prgm
Ogden, UT 84408-3905
Prgm Dir: Michael A Beard, EdD MT(ASCP)SBB
Tel: 801 626-6509
Med Dir: Dean Hammond, MD
Class Cap: 30   *Begins:* Sep Jan
Length: 24 mos   *Award:* Dipl, AAS
Tuition per yr: $1,863 res, $5,550 non-res

Salt Lake Community College

Clin Lab Tech/Med Lab Tech-AD Prgm
PO Box 30808
Salt Lake City, UT 84130
Prgm Dir: Karen A Brown, MS MT(ASCP) CLS
Tel: 801 581-3544   *Fax:* 801 581-4517
E-mail: karen_brown@medschool.med.utah.edu
Med Dir: Joseph A Knight, MD
Begins: Mar
Length: 24 mos   *Award:* Dipl, AAS
Tuition per yr: $1,446 res, $4,506 non-res
Evening or weekend classes available

Virginia

Northern Virginia Community College

Clin Lab Tech/Med Lab Tech-AD Prgm
8333 Little River Trnpk
Annandale, VA 22003
Prgm Dir: Judy A Horton, MS MT(ASCP)
Tel: 703 323-3418   *Fax:* 703 323-4576
Med Dir: Mary Paula Neuman, MD
Class Cap: 25   *Begins:* Aug
Length: 21 mos   *Award:* Dipl, AAS
Tuition per yr: $1,920 res, $6,294 non-res
Evening or weekend classes available

Thomas Nelson Community College

Clin Lab Tech/Med Lab Tech-AD Prgm
PO Box 9407
Hampton, VA 23670
Prgm Dir: Linda A Dezern, MS MT(ASCP)
Tel: 757 825-2812   *Fax:* 757 825-2951
E-mail: dezern@tncc.cc.va.us
Med Dir: Richard Clark, MD
Class Cap: 15   *Begins:* Aug
Length: 24 mos   *Award:* AAS
Tuition per yr: $1,913 res, $6,396 non-res
Evening or weekend classes available

J Sargeant Reynolds Community College

Clin Lab Tech/Med Lab Tech-AD Prgm
PO Box 85622
Richmond, VA 23285-5622
Prgm Dir: Lou Anne Manning, MS MT(ASCP)
Tel: 804 371-3253   *Fax:* 804 371-3311
E-mail: srmannl@jsr.cc.va.us
Med Dir: Richard H Carpenter, MD
Class Cap: 25   *Begins:* Aug
Length: 21 mos   *Award:* AAS
Tuition per yr: $1,991 res, $6,355 non-res
Evening or weekend classes available

Wytheville Community College

Clin Lab Tech/Med Lab Tech-AD Prgm
1000 E Main St
Wytheville, VA 24382
Prgm Dir: Betty V Craft, EdD MT(ASCP)
Tel: 540 223-4827   *Fax:* 540 223-4778
Med Dir: Andrew Williams, MD
Class Cap: 14   *Begins:* Aug
Length: 21 mos   *Award:* AAS
Tuition per yr: $2,456 res, $8,058 non-res

Washington

Pima Medical Institute - Seattle

Clin Lab Tech/Med Lab Tech-AD Prgm
1627 Eastlake Ave E
Seattle, WA 98102
Prgm Dir: Sonja Nehr-Kanet, MS, MT(ASCP)
Tel: 206 322-6100   *Fax:* 206 324-1985
Med Dir: Samuel Hammar, MD, FCCP
Class Cap: 15   *Begins:* Oct May
Length: 22 mos   *Award:* AAS
Tuition per yr: $8,260

Shoreline Community College

Clin Lab Tech/Med Lab Tech-AD Prgm
16101 Greenwood Ave N
Seattle, WA 98133
Prgm Dir: Linda L Brinkley, CLS(NCA)MT(ASCP)
Tel: 206 546-4710   *Fax:* 206 543-5826
Med Dir: Hector C Aldape, MD
Class Cap: 40   *Begins:* Sep
Length: 23 mos   *Award:* AAS
Tuition per yr: $1,853 res, $7,333 non-res
Evening or weekend classes available

Wenatchee Valley College

Clin Lab Tech/Med Lab Tech-AD Prgm
1300 Fifth St
Wenatchee, WA 98801
Prgm Dir: David C Abbott, CLS(NCA) MS
Tel: 509 662-1651
Med Dir: Gary Hannon, MD
Class Cap: 24   *Begins:* Sep
Length: 24 mos   *Award:* AAS
Tuition per yr: $1,800 res, $7,064 non-res

West Virginia

Fairmont State College

Clin Lab Tech/Med Lab Tech-AD Prgm
Locust Ave
Fairmont, WV 26554
Prgm Dir: Joan H Burns, MS MT(ASCP)
Tel: 304 367-4284   *Fax:* 304 366-4870
E-mail: jhb@fscvax.wvnet.edu
Med Dir: Cordell DeLaPena, MD
Class Cap: 14   *Begins:* Aug
Length: 22 mos   *Award:* AAS
Tuition per yr: $1,918 res, $4,428 non-res

Marshall University

Clin Lab Tech/Med Lab Tech-AD Prgm
Clinical Lab Science Dept
400 Hall Greer Blvd
Huntington, WV 25701
Prgm Dir: Bruce J Brown, EdD MS MT(ASCP)
Tel: 304 696-3188   *Fax:* 304 696-3243
E-mail: brownbru@marshall.edu
Med Dir: James R Morris, MD
Class Cap: 20   *Begins:* Aug
Length: 12 mos, 15 mos   *Award:* AAS
Tuition per yr: $3,282 res, $8,865 non-res
Evening or weekend classes available

Southern West Virginia Community College

Clin Lab Tech/Med Lab Tech-AD Prgm
Logan Campus/PO Box 2900
Mt Gay, WV 25637
Prgm Dir: Vernon R Elkins, BS MT(ASCP)
Tel: 304 792-4343   *Fax:* 304 792-7028
E-mail: vernone@swvcc.wvnet.edu
Med Dir: Carlos F DeLara, MD
Class Cap: 15   *Begins:* Aug
Length: 21 mos   *Award:* AD
Tuition per yr: $1,130 res, $3,950 non-res
Evening or weekend classes available

Programs

West Virginia Northern Community College
Clin Lab Tech/Med Lab Tech-AD Prgm
15th and Jacob Sts
Wheeling, WV 26003
Prgm Dir: Gary B Pickett, MS MT(ASCP)CLS
Tel: 304 233-5900, Ext 4409 *Fax:* 304 242-7695
E-mail: gpickett@nccvax.wynet.edu
Med Dir: Robert S Salisbury, MD
Class Cap: 16 *Begins:* Aug
Length: 20 mos *Award:* AD
Tuition per yr: $1,770 res, $1,770 non-res

Wisconsin

Chippewa Valley Technical College
Clin Lab Tech/Med Lab Tech-AD Prgm
620 W Clairemont Ave
Eau Claire, WI 54701
Prgm Dir: Patricia Griffin, MS MT(ASCP)
Tel: 715 833-6420 *Fax:* 715 833-6470
E-mail: pgriffin@mail.chippewa.tec.wi.us
Med Dir: Thomas W Hadley, MD
Class Cap: 24 *Begins:* Aug
Length: 21 mos *Award:* AS
Tuition per yr: $1,843 res, $14,220 non-res
Evening or weekend classes available

Northeast Wisconsin Technical College
Clin Lab Tech/Med Lab Tech-AD Prgm
2740 W Mason St/PO Box 19042
Green Bay, WI 54307-9042
Prgm Dir: Pat Moore-Cribb, MT(ASCP)
Tel: 414 498-6374 *Fax:* 414 498-5560
Med Dir: William Faller, MD FCAP
Class Cap: 17 *Begins:* Aug
Length: 21 mos *Award:* AS
Tuition per yr: $2,092 res, $11,689 non-res
Evening or weekend classes available

Western Wisconsin Technical College
Clin Lab Tech/Med Lab Tech-AD Prgm
304 N Sixth St
PO Box 908
La Crosse, WI 54602-0908
Prgm Dir: Patricia Cipriano, MT(ASCP)
Tel: 608 785-9169 *Fax:* 608 785-9194
E-mail: cipriano@a1.western.tec.wi.us
Med Dir: Martin J Smith, MD
Class Cap: 24 *Begins:* Aug
Length: 21 mos *Award:* AAS
Tuition per yr: $2,269 res, $12,838 non-res
Evening or weekend classes available

Madison Area Technical College
Clin Lab Tech/Med Lab Tech-AD Prgm
3550 Anderson St
Madison, WI 53704-2599
Prgm Dir: Mary Ann Nelson, BS MT(ASCP)
Tel: 608 246-6510 *Fax:* 608 246-6013
Med Dir: Stanley Inhorn, MD
Class Cap: 15 *Begins:* Aug Jan
Length: 18 mos *Award:* AAS
Tuition per yr: $2,778 res, $2,778 non-res

Milwaukee Area Technical College
Clin Lab Tech/Med Lab Tech-AD Prgm
700 W State St
Milwaukee, WI 53233
Prgm Dir: Dennis Schmidt, MS MT(ASCP)
Tel: 414 297-7142 *Fax:* 414 297-6851
E-mail: schmidtd@milwaukee.tec.wi.us
Med Dir: Erskine Tucker, MD
Class Cap: 24 *Begins:* Sep Jan
Length: 19 mos *Award:* AAS
Tuition per yr: $1,590 res, $10,634 non-res
Evening or weekend classes available

Clinical Lab Technician/ Medical Lab Technician- Certificate

California

Naval School of Hlth Sciences - San Diego
Clin Lab Tech/Med Lab Tech-C Prgm
San Diego, CA 92134-5291
Prgm Dir: Marjorie A Bianco, MT(ASCP)SBB MS
Tel: 619 532-7330 *Fax:* 619 532-7722
Med Dir: Robert W Sharpe, MC USN
Class Cap: 160 *Begins:* Quarterly
Length: 12 mos *Award:* Cert

Colorado

T H Pickens Technical Center
Clin Lab Tech/Med Lab Tech-C Prgm
500 Airport Blvd
Aurora, CO 80011
Prgm Dir: Mary Leslie Hutchinson, MA
   MT(ASCP) CLS
Tel: 303 344-4910 *Fax:* 303 340-1898
Med Dir: Paul Visconti, MD
Class Cap: 10 *Begins:* Aug Jan
Length: 12 mos *Award:* Cert
Tuition per yr: $2,016 res, $8,064 non-res

Florida

Sheridan Vocational Technical Center
Clin Lab Tech/Med Lab Tech-C Prgm
5400 Sheridan St
Hollywood, FL 33021
Prgm Dir: Phyllis Pacifico, EdD MT(ASCP)
Tel: 954 985-3220 *Fax:* 954 985-3229
Med Dir: William D Williams, MD
Class Cap: 30 *Begins:* Sep Feb
Length: 12 mos *Award:* Cert
Tuition per yr: $1,031 res, $5,633 non-res

David G Erwin Technical Center
Clin Lab Tech/Med Lab Tech-C Prgm
2010 E Hillsborough Ave
Tampa, FL 33610-8299
Prgm Dir: Carol A Mitchels, MT(ASCP) CLS
Tel: 813 231-1800 *Fax:* 813 231-1820
Med Dir: Glenn Hooper, MD
Class Cap: 24 *Begins:* July Feb
Length: 12 mos *Award:* Dipl
Tuition per yr: $683 res, $5,050 non-res

Georgia

Atlanta Area Technical School
Clin Lab Tech/Med Lab Tech-C Prgm
1560 Stewart Ave SW
Atlanta, GA 30310
Prgm Dir: Alma Jerrick, EdS MT(ASCP)
Tel: 404 756-3721   *Fax:* 404 756-0932
Med Dir: Nilda Winearski, MD
Class Cap: 40   *Begins:* Sep Apr
Length: 15 mos   *Award:* Dipl
Tuition per yr: $1,184 res, $1,184 non-res

North Georgia Technical Institute
Clin Lab Tech/Med Lab Tech-C Prgm
Hwy 197 N
PO Box 65
Clarkesville, GA 30523
Prgm Dir: Lauren Strader, MT(ASCP) MEd
Tel: 706 754-7757   *Fax:* 706 754-7777
E-mail: @adminl.clarkes.tec.ga.us
Med Dir: James Clay, MD
Class Cap: 15   *Begins:* Oct
Length: 18 mos   *Award:* Dipl
Tuition per yr: $1,008 res, $2,016 non-res
Evening or weekend classes available

De Kalb Technical Institute
Clin Lab Tech/Med Lab Tech-C Prgm
495 N Indian Creek Dr
Clarkston, GA 30021-2397
Prgm Dir: Sharon L Thatcher, EdS MT(ASCP)
Tel: 404 297-9522   *Fax:* 404 294-4234
E-mail: sharon@admin2.dekalb.tech.ga.us
Med Dir: William F McNeill, MD
Class Cap: 25   *Begins:* Oct
Length: 15 mos   *Award:* Dipl
Tuition per yr: $1,470 res, $2,730 non-res
Evening or weekend classes available

Macon Technical Institute
Clin Lab Tech/Med Lab Tech-C Prgm
3300 Macon Tech Dr
Macon, GA 31206
Prgm Dir: Laura H Kurish, MT(ASCP)
Tel: 912 757-3400   *Fax:* 912 757-3454
Med Dir: Robert S Donner, MD
Class Cap: 12   *Begins:* Oct
Length: 15 mos, 18 mos   *Award:* Dipl, AAT
Tuition per yr: $1,088

Lanier Technical Institute
Clin Lab Tech/Med Lab Tech-C Prgm
PO Box 58
Oakwood, GA 30566-0058
Prgm Dir: Kimberly A Holliday, MT(ASCP)
Tel: 770 531-6367   *Fax:* 770 531-6306
E-mail: khollida@mercury.gpeachnet.edu
Med Dir: Berton T Schaeffer, MD
Class Cap: 15   *Begins:* Oct
Length: 18 mos   *Award:* Dipl
Tuition per yr: $1,056 res, $2,112 non-res

Thomas Technical Institute
Clin Lab Tech/Med Lab Tech-C Prgm
15689 US HWY 19 N
Thomasville, GA 31792
Prgm Dir: Richard Miller, PhD MBA MT(ASCP), CLS(NCA)
Tel: 912 225-4078   *Fax:* 912 225-5289
E-mail: rmiller@ttin1.thomas.tec.ga.us
Med Dir: Jeff W Byrd, MD
Class Cap: 20   *Begins:* Sep
Length: 24 mos   *Award:* AAT
Tuition per yr: $1,008 res, $1,008 non-res

Okefenokee Technical Institute
Clin Lab Tech/Med Lab Tech-C Prgm
1701 Carswell Ave
Waycross, GA 31501
Prgm Dir: James J Peterson, MT(ASCP)
Tel: 912 287-6584   *Fax:* 912 287-4865
E-mail: jim@admin1.waycross.tech.ga.us
Med Dir: Michael E Stebler, MD
Class Cap: 14   *Begins:* Jul
Length: 15 mos   *Award:* Cert
Tuition per yr: $1,800
Evening or weekend classes available

Illinois

Southern Illinois Collegiate Common Mkt
Clin Lab Tech/Med Lab Tech-C Prgm
3213 S Park Ave
Herrin, IL 62948
Prgm Dir: Patricia M Luebke, BA MT(ASCP)
Tel: 618 993-5282
Class Cap: 32   *Begins:* Aug
Length: 18 mos   *Award:* AAS
Tuition per yr: $875 res, $3,100 non-res

Blessing Hospital
Clin Lab Tech/Med Lab Tech-C Prgm
1005 Broadway St
Quincy, IL 62301
Prgm Dir: Heather Ator, MT(ASCP)SM
Tel: 217 223-8400   *Fax:* 217 223-7032
Med Dir: Robert Merrick, MD
Class Cap: 8   *Begins:* Aug
Length: 12 mos   *Award:* Cert
Tuition per yr: $800
Evening or weekend classes available

Indiana

Lakeshore Med Laboratory Training Prgm
Clin Lab Tech/Med Lab Tech-C Prgm
402 Franklin St
PO Box 25
Michigan City, IN 46360-0025
Prgm Dir: Gina Watson, MT(ASCP)
Tel: 219 872-7032   *Fax:* 219 872-1453
Med Dir: Thomas H Roberts, MD
Class Cap: 12   *Begins:* Aug
Length: 12 mos   *Award:* Cert
Tuition per yr: $2,524

Kansas

Wichita Area Technical College
Clin Lab Tech/Med Lab Tech-C Prgm
324 N Emporia St
Wichita, KS 67202
Prgm Dir: Carolyn West, MT(ASCP)
Tel: 316 833-4370   *Fax:* 316 833-4332
Med Dir: Mary L Nielsen, MD
Class Cap: 15   *Begins:* Jan June
Length: 12 mos, 24 mos   *Award:* Dipl, AAS
Tuition per yr: $1,325 res, $8,160 non-res

Kentucky

Kentucky Tech Central Campus
Clin Lab Tech/Med Lab Tech-C Prgm
104 Vo Tech Rd
Lexington, KY 40517
Prgm Dir: Karman K Wheeler, BS MT(ASCP) SH
Tel: 606 255-8501
Med Dir: Valerie Mandina, MD
Class Cap: 15   *Begins:* Jan
Length: 15 mos   *Award:* Dipl
Tuition per yr: $600

Kentucky Tech/Jefferson State Campus
Clin Lab Tech/Med Lab Tech-C Prgm
800 W Chestnut St
Louisville, KY 40203
Prgm Dir: Catherine Cassaro, MBA MA MT(ASCP)
Tel: 502 595-4275   *Fax:* 502 595-2387
Med Dir: Joseph C Parker Jr, MD
Class Cap: 20   *Begins:* Aug
Length: 18 mos   *Award:* Dipl
Tuition per yr: $500 res, $1,000 non-res
Evening or weekend classes available

Madisonville Health Technology Center
Clin Lab Tech/Med Lab Tech-C Prgm
750 N Laffoon St
Madisonville, KY 42431
Prgm Dir: Karol Ann Conrad, MT(ASCP) SH MS
Tel: 502 824-7552   *Fax:* 502 824-7069
Med Dir: E E Kawas, MD
Class Cap: 12   *Begins:* Apr
Length: 15 mos   *Award:* Dipl
Tuition per yr: $775 res, $775 non-res
Evening or weekend classes available

Cumberland Valley Health Technology Ctr
Clin Lab Tech/Med Lab Tech-C Prgm
US 25E South PO Box 187
Pineville, KY 40977
Prgm Dir: Alice Fae Weiland, BS MT(ASCP) MEd
Tel: 606 337-3106   *Fax:* 606 337-5662
Med Dir: Ann Marshall, MD
Class Cap: 12   *Begins:* Aug
Length: 15 mos   *Award:* Dipl,Cert
Tuition per yr: $600 res, $1,200 non-res
Evening or weekend classes available

Louisiana

Louisiana Technical College
Clin Lab Tech/Med Lab Tech-C Prgm
PO Box 4909
Lafayette, LA 70502
Prgm Dir: Sallie Cooper, MBA MT(ASCP)
Tel: 318 262-5962 *Fax:* 318 262-5122
Med Dir: Joseph Brierre, MD
Begins: Aug Nov Mar May
Length: 18 mos *Award:* Dipl
Tuition per yr: $420 res, $840 non-res

Maryland

Naval School of Health Sciences - MD
Clin Lab Tech/Med Lab Tech-C Prgm
Technical Training Dept
Bethesda, MD 20889-5611
Prgm Dir: Kathleen L Nawn, CDR MSC USN
Tel: 301 295-0125 *Fax:* 301 295-0625
Med Dir: Jeffrey M Ogorzalek, CDR MC USN
Class Cap: 96 *Begins:* Oct Feb May Sep
Length: 12 mos *Award:* Cert

Massachusetts

Southeastern Technical Institute
Clin Lab Tech/Med Lab Tech-C Prgm
250 Foundry St
South Easton, MA 02375
Prgm Dir: Richard B Hamel, MT(ASCP)
Tel: 508 238-1860 *Fax:* 508 238-7266
Med Dir: George Lauro, MD
Class Cap: 20 *Begins:* Sep
Length: 12 mos *Award:* Cert
Tuition per yr: $1,000 res, $2,300 non-res

Minnesota

Alexandria Technical College
Clin Lab Tech/Med Lab Tech-C Prgm
1601 Jefferson St
Alexandria, MN 56308
Prgm Dir: Judith A Hoffman, MT(ASCP)
Tel: 320 762-0221
Med Dir: Gerald Obert, MD
Class Cap: 34 *Begins:* Sep
Length: 19 mos *Award:* Dipl
Tuition per yr: $1,674

Mayo Clinic/Mayo Foundation
Clin Lab Tech/Med Lab Tech-C Prgm
Sch Hlth Related Sciences
200 First St SW
Rochester, MN 55905
Prgm Dir: Joan T Converse, MA MT(ASCP)
Tel: 507 284-6008 *Fax:* 507 284-9758
E-mail: converse.joan@msgw.mayo.edu
Med Dir: Alvaro Pineda, MD
Class Cap: 24 *Begins:* Sep
Length: 21 mos *Award:* Cert, AS
Tuition per yr: $2,053 res, $4,106 non-res

Nevada

University of Nevada - Reno
Clin Lab Tech/Med Lab Tech-C Prgm
School of Medicine
300 Mackay Science Bldg
Reno, NV 89557-0046
Prgm Dir: Kenneth T Machara, PhD MT(ASCP)
Tel: 702 784-4846
Med Dir: Dennis A Mackey, MD
Begins: Aug
Length: 24 mos *Award:* Cert
Tuition per yr: $1,300 res, $4,300 non-res

New Jersey

Ocean County College
Clin Lab Tech/Med Lab Tech-C Prgm
Nursing and Health Technology
Ocean County College Dr
Toms River, NJ 08754
Prgm Dir: Linda Caltagirone, MS MT(ASCP)
Tel: 908 255-4000 *Fax:* 908 255-0418
E-mail: caltagir@pilot.njin.net
Med Dir: Stewart Miller, MD FCAP
Class Cap: 9 *Begins:* Aug
Length: 11 mos *Award:* Cert, AAS
Tuition per yr: $1,769 res, $2,079 non-res
Evening or weekend classes available

New York

Samaritan Medical Center
Clin Lab Tech/Med Lab Tech-C Prgm
830 Washington St
Watertown, NY 13601
Prgm Dir: Patricia Jaacks, MT(ASCP)
Tel: 315 785-4000 *Fax:* 315 785-4233
Med Dir: Joven G Kuan, MD
Class Cap: 10 *Begins:* Aug
Length: 12 mos *Award:* Cert

Ohio

Middletown Regional Hospital
Clin Lab Tech/Med Lab Tech-C Prgm
105 McKnight Dr
Middletown, OH 45044-8787
Prgm Dir: Jan E Schuster, MT(ASCP)
Tel: 513 420-5027 *Fax:* 513 420-5673
Med Dir: Barbara Steel, MD
Begins: Aug
Length: 12 mos *Award:* Cert

Pennsylvania

Chambersburg Hospital
Clin Lab Tech/Med Lab Tech-C Prgm
112 N Seventh St
Chambersburg, PA 17201
Prgm Dir: Virginia Regi, MT(ASCP)
Tel: 717 267-7970 *Fax:* 717 267-7127
Med Dir: Michael J Rupp, MD
Class Cap: 5 *Begins:* Jun
Length: 14 mos *Award:* Cert
Tuition per yr: $1,000
Evening or weekend classes available

Conemaugh Valley Memorial Hospital
Clin Lab Tech/Med Lab Tech-C Prgm
1086 Franklin St
Johnstown, PA 15905
Prgm Dir: Teresa A Palmer, MS MT(ASCP)SH
Tel: 814 534-9808 *Fax:* 814 534-3253
Med Dir: Vimal Mittal, MD
Class Cap: 12 *Begins:* Jul
Length: 12 mos *Award:* Cert
Tuition per yr: $2,500

Texas

Baptist Hospital, Orange
Clin Lab Tech/Med Lab Tech-C Prgm
608 Strickland
Orange, TX 77630
Prgm Dir: Jeanette Boehme, MT(ASCP)
Tel: 409 883-1137 *Fax:* 409 883-1176
Med Dir: Rolando Estrada-Gordillo, MD
Class Cap: 10 *Begins:* Aug Jan
Length: 12 mos *Award:* Cert

882 Training Group
Clin Lab Tech/Med Lab Tech-C Prgm
382 Training Squadron/BTL
917 Missile Rd/Ste 3
Sheppard AFB, TX 76311-2263
Prgm Dir: Maj Mark R Yager, MS MT(ASCP)
Tel: 817 676-3869 *Fax:* 817 676-3850
Med Dir: Anwar Kaleemullah, LtCol USAF MC
Class Cap: 448 *Begins:* Monthly
Length: 12 mos *Award:* Cert

Virginia

Centra Health Systems of Lynchburg
Clin Lab Tech/Med Lab Tech-C Prgm
3300 Rivermont Ave
Lynchburg, VA 24503
Prgm Dir: Robin L Smith, MEd BS MT(ASCP) SC
Tel: 804 947-4551 *Fax:* 804 947-4035
E-mail: robin.smith@centrahealth.com
Med Dir: James O Piggott, MD
Class Cap: 10 *Begins:* Aug
Length: 12 mos *Award:* Cert
Tuition per yr: $1,560
Evening or weekend classes available

Riverside Regional Med Ctr - Newport News
Clin Lab Tech/Med Lab Tech-C Prgm
12420 Warwick Blvd 6-G
Newport News, VA 23606
Prgm Dir: Barbara F Copeland, BS MT(ASCP)
Tel: 804 594-2722 *Fax:* 804 594-3063
Med Dir: Carol M Caplan, MD
Class Cap: 4 *Begins:* Jul
Length: 12 mos *Award:* Cert
Tuition per yr: $1,600 res, $1,900 non-res

Washington

Clover Park Technical College
Clin Lab Tech/Med Lab Tech-C Prgm
4500 Steilacoom Blvd SW
Tacoma, WA 98499-4098
Prgm Dir: Anne G O'Neil, MT(ASCP)
Tel: 206 589-5625 *Fax:* 206 589-5866
Med Dir: Sam J Insalaco, MD
Class Cap: 12 *Begins:* Mar
Length: 12 mos *Award:* Cert
Tuition per yr: $2,189

West Virginia

Dept of Veterans Affairs Medical Center
Clin Lab Tech/Med Lab Tech-C Prgm
200 Veterans Ave
Beckley, WV 25801
Prgm Dir: Beverley Jarrett, MS MT(ASCP)
Tel: 304 255-2121
Med Dir: Robert C Belding, MD
Begins: May
Length: 12 mos *Award:* Cert
Tuition per yr: $5,040

Bluefield Regional Medical Center
Clin Lab Tech/Med Lab Tech-C Prgm
500 Cherry St
Bluefield, WV 24701
Prgm Dir: Vickie L Cunningham, MS
  MT(ASCP)SH
Tel: 304 327-1596 *Fax:* 304 327-1591
Med Dir: Dennis I Pullins, MD
Class Cap: 6 *Begins:* Aug
Length: 12 mos *Award:* Cert
Tuition per yr: $1,500

Histologic Technician- Associate Degree

Delaware

Delaware Tech & Comm Coll - Wilmington
Histologic Technician-AD Prgm
Allied Hlth Dept
333 Shipley St
Wilmington, DE 19801
Prgm Dir: Mary Celene Kowalski, HT/HTL(ASCP)
Tel: 302 733-3661 *Fax:* 302 733-3686
Med Dir: A Clinton Hewes, MD
Class Cap: 6 *Begins:* Sep
Length: 21 mos *Award:* AAS
Tuition per yr: $1,146 res, $2,865 non-res
Evening or weekend classes available

Florida

Florida Community College - Jacksonville
Histologic Technician-AD Prgm
FCCJ N Campus
4501 Capper Rd
Jacksonville, FL 32218
Prgm Dir: Merry A Carter, MED MT(ASCP) SC
Tel: 904 766-6511 *Fax:* 904 766-6654
E-mail: mcarter@fccjvm.fcci.cc.fl.us
Med Dir: Nancy Lammert, MD
Class Cap: 10 *Begins:* Aug
Length: 24 mos *Award:* AS
Tuition per yr: $2,903 res, $10,959 non-res
Evening or weekend classes available

Maryland

Harford Community College
Histologic Technician-AD Prgm
401 Thomas Run Rd
Bel Air, MD 21014
Prgm Dir: Floyd M Grimm III, MEd
Tel: 410 836-4372 *Fax:* 410 836-4410
E-mail: fgrimm@harford.cc.md.us
Med Dir: Ramiro Lindado, MD
Begins: Sep
Length: 24 mos *Award:* AAS
Tuition per yr: $2,169 res, $3,441 non-res
Evening or weekend classes available

Minnesota

Medical Institute of Minnesota
Histologic Technician-AD Prgm
5503 Green Valley Dr
Bloomington, MN 55437
Prgm Dir: Anna Franklin, MT(ASCP)
Tel: 612 844-0064 *Fax:* 612 844-0671
Med Dir: Augustin Dalmasso, MD
Class Cap: 12 *Begins:* Jan Apr Jul Oct
Length: 21 mos *Award:* AAS
Tuition per yr: $7,275
Evening or weekend classes available

Fergus Falls Community College
Histologic Technician-AD Prgm
1414 College Way
Fergus Falls, MN 56537
Prgm Dir: Carol Bischof, HT(ASCP) MS
Tel: 218 739-7529 *Fax:* 218 739-7475
Med Dir: Greg Smith, MD
Class Cap: 6 *Begins:* Sep
Length: 18 mos *Award:* AS
Tuition per yr: $2,756 res, $5,299 non-res
Evening or weekend classes available

New York

SUNY Agric & Tech College at Cobleskill
Histologic Technician-AD Prgm
Rte 7
Cobleskill, NY 12043
Prgm Dir: Pamela Colony, PhD
Tel: 518 234-5417 *Fax:* 518 234-5333
E-mail: colonyp@cobleskill.edu
Med Dir: Russell E Newkirk, MD
Class Cap: 25 *Begins:* Aug Jan
Length: 24 mos *Award:* Dipl, AAS
Tuition per yr: $3,200 res, $8,300 non-res

Pennsylvania

Western Sch of Hlth & Business Careers
Histologic Technician-AD Prgm
421 Seventh Ave
Pittsburgh Campus
Pittsburgh, PA 15219-1907
Prgm Dir: Luigi M Mascio, BS HTL HT(ASCP)
Tel: 412 281-2600
Med Dir: H E Fenner, MD
Class Cap: 20 *Begins:* Sep Jan
Length: 15 mos *Award:* AST
Tuition per yr: $11,200 res, $11,200 non-res

Washington

Shoreline Community College
Histologic Technician-AD Prgm
16101 Greenwood Ave N
Seattle, WA 98133
Prgm Dir: Linda Brinkley, CLS(NCA)MT(ASCP)
Tel: 206 546-4710 *Fax:* 206 546-5826
Med Dir: Charles R Simrell, MD
Begins: Sep
Length: 23 mos *Award:* AAS
Tuition per yr: $1,853 res, $7,333 non-res

Wisconsin

Chippewa Valley Technical College
Histologic Technician-AD Prgm
620 W Clairemont Ave
Eau Claire, WI 54701
Prgm Dir: Patti Traphagan, HT(ASCP)
Tel: 715 833-6426 *Fax:* 715 835-6470
Med Dir: Thomas Hadley, MD
Class Cap: 16 *Begins:* Aug
Length: 20 mos *Award:* AS
Tuition per yr: $2,063 res, $13,800 non-res

Programs

Histologic Technician- Certificate

Alabama

Baptist Health System Inc
Histologic Technician-Cert Prgm
800 Montclair Rd
Birmingham, AL 35213
Prgm Dir: Patricia L Couch
Tel: 205 592-5389 *Fax:* 205 592-5646
Med Dir: George V Eisenhart, MD
Class Cap: 4 *Begins:* Jan
Length: 12 mos *Award:* Cert

Arkansas

Baptist Medical System
Histologic Technician-Cert Prgm
11900 Colonel Glenn Rd
Ste 1000
Little Rock, AR 72210-2820
Prgm Dir: Tamera J Quattlebaum, BS HT(ASCP)
Tel: 501 223-7412 *Fax:* 501 223-7406
Med Dir: Charles Sullivan, MD
Class Cap: 4 *Begins:* Jul
Length: 12 mos *Award:* Cert
Tuition per yr: $1,700

Colorado

Centura Health
Histologic Technician-Cert Prgm
2215 N Cascade Ave/PO Box 7021
Colorado Springs, CO 80933
Prgm Dir: Rose Virginia Brown, MEd MT(ASCP)
  CLS(NCA)
Tel: 719 776-5227 *Fax:* 719 776-5584
Med Dir: John Hegstrom, MD
Class Cap: 3 *Begins:* Aug
Length: 12 mos *Award:* Cert

Connecticut

Hartford Hospital
Histologic Technician-Cert Prgm
80 Seymour St
Hartford, CT 06115
Prgm Dir: Zoe Ann Durkin, MEd HT(ASCP)
Tel: 860 545-2611 *Fax:* 860 545-4250
Med Dir: Paul Cohen, MD
Class Cap: 6 *Begins:* Jan
Length: 12 mos *Award:* Cert
Tuition per yr: $2,000

Florida

Univ of Miami/Jackson Memorial Hosp
Histologic Technician-Cert Prgm
1611 NW 12th Ave
E Tower 2130
Miami, FL 33136
Prgm Dir: Bonnie M Cohen, HTL(ASCP)
Tel: 305 585-6044
Med Dir: Marie Valdes-Dapena, MD
Class Cap: 5 *Begins:* Sep
Length: 12 mos *Award:* Cert
Tuition per yr: $750

Georgia

St Joseph Hospital
Histologic Technician-Cert Prgm
5665 Peachtree-Dunwoody Rd NE
Atlanta, GA 30342
Prgm Dir: Kathleen Herris, HT/HTL(ASCP)
Tel: 404 851-7225 *Fax:* 404 851-7376
Med Dir: L David Stacy, MD
Class Cap: 4 *Begins:* Aug
Length: 12 mos *Award:* Cert

Illinois

Methodist Medical Center of Illinois
Histologic Technician-Cert Prgm
221 NE Glen Oak Ave
Peoria, IL 61636
Prgm Dir: Linda Hay, HT(ASCP)
Tel: 309 672-5994
Med Dir: Kathryn Kramer, MD
Begins: Jun
Length: 12 mos *Award:* Cert

St Francis Medical Center
Histologic Technician-Cert Prgm
530 NE Glen Oak Ave
Peoria, IL 61637
Prgm Dir: Cathy Moewe, MS MT(ASCP)CS
Tel: 309 655-3838 *Fax:* 309 655-7658
E-mail: camoewe@heartland.bradley.edu
Med Dir: Michael P Hayes, MD
Begins: Aug *Award:* Cert

Michigan

DMC University Laboratories
Histologic Technician-Cert Prgm
4707 St Antoine Blvd
Detroit, MI 48201
Prgm Dir: Patricia A Donner, HT/HTL(ASCP)
Tel: 313 745-0847 *Fax:* 313 993-8862
Med Dir: W Dwayne Lawrence, MD
Begins: Jan
Length: 6 mos *Award:* Cert

Hurley Medical Center
Histologic Technician-Cert Prgm
Number One Hurley Plaza
Flint, MI 48503
Tel: 810 257-9948 *Fax:* 810 762-7082
Med Dir: Willys Mueller, Jr, MD
Class Cap: 4 *Begins:* Jan Jul
Length: 6 mos *Award:* Cert
Tuition per yr: $990

Davenport College - Lansing
Histologic Technician-Cert Prgm
611 Hagadorn Rd
Mason, MI 48854-9330
Prgm Dir: Elizabeth Toy-Krummrey, MA
  HT(ASCP)
Tel: 517 676-1051, Ext 1357
Med Dir: Patricia K Senagore, MD
Class Cap: 6 *Begins:* Sep
Length: 20 mos *Award:* Cert

William Beaumont Hospital
Histologic Technician-Cert Prgm
3601 W Thirteen Mile Rd
Royal Oak, MI 48073-6769
Prgm Dir: Peggy A Wenk, BS HTL(ASCP)
Tel: 810 551-9079 *Fax:* 810 551-9054
Med Dir: Ali-Reza Armin, MD
Class Cap: 2 *Begins:* Sep
Length: 6 mos *Award:* Cert

Missouri

Trinity Lutheran Hospital
Histologic Technician-Cert Prgm
3030 Baltimore Ave
Kansas City, MO 64108
Prgm Dir: Marsha Danley, HT(ASCP)
Tel: 816 751-2430
Med Dir: Gerardo G Vergara, MD
Class Cap: 2 *Begins:* Feb
Length: 12 mos *Award:* Cert
Tuition per yr: $800

Truman Medical Center
Histologic Technician-Cert Prgm
2301 Holmes
Kansas City, MO 64108
Prgm Dir: Robert Burns, HT(ASCP)
Tel: 816 556-3228 *Fax:* 816 556-3942
Med Dir: Peter Kragel, MD
Class Cap: 3 *Begins:* Feb May
Length: 12 mos *Award:* Cert
Tuition per yr: $900

New Jersey

Cooper Hospital/University Medical Ctr
Histologic Technician-Cert Prgm
One Cooper Plaza
Camden, NJ 08103
Prgm Dir: Diana M Hullihen, BS MT(ASCP)
Tel: 609 342-2456 *Fax:* 609 342-9718
Med Dir: Edison Catalano, MD
Class Cap: 2 *Begins:* Sep
Length: 12 mos *Award:* Cert
Tuition per yr: $675

Mountainside Hospital
Histologic Technician-Cert Prgm
Bay and Highland Aves
Glen Ridge/Montclair, NJ 07042
Prgm Dir: Erika T Carlson, MT(ASCP)
Tel: 201 429-6176
Med Dir: Stephen C Kimler, MD
Class Cap: 2 *Begins:* Aug
Length: 12 mos *Award:* Cert
Tuition per yr: $1,000

Ohio

Columbus State Community College
Histologic Technician-Cert Prgm
550 E Spring St
Columbus, OH 43215
Prgm Dir: Beverly M Kovanda, PhD MT(ASCP)
Tel: 614 227-2608   *Fax:* 614 885-4966
Med Dir: Ben Mertens, MD
Class Cap: 12   *Begins:* Jun
Length: 12 mos   *Award:* Cert
Tuition per yr: $2,750 res, $7,296 non-res

Pennsylvania

Geisinger Medical Center
Histologic Technician-Cert Prgm
100 N Academy Ave
Danville, PA 17822
Prgm Dir: Alvin Swartzentruber, MT(ASCP)
Tel: 717 271-6700   *Fax:* 717 271-6105
Med Dir: Conrad Schuerch, MD
Class Cap: 2   *Begins:* Jul
Length: 12 mos   *Award:* Cert
Tuition per yr: $870

Conemaugh Valley Memorial Hospital
Histologic Technician-Cert Prgm
1086 Franklin St
Johnstown, PA 15905
Prgm Dir: Charles Shustrick, HT(ASCP)
Tel: 814 533-9797   *Fax:* 814 533-9372
Med Dir: Waheeb R Rizkalla, MD
Class Cap: 6   *Begins:* Aug
Length: 12 mos   *Award:* Cert
Tuition per yr: $2,500

Texas

Methodist Hospital
Histologic Technician-Cert Prgm
6565 Fannin
B154
Houston, TX 77030
Prgm Dir: Judy Jobe, MT(ASCP)
Tel: 713 790-2599   *Fax:* 713 793-7408
E-mail: jjobe@profsvcs.tmh.tm.edu
Med Dir: Richard Brown, MD
Class Cap: 2   *Begins:* Aug
Length: 12 mos   *Award:* Cert

Univ of Texas M D Anderson Cancer Ctr
Histologic Technician-Cert Prgm
1515 Holcombe Blvd
PO Box 85
Houston, TX 77030
Prgm Dir: Beverly Plocharski, HTL(ASCP)
Tel: 713 792-3118   *Fax:* 713 794-1695
Med Dir: Alberto G Ayala, MD
Class Cap: 4   *Begins:* Aug
Length: 12 mos   *Award:* Cert

University of Texas Health Science Ctr
Histologic Technician-Cert Prgm
Dept of Pathology
7703 Floyd Curl Dr
San Antonio, TX 78284
Prgm Dir: Margaret S Judge, HTL(ASCP)
Tel: 210 567-4057   *Fax:* 210 567-6729
E-mail: judge@uthscsa.edu
Med Dir: D Craig Allred, MD
Class Cap: 2   *Begins:* Aug
Length: 12 mos   *Award:* Cert

Wisconsin

St Joseph's Hospital
Histologic Technician-Cert Prgm
611 St Joseph Ave
Marshfield, WI 54449-1898
Prgm Dir: Virginia R Narlock, PhD CLS(NCA) MT(ASCP)
Tel: 715 387-7202   *Fax:* 715 387-7121
Med Dir: Kurt D Reed, MD
Class Cap: 4   *Begins:* Mar Sep
Length: 12 mos   *Award:* Cert

Histotechnologist

Illinois

St John's Hospital
Histotechnologst Prgm
800 E Carpenter
Springfield, IL 62769
Prgm Dir: Gilma Roncancio, MS MT(ASCP)
Tel: 217 544-6464   *Fax:* 217 535-3996
Med Dir: Donald Van Fossan, MD PhD
Begins: Jun
Length: 12 mos   *Award:* Cert
Tuition per yr: $3,000

Michigan

William Beaumont Hospital
Histotechnologist Prgm
3601 W 13 Mile Rd
Royal Oak, MI 48073-6769
Prgm Dir: Peggy Wenk, BS HTL(ASCP)
Tel: 810 551-9079   *Fax:* 810 551-9054
Med Dir: Ali-Reza Armin, MD
Class Cap: 4   *Begins:* Sep
Length: 12 mos   *Award:* BS

North Carolina

Presbyterian Hospital
Histotechnologist Prgm
PO Box 33549
Charlotte, NC 28233-3549
Prgm Dir: Jane Ingram, BS HTL(ASCP)
Tel: 704 384-7647   *Fax:* 704 384-7615
Med Dir: William K Poston Jr, MD
Class Cap: 4   *Begins:* Jan
Length: 12 mos   *Award:* Cert
Tuition per yr: $1,035

Programs

Pathologists' Assistant

Michigan

Wayne State University College of Pharmacy and Allied Health

Pathologists' Assistant Prgm
627 W Alexandrine
Detroit, MI 48801
Prgm Dir: Mary Louise Fritts-Williams, PhD
Tel: 313 577-2050
Med Dir: Nilsa Ramirez, MD
Begins: Aug
Length: 24 mos   *Award:* BS

North Carolina

Duke University Medical Ctr Department of Pathology

Pathologists' Assistant Prgm
Box 3712
Durham, NC 27710
Prgm Dir: James G Lewis, PhD
Tel: 919 684-2159
Med Dir: Alan Proia, MD
Begins: Aug
Length: 22 mos   *Award:* MS

Cytotechnologist

History

In the pioneer days of clinical pathology, it was the rare pathologist who did not have an assistant. These first technical "assistants," some of whom were trained by George N Papanicolaou, MD, famed American anatomist and cytologist, were always the product of an apprentice-type training. As their number and the number of apprentice programs grew, there was a need to certify that the apprentices had indeed learned their tasks well. The Board of Registry of the American Society of Clinical Pathologists (ASCP) offered the examination for the cytology technician for the first time in 1957.

Five years later, in 1962, the *Standards (Essentials) of an Acceptable School for the Cytotechnologist* were developed by the Cytology Committee of the ASCP and the ASCP Board of Schools and were adopted by the House of Delegates of the American Medical Association (AMA). Until 1975, representatives of the ASCP served on the Cytotechnology Review Committee of the National Accrediting Agency for Clinical Laboratory Sciences (NAACLS), which replaced the ASCP Board of Schools in 1974. In 1975, the American Society of Cytopathology (ASC) was recognized as the organization that would collaborate with the AMA Council on Medical Education (CME), and the ASC formed the Cytotechnology Programs Review Committee, which assumed the responsibilities formerly handled by NAACLS. In 1977, 1983, and 1992, the cytotechnology *Standards and Guidelines* were revised and adopted by the AMA CME and the ASC. In 1996, the *Essentials* were renamed *Standards* and adopted by the Committee on Accreditation of Allied Health Education Programs in conjunction with the CoA and sponsoring organizations.

Occupational Description

Cytology is the study of the structure and the function of cells. Cytotechnologists are specially trained technologists who work with pathologists to detect changes in body cells that may be important in the early diagnosis of cancer and other diseases. This is done primarily with the microscope to evaluate slide preparations of body cells for abnormalities in structure, indicating either benign or malignant conditions.

Job Description

Using special techniques, cytotechnologists prepare cellular samples for study under the microscope and assist in the diagnosis of disease by examining the samples. Cell specimens may be obtained from various body sites, such as the female reproductive tract, the oral cavity, the lung, or any body cavity shedding cells. Using the findings of cytotechnologists, the physician is then able in many instances to diagnose cancer and other diseases long before they can be detected by other methods. Cytologic techniques also can be used to detect diseases involving hormonal abnormalities and other pathological disease processes. In recent years, fine needles have been used to aspirate lesions, often deeply seated in the body, thus greatly enhancing the ability to diagnose tumors located in otherwise inaccessible sites.

Employment Characteristics

Most cytotechnologists work in hospitals or in commercial laboratories, while some prefer to work on research projects or to teach. Employment opportunities vary, depending on geographic location, experience, and ability. The demand for trained cytotechnologists varies by geographic area. According to the 1994 ASCP Wage and Vacancy Survey, entry-level salaries average $28,579.

Educational Programs

Length. The length of the program depends significantly on its organizational structure. In general, after completion of the prerequisite course work, at least 1 calendar year of structured professional instruction in cytotechnology is necessary to achieve program objectives and to establish entry-level competencies.

Prerequisites. Applicants should be well grounded in the biological sciences and in basic chemistry. This entails successful completion of at least 20 semester hours (30 quarter hours) in the biological sciences, chemistry courses equaling or exceeding 8 semester hours (12 quarter hours), and some mathematics.

Curriculum. The curriculum includes the historical background of cytology, cytology as applied in clinical medicine, and cytology in the evaluation of tumor cells obtained following spontaneous exfoliation or by needle aspiration biopsy. Other areas of study include anatomy, histology, embryology, cytochemistry, cytophysiology, endocrinology, and inflammatory diseases.

Standards. *Standards* are minimum educational standards developed and initially adopted in 1962 by the ASC in collaboration with the AMA. Each new program is assessed in accordance with the *Standards*, and established programs are reviewed periodically to determine whether they continue to meet the standards. The *Standards* are available on written request from the American Society of Cytopathology.

Inquiries

Accreditation

Requests for information on program accreditation, including the *Standards,* preparing the self-study report, and arranging a site visit, should be submitted to

American Society of Cytopathology
Cytotechnology Programs Review Committee
400 W 9th St/Ste 201
Wilmington, DE 19801
302 429-8802

Careers

Inquiries regarding careers and curriculum should be addressed to

American Society of Cytopathology
400 W 9th St/Ste 201
Wilmington, DE 19801
302 429-8802

Certification/Registration

Inquiries regarding certification may be addressed to

Board of Registry
PO Box 12270
Chicago, IL 60612

Cytotechnologist

Alabama

University of Alabama at Birmingham
Cytotechnologist Prgm
Sch of Hlth Related Professions
UAB Station-SHRP 381J
Birmingham, AL 35294-1270
Prgm Dir: Gunvanti Shah, SCT(ASCP) CMIAC
Tel: 205 934-3811   *Fax:* 205 975-7302
E-mail: shrp085@uabdpo.dpo.uab.edu
Med Dir: William Rodgers, MD
Class Cap: 12   *Begins:* Sep
Length: 12 mos   *Award:* Cert, BS
Tuition per yr: $3,840 res, $7,680 non-res
Evening or weekend classes available

Arkansas

Univ of Arkansas for Medical Sciences
Cytotechnologist Prgm
VA Med Ctr (UAMS/VAMC)
4301 W Markham/Slot 517
Little Rock, AR 72205
Prgm Dir: Wanda Culbreth, MA CT(ASCP)
Tel: 501 686-5618   *Fax:* 501 296-1184
Med Dir: Michael W Stanley, MD
Class Cap: 6   *Begins:* Jul
Length: 12 mos   *Award:* BS
Tuition per yr: $2,672 res, $6,672 non-res

California

Loma Linda University
Cytotechnologist Prgm
Dept of Clinical Laboratory Science
Loma Linda, CA 92350
Prgm Dir: Marlene Ota, CT(ASCP)
Tel: 909 824-4966   *Fax:* 909 824-4817
Med Dir: Darryl Heustis, MD
Class Cap: 6   *Begins:* Aug Sep
Length: 12 mos, 6 mos   *Award:* Cert, BS
Tuition per yr: $15,498 res, $15,498 non-res

Los Angeles County - USC Medical Center
Cytotechnologist Prgm
1200 N State St
Rm 16-638
Los Angeles, CA 90033
Prgm Dir: Carol A Carriere, CT(ASCP) CMIAC
Tel: 213 226-7212   *Fax:* 213 226-7476
Med Dir: S E Martin, MD PhD
Class Cap: 6   *Begins:* Aug
Length: 12 mos   *Award:* Cert

UCLA Center for Health Sciences
Cytotechnologist Prgm
10833 Le Conte Ave
Los Angeles, CA 90024-1732
Prgm Dir: Carole Williams, SCT(ASCP) CFIAC
Tel: 310 825-9102   *Fax:* 310 206-8108
E-mail: cwilliam@pathology.medsch.ucla.edu
Med Dir: Roberta K Nieberg, MD
Class Cap: 6   *Begins:* Aug
Length: 12 mos   *Award:* BS, MS
Tuition per yr: $930 res, $4,428 non-res

Connecticut

University of Connecticut Health Center

Cytotechnologist Prgm
263 Farmington Ave
Farmington, CT 06030
Prgm Dir: Nancy J Smith, MS SCT(ASCP)
Tel: 860 679-4215   *Fax:* 860 679-4334
E-mail: nsmith@nso1.uchc.edu
Med Dir: M Melinda Sanders, MD
Class Cap: 6   *Begins:* Aug
Length: 12 mos, 24 mos   *Award:* Dipl,Cert, BS
Tuition per yr: $3,900 res, $11,890 non-res

Florida

University Medical Center

Cytotechnologist Prgm
Univ of FL Hlth Sci Ctr
655 W Eighth St
Jacksonville, FL 32209
Prgm Dir: Shahla Masood, MD
Tel: 904 549-4668   *Fax:* 904 549-4629
Med Dir: Shahla Masood, MD
Class Cap: 6   *Begins:* Aug
Length: 12 mos   *Award:* Cert
Tuition per yr: $3,000 res, $4,000 non-res

Georgia

Grady Health System

Cytotechnologist Prgm
80 Butler St SE
PO Box 26095
Atlanta, GA 30335
Prgm Dir: Dean Willis, SCT(ASCP)
Tel: 404 616-3650   *Fax:* 404 616-9913
Med Dir: George Birdsong, MD
Class Cap: 4   *Begins:* Oct
Length: 12 mos   *Award:* Cert
Tuition per yr: $800

Illinois

Michael Reese Hospital

Cytotechnologist Prgm
2929 S Ellis Ave
Chicago, IL 60616-3390
Prgm Dir: Eleanor V Rabin, MD PhD
Tel: 312 791-2745
Med Dir: Enrique Beckmann, MD PhD
Class Cap: 8   *Begins:* Sep
Length: 12 mos   *Award:* Cert
Tuition per yr: $10,000

Indiana

Indiana University School of Medicine

Cytotechnologist Prgm
Medical Science Bldg
635 Barnhill Dr/Rm B029
Indianapolis, IN 46202-5120
Prgm Dir: William N Crabtree, MS SCT(ASCP)
Tel: 317 274-0040   *Fax:* 317 278-2018
Med Dir: Liang Che-Tao, MD
Class Cap: 8   *Begins:* Aug
Length: 12 mos   *Award:* Dipl, BS
Tuition per yr: $3,715 res, $12,400 non-res
Evening or weekend classes available

Iowa

Mercy Hospital Medical Center

Cytotechnologist Prgm
400 University
Des Moines, IA 50314-3190
Prgm Dir: Marty Boesenberg, SCT(ASCP)
Tel: 515 247-4466   *Fax:* 515 248-8810
Med Dir: Joy E Trueblood, MD
Class Cap: 4   *Begins:* Jul
Length: 12 mos   *Award:* Cert
Tuition per yr: $3,500

Kansas

University of Kansas Medical Center

Cytotechnologist Prgm
3901 Rainbow Blvd
Kansas City, KS 66160
Prgm Dir: Marilee Means, PhD SCT(ASCP)
Tel: 913 588-1179   *Fax:* 913 588-1195
E-mail: mmeans@kumc.edu
Med Dir: Paramjit Bhatia, MD
Class Cap: 4   *Begins:* Aug
Length: 12 mos   *Award:* BS
Tuition per yr: $2,252 res, $9,110 non-res

Kentucky

Pathology and Cytology Laboratories, Inc

Cytotechnologist Prgm
290 Big Run Rd
Lexington, KY 40503
Prgm Dir: Ivan Eads, MS SCT(ASCP)
Tel: 606 278-9513   *Fax:* 606 277-6063
Med Dir: Tamara L Sanderson, MD
Class Cap: 10   *Begins:* Aug
Length: 12 mos   *Award:* Cert, BS
Tuition per yr: $8,000 res, $8,000 non-res

University of Louisville

Cytotechnologist Prgm
K Wing Bldg/Rm #4042
Louisville, KY 40292
Prgm Dir: Mary Beth Adams, MEd SCT(ASCP)
Tel: 502 852-8295   *Fax:* 502 852-4597
E-mail: meadam01@ulkyvm.louisville.edu
Med Dir: Catherine L Sewell, MD
Class Cap: 8   *Begins:* Jan Aug
Length: 16 mos, 21 mos   *Award:* Cert, BHS
Tuition per yr: $3,705 res, $10,485 non-res

Maryland

Johns Hopkins Hospital

Cytotechnologist Prgm
600 N Wolfe St
412 Path Bldg
Baltimore, MD 21287
Prgm Dir: Yener S Erozan, MD
Tel: 410 955-1180   *Fax:* 410 955-3438
E-mail: yerozinepattlan.path.jfu.edu
Med Dir: Yener S Erozan, MD
Class Cap: 5   *Begins:* Sep
Length: 12 mos   *Award:* Cert
Tuition per yr: $7,000

Naval School of Health Sciences - MD

Cytotechnologist Prgm
Bethesda, MD 20889-5611
Prgm Dir: Gerald Frizzell, HMC USN SCT
Tel: 301 295-0733   *Fax:* 301 295-0621
E-mail: frizzell@nshao.med.navy.mil
Med Dir: Mazhar Rishi, MD, Major, USAF, MC
Class Cap: 12   *Begins:* Jul Mar
Length: 12 mos   *Award:* Cert

Massachusetts

Berkshire Medical Center

Cytotechnologist Prgm
725 North St
Pittsfield, MA 01201
Prgm Dir: Judith R Shaffer, SCT(ASCP) BS
Tel: 413 447-2590   *Fax:* 413 447-2097
Med Dir: Rebecca L Johnson, MD
Class Cap: 4   *Begins:* Sep
Length: 12 mos   *Award:* Cert
Tuition per yr: $3,500 res, $3,500 non-res

Michigan

DMC University Laboratories

Cytotechnologist Prgm
4201 St Antoine
Detroit, MI 48201
Prgm Dir: Ursula K Bedrossian, PhD MT CT(ASCP)
Tel: 313 745-4568   *Fax:* 313 993-0489
E-mail: bedrosian2@aol.com
Med Dir: Carlos Bedrossian, MD
Class Cap: 8   *Begins:* Sep
Length: 12 mos   *Award:* Cert, BS

Henry Ford Hospital

Cytotechnologist Prgm
2799 W Grand Blvd WC 608
Detroit, MI 48202
Prgm Dir: Sudha R Kini, MD
Tel: 313 876-2352   *Fax:* 313 876-2385
Med Dir: Sudha R Kini, MD
Class Cap: 5   *Begins:* Sep
Length: 12 mos   *Award:* Cert, BS
Tuition per yr: $2,000 res, $2,000 non-res

Minnesota

Mayo Clinic/Mayo Foundation

Cytotechnologist Prgm
Sch Hlth Related Sciences
200 First St SW
Rochester, MN 55905
Prgm Dir: Jill L Caudill, MEd SCT(ASCP)
Tel: 507 284-1142 *Fax:* 507 284-1599
E-mail: caudill.jill@mayo.edu
Med Dir: J R Goellner, MD
Class Cap: 6 *Begins:* Aug
Length: 12 mos *Award:* Cert
Tuition per yr: $2,500

Mississippi

University of Mississippi Medical Center

Cytotechnologist Prgm
2500 N State St
Jackson, MS 39216
Prgm Dir: Zelma Cason, SCT(ASCP)
Tel: 601 984-6358 *Fax:* 601 984-6768
E-mail: cason@shrp.umsmed.edu
Med Dir: Lucianno B Lemos, MD
Class Cap: 12 *Begins:* Aug
Length: 18 mos *Award:* Dipl, BS
Tuition per yr: $2,120 res, $4,579 non-res

Missouri

Truman Medical Center

Cytotechnologist Prgm
2301 Holmes St
Kansas City, MO 64108
Prgm Dir: Sandra McGuire, CT(ASCP)
Tel: 816 556-3960 *Fax:* 816 556-3942
Med Dir: Edward J Gutmann, MD
Class Cap: 4 *Begins:* Aug
Length: 12 mos *Award:* Cert
Tuition per yr: $6,000

Jewish Hosp-Coll of Nursing/Allied Hlth

Cytotechnologist Prgm
306 S Kingshighway Blvd
St Louis, MO 63110
Prgm Dir: Joan S Rossi, MA CT(ASCP)
Tel: 314 454-8655 *Fax:* 314 454-5239
Med Dir: Rosa Davila, MD
Class Cap: 12 *Begins:* June
Length: 12 mos *Award:* Cert, BS, CT
Tuition per yr: $10,000 res, $10,000 non-res

Nebraska

University of Nebraska Medical Center

Cytotechnologist Prgm
Pathology and Microbiology
Omaha, NE 68198
Prgm Dir: Karen A Allen, SCT(ASCP)
Tel: 402 559-7635 *Fax:* 402 559-6018
E-mail: kaallen@unmcvm.unmc.edu
Med Dir: Stanley J Radio, MD
Class Cap: 4 *Begins:* Aug
Length: 12 mos *Award:* Cert
Tuition per yr: $2,978 res, $7,358 non-res

Nevada

Associated Pathologists' Laboratories

Cytotechnologist Prgm
4230 S Burnham Ave
Las Vegas, NV 89119
Prgm Dir: Robert Gay, CT(ASCP)
Tel: 702 733-7866 *Fax:* 702 733-8941
Med Dir: David A Miller, MD
Class Cap: 10 *Begins:* Aug
Length: 12 mos *Award:* Cert
Tuition per yr: $5,500

New Jersey

Univ of Med & Dent of New Jersey

Cytotechnologist Prgm
Sch Hlth Related Professions
1776 Raritan Rd
Scotch Plains, NJ 07076
Prgm Dir: Cecilia B Vallejo, MD
Tel: 908 889-2424
Med Dir: Andrey Gritsman, MD
Class Cap: 8 *Begins:* Aug
Length: 12 mos *Award:* Cert, BS
Tuition per yr: $4,640 res, $6,187 non-res

New York

Albany Medical College

Cytotechnologist Prgm
47 New Scotland Ave/A81
Albany, NY 12208
Prgm Dir: Jean Taylor, MSEd SCT(ASCP)
Tel: 518 262-3938 *Fax:* 518 262-5927
Med Dir: Barbara McKenna, MD
Class Cap: 8 *Begins:* Sep
Length: 12 mos *Award:* Cert
Tuition per yr: $4,250

Bronx Lebanon Hospital Center

Cytotechnologist Prgm
1276 Fulton Ave
Bronx, NY 10456
Prgm Dir: Howard Panyu, MS CT(ASCP) MPA
Tel: 718 518-5169 *Fax:* 718 716-8242
Med Dir: Young J Choi, MD
Class Cap: 6 *Begins:* Sep
Length: 12 mos *Award:* Cert
Tuition per yr: $8,000

Memorial Sloan - Kettering Cancer Ctr

Cytotechnologist Prgm
1275 York Ave
New York, NY 10021
Prgm Dir: Rose Marie Gatscha, CT(ASCP)
Tel: 212 639-5902 *Fax:* 212 639-6318
E-mail: gatschar@mskcc.org
Med Dir: Patricia E Saigo, MD
Class Cap: 6 *Begins:* Aug
Length: 12 mos *Award:* Cert
Tuition per yr: $8,000 res, $8,000 non-res

New York Hospital

Cytotechnologist Prgm
525 E 68th St
New York, NY 10021
Prgm Dir: Frances Peteroski, SCT(ASCP)
Tel: 212 746-2808 *Fax:* 212 746-8624
Med Dir: June H Koizumi, MD
Begins: Sep
Length: 12 mos *Award:* Cert
Tuition per yr: $8,800

New York University Medical Center

Cytotechnologist Prgm
Bellevue Hospital
Cytopathology Dept 4S17D
New York, NY 10016
Prgm Dir: Angela I Shanerman, BA CT(ASCP)
Tel: 212 263-6455 *Fax:* 212 263-7649
Med Dir: Jerry Waisman, MD
Class Cap: 6 *Begins:* Aug
Length: 12 mos *Award:* Cert
Tuition per yr: $12,500 res, $12,500 non-res

SUNY School of Health Technology & Management

HSC Level 2-052
Stony Brook, NY 11794
Prgm Dir: Roberta Goodell, CT(ASCP)
Tel: 516 444-2403 *Fax:* 516 444-7621
Med Dir: Alan Heimann, MD
Class Cap: 4 *Award:* BS
Tuition per yr: $3,400 res, $8,300 non-res

SUNY Health Science Center at Syracuse

Cytotechnologist Prgm
750 E Adams St
Silverman Hall
Syracuse, NY 13210
Prgm Dir: Susan B Stowell, MA SCT(ASCP)
Tel: 315 464-6900 *Fax:* 315 464-6914
E-mail: towells@vax.cs.hscsyr.edu
Med Dir: Celeste Powers, MD
Class Cap: 10 *Begins:* Aug
Length: 12 mos *Award:* Dipl, BS
Tuition per yr: $5,237 res, $12,450 non-res

North Carolina

Univ of North Carolina at Chapel Hill

Cytotechnologist Prgm
Medical Allied Health Profs
CB 7120 Medical School Wing E
Chapel Hill, NC 27599-7120
Prgm Dir: Allen C Rinas, CT(ASCP)
Tel: 919 966-2339 *Fax:* 919 966-3678
E-mail: rinas@scc.unc.edu
Med Dir: Debra Novotny, MD
Class Cap: 5 *Begins:* Aug
Length: 12 mos *Award:* Cert

Central Piedmont Community College

Cytotechnologist Prgm
PO Box 35009
Charlotte, NC 28235
Prgm Dir: M Arlene Parrish, MS CT(ASCP)
Tel: 704 330-4084 *Fax:* 704 330-5930
Med Dir: Omar Idlibi, MD
Class Cap: 4 *Begins:* Aug
Length: 12 mos *Award:* Cert
Tuition per yr: $762 res, $6,040 non-res

East Carolina University
Cytotechnologist Prgm
Sch Allied Hlth Sciences
Dept of Clinical Lab Sciences
Greenville, NC 27858
Prgm Dir: Susan T Smith, PhD MT(ASCP)
Tel: 919 328-4417 *Fax:* 919 328-4470
E-mail: cjsmith@ecuvm.cis.ecu.edu
Med Dir: Jan F Silverman, MD
Class Cap: 6 *Begins:* Aug
Length: 21 mos *Award:* BS
Tuition per yr: $2,371 res, $12,634 non-res
Evening or weekend classes available

North Dakota

Univ of N Dakota Sch of Med and Hlth Sci
Cytotechnologist Prgm
PO Box 9037
Grand Forks, ND 58202-9037
Prgm Dir: Eric Thompson, SCT(ASCP)
Tel: 701 777-3011 *Fax:* 701 777-2311
E-mail: ethomso@mail.med.und.nodak.edu
Med Dir: Timothy L Wieland, MD
Class Cap: 6 *Begins:* Aug
Length: 12 mos *Award:* Cert, BS
Tuition per yr: $3,339 res, $8,184 non-res

Ohio

Akron General Medical Center
Cytotechnologist Prgm
400 Wabash Ave
Akron, OH 44307
Prgm Dir: Angela T Powell, MD
Tel: 330 384-6203 *Fax:* 330 384-6418
Med Dir: Angela T Powell, MD
Class Cap: 4 *Begins:* July
Length: 12 mos *Award:* Dipl,Cert, BS
Tuition per yr: $2,165 res, $2,165 non-res

St Luke's Medical Center
Cytotechnologist Prgm
11311 Shaker Blvd
Cleveland, OH 44104
Prgm Dir: Joseph A Boccia, MD
Tel: 216 368-7712
Med Dir: Joseph Boccia, MD
Class Cap: 4 *Begins:* Jun
Length: 12 mos *Award:* Cert, BA
Tuition per yr: $2,500 res, $2,500 non-res

St Elizabeth Health Center
Cytotechnologist Prgm
1044 Belmont Ave
Youngstown, OH 44501
Prgm Dir: Sue Herman, BS CT(ASCP)
Tel: 330 480-3459 *Fax:* 330 480-3459
Med Dir: Carl R Schaub, MD
Class Cap: 6 *Begins:* Jul
Length: 12 mos *Award:* Cert
Tuition per yr: $2,640

Oklahoma

University Hospitals
Cytotechnologist Prgm
PO Box 26307/EB400
Oklahoma City, OK 73126
Prgm Dir: Susan Townsend, MEd CT(ASCP)
Tel: 405 271-7732
Med Dir: Betty Jane McClellan, MD
Class Cap: 6 *Begins:* Sep
Length: 12 mos *Award:* Cert

Pennsylvania

Thomas Jefferson University
Cytotechnologist Prgm
130 S Ninth St/Ste 1924
Philadelphia, PA 19107-5233
Prgm Dir: Shirley E Greening, MS JD CT(ASCP)
Tel: 215 503-8561 *Fax:* 215 503-2189
E-mail: greenin1@jeflin.tju.edu
Med Dir: Ronald D Luff, MD
Class Cap: 32 *Begins:* Sep
Length: 12 mos, 20 mos *Award:* Cert, BS
Tuition per yr: $15,160 res, $15,160 non-res
Evening or weekend classes available

U Hlth Ctr Pittsburgh/Magee Women's Hosp
Cytotechnologist Prgm
Magee-Womens Hospital
300 Halket St
Pittsburgh, PA 15213
Prgm Dir: Anisa I Kanbour, MD
Tel: 412 641-4657 *Fax:* 412 641-1355
Med Dir: Anisa Kanbour, MD
Class Cap: 8 *Begins:* Jul
Length: 12 mos *Award:* Cert
Tuition per yr: $3,900 res, $3,900 non-res

Puerto Rico

University of Puerto Rico
Cytotechnologist Prgm
College of Allied Health
GPO Box 5067
San Juan, PR 00936
Prgm Dir: Ruth A Rodriguez, CT(ASCP)
Tel: 787 754-3536
Med Dir: Guillermo Villarmarzo, MD
Class Cap: 5 *Begins:* Aug
Length: 12 mos *Award:* Cert
Tuition per yr: $1,400 res, $3,000 non-res

Rhode Island

Our Lady of Fatima Hospital
Cytotechnologist Prgm
200 High Service Ave
North Providence, RI 02904
Prgm Dir: Ronald N Arpin III, BS CT(ASCP)
Tel: 401 456-3216 *Fax:* 401 456-3568
Med Dir: Salvatore R Allegra, MD
Class Cap: 8 *Begins:* Aug
Length: 11 mos *Award:* Cert, BS

Women & Infants' Hospital
Cytotechnologist Prgm
101 Dudley St
Providence, RI 02905
Prgm Dir: Naoma L Corvese, CT(ASCP) CFIAC
Tel: 401 453-7675 *Fax:* 401 453-7689
Med Dir: Stuart C Lauchlan, MB ChB
Class Cap: 8 *Begins:* Jul
Length: 12 mos *Award:* Cert, MS
Tuition per yr: $8,500 res, $8,500 non-res

South Carolina

Medical University of South Carolina
Cytotechnologist Prgm
Hlth Related Prof/Med Lab Sci
171 Ashley Ave
Charleston, SC 29425
Prgm Dir: E Blair Holladay, PhD CT(ASCP)
Tel: 803 792-3169 *Fax:* 803 792-3383
E-mail: holladab@muse.edu
Med Dir: Marshall Austin, MD PhD
Class Cap: 12 *Begins:* Aug
Length: 12 mos *Award:* Dipl, BS
Tuition per yr: $4,401 res, $12,822 non-res

South Dakota

LCM Pathologists PC
Cytotechnologist Prgm
1212 S Euclid Ave PO Box 5134
Sioux Falls, SD 57117-5134
Prgm Dir: Kathryn M Kairys, SCT(ASCP)
Tel: 605 333-1725 *Fax:* 605 333-1749
Med Dir: Richard D Schultz, MD
Class Cap: 6 *Begins:* Aug
Length: 12 mos *Award:* Cert
Tuition per yr: $3,500

Tennessee

Univ of Tennessee Med Ctr at Knoxville
Cytotechnologist Prgm
1924 Alcoa Hwy
Knoxville, TN 37920
Prgm Dir: Frederica Harrill, SCT(ASCP)
Tel: 423 544-9088 *Fax:* 423 544-6880
Med Dir: Stuart E VanMeter, MD
Class Cap: 4 *Begins:* Jan Jul
Length: 12 mos *Award:* Cert

University of Tennessee Memphis
Cytotechnologist Prgm
Coll of Allied Hlth Sciences
800 Madison Ave
Memphis, TN 38163
Prgm Dir: Barbara DuBray-Benstein, MS
  SCT(ASCP)
Tel: 901 448-6304 *Fax:* 901 448-7545
E-mail: bbenstein@utmem\.utmem.edu
Med Dir: Shamim Moinuddin, MD
Class Cap: 10 *Begins:* Jul
Length: 12 mos *Award:* BS
Tuition per yr: $4,151 res, $9,824 non-res

Texas

Brooke Army Medical Center

Cytotechnologist Prgm
US Army School
Dept of Pathology and ALS
Ft Sam Houston, TX 78234-6200
Prgm Dir: Hansa B Raval, MD
Tel: 210 916-9333
Med Dir: Hansa B Raval, MD
Class Cap: 25   *Begins:* Aug
Length: 12 mos   *Award:* Cert

Univ of Texas M D Anderson Cancer Ctr

Cytotechnologist Prgm
1515 Holcombe Blvd
PO Box 53
Houston, TX 77030
Prgm Dir: Christina M Alapat, MS CT(ASCP) IAC
Tel: 713 794-5877   *Fax:* 713 794-5664
Med Dir: Gregg A Staerkel, MD
Class Cap: 4   *Begins:* Aug
Length: 12 mos   *Award:* Cert
Tuition per yr: $1,000

University Hospital of San Antonio

Cytotechnologist Prgm
U of Texas Hlth Sciences Ctr
7703 Floyd Curl Dr
San Antonio, TX 78284
Prgm Dir: H Daniel Schantz, CT(ASCP) CMIAC
Tel: 210 567-6739   *Fax:* 210 567-2478
E-mail: schantz@uthscsa.edu
Med Dir: Philip T Valente, MD
Class Cap: 6   *Begins:* Aug
Length: 12 mos   *Award:* Cert
Tuition per yr: $1,000 res, $2,000 non-res

Utah

Univ of Utah Health Sciences Center

Cytotechnologist Prgm
ARUP Laboratory
500 Chipeta Way
Salt Lake City, UT 84108
Prgm Dir: Michael C Berry, BS CT(ASCP)
Tel: 801 581-5955   *Fax:* 801 583-2712
Med Dir: C Jay Marshall, MD
Class Cap: 4   *Begins:* Jun
Length: 12 mos   *Award:* Cert, BS
Tuition per yr: $3,350 res, $10,300 non-res

Vermont

Fletcher Allen Health Care

Cytotechnologist Prgm
111 Colchester Ave
Burlington, VT 05401
Prgm Dir: Sandra Giroux, SCT(ASCP) CMIAC
Tel: 802 656-5133   *Fax:* 802 656-3509
Med Dir: Matthew Zarka, MD
Class Cap: 7   *Begins:* Sep
Length: 12 mos   *Award:* Dipl,Cert, BS
Tuition per yr: $7,000 res, $7,000 non-res

Virginia

Old Dominion University

Cytotechnologist Prgm
Norfolk, VA 23529
Prgm Dir: Mohanraj Thomas, MS SCT(ASCP)
Tel: 757 683-3589, Ext 3016   *Fax:* 757 683-5028
E-mail: mxt100f@cranium.its.odu.edu
Med Dir: William Frable, MD
Class Cap: 12   *Begins:* Aug
Length: 12 mos   *Award:* BS
Tuition per yr: $5,670 res, $15,563 non-res
Evening or weekend classes available

Washington

Harborview Med Ctr - Univ of Washington

Cytotechnologist Prgm
325 Ninth Ave
Seattle, WA 98104
Prgm Dir: Rochelle Garcia, MD
Tel: 206 223-3145
Med Dir: Nancy Kiviat, MD
Class Cap: 4   *Begins:* Sep
Length: 12 mos   *Award:* Cert
Tuition per yr: $2,500 res, $2,500 non-res

West Virginia

Charleston Area Medical Center

Cytotechnologist Prgm
3200 MacCorkle Ave SE
Charleston, WV 25304
Prgm Dir: Carolyn H Stevens, CT(ASCP)
Tel: 304 348-5570   *Fax:* 304 348-4352
Med Dir: Michael R Cuadra, MD
Class Cap: 6   *Begins:* Jul
Length: 12 mos   *Award:* Cert, BS
Tuition per yr: $5,000

Cabell Huntington Hospital

Cytotechnologist Prgm
1340 Hal Greer Blvd
Huntington, WV 25701
Prgm Dir: Margene Smith, SCT(ASCP)
Tel: 304 526-2155   *Fax:* 304 526-2155
Med Dir: John P Sheils, MD
Class Cap: 4   *Begins:* Jun
Length: 12 mos   *Award:* Dipl, BS
Tuition per yr: $1,500 res, $1,500 non-res
Evening or weekend classes available

Wisconsin

State Laboratory of Hygiene

Cytotechnologist Prgm
UW Madison Health Science Ctr
465 Henry Mall
Madison, WI 53706
Prgm Dir: John E Shalkham, MA SCT(ASCP)
Tel: 608 262-2802   *Fax:* 608 265-6294
Med Dir: Stanley L Inhorn, MD
Class Cap: 18   *Begins:* Aug
Length: 12 mos   *Award:* Cert, BS
Tuition per yr: $3,600 res, $3,600 non-res

Marshfield Clinic

Cytotechnologist Prgm
1000 N Oak Ave
Marshfield, WI 54449
Prgm Dir: Virginia R Narlock, PhD MT(ASCP)
Tel: 715 387-7202   *Fax:* 715 387-7121
Med Dir: George M Rupp, MD
Class Cap: 4   *Begins:* Aug
Length: 12 mos   *Award:* Dipl, BS
Tuition per yr: $850 res, $850 non-res

Froedtert Memorial Lutheran Hospital

Cytotechnologist Prgm
9200 W Wisconsin Ave
Milwaukee, WI 53226
Prgm Dir: Lawrence J Clowry, MD
Tel: 414 257-6214   *Fax:* 414 257-7815
Med Dir: Lawrence J Clowry, MD
Class Cap: 4   *Begins:* Sep
Length: 12 mos   *Award:* Cert
Tuition per yr: $1,000 res, $1,000 non-res

Programs

Dental-Related Occupations

Dental Assistant

Occupational Description

The dental assistant increases the efficiency of the dental care team by aiding the dentist in the delivery of oral health care. The dental assistant performs a wide range of tasks requiring both interpersonal and technical skills. Routine duties range from aiding and educating patients to preparing dental instruments and performing administrative work.

Job Description

Dental assistants are responsible for helping patients feel comfortable before, during, and after treatment; assisting the dentist during treatment; taking and developing dental radiographs (x-rays); recording the patient's medical history and taking blood pressure, pulse, and temperature readings; preparing and sterilizing instruments and equipment for the dentist's use; providing patients with oral care instructions following such procedures as surgery or placement of a restoration (filling); teaching patients proper brushing and flossing techniques; making impressions of patients' teeth for study casts; and performing routine administrative and scheduling tasks, including using a personal computer, answering the telephone, and ordering supplies.

Employment Characteristics

Most of the more than 200,000 active dental assistants are employed by general dentists. In addition, dental specialists—such as orthodontists or oral and maxillofacial surgeons—employ dental assistants. Most assistants work chairside, although they may also participate in the business aspects of the practice. Besides dental offices, other practice settings available to dental assistants include schools and clinics (public health dentistry); hospitals (assisting dentists who are treating bedridden patients or in more elaborate dental procedures performed only in hospitals); dental school clinics; insurance companies (processing dental insurance claims); and vocational schools, technical institutes, community colleges, and universities (teaching others to be dental assistants).

The number of dental assistants, dental hygienists, and dental laboratory technicians employed by general dentists rose from an average of 3.3 positions per practice in 1986 to 4.0 positions in 1994. Since many dentists employ two or three dental assistants, employment opportunities in this field are excellent.

Dental assisting also offers both flexibility and stability. Approximately 27% of dental assistants work on a part-time basis, sometimes in more than one dental office, so assistants have considerable freedom to choose their own hours. As of 1996, dental assistants had been working in their current practices for an average of 6 years.

The salary of a dental assistant varies, depending on the responsibilities associated with the specific position, the individual training, and the geographic location of employment. The average national wage of a dental assistant in 1994 was $9.90 per hour.

In addition to salary, many dental assistants receive benefit packages from their employers that may include health and disability insurance coverage, dues for membership in professional organizations, allowance for uniforms, and paid vacations.

Employment Outlook

According to the 1993-94 edition of the *Occupational Outlook Handbook*, published by the US Department of Labor's Bureau of Labor Statistics, employment of dental assistants is expected to grow at the average rate for all occupations through the year 2000. Most areas of the country are currently reporting shortages of dental assistants. Owing to the success of preventive dentistry in reducing the incidence of oral disease, senior citizens—a growing population—will retain their teeth longer and will be even more aware of the importance of regular dental care.

Educational Programs

Length. Nine to 11 months.

Prerequisites. High school diploma or equivalent.

Certification. Dental assistants who pass an examination administered by the Dental Assisting National Board, Inc, may use the designation of Certified Dental Assistant (CDA). Dental assistants are eligible to take the examination if they have completed a dental assisting program accredited by the Commission on Dental Accreditation or have completed 2 years of full-time work experience as dental assistants. State regulations vary, and some states offer registration or licensure in addition to this national certification program.

Standards. *The Accreditation Standards for Dental Assisting Education Programs* have been developed (1) to protect the public, (2) to serve as a guide for dental assisting program development, (3) to serve as a stimulus for the improvement of established programs, and (4) to provide criteria for the evaluation of new and established programs. Accreditation by the Commission on Dental Accreditation requires that a dental assisting program meet the national standards set forth by the Commission, which represent the minimum requirements for accreditation.

Accreditation history. In 1957, the Council on Dental Education sponsored the first national workshop on dental assisting. Practicing dentists, dental educators, and dental assistants made recommendations for the education and certification of dental assistants. These recommendations were considered in developing the first *Requirements for an Accredited Program in Dental Assisting Education*, which were approved by the House of Delegates of the American Dental Association in 1960.

Prior to 1960, the American Dental Assistants Association (ADAA) approved courses of training for dental assistants, varying in length from 104 clock hours to 2 academic years. Subsequent to the adoption in 1960 of the first accreditation standards, the Council on Dental Education granted provisional approval to those programs approved by the ADAA that were at least 1 academic year in length until site visits could be conducted. Thus 26 programs appeared on the first list of accredited dental assisting programs published in 1961.

The accreditation standards have been revised four times—in 1969, 1973, 1979, and 1991—to reflect the dental profession's changing needs and educational trends. The communities of interest provided input into the latest revision of the standards through an ad hoc committee, open hearings, and review of and comment on two drafts of the proposed revision of the standards. Prior to approving the revised standards in December 1991, the Commission carefully considered comments received from all sources. The revised accreditation standards were implemented in January 1993.

Miscellaneous Facts

- The 237 dental assisting education programs in the United States accredited by the American Dental Association's Commission on Dental Accreditation enrolled 7,210 students in 1995-1996.

- Approximately 98% of the students enrolled in dental assisting programs were women in 1995-1996.
- Minority students represented approximately 22% of enrollees in dental assisting programs in 1995-1996.
- Excellent career opportunities exist for nontraditional dental assisting students, including those over 23 years of age, seeking career change or job reentry after a period of unemployment, or from a culturally diverse background. Many dental assisting education programs offer more flexible program designs that meet the needs of nontraditional students by offering a variety of educational options, such as part-time or evening hours.

Dental Hygienist

Occupational Description

Dental hygienists work with dentists in the delivery of dental care to patients. Hygienists use their knowledge and clinical skills to provide dental care to patients and their interpersonal skills to motivate and instruct patients on methods to prevent oral disease and maintain oral health.

Job Description

Although the range of services performed by dental hygienists varies from state to state, patient services rendered by dental hygienists frequently include
- performing patient screening procedures, such as reviewing health and dental history and taking blood pressure, pulse, and temperature;
- taking and developing dental radiographs (x-rays);
- removing calculus and plaque (hard and soft deposits) from teeth;
- applying preventive materials to teeth (eg, sealants and fluorides);
- teaching patients appropriate oral hygiene techniques;
- counseling patients regarding good nutrition and its impact on oral health;
- making impressions of patients' teeth for study casts; and
- performing office management activities.

Employment Characteristics

Most of the approximately 100,000 active dental hygienists in the United States today are employed by general dentists. Additionally, dental specialists (such as periodontists or pediatric dentists) employ dental hygienists. Most hygienists work chairside, although they often participate in the business aspects of the practice.

Dental hygienists also may be employed to provide dental hygiene services for patients in hospitals, nursing homes, and public health clinics. Depending on the level of education and experience they have achieved, dental hygienists also can apply their skills and knowledge to other career activities, such as teaching hygiene students. Research, office management, and business administration are other options. In addition, employment opportunities may be available with companies that market dentally related materials and equipment.

The total number of dental hygienists, dental assistants, and dental laboratory technicians employed by general dentists rose from an average of 3.3 positions per practice in 1986 to 4.0 positions in 1994. Because approximately 63% of general dentists employ at least one dental hygienist, and 37% employ two or more hygienists, employment opportunities in this field are excellent.

As a career, dental hygiene also offers both stability and flexibility. As of 1996, for example, dental hygienists had been working in their current practices for an average of 6.2 years. Many hygienists also have considerable freedom to choose their own hours and to undertake a full- or part-time schedule with evening or weekend hours.

The salary of a dental hygienist varies, depending on the responsibilities associated with the specific position, the geographic location of employment, and the type of practice or other setting in which the hygienist works. The average national wage of a full-time dental hygienist in 1994 was $19.80 per hour. Hygienists who work part-time averaged $23.70 per hour.

In addition, many dental hygienists receive benefit packages from their dentist/employers, which may include health insurance coverage, dues for membership in professional organizations, paid vacations and sick leave, and tuition assistance for continuing education.

Employment Outlook

According to the 1993-94 edition of the *Occupational Outlook Handbook* and the *Monthly Labor Review*, published by the US Department of Labor's Bureau of Labor Statistics, dental hygiene will continue to be among the top 10 growth disciplines in the health care professions through the year 2005. Some areas of the country are currently reporting shortages of dental hygienists.

Owing to the success of preventive dentistry in reducing the incidence of oral disease, senior citizens—a growing population—will retain their teeth longer and will be even more aware of the importance of regular dental care.

Educational Programs

Length. The majority of community college-based dental hygiene programs offer a 2-year associate degree. University-based dental hygiene programs may offer baccalaureate and master's degrees, which generally require at least 2 years of further schooling.

Prerequisites. Admission requirements vary, depending on the institution. High school-level courses such as health, biology, psychology, chemistry, mathematics, and speech will be beneficial in a dental hygiene career. Many programs prefer individuals who have completed at least 1 year of college, and some baccalaureate degree programs require applicants to have completed 2 years of college.

Curriculum. Dental hygiene education programs provide supervised patient care experiences. Programs also include courses in the liberal arts (English, speech, sociology, and psychology); basic sciences (anatomy, microbiology, and pathology); and clinical sciences (dental hygiene, radiology, and dental materials). After completing a dental hygiene program, dental hygienists can pursue additional training in such areas as education, business administration, basic sciences, and public health.

Licensure. Dental hygienists are licensed by each state to provide dental hygiene care and patient education. Eligibility for state licensure usually includes graduation from a Commission-accredited dental hygiene education program. In addition to requiring a passing score on the state-authorized licensure examination, which tests candidates' clinical dental hygiene skills as well as their knowledge of dental hygiene and related subjects, almost all states require candidates for licensure to obtain a passing score on the Dental Hygiene National Board Examination (a comprehensive written examination).

Upon receipt of their license, dental hygienists may use "RDH," signifying Registered Dental Hygienist, after their name.

Standards. *Accreditation Standards for Dental Hygiene Education Programs* (a revision of *Requirements and Guidelines for Accredited Dental Hygiene Education Programs*) were developed (1) to protect the public welfare, (2) to serve as a guide for dental hygiene program development, (3) to serve as a stimulus for the improvement of established programs, and (4) to provide criteria for the evaluation of new and established programs. To be accredited by the Commission on Dental Accreditation, a dental hygiene program must meet the national standards set forth by the Commission, which represent the minimum requirements for accreditation, stated in terms that allow an institution flexibility in the development of an educational program.

Accreditation history. The first dental hygiene accreditation standards were developed by three groups: the American Dental Hygienists' Association, the National Association of Dental Examiners, and the American Dental Association's Council on Dental Education. The standards were submitted to and approved by the American Dental Association House of Delegates in 1947, 5 years prior to the launching of the dental hygiene accreditation program in 1952. The first list of accredited dental hygiene programs was published in 1953, with 21 programs. Since then the standards for accreditation have been revised four times—in 1969, 1973, 1979, and 1991.

The communities of interest provided input into the latest revision of the standards through an ad hoc committee, open hearings, and review of and comment on two drafts of the proposed revised standards. Prior to approving the revised standards in December 1991, the Commission carefully considered comments received from all sources. The revised accreditation standards were implemented in January 1993.

Miscellaneous facts

- The United States has approximately 223 dental hygiene education programs accredited by the American Dental Association's Commission on Dental Accreditation.
- Approximately 97% of the students enrolled in dental hygiene programs in 1995-1996 were women.
- Minority students represented approximately 11% of enrollees in dental hygiene programs in 1995-1996.
- Excellent career opportunities exist for nontraditional dental hygiene students, who might meet one or more of the following criteria: over 23 years of age, seeking career change or job re-entry after a period of unemployment, or from a culturally diverse background. Some dental hygiene education programs offer more flexible program designs that meet the needs of nontraditional students by offering a variety of educational options, such as part-time or evening hours.

Dental Laboratory Technician

Occupational Description

Dental laboratory technicians make dental prostheses—replacements for natural teeth, including dentures and crowns. The hallmarks of the qualified dental laboratory technician are skill in using small hand instruments, accuracy, artistic ability, and attention to detail to create practical, esthetically pleasing teeth replacements.

Job Description

Dental laboratory technicians seldom interact directly with patients; rather, they work with dentists by following detailed written instructions to make dental prostheses, which are replacements for natural teeth that enable people who have lost some or all of their teeth to eat, chew, talk, and smile in a manner similar to the way they did before. The dental technician uses impressions (molds) of the patient's teeth or oral soft tissues to create full dentures, removable partial dentures or fixed bridges, crowns, caps, and orthodontic appliances and splints.

Dental technicians use sophisticated instruments and equipment and work with a variety of materials for replacing damaged or missing tooth structure, including waxes, plastics, precious and nonprecious alloys, stainless steel, and porcelain.

Employment Characteristics

Most of the more than 60,000 active dental laboratory technicians in the United States today work in commercial dental laboratories, which on average employ between three to five technicians. In addition, some dentists employ dental technicians in their private dental offices. Other employment opportunities for dental technicians include dental schools, hospitals, the military, and companies that manufacture dental prosthetic materials. Dental laboratory technician education programs also offer teaching positions for qualified technicians.

The starting salary of a dental technician is approximately $20,000 and varies depending on the responsibilities associated with the specific position and the geographic location of employment. In addition to salary, many dental technicians receive benefit packages from their employers, which may include health and disability insurance coverage, reimbursement for continuing education programs, and paid vacations and holidays.

Employment Outlook

Since most dentists use laboratory services, employment opportunities in this field are excellent. Owing to the success of preventive dentistry in reducing the incidence of oral disease, senior citizens— a growing population—will retain their teeth longer and will require more sophisticated prostheses for longer periods, thus increasing the demand for dental laboratory services.

Educational Programs

Length. Most dental laboratory technicians receive their education and training through a 2-year program at a community college, vocational school, technical college, or dental school, for which they may receive a certificate or an associate degree.

Prerequisites. High school diploma or its equivalent, although the Commission strongly encourages formal college-level education.

Certification. Dental laboratory technicians can become certified by passing an examination, administered by the National Board for Certification in Dental Laboratory Technology, that evaluates their technical skills and knowledge. Passing this examination qualifies a dental technician to use the designation Certified Dental Technician (CDT). CDTs specialize in one or more of five areas: complete dentures, partial dentures, crowns and bridges, ceramics, and orthodontics.

Dental technicians are eligible to take the examination if they have completed a dental laboratory technology program accredited by the Commission on Dental Accreditation and have 2 years of professional experience or have completed 5 years of work experience as dental technicians and passed a comprehensive examination.

Standards. *Accreditation Standards for Dental Laboratory Technology Education Programs* have been developed (1) to protect the public welfare, (2) to serve as a guide for dental laboratory technology education program development, (3) to serve as a stimulus for the improvement of established programs, and (4) to provide criteria for the evaluation of new and established programs. To be accredited by the Commission on Dental Accreditation, a dental laboratory technology program must meet the national standards set forth by the Commission, which represent the minimum requirements for accreditation.

Accreditation History. The first educational standards for the education of dental laboratory technicians, adopted by the American Dental Association House of Delegates in 1946, were rescinded and revised in 1957. Since then the accreditation standards have been revised four times—in 1967, 1973, 1979, and 1991—to reflect the changing needs and educational trends of the dental profession and laboratory industry.

The communities of interest provided input into the latest revision of the standards through an ad hoc committee, open hearings at annual meetings of the National Association of Dental Laboratories and American Association of Dental Schools, and review of and comment on drafts of the proposed revision of the standards. Prior to approving the revised standards in December 1991, the Commission carefully considered comments received from all sources. The revised accreditation standards were implemented in January 1993.

Miscellaneous facts

- In 1995, 798 first-year dental laboratory technician students were enrolled in the approximately 40 dental technology education programs in the United States accredited by the American Dental Association's Commission on Dental Accreditation.
- Dental technology presents equal career opportunities for women and men. In 1995-1996, 46% of the students enrolled in dental technology programs were women, 54% were men.
- Minority students represented approximately 38% of enrollees in dental technology programs in 1995-1996.
- Excellent career opportunities exist for nontraditional dental technology students, who might meet one or more of the following criteria: over 23 years of age; seeking career change or job reentry after a period of unemployment; or from a culturally diverse background.

Inquiries

Accreditation

Inquiries regarding accreditation should be addressed to

Commission on Dental Accreditation
American Dental Association
211 E Chicago Ave
Chicago, IL 60611-2678
312 440-2718
312 440-2915 Fax
Internet: http://www.ada.org

Careers

Inquiries regarding careers and curriculum should be addressed to

American Dental Association
Department of Career Guidance
211 E Chicago Ave
Chicago IL 60611-2678
800 621-8099, ext 4653
Internet: http://www.ada.org

American Association of Dental Schools
1625 Massachusetts Ave, NW
Washington, DC 20036
202 667-9433

American Dental Assistants Association
203 N LaSalle St
Chicago, IL 60601
312 541-1550

American Dental Hygienists' Association
444 N Michigan Ave/Ste 3400
Chicago IL 60611
312 440-8900

Laboratory Conference Section Board of the American Dental Trade Association (ADTA)
4222 King St W
Alexandria, VA 22302
703 379-7755

National Association of Dental Laboratories
555 E Braddock Rd
Alexandria, VA 22314-2106
703 683-5263

Certification/Registration

Inquiries on certification may be directed to

Dental Assisting National Board, Inc
216 E Ontario St
Chicago, IL 60611
312 642-3368

National Board for Certification in Dental Laboratory Technology
555 Braddock Rd
Alexandria, VA 22314-2106
703 683-5263

Dental Assistant

Alabama

James Faulkner State Community College
Dental Assistant Prgm
1900 Hwy 31 S
Bay Minette, AL 36507-2619
Prgm Dir: Betty Hardin
Tel: 334 580-2110   *Fax:* 334 580-2253
Class Cap: 30   *Begins:* Sep
Length: 11 mos, 13 mos   *Award:* Cert, AAS
Tuition per yr: $2,447 res, $4,372 non-res

Bessemer State Technical College
Dental Assistant Prgm
Highway 11 S/PO Box 308
Bessemer, AL 35021
Prgm Dir: D Smith
Tel: 205 428-6391   *Fax:* 205 424-5119
Class Cap: 22   *Begins:* Sep
Length: 12 mos   *Award:* Dipl
Tuition per yr: $1,440 res, $2,880 non-res
Evening or weekend classes available

University of Alabama at Birmingham
Dental Assistant Prgm
1919 Seventh Ave/S Box 59
Birmingham, AL 35294
Prgm Dir: V Holmes
Tel: 205 934-7016
Class Cap: 25
Length: 9 mos   *Award:* Cert
Tuition per yr: $2,179 res, $2,742 non-res

John Calhoun State Community College
Dental Assistant Prgm
PO Box 2216
Decatur, AL 35609-2216
Prgm Dir: Patricia Stueck
Tel: 205 306-2812   *Fax:* 205 306-2885
Class Cap: 30   *Begins:* Sep
Length: 10 mos, 13 mos   *Award:* Cert, AAS
Tuition per yr: $2,742 res, $4,038 non-res
Evening or weekend classes available

Wallace State College
Dental Assistant Prgm
PO Box 2000
Hanceville, AL 35077-2000
Prgm Dir: L Hypes
Tel: 205 352-2090   *Fax:* 205 352-8380
Med Dir: Douglas Allen
Class Cap: 25   *Begins:* Sep
Length: 24 mos   *Award:* Cert, AAS
Tuition per yr: $2,060 res, $4,120 non-res
Evening or weekend classes available

H Councill Trenholm State Technical College
Dental Assistant Prgm
1225 Air Base Blvd
Montgomery, AL 36108
Prgm Dir: E Allen
Tel: 334 832-9000   *Fax:* 334 832-9797
Class Cap: 20
Length: 12 mos, 18 mos   *Award:* Cert
Tuition per yr: $2,558 res, $3,899 non-res

Alaska

University of Alaska Anchorage
Dental Assistant Prgm
3211 Providence Dr/AHS 124
Anchorage, AK 99508-8371
Prgm Dir: N Bish
Tel: 907 786-1637   *Fax:* 907 786-1722
Class Cap: 15   *Begins:* Aug Sep
Length: 8 mos   *Award:* Cert
Tuition per yr: $2,520 res, $7,560 non-res

Arizona

Phoenix College
Dental Assistant Prgm
1202 W Thomas Rd
Phoenix, AZ 85013
Prgm Dir: Janet Wilburn
Tel: 602 285-7327   *Fax:* 602 285-7700
Class Cap: 24   *Begins:* Aug
Length: 8 mos   *Award:* Cert, AAS
Tuition per yr: $1,953 res, $6,828 non-res

Pima County Community College
Dental Assistant Prgm
2202 W Anklam Rd
Tucson, AZ 85709
Prgm Dir: Barbara Crowley
Tel: 520 884-6916
Class Cap: 30   *Begins:* Aug
Length: 8 mos   *Award:* Cert, AA
Tuition per yr: $2,471 res, $5,380 non-res

Arkansas

Cotton Boll Technical Institute
Dental Assistant Prgm
Box 36
Burdette, AR 72321
Prgm Dir: Tammie C Campbell
Tel: 501 763-1486   *Fax:* 501 763-1496
Class Cap: 18   *Begins:* Aug
Length: 11 mos   *Award:* Cert
Tuition per yr: $900

Pulaski Technical College
Dental Assistant Prgm
3000 W Scenic Dr
North Little Rock, AR 72118-3399
Prgm Dir: D Davis
Tel: 501 771-1000   *Fax:* 501 771-2844
Class Cap: 26   *Begins:* Aug
Length: 9 mos   *Award:* Dipl
Tuition per yr: $984 res, $2,635 non-res

California

College of Alameda
Dental Assistant Prgm
555 Atlantic Ave
Alameda, CA 94501
Prgm Dir: Y Carter
Tel: 510 748-2262   *Fax:* 510 769-6019
Class Cap: 40
Length: 9 mos   *Award:* Cert
Tuition per yr: $1,102 res, $4,872 non-res

Orange Coast College
Dental Assistant Prgm
2701 Fairview Rd
Costa Mesa, CA 92628-0120
Prgm Dir: J Rose, MA CDA RDA
Tel: 714 432-5565   *Fax:* 714 432-5609
Class Cap: 30   *Begins:* Aug
Length: 9 mos   *Award:* Cert, AA
Tuition per yr: $351 res, $3,429 non-res

Cypress College
Dental Assistant Prgm
9200 Valley View St
Cypress, CA 90630
Prgm Dir: Ina M Rydalch
Tel: 562 421-0988
Class Cap: 32   *Begins:* Aug
Length: 9 mos   *Award:* Cert
Tuition per yr: $1,279 res, $4,149 non-res

College of the Redwoods
Dental Assistant Prgm
Tompkins Hill Rd
Eureka, CA 95501
Prgm Dir: Karen Sperry
Tel: 707 445-6904   *Fax:* 707 441-5943
Class Cap: 30   *Begins:* Aug
Length: 9 mos   *Award:* Cert, AS
Tuition per yr: $1,512 res, $5,626 non-res

Citrus College
Dental Assistant Prgm
1000 W Foothill
Glendora, CA 91740
Prgm Dir: J Dold
Tel: 818 914-8727
Class Cap: 35   *Begins:* Aug Oct Jan
Length: 9 mos   *Award:* Cert
Tuition per yr: $1,188 res, $602 non-res

Chabot College
Dental Assistant Prgm
25555 Hesperian Blvd
Hayward, CA 94545
Prgm Dir: Linda Zweifel, CDA RDA RDH BS
Tel: 510 786-6951   *Fax:* 510 782-9315
Class Cap: 40   *Begins:* Aug
Length: 9 mos   *Award:* Cert, AA
Evening or weekend classes available

College of Marin
Dental Assistant Prgm
College Ave
Kentfield, CA 94904
Prgm Dir: B Cancilla
Tel: 415 485-9327   *Fax:* 415 485-0135
Class Cap: 24   *Begins:* Aug
Length: 10 mos, 19 mos   *Award:* Cert
Tuition per yr: $501 res, $5,082 non-res
Evening or weekend classes available

Hacienda LaPuente Unified School Dist
Dental Assistant Prgm
15540 E Fairgrove Ave
La Puente, CA 91744
Prgm Dir: G Richardson, CDA RDA
Tel: 818 855-3160   *Fax:* 818 855-3833
Class Cap: 70
Length: 12 mos   *Award:* Cert
Tuition per yr: $588 res, $588 non-res

Foothill College
Dental Assistant Prgm
12345 El Monte Rd
Los Altos Hills, CA 94022
Prgm Dir: C Miyasaki-Ching
Tel: 415 949-7351 *Fax:* 415 949-7375
Class Cap: 24
Length: 9 mos *Award:* Cert
Tuition per yr: $1,718 res, $5,118 non-res
Evening or weekend classes available

East Los Angeles Occupational Center
Dental Assistant Prgm
2100 Marengo St
Los Angeles, CA 90033
Prgm Dir: Ben Avila
Tel: 213 223-1283 *Fax:* 213 223-6365
Class Cap: 30
Length: 10 mos *Award:* Cert
Tuition per yr: $395

Modesto Junior College
Dental Assistant Prgm
435 College Ave
Modesto, CA 95350
Prgm Dir: R Keach
Tel: 209 575-6367
Class Cap: 32
Length: 9 mos *Award:* Cert
Tuition per yr: $1,370 res, $5,330 non-res

Monterey Peninsula College
Dental Assistant Prgm
980 Fremont Ave
Monterey, CA 93940
Prgm Dir: Patricia A Lewis
Tel: 408 646-4137 *Fax:* 408 645-1353
Class Cap: 32 *Begins:* Aug
Length: 8 mos *Award:* Cert, AS
Tuition per yr: $416 res, $3,488 non-res
Evening or weekend classes available

Cerritos College
Dental Assistant Prgm
11110 E Alondra Blvd
Norwalk, CA 90650
Prgm Dir: J Failor
Tel: 310 860-2451 *Fax:* 310 467-5077
Class Cap: 45 *Begins:* Aug
Length: 11 mos *Award:* Cert
Tuition per yr: $1,117 res, $4,349 non-res

Pasadena City College
Dental Assistant Prgm
1570 E Colorado Blvd
Pasadena, CA 91106
Prgm Dir: A Pendleton
Tel: 818 585-7542 *Fax:* 818 585-7912
Class Cap: 9 *Begins:* Aug
Length: 18 mos *Award:* Cert, AS
Tuition per yr: $403 res, $3,627 non-res

Diablo Valley College
Dental Assistant Prgm
321 Golf Club Rd
Pleasant Hill, CA 94523
Prgm Dir: Marylou Pineda, CDA RDA MA
Tel: 510 685-1230, Ext 351 *Fax:* 510 685-1551
Class Cap: 24 *Begins:* Aug
Length: 9 mos *Award:* Cert, AA
Tuition per yr: $527 res, $8,100 non-res
Evening or weekend classes available

Chaffey Community College
Dental Assistant Prgm
5885 Haven Ave
Rancho Cucamonga, CA 91737-3002
Prgm Dir: M Graham
Tel: 909 941-2189 *Fax:* 909 941-2783
Class Cap: 55 *Begins:* Aug Jan
Length: 9 mos, 18 mos *Award:* Cert, AS
Tuition per yr: $954 res, $3,821 non-res

Sacramento City College
Dental Assistant Prgm
3835 Freeport Blvd
Sacramento, CA 95822
Prgm Dir: M Dunne
Tel: 916 558-2650 *Fax:* 916 441-4142
Class Cap: 32 *Begins:* Aug
Length: 10 mos *Award:* Cert
Tuition per yr: $1,360 res, $3,885 non-res

San Diego Mesa College
Dental Assistant Prgm
7250 Mesa College Dr
San Diego, CA 92111-2697
Prgm Dir: Philomena Lindsay, MEd CDA RDA
Tel: 619 627-2697
Class Cap: 30 *Begins:* Aug
Length: 10 mos, 24 mos *Award:* Cert, AS

City College of San Francisco
Dental Assistant Prgm
50 Phelan Ave
San Francisco, CA 94112
Prgm Dir: A Nelson
Tel: 415 239-3479
Class Cap: 40 *Begins:* Aug
Length: 9 mos *Award:* Cert, AA
Tuition per yr: $1,044 res, $4,615 non-res

San Jose City College
Dental Assistant Prgm
2100 Moorpark Ave
San Jose, CA 95128
Prgm Dir: P Wilson
Tel: 408 288-3712 *Fax:* 408 275-9386
E-mail: pwilson@jeced.cc.ca.us
Class Cap: 35 *Begins:* Aug Jan
Length: 11 mos *Award:* Cert, AS
Tuition per yr: $1,105 res, $4,570 non-res

Palomar Community College
Dental Assistant Prgm
1140 W Mission Rd
San Marcos, CA 92069
Prgm Dir: J Landmesser, CDA RDA BA
Tel: 619 744-1150, Ext 2573 *Fax:* 619 744-8123
Class Cap: 25 *Begins:* Aug
Length: 10 mos *Award:* Cert, AA
Tuition per yr: $1,245 res, $6,413 non-res

College of San Mateo
Dental Assistant Prgm
1700 W Hillsdale Blvd
San Mateo, CA 94402-3795
Prgm Dir: Elizabeth Bassi
Tel: 415 574-6212
Class Cap: 30 *Begins:* Aug
Length: 9 mos *Award:* Cert, AA
Tuition per yr: $1,144

Contra Costa College
Dental Assistant Prgm
2600 Mission Bell Dr
San Pablo, CA 94806
Prgm Dir: S Everhart
Tel: 510 235-7800, Ext 265
Class Cap: 30 *Begins:* Jun
Length: 11 mos *Award:* Cert, AA
Tuition per yr: $1,821 res, $6,609 non-res

Santa Rosa Junior College
Dental Assistant Prgm
1501 Mendocino Ave
Santa Rosa, CA 95401
Prgm Dir: D Bird
Tel: 707 527-4447 *Fax:* 707 527-4426
E-mail: dbird@floyd.santarosa.edu
Begins: Aug
Length: 12 mos *Award:* Cert
Tuition per yr: $975 res, $5,317 non-res
Evening or weekend classes available

Colorado

T H Pickens Technical Center
Dental Assistant Prgm
500 Airport Rd
Aurora, CO 80011
Prgm Dir: Denese Cranga, MA CDA EFDA
Tel: 303 344-4910
Class Cap: 20 *Begins:* Aug
Length: 12 mos *Award:* Cert
Tuition per yr: $1,936 res, $4,809 non-res

Pikes Peak Community College
Dental Assistant Prgm
5765 S Academy Blvd
Colorado Springs, CO 80906
Prgm Dir: Anne Maestas
Tel: 719 540-7474 *Fax:* 719 540-7461
Class Cap: 30 *Begins:* Aug
Length: 8 mo , 16 mos *Award:* Cert, AAS
Tuition per yr: $4,565 res, $15,340 non-res
Evening or weekend classes available

Emily Griffith Opportunity School
Dental Assistant Prgm
1250 Welton St
Denver, CO 80204
Prgm Dir: Sindi Pillers
Tel: 303 575-4737
Class Cap: 20 Begins: Sep Jan
Length: 10 mos *Award:* Cert
Tuition per yr: $950 res, $2,350 non-res

Front Range Comm College - Ft Collins
Dental Assistant Prgm
Larimer Campus/PO Box 270490
Fort Collins, CO 80527
Prgm Dir: A Jansen
Tel: 303 226-2500 *Fax:* 303 825-6819
E-mail: fr_arlis@cccs.ccco.edu
Class Cap: 24 *Begins:* Aug Jan
Length: 10 mos, 22 mos *Award:* Cert
Tuition per yr: $2,803 res, $10,984 non-res
Evening or weekend classes available

Programs

Pueblo Community College

Dental Assistant Prgm
900 W Orman Ave
TE Rm 137
Pueblo, CO 81004
Prgm Dir: Janet Trujillo
Tel: 719 549-3263 *Fax:* 719 549-3136
Class Cap: 15 *Begins:* Sep
Length: 9 mos *Award:* Cert, AAS
Tuition per yr: $2,807 res, $11,006 non-res
Evening or weekend classes available

Front Range Comm College - Westminster

Dental Assistant Prgm
3645 W 112th Ave
Westminster, CO 80030
Prgm Dir: J Strauss
Tel: 303 404-5212 *Fax:* 303 404-2178
Class Cap: 30 *Begins:* Aug Jan March
Length: 11 mos, 24 mos *Award:* Cert
Tuition per yr: $3,628 res, $10,919 non-res
Evening or weekend classes available

Connecticut

Tunxis Community Technical College

Dental Assistant Prgm
271 Scott Swamp Rd
Farmington, CT 06032-3187
Prgm Dir: S Seaver
Tel: 203 679-9636 *Fax:* 203 676-8906
Class Cap: 40 *Begins:* Aug
Length: 10 mos *Award:* Cert
Tuition per yr: $1,722 res, $4,842 non-res

Eli Whitney Regional Voc Tech School

Dental Assistant Prgm
71 Jones Rd
Hamden, CT 06514
Prgm Dir: A Longo
Tel: 203 397-4037 *Fax:* 203 397-4129
Class Cap: 20
Length: 9 mos *Award:* Cert
Tuition per yr: $685 res, $8,347 non-res

A I Prince Regional Vocational Technical

Dental Assistant Prgm
500 Bookfield St
Hartford, CT 06106
Prgm Dir: M Willis
Tel: 860 246-8594 *Fax:* 860 951-1529
Class Cap: 20
Length: 9 mos *Award:* Cert
Tuition per yr: $685 res, $8,347 non-res

Briarwood College

Dental Assistant Prgm
2279 Mount Vernon Rd
Southington, CT 06489
Prgm Dir: J Foley
Tel: 860 628-4751, Ext 20 *Fax:* 860 628-6444
Class Cap: 14 *Begins:* Sep
Length: 9 mos *Award:* Dipl
Tuition per yr: $12,308
Evening or weekend classes available

Windham Regional Vocational Tech School

Dental Assistant Prgm
210 Birch St
Willimantic, CT 06226
Prgm Dir: M Hammel
Tel: 860 456-3789 *Fax:* 860 450-0630
Class Cap: 18
Length: 9 mos *Award:* Cert
Tuition per yr: $685 res, $8,342 non-res

District of Columbia

M M Washington Career High School

Dental Assistant Prgm
27 O Street NW
Washington, DC 20001
Prgm Dir: Maria O Melchor
Tel: 202 673-7478 *Fax:* 202 673-7229
Class Cap: 30
Length: 9 mos *Award:* Cert
Tuition per yr: $4,458 res, $7,558 non-res

Florida

Manatee Area Vocational-Technical Center

Dental Assistant Prgm
5603 34th St W
Bradenton, FL 34210
Prgm Dir: Kathleen Matthews, CDA
Tel: 941 751-7937 *Fax:* 941 751-7927
E-mail: kpxq6da@prodigy.com
Class Cap: 32 *Begins:* Aug
Length: 11 mos *Award:* Cert
Tuition per yr: $576 res, $576 non-res

Brevard Community College

Dental Assistant Prgm
1519 Clearlake Rd
Cocoa, FL 32922
Prgm Dir: C Cameron
Tel: 407 632-1111 *Fax:* 407 634-3731
E-mail: cameron.c@a1.brevard.cc.flus
Class Cap: 16
Length: 9 mos *Award:* Cert
Tuition per yr: $1,542 res, $2,234 non-res

Daytona Beach Community College

Dental Assistant Prgm
1200 International Speedway
Daytona Beach, FL 32114
Prgm Dir: Mary E Pryor, DDS
Tel: 904 255-8131, Ext 2082 Fax: 904 255-4491
Class Cap: 48
Length: 10 mos *Award:* Cert
Tuition per yr: $894 res, $3,009 non-res

Broward Community College

Dental Assistant Prgm
3501 SW Davie Rd
Ft Lauderdale, FL 33314
Prgm Dir: J Moskowitz
Tel: 954 475-6904 *Fax:* 954 473-9037
Class Cap: 32 *Begins:* Aug
Length: 10 mos *Award:* Cert
Tuition per yr: $1,983 res, $4,256 non-res

Indian River Community College

Dental Assistant Prgm
3209 Virginia Ave
Ft Pierce, FL 34981-5599
Prgm Dir: K Allen
Tel: 561 462-4480 *Fax:* 561 462-4796
Class Cap: 16 *Begins:* Aug
Length: 10 mos *Award:* Cert
Tuition per yr: $2,997 res, $5,661 non-res

Santa Fe Community College

Dental Assistant Prgm
3000 NW 83rd St
Bldg W201E
Gainesville, FL 32606
Prgm Dir: Dana Rafferty Parker, DMD MEd
Tel: 352 395-5705 Fax: 352 395-5711
Class Cap: 30 *Begins:* Aug
Length: 10 mos *Award:* Cert
Tuition per yr: $2,920 res, $4,765 non-res

Palm Beach Community College

Dental Assistant Prgm
4200 Congress Ave
Lake Worth, FL 33461
Prgm Dir: C Hanson
Tel: 561 439-8095 *Fax:* 561 439-8314
Class Cap: 25
Length: 9 mos *Award:* Cert
Tuition per yr: $1,982 res, $5,320 non-res

Lindsey Hopkins Tech Education Center

Dental Assistant Prgm
750 NW 20th St
Miami, FL 33127
Prgm Dir: F Slavichak, DDS
Tel: 305 324-6070 *Fax:* 305 324-6249
Class Cap: 40 *Begins:* Apr Sep
Length: 12 mos *Award:* Cert
Tuition per yr: $558 res, $4,196 non-res

R Morgan Vocational Technical Institute

Dental Assistant Prgm
18180 SW 122nd Ave
Miami, FL 33177
Prgm Dir: Thomas B Connell, DDS
Tel: 305 253-9920 *Fax:* 305 253-3023
Class Cap: 15
Length: 11 mos *Award:* Cert
Tuition per yr: $1,349

J Walker Vocational Technical Center

Dental Assistant Prgm
3702 Estey Ave
Naples, FL 33942-4498
Prgm Dir: M Reback
Tel: 941 643-0919 *Fax:* 941 643-7462
Class Cap: 15 *Begins:* Aug Jan
Length: 12 mos *Award:* Cert
Tuition per yr: $1,008 res, $5,412 non-res
Evening or weekend classes available

Orlando Technical Education Centers

Dental Assistant Prgm
301 W Amelia St
Orlando, FL 32801
Prgm Dir: R Walls
Tel: 407 246-7060, Ext 4835 *Fax:* 407 317-3372
Class Cap: 50 *Begins:* Aug Jan
Length: 10 mos *Award:* Cert
Tuition per yr: $1,269
Evening or weekend classes available

Southern College

Dental Assistant Prgm
5600 Lake Underhill Rd
Orlando, FL 32807
Prgm Dir: Carole Falkner
Tel: 407 273-1000   *Fax:* 407 273-0492
Class Cap: 15
Length: 24 mos   *Award:* AS
Tuition per yr: $5,850
Evening or weekend classes available

Gulf Coast Community College

Dental Assistant Prgm
5230 W Hwy 98
Panama City, FL 32401
Prgm Dir: G Daugherty II, DDS MS
Tel: 904 872-3829
Class Cap: 24   *Begins:* Aug
Length: 10 mos, 24 mos   *Award:* Cert
Tuition per yr: $2,200 res, $4,800 non-res
Evening or weekend classes available

Pensacola Junior College

Dental Assistant Prgm
5555 W Hwy 98
Pensacola, FL 32507
Prgm Dir: J Ponson
Tel: 904 484-2245   *Fax:* 904 484-2365
Class Cap: 24   *Begins:* Aug
Length: 10 mos   *Award:* Cert
Tuition per yr: $605 res, $1,099 non-res

Charlotte Vocational Technical Center

Dental Assistant Prgm
18300 Toledo Blade Blvd
Port Charlotte, FL 33948-3399
Prgm Dir: Cathy Geoyger
Tel: 941 629-6819   *Fax:* 941 629-2058
Class Cap: 32   *Begins:* Aug
Length: 11 mos   *Award:* Cert
Tuition per yr: $612 res, $1,224 non-res

Pinellas Tech Educ Ctr - St Petersburg

Dental Assistant Prgm
901 34th St S
St Petersburg, FL 33711
Prgm Dir: B Thomas
Tel: 800 893-2500   *Fax:* 813 893-2776
Class Cap: 24
Length: 12 mos   *Award:* Dipl
Tuition per yr: $937 res, $5,324 non-res

Tallahassee Community College

Dental Assistant Prgm
444 Appleyard Dr
Tallahassee, FL 32304
Prgm Dir: Cynthia R Biron, RDH MA
Tel: 904 488-9200   *Fax:* 904 487-7028
Class Cap: 30   *Begins:* May
Length: 13 mos   *Award:* Cert
Tuition per yr: $829 res, $2,723 non-res
Evening or weekend classes available

David G Erwin Technical Center

Dental Assistant Prgm
2010 E Hillsborough Ave
Tampa, FL 33610
Prgm Dir: P Spoto
Tel: 813 231-1800   *Fax:* 813 231-1820
Class Cap: 7
Length: 12 mos   *Award:* Dipl
Tuition per yr: $550 res, $4,070 non-res

Georgia

Albany Technical Institute

Dental Assistant Prgm
1021 Lowe Rd
Albany, GA 31708
Prgm Dir: P Ryals
Tel: 912 430-3500   *Fax:* 912 430-5115
Class Cap: 25   *Begins:* Oct Mar
Length: 12 mos   *Award:* Dipl
Tuition per yr: $1,520

Augusta Technical Institute

Dental Assistant Prgm
3116 Deans Bridge Rd
Augusta, GA 30906
Prgm Dir: Barbara Nelms-Williams
Tel: 706 771-4179   *Fax:* 706 771-4181
E-mail: bwilliam@aug.tec.ga.us
Class Cap: 23   *Begins:* Sep Mar
Length: 15 mos   *Award:* Dipl
Tuition per yr: $1,100 res, $2,200 non-res

Gwinnett Technical Institute

Dental Assistant Prgm
5150 Sugarloaf Pkwy
Lawrenceville, GA 30246-1505
Prgm Dir: S Powell, PhD
Tel: 770 962-7580   *Fax:* 770 962-7985
Class Cap: 20
Length: 10 mos   *Award:* Dipl
Tuition per yr: $1,200 res, $1,936 non-res

Medix School

Dental Assistant Prgm
2480 Windy Hill Rd
Marietta, GA 30067
Prgm Dir: V Turry
Tel: 770 980-0002   *Fax:* 770 980-0811
Class Cap: 350
Length: 9 mos   *Award:* Cert
Tuition per yr: $7,740 res, $7,740 non-res
Evening or weekend classes available

Lanier Technical Institute

Dental Assistant Prgm
PO Box 58
Oakwood, GA 30566
Prgm Dir: S Kirk
Tel: 770 531-6370   *Fax:* 770 531-6426
E-mail: skirk@admin1.anier.tec.ga.us
Class Cap: 20   *Begins:* Sep Oct
Length: 12 mos   *Award:* Dipl
Tuition per yr: $1,893 res, $2,949 non-res
Evening or weekend classes available

Savannah Technical Institute

Dental Assistant Prgm
5717 White Bluff Rd
Savannah, GA 31405-5594
Prgm Dir: Marcia P Jones
Tel: 912 351-4562   *Fax:* 912 352-4362
Class Cap: 20   *Begins:* Oct
Length: 12 mos   *Award:* Dipl
Tuition per yr: $1,104 res, $2,112 non-res
Evening or weekend classes available

Idaho

Boise State University

Dental Assistant Prgm
College of Technology
1910 University
Boise, ID 83725
Prgm Dir: Bonnie Imbs
Tel: 208 385-1541   *Fax:* 208 385-3155
Class Cap: 24   *Begins:* Sep
Length: 9 mos   *Award:* Cert
Tuition per yr: $2,356 res, $5,406 non-res

Illinois

John A Logan College

Dental Assistant Prgm
Rural Rte 2
Carterville, IL 62918
Prgm Dir: S Bryan
Tel: 618 985-3741   *Fax:* 618 985-2248
Class Cap: 25   *Begins:* Aug
Length: 10 mos   *Award:* Cert
Tuition per yr: $1,472 res, $3,786 non-res

Kaskaskia College

Dental Assistant Prgm
27210 College Rd
Centralia, IL 62801
Prgm Dir: N Nollman
Tel: 618 532-1981   *Fax:* 618 532-1990
Class Cap: 36   *Begins:* Aug
Length: 8 mos   *Award:* Cert
Tuition per yr: $1,241 res, $3,138 non-res

Parkland College

Dental Assistant Prgm
2400 W Bradley
Champaign, IL 61821
Prgm Dir: K Castongue
Tel: 217 351-2284   *Fax:* 217 373-3830
E-mail: kcstongue@parkland.cc.il.us
Class Cap: 18   *Begins:* Aug
Length: 10 mos   *Award:* Cert
Tuition per yr: $1,710 res, $5,552 non-res
Evening or weekend classes available

Morton College

Dental Assistant Prgm
3801 S Central Ave
Cicero, IL 60804
Prgm Dir: F Holbrook
Tel: 708 656-8000   *Fax:* 708 656-3297
Class Cap: 20   *Begins:* Aug
Length: 8 mos   *Award:* Cert
Tuition per yr: $1,954 res, $4,892 non-res

Illinois Central College

Dental Assistant Prgm
210 SW Adams
East Peoria, IL 61635-0001
Prgm Dir: D Daniels
Tel: 309 999-4668
Class Cap: 15
Length: 12 mos   *Award:* Cert
Tuition per yr: $1,800
Evening or weekend classes available

Elgin Community College
Dental Assistant Prgm
1700 Spartan Dr
Elgin, IL 60123
Prgm Dir: M Westerhoff
Tel: 847 888-7351   *Fax:* 847 622-0395
Med Dir: Mary Ann Vaca
Class Cap: 24   *Begins:* Aug Jan Jun
Length: 11 mos   *Award:* Cert
Tuition per yr: $1,442 res, $6,924 non-res
Evening or weekend classes available

Lewis & Clark Community College
Dental Assistant Prgm
5800 Godfrey Rd
Godfrey, IL 62035
Prgm Dir: C Pero-Fox
Tel: 618 466-3411   *Fax:* 618 466-9271
Class Cap: 24
Length: 9 mos   *Award:* Cert
Tuition per yr: $1,406 res, $5,148 non-res

Illinois Valley Community College
Dental Assistant Prgm
815 N Orlando Smith Ave
Oglesby, IL 61348-9691
Prgm Dir: P Pearson
Tel: 815 224-2720, Ext 359   *Fax:* 815 224-3033
E-mail: pearson@rs6000.ivcc.edu
Class Cap: 22   *Begins:* Aug Jan
Length: 9 mos   *Award:* Cert
Tuition per yr: $1,395 res, $5,658 non-res

Indiana

University of Southern Indiana
Dental Assistant Prgm
8600 University Blvd
Evansville, IN 47712
Prgm Dir: L Matheson
Tel: 812 464-1778   *Fax:* 812 465-7092
E-mail: lmatheso.usc@smtp.usi.edu
Class Cap: 30   *Begins:* Aug
Length: 8 mo , 16 mos   *Award:* Cert, AAS
Tuition per yr: $3,660 res, $8,590 non-res
Evening or weekend classes available

Indiana Univ/Purdue Univ Ft Wayne
Dental Assistant Prgm
2101 Coliseum Blvd E
Fort Wayne, IN 46805
Prgm Dir: J Beard
Tel: 219 481-6837   *Fax:* 219 481-6083
E-mail: 1#-beard@smtplink.ipfw.indiana.edu
Class Cap: 24   *Begins:* Aug
Length: 8 mo , 16 mos   *Award:* Cert
Tuition per yr: $3,285 res, $7,863 non-res
Evening or weekend classes available

Indiana University Northwest
Dental Assistant Prgm
3223 Broadway
Gary, IN 46409
Prgm Dir: K Hinshaw
Tel: 219 980-6721   *Fax:* 219 981-4249
E-mail: khinshaw@iunhaw1.indiana.edu
Class Cap: 18   *Begins:* Aug
Length: 9 mos   *Award:* Cert
Tuition per yr: $1,530 res, $3,388 non-res

Indiana University School of Medicine
Dental Assistant Prgm
1121 W Michigan St
Indianapolis, IN 46202-5186
Prgm Dir: P Spencer
Tel: 317 274-4407
Class Cap: 30
Length: 8 mos   *Award:* Cert
Tuition per yr: $4,119

Professional Careers Institute
Dental Assistant Prgm
2611 Waterfront Pkwy E Dr
Indianapolis, IN 46421
Prgm Dir: Lisa Hutt-Smith
Tel: 317 299-6001
Length: 8 mos   *Award:* Dipl, AA
Tuition per yr: $6,252 res, $6,252 non-res

Ivy Tech State Coll - Lafayette
Dental Assistant Prgm
3208 Ross Rd/Box 6299
Lafayette, IN 47903
Prgm Dir: J Buckles
Tel: 317 477-9205
Class Cap: 24   *Begins:* Aug
Length: 12 mos   *Award:* Cert
Tuition per yr: $2,631 res, $4,792 non-res

Indiana University - South Bend
Dental Assistant Prgm
1700 Mishawaka Ave
South Bend, IN 46634
Prgm Dir: Barbara Pasionek-Wieczorek
Tel: 219 237-4152
Class Cap: 30   *Begins:* Aug Jan
Length: 8 mos   *Award:* Cert, AA
Tuition per yr: $4,620 res, $9,915 non-res

Iowa

Des Moines Area Community College
Dental Assistant Prgm
2006 Ankeny Blvd
Ankeny, IA 50021
Prgm Dir: Deborah P Bell
Tel: 515 964-6308   *Fax:* 515 964-6440
Class Cap: 36
Length: 11 mos   *Award:* Dipl
Tuition per yr: $2,604 res, $4,606 non-res

Kirkwood Community College
Dental Assistant Prgm
6301 Kirkwood Blvd SW
PO Box 2068
Cedar Rapids, IA 52406-9973
Prgm Dir: P Hanson
Tel: 319 398-5560   *Fax:* 319 398-1293
Class Cap: 36   *Begins:* Aug
Length: 11 mos, 15 mos   *Award:* Dipl
Tuition per yr: $2,448 res, $4,895 non-res

Iowa Western Community College
Dental Assistant Prgm
2700 College Rd/Box 4C
Council Bluffs, IA 51502
Prgm Dir: J Miller
Tel: 712 325-3351   *Fax:* 712 325-3717
Class Cap: 20   *Begins:* Aug
Length: 20 mos   *Award:* Dipl
Tuition per yr: $3,306 res, $4,377 non-res

Marshalltown Community College
Dental Assistant Prgm
3700 S Ctr St
Marshalltown, IA 50158
Prgm Dir: Mary Croker
Tel: 515 752-7106   *Fax:* 515 754-1445
E-mail: mlcroker@iavalley.cc.ia.us
Class Cap: 22   *Begins:* Aug
Length: 10 mos   *Award:* Dipl
Tuition per yr: $2,842 res, $5,684 non-res

Northeast Iowa Community College
Dental Assistant Prgm
10250 Sundown Rd
Peosta, IA 52068
Prgm Dir: G Kluesner
Tel: 800 728-7367   *Fax:* 319 556-5058
E-mail: kluesneg@nicc.co.ia.us
Class Cap: 25   *Begins:* Aug
Length: 11 mos   *Award:* Dipl
Tuition per yr: $2,666 res, $3,732 non-res
Evening or weekend classes available

Western Iowa Tech Community College
Dental Assistant Prgm
4647 Stone Ave/PO Box 265
Sioux City, IA 51102
Prgm Dir: J Erickson
Tel: 712 274-8733   *Fax:* 712 274-6412
Class Cap: 24   *Begins:* Aug
Length: 11 mos   *Award:* Dipl
Tuition per yr: $3,490 res, $5,996 non-res

Hawkeye Community College
Dental Assistant Prgm
1501 E Orange Rd/Box 8015
Waterloo, IA 50704
Prgm Dir: S Van Syoc
Tel: 319 296-2320
Class Cap: 24   *Begins:* Aug
Length: 11 mos   *Award:* Dipl
Tuition per yr: $4,285 res, $7,299 non-res

Kansas

Flint Hills Technical School
Dental Assistant Prgm
3301 W 18th Ave
Emporia, KS 66801
Prgm Dir: P Fleming
Tel: 316 343-2300
Class Cap: 20   *Begins:* Aug
Length: 9 mos   *Award:* Dipl
Tuition per yr: $1,675

Salina Area Vocational Technical School
Dental Assistant Prgm
2562 Scanlan Ave
Salina, KS 67401
Tel: 913 827-0134
Class Cap: 18   *Begins:* Aug
Length: 9 mos   *Award:* Cert
Tuition per yr: $1,076 res, $1,076 non-res

Wichita Area Technical College
Dental Assistant Prgm
324 N Emporia
Wichita, KS 67202
Prgm Dir: M Mitchell
Tel: 316 833-4370   *Fax:* 316 833-4332
Class Cap: 16   *Begins:* Aug
Length: 9 mo , 24 mos   *Award:* Dipl, AAS
Tuition per yr: $999 res, $6,660 non-res

Kentucky

Bowling Green State Voc Tech School

Dental Assistant Prgm
1845 Loop Dr
Bowling Green, KY 42101-3601
Prgm Dir: Wendi Hulsey
Tel: 502 746-7461   *Fax:* 502 746-7466
Class Cap: 15   *Begins:* Aug
Length: 10 mos   *Award:* Dipl
Tuition per yr: $975 res, $1,475 non-res

Kentucky Tech Central Campus

Dental Assistant Prgm
104 Vo-Technical Rd
Lexington, KY 40511-1020
Prgm Dir: S Begley, ROH CDA
Tel: 606 246-2400   *Fax:* 606 246-2417
Class Cap: 15   *Begins:* Aug Jan
Length: 10 mos   *Award:* Dipl
Tuition per yr: $1,085
Evening or weekend classes available

West Kentucky Tech

Dental Assistant Prgm
PO Box 7408/Blandville Rd
Paducah, KY 42002-7408
Prgm Dir: Darlene Carter
Tel: 502 554-4991   *Fax:* 502 554-9754
Class Cap: 12   *Begins:* Aug
Length: 11 mos   *Award:* Dipl
Tuition per yr: $600 res, $1,200 non-res
Evening or weekend classes available

Maine

University of Maine - Bangor

Dental Assistant Prgm
Lincoln Hall
29 Texas Ave
Bangor, ME 04401-4324
Prgm Dir: D Graham Olsen
Tel: 207 581-6056   *Fax:* 207 581-6075
E-mail: dolsen@maine.maine.edu
Class Cap: 12   *Begins:* Sep
Length: 9 mos   *Award:* Cert
Tuition per yr: $3,510 res, $9,360 non-res

Maryland

Medix School

Dental Assistant Prgm
1017 York Rd
Towson, MD 21204
Prgm Dir: R Caplan
Tel: 410 337-5155   *Fax:* 410 337-5104
Length: 8 mos   *Award:* Dipl
Tuition per yr: $6,225

Massachusetts

Massasoit Community College

Dental Assistant Prgm
Massasoit Community College
900 Randolph St
Canton, MA 02021
Prgm Dir: M Frohn
Tel: 617 821-2222
Class Cap: 20
Length: 8 mos   *Award:* Cert
Tuition per yr: $2,844
Evening or weekend classes available

Northern Essex Community College

Dental Assistant Prgm
45 Franklin St
Lawrence, MA 01840
Prgm Dir: K Hamidiani
Tel: 508 688-3181, Ext 4330   *Fax:* 508 683-1667
Class Cap: 20   *Begins:* Sep
Length: 9 mos   *Award:* Cert
Tuition per yr: $3,204 res, $8,706 non-res
Evening or weekend classes available

Middlesex Community College - Lowell

Dental Assistant Prgm
33 Kearney Square
Lowell, MA 01852
Prgm Dir: M Jacobs-Bloy
Tel: 508 656-3200   *Fax:* 508 656-3078
Class Cap: 20   *Begins:* Sep
Length: 9 mos   *Award:* Cert
Tuition per yr: $3,290 res, $3,614 non-res

Mt Ida College

Dental Assistant Prgm
777 Dedham St
Newton Centre, MA 02159
Prgm Dir: Kathleen Held
Tel: 617 969-4562
Class Cap: 20   *Begins:* Sep
Length: 8 mos   *Award:* Cert
Tuition per yr: $11,590 res, $11,590 non-res

Charles H McCann Technical School

Dental Assistant Prgm
Hodges Crossroad
North Adams, MA 01247
Prgm Dir: D Traversa
Tel: 413 663-5383   *Fax:* 413 664-9424
Class Cap: 18   *Begins:* Sep
Length: 10 mos   *Award:* Cert
Tuition per yr: $459 res, $7,858 non-res

Southeastern Technical Institute

Dental Assistant Prgm
250 Foundry St
South Easton, MA 02375
Prgm Dir: A Beaudoin
Tel: 508 238-1860
Length: 9 mos   *Award:* Dipl
Tuition per yr: $1,625 res, $2,625 non-res

Springfield Technical Community College

Dental Assistant Prgm
One Armory Square
Springfield, MA 01105
Prgm Dir: Carol A Giaquinto
Tel: 413 781-7822
Class Cap: 25   *Begins:* Sep Jun
Length: 12 mos, 16 mos   *Award:* Cert
Tuition per yr: $5,175 res, $9,175 non-res
Evening or weekend classes available

Worcester Technical Institute

Dental Assistant Prgm
251 Belmont St
Worcester, MA 01605
Prgm Dir: A Nichols
Tel: 508 799-1945   *Fax:* 508 799-1932
Class Cap: 12   *Begins:* Aug
Length: 9 mos   *Award:* Cert
Tuition per yr: $1,600 res, $2,000 non-res

Michigan

Washtenaw Community College

Dental Assistant Prgm
4800 E Huron River Dr
Ann Arbor, MI 48106
Prgm Dir: Betty Finkbeiner
Tel: 313 973-3332   *Fax:* 313 973-5414
Class Cap: 24   *Begins:* Sep
Length: 12 mos   *Award:* Cert
Tuition per yr: $2,400 res, $3,160 non-res

Lake Michigan College

Dental Assistant Prgm
2755 E Napier
Benton Harbor, MI 49022
Prgm Dir: D Burch
Tel: 616 927-8100   *Fax:* 616 927-6585
E-mail: burch@raptor.lmc.cc.mi.us
Class Cap: 20   *Begins:* Varies
Length: 12 mos, 24 mos   *Award:* Cert, AAS
Tuition per yr: $2,676 res, $3,136 non-res
Evening or weekend classes available

Wayne County Community College

Dental Assistant Prgm
8551 Greenfield/Rm 310
Detroit, MI 48228
Prgm Dir: J Nyquist
Tel: 313 943-4055   *Fax:* 313 943-4025
Class Cap: 15
Length: 11 mos   *Award:* Cert
Tuition per yr: $2,646 res, $3,738 non-res
Evening or weekend classes available

Charles Stewart Mott Community College

Dental Assistant Prgm
1401 E Court St
Flint, MI 48503
Prgm Dir: D Boersema
Tel: 810 762-0496
Class Cap: 20   *Begins:* Sep
Length: 9 mos   *Award:* Cert, AA
Tuition per yr: $5,151 res, $8,992 non-res

Grand Rapids Community College

Dental Assistant Prgm
143 Bostwick St NE
Grand Rapids, MI 49503
Prgm Dir: M Campo
Tel: 616 771-4225   *Fax:* 616 771-4234
Class Cap: 16
Length: 12 mos   *Award:* Cert
Tuition per yr: $2,322 res, $3,913 non-res

Programs

Lansing Community College
Dental Assistant Prgm
PO Box 40010
Lansing, MI 48901-7210
Prgm Dir: S Deck, ROH MS
Tel: 517 483-1457
Class Cap: 18   *Begins:* Aug
Length: 9 mos   *Award:* Cert
Tuition per yr: $1,500 res, $3,535 non-res

Northwestern Michigan College
Dental Assistant Prgm
1701 E Front St
Traverse City, MI 49684
Prgm Dir: Sallie Donovan
Tel: 616 922-1240
Class Cap: 25   *Begins:* Aug
Length: 16 mos   *Award:* AA
Tuition per yr: $2,299 res, $3,756 non-res

Delta College
Dental Assistant Prgm
University Center, MI 48710
Prgm Dir: P Jernstadt
Tel: 517 686-9428
Class Cap: 28   *Begins:* Aug
Length: 8 mos   *Award:* Cert, AAS
Tuition per yr: $3,395 res, $5,600 non-res

Minnesota

Northwest Technical Coll - Bemidji
Dental Assistant Prgm
905 Grant Ave SE
Bemidji, MN 56601
Prgm Dir: J Damp
Tel: 218 755-4270   *Fax:* 218 755-4289
Class Cap: 24
Length: 11 mos   *Award:* Dipl
Tuition per yr: $3,215 res, $5,794 non-res

Normandale Community College
Dental Assistant Prgm
9700 France Ave S
Bloomington, MN 55431
Prgm Dir: Geneva Middleton
Tel: 612 832-6339   *Fax:* 612 832-6571
E-mail: gmiddleton@nr.cc.mn.us
Class Cap: 24   *Begins:* Sep
Length: 10 mos   *Award:* Cert
Tuition per yr: $3,000 res, $5,380 non-res
Evening or weekend classes available

Central Lakes College
Dental Assistant Prgm
300 Quince St
Brainerd, MN 56401
Prgm Dir: Leann Schoenle
Tel: 218 825-2117
Class Cap: 24   *Begins:* Sep
Length: 11 mos   *Award:* Dipl, AA
Tuition per yr: $1,843 res, $3,123 non-res

Minnesota School of Business - Brooklyn Ctr
Dental Assistant Prgm
6120 Earle Brown Dr
Brooklyn Center, MN 55430
Prgm Dir: Lynn Melin
Tel: 612 566-7777   *Fax:* 612 566-7030
Class Cap: 43   *Begins:* Quarterly
Length: 12 mos, 21 mos   *Award:* Dipl, AAS
Evening or weekend classes available

Hennepin Technical College
Dental Assistant Prgm
9000 Brooklyn Blvd
Brooklyn Park, MN 55445
Prgm Dir: S Thaemert
Tel: 612 550-2118   *Fax:* 612 550-2119
Class Cap: 30   *Begins:* Sep Mar
Length: 12 mos   *Award:* Dipl, AAS
Tuition per yr: $2,855 res, $5,709 non-res
Evening or weekend classes available

Minnesota West Comm and Tech College
Dental Assistant Prgm
1011 First St W
Canby, MN 56220
Prgm Dir: Mary Boulton
Tel: 507 223-7252   *Fax:* 507 223-5291
Class Cap: 21   *Begins:* Sep
Length: 11 mos   *Award:* Dipl, AAS
Tuition per yr: $3,029 res, $5,493 non-res

Duluth Business Univ/MN Sch of Business
Dental Assistant Prgm
412 W Superior St
Duluth, MN 55802
Prgm Dir: Kathleen Sannes
Tel: 218 722-3361
Class Cap: 50   *Begins:* Quarterly
Length: 15 mos, 21 mos   *Award:* Dipl
Tuition per yr: $11,000
Evening or weekend classes available

Hibbing Community College
Dental Assistant Prgm
2900 E Beltline
Hibbing, MN 55747
Prgm Dir: A Badanjak
Tel: 218 262-7242   *Fax:* 218 262-7222
Class Cap: 32
Length: 9 mos   *Award:* Dipl
Tuition per yr: $3,127 res, $5,129 non-res

Lakeland Medical Dental Academy
Dental Assistant Prgm
1402 W Lake St
Minneapolis, MN 55408
Prgm Dir: R Anderson
Tel: 612 827-5656   *Fax:* 612 827-3833
Class Cap: 60   *Begins:* Jan Mar Jun Sep
Length: 12 mos   *Award:* Dipl, AAS
Tuition per yr: $6,525 res, $6,525 non-res
Evening or weekend classes available

Minneapolis Technical College
Dental Assistant Prgm
1501 Hennepin Ave S/Rm 403B
Minneapolis, MN 55403
Prgm Dir: K Lapham
Tel: 612 370-9472   Fax: 612 370-9428
Class Cap: 18   Begins: Sep Mar
Length: 12 mos   *Award:* Dipl, Cert
Tuition per yr: $2,854 res, $5,298 non-res

Northwest Technical Coll - Moorhead
Dental Assistant Prgm
1900 28th Ave S
Moorhead, MN 56560-4899
Prgm Dir: P Humphrey
Tel: 218 299-6522   *Fax:* 218 236-0342
Class Cap: 24   *Begins:* Sep
Length: 12 mos   *Award:* Dipl
Tuition per yr: $2,905 res, $5,733 non-res
Evening or weekend classes available

South Central Technical College
Dental Assistant Prgm
1920 Lee Blvd
North Mankato, MN 56002-1920
Prgm Dir: K Metz
Tel: 507 389-5846   *Fax:* 507 389-5850
Class Cap: 25   *Begins:* Aug
Length: 11 mos   *Award:* Cert, AAS
Tuition per yr: $3,982 res, $6,589 non-res
Evening or weekend classes available

Rochester Community and Technical College
Dental Assistant Prgm
1926 College View Rd SE
Rochester, MN 55904
Prgm Dir: Bonnie Crawford
Tel: 507 280-3149
Class Cap: 36   *Begins:* Sep
Length: 11 mos   *Award:* Dipl
Tuition per yr: $3,400 res, $5,928 non-res

Dakota County Technical College
Dental Assistant Prgm
1300 145th St E
Rosemont, MN 55068
Prgm Dir: Diana Sullivan
Tel: 612 423-8483
Class Cap: 45   *Begins:* Sep
Length: 9 mos   *Award:* Dipl
Tuition per yr: $3,553 res, $3,553 non-res

St Cloud Technical College
Dental Assistant Prgm
1540 Northway Dr
Saint Cloud, MN 56303-1240
Prgm Dir: K Brown
Tel: 320 654-5031   *Fax:* 320 654-5981
E-mail: khb@cloud.tec.mn.us
Class Cap: 20   *Begins:* Sep
Length: 12 mos   *Award:* Cert, AAS
Tuition per yr: $2,991 res, $5,511 non-res
Evening or weekend classes available

Century Community and Technical College
Dental Assistant Prgm
3300 Century Ave N
White Bear Lake, MN 55110
Prgm Dir: D Bruns
Tel: 612 779-1771   *Fax:* 612 779-5779
Length: 15 mos   *Award:* Dipl
Tuition per yr: $3,509 res, $6,081 non-res

Mississippi

Pearl River Community College
Dental Assistant Prgm
5448 US Hwy 49 S
Hattiesburg, MS 39401
Prgm Dir: E Addison
Tel: 601 544-7722   *Fax:* 601 545-2976
Class Cap: 12   *Begins:* Aug
Length: 12 mos   *Award:* Dipl,Cert
Tuition per yr: $2,235
Evening or weekend classes available

Hinds Community College District
Dental Assistant Prgm
1750 Chadwick Dr
Jackson, MS 39204
Prgm Dir: Richard Gavant
Tel: 601 371-3526
Class Cap: 24   Begins: Aug Jan
Length: 9 mos   *Award:* Cert, AA
Tuition per yr: $2,450 res, $5,226 non-res

Missouri

Nichols Career Center
Dental Assistant Prgm
609 Union St
Jefferson City, MO 65101
Prgm Dir: P Noirfalise
Tel: 573 659-3112
Class Cap: 16
Length: 9 mos   *Award:* Dipl
Tuition per yr: $3,500 res, $3,500 non-res

Mineral Area College
Dental Assistant Prgm
PO Box 1000
Park Hills, MO 63601
Prgm Dir: D Eck
Tel: 573 431-4593   *Fax:* 573 431-2321
Class Cap: 16   *Begins:* Aug
Length: 12 mos   *Award:* Cert
Tuition per yr: $3,140 res, $3,860 non-res

Ozarks Technical Community College
Dental Assistant Prgm
1417 N Jefferson
Springfield, MO 65802
Prgm Dir: S Wood
Tel: 417 895-7124   *Fax:* 417 895-7161
Class Cap: 22   *Begins:* Aug
Length: 9 mos   *Award:* Cert
Tuition per yr: $2,881 res, $4,731 non-res
Evening or weekend classes available

East Central College
Dental Assistant Prgm
Box 529 Hwy 50 & Prairie Dell
Union, MO 63084
Prgm Dir: B Scott
Tel: 314 583-5193   *Fax:* 314 583-6637
Med Dir: Pat O'Conner
Class Cap: 30
Length: 8 mos   *Award:* Cert
Tuition per yr: $2,261 res, $4,065 non-res

Montana

Montana State Univ Coll of Technology
Dental Assistant Prgm
2100 16th Ave S
Great Falls, MT 59405
Prgm Dir: A Buer
Tel: 406 771-4351   *Fax:* 406 771-4317
E-mail: zgf6008@maia.oscs.montana.edu
Class Cap: 24
Length: 12 mos   *Award:* Cert
Tuition per yr: $2,376 res, $5,590 non-res

Salish Kootenai College
Dental Assistant Prgm
Box 117
Pablo, MT 59855
Prgm Dir: Garry Pitts, DDS MPH
Tel: 406 675-4800   *Fax:* 406 675-4801
E-mail: garry_pitts@skc.edu
Class Cap: 20   *Begins:* Varies
Length: 12 mos   *Award:* Cert, AAS
Tuition per yr: $5,215 res, $11,275 non-res

Nebraska

Central Community College
Dental Assistant Prgm
PO Box 1024
Hastings, NE 68902-1024
Prgm Dir: M Cecil
Tel: 402 461-2467   *Fax:* 402 461-2454
E-mail: cechdea@cccadm.gi.cccneb.edu
Begins: Varies
Length: 10 mos   *Award:* Dipl
Tuition per yr: $1,722 res, $2,533 non-res

Southeast Community College
Dental Assistant Prgm
8800 O St
Lincoln, NE 68520
Prgm Dir: S Asher
Tel: 402 437-2740   *Fax:* 402 437-2404
Class Cap: 30   *Begins:* Oct Jan Apr Jul
Length: 12 mos   *Award:* Dipl
Tuition per yr: $1,938 res, $2,318 non-res
Evening or weekend classes available

Mid Plains Community College
Dental Assistant Prgm
1101 Halligan Dr
North Platte, NE 69101
Prgm Dir: R White
Tel: 308 532-8740   *Fax:* 308 532-8494
Class Cap: 15   *Begins:* Aug
Length: 11 mos   *Award:* Dipl
Tuition per yr: $1,373 res, $1,449 non-res

Metropolitan Community College
Dental Assistant Prgm
PO Box 3777
Omaha, NE 68103-0777
Prgm Dir: Karen Finley
Tel: 402 449-8510
Class Cap: 30   *Begins:* Sep
Length: 11 mos   *Award:* Cert, AA
Tuition per yr: $1,891 res, $2,260 non-res

Omaha College of Health Careers
Dental Assistant Prgm
10845 Harney St
Omaha, NE 68154-2655
Prgm Dir: T Watson
Tel: 402 333-1400   *Fax:* 402 333-4588
Class Cap: 15
Length: 9 mos   *Award:* Dipl
Tuition per yr: $6,772

Nevada

Truckee Meadows Community College
Dental Assistant Prgm
7000 Dandini Blvd
Reno, NV 89512-3999
Prgm Dir: S Christine Wagner
Tel: 702 673-7115   *Fax:* 702 673-7034
Class Cap: 25   *Begins:* Aug
Length: 10 mos, 18 mos   *Award:* Cert, AS
Tuition per yr: $1,847 res, $4,007 non-res

New Hampshire

New Hampshire Technical Institute
Dental Assistant Prgm
11 Institute Dr
Concord, NH 03301-7412
Prgm Dir: Sue Ellen Casey
Tel: 603 225-1844   *Fax:* 603 225-1895
Class Cap: 24   *Begins:* Aug
Length: 11 mos   *Award:* Dipl
Tuition per yr: $3,416 res, $7,178 non-res

New Jersey

Camden County College
Dental Assistant Prgm
PO Box 200
Blackwood, NJ 08012
Prgm Dir: C Hewitt, CDA RDA BS/MCA
Tel: 609 227-7200, Ext 4471   *Fax:* 609 374-4880
Class Cap: 30
Length: 8 mos   *Award:* Cert, AAS
Tuition per yr: $2,912 res, $3,060 non-res
Evening or weekend classes available

Cumberland County Technical Education Center
Dental Assistant Prgm
601 Bridgeton Ave
Bridgeton, NJ 08302
Prgm Dir: Judith Zirkle, CDA RDA
Tel: 609 451-9000   *Fax:* 609 451-8487
E-mail: cctenj@algorithms.com
Begins: Sep
Length: 10 mos
Tuition per yr: $1,025

Atlantic County Vocational Tech School
Dental Assistant Prgm
5080 Atlantic Ave
Mays Landing, NJ 08330
Prgm Dir: S White
Tel: 609 625-2249   *Fax:* 609 625-8622
Class Cap: 15   *Begins:* Sep
Length: 10 mos   *Award:* Cert
Tuition per yr: $2,045

Univ of Med & Dent of New Jersey
Dental Assistant Prgm
65 Bergen St
Newark, NJ 07107-3006
Prgm Dir: C Drew, EdD
Tel: 201 982-4279
Class Cap: 24
Length: 10 mos   *Award:* Cert
Tuition per yr: $2,448 res, $4,896 non-res

Programs

Technical Institute of Camden County
Dental Assistant Prgm
343 Berlin-Cross Keys Rd
Sicklerville, NJ 08081-9709
Prgm Dir: T Stallone
Tel: 609 767-7000
Class Cap: 25
Length: 9 mos   *Award:* Dipl
Tuition per yr: $880 res, $2,780 non-res
Evening or weekend classes available

Berdan Institute
Dental Assistant Prgm
265 Rte 46 W
Totowa, NJ 07512
Prgm Dir: A Germann
Tel: 201 256-3444   *Fax:* 201 256-0816
Class Cap: 25
Length: 9 mos   *Award:* Cert
Tuition per yr: $7,140
Evening or weekend classes available

New Mexico

University of New Mexico - Gallup/IHS
Dental Assistant Prgm
200 College Rd
Gallup, NM 87301
Prgm Dir: Jean Martinez-Welles
Length: 9 mos   *Award:* Cert, AA
Tuition per yr: $2,464 res, $3,724 non-res

New York

SUNY Educational Opportunity Center
Dental Assistant Prgm
465 Washington St
Buffalo, NY 14203
Prgm Dir: N Robinson
Tel: 716 849-6725   *Fax:* 716 849-6755
Class Cap: 32   *Begins:* Sep May
Length: 9 mos   *Award:* Cert

New York University
Dental Assistant Prgm
345 E 24th St
New York, NY 10010
Prgm Dir: J Cleary
Tel: 212 998-9777   *Fax:* 212 995-4085
E-mail: cleary@is2.nyu.edu
Class Cap: 100   *Begins:* Sep Feb
Length: 10 mos   *Award:* Cert
Tuition per yr: $8,077
Evening or weekend classes available

North Carolina

Asheville Buncombe Technical Comm Coll
Dental Assistant Prgm
340 Victoria Rd
Asheville, NC 28801
Prgm Dir: S Tate
Tel: 704 254-1921   *Fax:* 704 251-6355
Class Cap: 26   *Begins:* Sep
Length: 12 mos   *Award:* Dipl
Tuition per yr: $776 res, $6,054 non-res

Univ of North Carolina at Chapel Hill
Dental Assistant Prgm
367 Old Dental Bldg/CB 7450
Chapel Hill, NC 27599-7450
Prgm Dir: J Jenzano
Tel: 919 966-2800   *Fax:* 919 966-6761
E-mail: jenzane.decology@mhs.unc.edu
Class Cap: 25   *Begins:* Aug
Length: 10 mos   *Award:* Cert
Tuition per yr: $450 res, $450 non-res

Central Piedmont Community College
Dental Assistant Prgm
1201 Elizabeth Ave/Kings Dr
Charlotte, NC 28204
Prgm Dir: Marilyn M Wright
Tel: 704 330-5951   *Fax:* 704 330-6947
Class Cap: 28   *Begins:* Sep
Length: 12 mos   *Award:* Dipl
Tuition per yr: $2,224 res, $7,522 non-res

Fayetteville Technical Community College
Dental Assistant Prgm
2201 Hull Rd/PO Box 35236
Fayetteville, NC 28303
Prgm Dir: D McGrath, BS CDA
Tel: 910 678-8280   *Fax:* 910 484-6600
E-mail: dmcgrath@pst.faytech.cc.nc.us
Class Cap: 35   *Begins:* Sep
Length: 10 mos   *Award:* Dipl
Tuition per yr: $742 res, $6,020 non-res

Wayne Community College
Dental Assistant Prgm
Caller Box 8002
Goldsboro, NC 27530
Prgm Dir: C McCullen
Tel: 919 735-5151   *Fax:* 919 736-3204
E-mail: conniem@wcc.wayne.cc.nc.us
Med Dir: Sue Brambaugh
Class Cap: 24   *Begins:* Aug
Length: 12 mos   *Award:* Dipl
Tuition per yr: $778 res, $6,056 non-res

Alamance Community College
Dental Assistant Prgm
PO Box 8000
Graham, NC 27253-8000
Prgm Dir: Margaret Hooper
Tel: 910 578-2002   *Fax:* 910 578-1987
Class Cap: 30   *Begins:* Sep
Length: 8 mos   *Award:* Dipl
Tuition per yr: $1,620 res, $6,898 non-res

Coastal Carolina Community College
Dental Assistant Prgm
444 Western Blvd
Jacksonville, NC 28546
Prgm Dir: E Beall
Tel: 910 938-6276   *Fax:* 910 455-7027
Class Cap: 24   *Begins:* Sep
Length: 12 mos   *Award:* Dipl
Tuition per yr: $742 res, $6,020 non-res

Guilford Technical Community College
Dental Assistant Prgm
PO Box 309
Jamestown, NC 27282
Prgm Dir: Lynda Snider
Tel: 910 334-4822
Class Cap: 36   *Begins:* Sep
Length: 11 mos   *Award:* Dipl
Tuition per yr: $2,160 res, $7,460 non-res

Western Piedmont Community College
Dental Assistant Prgm
1001 Burkemont Ave
Morgantown, NC 28655
Prgm Dir: Naomi Smith
Tel: 704 438-6130
Class Cap: 16   *Begins:* Sep
Length: 10 mos   *Award:* Dipl
Tuition per yr: $1,866 res, $7,120 non-res

Wake Technical Community College
Dental Assistant Prgm
9101 Fayetteville Rd
Raleigh, NC 27603-5696
Prgm Dir: Sandra L Lytle
Tel: 919 231-4500   *Fax:* 919 779-3360
Class Cap: 24   *Begins:* Sep
Length: 12 mos   *Award:* Dipl

Rowan-Cabarrus Community College
Dental Assistant Prgm
PO Box 1595
Salisbury, NC 28144
Prgm Dir: L Kamp
Tel: 704 637-0760, Ext 375   *Fax:* 704 642-0750
Class Cap: 18
Length: 11 mos   *Award:* Dipl
Tuition per yr: $1,471 res, $6,749 non-res

Wilkes Community College
Dental Assistant Prgm
PO Box 120
Wilkesboro, NC 28697-0120
Prgm Dir: D Billings
Tel: 910 838-6253   *Fax:* 910 838-6277
Class Cap: 15   *Begins:* Sep
Length: 12 mos   *Award:* Dipl
Tuition per yr: $742 res, $6,020 non-res
Evening or weekend classes available

Cape Fear Community College
Dental Assistant Prgm
411 N Front St
Wilmington, NC 28401-3993
Prgm Dir: N Keller
Tel: 910 251-6943   *Fax:* 910 251-6945
Class Cap: 12   *Begins:* Sep
Length: 11 mos   *Award:* Dipl
Tuition per yr: $1,549 res, $6,827 non-res

North Dakota

Interstate Business College
Dental Assistant Prgm
2720 32nd Ave SW
Fargo, ND 58103
Prgm Dir: L Aadland
Tel: 701 232-2477   *Fax:* 701 232-5963
Class Cap: 28   *Begins:* Sep
Length: 12 mos   *Award:* Dipl
Tuition per yr: $9,300

North Dakota State College of Science
Dental Assistant Prgm
College of Science
Wahpeton, ND 58076
Prgm Dir: S Swanson
Tel: 701 671-2333
E-mail: suswanso@plains.nodak.edu
Class Cap: 18   *Begins:* Aug
Length: 10 mos   *Award:* Cert
Tuition per yr: $1,976 res, $5,101 non-res

Ohio

Cuyahoga Community College

Dental Assistant Prgm
2900 Community College Ave
Cleveland, OH 44115
Prgm Dir: M Gerosky
Tel: 216 987-4494 *Fax:* 216 987-4386
E-mail: mary-lou.gerosky@tri-c.cc.oh.us
Class Cap: 20 *Begins:* Sep
Length: 8 mos *Award:* Cert
Tuition per yr: $2,079 res, $2,808 non-res
Evening or weekend classes available

Jefferson Community College

Dental Assistant Prgm
4000 Sunset Blvd
Steubenville, OH 43952
Prgm Dir: D Robinson
Tel: 614 264-5591 *Fax:* 614 264-1335
Class Cap: 24 *Begins:* Aug
Length: 10 mos *Award:* Cert, AAS
Tuition per yr: $2,337 res, $2,542 non-res
Evening or weekend classes available

Youngstown Pub Sch/Choffin Career Center

Dental Assistant Prgm
O W Wood St/Box 550
Youngstown, OH 44501
Prgm Dir: Paula J Oliver
Tel: 330 744-8749 *Fax:* 330 539-0801
Class Cap: 24
Length: 9 mos *Award:* Cert
Tuition per yr: $2,935

Oklahoma

Rose State College

Dental Assistant Prgm
6420 SE 15th St
Midwest City, OK 73110
Prgm Dir: Janet Turley
Tel: 405 733-7336 *Fax:* 405 736-0338
Class Cap: 12 *Begins:* Aug
Length: 8 mos *Award:* Cert, AAS
Tuition per yr: $1,365 res, $3,465 non-res
Evening or weekend classes available

Oregon

Linn-Benton Community College

Dental Assistant Prgm
6500 SW Pacific Blvd
Albany, OR 97321
Prgm Dir: Sharon Billetter
Tel: 541 928-2361 *Fax:* 541 917-4508
E-mail: paulsj@gw.lbcc.cc.or.us
Class Cap: 25 *Begins:* Sep
Length: 11 mos *Award:* Cert
Tuition per yr: $2,135 res, $7,442 non-res

Lane Community College

Dental Assistant Prgm
4000 E 30th
Eugene, OR 97405
Prgm Dir: Elizabeth Webb
Tel: 541 747-4501
Class Cap: 30 *Begins:* Sep
Length: 9 mos *Award:* Cert, AA
Tuition per yr: $3,042 res, $7,277 non-res

Blue Mountain Community College

Dental Assistant Prgm
2411 NW Carden
Pendleton, OR 97801
Prgm Dir: Crystal D Patton-Doherty
Tel: 541 278-5876 *Fax:* 541 276-6119
E-mail: cpatton@bmcc.cc.or.us
Class Cap: 17 *Begins:* Sep
Length: 9 mos *Award:* Cert
Tuition per yr: $1,728 res, $5,376 non-res
Evening or weekend classes available

CollegeAmerica

Dental Assistant Prgm
921 SW Washington/Rm 200
Portland, OR 97205
Prgm Dir: Marcella McClain
Tel: 503 242-9000 *Fax:* 503 222-3801
Class Cap: 40 *Begins:* Monthly
Length: 9 mos *Award:* Dipl
Tuition per yr: $9,700
Evening or weekend classes available

ConCorde Career Institute

Dental Assistant Prgm
1827 NE 44th Ave
Portland, OR 97213
Tel: 503 281-4181

Portland Community College

Dental Assistant Prgm
PO Box 19000
Portland, OR 97219-0990
Prgm Dir: A Jackson
Tel: 503 244-6111 *Fax:* 503 977-4869
E-mail: ajackson@pcc.edu
Class Cap: 45 *Begins:* Sep
Length: 8 mos *Award:* Cert
Tuition per yr: $1,680 res, $6,000 non-res

Chemeketa Community College

Dental Assistant Prgm
4000 Lancaster Dr NE
Salem, OR 97309
Prgm Dir: Joyce Vaughan
Tel: 503 399-5269 *Fax:* 503 399-5496
E-mail: joycev@chemek.cc.01.us
Class Cap: 30 *Begins:* Sep
Length: 8 mos *Award:* Cert
Tuition per yr: $1,768 res, $6,240 non-res
Evening or weekend classes available

Pennsylvania

Harcum College

Dental Assistant Prgm
Montgomery Ave
Bryn Mawr, PA 19010
Prgm Dir: D Cavallucci
Tel: 610 526-6109 *Fax:* 610 526-6031
Class Cap: 25 *Begins:* Aug
Length: 8 mos *Award:* Cert
Tuition per yr: $16,790 res, $11,710 non-res
Evening or weekend classes available

Harrisburg Area Community College

Dental Assistant Prgm
One Hacc Dr
Harrisburg, PA 17110-2999
Prgm Dir: D Nickey
Tel: 717 780-2396 *Fax:* 717 780-2551
Class Cap: 18
Length: 10 mos *Award:* Cert
Tuition per yr: $2,400 res, $4,500 non-res

Manor Junior College

Dental Assistant Prgm
700 Fox Chase Rd
Jenkintown, PA 19046-3399
Prgm Dir: Diane Meehan, CDA
Tel: 215 885-2360 *Fax:* 215 885-6084
Class Cap: 18 *Begins:* Sep Jan
Length: 19 mos *Award:* Cert, AS
Tuition per yr: $1,160 res, $7,860 non-res
Evening or weekend classes available

Luzerne County Community College

Dental Assistant Prgm
1333 S Prospect St
Nanticoke, PA 18634-3899
Prgm Dir: Lisa Rowley, CDA RDH MS
Tel: 717 740-0448 *Fax:* 717 740-0265
Class Cap: 20
Length: 9 mos, 18 mos *Award:* Cert, AAS
Tuition per yr: $1,643 res, $4,929 non-res

Community College of Philadelphia

Dental Assistant Prgm
1700 Spring Garden St
Philadelphia, PA 19130
Prgm Dir: R Lynn
Tel: 215 751-8428 *Fax:* 215 751-8937
Class Cap: 36
Length: 10 mos *Award:* Cert
Tuition per yr: $2,898 res, $5,658 non-res
Evening or weekend classes available

Median School of Allied Health Careers

Dental Assistant Prgm
125 Seventh St
Pittsburgh, PA 15222-3400
Prgm Dir: Joan Ritchex, CDA
Tel: 412 391-0422
Class Cap: 25 *Begins:* Apr Sep
Length: 9 mos *Award:* Dipl
Tuition per yr: $5,400

Puerto Rico

University of Puerto Rico

Dental Assistant Prgm
GPO Box 5067
San Juan, PR 00936
Prgm Dir: Angel Rafael Aja
Tel: 787 758-2525
Class Cap: 25
Length: 9 mos *Award:* AA, BA
Tuition per yr: $2,796

Rhode Island

Community College of Rhode Island
Dental Assistant Prgm
Louisquisset Pike
Lincoln, RI 02865
Prgm Dir: D Medas Patton
Tel: 401 333-7252
Class Cap: 30　*Begins:* Sep
Length: 8 mos　*Award:* Cert
Tuition per yr: $1,566 res, $4,584 non-res

South Carolina

Aiken Technical College
Dental Assistant Prgm
PO Drawer 696
Aiken, SC 29802
Prgm Dir: Amelia Capers
Tel: 803 593-9231
Class Cap: 24　*Begins:* Aug
Length: 11 mos　*Award:* Dipl, AA
Tuition per yr: $2,462 res, $2,834 non-res

Trident Technical College
Dental Assistant Prgm
PO Box 118067
Charleston, SC 29423-8067
Prgm Dir: D Jennings, DMD
Tel: 803 569-6449　*Fax:* 803 569-6585
Class Cap: 24　*Begins:* Aug
Length: 8 mos　*Award:* Dipl
Tuition per yr: $2,436 res, $3,444 non-res

Midlands Technical College
Dental Assistant Prgm
PO Box 2408
Columbia, SC 29202
Prgm Dir: M Marchant
Tel: 803 822-3453　*Fax:* 803 822-3079
Class Cap: 24　*Begins:* Aug
Length: 12 mos　*Award:* Dipl
Tuition per yr: $1,533 res, $2,635 non-res

Florence-Darlington Technical College
Dental Assistant Prgm
PO Box 100548
Florence, SC 29501-0548
Prgm Dir: M Hewitt
Tel: 803 661-8023　*Fax:* 803 661-8306
Class Cap: 18　*Begins:* Aug
Length: 11 mos　*Award:* Dipl
Tuition per yr: $1,650 res, $1,875 non-res

Greenville Technical College
Dental Assistant Prgm
PO Box 5616
Greenville, SC 29606-5616
Prgm Dir: J.S. Demosthenes
Tel: 864 250-8286　*Fax:* 864 250-8462
E-mail: demostjsd@gvltec.edu
Class Cap: 25　*Begins:* Aug
Length: 12 mos　*Award:* Dipl
Tuition per yr: $1,575 res, $2,520 non-res

Tri-County Technical College
Dental Assistant Prgm
PO Box 587
Pendleton, SC 29670
Prgm Dir: J Trypack
Tel: 864 646-8361　*Fax:* 864 646-8256
Class Cap: 16　*Begins:* Aug
Length: 12 mos　*Award:* Dipl
Tuition per yr: $1,350 res, $1,638 non-res
Evening or weekend classes available

York Technical College
Dental Assistant Prgm
452 S Anderson Rd
Rock Hill, SC 29730
Prgm Dir: Deedee Mclain-Smith, RCM MS
Tel: 803 327-8039　*Fax:* 803 327-8059
E-mail: dsmith@york.tec.sc.us
Class Cap: 20
Length: 12 mos　*Award:* Dipl
Tuition per yr: $1,296 res, $1,548 non-res
Evening or weekend classes available

Spartanburg Technical College
Dental Assistant Prgm
PO Drawer 4386
Highway I-85
Spartanburg, SC 29305-4386
Prgm Dir: L Walker
Tel: 864 591-3872　*Fax:* 864 591-3708
E-mail: walkerL@aol.com@smtp@stc
Class Cap: 22　*Begins:* Aug
Length: 12 mos　*Award:* Dipl
Tuition per yr: $1,500 res, $1,825 non-res
Evening or weekend classes available

South Dakota

Lake Area Technical Institute
Dental Assistant Prgm
230 11th St NE
Watertown, SD 57201
Prgm Dir: R Bradberry
Tel: 605 886-5872　*Fax:* 605 882-6299
Class Cap: 35　*Award:* Dipl
Tuition per yr: $1,975

Tennessee

Chattanooga State Technical Comm College
Dental Assistant Prgm
4501 Amnicola Hwy
Chattanooga, TN 37406-1097
Prgm Dir: W Johnson
Tel: 423 634-7711　*Fax:* 423 634-3071
Class Cap: 24　*Begins:* Aug
Length: 8 mos　*Award:* Cert
Tuition per yr: $994 res, $3,920 non-res

East Tennessee State University
Dental Assistant Prgm
1000 West E St
Elizabethton, TN 37643
Prgm Dir: Victor Hopson
Tel: 423 547-4911
Class Cap: 12　*Begins:* Aug
Length: 11 mos　*Award:* Cert, BA
Tuition per yr: $3,392 res, $9,587 non-res

Volunteer State Community College
Dental Assistant Prgm
Nashville Pike
Gallatin, TN 37066
Prgm Dir: Judith Harrison
Tel: 615 741-3215
Class Cap: 24　*Begins:* Sep
Length: 10 mos　*Award:* Cert, AA
Tuition per yr: $2,346 res, $5,304 non-res

Tennessee Technical Center - Knoxville
Dental Assistant Prgm
1100 Liberty St
Knoxville, TN 37919
Prgm Dir: M Vaughn
Tel: 423 546-5567　*Fax:* 423 971-4474
Class Cap: 30　*Begins:* Oct
Length: 11 mos　*Award:* Dipl
Tuition per yr: $1,324

Tennessee Technology Center - Memphis
Dental Assistant Prgm
550 Alabama
Memphis, TN 38105
Prgm Dir: Carolyn Roach
Tel: 901 543-6143　*Fax:* 901 543-6197
Class Cap: 20　*Begins:* Apr Oct
Length: 9 mos　*Award:* Dipl
Tuition per yr: $1,600

Texas

Del Mar College
Dental Assistant Prgm
Baldwin and Ayers Sts
Corpus Christi, TX 78404
Prgm Dir: Earl Williams
Tel: 512 886-1358
Class Cap: 24　*Begins:* Aug
Length: 10 mos　*Award:* Cert, AA
Tuition per yr: $965 res, $2,165 non-res

Grayson County College
Dental Assistant Prgm
6101 Grayson Dr
Denison, TX 75020-8299
Prgm Dir: M Broomfield
Tel: 903 786-4469　*Fax:* 903 463-8779
Class Cap: 16　*Begins:* Aug
Length: 11 mos　*Award:* Cert
Tuition per yr: $1,200 res, $1,360 non-res

El Paso Community College
Dental Assistant Prgm
PO Box 20500
El Paso, TX 79998
Prgm Dir: S Dickinson
Tel: 915 534-4065　*Fax:* 915 534-3445
Class Cap: 10　*Begins:* Jun
Length: 12 mos, 24 mos　*Award:* Cert, AAS
Tuition per yr: $1,005 res, $4,020 non-res
Evening or weekend classes available

Houston Community College Central
Dental Assistant Prgm
3100 Shenandoah
Houston, TX 77021
Prgm Dir: R Perez
Tel: 713 746-5335　*Fax:* 713 718-7401
Class Cap: 24　*Begins:* Aug
Length: 2 mos　*Award:* Cert
Tuition per yr: $1,176 res, $1,974 non-res

San Antonio College

Dental Assistant Prgm
1300 San Pedro Ave
San Antonio, TX 78212-4299
Prgm Dir: Stella Lovato
Tel: 210 733-2572 *Fax:* 210 733-2907
Class Cap: 24 *Begins:* Aug Jan May
Length: 12 mos *Award:* Cert, AAS
Tuition per yr: $1,500 res, $6,470 non-res

882 Training Group

Dental Assistant Prgm
Sheppard AFB, TX 76311-2246
Prgm Dir: Richard Hiraki, LtC
Tel: 800 676-6932 *Fax:* 817 676-6928
E-mail: hiraki@win.spd.ated.af mil
Class Cap: 28 *Begins:* Varies
Length: 2 mos *Award:* Cert

Texas State Technical College

Dental Assistant Prgm
3801 Campus Dr
Waco, TX 76705
Prgm Dir: Margaret Dickenson, CDA
Tel: 254 867-4864 *Fax:* 254 867-3968
Class Cap: 146 *Begins:* Varies
Length: 12 mos *Award:* Cert
Tuition per yr: $1,440

Utah

American Inst of Med/Dental Tech

Dental Assistant Prgm
1675 N Freedom Blvd/Bldg 9A
Provo, UT 84604
Prgm Dir: C Ivers
Tel: 801 377-2900 *Fax:* 801 375-3077
Class Cap: 40 *Begins:* Sep Jan Mar
Length: 8 mos *Award:* Dipl
Tuition per yr: $3,795

Provo College

Dental Assistant Prgm
1450 W 820 N
Provo, UT 84601
Prgm Dir: Judy Simpson
Tel: 801 375-1861
Class Cap: 120 *Begins:* Jan Mar Jul Sep
Length: 11 mos *Award:* Dipl
Tuition per yr: $6,000

Vermont

Essex Technical Center

Dental Assistant Prgm
3 Educational Dr
Essex Junction, VT 05452
Prgm Dir: B Shannon
Tel: 802 879-4832 *Fax:* 802 879-5593
Class Cap: 28
Length: 9 mos *Award:* Dipl
Tuition per yr: $7,357 res, $7,357 non-res

Virginia

Old Dominion University

Dental Assistant Prgm
G W Hirschfeld School
Norfolk, VA 23529-0499
Prgm Dir: Ester Andrews, CDA,RDA,RDH,MA
Tel: 757 683-5231 *Fax:* 757 683-5239
E-mail: ekaf@giraffe.tech.odu.edu
Class Cap: 32 *Begins:* Aug
Length: 8 mos *Award:* Cert
Tuition per yr: $4,900 res, $4,900 non-res

Tidewater Technical

Dental Assistant Prgm
1760 E Little Creek Rd
Norfolk, VA 23518
Prgm Dir: Allen S Bridge, DDS
Tel: 757 588-2121 *Fax:* 757 583-9017
Class Cap: 10 *Begins:* Monthly
Length: 12 mos *Award:* Dipl
Tuition per yr: $8,160
Evening or weekend classes available

J Sargeant Reynolds Community College

Dental Assistant Prgm
PO Box 85622
Richmond, VA 23285-5622
Prgm Dir: D Graybeal
Tel: 804 786-4380
Begins: Aug
Length: 11 mos *Award:* Cert
Tuition per yr: $2,762 res, $7,843 non-res
Evening or weekend classes available

Computer Dynamics Institute

Dental Assistant Prgm
400 S Witchduck Rd #10
Virginia Beach, VA 23462
Prgm Dir: N Daniel
Tel: 757-490-1234
Class Cap: 12 *Begins:* Jan Apr Jul Oct
Length: 9 mo , 14 mos *Award:* Dipl
Tuition per yr: $7,050 res, $7,050 non-res
Evening or weekend classes available

Wytheville Community College

Dental Assistant Prgm
1000 E Main St
Wytheville, VA 24382
Prgm Dir: P Bradshaw
Tel: 540 223-4830 *Fax:* 540 223-4778
Class Cap: 20
Length: 8 mos *Award:* Cert
Tuition per yr: $2,802 res, $7,653 non-res

Washington

Bellingham Technical College

Dental Assistant Prgm
3028 Lindbergh Ave
Bellingham, WA 98225
Prgm Dir: K Hulbert
Tel: 360 738-3105 *Fax:* 360 676-3798
E-mail: jshuler@belltc.ctc.edu
Class Cap: 19
Length: 11 mos *Award:* Cert
Tuition per yr: $2,188
Evening or weekend classes available

Highline Community College

Dental Assistant Prgm
PO Box 98000
Des Moines, WA 98198-9800
Prgm Dir: Carol Cologerou
Tel: 206 878-3710
Class Cap: 24 *Begins:* Sep
Length: 10 mos *Award:* Cert, AA
Tuition per yr: $2,489 res, $7,594 non-res

Lake Washington Technical College

Dental Assistant Prgm
11605 132nd Ave NE
Kirkland, WA 98034
Prgm Dir: Ellen Williams
Tel: 206 828-5600
Class Cap: 30 *Begins:* Mar Sep
Length: 1 mo *Award:* Cert
Tuition per yr: $3,488

South Puget Sound Community College

Dental Assistant Prgm
2011 Mottman Rd
Olympia, WA 98502
Prgm Dir: Joan Martin
Tel: 360 754-7711, Ext 295
Class Cap: 28 *Begins:* Sep
Length: 14 mos *Award:* Cert, AA
Tuition per yr: $1,645 res, $4,277 non-res

Renton Technical College

Dental Assistant Prgm
3000 NE 4th St
Renton, WA 98056
Prgm Dir: Kathy Leviton
Tel: 206 235-2352
Class Cap: 44 *Begins:* Jan Sep
Length: 9 mos *Award:* Cert
Tuition per yr: $2,236

Spokane Community College

Dental Assistant Prgm
N 1810 Greene St MS 2090
Spokane, WA 99207
Prgm Dir: D Phinney
Tel: 509 533-7300 *Fax:* 509 533-8621
E-mail: jphinney@etc.edu
Class Cap: 42
Length: 9 mos *Award:* Cert
Tuition per yr: $2,146 res, $5,944 non-res
Evening or weekend classes available

Bates Technical College

Dental Assistant Prgm
1101 S Yakika Ave
Tacoma, WA 98405
Prgm Dir: D Dailey
Tel: 206 596-1563
Class Cap: 45
Length: 11 mos *Award:* Cert
Tuition per yr: $2,884
Evening or weekend classes available

Clover Park Technical College

Dental Assistant Prgm
4500 Steilacoom Blvd SW
Tacoma, WA 98498-4098
Prgm Dir: K Rasmussen
Tel: 206 589-5742 *Fax:* 206 589-5866
Class Cap: 60 *Begins:* Sep Feb Apr
Length: 11 mos *Award:* Dipl
Tuition per yr: $3,243
Evening or weekend classes available

Programs

Wisconsin

Fox Valley Technical College
Dental Assistant Prgm
1825 Bluemound Dr
Appleton, WI 54913
Prgm Dir: Harold Peaslee
Tel: 414 735-5666
Class Cap: 25   *Begins:* Jan Sep
Length: 9 mos   *Award:* Dipl, AA
Tuition per yr: $2,801 res, $12,790 non-res

Lakeshore Technical College
Dental Assistant Prgm
1290 North Ave
Cleveland, WI 53015
Prgm Dir: P Carter-Diers
Tel: 414 458-4183   *Fax:* 414 693-8955
Class Cap: 30   *Begins:* Aug
Length: 10 mos   *Award:* Dipl
Tuition per yr: $2,225 res, $11,295 non-res

Northeast Wisconsin Technical College
Dental Assistant Prgm
2740 W Mason St/PO Box 19042
Green Bay, WI 54307-9042
Prgm Dir: Deborah L Hardy, RDH MS
Tel: 414 498-5451   *Fax:* 414 498-5673
E-mail: deborah?hardy@mail.northeast.tec.wi.us
Class Cap: 15   *Begins:* Aug Jan
Length: 8 mos   *Award:* Dipl
Tuition per yr: $2,844 res, $10,200 non-res

Blackhawk Technical College
Dental Assistant Prgm
6004 Prairie Rd
Janesville, WI 53547
Prgm Dir: Lois Swanson
Tel: 608 757-7732   *Fax:* 608 757-9407
Class Cap: 24   *Begins:* Aug
Length: 9 mos   *Award:* Dipl
Tuition per yr: $2,033 res, $12,345 non-res

Gateway Technical College
Dental Assistant Prgm
3520 30th Ave
Kenosha, WI 53144-1690
Prgm Dir: A Lopiccolo
Tel: 414 656-6900   *Fax:* 414 656-8966
Class Cap: 18   *Begins:* Aug
Length: 9 mos   *Award:* Dipl
Tuition per yr: $2,239 res, $12,993 non-res

Western Wisconsin Technical College
Dental Assistant Prgm
Sixth and Vine Sts
La Crosse, WI 54601
Prgm Dir: E Ferguson
Tel: 608 785-9137   *Fax:* 608 785-9194
E-mail: ferguson@al.wester.tec.wi.us
Class Cap: 24   *Begins:* Aug
Length: 10 mos   *Award:* Dipl
Tuition per yr: $2,486 res, $11,002 non-res
Evening or weekend classes available

Madison Area Technical College
Dental Assistant Prgm
3550 Anderson St/Rm 320A
Madison, WI 53704
Prgm Dir: Nancy Bingham
Tel: 608 246-6754   *Fax:* 608 246-6013
Class Cap: 30   *Begins:* Aug
Length: 9 mos   *Award:* Dipl
Tuition per yr: $2,311

Wyoming

Sheridan College
Dental Assistant Prgm
3059 Coffeen Ave
Whitney Bldg
Sheridan, WY 82801
Prgm Dir: C Foster
Tel: 307 674-6446
Class Cap: 15   *Begins:* Aug
Length: 11 mos   *Award:* Cert
Tuition per yr: $1,293 res, $3,445 non-res

Dental Hygienist

Alabama

Wallace State College
Dental Hygienist Prgm
PO Box 2000
Hanceville, AL 35077-2000
Prgm Dir: Lisa Hypes
Tel: 205 352-8328   *Fax:* 205 352-8380
Med Dir: Doug Allen, MD
Class Cap: 24   *Begins:* Sep
Length: 19 mos   *Award:* AS
Tuition per yr: $1,740 res, $3,480 non-res
Evening or weekend classes available

Alaska

University of Alaska Anchorage
Dental Hygienist Prgm
3211 Providence Dr/AHS 124
Anchorage, AK 99508-8371
Prgm Dir: Susan Luethge, RDH MS
Tel: 907 786-1701   *Fax:* 907 786-1722
Class Cap: 12   *Begins:* Aug
Length: 16 mos   *Award:* AS
Tuition per yr: $10,006 res, $17,010 non-res
Evening or weekend classes available

Arizona

Northern Arizona University
Dental Hygienist Prgm
Box 15065
Flagstaff, AZ 86011-5065
Prgm Dir: S Peterson- Mansfield, AOH EdD
Tel: 520 523-7447   *Fax:* 520 523-4315
E-mail: susan.mansfield@nau.edu
Class Cap: 26   *Begins:* Aug
Length: 26 mos   *Award:* BS, DH
Tuition per yr: $2,000 res, $7,100 non-res

Phoenix College
Dental Hygienist Prgm
1202 W Thomas Rd
Phoenix, AZ 85013
Prgm Dir: Kristen Anderson
Tel: 602 285-7320
Class Cap: 24
Length: 16 mos   *Award:* AAS
Tuition per yr: $4,384 res, $10,444 non-res

Pima County Community College
Dental Hygienist Prgm
2202 W Anklam Rd
Tuscon, AZ 85709
Prgm Dir: J Flieger
Tel: 520 884-6916
Class Cap: 24 *Begins:* Sep
Length: 20 mos *Award:* AS
Evening or weekend classes available

Arkansas

University of Arkansas & VA Medical Ctr
Dental Hygienist Prgm
4301 W Markham St
Little Rock, AR 72205
Prgm Dir: Virginia Goral
Tel: 501 686-5733
Class Cap: 30 *Begins:* Aug
Length: 16 mos *Award:* BA
Tuition per yr: $3,642 res, $4,140 non-res

California

Cabrillo College
Dental Hygienist Prgm
6500 Soquel Dr
Aptos, CA 95003
Prgm Dir: Barbara Paige
Tel: 408 479-6472
E-mail: bapaige@cabrillo.cc.ca.us
Class Cap: 22 *Begins:* Aug
Length: 17 mos *Award:* AS
Tuition per yr: $455 res, $3,815 non-res
Evening or weekend classes available

West Los Angeles College
Dental Hygienist Prgm
4800 Freshman Dr
Culver City, CA 90230
Prgm Dir: Ulla E Lemborn
Tel: 310 287-4242 *Fax:* 310 841-0396
E-mail: lemboru@laccd.cc.ca.us
Begins: Aug
Length: 18 mos *Award:* AS
Tuition per yr: $4,000 res, $10,680 non-res

Cypress College
Dental Hygienist Prgm
9200 Valley View St
Cypress, CA 90630
Prgm Dir: Ina Rydalch, RDH MA
Tel: 310 826-2710 *Fax:* 310 421-0988
Class Cap: 16
Length: 18 mos *Award:* Cert, AA
Tuition per yr: $3,063 res, $8,906 non-res
Evening or weekend classes available

Fresno City College
Dental Hygienist Prgm
1101 E University
Fresno, CA 93741
Prgm Dir: Thomas Ray Davies, DDS
Tel: 209 442-8212 *Fax:* 209 244-2626
Class Cap: 30 *Begins:* Aug
Length: 18 mos *Award:* AS
Tuition per yr: $4,696

Chabot College
Dental Hygienist Prgm
25555 Hesperian Blvd
Hayward, CA 94545
Prgm Dir: Linda Zweifel, CDA RDA RDH BS
Tel: 510 786-6951 *Fax:* 510 782-9315
Class Cap: 18 *Begins:* Aug
Length: 24 mos *Award:* AS
Evening or weekend classes available

Loma Linda University
Dental Hygienist Prgm
School of Dentistry
Loma Linda, CA 92350
Prgm Dir: K Simpson
Tel: 909 824-4631 *Fax:* 909 824-4822
Class Cap: 42 *Begins:* Sep
Length: 21 mos *Award:* BS
Tuition per yr: $12,850

Foothill College
Dental Hygienist Prgm
12345 El Monte Rd
Los Altos Hills, CA 94022
Prgm Dir: Cara Miyasaki
Tel: 415 949-7351 *Fax:* 415 947-9788
Class Cap: 24
Length: 18 mos *Award:* AS
Tuition per yr: $7,407 res, $16,854 non-res

University of Southern California
Dental Hygienist Prgm
University Park MC0641
Los Angeles, CA 90089-0641
Prgm Dir: William Crawford, DDS
Tel: 213 740-1072
Class Cap: 52
Length: 19 mos *Award:* BA
Tuition per yr: $23,027

Cerritos College
Dental Hygienist Prgm
11110 E Alondra Blvd
Norwalk, CA 90650
Prgm Dir: I Zive
Tel: 310 860-2451, Ext 2557 *Fax:* 310 467-5077
Class Cap: 24 *Begins:* Aug
Length: 19 mos *Award:* AS
Tuition per yr: $364 res, $3,192 non-res
Evening or weekend classes available

Pasadena City College
Dental Hygienist Prgm
1570 E Colorado Blvd
Pasadena, CA 91106
Prgm Dir: J Porush
Tel: 818 585-7537 *Fax:* 818 585-7912
Class Cap: 18 *Begins:* Aug
Length: 18 mos *Award:* AS

Diablo Valley College
Dental Hygienist Prgm
321 Golf Club Rd
Pleasant Hill, CA 94523
Prgm Dir: Barbara Heckman
Tel: 510 685-1230
Class Cap: 20 *Begins:* Aug
Length: 20 mos *Award:* Cert, AA
Tuition per yr: $2,444 res, $5,472 non-res

Sacramento City College
Dental Hygienist Prgm
3835 Freeport Blvd
Sacramento, CA 95822
Prgm Dir: M Dunne
Tel: 916 558-2650 *Fax:* 916 441-4142
Class Cap: 24 *Begins:* Aug
Length: 20 mos *Award:* AS
Tuition per yr: $3,050 res, $10,910 non-res

University of California - San Francisco
Dental Hygienist Prgm
Div of Dental Hygiene
PO Box 0754
San Francisco, CA 94143
Prgm Dir: D Perry
Tel: 415 476-9884 *Fax:* 415 476-9884
E-mail: dperry@itsq.ucsf.edu
Class Cap: 18 *Begins:* Sep
Length: 19 mos *Award:* Dipl, BS
Tuition per yr: $4,184 res, $8,394 non-res

Taft College
Dental Hygienist Prgm
29 Emmons Park Dr/Box 1437
Taft, CA 93268
Prgm Dir: Stacy Eastman
Tel: 805 765-4384
Class Cap: 24 *Begins:* Aug
Length: 17 mos *Award:* AS
Tuition per yr: $1,948 res, $4,443 non-res

Colorado

Community College of Denver
Dental Hygienist Prgm
Bldg 753/960 Xanthia St
Denver, CO 80220
Tel: 303 364-4821 *Fax:* 303 364-4836
Class Cap: 18 *Begins:* Aug *Award:*
Evening or weekend classes available

University of Colorado Hlth Science Ctr
Dental Hygienist Prgm
Medical Ctr
4200 E Ninth Ave
Denver, CO 80262
Prgm Dir: G Cross-Poline
Tel: 303 270-8017 *Fax:* 303 315-8299
E-mail: gail.poline@uchsc.edu
Class Cap: 20 *Begins:* Jul
Length: 12 mos *Award:* BS
Tuition per yr: $13,203 res, $30,491 non-res
Evening or weekend classes available

Pueblo Community College
Dental Hygienist Prgm
415 Harrison Ave
Pueblo, CO 81004
Prgm Dir: K Learned
Tel: 719 549-3286 *Fax:* 719 549-3136
Class Cap: 16 *Begins:* Sep
Length: 20 mos *Award:* AAS
Tuition per yr: $2,528 res, $10,520 non-res
Evening or weekend classes available

Colorado Northwestern Community College
Dental Hygienist Prgm
500 Kennedy Dr
Rangley, CO 81648
Prgm Dir: C Crookston
Tel: 970 675-3248   *Fax:* 970 675-3330
E-mail: ccrookston@cncc.cc.co.us
Class Cap: 20   *Begins:* Aug
Length: 18 mos   *Award:* AAS
Evening or weekend classes available

Connecticut

Univ of Bridgeport/Fones School
Dental Hygienist Prgm
30 Hazel St
Bridgeport, CT 06601
Prgm Dir: Jocelyne D Poisson
Tel: 203 576-4138   *Fax:* 203 576-4220
Class Cap: 40   *Begins:* Sep
Length: 9 mos   *Award:* AS
Tuition per yr: $14,390 res, $14,390 non-res

Tunxis Community Technical College
Dental Hygienist Prgm
271 Scott Swamp Rd
Farmington, CT 06032-3187
Prgm Dir: M Bencivengo
Tel: 203 679-9667   *Fax:* 203 676-8906
Class Cap: 32   *Begins:* Sep
Length: 9 mos   *Award:* AS
Tuition per yr: $1,722 res, $4,842 non-res

University of New Haven
Dental Hygienist Prgm
300 W Orange Ave
West Haven, CT 06516
Prgm Dir: Jeanne Maloney
Tel: 203 931-6025
Class Cap: 30   *Begins:* Sep
Length: 26 mos   *Award:* AS, BA
Tuition per yr: $11,720

Delaware

Delaware Tech & Comm Coll - Wilmington
Dental Hygienist Prgm
333 Shipley St
Wilmington, DE 19801
Prgm Dir: J Hall
Tel: 302 657-5177   *Fax:* 302 577-2548
Class Cap: 23   *Begins:* Aug
Length: 21 mos   *Award:* AS
Tuition per yr: $6,453 res, $10,928 non-res
Evening or weekend classes available

District of Columbia

Howard University
Dental Hygienist Prgm
600 W St NW
Washington, DC 20059
Prgm Dir: Marie Frazier-Kelley
Tel: 202 806-0079
Class Cap: 18   Begins: Aug
Length: 18 mos   *Award:* Cert, BA
Tuition per yr: $8,879 res, $8,359 non-res

Florida

Brevard Community College
Dental Hygienist Prgm
1519 Clearlake Rd
Cocoa, FL 32922
Prgm Dir: J Raulerson
Tel: 407 632-1111   *Fax:* 407 634-3731
E-mail: raulerson.j@a1.brevard.cc.fl.us
Class Cap: 12
Length: 16 mos   *Award:* AS
Tuition per yr: $5,470 res, $8,340 non-res
Evening or weekend classes available

Daytona Beach Community College
Dental Hygienist Prgm
1200 International Speedway Blvd
Daytona Beach, FL 32114
Prgm Dir: Mary E Pryor, DDS
Tel: 904 255-8131   *Fax:* 904 254-4491
Class Cap: 15   *Begins:* Jan
Length: 20 mos   *Award:* Dipl, AAS
Tuition per yr: $3,347 res, $12,594 non-res
Evening or weekend classes available

Broward Community College
Dental Hygienist Prgm
3501 SW Davie Rd
Ft Lauderdale, FL 33314
Prgm Dir: Abby Brodie
Tel: 954 475-6563   *Fax:* 954 473-9037
Class Cap: 16   *Begins:* Aug
Length: 12 mos   *Award:* AS
Tuition per yr: $3,608 res, $8,164 non-res
Evening or weekend classes available

Edison Community College
Dental Hygienist Prgm
8099 College Pkwy SW
Ft Meyers, FL 33919
Prgm Dir: J Hillis
Tel: 941 489-9109   *Fax:* 941 489-9037
E-mail: jhillis@edison.cc.fl.us
Class Cap: 12   *Begins:* Jan
Length: 24 mos   *Award:* AS
Tuition per yr: $3,941 res, $6,916 non-res
Evening or weekend classes available

Indian River Community College
Dental Hygienist Prgm
3209 Virginia Ave
Ft Pierce, FL 34981-5599
Prgm Dir: M Ferguson, EdD
Tel: 407 462-4700   *Fax:* 407 462-4203
Class Cap: 8
Length: 16 mos   *Award:* AS
Tuition per yr: $5,375 res, $14,075 non-res
Evening or weekend classes available

Santa Fe Community College
Dental Hygienist Prgm
3000 NW 83rd St
Bldg W201E
Gainesville, FL 32606
Prgm Dir: Dana Rafferty Parker, DMD MEd
Tel: 352 395-5705   Fax: 352-395-5711
Class Cap: 24   *Begins:* Aug Jan May
Length: 13 mos, 20 mos   *Award:* Dipl, AS
Tuition per yr: $6,400 res, $15,276 non-res

Florida Community College - Jacksonville
Dental Hygienist Prgm
4501 Capper Rd
Jacksonville, FL 32218
Prgm Dir: J Lekas
Tel: 904 766-6573   *Fax:* 904 766-6654
Class Cap: 22   *Begins:* Aug
Length: 20 mos   *Award:* AS
Tuition per yr: $1,490 res, $5,624 non-res

Palm Beach Community College
Dental Hygienist Prgm
4200 Congress Ave
Lake Worth, FL 33461
Prgm Dir: N Macpherson
Tel: 561 439-8098   *Fax:* 561 439-3531
Class Cap: 32   *Begins:* Aug
Length: 21 mos   *Award:* AS
Tuition per yr: $1,187 res, $4,414 non-res
Evening or weekend classes available

Miami-Dade Community College
Dental Hygienist Prgm
Medical Ctr Campus
950 NW 20th St
Miami, FL 33127
Prgm Dir: S Kass
Tel: 305 237-4029   *Fax:* 305 237-4278
Class Cap: 50   *Begins:* Aug
Length: 19 mos   *Award:* AS
Tuition per yr: $4,693 res, $11,209 non-res
Evening or weekend classes available

Pasco-Hernando Community College
Dental Hygienist Prgm
10230 Ridge Rd
New Port Richey, FL 34654-5199
Prgm Dir: H Summers
Tel: 813 847-2727   *Fax:* 813 816-3300
Class Cap: 6
Length: 11 mos   *Award:* AS
Tuition per yr: $4,795 res, $12,135 non-res
Evening or weekend classes available

Valencia Community College
Dental Hygienist Prgm
1800 S Kirkman Rd
Orlando, FL 32811
Prgm Dir: Susan Meade
Tel: 407 299-5000   *Fax:* 407 293-8839
Class Cap: 30   *Begins:* Aug
Length: 15 mos   *Award:* AS
Tuition per yr: $6,039 res, $14,008 non-res
Evening or weekend classes available

Gulf Coast Community College
Dental Hygienist Prgm
5230 W Hwy 98
Panama City, FL 32114
Tel: 904 872-3827

Pensacola Junior College
Dental Hygienist Prgm
5555 W Hwy 98
Pensacola, FL 32507
Prgm Dir: L Fazio
Tel: 904 484-2244   *Fax:* 904 484-2365
Class Cap: 50
Length: 16 mos   *Award:* AS
Tuition per yr: $6,558 res, $14,825 non-res
Evening or weekend classes available

St Petersburg Junior College

Dental Hygienist Prgm
PO Box 13489
St Petersburg, FL 33733
Prgm Dir: T Grzesikowski
Tel: 813 341-3671   *Fax:* 813 341-3744
E-mail: grzesikowskit@email.spjc.cc.fl.us
Class Cap: 36   *Begins:* May
Length: 24 mos   *Award:* AS
Tuition per yr: $1,989 res, $7,133 non-res
Evening or weekend classes available

Tallahassee Community College

Dental Hygienist Prgm
444 Appleyard Dr
Tallahassee, FL 32304
Prgm Dir: C Biron
Tel: 904 922-8142
Class Cap: 60
Length: 24 mos   *Award:* AS
Tuition per yr: $6,313 res, $14,569 non-res

Georgia

Darton College

Dental Hygienist Prgm
2400 Gillionville Rd
Albany, GA 31707
Prgm Dir: S Marshall
Tel: 912 430-6840   *Fax:* 912 430-6910
E-mail: smarshal@dmail.dartnet.peachnet.edu
Class Cap: 30   *Begins:* Sep
Length: 22 mos   *Award:* AS
Tuition per yr: $1,600 res, $6,552 non-res
Evening or weekend classes available

Medical College of Georgia

Dental Hygienist Prgm
1120 15th St
Augusta, GA 30912
Prgm Dir: G Winkley
Tel: 706 721-2938   *Fax:* 706 721-8857
Class Cap: 28   *Begins:* Aug
Length: 19 mos   *Award:* AS, BS
Tuition per yr: $10,171 res, $19,033 non-res

Columbus State University

Dental Hygienist Prgm
4225 University Ave
Columbus, GA 31907-2079
Prgm Dir: A Derouen
Tel: 706 568-2242   *Fax:* 706 568-2084
E-mail: Derouen_allice@colstate.edu
Class Cap: 22   *Begins:* Sep
Length: 18 mos   *Award:* AS
Tuition per yr: $2,460 res, $7,632 non-res
Evening or weekend classes available

Carroll Technical Institute

Dental Hygienist Prgm
4600 Timber Ridge Dr
Douglasville, GA 30135
Tel: 770 947-7300

DeKalb College

Dental Hygienist Prgm
2101 Womack Rd
Dunwoody, GA 30338
Prgm Dir: R Karelitz
Tel: 770 551-3096   *Fax:* 770 604-3797
E-mail: rkarelit@dekalb.dc.peachnet.edu
Class Cap: 26   *Begins:* Sep
Length: 21 mos   *Award:* AS
Tuition per yr: $1,592 res, $5,232 non-res
Evening or weekend classes available

Macon College

Dental Hygienist Prgm
100 College Station Dr
Macon, GA 31297
Prgm Dir: S Bailey
Tel: 912 471-2738   *Fax:* 912 471-2753
E-mail: sbailey@cennet.mc.peachnet.edu
Class Cap: 18   *Begins:* Jun Sep
Length: 15 mos   *Award:* AS
Tuition per yr: $1,556 res, $5,428 non-res
Evening or weekend classes available

Clayton State College

Dental Hygienist Prgm
5900 N Lee St
Morrow, GA 30260
Prgm Dir: L Tebbe
Tel: 770 961-3596   *Fax:* 770 961-3639
E-mail: internettebbe@cc.cs.peachnet.edu
Class Cap: 36   *Begins:* Sep
Length: 17 mos   *Award:* AS
Tuition per yr: $2,286 res, $6,789 non-res
Evening or weekend classes available

Lanier Technical Institute

Dental Hygienist Prgm
PO Box 58
Oakwood, GA 30566
Prgm Dir: Heather Mapp
Tel: 770 531-6368   *Fax:* 770 531-6306
Class Cap: 14
Length: 18 mos   *Award:* AS
Tuition per yr: $6,435 res, $10,835 non-res

Armstrong Atlantic State University

Dental Hygienist Prgm
11935 Abercorn St
Savannah, GA 31419-1997
Prgm Dir: Barbara Tanenbaum
Tel: 912 927-5308   *Fax:* 912 921-7466
E-mail: barbara-tenenbaum@
   mailgate.armstrong.edu
Class Cap: 28   *Begins:* Sep
Length: 21 mos, 42 mos   *Award:* AS, BS
Tuition per yr: $1,836 res, $5,715 non-res
Evening or weekend classes available

Hawaii

University of Hawaii at Manoa

Dental Hygienist Prgm
2445 Campus Rd/Rm 200-B
Honolulu, HI 96822
Prgm Dir: Carolyn Kuba
Tel: 808 956-8821
Class Cap: 18   *Begins:* Aug
Length: 17 mos   *Award:* Cert, BA
Tuition per yr: $4,964 res, $8,158 non-res

Idaho

Idaho State University

Dental Hygienist Prgm
741 S 8th St
Pocatello, ID 83209
Prgm Dir: D Bowen
Tel: 208 236-2811   *Fax:* 208 236-4071
E-mail: bowedeni@isu.edu
Class Cap: 30
Length: 16 mos   *Award:* BS
Tuition per yr: $8,337 res, $17,333 non-res

Illinois

Southern Illinois Univ at Carbondale

Dental Hygienist Prgm
College of Applied Sciences and Arts
Mail Code 6615
Carbondale, IL 62901
Prgm Dir: Shirley M Beaver, RDH PhD
Tel: 618 453-7213   *Fax:* 618 453-7286
E-mail: sheaven@si4.edu
Class Cap: 36   *Begins:* Aug
Length: 18 mos, 32 mos   *Award:* AAS , BS
Tuition per yr: $6,010 res, $14,330 non-res

Parkland College

Dental Hygienist Prgm
2400 W Bradley
Champaign, IL 61821
Prgm Dir: J Henthorn
Tel: 217 351-2224
Class Cap: 38
Length: 20 mos   *Award:* AAS
Tuition per yr: $2,099 res, $6,072 non-res

Kennedy-King College/University of Illinois

Dental Hygienist Prgm
6800 S Wentworth Ave
Chicago, IL 60621
Prgm Dir: Debra B Morrissette, DDS
Tel: 773 602-5229   *Fax:* 773 996-1022
Class Cap: 30   *Begins:* Jun
Length: 24 mos   *Award:* AAS

Prairie State College

Dental Hygienist Prgm
202 S Halsted
Chicago Heights, IL 60411
Prgm Dir: B Gorbitz
Tel: 708 709-3714   *Fax:* 708 709-3777
Class Cap: 32   *Begins:* Jun
Length: 24 mos   *Award:* AS
Tuition per yr: $6,913 res, $15,685 non-res
Evening or weekend classes available

Illinois Central College

Dental Hygienist Prgm
One College Dr
East Peoria, IL 61635
Prgm Dir: J Servie
Tel: 309 999-4662   *Fax:* 309 673-9626
Class Cap: 24   *Begins:* Aug
Length: 18 mos   *Award:* AAS
Tuition per yr: $1,420 res, $3,148 non-res
Evening or weekend classes available

Programs

Lewis & Clark Community College
Dental Hygienist Prgm
5800 Godfrey Rd
Godfrey, IL 62035
Prgm Dir: M Singley
Tel: 618 466-3411 *Fax:* 618 466-9271
E-mail: singleyrdh@aol.com
Class Cap: 24 *Begins:* Aug
Length: 16 mos *Award:* AAS
Tuition per yr: $1,240 res, $4,199 non-res
Evening or weekend classes available

Lake Land College
Dental Hygienist Prgm
5001 Lake Land Blvd
Mattoon, IL 61938-9366
Prgm Dir: M Jorstad
Tel: 217 234-5203 *Fax:* 217 258-5253
E-mail: mjorstad@lakeland.cc.il.us
Class Cap: 30
Length: 16 mos *Award:* AS
Tuition per yr: $1,424 res, $2,738 non-res
Evening or weekend classes available

William Rainey Harper College
Dental Hygienist Prgm
1200 W Algonquin Rd
Palatine, IL 60067
Prgm Dir: M Holt
Tel: 847 925-6474
Class Cap: 36 *Begins:* Jun
Length: 24 mos, 36 mos *Award:* AAS
Tuition per yr: $3,444 res, $5,378 non-res

Indiana

University of Southern Indiana
Dental Hygienist Prgm
8600 University Blvd
Evansville, IN 47712
Prgm Dir: D Carl
Tel: 812 464-1707 *Fax:* 812 465-7092
E-mail: dcarl.ucs@smtp.usi.edu
Class Cap: 12 *Begins:* Aug
Length: 16 mos *Award:* AS
Tuition per yr: $2,880 res, $7,029 non-res
Evening or weekend classes available

Indiana Univ/Purdue Univ Ft Wayne
Dental Hygienist Prgm
2101 Coliseum Blvd E
Fort Wayne, IN 46805
Prgm Dir: Elaine S Foley
Tel: 219 481-6837 *Fax:* 219 481-6083
E-mail: foley@smtplnk.ipfw.indiana.edu
Class Cap: 24 *Begins:* Aug
Length: 18 mos *Award:* AS
Tuition per yr: $4,595 res, $8,385 non-res
Evening or weekend classes available

Indiana University Northwest
Dental Hygienist Prgm
3223 Broadway
Gary, IN 46409
Prgm Dir: K Hinshaw
Tel: 219 980-6721 *Fax:* 219 981-4249
E-mail: khinshaw@iunhaw1.indiana.edu
Class Cap: 24 *Begins:* Aug
Length: 16 mos *Award:* AS
Tuition per yr: $3,060 res, $4,776 non-res
Evening or weekend classes available

Indiana University School of Medicine
Dental Hygienist Prgm
1121 W Michigan St
Indianapolis, IN 46202-5186
Prgm Dir: Evelyn R Oldsen
Tel: 317 274-7801 *Fax:* 317 274-2419
E-mail: e.oldsen@iusd.iupui.edu
Class Cap: 50 *Begins:* Aug
Length: 18 mos *Award:* AS
Tuition per yr: $2,962 res, $9,092 non-res
Evening or weekend classes available

Indiana University - South Bend
Dental Hygienist Prgm
1700 Mishawaka Ave
South Bend, IN 46634
Prgm Dir: N Yokom
Tel: 219 237-4154 *Fax:* 219 237-4854
E-mail: nyokom@vines.iusb.edu
Class Cap: 36 *Begins:* Sep
Length: 16 mos *Award:* AS
Tuition per yr: $2,798 res, $3,653 non-res
Evening or weekend classes available

Iowa

Des Moines Area Community College
Dental Hygienist Prgm
2006 Ankeny Blvd
Ankeny, IA 50021
Prgm Dir: S Leggett
Tel: 515 964-6406 *Fax:* 515 964-6440
Class Cap: 20
Length: 19 mos *Award:* AS
Tuition per yr: $2,401 res, $4,802 non-res

Hawkeye Community College
Dental Hygienist Prgm
1501 E Orange Rd/Box 8015
Waterloo, IA 50704
Prgm Dir: S Van Syoc
Tel: 319 296-2320
Class Cap: 24 *Begins:* Aug
Length: 44 mos *Award:* Dipl
Tuition per yr: $4,285 res, $7,299 non-res

Kansas

Johnson County Community College
Dental Hygienist Prgm
12345 College Blvd
Overland Park, KS 66210-1299
Prgm Dir: M Biethman, RDH MS
Tel: 913 469-8500, Ext 3243 *Fax:* 913 469-2518
E-mail: mbieth@jcccnet.johnco.cc.ks.us
Class Cap: 26 *Begins:* Aug
Length: 24 mos *Award:* AS
Tuition per yr: $1,978 res, $5,246 non-res
Evening or weekend classes available

Wichita State University
Dental Hygienist Prgm
1845N Fairmount
Wichita, KS 67260-0144
Prgm Dir: S Lavigne
Tel: 316 978-3614 *Fax:* 316 978-3025
E-mail: lavigne@chp.twsu.edu
Class Cap: 32 *Begins:* Aug
Length: 16 mos *Award:* AS
Tuition per yr: $2,568 res, $8,886 non-res
Evening or weekend classes available

Kentucky

Western Kentucky University
Dental Hygienist Prgm
Academic Complex/Rm 207
Bowling Green, KY 42101
Prgm Dir: D Schutte
Tel: 502 745-2427 *Fax:* 502 745-6869
E-mail: schutte.doug@wru.edu
Class Cap: 24 *Begins:* Aug
Length: 17 mos, 33 mos *Award:* Dipl, AS, BS
Tuition per yr: $1,910 res, $2,710 non-res
Evening or weekend classes available

Maysville Comm Coll/N Kentucky Univ
Dental Hygienist Prgm
Hankins Hall
1401 Dixie Hwy
Covington, KY 41011
Prgm Dir: Jill Porter
Tel: 606 886-3863
Class Cap: 14 *Begins:* Jun
Length: 20 mos *Award:* AS
Tuition per yr: $1,158 res, $2,138 non-res

Elizabethtown Community College
Dental Hygienist Prgm
Elizabethtown, KY 42701
Prgm Dir: Lesa Kim Dean, RDH MS
Tel: 502 737-2446
Class Cap: 14 *Begins:* Aug
Length: 24 mos *Award:* AAS
Tuition per yr: $1,080 res, $3,000 non-res

Lexington Community College
Dental Hygienist Prgm
Cooper Dr/Oswald Bldg
Lexington, KY 40506
Prgm Dir: C Lawrence Chiswell, DMD MS Ed
Tel: 606 257-1213 *Fax:* 606 257-4339
E-mail: lcchis00@pop.uky.edu
Class Cap: 24 *Begins:* May
Length: 24 mos *Award:* AAS
Tuition per yr: $2,850 res, $7,704 non-res
Evening or weekend classes available

University of Louisville
Dental Hygienist Prgm
School of Dentistry
Louisville, KY 40292
Prgm Dir: Teresa Butler
Tel: 502 852-1278
Class Cap: 30 *Begins:* Aug
Length: 20 mos *Award:* AS, BA
Tuition per yr: $3,340 res, $7,700 non-res

Louisiana

Northeast Louisiana University
Dental Hygienist Prgm
700 University Ave
Monroe, LA 71209
Prgm Dir: Beverly B Jarrell
Tel: 318 342-1619 *Fax:* 318 342-1687
E-mail: aljarrell@alpha.nlu.edu
Class Cap: 24 *Begins:* Aug
Length: 15 mos, 30 mos *Award:* AS, BS
Tuition per yr: $1,926 res, $4,326 non-res
Evening or weekend classes available

Louisiana State University

Dental Hygienist Prgm
1100 Florida Ave
New Orleans, LA 70119
Prgm Dir: N Cline
Tel: 504 619-8530   *Fax:* 504 619-8740
Class Cap: 32   *Begins:* Aug
Length: 16 mos   *Award:* AS, BS
Tuition per yr: $1,800 res, $3,100 non-res

Maine

University of Maine - Bangor

Dental Hygienist Prgm
Lincoln Hall
29 Texas Ave
Bangor, ME 04401-4324
Prgm Dir: Dawn Bearor
Tel: 207 581-6053   *Fax:* 207 581-6075
E-mail: bearor@maine.maine.edu
Class Cap: 24   *Begins:* Sep
Length: 27 mos   *Award:* AS
Tuition per yr: $3,510 res, $9,300 non-res

University of New England

Dental Hygienist Prgm
Westbrook College Campus
716 Stevens Ave
Portland, ME 04103
Prgm Dir: E Beaulieu
Tel: 207 797-7261   *Fax:* 207 797-7225
Class Cap: 50   *Begins:* Sep Jan
Length: 18 mos   *Award:* AS, BS
Tuition per yr: $11,650 res, $11,650 non-res

Maryland

Baltimore City Community College

Dental Hygienist Prgm
2901 Liberty Heights Ave
Baltimore, MD 21215
Prgm Dir: G Riley, RDH BS MEd
Tel: 410 462-7713
Class Cap: 30   *Begins:* Sep
Length: 16 mos   *Award:* AS, AAS
Tuition per yr: $2,604 res, $2,796 non-res
Evening or weekend classes available

University of Maryland

Dental Hygienist Prgm
666 W Baltimore St
Baltimore, MD 21201
Prgm Dir: L Devore
Tel: 410 706-7773   *Fax:* 410 706-0349
E-mail: led001@dental3.umd.edu
Class Cap: 22   *Begins:* Sep
Length: 18 mos, 24 mos   *Award:* BS, MS
Tuition per yr: $2,813 res, $8,905 non-res
Evening or weekend classes available

Allegany College of Maryland

Dental Hygienist Prgm
12401 Willowbrook Rd SE
Cumberland, MD 21502-2596
Prgm Dir: J Steven Skupas
Tel: 301 724-7700
Class Cap: 40   *Begins:* Sep
Length: 18 mos   *Award:* AS
Tuition per yr: $4,626 res, $6,236 non-res

Massachusetts

Forsyth School

Dental Hygienist Prgm
140 The Fenway
Boston, MA 02115
Prgm Dir: Linda Hanlon
Tel: 617 262-5200   *Fax:* 617 262-4021
E-mail: lhanlon@forsyth.org
Class Cap: 48   *Begins:* Sep
Length: 18 mos, 36 mos   *Award:* Cert, AS, BS
Tuition per yr: $12,590

Bristol Community College

Dental Hygienist Prgm
777 Elsbree St
Fall River, MA 02720
Prgm Dir: Bernice K Fastoso, RDH MEd
Tel: 508 678-2811
E-mail: bfastoso@bristol.mass.edu
Class Cap: 22   *Begins:* Sep
Length: 15 mos   *Award:* AS
Tuition per yr: $8,537 res, $19,193 non-res

Middlesex Community College - Lowell

Dental Hygienist Prgm
33 Kearney Square
Lowell, MA 01852
Prgm Dir: JoAnne Lamoureux
Tel: 508 656-3064   *Fax:* 508 656-3078
Class Cap: 32   *Begins:* Sep
Length: 16 mos   *Award:* AS
Tuition per yr: $5,530 res, $5,870 non-res
Evening or weekend classes available

Springfield Technical Community College

Dental Hygienist Prgm
One Armory Square
Springfield, MA 01105
Prgm Dir: D Ryan
Tel: 413 781-7822   *Fax:* 413 781-5805
Class Cap: 20
Length: 15 mos   *Award:* AS
Tuition per yr: $10,033 res, $20,393 non-res

Cape Cod Community College

Dental Hygienist Prgm
Rte 132
West Barnstable, MA 02668
Prgm Dir: Suzanne M Box
Tel: 508 362-2131, Ext 4376   *Fax:* 508 375-4020
Class Cap: 14   *Begins:* Sep
Length: 18 mos   *Award:* AS
Tuition per yr: $1,044 res, $2,964 non-res

Quinsigamond Community College

Dental Hygienist Prgm
670 W Boylston St
Worcester, MA 01606
Prgm Dir: A Iverson
Tel: 508 854-4282
Class Cap: 20   *Begins:* Sep
Length: 16 mos   *Award:* AS
Tuition per yr: 3,935 res, $6,895 non-res

Michigan

University of Michigan

Dental Hygienist Prgm
1011 N University
Ann Arbor, MI 48109
Prgm Dir: W Kerschbaum
Tel: 313 763-3392   *Fax:* 313 763-5503
E-mail: wendyed@umich.edu
Class Cap: 36   *Begins:* Sep
Length: 14 mos   *Award:* BS
Tuition per yr: $5,890 res, $18,630 non-res

Kellogg Community College

Dental Hygienist Prgm
450 North Ave
Battle Creek, MI 49016
Prgm Dir: A Brebner
Tel: 616 965-3931, Ext 2300   *Fax:* 616 965-4133
Med Dir: Robert L Houghtaling, DDS
Class Cap: 20   *Begins:* Aug
Length: 18 mos   *Award:* AAS
Tuition per yr: $1,956 res, $4,879 non-res

Ferris State University

Dental Hygienist Prgm
200 Ferris Dr
Big Rapids, MI 49307-2740
Prgm Dir: Eve Sidney
Tel: 616 592-2279   *Fax:* 616 592-3788
E-mail: esidney@music.ferris.edu
Class Cap: 66
Length: 21 mos   *Award:* AS
Tuition per yr: $3,630 res, $5,445 non-res

University of Detroit Mercy

Dental Hygienist Prgm
2985 E Jefferson Ave
Detroit, MI 48207-4282
Prgm Dir: Judy Kwapis-Jaeger
Tel: 313 446-1872
Class Cap: 30   *Begins:* Aug
Length: 19 mos   *Award:* Cert, BA
Tuition per yr: $13,700 res, $13,700 non-res

Wayne County Community College

Dental Hygienist Prgm
8551 Greenfield/Rm 310
Detroit, MI 48228
Prgm Dir: J Nyquist
Tel: 313 943-4055   *Fax:* 313 943-4025
Class Cap: 24
Length: 15 mos   *Award:* AS
Tuition per yr: $14,700 res, $17,000 non-res
Evening or weekend classes available

Charles Stewart Mott Community College

Dental Hygienist Prgm
1401 E Court St
Flint, MI 48503
Prgm Dir: M Nicolai
Tel: 810 762-0495
Class Cap: 40   *Begins:* Sep
Length: 16 mos   *Award:* AS
Tuition per yr: $2,362 res, $2,458 non-res
Evening or weekend classes available

Programs

Grand Rapids Community College
Dental Hygienist Prgm
143 Bostwick St NE
Grand Rapids, MI 49503
Prgm Dir: M Campo
Tel: 616 771-4239   *Fax:* 616 771-4234
Class Cap: 32   *Begins:* Aug
Length: 16 mos   *Award:* AS
Tuition per yr: $2,538 res, $4,277 non-res
Evening or weekend classes available

Kalamazoo Valley Community College
Dental Hygienist Prgm
6767 West O Ave/Box 4070
Kalamazoo, MI 49003-4070
Prgm Dir: W Scott
Tel: 616 372-5267   *Fax:* 616 372-5458
Class Cap: 24   *Begins:* Aug
Length: 19 mos   *Award:* AAS
Tuition per yr: $1,641 res, 4,149 non-res
Evening or weekend classes available

Lansing Community College
Dental Hygienist Prgm
PO Box 40010
Lansing, MI 48901-7210
Prgm Dir: S Deck
Tel: 517 483-1457
Class Cap: 18   *Begins:* Aug
Length: 16 mos   *Award:* Dipl, AAS
Tuition per yr: $860 res, $2,120 non-res

Baker College of Port Huron
Dental Hygienist Prgm
3403 Lapeer Rd
Port Huron, MI 48060
Tel: 810 985-7000

Delta College
Dental Hygienist Prgm
University Center, MI 48710
Prgm Dir: Virginia Przygocki
Tel: 517 686-9383
Class Cap: 18
Length: 17 mos   *Award:* AAS
Tuition per yr: $2,190 res, $4,000 non-res

Oakland Community College - Waterford
Dental Hygienist Prgm
7350 Cooley Lake Rd
Waterford, MI 48327
Prgm Dir: Mary Bogucki
Tel: 810 360-3025
Class Cap: 30   *Begins:* Sep
Length: 17 mos   *Award:* AS
Tuition per yr: $2,870 res, $4,288 non-res

Minnesota

Normandale Community College
Dentla Hygienist Prgm
9700 France Ave S
Bloomington, MN 55431
Prgm Dir: Geneva E Middleton
Tel: 612 832-6366   *Fax:* 612 832-6571
E-mail: g.middleton@nr.cc.mn.us
Class Cap: 32   *Begins:* Sep
Length: 19 mos   *Award:* AS
Tuition per yr: $2,700 res, $4,590 non-res
Evening or weekend classes available

Lake Superior College
Dental Hygienist Prgm
2101 Trinity Rd
Duluth, MN 55811
Prgm Dir: K Griffin
Tel: 218 733-5938   *Fax:* 218 723-4921
Class Cap: 20   *Begins:* Sep
Length: 18 mos   *Award:* AAS
Tuition per yr: $5,385 res, $8,622 non-res
Evening or weekend classes available

Mankato State University
Dental Hygienist Prgm
Box 8400/PO Box 81
Mankato, MN 56002-8400
Prgm Dir: Nancy Geistfeld
Tel: 507 389-5845
Class Cap: 48
Length: 24 mos   *Award:* AS, BA
Tuition per yr: $3,810 res, $5,971 non-res

University of Minnesota - Twin Cities
Dental Hygienist Prgm
9-436 Moos Tower
Minneapolis, MN 55455
Prgm Dir: K Newell
Tel: 612 625-9121   *Fax:* 612 626-2652
E-mail: newel001@maroon.tc.uma.edu
Class Cap: 36   *Begins:* Sep
Length: 24 mos   *Award:* BS
Tuition per yr: $4,811 res, $13,277 non-res

Northwest Technical Coll - Moorhead
Dental Hygienist Prgm
1900 28th Ave S
Moorehead, MN 56560-4809
Tel: 218 299-6560

Rochester Community and Technical College
Dental Hygienist Prgm
851 30th Ave SE
Rochester, MN 55904
Prgm Dir: Anne M Niccolai, RDH MS
Tel: 507 280-3114   *Fax:* 507 280-2970
Class Cap: 18   *Begins:* Jun
Length: 18 mos   *Award:* AAS
Tuition per yr: $2,629 res, $5,258 non-res
Evening or weekend classes available

St Cloud Technical College
Dental Hygienist Prgm
1540 Northway Dr
Saint Cloud, MN 56303-1240
Prgm Dir: Barbara L Henke-Meyer, RDH
Tel: 320 654-5906   *Fax:* 320 654-5981
Class Cap: 14
Length: 18 mos   *Award:* AS
Tuition per yr: $1,800

Century Community and Technical College
Dental Hygienist Prgm
3300 Century Ave N
White Bear Lake, MN 55110
Prgm Dir: P Flaherty
Tel: 612 779-2351
Class Cap: 24
Length: 21 mos   *Award:* AS
Tuition per yr: $4,351 res, $7,498 non-res

Mississippi

Northeast Mississippi Community College
Dental Hygienist Prgm
Community College
Booneville, MS 38829
Prgm Dir: Jocelyn Cain
Tel: 601 728-7751
Class Cap: 15   *Begins:* Aug
Length: 18 mos   *Award:* AS
Tuition per yr: $1,413 res, $2,223 non-res

Pearl River Community College
Dental Hygienist Prgm
5448 US Hwy 49 S
Hattiesburg, MS 39401
Prgm Dir: Stanley L Hill, OMD
Tel: 601 544-7722   *Fax:* 601 545-2976
Class Cap: 16   *Begins:* Aug
Length: 21 mos   *Award:* AS
Tuition per yr: $2,945
Evening or weekend classes available

University of Mississippi Medical Center
Dental Hygienist Prgm
2500 N State St
Jackson, MS 39216-4505
Prgm Dir: S Daniel
Tel: 601 984-6310   *Fax:* 601 984-6344
E-mail: daniel@shrp.umsmed.edu
Class Cap: 21   *Begins:* Aug
Length: 18 mos   *Award:* BS
Tuition per yr: $1,196 res, $4,815 non-res
Evening or weekend classes available

Meridian Community College
Dental Hygienist Prgm
910 Hwy 19 N
Meridian, MS 39307
Prgm Dir: William Lindsay
Tel: 601 484-8751   *Fax:* 601 482-3936
Class Cap: 12
Length: 18 mos   *Award:* AA
Tuition per yr: $1,440 res, $2,000 non-res

Missouri

Missouri Southern State College
Dental Hygienist Prgm
Newman and Duquesne Rds
Joplin, MO 64801
Prgm Dir: S Scorse
Tel: 417 625-9379
Class Cap: 40
Length: 17 mos   *Award:* AS
Tuition per yr: $8,641 res, $13,697 non-res
Evening or weekend classes available

University of Missouri - Kansas City
Dental Hygienist Prgm
650 E 25th St
Kansas City, MO 64108
Prgm Dir: P Overman
Tel: 816 235-2051   *Fax:* 816 235-2157
E-mail: overmanp@smtpgate.ssb.umkc.edu
Class Cap: 24   *Begins:* Aug
Length: 20 mos, 32 mos   *Award:* BS
Tuition per yr: $10,745 res, $24,190 non-res
Evening or weekend classes available

St Louis Comm College at Forest Park
Dental Hygienist Prgm
5600 Oakland Ave
St Louis, MO 63110
Prgm Dir: Pat Heaton, RDH MA
Tel: 314 644-9330   *Fax:* 314 644-9752
Class Cap: 32   *Begins:* Aug
Length: 17 mos   *Award:* AAS
Tuition per yr: $1,260 res, $1,590 non-res
Evening or weekend classes available

Nebraska

Central Community College
Dental Hygienist Prgm
PO Box 1024
Hastings, NE 68902-1024
Prgm Dir: W Cloet
Tel: 402 461-2468   *Fax:* 402 461-2454
E-mail: clohdeh@cccadm.gi.cccneb.edu
Class Cap: 15   *Begins:* Sep
Length: 16 mos   *Award:* AS
Tuition per yr: $1,476 res, $2,171 non-res
Evening or weekend classes available

University of Nebraska
Dental Hygienist Prgm
40th and Holdrege Sts
Lincoln, NE 68583-0740
Prgm Dir: Gwen Hlava
Tel: 402 472-1433
Class Cap: 20   Begins: Aug
Length: 18 mos   *Award:* BA
Tuition per yr: $4,787 res, $9,256 non-res

Nevada

Community College of Southern Nevada
Dental Hygienist Prgm
6375 W Charleston Blvd
Las Vegas, NV 89102
Prgm Dir: Adele Koot, RDH EdD
Tel: 702 651-5594   *Fax:* 702 258-5084
E-mail: koot@ccsn.nevada.edu
Class Cap: 30   *Begins:* Sep
Length: 16 mos   *Award:* AAS
Tuition per yr: $1,095 res, $2,795 non-res

New Hampshire

New Hampshire Technical Institute
Dental Hygienist Prgm
11 Institute Dr
Concord, NH 03301-7412
Prgm Dir: C Hartnett
Tel: 603 225-1833
Class Cap: 56
Length: 16 mos   *Award:* AS
Tuition per yr: $7,327 res, $15,125 non-res

New Jersey

Camden County College
Dental Hygienist Prgm
PO Box 200
Blackwood, NJ 08012
Prgm Dir: C Boos
Tel: 609 227-7200
Class Cap: 22
Length: 16 mos   *Award:* AS
Tuition per yr: $7,770 res, $8,250 non-res

Middlesex County College
Dental Hygienist Prgm
153 Mill Rd/Box 3050
Edison, NJ 08818
Prgm Dir: E Buscemi
Tel: 908 906-2580
Class Cap: 30   *Begins:* Sep
Length: 15 mos   *Award:* AAS
Tuition per yr: $5,993 res, $2,965 non-res

Bergen Community College
Dental Hygienist Prgm
400 Paramus Rd
Paramus, NJ 07652
Prgm Dir: E Satin
Tel: 201 447-7937   *Fax:* 201 447-7127
Class Cap: 36   *Begins:* Sep
Length: 18 mos   *Award:* AAS
Tuition per yr: $2,955 res, $5,910 non-res
Evening or weekend classes available

Univ of Med & Dent of New Jersey
Dental Hygienist Prgm
1776 Raritan Rd
Scotch Plains, NJ 07076
Prgm Dir: Carolyn K Breen
Tel: 201 982-5453
E-mail: breen@umdnj.edu
Class Cap: 40   *Begins:* Jan
Length: 20 mos   *Award:* Dipl, AAS
Tuition per yr: $6,260 res, $13,160 non-res
Evening or weekend classes available

New Mexico

University of New Mexico
Dental Hygienist Prgm
2320 Tucker NE
Albuquerque, NM 87131-1391
Prgm Dir: Demetra Logothethis
Tel: 505 277-4513   *Fax:* 505 277-5584
Class Cap: 27   *Begins:* Aug
Length: 16 mos   *Award:* AS, BS
Tuition per yr: $1,036 res, $3,911 non-res
Evening or weekend classes available

New York

Broome Community College
Dental Hygienist Prgm
PO Box 1017
Binghamton, NY 13902
Prgm Dir: D Walsh
Tel: 607 778-5149   *Fax:* 607 778-5345
Class Cap: 40
Length: 15 mos   *Award:* AS
Tuition per yr: $2,168 res, $4,336 non-res

Hostos Community College of CUNY
Dental Hygienist Prgm
475 Grand Concourse
Bronx, NY 10451
Prgm Dir: S James
Tel: 718 518-4234   Fax: 718 518-4294
Class Cap: 40
Length: 14 mos   *Award:* AAS
Tuition per yr: $1,250 res, $1,538 non-res

CUNY New York City Technical College
Dental Hygienist Prgm
300 Jay St
Brooklyn, NY 11201
Prgm Dir: J Schwartz
Tel: 718 260-5070   *Fax:* 718 260-5995
Class Cap: 48   *Begins:* Sep
Length: 56 mos   *Award:* AS
Tuition per yr: $6,310 res, $11,540 non-res
Evening or weekend classes available

SUNY at Farmingdale
Dental Hygienist Prgm
Rte 110
Farmingdale, NY 11735
Prgm Dir: J Friedman, RDH PD
Tel: 516 420-2060   *Fax:* 516 420-2582
E-mail: friedmjm@bnyfarva.cc.farmingdale.edu
Class Cap: 50   *Begins:* Sep
Length: 15 mos, 23 mos   *Award:* AS
Tuition per yr: $8,220 res, $15,820 non-res
Evening or weekend classes available

Orange County Community College
Dental Hygienist Prgm
115 South St
Middletown, NY 10940
Prgm Dir: R Smith
Tel: 914 341-4306   *Fax:* 914 343-1228
E-mail: rsmith@mail.sunyorange.edu
Class Cap: 20   *Begins:* Sep Jan
Length: 15 mos   *Award:* AAS
Tuition per yr: $2,100 res, $4,200 non-res
Evening or weekend classes available

New York University
Dental Hygienist Prgm
345 E 24th St
New York, NY 10010
Prgm Dir: Cheryl Westphal
Tel: 212 998-9390
Class Cap: 180   *Begins:* Sep
Length: 15 mos   *Award:* AS, BA
Tuition per yr: $20,200 res, $20,200 non-res

Monroe Community College
Dental Hygienist Prgm
1000 E Henrietta Rd
Rochester, NY 14623
Prgm Dir: D Lawrence
Tel: 716 292-2000
Class Cap: 54
Length: 15 mos   *Award:* AS
Tuition per yr: $2,410 res, $4,820 non-res
Evening or weekend classes available

Programs

Onondaga Community College

Dental Hygienist Prgm
4941 Onondaga Rd
Syracuse, NY 13215
Prgm Dir: Judy Lambert
Tel: 315 469-2462   *Fax:* 315 469-2593
Class Cap: 40   *Begins:* Aug
Length: 18 mos   *Award:* AS
Tuition per yr: $2,450 res, $4,900 non-res
Evening or weekend classes available

Hudson Valley Community College

Dental Hygienist Prgm
80 Vandenburgh Ave
Troy, NY 12180
Prgm Dir: C Davis
Tel: 518 279-7437   *Fax:* 518 270-7471
Class Cap: 60
Length: 16 mos   *Award:* AS
Tuition per yr: $1,410 res, $3,620 non-res
Evening or weekend classes available

Erie Community College - City Campus

Dental Hygienist Prgm
6205 Main St
Williamsville, NY 14221-7095
Prgm Dir: J Sowinski, DDS MS
Tel: 716 851-1390   *Fax:* 716 851-1429
Class Cap: 56   *Begins:* Sep Jan
Length: 18 mos, 27 mos   *Award:* AAS
Tuition per yr: $4,500 res, $9,000 non-res
Evening or weekend classes available

North Carolina

Asheville Buncombe Technical Comm Coll

Dental Hygienist Prgm
340 Victoria Rd
Asheville, NC 28801
Prgm Dir: S Tate
Tel: 704 254-1921   *Fax:* 704 251-6355
Class Cap: 16   *Begins:* Sep
Length: 21 mos   *Award:* AS
Tuition per yr: $3,385 res, $10,598 non-res

Univ of North Carolina at Chapel Hill

Dental Hygienist Prgm
Allied Dental Education Prgms
367 Old Dental Bldg/CB #7450
Chapel Hill, NC 27599-7450
Prgm Dir: Joyce N Jenzano
Tel: 919 966-2800   *Fax:* 919 966-6761
E-mail: jenzano.decology@mhs.unc.edu
Class Cap: 28   *Begins:* Aug
Length: 18 mos   *Award:* Cert, BS
Tuition per yr: $1,386 res, $9,918 non-res

Central Piedmont Community College

Dental Hygienist Prgm
1201 Elizabeth Ave/Kings Dr
Charlotte, NC 28204
Prgm Dir: Marilyn Wright
Tel: 704 342-6431
Class Cap: 22   *Begins:* Sep
Length: 22 mos   *Award:* AS
Tuition per yr: $1,567 res, $6,185 non-res

Fayetteville Technical Community College

Dental Hygienist Prgm
2201 Hull Rd/PO Box 35236
Fayetteville, NC 28303
Prgm Dir: R Mumford, DMD MPH
Tel: 910 678-8254   *Fax:* 910 484-6600
E-mail: rmumford@post.faytech.cc.nc.us
Class Cap: 30
Length: 21 mos   *Award:* AS
Tuition per yr: $742 res, $6,020 non-res

Wayne Community College

Dental Hygienist Prgm
Caller Box 8002
Goldsboro, NC 27530
Prgm Dir: A Edmundson
Tel: 919 735-5151   *Fax:* 919 736-3204
E-mail: anna@wcc.wayne.cc.nc.us
Class Cap: 24   *Begins:* Aug
Length: 21 mos   *Award:* AS
Tuition per yr: $584 res, $4,542 non-res

Coastal Carolina Community College

Dental Hygienist Prgm
444 Western Blvd
Jacksonville, NC 28540
Prgm Dir: Barbara Branche
Tel: 910 938-6270   *Fax:* 910 455-7027
Class Cap: 24
Length: 17 mos   *Award:* AS
Tuition per yr: $3,927 res, $13,164 non-res
Evening or weekend classes available

Guilford Technical Community College

Dental Hygienist Prgm
PO Box 309
Jamestown, NC 27282
Prgm Dir: Beverly Carson
Tel: 910 334-4822
Class Cap: 30   Begins: Sep
Length: 19 mos   *Award:* AS
Tuition per yr: $2,167 res, $6,785 non-res

North Dakota

North Dakota State College of Science

Dental Hygienist Prgm
College of Science
Wahpeton, ND 58076
Prgm Dir: S Swanson
Tel: 701 671-2333
E-mail: suswanso@plains.nodak.edu
Class Cap: 28   *Begins:* Aug
Length: 20 mos   *Award:* AS
Tuition per yr: $2,239 res, $5,684 non-res

Ohio

Univ of Cincinnati

Dental Hygienist Prgm
Raymond Walters College
9555 Plainfield Rd
Cincinnati, OH 45236
Prgm Dir: P Frese
Tel: 513 745-5635   *Fax:* 513 792-8623
E-mail: fresepa@ucrwcu.rwc.uc.edu
Class Cap: 32
Length: 15 mos   *Award:* AAS
Tuition per yr: $6,678 res, $16,842 non-res
Evening or weekend classes available

Cuyahoga Community College

Dental Hygienist Prgm
2900 Community College Ave
Cleveland, OH 44115
Prgm Dir: M Gerosky
Tel: 216 987-4494   *Fax:* 216 987-4386
E-mail: mary-lou.gerosky@tri-c.cc.oh.us
Class Cap: 25   *Begins:* Sep
Length: 17 mos   *Award:* AS
Tuition per yr: $4,120 res, $10,914 non-res
Evening or weekend classes available

Ohio State University

Dental Hygienist Prgm
305 W 12th Ave
Columbus, OH 43210
Prgm Dir: Cheryl DeVore
Tel: 614 292-2228   *Fax:* 614 292-8013
E-mail: devore.2@osu.edu
Med Dir: Heary V Fields, DDS MS MSD
Class Cap: 35   *Begins:* Sep
Length: 36 mos   *Award:* Dipl, BS
Tuition per yr: $10,404 res, $31,005 non-res
Evening or weekend classes available

Sinclair Community College

Dental Hygienist Prgm
444 W Third St
Dayton, OH 45402
Prgm Dir: R Skinner
Tel: 513 226-2779   *Fax:* 513 449-5192
E-mail: ltaylor@cleo.sinclair.edu
Class Cap: 35   *Begins:* Sep
Length: 27 mos   *Award:* AS
Tuition per yr: $1,922 res, $2,914 non-res
Evening or weekend classes available

Lakeland Community College

Dental Hygienist Prgm
7700 Clocktower Dr
Kirtland, OH 44094-5198
Prgm Dir: C Patterson
Tel: 216 953-7190   *Fax:* 216 975-4733
Class Cap: 20   *Begins:* Sep
Length: 17 mos   *Award:* AS
Tuition per yr: $2,877 res, $3,529 non-res

Lima Technical College

Dental Hygienist Prgm
4240 Campus Dr
Lima, OH 45804
Prgm Dir: L Lesher
Tel: 419 995-8380   *Fax:* 419 995-8818
E-mail: lesherl@ltc.tec.oh.us
Class Cap: 28   *Begins:* Sep
Length: 17 mos   *Award:* AS
Tuition per yr: $3,022 res, $6,044 non-res
Evening or weekend classes available

Shawnee State University

Dental Hygienist Prgm
940 Second St
Portsmouth, OH 45662
Prgm Dir: J Kadel
Tel: 614 355-2216   *Fax:* 614 355-2354
E-mail: jkadel@shanner.edu
Class Cap: 24   *Begins:* Sep
Length: 17 mos   *Award:* AS
Tuition per yr: $3,780 res, $6,182 non-res
Evening or weekend classes available

Owens Community College

Dental Hygienist Prgm
PO Box 10,000
Toledo, OH 43699
Prgm Dir: T Palmateer, RDN BHS
Tel: 419 661-7374   *Fax:* 419 661-7665
E-mail: tpalmateer@owens.cc.oh.us
Class Cap: 32   *Begins:* Jun
Length: 20 mos   *Award:* AS
Tuition per yr: $1,975 res, $4,792 non-res
Evening or weekend classes available

Youngstown State University

Dental Hygienist Prgm
Dept of Health Professions
1 University Plaza
Youngstown, OH 44555
Prgm Dir: Maureen Vendemia, RDH
Tel: 330 742-1766   *Fax:* 330 742-2921
Class Cap: 28   *Begins:* Sep
Length: 17 mos   *Award:* AAS
Tuition per yr: $3,266 res, $4,986 non-res
Evening or weekend classes available

Oklahoma

Rose State College

Dental Hygienist Prgm
6420 SE 15th St
Midwest City, OK 73110
Prgm Dir: Janet Turley
Tel: 405 733-7336   *Fax:* 405 736-0338
Class Cap: 12   *Begins:* Aug
Length: 8 mos   *Award:* AAS
Tuition per yr: $1,209 res, $2,069 non-res
Evening or weekend classes available

Univ of Oklahoma Health Sciences Center

Dental Hygienist Prgm
PO Box 26901
Oklahoma City, OK 73190
Prgm Dir: Pat Nunn, RDH MS
Tel: 405 271-4435   *Fax:* 405 271-3423
E-mail: pat_nunn@uokhsc.edu
Class Cap: 24   *Begins:* Aug
Length: 16 mos   *Award:* BS
Tuition per yr: $1,456 res, $4,690 non-res

Tulsa Community College

Dental Hygienist Prgm
909 S Boston Ave
MP 458
Tulsa, OK 74119-2094
Prgm Dir: C Matthies
Tel: 918 631-7023   *Fax:* 918 595-7298
E-mail: cmatthi@vm.tulsa.cc.ok.us
Class Cap: 14   *Begins:* Aug
Length: 16 mos   *Award:* AS
Tuition per yr: $5,844
Evening or weekend classes available

Oregon

Lane Community College

Dental Hygienist Prgm
4000 E 30th
Eugene, OR 97405
Prgm Dir: S Hagan
Tel: 541 747-4501   *Fax:* 541 744-4151
E-mail: hagans@lanecc.edu
Class Cap: 20
Length: 17 mos   *Award:* AS
Evening or weekend classes available

Mt Hood Community College

Dental Hygienist Prgm
26000 SE Stark St
Gresham, OR 97030
Prgm Dir: T Tong
Tel: 503 667-7691   *Fax:* 503 492-6005
Class Cap: 16   *Begins:* Sep
Length: 17 mos   *Award:* AS
Tuition per yr: $1,485 res, $5,875 non-res

Oregon Institute of Technology

Dental Hygienist Prgm
3201 Campus Dr
Klamath Falls, OR 97601
Prgm Dir: J Torres
Tel: 541 885-1366   *Fax:* 541 885-1849
E-mail: torresjadit.dsshe.edu
Class Cap: 32   *Begins:* Sep
Length: 27 mos, 36 mos   *Award:* AS, BS
Tuition per yr: $3,129 res, $10,065 non-res
Evening or weekend classes available

Oregon Health Sciences University

Dental Hygienist Prgm
3181 SW Sam Jackson Park Rd SD-3
Portland, OR 97201-3098
Prgm Dir: Margaret M Ryan
Tel: 503 494-8502   *Fax:* 503 494-4666
Class Cap: 36
Length: 18 mos   *Award:* BS
Tuition per yr: $4,788 res, $9,354 non-res

Portland Community College

Dental Hygienist Prgm
PO Box 19000
Portland, OR 97219-0990
Prgm Dir: Anne Jackson
Tel: 503 977-4235   *Fax:* 503 977-4869
E-mail: ajackson@pcc.edu
Class Cap: 18   *Begins:* Sep
Length: 18 mos   *Award:* Cert, AS
Tuition per yr: $1,368 res, $4,788 non-res
Evening or weekend classes available

Pennsylvania

Northampton Community College

Dental Hygienist Prgm
3835 Green Pond Rd
Bethlehem, PA 18017
Prgm Dir: Terry Sigal Greene
Tel: 610 861-5440   *Fax:* 610 861-8577
E-mail: psg@pmail.nrhmcc.pa.us
Class Cap: 46   *Begins:* Aug
Length: 15 mos   *Award:* AAS
Tuition per yr: $5,040

Montgomery County Community College

Dental Hygienist Prgm
340 DeKalb Pike/227 Science Center
Blue Bell, PA 19422-0758
Prgm Dir: Victoria Bastecki-Perez, RDH EdD
Tel: 215 641-6483   *Fax:* 215 641-6467
E-mail: vbasteck@admin.mc3.edu
Class Cap: 20   *Begins:* Sep
Length: 16 mos   *Award:* AS
Tuition per yr: $2,391 res, $4,756 non-res
Evening or weekend classes available

Harcum College

Dental Hygienist Prgm
750 Montgomery Ave
Bryn Mawr, PA 19010
Prgm Dir: J Byrnes-Ziegler
Tel: 610 526-6110   *Fax:* 610 526-6031
Class Cap: 32
Length: 15 mos   *Award:* AS
Tuition per yr: $8,310 res, $8,310 non-res

Harrisburg Area Community College

Dental Hygienist Prgm
One HACC Dr
Harrisburg, PA 17110-2999
Prgm Dir: M Mattox
Tel: 717 780-2419   *Fax:* 717 236-0709
Class Cap: 22   *Begins:* Jun
Length: 20 mos   *Award:* AA
Tuition per yr: $2,330 res, $4,660 non-res
Evening or weekend classes available

Manor Junior College

Dental Hygienist Prgm
700 Fox Chase
Jenkintown, PA 19046-3396
Tel: 215 885-2360   *Fax:* 215 576-6564
Class Cap: 14   *Begins:* Jun Sep
Length: 24 mos   *Award:* AS
Tuition per yr: $11,660 res, $7,860 non-res
Evening or weekend classes available

Luzerne County Community College

Dental Hygienist Prgm
1333 S Prospect St
Nanticoke, PA 18634-3899
Prgm Dir: Lisa Rowley, CDA RDH MS
Tel: 717 829-7447   *Fax:* 717 740-0265
Class Cap: 24   *Begins:* Jun
Length: 24 mos   *Award:* AAS
Tuition per yr: $2,332 res, $6,996 non-res

Community College of Philadelphia

Dental Hygienist Prgm
1700 Spring Garden St
Philadelphia, PA 19130
Prgm Dir: R Lynn
Tel: 215 751-8428   *Fax:* 215 751-8937
Class Cap: 36
Length: 14 mos   *Award:* AS
Tuition per yr: $3,174 res, $6,348 non-res
Evening or weekend classes available

University of Pittsburgh

Dental Hygienist Prgm
B-23 Salk Hall
Pittsburgh, PA 15261
Prgm Dir: Angelina Riccelli
Tel: 412 648-8432
Class Cap: 46   Begins: Aug
Length: 21 mos   *Award:* Cert, BA
Tuition per yr: $8,221 res, $15,165 non-res

Programs

Pennsylvania College of Technology
Dental Hygienist Prgm
1 College Ave
Williamsport, PA 17701
Prgm Dir: K Morr
Tel: 717 327-4500
Begins: Aug
Length: 16 mos   *Award:* AS
Tuition per yr: $8,352 res, $8,662 non-res
Evening or weekend classes available

Westmoreland County Community College
Dental Hygienist Prgm
Armbrust Rd
Youngwood, PA 15697-1895
Prgm Dir: Angela S Rinchuse, RDH MEd
Tel: 412 925-4163   *Fax:* 412 925-5808
Class Cap: 32   *Begins:* Aug
Length: 21 mos   *Award:* AAS
Tuition per yr: $1,978 res, $3,956 non-res
Evening or weekend classes available

Puerto Rico

University of Puerto Rico
Dental Hygienist Prgm
GPO Box 5067
San Juan, PR 00936
Prgm Dir: Blanca Rodriguez
Tel: 787 758-2525
Class Cap: 20   Begins: Aug
Length: 10 mos   *Award:* AS, BA
Tuition per yr: $3,562

Rhode Island

Community College of Rhode Island
Dental Hygienist Prgm
Louisquisset Pike
Lincoln, RI 02865
Prgm Dir: Cathy Patterson
Tel: 216 953-7190
Class Cap: 24   *Begins:* Sep
Length: 15 mos   *Award:* AS
Tuition per yr: $2,951 res, $5,911 non-res

South Carolina

Trident Technical College
Dental Hygienist Prgm
PO Box 118067
Charleston, SC 29423-8067
Prgm Dir: B Ankersen
Tel: 803 569-6439   *Fax:* 803 569-6585
E-mail: zpankersenb@trident.tec.sc.us
Class Cap: 24   *Begins:* Aug
Length: 21 mos   *Award:* AS
Tuition per yr: $2,545 res, $2,810 non-res
Evening or weekend classes available

Midlands Technical College
Dental Hygienist Prgm
PO Box 2408
Columbia, SC 29202
Prgm Dir: M Hanks
Tel: 803 822-3451   *Fax:* 803 822-3079
Class Cap: 36   *Begins:* Aug
Length: 15 mos   *Award:* AS
Tuition per yr: $1,120 res, $2,116 non-res
Evening or weekend classes available

Florence-Darlington Technical College
Dental Hygienist Prgm
PO Box 100548
Florence, SC 29501-0548
Prgm Dir: M Hewitt
Tel: 803 661-8023   *Fax:* 803 661-8306
Class Cap: 18   *Begins:* Aug
Length: 19 mos   *Award:* AS
Tuition per yr: $1,650 res, $1,875 non-res

Greenville Technical College
Dental Hygienist Prgm
PO Box 5616
Greenville, SC 29606-5616
Prgm Dir: J S Demosthenes
Tel: 864 250-8286   *Fax:* 864 250-8462
E-mail: demostjsd@gultec.edu
Class Cap: 24   *Begins:* Jan Aug
Length: 28 mos   *Award:* AS
Tuition per yr: $1,575 res, $1,710 non-res

York Technical College
Dental Hygienist Prgm
452 S Anderson Rd
Rock Hill, SC 29730
Prgm Dir: Deedee M Smith, RDH MS
Tel: 803 327-8039   *Fax:* 803 327-8059
E-mail: dsmith@york.tec.sc.us
Class Cap: 20   *Begins:* Aug
Length: 23 mos   *Award:* AS
Tuition per yr: $1,296 res, $1,548 non-res
Evening or weekend classes available

South Dakota

University of South Dakota
Dental Hygienist Prgm
E Hall 414/E Clark St
Vermillion, SD 57069
Prgm Dir: Ann Brunick, RDH MS
Tel: 605 677-5379   *Fax:* 605 677-5638
E-mail: abrunick@sandance.usd.edu
Class Cap: 32   *Begins:* Varies
Length: 16 mos   *Award:* AS
Tuition per yr: $3,171 res, $7,196 non-res

Tennessee

Chattanooga State Technical Comm College
Dental Hygienist Prgm
4501 Amnicola Hwy
Chattanooga, TN 37406-1097
Prgm Dir: W Johnson
Tel: 423 697-4444   *Fax:* 423 634-3071
Class Cap: 18   *Begins:* Aug
Length: 16 mos   *Award:* AS
Tuition per yr: $994 res, $3,920 non-res
Evening or weekend classes available

East Tennessee State University
Dental Hygienist Prgm
PO Box 70690
Johnson City, TN 37614-0690
Prgm Dir: Rebecca L Nunley, DDS
Tel: 423 439-4497   *Fax:* 423 439-5238
Class Cap: 26   *Begins:* Aug
Length: 19 mos   *Award:* AAS
Tuition per yr: $3,129 res, $9,633 non-res

University of Tennessee Memphis
Dental Hygienist Prgm
822 Beale St/Rm 321E
Memphis, TN 38163
Prgm Dir: M Gaston
Tel: 901 448-6230
E-mail: mgaston@utmem1.utmem.edu
Class Cap: 34   *Begins:* Sep
Length: 16 mos   *Award:* BS
Tuition per yr: $6,952 res, $4,336 non-res

Tennessee State University
Dental Hygienist Prgm
3500 John A Merritt Blvd
Nashville, TN 37209-1561
Prgm Dir: Marian W Patton, RDH EdD
Tel: 615 320-3565   *Fax:* 615 963-5836
Class Cap: 30   *Begins:* Aug
Length: 16 mos   *Award:* AS, AAS
Tuition per yr: $1,916 res, $6,252 non-res
Evening or weekend classes available

Roane State Community College
Dental Hygienist Prgm
728 Emory Valley Rd
Oak Ridge, TN 37830
Prgm Dir: M Curran
Tel: 423 481-3469   *Fax:* 423 483-0447
Class Cap: 12   *Begins:* Aug
Length: 19 mos   *Award:* AS
Tuition per yr: $1,424 res, $4,206 non-res
Evening or weekend classes available

Texas

Amarillo College
Dental Hygienist Prgm
PO Box 447
Amarillo, TX 79178
Prgm Dir: Clara Hall Oldham, PhD
Tel: 806 354-6056   *Fax:* 806 354-6096
E-mail: choldham@actx.edu
Class Cap: 20
Length: 18 mos   *Award:* AAS
Tuition per yr: $4,886 res, $6,926 non-res

Lamar Univ Institute of Tech - Beaumont
Dental Hygienist Prgm
PO Box 10061
Beaumont, TX 77710
Prgm Dir: B Reynard
Tel: 409 880-8858   *Fax:* 409 880-8955
Class Cap: 30
Length: 30 mos   *Award:* AS
Tuition per yr: $6,145 res, $14,276 non-res

Bee County College

Dental Hygienist Prgm
3800 Charco Rd
Beeville, TX 78102
Prgm Dir: A Pickett
Tel: 512 358-1104 *Fax:* 512 358-3971
Class Cap: 25
Length: 16 mos *Award:* AS
Tuition per yr: $464 res, $812 non-res

Howard College

Dental Hygienist Prgm
1001 Birdwell Ln
Big Spring, TX 79720
Prgm Dir: Robert Patterson, DDS
Tel: 915 264-5075
Class Cap: 16 *Begins:* Sep
Length: 18 mos *Award:* AS
Tuition per yr: $3,812 res, $4,612 non-res

Del Mar College

Dental Hygienist Prgm
Baldwin and Ayers Sts
Corpus Christi, TX 78404
Prgm Dir: Earl Williams
Tel: 512 886 1356
Class Cap: 18 *Begins:* Aug
Length: 16 mos *Award:* AS
Tuition per yr: $655 res, $1,570 non-res

Baylor University Medical Center

Dental Hygienist Prgm
PO Box 660677
Dallas, TX 75266-0677
Prgm Dir: J Dewald
Tel: 214 828-8341 *Fax:* 214 828-8346
Class Cap: 30
Length: 21 mos *Award:* BS
Tuition per yr: $1,194 res, $8,288 non-res

Texas Woman's University

Dental Hygienist Prgm
Box 425796/TWU Station
Denton, TX 76204
Prgm Dir: Nancy Glick, PhD
Tel: 817 898-2871 *Fax:* 817 898-2869
E-mail: d_glick@twu.edu
Class Cap: 24 *Begins:* Aug
Length: 17 mos *Award:* BS
Tuition per yr: $1,890 res, $8,034 non-res
Evening or weekend classes available

El Paso Community College

Dental Hygienist Prgm
PO Box 20500
El Paso, TX 79998
Prgm Dir: Tena Liley, RDH MS
Tel: 915 534-4064 *Fax:* 915 534-4114
Class Cap: 16 *Begins:* Aug
Length: 22 mos *Award:* AAS
Tuition per yr: $3,878 res, $8,480 non-res

Univ of Texas Hlth Sci Ctr at Houston

Dental Hygienist Prgm
PO Box 20068
Houston, TX 77225
Prgm Dir: Nina Bay Infante, RDH MS
Tel: 713 792-4084 *Fax:* 713 500-4100
E-mail: nyay@bite.db.uth.tmc.edu
Class Cap: 35 *Begins:* Aug
Length: 16 mos *Award:* Cert
Tuition per yr: $1,120 res, $8,610 non-res

Tarrant Junior College

Dental Hygienist Prgm
828 Harwood Rd
Hurst, TX 76054
Prgm Dir: Barbara Shearer
Tel: 817 515-6640 *Fax:* 817 515-6601
Class Cap: 24 *Begins:* Jul
Length: 16 mos *Award:* AS
Tuition per yr: $5,956 res, $14,199 non-res
Evening or weekend classes available

Univ of Texas Hlth Sci Ctr at San Antonio

Dental Hygienist Prgm
7703 Floyd Curl Dr
San Antonio, TX 78284-7904
Prgm Dir: J Wallace
Tel: 210 567-3030 *Fax:* 210 567-3048
E-mail: wallacej@uthscsa.edu
Class Cap: 32 *Begins:* Aug
Length: 21 mos *Award:* Cert
Tuition per yr: $1,056 res, $8,184 non-res

Tyler Junior College

Dental Hygienist Prgm
PO Box 9020
Tyler, TX 75711
Prgm Dir: Elizabeth Wimberly
Tel: 903 510-2341 *Fax:* 903 510-2330
Class Cap: 52
Length: 16 mos *Award:* AS
Tuition per yr: $4,315 res, $5,735 non-res

Wharton County Junior College

Dental Hygienist Prgm
911 Boling Hwy
Wharton, TX 77488
Prgm Dir: Leigh Ann Collins
Tel: 409 532-6398 *Fax:* 409 532-6489
Class Cap: 28 *Begins:* Aug
Length: 24 mos *Award:* AAS
Tuition per yr: $455 res, $1,820 non-res
Evening or weekend classes available

Midwestern State University

Dental Hygienist Prgm
3410 Taft
Wichita Falls, TX 76308-2099
Prgm Dir: B Debois
Tel: 817 689-4480
Class Cap: 14 *Begins:* Sep
Length: 16 mos *Award:* BS
Tuition per yr: $1,800 res, $8,200 non-res
Evening or weekend classes available

Utah

Weber State University

Dental Hygienist Prgm
3750 University Circle
Ogden, UT 84408-1601
Prgm Dir: Bonnie Branson, RDH PhD
Tel: 801 626-6130 *Fax:* 801 626-7304
E-mail: bbranson@weber.edu
Class Cap: 30 *Begins:* Sep
Length: 15 mos *Award:* AS
Tuition per yr: $7,176 res, $12,354 non-res
Evening or weekend classes available

Vermont

University of Vermont

Dental Hygienist Prgm
Rowell Bldg/Rm 002
Burlington, VT 05405
Prgm Dir: C Hill
Tel: 802 656-2587 *Fax:* 802 656-8440
E-mail: chill@cosmos.uvm.edu
Class Cap: 25 *Begins:* Sep
Length: 16 mos *Award:* AS
Tuition per yr: $6,732 res, $6,824 non-res
Evening or weekend classes available

Virginia

Northern Virginia Community College

Dental Hygienist Prgm
8333 Little River Tnpk
Annandale, VA 22003
Prgm Dir: E Tynan
Tel: 703 323-3436
Class Cap: 21 *Begins:* Aug
Length: 20 mos *Award:* AS
Tuition per yr: $1,680 res, $5,507 non-res

Old Dominion University

Dental Hygienist Prgm
Norfolk, VA 23529-0499
Prgm Dir: Deanne Shuman
Tel: 757 683-3338 *Fax:* 757 683-5239
E-mail: dsa100u@giraffe.tech.odu.edu
Class Cap: 48 *Begins:* Aug
Length: 19 mos *Award:* BS
Tuition per yr: $15,960 res, $41,400 non-res
Evening or weekend classes available

Med Coll of VA/Virginia Commonwealth U

Dental Hygienist Prgm
School of Dentistry
PO Box 980566
Richmond, VA 23298
Prgm Dir: J Scharer
Tel: 804 828-9096 *Fax:* 804 828-4913
E-mail: jscharer@den1.den.vcu.edu
Class Cap: 18 *Begins:* Aug
Length: 19 mos *Award:* BS
Tuition per yr: $4,387 res, $12,312 non-res
Evening or weekend classes available

Virginia Western Community College

Dental Hygienist Prgm
3095 Colonial Ave SW
Roanoke, VA 24038
Prgm Dir: A Hutcherson
Tel: 540 857-7206 *Fax:* 540 857-7544
Class Cap: 18 *Begins:* Aug
Length: 19 mos *Award:* AAS
Tuition per yr: $2,192 res, $7,222 non-res
Evening or weekend classes available

Wytheville Community College

Dental Hygienist Prgm
1000 E Main St
Wytheville, VA 24382
Prgm Dir: P Bradshaw
Tel: 540 223-4830 *Fax:* 540 223-4778
Class Cap: 20 *Begins:* Aug
Length: 16 mos *Award:* AS
Tuition per yr: $5,532 res, $13,518 non-res

Programs

Washington

Lake Washington Technical College
Dental Hygienist Prgm
11605 132nd Ave NE
Kirkland, WA 98034
Prgm Dir: Ellen Williams, RDH MS
Tel: 206 828-5600 *Fax:* 206 828-5648
E-mail: ewillia@mailnet.etc.edu
Class Cap: 12 *Begins:* Sep
Length: 22 mos *Award:* AAS
Tuition per yr: $7,351
Evening or weekend classes available

Shoreline Community College
Dental Hygienist Prgm
16101 Greenwood Ave
North Seattle, WA 98133
Prgm Dir: B Renshaw
Tel: 206 546-4709 *Fax:* 206 546-5830
Class Cap: 24 *Begins:* Sep
Length: 20 mos *Award:* AA, AS
Tuition per yr: $8,036 res, $19,171 non-res
Evening or weekend classes available

East Washington University
Dental Hygienist Prgm
Paulsen Bldg/Rm 252
Spokane, WA 99201
Prgm Dir: G Orton
Tel: 509 623-4309 *Fax:* 509 623-4318
E-mail: gorton@ewu.edu
Class Cap: 24 *Begins:* Sep
Length: 29 mos *Award:* BS
Tuition per yr: $2,550 res, $8,736 non-res

Pierce College
Dental Hygienist Prgm
9401 Farwest Dr SW
Tacoma, WA 98498
Prgm Dir: Sharon S Golightly, RDH MS
Tel: 206 964-6661
Class Cap: 20
Length: 20 mos *Award:* AS
Tuition per yr: $7,812 res, $15,160 non-res

Clark College
Dental Hygienist Prgm
1800 E McLoughlin Blvd
Vancouver, WA 98663
Prgm Dir: G Liberman
Tel: 206 699-0474
Class Cap: 29
Length: 17 mos *Award:* AS
Tuition per yr: $7,641 res, $16,998 non-res

Yakima Valley Community College
Dental Hygienist Prgm
16th Ave/Nob Hill Blvd
Yakima, WA 98907
Prgm Dir: P Hakala
Tel: 509 574-4918 *Fax:* 509 574-6875
Class Cap: 18 *Begins:* Sep
Length: 18 mos *Award:* AS
Tuition per yr: $2,862 res, $11,082 non-res
Evening or weekend classes available

West Virginia

West Virginia Institute of Technology
Dental Hygienist Prgm
Montgomery, WV 25136
Prgm Dir: Michelle G Klenk, RDH EdD
Tel: 304 442-3222 *Fax:* 304 442-3245
Class Cap: 22 *Begins:* Aug
Length: 18 mos *Award:* AS
Tuition per yr: $6,039 res, $11,379 non-res

West Virginia University
Dental Hygienist Prgm
Health Science Ctr N
PO Box 9425
Morgantown, WV 26506-9425
Prgm Dir: B Komives-Norris
Tel: 304 293-3417 *Fax:* 304 293-2859
E-mail: bkomives@wvuvphs1.hsc.wvu.edu
Class Cap: 20
Length: 32 mos *Award:* BS
Tuition per yr: $2,794 res, $8,702 non-res
Evening or weekend classes available

West Liberty State College
Dental Hygienist Prgm
West Liberty, WV 26074
Prgm Dir: Carol L Frum, RDH MA
Tel: 304 336-8030 *Fax:* 304 336-8285
E-mail: healdsam@wlsuaxwvnet.edu
Class Cap: 42 *Begins:* Aug
Length: 18 mos *Award:* AS
Tuition per yr: $2,020 res, $5,460 non-res

Wisconsin

Northeast Wisconsin Technical College
Dental Hygienist Prgm
2740 W Mason St/PO Box 19042
Green Bay, WI 54307-9042
Prgm Dir: Deborah L Hardy, RDH MS
Tel: 414 498-5451 *Fax:* 414 498-5673
E-mail: hardydl@nwtc.tec.wi.us
Class Cap: 24 *Begins:* Jun Aug Jan
Length: 17 mos *Award:* AS
Tuition per yr: $7,237 res, $24,573 non-res

Madison Area Technical College
Dental Hygienist Prgm
3550 Anderson St
Madison, WI 53704
Prgm Dir: E Lynn Goetsch, RDH MS
Tel: 608 258-2470 *Fax:* 608 258-2480
E-mail: egoetsch@madison.tec.wi.us
Class Cap: 36
Length: 18 mos *Award:* AS
Tuition per yr: $5,897

Marquette University
Dental Hygienist Prgm
604 N 16th St
Milwaukee, WI 53233
Prgm Dir: Kim L Autio Halula, RDH MS
Tel: 414 288-7153 *Fax:* 414 288-3126
Class Cap: 24
Length: 48 mos *Award:* BS
Tuition per yr: $14,710 res, $14,710 non-res

Milwaukee Area Technical College
Dental Hygienist Prgm
700 W State St
Milwaukee, WI 53233
Prgm Dir: G Bohlman
Tel: 414 297-7123 *Fax:* 414 297-6851
E-mail: bohlmang@milwaukee.tec.wi.us
Class Cap: 48 *Begins:* Aug
Length: 18 mos *Award:* AS
Tuition per yr: $1,590 res, $12,225 non-res

Waukesha County Technical College
Dental Hygienist Prgm
800 Main St
Pewaukee, WI 53072
Prgm Dir: Liz Kaz, MS
Tel: 414 691-5224 *Fax:* 414 691-5451
Med Dir: Sheila Strock, DDS
Class Cap: 18 *Begins:* Aug
Length: 24 mos *Award:* AS
Tuition per yr: $4,410 res, $24,850 non-res
Evening or weekend classes available

Northcentral Technical College
Dental Hygienist Prgm
1000 Campus Dr
Wausau, WI 54401
Prgm Dir: S Budjac
Tel: 715 675-3331, Ext 4487 *Fax:* 715 675-3772
E-mail: budjae?ntc@mail.northcentral.tec.wi.us
Class Cap: 54 *Begins:* Aug
Length: 18 mos, 27 mos *Award:* AS
Tuition per yr: $1,880 res, $28,440 non-res

Wyoming

Laramie County Community College
Dental Hygienist Prgm
1400 E College Dr
Cheyenne, WY 82007
Prgm Dir: Bette Buchanan
Tel: 307 778-1386 *Fax:* 307 778-1399
Class Cap: 16 *Begins:* Aug
Length: 16 mos *Award:* AS
Tuition per yr: $992 res, $2,640 non-res

Sheridan College
Dental Hygienist Prgm
3059 Coffeen Ave
Sheridan, WY 82801
Prgm Dir: Constance R Sharuga, RDH PhD
Tel: 307 674-6446 *Fax:* 307 674-4293
E-mail: csharuga@generals.sc.wheen.edu
Class Cap: 24 *Begins:* Aug
Length: 16 mos *Award:* AS
Tuition per yr: $992 res, $2,640 non-res

Dental Laboratory Technician

Alabama

H Councill Trenholm State Technical College
Dental Lab Technician Prgm
1225 Air Base Blvd
Montgomery, AL 36108
Prgm Dir: David Cawley
Tel: 334-286-0879
Class Cap: 12 *Begins:* Sep
Length: 20 mos *Award:* AA
Tuition per yr: $1,585 res, $1,585 non-res

Arizona

Pima County Community College
Dental Lab Technician Prgm
2202 W Anklam Rd/HRP 220
Tucson, AZ 85709-0080
Prgm Dir: R Douglas
Tel: 602 884-6916
E-mail: rdouglas@pimacc.pima.edu
Class Cap: 16 *Begins:* Aug
Length: 18 mos *Award:* AS
Tuition per yr: $724 res, $4,596 non-res

California

Los Angeles City College
Dental Lab Technician Prgm
855 N Vermont Ave
Los Angeles, CA 90029
Prgm Dir: Dana Cohen
Tel: 213 953-4236
Class Cap: 24 *Begins:* Jan Aug
Length: 18 mos *Award:* Cert, AA
Tuition per yr: $970 res, $3,619 non-res

Pasadena City College
Dental Lab Technician Prgm
1570 E Colorado Blvd
Pasadena, CA 91106
Prgm Dir: Anita Bobich
Tel: 818 585-7200
E-mail: zadar@aol.com
Class Cap: 26 *Begins:* Aug
Length: 18 mos *Award:* Cert, AS
Tuition per yr: $1,212 res, $2,596 non-res

Naval School of Dental Technology
Dental Lab Technician Prgm
4170 Norman Scott Rd
San Diego, CA 92136-5597
Prgm Dir: E Ibarra
Tel: 619 556-7987 *Fax:* 619 556-8266
Class Cap: 25 *Begins:* Jan Apr Jun Oct
Length: 12 mos *Award:* Cert

Florida

McFatter Vocational Technical Center
Dental Lab Technician Prgm
6500 Nova Dr
Davie, FL 33317
Prgm Dir: H Jung
Tel: 954 370-8324 *Fax:* 954 370-1647
Class Cap: 26 *Begins:* Varies
Length: 16 mos *Award:* Cert
Tuition per yr: $1,283 res, $2,381 non-res

Indian River Community College
Dental Lab Technician Prgm
3209 Virginia Ave
Ft Pierce, FL 34981-5599
Prgm Dir: Anthony Valvano
Tel: 407 462-4700
Class Cap: 16 *Begins:* Aug
Length: 18 mos *Award:* AS
Tuition per yr: $2,885 res, $10,013 non-res

Lindsey Hopkins Tech Education Center
Dental Lab Technician Prgm
750 NW 20th St
Miami, FL 33127
Prgm Dir: F Slavichak, DDS
Tel: 305 324-6070 *Fax:* 305 324-6249
Class Cap: 64 *Begins:* Sep Jan
Length: 24 mos *Award:* Cert
Tuition per yr: $558 res, $4,196 non-res

Southern College
Dental Lab Technician Prgm
5600 Lake Underhill Rd
Orlando, FL 32807
Prgm Dir: J Mac Donald, CDT AS
Tel: 407 273-1000 *Fax:* 407 273-0492
Class Cap: 60 *Begins:* Bi-annual
Length: 24 mos *Award:* AS
Tuition per yr: $7,151 res, $7,151 non-res
Evening or weekend classes available

Georgia

Atlanta Area Technical School
Dental Lab Technician Prgm
1560 Stewart Ave SW
Atlanta, GA 30310
Prgm Dir: L Storey, CDT
Tel: 404 756-3724 *Fax:* 404 756-0932
Class Cap: 20 *Begins:* Mar Sep
Length: 18 mos *Award:* Dipl,Cert
Tuition per yr: $1,359 res, $1,632 non-res

Gwinnett Technical Institute
Dental Lab Technician Prgm
1250 Atkinson Rd/Box 1505
Lawrenceville, GA 30246-1505
Prgm Dir: Wallis Turner
Tel: 770 962-7580, Ext 175
Class Cap: 20 *Begins:* Sep
Length: 20 mos *Award:* Dipl, AA
Tuition per yr: $1,345 res, $2,101 non-res

Idaho

Idaho State University
Dental Lab Technician Prgm
Dental Lab Tech Box 8380
Pocatello, ID 83209-8380
Prgm Dir: G George
Tel: 208 236-3141 *Fax:* 208 236-4641
Class Cap: 8 *Begins:* Aug
Length: 20 mos *Award:* Dipl, AAS
Tuition per yr: $2,400 res, $8,770 non-res

Illinois

Southern Illinois Univ at Carbondale
Dental Lab Technician Prgm
College of Technical Careers
Carbondale, IL 62901
Prgm Dir: Dennis Laake
Tel: 618 453-7215 *Fax:* 618 453-7286
Class Cap: 35 *Begins:* Aug
Length: 16 mos *Award:* AAS
Tuition per yr: $2,550 res, $7,650 non-res

Triton College
Dental Lab Technician Prgm
2000 N Fifth Ave
River Grove, IL 60171
Prgm Dir: A Mc Kinnor
Tel: 708 456-0300
Class Cap: 40
Length: 20 mos *Award:* Cert
Tuition per yr: $2,140 res, $6,630 non-res

Indiana

Indiana Univ/Purdue Univ Ft Wayne
Dental Lab Technician Prgm
2101 Coliseum Blvd E
Fort Wayne, IN 46805
Prgm Dir: C Champion
Tel: 219 481-6837 *Fax:* 219 481-6083
Class Cap: 15 *Begins:* Aug
Length: 18 mos *Award:* AS
Tuition per yr: $7,926 res, $15,752 non-res

Iowa

Kirkwood Community College
Dental Lab Technician Prgm
6301 Kirkwood Blvd SW
PO Box 2068
Cedar Rapids, IA 52406-9973
Prgm Dir: B Mitchell
Tel: 319 398-5400 *Fax:* 319 398-1293
E-mail: jbmitche@kirkwood.cc.ia.us
Class Cap: 15 *Begins:* Aug
Length: 18 mos *Award:* AAS
Tuition per yr: $2,557 res, $5,115 non-res
Evening or weekend classes available

Programs

Kentucky

Lexington Community College
Dental Lab Technician Prgm
Cooper Dr/Oswald Bldg
Lexington, KY 40506
Prgm Dir: Arthur A Dameron
Tel: 606 257-6142
E-mail: artdame@pop.uky.edu
Class Cap: 18   *Begins:* Aug
Length: 20 mos   *Award:* AAS
Tuition per yr: $1,956 res, $5,196 non-res

Louisiana

Louisiana State University
Dental Lab Technician Prgm
1100 Florida Ave
New Orleans, LA 70119
Prgm Dir: R Schiele
Tel: 504 619-8684   *Fax:* 504 619-8740
Class Cap: 12   *Begins:* Jul
Length: 20 mos, 30 mos   *Award:* Dipl, AS
Tuition per yr: $2,797 res, $5,297 non-res

Massachusetts

Middlesex Community College - Lowell
Dental Lab Technician Prgm
33 Kearney Square
Lowell, MA 01852
Prgm Dir: J Kessler
Tel: 508 656-3056   *Fax:* 508 656-3078
Class Cap: 15   *Begins:* Sep
Length: 18 mos   *Award:* AS
Tuition per yr: $7,113 res, $15,993 non-res
Evening or weekend classes available

Michigan

Ferris State University
Dental Lab Technician Prgm
200 Ferris Dr
Big Rapids, MI 49307-2740
Prgm Dir: D Harrison
Tel: 616 592-2261   *Fax:* 616 592-3788
E-mail: harrison@alh01.ferris.edu
Class Cap: 20   *Begins:* Aug
Length: 18 mos   *Award:* AS
Tuition per yr: $3,630 res, $5,445 non-res

Minnesota

Century Community and Technical College
Dental Lab Technician Prgm
3300 Century Ave N
White Bear Lake, MN 55110
Prgm Dir: L Pole
Tel: 612 770-2351
Length: 16 mos   *Award:* Dipl
Tuition per yr: $3,868 res, $7,385 non-res

Nebraska

Central Technical Community College
Dental Lab Technician Prgm
PO Box 1024
Hastings, NE 68902-1024
Prgm Dir: P Cecil
Tel: 402 461-2466   *Fax:* 402 461-2454
E-mail: cechdel@cccadm.gi.cccneb.edu
Class Cap: 15
Length: 24 mos   *Award:* AAS
Tuition per yr: $1,273 res, $1,872 non-res

New York

CUNY New York City Technical College
Dental Lab Technician Prgm
300 Jay St
Brooklyn, NY 11201
Prgm Dir: Nicholas Manos
Tel: 718 260-5137   *Fax:* 718 260-5995
Class Cap: 40   *Begins:* Sep Jan
Length: 14 mos   *Award:* AAS
Tuition per yr: $3,200 res, $7,800 non-res

Erie Community College - City Campus
Dental Lab Technician Prgm
4041 Southwestern Blvd
Orchard Park, NY 14127-2199
Prgm Dir: Marvin Herman, MD
Tel: 716 851-1759   *Fax:* 716 851-1629
E-mail: herman@sstaff.sunyerie.edu
Class Cap: 32   *Begins:* Sep
Length: 21 mos   *Award:* AAS
Tuition per yr: $2,500 res, $5,000 non-res
Evening or weekend classes available

North Carolina

Durham Technical Community College
Dental Lab Technician Prgm
1637 Lawson St
Durham, NC 27703
Prgm Dir: M Patrick
Tel: 919 686-3399   *Fax:* 919 686-3693
Class Cap: 24
Length: 19 mos   *Award:* AAS
Tuition per yr: $794 res, $6,072 non-res
Evening or weekend classes available

Ohio

Cuyahoga Community College
Dental Lab Technician Prgm
2900 Community College Ave
Cleveland, OH 44115
Prgm Dir: Mary Lou Gerosky
Tel: 216 987-4377   *Fax:* 216 987-4386
E-mail: mary.lou.gerosky@tric.cc.oh.us
Class Cap: 20   *Begins:* Sep
Length: 16 mos   *Award:* Cert
Tuition per yr: $2,079 res, $2,808 non-res
Evening or weekend classes available

Columbus State Community College
Dental Lab Technician Prgm
550 E Spring St/Box 1609
Columbus, OH 43215
Prgm Dir: C Narcross
Tel: 614 227-2547   *Fax:* 614 227-5144
E-mail: cnarcros@cougar.colstate.cc.oh.us
Class Cap: 25   *Begins:* Sep
Length: 21 mos   *Award:* AS
Tuition per yr: $3,036 res, $6,300 non-res

Oregon

Portland Community College
Dental Lab Technician Prgm
PO Box 19000
Portland, OR 97219-0990
Prgm Dir: Anne Jackson
Tel: 503 244-6111   *Fax:* 503 977-4869
E-mail: ajackson@pcc.edu
Class Cap: 24   *Begins:* Sep
Length: 18 mos   *Award:* Cert, AAS
Tuition per yr: $1,368 res, $4,788 non-res

Tennessee

East Tennessee State University
Dental Lab Technician Prgm
1000 West E St
Elizabethton, TN 37643
Prgm Dir: Victor Hopson
Tel: 423 547-4911
Class Cap: 10   *Begins:* Aug
Length: 19 mos   *Award:* AA, BS
Tuition per yr: $2,780 res, $7,943 non-res

Texas

Army Medical Dept Center and School
Dental Lab Technician Prgm
Dept of Dental Science/3151 Scott Rd
COMDT AHS/Attn: MCCS HDL Col Netti
Ft Sam Houston, TX 78234-6134
Prgm Dir: Charles Netti
Tel: 210 221-8003   *Fax:* 210 221-8698
Class Cap: 56
Length: 6 mos   *Award:* Dipl

Univ of Texas Hlth Sci Ctr at San Antonio
Dental Lab Technician Prgm
7703 Floyd Curl Dr
San Antonio, TX 78284-7914
Prgm Dir: R Davis
Tel: 210 567-3056   *Fax:* 210 567-3061
E-mail: davisr0@uthscsa.edu
Class Cap: 24
Length: 16 mos   *Award:* Cert, BS
Tuition per yr: $3,954 res, $14,270 non-res

882 Training Group
Dental Lab Technician Prgm
Sheppard AFB, TX 76311-2246
Prgm Dir: Douglas Wasson, LtC
Tel: 817 676-6967   *Fax:* 817 676-6928
E-mail: wasson@win.spd.aetc.af.mil
Class Cap: 16   *Begins:* Varies
Length: 6 mos   *Award:* Cert

Virginia

J Sargeant Reynolds Community College
Dental Lab Technician Prgm
PO Box 85622
Richmond, VA 23285-5622
Prgm Dir: Ernie Wolfe
Tel: 804 786-6931
Class Cap: 20   *Begins:* Aug
Length: 19 mos   *Award:* AA
Tuition per yr: $2,497 res, $3,919 non-res

Washington

Bates Technical College
Dental Lab Technician Prgm
1101 S Yakima Ave
Tacoma, WA 98405
Prgm Dir: Raymond Marostica
Tel: 206 596-1577   *Fax:* 206 596-1540
E-mail: rmarosti@ctc.ctc.edu
Class Cap: 18   *Begins:* Varies
Length: 11 mos   *Award:* Cert, AT
Tuition per yr: $1,917 res, $1,917 non-res
Evening or weekend classes available

Wisconsin

Milwaukee Area Technical College
Dental Lab Technician Prgm
700 W State St
Milwaukee, WI 53233
Prgm Dir: P Godin, CDT
Tel: 414 297-7134   *Fax:* 414 297-7990
E-mail: godinp@milwaukee.tec.wi.us
Class Cap: 24   *Begins:* Aug
Length: 16 mos   *Award:* AAS
Tuition per yr: $5,275
Evening or weekend classes available

Diagnostic Medical Sonographer

History

In 1972, the American Society of Ultrasound Technical Specialists (ASUTS) appointed a committee to explore the mechanism of accreditation of educational programs for the ultrasound technical specialist through the American Medical Association (AMA) Council on Medical Education (CME). In October 1973, members of ASUTS (now known as the Society of Diagnostic Medical Sonographers) met with a representative from the AMA Department of Health Manpower and initiated activities to receive formal recognition as an occupation. One year later the occupation of diagnostic medical sonography received recognition by the AMA.

From 1974 to 1979, the *Standards (Essentials) of an Accredited Educational Program for the Diagnostic Medical Sonographer* were developed. Because of the multidisciplinary nature of diagnostic ultrasound, many interested medical and allied health organizations collaborated in drafting the *Standards*, which were formally adopted by the following organizations: the American College of Cardiology (withdrew as a sponsoring organization in 1983; resumed sponsorship in 1986), American College of Radiology, American Institute of Ultrasound in Medicine, AMA, American Society of Echocardiography, American Society of Radiologic Technologists, Society of Diagnostic Medical Sonographers, and Society of Nuclear Medicine (withdrew as a sponsoring organization in 1981). These organizations, with the exception of the AMA and the Society of Nuclear Medicine, and the addition of the Society of Vascular Technology in 1993, currently sponsor the Joint Review Committee on Education in Diagnostic Medical Sonography. New *Standards* were adopted in 1996 and will be used exclusively beginning January 1, 1998. Programs undergoing evaluation prior to January 1, 1998 may continue to use the 1987 *Standards* if they choose. Educational programs were first accredited in January 1982.

Occupational Description

The diagnostic medical sonographer provides patient services using medical ultrasound under the supervision of a physician responsible for the use and interpretation of ultrasound procedures. The sonographer assists the physician in gathering sonographic data necessary to diagnose a variety of conditions and diseases.

Job Description

The sonographer provides patient services in a variety of medical settings in which the physician is responsible for the use and interpretation of ultrasound procedures. In assisting physicians in gathering sonographic data, the diagnostic medical sonographer is able to obtain, review, and integrate pertinent patient history and supporting clinical data to facilitate optimum diagnostic results; perform appropriate procedures and record anatomical, pathological, and/or physiological data for interpretation by a physician; record and process sonographic data and other pertinent observations made during the procedure for presentation to the interpreting physician; exercise discretion and judgment in the performance of sonographic services; provide patient education related to medical ultrasound; and promote principles of good health.

Employment Characteristics

Diagnostic medical sonographers may be employed in hospitals, clinics, private offices, and industry. There is also a need for suitably qualified educators, researchers, and administrators. The demand for sonographers continues to exceed the supply. The supply and demand ratio affects salaries, depending on experience and responsibilities.

Programs

According to the Society of Diagnostic Medical Sonographers, the 1995 salary for diagnostic medical sonographers with less than 1 year of experience was $29,800.

Educational Programs

Length. Programs may be 1, 2, or 4 years, depending on program design, objectives, and the degree or certificate awarded.

Prerequisites. Applicants to a 1-year program must possess qualifications in a clinically related allied health profession. Applicants to 2-year programs must be high school graduates (or equivalent) with an educational background in basic science and physics.

Curriculum. Curricula of accredited programs include physical sciences, applied biological sciences, patient care, clinical medicine, applications of ultrasound, instrumentation, related diagnostic procedures, and image evaluation. A plan for well-structured, competency-based clinical education is an essential part of the curriculum of all sonography programs.

Standards. *Standards* are national educational standards adopted by the several collaborating organizations. Each applicant is assessed in accordance with the *Standards*, and accredited programs are periodically reviewed to determine continuing compliance.

Inquiries

Accreditation

Requests for information on program accreditation, including *Standards,* preparing the self-study report, and arranging a site visit, should be submitted to

Joint Review Committee on Education in
  Diagnostic Medical Sonography
7108-C S Alton Way/Ste 150
Englewood, CO 80112-2106
303 741-3533

Careers

Inquiries regarding careers and curriculum should be addressed to

Society of Diagnostic Medical Sonographers
12770 Coit Rd/Ste 508
Dallas, TX 75251-1319
214 239-7367

Certification/Registration

Inquiries regarding certification should be addressed to

American Registry of Diagnostic Medical Sonographers
600 Jefferson Plaza/Ste 360
Rockville, MD 20852-1150
301 738-8401

Diagnostic Medical Sonographer

Alabama

Wallace State College
Diagnostic Med Sonographer Prgm
PO Box 2000
Hanceville, AL 35077-2000
Prgm Dir: Janet E Money, RDMS CNMT ARRT
Tel: 205 352-2090 *Fax:* 205 352-8228
Med Dir: J Lanett Varnell, MD
Class Cap: 25 *Begins:* Sep
Length: 24 mos *Award:* AD
Tuition per yr: $1,746 res, $3,492 non-res
Evening or weekend classes available

Arizona

Gateway Community College
Diagnostic Med Sonographer Prgm
108 N 40th St
Phoenix, AZ 85034
Prgm Dir: Kathleen Murphy
Tel: 602 392-5145 *Fax:* 602 392-5329
Med Dir: John Crowe, MD
Class Cap: 15 *Begins:* Aug
Length: 18 mos *Award:* Cert, AS
Tuition per yr: $1,500 res, $4,500 non-res

Pima Medical Institute - Tucson
Diagnostic Med Sonographer Prgm
3350 E Grant
Tucson, AZ 85716
Prgm Dir: Carl R Johnson
Tel: 520 326-1600 *Fax:* 520 795-3463
Med Dir: Fred Brickman
Class Cap: 12 *Begins:* Sep
Length: 12 mos *Award:* Cert
Tuition per yr: $7,754 res, $7,754 non-res

California

Orange Coast College
Diagnostic Med Sonographer Prgm
2701 Fairview Rd
Costa Mesa, CA 92628
Prgm Dir: Joan M Clasby, BVE RDMS
Tel: 714 432-5893 *Fax:* 714 432-5534
Med Dir: Robert Reinke, MD
Class Cap: 18 *Begins:* Aug
Length: 24 mos *Award:* Cert, AA
Tuition per yr: $429 res, $3,960 non-res

Loma Linda University
Diagnostic Med Sonographer Prgm
Sch of Allied Hlth Profs
Loma Linda, CA 92350
Prgm Dir: Marie DeLange, BS RT RDMS
Tel: 909 824-4931 *Fax:* 909 824-4166
Med Dir: Glenn A Rouse, MD
Class Cap: 10 *Begins:* Sep
Length: 24 mos *Award:* Cert
Tuition per yr: $5,950 res, $5,950 non-res

Colorado

Penrose-St Francis Health System
Diagnostic Med Sonographer Prgm
School of Sonography at Penrose Hosp
2215 N Cascade Ave/PO Box 7021
Colorado Springs, CO 80933
Prgm Dir: Anna S Worley, BS RDMS RVT
Tel: 719 776-5245   *Fax:* 719 776-5461
Med Dir: James Borgstede, MD
Class Cap: 6   *Begins:* Sep
Length: 18 mos   *Award:* Cert
Tuition per yr: $3,000 res, $3,000 non-res

University of Colorado Hlth Science Ctr
Diagnostic Med Sonographer Prgm
Dept of Ultrasound/Box C-277
4200 E 9th Ave
Denver, CO 80262
Prgm Dir: Carolyn T Coffin, BS RT RDMS RVT
Tel: 303 270-5255   *Fax:* 303 372-6271
E-mail: coffin-c@defiance.uchsc.edu
Med Dir: Elizabeth R Stamm, MD
Class Cap: 10   *Begins:* Sep
Length: 12 mos   *Award:* Cert
Tuition per yr: $3,000 res, $3,000 non-res

Delaware

Delaware Tech & Comm Coll - Wilmington
Diagnostic Med Sonographer Prgm
333 Shipley St
Wilmington, DE 19801
Prgm Dir: Ronald Veasey, RDMS AS
Tel: 302 428-6395   *Fax:* 302 428-2691
Med Dir: Howard M Levy, MD
Class Cap: 9   *Begins:* Jun
Length: 24 mos   *Award:* AAS
Tuition per yr: $1,890 res, $4,725 non-res
Evening or weekend classes available

District of Columbia

George Washington University Med Ctr
Diagnostic Med Sonographer Prgm
2300 K St NW/#208 D
Washington, DC 20037
Prgm Dir: Catheeja Ismail, BA RDMS
Tel: 202 994-8697   *Fax:* 202 994-1299
E-mail: cismail@gwis2.circ.gwu.edu
Med Dir: Michael C Hill, MD
Class Cap: 9   *Begins:* Aug
Length: 21 mos   *Award:* BS
Tuition per yr: $13,000 res, $13,000 non-res

Florida

Broward Community College
Diagnostic Med Sonographer Prgm
3501 SW Davie Rd
Ft Lauderdale, FL 33314
Prgm Dir: Sharon Calton, MS RDMS RDCS
Tel: 954 475-6918   *Fax:* 954 473-9037
Med Dir: Stuart Hantman, MD
Begins: May
Length: 24 mos   *Award:* AS
Tuition per yr: $1,400 res, $5,600 non-res

Miami-Dade Community College/Jackson Mem Hosp Consortium
Diagnostic Med Sonographer Prgm
Medical Center Campus
950 NW 20th St
Miami, FL 33127
Prgm Dir: Joseph Schnetzer, MS RDMS RDCS
Tel: 305 237-4245   *Fax:* 305 237-4116
E-mail: schnetj@mdcc.edu
Med Dir: Javier Casillas, MD
Class Cap: 15   *Begins:* Aug
Length: 24 mos   *Award:* Dipl, AS
Tuition per yr: $1,444 res, $5,075 non-res
Evening or weekend classes available

Florida Hospital Coll of Health Sciences
Diagnostic Med Sonographer Prgm
800 Lake Estelle Dr
Orlando, FL 32803
Prgm Dir: Charlotte G Henningsen, MS RT RDMS
Tel: 407 895-5733   *Fax:* 407 895-7680
Med Dir: Gregory A Logsdon, MD
Class Cap: 32   *Begins:* Aug
Length: 12 mos, 24 mos   *Award:* Cert, AS
Tuition per yr: $4,000

Minnesota Riverland Tech Coll-Faribault
Diagnostic Med Sonographer Prgm
800 Lake Estelle Dr
Orlando, FL 32803
Prgm Dir: Charlotte G Henningsen, MS RT RDMS
Tel: 407 895-5733   *Fax:* 407 895-7680
Med Dir: Gregory A Logsdon, MD
Class Cap: 16   *Begins:* Aug
Length: 12 mos, 24 mos   *Award:* Cert, AS
Tuition per yr: $4,000

Valencia Community College
Diagnostic Med Sonographer Prgm
925 S Orange Ave
Orlando, FL 32806
Prgm Dir: Sue Ellison, AA RT(R) RDMS
Tel: 407 841-5111, Ext 6971   *Fax:* 407 423-3204
Med Dir: Lennard D Greenbaum, MD
Class Cap: 5   *Begins:* Aug
Length: 24 mos   *Award:* AS
Tuition per yr: $1,617 res, $5,698 non-res
Evening or weekend classes available

Hillsborough Community College
Diagnostic Med Sonographer Prgm
PO Box 30030
Tampa, FL 33630-3030
Prgm Dir: Susan Zeiter, RDMS
Tel: 813 782-8829   *Fax:* 813 253-7400
Med Dir: Richard E Schwab, MD
Class Cap: 28   *Begins:* Aug
Length: 12 mos, 24 mos   *Award:* Cert, AS
Tuition per yr: $1,049 res, $3,908 non-res
Evening or weekend classes available

Georgia

Grady Health System
Diagnostic Med Sonographer Prgm
80 Butler St SE
PO Box 26095
Atlanta, GA 30335
Prgm Dir: Tami J Daniels, BS RT(R) RDMS
Tel: 404 616-5032   *Fax:* 404 616-3512
Med Dir: Frederick B Murphy, MD
Class Cap: 7   *Begins:* Oct
Length: 12 mos   *Award:* Cert
Tuition per yr: $3,200

Medical College of Georgia
Diagnostic Med Sonographer Prgm
AE-1003
Augusta, GA 30912-0600
Prgm Dir: Lynn Reyes, BS RDMS RDCS
Tel: 706 721-3691   *Fax:* 706 721-8293
E-mail: lreyes@mail.meg.edu
Med Dir: Sathyanarayna, MD
Class Cap: 11   *Begins:* Sep
Length: 12 mos, 22 mos   *Award:* Cert, BS
Tuition per yr: $3,084 res, $8,800 non-res
Evening or weekend classes available

Illinois

Wilbur Wright College
Diagnostic Med Sonographer Prgm
4300 N Narragansett Ave
Chicago, IL 60634
Prgm Dir: Dennis M King, MHS RT(R)
Tel: 312 481-8887   *Fax:* 312 481-8892
E-mail: dking@ccc.edu
Med Dir: Martin Lipton, MD
Class Cap: 33   *Begins:* Sep
Length: 14 mos, 26 mos   *Award:* Cert, AAS
Tuition per yr: $1,513

Triton College
Diagnostic Med Sonographer Prgm
2000 N Fifth Ave
River Grove, IL 60171
Prgm Dir: Debra L Krukowski, RDMS
Tel: 708 456-0300   *Fax:* 708 583-3121
Med Dir: S Asokan, MD
Class Cap: 31   *Begins:* Sep
Length: 21 mos   *Award:* AAS
Tuition per yr: $891 res, $2,491 non-res

Iowa

University of Iowa Hospitals and Clinics
Diagnostic Med Sonographer Prgm
Radiology Dept/C726 GH
200 Hawkins Dr
Iowa City, IA 52242-1077
Prgm Dir: Stephanie Ellingson, BA RDMS RVT
Tel: 319 356-4871   *Fax:* 319 353-6769
E-mail: stephanie-ellingson@uiowa.edu
Med Dir: Yutaka Sato, MD
Class Cap: 7   *Begins:* Sep
Length: 12 mos   *Award:* Cert
Tuition per yr: $2,000 res, $2,500 non-res

Programs

Kentucky

West Kentucky Tech

Diagnostic Med Sonographer Prgm
Blandville Rd
PO Box 7408
Paducah, KY 42002-7408
Prgm Dir: Alice R Vaughn, BS RT(R) RDMS
Tel: 502 554-6229 *Fax:* 502 554-6227
Med Dir: Danny R Hatfield, MD
Class Cap: 11 *Begins:* Aug
Length: 11 mos *Award:* Dipl
Tuition per yr: $500 res, $1,000 non-res
Evening or weekend classes available

Louisiana

Alton Ochsner Medical Foundation

Diagnostic Med Sonographer Prgm
1516 Jefferson Hwy
New Orleans, LA 70123-3335
Prgm Dir: Benita Barthel, RDMS
Tel: 504 842-3481 *Fax:* 504 842-2459
Med Dir: Christopher R Merritt, MD
Class Cap: 3 *Begins:* Jul
Length: 12 mos *Award:* Cert

Maryland

Johns Hopkins Hospital

Diagnostic Med Sonographer Prgm
Radiology Admin B-179
600 N Wolfe St
Baltimore, MD 21287
Prgm Dir: Jan Bloomer, AS RT RDMS
Tel: 410 955-6198 *Fax:* 410 955-0059
E-mail: jlbloome@rad.jhu.edu
Med Dir: Ulrike Hamper, MD
Class Cap: 11 *Begins:* Jul
Length: 13 mos *Award:* Cert
Tuition per yr: $4,000 res, $4,000 non-res
Evening or weekend classes available

University of Maryland Baltimore County

Diagnostic Med Sonographer Prgm
UMBC
1000 Hilltop Circle
Baltimore, MD 21250
Prgm Dir: Janice Dolk, MA RT(R) RDMS
Tel: 410 455-2758 *Fax:* 410 455-1115
E-mail: dolk@umbc.edu
Med Dir: Roger C Sanders, MD
Class Cap: 22 *Begins:* Aug
Length: 14 mos *Award:* Cert
Tuition per yr: $6,500 res, $6,500 non-res
Evening or weekend classes available

Montgomery College

Diagnostic Med Sonographer Prgm
7600 Takoma Ave
Takoma Park, MD 20912
Prgm Dir: Linda Zanin, MA RDMS
Tel: 301 650-1431
Med Dir: Kathleen Cantwell, MD
Class Cap: 17 *Begins:* Sep
Length: 18 mos, 23 mos *Award:* Cert, AAS
Tuition per yr: $1,296 res, $4,800 non-res
Evening or weekend classes available

Massachusetts

Middlesex Community College - Bedford

Diagnostic Med Sonographer Prgm
Springs Rd
Bedford, MA 01730
Prgm Dir: Thomas Walsh, MA RDMS
Tel: 617 280-3983
Med Dir: Jorge Merino de Villasante, MD
Class Cap: 20 *Begins:* Sep
Length: 24 mos *Award:* AS
Tuition per yr: $2,010 res, $5,682 non-res

Michigan

Henry Ford Hospital

Diagnostic Med Sonographer Prgm
2799 W Grand Blvd
Detroit, MI 48202
Prgm Dir: Michael Moffatt, MA RDMS
Tel: 313 876-3526 *Fax:* 313 876-9480
Med Dir: Wayne Wolfson, MD
Class Cap: 10 *Begins:* Jul
Length: 14 mos *Award:* Cert
Tuition per yr: $1,000

Jackson Community College

Diagnostic Med Sonographer Prgm
2111 Emmons Rd
Jackson, MI 49201
Prgm Dir: Lynne Schreiber, MS RDMS RT(R)
Tel: 517 787-0800 *Fax:* 517 789-1633
Med Dir: Richard McLeary, MD
Class Cap: 20 *Begins:* May
Length: 18 mos *Award:* AS
Tuition per yr: $1,376 res, $1,728 non-res
Evening or weekend classes available

Oakland Community College

Diagnostic Med Sonographer Prgm
22322 Rutland Dr
Southfield, MI 48075
Prgm Dir: Carolyn E Nacy, RDMS
Tel: 810 552-2610 *Fax:* 810 552-2661
Med Dir: Shazed Sadiq, MD
Class Cap: 22 *Begins:* May
Length: 24 mos *Award:* AD
Tuition per yr: $1,564 res, $2,652 non-res
Evening or weekend classes available

Providence Hospital and Medical Centers

Diagnostic Med Sonographer Prgm
16001 W Nine Mile Rd
Southfield, MI 48037
Prgm Dir: Janette Jablonski, RDMS RDCS
Tel: 810 424-5385 *Fax:* 810 424-5395
Med Dir: John E Temple, MD
Class Cap: 8 *Begins:* Jul
Length: 15 mos *Award:* Dipl
Tuition per yr: $1,200 res, $1,200 non-res

Minnesota

Mayo Clinic/Mayo Foundation

Diagnostic Med Sonographer Prgm
200 First St SW
Rochester, MN 55905
Prgm Dir: Kathryn Kuntz, RT RDMS RVT
Tel: 507 284-2511 *Fax:* 507 284-0656
E-mail: kuntz.kathryn@mayo.edu
Med Dir: Eric Lantz, MD
Class Cap: 15 *Begins:* Sep
Length: 15 mos *Award:* Cert
Tuition per yr: $1,500

College of St Catherine

Diagnostic Med Sonographer Prgm
601 25th Ave South
St Paul, MN 55454
Prgm Dir: Dick Mabbs, BA RVT ROMS
Tel: 612 690-7889 *Fax:* 612 670-7849
E-mail: dvmabbs@alex.stka.edu
Med Dir: Beverly Trombley, MD
Class Cap: 10 *Begins:* Jul
Length: 13 mos, 24 mos *Award:* Cert, AAS
Tuition per yr: $13,120

Missouri

St Louis Comm College at Forest Park

Diagnostic Med Sonographer Prgm
5600 Oakland Ave
St Louis, MO 63110
Prgm Dir: Beth Anderhub, MEd RT RDMS
Tel: 314 644-9399 *Fax:* 314 644-9752
Med Dir: Richard Schulz, MD
Class Cap: 29 *Begins:* Aug
Length: 12 mos *Award:* Cert
Tuition per yr: $1,344 res, $1,696 non-res
Evening or weekend classes available

Nebraska

NE Methodist Coll Nursing & Allied Hlth

Diagnostic Med Sonographer Prgm
8501 W Dodge Rd
Omaha, NE 68114
Prgm Dir: Patricia Sullivan, MA RDMS RT
Tel: 402 354-4851 *Fax:* 402 354-8875
Med Dir: Kevin Cawley, MD
Class Cap: 5 *Begins:* May
Length: 24 mos *Award:* AS
Tuition per yr: $7,100 res, $8,900 non-res
Evening or weekend classes available

University of Nebraska Medical Center

Diagnostic Med Sonographer Prgm
Radiology Dept/Ultrasound
600 S 42nd St
Omaha, NE 68198-1045
Prgm Dir: Cheri R Fisher, BS RT(R) RDMS
Tel: 402 559-8106 *Fax:* 402 559-9408
E-mail: cfisher@mail.unmc.edu
Med Dir: Joseph C Anderson, MD
Class Cap: 6 *Begins:* Aug
Length: 12 mos *Award:* BS
Tuition per yr: $2,850 res, $7,752 non-res
Evening or weekend classes available

New Jersey

Elizabeth General Medical Center
Diagnostic Med Sonographer Prgm
925 E Jersey St
Elizabeth, NJ 07201
Prgm Dir: Harry H Holdorf, MPA RT RDMS
Tel: 908 965-7390 *Fax:* 908 629-8219
Med Dir: Robert Silbey, MD FACR
Class Cap: 16 *Begins:* Sep
Length: 12 mos *Award:* Dipl
Tuition per yr: $6,000 res, $6,000 non-res

Univ of Med & Dent of New Jersey
Diagnostic Med Sonographer Prgm
Sch Hlth Related Professions
65 Bergen St
Newark, NJ 07107-3006
Prgm Dir: Cynthia Silkowski, BA RDMS RVT
Tel: 201 597-0156 *Fax:* 201 597-0162
E-mail: silkowey@umdnj.edu
Med Dir: Alan G Dembner, MD
Class Cap: 19 *Begins:* May
Length: 15 mos, 48 mos *Award:* Cert, BA, BS
Tuition per yr: $6,533 res, $8,689 non-res

Bergen Community College
Diagnostic Med Sonographer Prgm
400 Paramus Rd
Paramus, NJ 07652-1595
Prgm Dir: Katherine Benz- Campbell, BS RDMS
Tel: 201 447-7178 *Fax:* 201 612-8225
Med Dir: Frederick P Ayers, MD
Class Cap: 12 *Begins:* Sep
Length: 23 mos *Award:* AAS
Tuition per yr: $2,305 res, $5,611 non-res
Evening or weekend classes available

Gloucester County College
Diagnostic Med Sonographer Prgm
1400 Tanyard Rd
Sewell, NJ 08080
Prgm Dir: Michael Keith, RD MS
Tel: 609 468-5000 *Fax:* 609 464-8463
Med Dir: Joseph Centerne, MD
Class Cap: 14 *Begins:* Sep
Length: 21 mos *Award:* AAS
Tuition per yr: $1,700 res, $6,800 non-res
Evening or weekend classes available

New Mexico

Univ of New Mexico School of Medicine
Diagnostic Med Sonographer Prgm
Basic Med Sciences - Box 710
Albuquerque, NM 87131-5656
Prgm Dir: Rebecca Hall, PhD RDMS
Tel: 505 277-5254 *Fax:* 505 277-7011
E-mail: rebecca_hall@somasf.unm.edu
Med Dir: Michael Williamson, MD
Class Cap: 8 *Begins:* Aug
Length: 18 mos *Award:* Cert
Tuition per yr: $3,368 res, $8,360 non-res

New York

SUNY Health Science Center - Brooklyn
Diagnostic Med Sonographer Prgm
Coll Hlth Related Professions
450 Clarkson Ave
Brooklyn, NY 11203
Prgm Dir: Linda M Chase, BS RDMS
Tel: 718 270-7764 *Fax:* 718 270-7751
E-mail: lchase@netmail.hscbklyn.edu
Med Dir: Harris L Cohen, MD
Class Cap: 28 *Begins:* Sep
Length: 24 mos *Award:* BS
Tuition per yr: $4,496 res, $11,068 non-res

New York University Medical Center
Diagnostic Med Sonographer Prgm
Basic Science Bldg
342 E 26th St
New York, NY 10010
Prgm Dir: Kerry Weinberg, MPA RT RDCS RDM
Tel: 212 263-6644 *Fax:* 212 779-1493
Med Dir: Joseph Yee, MD
Class Cap: 40 *Begins:* Sep Feb
Length: 12 mos *Award:* Cert
Tuition per yr: $8,990 res, $8,990 non-res

Western Suffolk BOCES
Diagnostic Med Sonographer Prgm
Northport VA Med Ctr
Middleville Rd/Bldg 62
Northport, NY 11768
Prgm Dir: Claudia Freeman, BS RDMS RDCS
Tel: 516 261-4400
Med Dir: Paul Bonheim, MD
Class Cap: 24 *Begins:* Jul
Length: 24 mos *Award:* Cert
Tuition per yr: $2,800

Rochester Institute of Technology
Diagnostic Med Sonographer Prgm
85 Lomb Memorial Dr
Rochester, NY 14623-5603
Prgm Dir: Hamad Ghazle, BS MS RDMS
Tel: 716 475-2241 *Fax:* 716 475-5766
E-mail: hhgscl@rit.edu
Med Dir: Peter G Gleason, MD
Begins: Sep
Length: 12 mos, 48 mos *Award:* Cert, BS
Tuition per yr: $15,375

Hudson Valley Community College
Diagnostic Med Sonographer Prgm
80 Vandenburgh Ave
Troy, NY 12180
Prgm Dir: Sheila Hughes, BPS LRT RDMS
Tel: 518 270-7123 *Fax:* 518 270-7542
Med Dir: Ronald Karo, MD
Class Cap: 18 *Begins:* Aug
Length: 12 mos *Award:* Cert
Tuition per yr: $3,000 res, $6,000 non-res

North Carolina

Pitt Community College
Diagnostic Med Sonographer Prgm
PO Drawer 7007
Greenville, NC 27835-7007
Prgm Dir: Lyn M Jacobson, RDMS
Tel: 919 321-4254 *Fax:* 919 321-4451
Med Dir: William S Trought, MD
Class Cap: 12 *Begins:* Sep
Length: 12 mos, 24 mos *Award:* Dipl, AS
Tuition per yr: $758 res, $6,022 non-res
Evening or weekend classes available

Caldwell Comm College & Tech Institute
Diagnostic Med Sonographer Prgm
1000 Hickory Blvd
Hudson, NC 28638
Prgm Dir: Kimberlee B Watts, BS RDMS
Tel: 704 726-2322 *Fax:* 704 726-2216
Med Dir: Philip Howerton, MD
Class Cap: 8 *Begins:* Aug
Length: 12 mos, 24 mos *Award:* Dipl, AAS
Tuition per yr: $800 res, $6,500 non-res

Forsyth Technical Community College
Diagnostic Med Sonographer Prgm
2100 Silas Creek Pkwy
Winston-Salem, NC 27103
Prgm Dir: Anne Conner-Day, RDMS
Tel: 910 723-0371 *Fax:* 910 748-9395
Med Dir: Neal Wolfman, MD
Class Cap: 10 *Begins:* Sep
Length: 24 mos *Award:* AAS
Tuition per yr: $742 res, $6,020 non-res
Evening or weekend classes available

Ohio

Aultman Hospital
Diagnostic Med Sonographer Prgm
2600 Sixth St SW
Canton, OH 44710
Prgm Dir: Cynthia Peterson, RT RDMS
Tel: 330 438-6205 *Fax:* 330 438-9811
Med Dir: Samuel L Hissong, MD
Class Cap: 4 *Begins:* Jul
Length: 12 mos *Award:* Dipl,Cert
Tuition per yr: $2,500

Lorain County Community College
Diagnostic Med Sonographer Prgm
1005 N Abbe Rd
Elyria, OH 44035
Prgm Dir: Craig Peneff, AAS RDMS
Tel: 216 366-4015 *Fax:* 216 366-4116
E-mail: cpens@aol.com
Med Dir: Cathy Miller, MD
Class Cap: 16 *Begins:* Sep
Length: 21 mos *Award:* Dipl, AAS
Tuition per yr: $2,982 res, $3,542 non-res
Evening or weekend classes available

Programs

Kettering College of Medical Arts

Diagnostic Med Sonographer Prgm
3737 Southern Blvd
Kettering, OH 45429
Prgm Dir: Linda W Ontko, MS RDMS
Tel: 513 296-7201 *Fax:* 513 296-4238
Med Dir: Theodore R Miller, MD
Class Cap: 15 *Begins:* Aug
Length: 22 mos *Award:* Dipl, AS
Tuition per yr: $7,380

Central Ohio Technical College

Diagnostic Med Sonographer Prgm
1179 University Dr
Newark, OH 43055-1767
Prgm Dir: Joyce Grube, BS RDMS
Tel: 614 366-9274 *Fax:* 614 366-5047
Med Dir: Owen Lee, MD
Class Cap: 19 *Begins:* Sep
Length: 12 mos, 24 mos *Award:* Cert, AAS
Tuition per yr: $2,954 res, $6,134 non-res

Owens Community College

Diagnostic Med Sonographer Prgm
PO Box 10,000/Oregon Rd
Toledo, OH 43699-1947
Prgm Dir: Pamela Butler, RDMS RT(R)
Tel: 419 661-7261 *Fax:* 419 661-7665
E-mail: pbutler@owens.cc.oh.us
Med Dir: Parag Parikh, MD
Class Cap: 10 *Begins:* Jun Jan
Length: 16 mos, 24 mos *Award:* AAS
Tuition per yr: $2,060 res, $3,860 non-res
Evening or weekend classes available

Oklahoma

Univ of Oklahoma Health Sciences Center

Diagnostic Med Sonographer Prgm
PO Box 26901
Oklahoma City, OK 73190
Prgm Dir: Jean Lea Spitz, MPH RDMS
Tel: 405 271-6477 *Fax:* 405 271-1424
E-mail: jean-spitz@uokhsc.edu
Med Dir: Jay Harold, MD
Class Cap: 20 *Begins:* Aug
Length: 48 mos *Award:* BS
Tuition per yr: $2,777 res, $7,866 non-res
Evening or weekend classes available

Pennsylvania

Lancaster Institute for Health Education

Diagnostic Med Sonographer Prgm
143 Lemon St
Lancaster, PA 17602
Prgm Dir: Robert M Hess, BS RDMS
Tel: 717 290-4900 *Fax:* 717 290-5907
Med Dir: Rebecca G Pennell, MD
Class Cap: 5 *Begins:* Jul
Length: 12 mos *Award:* Cert, AST
Tuition per yr: $4,250 res, $4,250 non-res

Comm Coll of Allegheny Cnty-Boyce Campus

Diagnostic Med Sonographer Prgm
595 Beatty Rd
Community College of Allegheny County
Monroeville, PA 15146
Prgm Dir: Lynn Gigandet, MSEd RDMS
Tel: 412 325-6731 *Fax:* 412 325-6799
E-mail: lgigande@ccac.edu
Med Dir: Ave Bocher, MD
Class Cap: 30 *Begins:* Aug
Length: 20 mos *Award:* AS
Tuition per yr: $2,048 res, $4,080 non-res
Evening or weekend classes available

Thomas Jefferson University

Diagnostic Med Sonographer Prgm
130 S Ninth St/Rm 1004
Philadelphia, PA 19107
Prgm Dir: A D Herbert Jr, MS RT(R) LRT
Tel: 215 503-6678 *Fax:* 215 503-1031
E-mail: herber1@jeflin.tju.edu
Med Dir: Barry Goldberg, MD
Class Cap: 58 *Begins:* Sep
Length: 48 mos *Award:* BS
Tuition per yr: $13,800

Western Sch of Hlth & Business Careers

Diagnostic Med Sonographer Prgm
327 5th Ave
Pittsburgh, PA 15222
Prgm Dir: Lynda Miller, AS RDMS
Tel: 412 281-2600 *Fax:* 412 281-0319
Med Dir: Edward Urbanik, MD
Class Cap: 10 *Begins:* Sep
Length: 12 mos, 24 mos *Award:* Dipl, AST
Tuition per yr: $9,800

Rhode Island

Rhode Island Hospital

Diagnostic Med Sonographer Prgm
593 Eddy St
Providence, RI 02902
Prgm Dir: Jack Grusmark, RDMS
Tel: 401 444-5309
Med Dir: Francis Scola, MD
Begins: Sep
Length: 13 mos *Award:* Cert
Tuition per yr: $3,500

Tennessee

Chattanooga State Technical Comm College

Diagnostic Med Sonographer Prgm
407-B Chestnut St
Chattanooga, TN 37402
Prgm Dir: Jody Arnold, BS RDMS RT(R)
Tel: 423 634-7716 *Fax:* 423 634-7706
E-mail: arnold@cstcc.cc.tn.us
Med Dir: Kenneth Rule, MD
Class Cap: 25 *Begins:* Aug
Length: 12 mos *Award:* Cert
Tuition per yr: $1,449 res, $5,628 non-res

Baptist Memorial Health Care Systems

Diagnostic Med Sonographer Prgm
1003 Monroe/3rd Fl
Memphis, TN 38104
Prgm Dir: Sandra Hagen, BA RDMS RDCS
Tel: 901 227-5006 *Fax:* 901 227-4311
Med Dir: James E Machin
Class Cap: 10 *Begins:* Sep
Length: 12 mos *Award:* Cert
Tuition per yr: $5,000

Texas

Austin Community College

Diagnostic Med Sonographer Prgm
1020 Grove Blvd
Austin, TX 78741-3300
Prgm Dir: Regina Swearengin, AAS RDMS
Tel: 512 223-6286 *Fax:* 512 369-6700
Med Dir: Mark B Gray, MD
Begins: Aug
Length: 12 mos *Award:* Cert
Tuition per yr: $1,284 res, $4,722 non-res

Del Mar College

Diagnostic Med Sonographer Prgm
Corpus Christi, TX 78404
Prgm Dir: Robert J Cooper, MS RTR RDMS
Tel: 512 886-1101 *Fax:* 512 886-1598
Med Dir: Kenneth R Cook, MD
Class Cap: 7 *Begins:* Aug
Length: 12 mos, 24 mos *Award:* Cert, AAS
Tuition per yr: $1,000 res, $1,500 non-res
Evening or weekend classes available

El Centro College

Diagnostic Med Sonographer Prgm
Main and Lamar Sts
Dallas, TX 75202
Prgm Dir: Jan Bryant, MS RDMS
Tel: 214 746-2303 *Fax:* 214 860-2268
E-mail: jdb5529@dcccd.edu
Med Dir: Bill Waters, MD
Class Cap: 10 *Begins:* Aug
Length: 12 mos, 24 mos *Award:* Cert, AD
Tuition per yr: $849 res, $1,362 non-res
Evening or weekend classes available

El Paso Community College

Diagnostic Med Sonographer Prgm
PO Box 20500
El Paso, TX 79998
Prgm Dir: Nora M Balderas, BS RT(R) RDMS
Tel: 915 534-4108 *Fax:* 915 534-4114
Med Dir: William Sullivan, MD
Class Cap: 6 *Begins:* Jul
Length: 13 mos *Award:* Cert
Tuition per yr: $855 res, $3,940 non-res

Virginia

Tidewater Community College

Diagnostic Med Sonographer Prgm
1700 College Cresent
Virginia Beach, VA 23456
Prgm Dir: Felicia Jones, BS RDMS RVT
Tel: 804 427-7271 *Fax:* 804 427-1338
E-mail: felicia@exis.net
Med Dir: William Richie, MD
Class Cap: 14 *Begins:* Aug
Length: 12 mos *Award:* Cert
Tuition per yr: $2,184 res, $6,777 non-res

Washington

Bellevue Community College

Diagnostic Med Sonographer Prgm
3000 Landerholm Circle SE/Rm B243
Bellevue, WA 98009-2037
Prgm Dir: Joan P Baker, MSR RDMS
Tel: 206 641-2316 *Fax:* 206 603-4193
Med Dir: Diane Engelbrecht, MD
Class Cap: 25 *Begins:* Sep
Length: 24 mos *Award:* AA
Tuition per yr: $1,928 res, $7,408 non-res
Evening or weekend classes available

Seattle University

Diagnostic Med Sonographer Prgm
Broadway and Madison
Seattle, WA 98122-4460
Prgm Dir: Andrea C Skelly, BS RDMS
Tel: 206 296-5960 *Fax:* 206 296-6429
E-mail: askelly@seattleu.edu
Med Dir: Frank H Allen, MD
Class Cap: 25 *Begins:* Sep
Length: 48 mos *Award:* BS
Tuition per yr: $13,635

West Virginia

College of West Virginia

Diagnostic Med Sonographer Prgm
PO Box AG
Beckley, WV 25801
Prgm Dir: Mousa Hdeib, MD RDMS RVT
Tel: 304 253-7351 *Fax:* 304 253-0789
E-mail: mhdeib@cwy
Med Dir: Maurice Bassalli, MD
Class Cap: 22 *Begins:* May
Length: 12 mos, 24 mos *Award:* Cert, AAS , BS
Tuition per yr: $9,275 res, $9,275 non-res
Evening or weekend classes available

West Virginia University Hospitals, Inc

Diagnostic Med Sonographer Prgm
PO Box 6401
Morgantown, WV 26506
Prgm Dir: Debra L Williams, MS RDMS RT(R)
Tel: 304 598-4254 *Fax:* 304 598-4072
Med Dir: Charlotte Dillis
Begins: Jul
Length: 12 mos *Award:* Cert
Tuition per yr: $1,800

Wisconsin

Chippewa Valley Technical College

Diagnostic Med Sonographer Prgm
620 W Clairemont Ave
Eau Claire, WI 54701
Prgm Dir: Corey Weinfurtner, RDMS
Tel: 715 833-6420 *Fax:* 715 833-6470
E-mail: cweinfurtner@mail.chippewa.tec.wi.us
Med Dir: Thomas Edwards, MD
Class Cap: 16 *Begins:* Aug
Length: 12 mos, 24 mos *Award:* Cert, AD
Tuition per yr: $1,590 res, $12,224 non-res

University of Wisconsin Hosp & Clinics

Diagnostic Med Sonographer Prgm
Dept of Radiology
600 Highland Ave
Madison, WI 53792
Prgm Dir: John A Parks, BA RDMS
Tel: 608 263-9033 *Fax:* 608 262-0907
Med Dir: Myron A Pozniak, MD
Class Cap: 6 *Begins:* Apr Jan
Length: 15 mos, 24 mos *Award:* Dipl
Tuition per yr: $1,725 res, $2,100 non-res

St Francis Hospital

Diagnostic Med Sonographer Prgm
3237 S 16th St
Milwaukee, WI 53215
Prgm Dir: Stephanie Maass, RT RDMS RDCS
Tel: 414 647-5512
Med Dir: Clifford S Liddle, MD
Class Cap: 4 *Begins:* Sep
Length: 12 mos *Award:* Cert
Tuition per yr: $1,000

St Luke's Medical Center

Diagnostic Med Sonographer Prgm
2900 W Oklahoma Ave
Milwaukee, WI 53215
Prgm Dir: Jean M Schultz, BS RDMS
Tel: 414 649-6689 *Fax:* 414 649-7981
Med Dir: James Rankin, MD
Class Cap: 10 *Begins:* Jun
Length: 14 mos *Award:* Cert
Tuition per yr: $1,500 res, $1,500 non-res

St Mary's Hospital

Diagnostic Med Sonographer Prgm
2323 N Lake Dr
Milwaukee, WI 53201
Prgm Dir: Joseph B Morton, RDMS BS RT
Tel: 414 291-1156 *Fax:* 414 291-1720
Med Dir: Henry J Bradley, MD
Class Cap: 3 *Begins:* Oct
Length: 12 mos *Award:* Cert
Tuition per yr: $1,200

Dietetics

History

Founded in 1917, The American Dietetic Association (ADA) is the largest organization of food and nutrition professionals promoting optimal nutrition to improve public health and well-being. The early leaders laid a strong foundation for dietetics education. In 1923, the first plans for courses for student dietitians were discussed. By 1928, a list of hospitals with the approved course for student dietitians in hospitals was published. The approved course required that students have a baccalaureate degree with a major in foods and nutrition and receive at least 6 months' training in a hospital under the supervision of a dietitian.

As the number of programs increased, the need for evaluating the quality of the course became evident. In 1929, it was determined that a committee of three association members would conduct site visits every 2 years.

From 1932 until 1987, recommended academic requirements for entering dietetic internships were published and periodically revised to reflect practice needs. In 1987, the Knowledge Requirements for Dietitians were implemented under the Standards of Education, the minimum criteria to be met by all dietetics education programs.

In 1991 and 1994, the Standards of Education were updated to reflect role delineation studies and environmental changes affecting dietetics practice and to clarify and streamline the criteria and documentation required for accreditation and approval. Programs approved as meeting the Knowledge Requirements for Entry-Level Dietitians were designated Didactic Programs in Dietetics (DPD). Programs were encouraged to continually update their curricula based on current practice in dietetics.

As academic requirements changed, so did the types of programs offered. In 1962, the first Coordinated Undergraduate Program was developed. As an accredited program, it integrated experiential and academic components in an undergraduate curriculum. In 1987, the Standards of Education allowed for the approval of Preprofessional Practice Programs (AP4s) as an alternative to Dietetic Internships.

In the early 1970s, the ADA membership voiced a need for support personnel at the associate degree level. In 1974, Essentials were published for approving dietetic technician programs for food service management and nutrition care dietetic technicians.

In an effort to maintain appropriate standards for program review, the ADA became involved in program accreditation. In 1974, the ADA was first recognized by the US Department of Health, Education, and Welfare, now the US Department of Education (ED), as the accrediting agency for Dietetic Internships and Coordinated Undergraduate Programs. At the same time, COPA, now the Commission on Recognition of Postsecondary Accreditation (CORPA), also recognized the ADA as an accrediting agency for Coordinated Undergraduate Programs, and later Dietetic Internships. In 1988, postbaccalaureate Coordinated Programs were recognized as accredited by COPA.

In 1994, accreditation of Dietetic Technician and Preprofessional Practice Programs (AP4s), in addition to Coordinated Programs and Dietetic Internships, was implemented. As AP4s are phased into the accreditation process, they are designated Dietetic Internships.

In 1994, the ADA bylaws were amended to demonstrate the administrative autonomy of the body charged with accreditation. The ADA's accrediting body is now the Commission on Accreditation/Approval for Dietetics Education (CAADE).

Dietetic Technician

Occupational/Job Description

Dietetic technicians assist in shaping the public's food choices and provide nutrition assessment and counseling to persons with illnesses or injuries. Technicians often screen patients to identify nutrition problems, provide patient education and counseling to individuals and groups, develop menus and recipes, supervise food service personnel, purchase food, and monitor inventory and food quality. Dietetic technicians also use computer skills for tasks ranging from inputting inventory and payroll to charting patients' nutritional progress.

Employment Characteristics

As an integral part of the nutrition care team, dietetic technicians work with registered dietitians in a number of different settings, such as hospitals, public health nutrition programs, and long-term care facilities. Technicians also work in child nutrition and school lunch programs, community wellness centers, health clubs, nutrition programs for the elderly, food companies, restaurants, and food service management.

According to the ADA's 1995 membership database, of those registered dietetic technicians who have been employed full time in their current primary position for 1 to 5 years, 23% report annual gross incomes of less than $20,000, 62% report incomes between $20,000 and $30,000, and 12% report incomes between $30,000 and $40,000. Salary levels may vary based on location, scope of responsibility, and supply of job applicants.

Educational Programs

Length. Two years (associate degree), combining classroom and supervised practical experience, at a regionally accredited college or university. After completing this program, individuals are eligible to take the registration examination for dietetic technicians. Those who pass the exam become Dietetic Technicians, Registered, and can use the initials "DTR" after their names.
Prerequisites. Applicants must have a high school diploma or equivalency and must meet institutional entrance requirements.
Curriculum. Didactic instruction and a minimum of 450 hours of supervised practice experiences make up the curriculum. Food, nutrition, and management courses are emphasized, supported by the sciences, especially biology, anatomy, and chemistry. Math, English, sociology, psychology, communications, and business courses are also important.
Standards. The Standards of Education, revised in 1994, are minimum educational standards adopted by CAADE. Each new program is assessed in accordance with these Standards, and existing programs are periodically reviewed to determine whether they remain in compliance.

Dietitian/Nutritionist

Occupational/Job Description

Dietetics is the science of applying food and nutrition to health. Dietitians and nutritionists integrate and apply the principles derived from the sciences of food, nutrition, biochemistry, physiology, food management, and behavior to achieve and maintain the health status of the public they serve.

Employment Characteristics

Dietitians and nutritionists work in a variety of settings:

Clinical dietitians are a vital part of the medical team in hospitals, nursing homes, health maintenance organizations, and other health care facilities. As a key member of the health care team, the clinical dietitian provides medical nutrition therapy and the use of specific nutrition services to treat chronic conditions, illnesses, or injuries. Opportunities for advancement are available by choosing a particular area of nutrition practice, such as diabetes, heart disease, or pediatrics, or by expanding into hospital administration.

Community dietitians work in public and home health agencies, day care centers, health and recreation clubs, and in government-funded programs that feed and counsel families, the elderly, pregnant women, children, and individuals with special needs. Wherever proper nutrition can help improve quality of life, community dietitians reach out to the public to teach, monitor, and advise.

Educator dietitians work in colleges, universities, and community or technical schools, teaching future doctors, nurses, dietitians, and dietetic technicians the sophisticated science of foods and nutrition.

Research dietitians work in government agencies, food and pharmaceutical companies, and in major universities and medical centers. They conduct or direct experiments to answer critical nutrition questions, study alternative foods, and help modify dietary recommendations for the public.

Consultant dietitians work full- or part-time, usually under contract with a health care facility or in their own private practice. Consultant dietitians in private practice perform nutrition screening and assessment of their own clients and those referred to them by physicians. They offer advice on weight loss, cholesterol reduction, and a variety of other diet-related concerns. Those under contract with health care facilities often consult with food service managers, providing expertise on sanitation and safety procedures, budgeting, and portion control. Other clients include athletes and nursing home residents.

Management dietitians work in health care institutions, schools, cafeterias, and restaurants, playing a key role where food is served. They are responsible for personnel management, menu planning, budgeting, and purchasing.

Business dietitians work in food- and nutrition-related industries. They work in such areas as product development, sales, marketing, advertising, public relations, and purchasing.

According to the ADA's 1995 membership database, of those registered dietitians who have been employed full time in dietetics for 1 to 5 years after registration, 63% report annual gross incomes between $25,000 and $35,000, and 24% report incomes between $35,000 and $45,000. Salary levels may vary with location, scope of responsibility, and supply of job applicants.

Employment Outlook

According to the US Bureau of Labor Statistics, employment of dietitians is expected to grow faster than the average profession through the year 2000, especially in the community, consulting, and business areas.

Educational Programs

Length. The professional component is a minimum of 2 years at the baccalaureate or master's degree level. Postbaccalaureate supervised practice programs vary from 6 months to 2 years, depending on study design and integration in a graduate program. Following completion of academic and supervised practice requirements, individuals are eligible to take a national certification examination for registered dietitians. Many states also regulate dietitians and nutritionists.

Prerequisites. Variable for programs at the baccalaureate and master's levels, depending on the degree offered and institutional requirements. Applicants to postbaccalaureate supervised practice programs must have completed a baccalaureate degree and CAADE-approved didactic coursework.

Curriculum. The *Coordinated Program in Dietetics (CP)-Accredited*:

- an academic program in a regionally accredited college or university culminating in a minimum of a baccalaureate degree;
- provides didactic instruction and a minimum of 900 hours of supervised practice experiences, which may be planned concurrently with or following the didactic component;
- enables graduates to establish eligibility to write the registration examination for dietitians.

The *Didactic Program in Dietetics (DPD)-Approved*:

- an academic program in a regionally accredited college or university culminating in a minimum of a baccalaureate degree;
- enables graduates to apply for a supervised practice program leading to eligibility to write the registration examination for dietitians.

Dietetic Internship (DI)-Accredited/Preprofessional Practice Programs (AP4)-Approved:

- a supervised practice program sponsored by a health care facility, college or university, federal or state agency, business, or corporation;
- provides a minimum of 900 hours of supervised practice experiences;
- follows completion of CAADE-approved Didactic Program in Dietetics and a baccalaureate degree;
- may be full-time or part-time completed within a 2-year period;
- enables graduates to establish eligibility to write the registration examination for dietitians.

Didactic curriculum requirements focus on food, nutrition, and management, supported by the sciences—physical and biological, behavioral and social—as well as business and communication. The supervised practice curriculum provides experiences to develop the skills and competence to practice dietetics.

Standards. The Standards of Education, revised in 1994, are minimum educational standards adopted by the CAADE. Each new program is assessed in accordance with these Standards, and existing programs are periodically reviewed to determine whether they remain in compliance.

Inquiries

Accreditation

Requests for information on program accreditation or approval, including the Standards of Education, preparing the self-study application, and arranging a site visit, should be addressed to

Education and Accreditation Team
Commission on Accreditation/Approval for Dietetics Education
The American Dietetic Association
216 W Jackson Blvd
Chicago, Illinois 60606-6995
312 899-0040, ext 4876
E-mail: education@eatright.org

Careers

Inquiries regarding careers in dietetics and nutrition should be addressed to

Networks Team
The American Dietetic Association
216 W Jackson Blvd
Chicago, Illinois 60606-6995
312 899-0040, ext 4897

Certification/Registration

Inquiries regarding dietitian and dietetic technician registration should be addressed to

Commission on Dietetic Registration
216 W Jackson Blvd
Chicago, Illinois 60606-6995
312 899-0040, ext 4849

Accredited and Approved Programs

The Directory of Dietetics Programs includes complete listings of CAADE-accredited dietetic internships and coordinated programs, CAADE-approved preprofessional practice programs and didactic programs, and CAADE-accredited/approved dietetic technician programs. Also included are listings of advanced degree and specialty practice education programs. (Catalog number 0416; price $15 nonmember, $12.75 member, plus shipping and handling.) Orders should be addressed to

Customer Service Team
The American Dietetic Association
216 W Jackson Blvd
Chicago, Illinois 60606-6995
800 745-0775
312 899-4899 Fax

A list of accredited and approved programs is also available on the ADA Home Page on the World Wide Web. The URL is http://www.eatright.org/caade.html

Dietitian/Nutritionist

Alabama

Auburn University

Dietetics-Didactic Prgm
Nutrition and Food Science
328 Spidle Hall
Auburn, AL 36849-5605
Prgm Dir: Robin B Fellers, PhD RD LD
Tel: 334 844-4261

Samford University

Dietetics-Didactic Prgm
Family and Consumer Educ
800 Lakeshore Dr
Birmingham, AL 35229-2239
Prgm Dir: Patricia C Hart, PhD RD LD
Tel: 205 870-2930

University of Alabama at Birmingham

Dietetic Internship Prgm
Dept of Nutrition Sciences
Webb Bldg Rm 256
Birmingham, AL 35294
Prgm Dir: Rebecca L Bradley, MA RD
Tel: 205 934-3006

Oakwood College

Preprofessional Practice Prgm
Family and Consumer Science
Huntsville, AL 35896
Prgm Dir: Donna Smith, MPH RD
Tel: 205 726-7230

Oakwood College

Dietetics-Didactic Prgm
Family and Consumer Science
Huntsville, AL 35896
Prgm Dir: Donna Smith, MPH RD LD
Tel: 205 726-7230

Jacksonville State University

Dietetics-Didactic Prgm
Family and Consumer Sciences
Mason Hall
Jacksonville, AL 36265
Prgm Dir: Debra K Goodwin, MA RD
Tel: 205 782-5054

University of Montevallo

Dietetics-Didactic Prgm
Family and Consumer Sciences
Station 6385
Montevallo, AL 35115-6000
Prgm Dir: Gayl J Canfield, PhD RD LD
Tel: 205 665-6385

Alabama A & M University

Dietetics-Didactic Prgm
Nutrition & Hospitality Mgmt
Div of Home Econ/PO Box 639
Normal, AL 35762-0639
Prgm Dir: Ann P Warren, MS RD LD
Tel: 205 851-5440

University of Alabama

Dietetics-Coordinated Prgm
Human Nutrition & Hosp Mgmt
PO Box 870158
Tuscaloosa, AL 35487-0158
Prgm Dir: Patricia A M Hodges, EdD RD
Tel: 205 348-6157

University of Alabama

Dietetics-Didactic Prgm
Human Nutrition & Hosp Mgmt
Box 870158
Tuscaloosa, AL 35487-0158
Prgm Dir: Kathleen Stitt, PhD RD
Tel: 205 348-6157

Tuskegee University

Dietetics-Didactic Prgm
Dept of Home Economics
202 Washington Hall
Tuskegee, AL 36088
Prgm Dir: Beatrice W Phillips, EdD RD LD
Tel: 205 727-8331

Alaska

University of Alaska Anchorage

Preprofessional Practice Prgm
3211 Providence Dr
Anchorage, AK 99508
Prgm Dir: Nancy Overpeck, EdD RD
Tel: 907 786-6414

Arizona

Northern Arizona University

Dietetics-Didactic Prgm
Food and Nutrition Science
NAU Box 15095
Flagstaff, AZ 86011-5095
Prgm Dir: Leslie A Hildebrandt, PhD RD
Tel: 602 523-6164

Focus on Nutrition

Preprofessional Practice Prgm
Ste 26-113
3923 E Thunderbird Rd
Phoenix, AZ 85032
Prgm Dir: Susan Grogan, MA RD
Tel: 602 788-7096

Paradise Valley Unified School District

Preprofessional Practice Prgm
20621 N 32nd St
Phoenix, AZ 85024
Prgm Dir: Kathleen Glindmeier, MBA RD
Tel: 602 493-6330

Yavapai County Health Department

Dietetic Internship Prgm
930 Division St
Prescott, AZ 86301
Prgm Dir: Judy S Lee-Norris, MPH RD
Tel: 520 771-3138

Walter O Boswell Memorial Hospital

Preprofessional Practice Prgm
10401 W Thunderbird Blvd
Sun City, AZ 85372
Prgm Dir: Angelica Hathorn, MS RD
Tel: 602 977-7211

Arizona State University

Preprofessional Practice Prgm
Fam Resources & Human Devel
Tempe, AZ 85287-2502
Prgm Dir: Rose Martin, MS RD
Tel: 602 965-7034

Arizona State University

Dietetics-Didactic Prgm
Family Resources & Human Dev
Box 872502
Tempe, AZ 85287-2502
Prgm Dir: Linda A Vaughan, PhD RD
Tel: 602 965-7731

Maricopa County Dept of Public Health

Preprofessional Practice Prgm
Office of Nutrition Services
1414 W Broadway Ste 237
Tempe, AZ 85282
Prgm Dir: Shirley K Strembel, MS RD
Tel: 602 966-3090

Carondelet St Mary's Hospital

Preprofessional Practice Prgm
Morrisons Custom Mgmt Co
1601 W St Mary's Rd
Tucson, AZ 85745
Prgm Dir: Mary J Marian, MS RD CNSD
Tel: 520 622-5833

Univ Medical Center/Univ of Arizona

Dietetic Internship Prgm
Food Nutrition and Environmental Svcs
1501 N Campbell Ave
Tucson, AZ 85724-0001
Prgm Dir: Katherine K Duncan, MS RD
Tel: 520 694-4416

University of Arizona

Dietetics-Didactic Prgm
Nutrition and Food Science
Tucson, AZ 85721
Prgm Dir: Edward T Sheehan, PhD RD
Tel: 520 621-1449

Arkansas

Ouachita Baptist University

Dietetics-Didactic Prgm
Family and Consumer Sciences
PO Box 3713
Arkadelphia, AR 71998-0001
Prgm Dir: Stacy L Freeman, MS RD LD
Tel: 501 245-5542

University of Central Arkansas

Dietetics-Didactic Prgm
Family and Consumer Sciences
McAlister Hall 100
Conway, AR 72035
Prgm Dir: Mary Harlan, EdD RD LD
Tel: 501 450-5950

University of Central Arkansas

Dietetic Internship Prgm
Family Consumer Sciences
McAlister Hall
Conway, AR 72035
Prgm Dir: Melissa Shock, PhD RD
Tel: 501 450-5950

University of Arkansas Main Campus

Dietetics-Didactic Prgm
Human Environmental Sciences
118 Home Economics Bldg
Fayetteville, AR 72701
Prgm Dir: Jamie Dollahite, PhD RD
Tel: 501 575-4305

Univ of Arkansas for Medical Sciences

Dietetic Internship Prgm
Veterans Affairs Med Ctr
4301 W Markham St
LIttle Rock, AR 72205-7199
Prgm Dir: Christine R Anderson, PhD RD
Tel: 501 686-6166

University of Arkansas at Pine Bluff

Dietetics-Didactic Prgm
Dept of Home Economics
PO Box 4971
Pine Bluff, AR 71611
Prgm Dir: Lucille Meadows, MS RD
Tel: 501 543-8817

Harding University Main Campus

Dietetics-Didactic Prgm
Family and Consumer Sciences
900 E Ctr Ave Box 2233
Searcy, AR 72149-0001
Prgm Dir: Lisa Ritchie, MSE RD LD
Tel: 501 279-4472

California

Pacific Union College

Dietetics-Didactic Prgm
Family and Consumer Sciences
Angwin, CA 94508-6694
Prgm Dir: Diane L Fletcher, EdD RD CFCS
Tel: 707 965-6694

University of California Berkeley

Preprofessional Practice Prgm
Dept of Nutritional Sciences
119 Morgan Hall
Berkeley, CA 94720
Prgm Dir: Nancy R Hudson, MS RD
Tel: 510 642-4090

University of California Berkeley

Dietetic Internship Prgm
School of Public Health
129 Morgan Hall-3104
Berkeley, CA 94720-3104
Prgm Dir: Mary Mead, MEd RD
Tel: 510 642-0980

University of California Berkeley

Dietetics-Didactic Prgm
Dept of Nutritional Sciences
119 Morgan Hall
Berkeley, CA 94720
Prgm Dir: Nancy R Hudson, MS RD
Tel: 510 642-4090

California State University - Chico

Dietetic Internship Prgm
Nutrition & Food Sciences
Dept of Biological Sciences
Chico, CA 95929-0515
Prgm Dir: Barbara A Kirks, MPH EdD RD
Tel: 916 898-6805

Programs

California State University - Chico
Dietetics-Didactic Prgm
Dept of Biological Sciences
Tehama Hall 124
Chico, CA 95929-0515
Prgm Dir: Faye C Johnson, EdD RD
Tel: 916 898-6805

University of California - Davis
Dietetics-Didactic Prgm
Dept of Nutrition
Davis, CA 95616-8669
Prgm Dir: Francene Steinberg, PhD
Tel: 916 752-2666

California State University - Fresno
Dietetics-Didactic Prgm
Ecology Food Sci & Nutrition
5300 N Campus Dr
Fresno, CA 93740-0017
Prgm Dir: Sandra S Witte, PhD RD
Tel: 209 278-2043

Comm Hospital of Central California
Dietetic Internship Prgm
Fresno VA
Nutrition & Food Services
Fresno & R Sts/PO Box 1232
Fresno, CA 93715-1232
Prgm Dir: Christine A Pickett, MS RD
Tel: 209 442-3946

Uni Health America/Glendale Mem Hosp
Dietetic Internship Prgm
1420 S Central Ave
Glendale, CA 91204-2594
Prgm Dir: Teresa Bush-Zurn, MA RD
Tel: 818 502-2334

Public Health Foundation
Dietetic Internship Prgm
WIC Program
12781 Schabarum Ave
Irwindale, CA 91706-6802
Prgm Dir: Robin Evans, MPH RD
Tel: 818 856-6376

Loma Linda University
Preprofessional Practice Prgm
Schl of Pub Hlth Nutri Dept
Nichol Hall-Rm 1102
Loma Linda, CA 92350
Prgm Dir: Elaine Fleming, MPH RD LD
Tel: 909 824-4598

Loma Linda University
Dietetics-Coordinated Prgm
School of Allied Health Profs
Dept of Nutrition & Dietetics
Loma Linda, CA 92350
Prgm Dir: Bert Connell, PhD RD
Tel: 909 824-4593

California State University - Long Beach
Dietetic Internship Prgm
Family and Consumer Sciences
1250 N Bellflower Blvd
Long Beach, CA 90840-0501
Prgm Dir: Jacqueline D Lee, PhD RD
Tel: 310 985-4494

California State University - Long Beach
Dietetics-Didactic Prgm
Family and Consumer Sciences
1250 Bellflower Blvd
Long Beach, CA 90840-0501
Prgm Dir: Jacqueline Lee, PhD RD
Tel: 310 985-4545

California State University - Los Angeles
Dietetics-Coordinated Prgm
Health & Nutritional Sciences
5151 State University Dr
Los Angeles, CA 90032-8172
Prgm Dir: Laura L Calderon, DrPH RD
Tel: 213 343-5439

California State University - Los Angeles
Dietetics-Didactic Prgm
Health & Nutritional Sciences
5151 State University Dr
Los Angeles, CA 90032-8172
Prgm Dir: Joyce Gota, MA RD
Tel: 213 343-5439

Charles R Drew Univ of Med & Science
Dietetics-Coordinated Prgm
College of Allied Health
1621 E 120th St
Los Angeles, CA 90059-3025
Prgm Dir: Mable Everette, MPH RD FADA
Tel: 213 563-4811

Children's Hospital of Los Angeles
Preprofessional Practice Prgm
Child Devel & Devel Disorders
Mailstop 53/PO Box 54700
Los Angeles, CA 90054-0700
Prgm Dir: Anne Bradford Harris, MS RD
Tel: 213 669-2300

Los Angeles County - USC Medical Center
Dietetic Internship Prgm
1200 N State St Rm 1833
Los Angeles, CA 90033-4525
Prgm Dir: Elizabeth H Ma, MS RD
Tel: 213 226-6901

Veterans Affairs Med Ctr W Los Angeles
Dietetic Internship Prgm
Nutrition & Food (120G)
1301 Wilshire Blvd
Los Angeles, CA 90073
Prgm Dir: Jenna Mason, MPH RD
Tel: 310 268-3120

Pepperdine University
Dietetics-Didactic Prgm
Natural Science Div
Malibu, CA 90263
Prgm Dir: June R Palacio, PhD RD
Tel: 310 456-4339

ARAMARK Healthcare Support Services
Preprofessional Practice Prgm
477 Devlin Rd Ste 108
Napa, CA 94558
Prgm Dir: Aladina B Capacioli, MS RD
Tel: 707 254-1130

Napa State Hospital
Dietetic Internship Prgm
2100 Napa Vallejo Hwy
Napa, CA 94558-6293
Prgm Dir: Debbie Chinn Davis, MS RD
Tel: 707 253-5428

California State University - Northridge
Dietetic Internship Prgm
Family Environmental Sciences
18111 Nordhoff St
Northridge, CA 91330-8308
Prgm Dir: Elaine M Blyler, MS RD FAAD
Tel: 818 885-3907

California State University - Northridge
Dietetics-Didactic Prgm
Family Environmental Sciences
18111 Nordhoff St
Northridge, CA 91330-8308
Prgm Dir: Christine H Smith, PhD RD
Tel: 818 667-3051

Patton State Hospital
Dietetic Internship Prgm
3102 E Highland Ave
Patton, CA 92369
Prgm Dir: Dolores Otto-Moreno, MPH RD
Tel: 909 425-7297

California State Polytechnic University
Dietetics-Didactic Prgm
Foods and Nutrition Dept
3801 W Temple Ave
Pomona, CA 91768-2557
Prgm Dir: Cheryl L Loggins, MS RD
Tel: 909 869-2168

California State Polytechnic University
Dietetic Internship Prgm
Foods & Nutri/Home Economics
3801 W Temple Ave
Pomona, CA 91768-2557
Prgm Dir: Kara Caldwell-Freeman, DrHSc RD
Tel: 909 869-2163

Porterville Development Center
Dietetic Internship Prgm
PO Box 2000
Porterville, CA 93258-2000
Prgm Dir: Michelle Smither, MS RD
Tel: 209 782-2753

California State University - Sacramento
Dietetics-Didactic Prgm
Human Environmental Sciences
6000 J St
Sacramento, CA 95819-6053
Prgm Dir: Carol Redard, PhD RD
Tel: 916 278-5339

California State Univ - San Bernardino
Dietetics-Didactic Prgm
Hlth Science & Human Ecology
5500 University Pkwy
San Bernardino, CA 92407-2318
Prgm Dir: Dorothy C Chen, PhD RD
Tel: 909 880-5340

San Diego State University
Dietetic Internship Prgm
Exercise and Nutrition Sciences
5300 Campanile Dr
San Diego, CA 92182-7251
Prgm Dir: Cindy L Swann, MS RD
Tel: 619 594-1341

San Diego State University

Dietetics-Didactic Prgm
Exercise and Nutrition Sciences
San Diego, CA 92182-7251
Prgm Dir: Audrey Spindler, PhD RD CNS
Tel: 619 594-3045

Veterans Affairs San Diego Healthcare System

Dietetic Internship Prgm
Dietetic Service (120)
3350 La Jolla Village Dr
San Diego, CA 92161-0002
Prgm Dir: Jana D Kelley, MS RD
Tel: 619 552-8585

San Francisco State University

Dietetics-Didactic Prgm
Cons & Fam Studies/Dietetics
1600 Holloway Ave
San Francisco, CA 94132-1722
Prgm Dir: Janet Sim, EdD RD
Tel: 415 338-1750

San Francisco State University

Dietetic Internship Prgm
Cons & Fam Studies/Dietetics
Burk Hall 1600 Holloway Ave
San Francisco, CA 94132-1722
Prgm Dir: Randee L Reidy, MS RD
Tel: 415 338-1219

University of California - San Francisco

Dietetic Internship Prgm
Medical Center
Box 0212 Rm M-294
San Francisco, CA 94143
Prgm Dir: Carol Porter, PhD RD
Tel: 415 476-1461

San Jose State University

Dietetics-Didactic Prgm
Nutrition & Food Science
San Jose, CA 95192-0058
Prgm Dir: Nancy C Lu, PhD RD
Tel: 408 924-3109

San Jose State University

Preprofessional Practice Prgm
Nutrition Food & Science
One Washington Square
San Jose, CA 95192-0058
Prgm Dir: Kathryn P Sucher, ScD RD
Tel: 408 924-3104

California Polytechnic State University

Dietetics-Didactic Prgm
Food Science & Nutrition
San Luis Obispo, CA 93407
Prgm Dir: Kathleen A McBurney, RD DrPH
Tel: 805 756-6126

Olive View/UCLA Medical Center

Dietetic Internship Prgm
Dept of Food and Nutrition
14445 Olive View Dr Rm 1C112
Sylmar, CA 91342-1438
Prgm Dir: Sohair Saad, MS RD CNSD
Tel: 818 364-4224

Colorado

Penrose-St Francis Health System

Dietetic Internship Prgm
Nutrition Services
PO Box 7021
Colorado Springs, CO 80933-7021
Prgm Dir: Yvonne Steinhour, MPH RD
Tel: 719 776-5863

Tri-County Health Nutrition Services

Dietetic Internship Prgm
4857 S Broadway
Englewood, CO 80110-6894
Prgm Dir: Anne E Bennett, MPH RD
Tel: 303 761-1340

Colorado State University

Dietetic Internship Prgm
Food Sci & Human Nutrition
Ft Collins, CO 80523
Prgm Dir: Mary A Harris, PhD RD
Tel: 970 491-5093

Colorado State University

Dietetics-Didactic Prgm
Food Sci & Human Nutrition
Gifford Bldg 205
Ft Collins, CO 80523
Prgm Dir: Mary A Harris, PhD RD
Tel: 970 491-7462

University of Northern Colorado

Dietetic Internship Prgm
Community Health & Nutrition
Gunter 2400
Greeley, CO 80639
Prgm Dir: Naomi Benell, MS RD
Tel: 970 351-1769

University of Northern Colorado

Dietetics-Didactic Prgm
Community Health & Nutrition
Gunter 232
Greeley, CO 80639
Prgm Dir: Sherrie B Frye, PhD RD
Tel: 970 351-1705

Connecticut

Danbury Hospital

Preprofessional Practice Prgm
24 Hospital Ave
Danbury, CT 06810-6099
Prgm Dir: Linda Sue Taub, MS RD
Tel: 203 797-7394

Yale-New Haven Hospital

Dietetic Internship Prgm
Nutritional Services
20 York St GBB
New Haven, CT 06504
Prgm Dir: Deborah F Flanel, MS RD FADA CD-N
Tel: 203 785-5074

University of Connecticut

Dietetics-Coordinated Prgm
School of Allied Health Profs
358 Mansfield Rd U-101
Storrs, CT 06269-2101
Prgm Dir: Sandra M Affenito, PhD RD
Tel: 860 486-1588

University of Connecticut

Dietetics-Didactic Prgm
Nutritional Sciences U-17
3624 Horsebarn Rd Extension
Storrs, CT 06269
Prgm Dir: Ellen L Shanley, MBA RD
Tel: 860 486-0119

University of Connecticut

Dietetic Internship Prgm
Allied Health Professions
358 Mansfield Rd U-101
Storrs, CT 06269-2101
Prgm Dir: Sandra Affenito, PhD RD
Tel: 860 486-0016

Saint Joseph College

Dietetic Internship Prgm
Nutrition and Family Studies
1678 Asylum Ave
West Hartford, CT 06117-2700
Prgm Dir: Donna W Corcoran, MS RD
Tel: 860 232-4571

Saint Joseph College

Dietetics-Didactic Prgm
Nutrition and Family Studies
1678 Asylum Ave
West Hartford, CT 06117-2700
Prgm Dir: Margery Lawrence, PhD RD
Tel: 203 232-4571

Saint Joseph College

Dietetics-Coordinated Prgm
Nutrition and Family Studies
1678 Asylum Ave
West Hartford, CT 06117-2700
Prgm Dir: Margaret E Gaughan, PhD RD
Tel: 203 232-4571

University of New Haven

Dietetics-Didactic Prgm
Hotel Rest & Tourism Admin
300 Orange Ave
West Haven, CT 06516-1916
Prgm Dir: Beverly Bentivegna, MEd RD
Tel: 203 932-7413

Delaware

Delaware State University

Dietetics-Didactic Prgm
Dept of Home Economics
1200 N Dupont Hwy
Dover, DE 19901-2277
Prgm Dir: Maggie Clausell, PhD RD
Tel: 302 739-4964

University of Delaware

Dietetics-Didactic Prgm
Dept of Nutrition & Dietetics
331 Alison Hall
Newark, DE 19716-3301
Prgm Dir: Connie E Vickery, PhD RD
Tel: 302 831-2798

University of Delaware

Dietetic Internship Prgm
Nutrition & Dietetics
315 Alison Hall
Newark, DE 19716
Prgm Dir: Charlene Hamilton, PhD RD
Tel: 302 831-1677

District of Columbia

Howard University
Dietetics-Coordinated Prgm
6th and Bryant Sts NW
Annex I Rm 343
Washington, DC 20059
Prgm Dir: Thelma B Baker, PhD RD LD
Tel: 202 806-6238

Marriott Corp/Marriott Hlthcare Mid-Atlantic
Dietetic Internship Prgm
Dept 877.11
One Marriott Dr
Washington, DC 20058
Prgm Dir: Linda Marmer, MS MBA RD LD
Tel: 301 380-3936

University of the District of Columbia
Dietetics-Didactic Prgm
Bldg 44 Rm 203E
4200 Connecticut Ave NW
Washington, DC 20008-1173
Prgm Dir: Prema Ganganna, PhD RD LD
Tel: 202 274-5516

Walter Reed Army Medical Center
Dietetic Internship Prgm
Education & Research Div
Nutrition Care Directorate
Washington, DC 20307-5001
Prgm Dir: Cheryl A Hostetler, MS RD LD
Tel: 202 782-0387

Florida

University of Florida
Dietetics-Didactic Prgm
Food Sci & Human Nutrition
359 FSB
Gainesville, FL 32611
Prgm Dir: Laura K Guyer, PhD RD
Tel: 352 392-1991

University of Florida
Dietetic Internship Prgm
Food Sci & Human Nutrition
359 FSB
Gainesville, FL 32611
Prgm Dir: Laura K Guyer, PhD RD LD
Tel: 352 392-1991

St Luke's Hosp/Mayo Clinic Jacksonville
Dietetic Internship Prgm
4201 Belfort Rd
Jacksonville, FL 32216-1431
Prgm Dir: Nell E Robinson, MS RD LD
Tel: 904 296-3733

University of North Florida
Dietetics-Didactic Prgm
College of Health
4567 St Johns Bluff Rd S
Jacksonville, FL 32224-2645
Prgm Dir: Judith C Rodriguez, PhD RD LD
Tel: 904 646-2840

University of North Florida
Preprofessional Practice Prgm
College of Health
4567 St Johns Bluff Rd S
Jacksonville, FL 32224-2646
Prgm Dir: Judith C Rodriguez, PhD RD
Tel: 904 646-2840

Florida International University
Dietetics-Coordinated Prgm
Dept of Dietetics & Nutrition
Health Bldg Rm 201/Univ Park
Miami, FL 33199
Prgm Dir: Susan P Himburg, PhD RD LD
Tel: 305 348-2878

Florida International University
Dietetic Internship Prgm
Dietetics & Nutrition
University Park HB 206
Miami, FL 33199
Prgm Dir: Amy Jaffe, MS RD LD
Tel: 305 348-2878

Florida International University
Dietetics-Didactic Prgm
Dietetics & Nutrition
University Park HB 208
Miami, FL 33199
Prgm Dir: Michele W Keane, PhD RD
Tel: 305 348-2878

HRS Pasco County Public Health Unit
Dietetic Internship Prgm
Nutrition Div
10841 Little Rd
New Port Richey, FL 34654-2533
Prgm Dir: Clara H Lawhead, MS RD LD
Tel: 813 869-3900

Sarasota Memorial Hospital
Dietetic Internship Prgm
Food & Nutrition Services
1700 S Tamiami Trail
Sarasota, FL 34239-3555
Prgm Dir: Sharon J Peachey, MS RD LD
Tel: 813 917-1080

Florida State University
Dietetics-Didactic Prgm
Nutri Food & Movement Sciences
College of Human Sciences
Tallahassee, FL 32306-2033
Prgm Dir: Jodee Dorsey, PhD RD LDN
Tel: 904 644-4794

Florida State University
Preprofessional Practice Prgm
Nutri Food & Movement Sciences
215 Johnston Bldg
Tallahassee, FL 32306-2033
Prgm Dir: Laura R Cook, PhD RD LD
Tel: 904 644-1828

James A Haley Veteran's Hospital
Dietetic Internship Prgm
13000 N Bruce B Downs Blvd
Tampa, FL 33612-4745
Prgm Dir: Anne E Brezina, MEd RD
Tel: 813 972-2000

Georgia

University of Georgia
Dietetics-Didactic Prgm
Dept of Foods & Nutrition
Dawson Hall
Athens, GA 30602
Prgm Dir: Joan Fischer, PhD RD LD
Tel: 706 542-7983

University of Georgia
Preprofessional Practice Prgm
Dept of Foods & Nutrition
Dawson Hall
Athens, GA 30602
Prgm Dir: Marian Wang, PhD RD
Tel: 706 542-4908

Div of Pub Hlth/Georgia Dept of Hum
Dietetic Internship Prgm
Office of Nutrition Ste 8-413
2 Peachtree St NW
Atlanta, GA 30303-3186
Prgm Dir: Frances Hanks Cook, MA RD LD
Tel: 404 657-6012

Georgia State University
Dietetics-Didactic Prgm
Dept of Nutrition & Dietetics
University Plaza PO Box 873
Atlanta, GA 30303-3083
Prgm Dir: Christine Rosenbloom, PhD RD
Tel: 404 651-1102

Georgia State University
Dietetic Internship Prgm
Dept of Nutrition & Dietetics
University Plaza
Atlanta, GA 30303-3083
Prgm Dir: Delia H Baxter, PhD RD LD
Tel: 404 651-1108

Emory University Hospital
Dietetic Internship Prgm
Food & Nutrition Services
1364 Clifton Rd NE
Atlanta, GA 30322-1104
Prgm Dir: Deborah J Clegg, MS RD LD
Tel: 404 657-6012

Augusta Area Dietetic Internship
Dietetic Internship Prgm
University Hospital
1350 Walton Way (10)
Augusta, GA 30901-2629
Prgm Dir: Jeanne H Bingham, MS RD LD
Tel: 706 774-8897

Fort Valley State College
Dietetics-Didactic Prgm
Family & Consumer Sciences
805 State College Dr
Fort Valley, GA 31030-3242
Prgm Dir: Sharon K Hunt, MS RD
Tel: 912 825-6234

Life College
Dietetics-Didactic Prgm
Dept of Nutrition
1269 Barclay Circle
Marietta, GA 30060-2903
Prgm Dir: Maria Boyle, PhD RD
Tel: 404 424-0554

Southern Regional Medical Center
Dietetic Internship Prgm
11 Upper Riverdale Rd SW
Riverdale, GA 30274-2600
Prgm Dir: Jaleh Dehpahlavan, MMSc RD LD
CNSD
Tel: 770 991-8053

Georgia Southern University
Dietetics-Didactic Prgm
Family & Consumer Sciences
Box 8034
Statesboro, GA 30460
Prgm Dir: Elfrieda F Brown, MS RD
Tel: 912 681-5345

Hawaii

University of Hawaii at Manoa
Dietetic Internship Prgm
School of Public Health
1960 EW Rd D-104J
Honolulu, HI 96822-2319
Prgm Dir: Carol I Waslien, PhD RD
Tel: 808 956-5745

University of Hawaii at Manoa
Dietetics-Didactic Prgm
Food Sci & Human Nutrition
Miller Hall 12/2515 Campus Rd
Honolulu, HI 96822-2218
Prgm Dir: Anne Caprio Shovic, PhD RD
Tel: 808 956-3847

Idaho

University of Idaho
Dietetics-Coordinated Prgm
Family and Consumer Science
College of Agriculture
Moscow, ID 83844-3183
Prgm Dir: Kathe A Gabel, PhD RD
Tel: 208 885-6026

Idaho State University
Dietetic Internship Prgm
Health & Nutrition Sciences
Campus Box 8109
Pocatello, ID 83209-8109
Prgm Dir: Patricia Z Marinicic, MS RD
Tel: 208 236-2729

Idaho State University
Dietetics-Didactic Prgm
Health & Nutrition Science
Campus Box 8109
Pocatello, ID 83209-8109
Prgm Dir: Mary Dundas, PhD RD LDN
Tel: 208 236-2729

Illinois

Southern Illinois Univ at Carbondale
Dietetic Internship Prgm
Food & Nutrition
Mailcode 4317
Carbondale, IL 62901-4317
Prgm Dir: Carol J Boushey, PhD MPH RD
Tel: 618 453-5193

Southern Illinois Univ at Carbondale
Dietetics-Didactic Prgm
Animal Sci Food & Nutrition
Mailcode 4317
Carbondale, IL 62901-4317
Prgm Dir: Sara Long Anderson, PhD RD
Tel: 618 453-7512

Eastern Illinois University
Dietetic Internship Prgm
Family & Consumer Sciences
Charleston, IL 61920
Prgm Dir: Ruth M Dow, PhD RD LD FADA
Tel: 217 581-3223

Eastern Illinois University
Dietetics-Didactic Prgm
Family & Consumer Sciences
Charleston, IL 61920-3099
Prgm Dir: Ruth M Dow, PhD RD LD FADA
Tel: 217 581-3223

Loyola University of Chicago
Dietetics-Didactic Prgm
Dept of Food & Nutrition
6525 N Sheridan Rd
Chicago, IL 60626-5311
Prgm Dir: Tracey L Carlyle, MS RD
Tel: 773 508-8299

Loyola University of Chicago
Dietetic Internship Prgm
Dept of Food and Nutrition
6525 N Sheridan Rd
Chicago, IL 60626-5311
Prgm Dir: Joanna Kouba, MS RD
Tel: 773 508-8298

Rush University
Dietetic Internship Prgm
Rush-Presbyterian St Lukes Med Ctr
1653 W Congress Pkwy
Chicago, IL 60612-3864
Prgm Dir: Mary B Gregoire, PhD RD LD
Tel: 312 942-5929

Univ of Illinois at Chicago
Dietetics-Coordinated Prgm
Human Nutrition and Dietetics
1919 W Taylor St (M/C 517)
Chicago, IL 60612-7256
Prgm Dir: Carol L Braunschweig, PhD RD
Tel: 312 996-1209

Northern Illinois University
Dietetic Internship Prgm
Family Consumer and Nutri Sciences
DeKalb, IL 60115-2854
Prgm Dir: Lucy Robinson, MS RD
Tel: 815 753-6386

Northern Illinois University
Dietetics-Didactic Prgm
Family Consumer and Nutri Sciences
Wirtz 209
DeKalb, IL 60115-2854
Prgm Dir: Joan E Quinn, MEd RD
Tel: 815 753-6384

Ingalls Memorial Hospital
Dietetic Internship Prgm
One Ingalls Dr
Harvey, IL 60426
Prgm Dir: Mary Keith Vaughn, MA RD
Tel: 708 333-2300

Edward Hines Jr VA Hospital
Dietetic Internship Prgm
Nutrition and Food Service (120D)
Hines, IL 60141
Prgm Dir: Sharon Foley, MS RD
Tel: 708 216-2343

Olivet Nazarene University
Dietetics-Didactic Prgm
Family & Consumer Sciences
PO Box 592
Kankakee, IL 60901-0592
Prgm Dir: Janice Dowell, MHS RD
Tel: 815 939-5398

Illinois Benedictine College
Dietetics-Didactic Prgm
Dept of Biological Sciences
5700 College Rd
Lisle, IL 60532-2851
Prgm Dir: Catherine Stein, MS RD LD
Tel: 630 829-6534

Western Illinois University
Dietetics-Didactic Prgm
Family & Consumer Sciences
Macomb, IL 61455
Prgm Dir: Karen R Greathouse, PhD RD
Tel: 309 298-1581

Illinois State University
Dietetics-Didactic Prgm
Family and Consumer Sciences
Campus Box 5060
Normal, IL 61790-5060
Prgm Dir: Robert W Cullen, PhD RD
Tel: 309 438-8850

Illinois State University
Dietetic Internship Prgm
Family and Consumer Sciences
Room 144, Turner Hall
Normal, IL 61790-5060
Prgm Dir: Nweze Nnakwe, PhD RD
Tel: 309 438-5037

Bradley University
Dietetics-Didactic Prgm
Family and Consumer Science
Bradley Hall 221
Peoria, IL 61625
Prgm Dir: Jeannette Davidson, PhD RD
Tel: 309 677-2436

St Francis Medical Center
Dietetic Internship Prgm
530 NE Glen Oak Ave
Peoria, IL 61637-0001
Prgm Dir: Mei-Ling Lin, MS RD
Tel: 309 655-3707

Rosary College
Dietetics-Didactic Prgm
Dept of Nutrition Sciences
7900 W Division St
River Forest, IL 60305-1066
Prgm Dir: Judith Beto, PhD RD
Tel: 708 524-6906

St John's Hospital
Dietetic Internship Prgm
800 E Carpenter St
Springfield, IL 62769
Prgm Dir: Sara A Lopinski, MS RD
Tel: 217 544-6464

Programs

Univ of Illinois at Urbana - Champaign
Dietetics-Didactic Prgm
Foods & Nutri Bevier Hall-345
905 S Goodwin Ave
Urbana, IL 61801-3852
Prgm Dir: Karen L Plawecki, MS RD
Tel: 217 244-2884

Indiana

Indiana University - Bloomington
Dietetics-Didactic Prgm
Applied Health Science
HPER 116
Bloomington, IN 47405-4801
Prgm Dir: Alice K Lindeman, PhD RD
Tel: 812 855-6437

Purdue University-Calumet
Preprofessional Practice Prgm
Dept of Behavioral Sciences
Hammond, IN 46323-2094
Prgm Dir: Rita A Fields, MS RD
Tel: 219 989-2716

Indiana University School of Medicine
Dietetic Internship Prgm
Clinical Bldg 555A
541 N Clinical Dr
Indianapolis, IN 46202-5111
Prgm Dir: Jacquelynn O'Palka, PhD RD
Tel: 317 278-0934

Marian College
Dietetics-Didactic Prgm
Nursing & Nutrition Sciences
3200 Cold Springs Rd
Indianapolis, IN 46222-1997
Prgm Dir: Catherine Strain, MS RD
Tel: 317 929-0346

Ball Memorial Hospital
Dietetic Internship Prgm
Dept of Dietetics
2401 University Ave
Muncie, IN 47303-3499
Prgm Dir: Mary D Snell, MS RD
Tel: 317 747-3273

Ball State University
Preprofessional Practice Prgm
Family & Consumer Sciences
150 Practical Arts Complex
Muncie, IN 47306
Prgm Dir: Carmen Margenau, MS RD
Tel: 317 285-5931

Ball State University
Dietetics-Didactic Prgm
Family and Consumer Sciences
Muncie, IN 47306-0250
Prgm Dir: Judith Burns Lowe, MA RD
Tel: 317 285-5931

Indiana State University
Dietetics-Coordinated Prgm
Family and Consumer Sciences
Terre Haute, IN 47809
Prgm Dir: Judith C Byrne, EdD RD
Tel: 812 237-3309

Purdue University
Dietetics-Didactic Prgm
Dept of Foods and Nutrition
1264 Stone Hall
West Lafayette, IN 47907-1264
Prgm Dir: Olivia Bennett Wood, MPH RD
Tel: 317 494-8238

Purdue University
Dietetics-Coordinated Prgm
Dept of Foods and Nutrition
1264 Stone Hall
West Lafayette, IN 47907-1264
Prgm Dir: Louise W Peck, PhD RD
Tel: 317 494-8236

Iowa

Iowa State University
Dietetic Internship Prgm
Food Sci & Human Nutrition
1127 HNS Bldg
Ames, IA 50011-4436
Prgm Dir: Mary Jane Oakland, PhD RD LD
Tel: 515 294-2536

Iowa State University
Dietetics-Didactic Prgm
Food Sci & Human Nutrition
1104 Human Nutrition Ctr
Ames, IA 50011
Prgm Dir: Jean A Anderson, MS RD LD
Tel: 515 294-7316

University of Northern Iowa
Dietetics-Didactic Prgm
Design Fam & Cons Sciences
235 Latham Hall
Cedar Falls, IA 50614-0332
Prgm Dir: Joanne Spaide, PhD RD LD
Tel: 319 273-2814

University of Iowa Hospitals and Clinics
Dietetic Internship Prgm
200 Hawkins Dr
W146GH
Iowa City, IA 52242-1051
Prgm Dir: Joetta M Redlin, MS RD LD
Tel: 319 356-7272

Kansas

University of Kansas Medical Center
Dietetic Internship Prgm
Dept of Dietetics & Nutrition
3901 Rainbow Blvd
Kansas City, KS 66160-7250
Prgm Dir: Norma Winn, MS RD LD
Tel: 913 588-5355

Kansas State University
Dietetics-Coordinated Prgm
Hotel Rest Inst Mgmt & Diet
Justin Hall 103
Manhattan, KS 66506-1404
Prgm Dir: Deborah Canter, PhD RD
Tel: 913 532-5521

Kansas State University
Dietetics-Didactic Prgm
Food & Nutrition/HRIMD
Justin Hall 103
Manhattan, KS 66506-1404
Prgm Dir: Rebecca Gould, PhD RD
Tel: 913 532-2207

Kentucky

Berea College
Dietetics-Didactic Prgm
Child & Family Studies
CPO 2319
Berea, KY 40404
Prgm Dir: Janice B Blythe, PhD RD
Tel: 606 986-9341

Western Kentucky University
Dietetics-Didactic Prgm
Academic Complex 302F
One Big Red Way
Bowling Green, KY 42101-3576
Prgm Dir: Danita Saxon Kelley, PhD RD
Tel: 502 745-4352

Univ of Kentucky Chandler Med Ctr
Dietetic Internship Prgm
H-36 Dietetics & Nutrition
800 Rose St
Lexington, KY 40536-0084
Prgm Dir: Toni Gardner, MS RD
Tel: 606 323-5152

University of Kentucky
Dietetics-Didactic Prgm
Nutrition & Food Science
HES 212 Erikson Hall
Lexington, KY 40506-0050
Prgm Dir: Myrna M Wesley, MS RD CN CFCS
Tel: 606 257-7796

University of Kentucky
Preprofessional Practice Prgm
Human Environmental Sciences
204 Funkhouser Bldg
Lexington, KY 40506-1031
Prgm Dir: Pamela S McMahon, PhD RD
Tel: 606 257-1031

University of Kentucky
Dietetics-Coordinated Prgm
Nutrition and Food Science
218 Funkhouser
Lexington, KY 40506-0054
Prgm Dir: Pamela S McMahon, PhD RD
Tel: 606 257-1031

Spalding University
Dietetic Internship Prgm
851 S Fourth St
Louisville, KY 40203-2115
Prgm Dir: Kathy Rapp, MBA RD
Tel: 502 585-9911

Morehead State University
Preprofessional Practice Prgm
Dept of Home Economics
UPO Box 889
Morehead, KY 40351
Prgm Dir: Marilyn Y Sampley, PhD RD
Tel: 606 783-2966

Morehead State University
Dietetics-Didactic Prgm
Dept of Home Economics
PO Box 889
Morehead, KY 40351-0889
Prgm Dir: Marilyn Y Sampley, PhD RD LD CN
Tel: 606 783-2967

Murray State University
Dietetics-Didactic Prgm
Family & Consumer Studies
Murray, KY 42071
Prgm Dir: Sally T DuFord, PhD RD
Tel: 502 762-6958

Eastern Kentucky University
Dietetics-Didactic Prgm
Human Environmental Sciences
102 Burrier
Richmond, KY 40475
Prgm Dir: Sara Sutton, MS RD
Tel: 606 622-3445

Eastern Kentucky University
Dietetic Internship Prgm
Human Environmental Sciences
102 Burrier Bldg
Richmond, KY 40475
Prgm Dir: Margaret Ann McCarthy, MPH RD
Tel: 606 622-1172

Louisiana

Louisiana State Univ and A & M College
Dietetic Internship Prgm
School of Human Ecology
125 Human Ecology Bldg
Baton Rouge, LA 70803-4301
Prgm Dir: Evelina Cross, PhD RD LDN
Tel: 504 388-2406

Louisiana State Univ and A & M College
Dietetics-Didactic Prgm
School of Human Ecology
Baton Rouge, LA 70803-4300
Prgm Dir: Jo Ann Puls, MS RD LDN
Tel: 504 388-1537

Southern Univ and A & M College
Dietetics-Didactic Prgm
Agriculture & Home Econ
Box 11342
Baton Rouge, LA 70813-1342
Prgm Dir: Bernestine B McGee, PhD RD LDN
Tel: 504 771-4660

Southern Univ and A & M College
Preprofessional Practice Prgm
PO Box 11342
Baton Rouge, LA 70813-1342
Prgm Dir: Bernestine B McGee, PhD RD LDN
Tel: 504 771-4660

North Oaks Health System
Dietetic Internship Prgm
Nutritional Services
PO Box 2668
Hammond, LA 70404-2668
Prgm Dir: Carolyn Major, MA RD LDN
Tel: 504 543-6606

University of Southwestern Louisiana
Dietetics-Didactic Prgm
Coll of Applied Life Sciences
Sch of Human Res/Box 40399
Lafayette, LA 70504-0399
Prgm Dir: Bernice O Adeleye, PhD RD
Tel: 318 482-5724

University of Southwestern Louisiana
Dietetic Internship Prgm
School of Human Resources
PO Box 40399
Lafayette, LA 70504-0399
Prgm Dir: Rachel M Fournet, PhD LDN RD
Tel: 318 482-5724

McNeese State University
Dietetic Internship Prgm
PO Box 92820 MSU
Lake Charles, LA 70609
Prgm Dir: Debra Hollingsworth, PhD LDN RD
Tel: 318 475-5684

McNeese State University
Dietetics-Didactic Prgm
PO Box 92820
Lake Charles, LA 70609
Prgm Dir: Yvette M LeBlanc, MS RD LDN
Tel: 318 475-5685

Ochsner School of Allied Health Sciences
Dietetic Internship Prgm
BH 332/1516 Jefferson Hwy
New Orleans, LA 70121
Prgm Dir: Penny Rodriguez, MHA RD
Tel: 504 842-3267

Touro Infirmary School of Med Tech
Dietetic Internship Prgm
1401 Foucher St
New Orleans, LA 70115-3515
Prgm Dir: Patricia Fitzpatrick, MA LDN RD
Tel: 504 897-8320

Tulane University
Preprofessional Practice Prgm
Pub Hlth and Tropical Med
1430 Tulane Ave
New Orleans, LA 70112-2699
Prgm Dir: Ann B Metzinger, DrPH LDN RD
Tel: 504 588-5371

Louisiana Tech University
Dietetics-Didactic Prgm
College of Human Ecology
PO Box 3167
Ruston, LA 71272
Prgm Dir: Alice E Hunt, PhD RD LDN
Tel: 318 257-3043

Louisiana Tech University
Dietetic Internship Prgm
College of Human Ecology
PO Box 3167
Ruston, LA 71272
Prgm Dir: Dawn Erickson, MPH LDN RD
Tel: 318 257-3043

Nicholls State University
Dietetics-Didactic Prgm
Family & Consumer Sciences
Box 2014
Thibodaux, LA 70310
Prgm Dir: Colette Leistner, PhD RD
Tel: 504 448-4732

Maine

University of Maine - Orono
Dietetics-Didactic Prgm
Food Sci & Human Nutrition
5749 Merrill Hall Rm 23
Orono, ME 04469-5749
Prgm Dir: Adrienne A White, PhD RD
Tel: 207 581-3134

University of Maine - Orono
Dietetic Internship Prgm
Food Sci & Human Nutrition
5749 Merrill Hall Rm 23
Orono, ME 04469-5749
Prgm Dir: Adrienne A White, PhD RD
Tel: 207 581-3134

Maryland

Malcolm Grow USAF Medical Center
Dietetic Internship Prgm
89th Medical Support System
1050 W Perimeter Rd
Andrews AFB, MD 20762-6600
Prgm Dir: Denise K Black, MS RD
Tel: 301 981-3901

Maryland Dept of Hlth & Mental Hygiene
Dietetic Internship Prgm
Div of Dietetic Service
6 St Paul St Ste 1301
Baltimore, MD 21202
Prgm Dir: Ruby MacDonnell, MS RD LD
Tel: 410 767-8440

Mercy Medical Center
Dietetic Internship Prgm
Nutrition & Food Services
301 Saint Paul Pl
Baltimore, MD 21202-2165
Prgm Dir: Mary Ellen Beazley, MS RD LD
Tel: 410 332-9307

Morgan State University
Dietetics-Didactic Prgm
Human Ecology Key Bldg 52
Coldspring Ln & Hillen Rd
Baltimore, MD 21239-4098
Prgm Dir: Arleen B Tate, MS RD LD
Tel: 410 319-3905

University of Maryland Medical System
Dietetic Internship Prgm
Food & Nutrition Services
22 S Greene St
Baltimore, MD 21201-1544
Prgm Dir: Laura K Wohlberg, MS RD LD
Tel: 410 328-2561

National Institutes of Health
Dietetic Internship Prgm
Clinic Ctr Nutri Dept Bldg 10
Rm BIS-234/10 Ctr Dr MSC 1078
Bethesda, MD 20892-1078
Prgm Dir: Elaine J Ayres, MS RD LD
Tel: 301 496-3311

Univ of Maryland at College Park

Dietetics-Didactic Prgm
Nutrition & Food Science
College Park, MD 20742-7521
Prgm Dir: Suzanne R Curtis, PhD RD
Tel: 301 405-4532

University of Maryland Eastern Shore

Preprofessional Practice Prgm
Dept of Human Ecology
Princess Anne, MD 21853
Prgm Dir: Bettie Wright Blakely, MS RD
Tel: 410 651-6066

University of Maryland Eastern Shore

Dietetics-Didactic Prgm
Dept of Human Ecology
Princess Anne, MD 21853-1299
Prgm Dir: Bettie Blakely, MS RD
Tel: 410 651-6066

Massachusetts

University of Massachusetts - Amherst

Dietetic Internship Prgm
Div of Continuing Education
608 Goodell Bldg Box 33260
Amherst, MA 01003-3260
Prgm Dir: Alice E Szlosek, MS RD
Tel: 413 545-2484

University of Massachusetts - Amherst

Dietetics-Didactic Prgm
Dept of Nutrition Box 31420
Chenoweth Laboratory
Amherst, MA 01003-1420
Prgm Dir: Alice E Szlosek, MS RD
Tel: 413 545-0740

Beth Israel Deaconess Healthcare

Dietetic Internship Prgm
330 Brookline Ave
Boston, MA 02215-5491
Prgm Dir: Terri Lee Smith, MA RD
Tel: 617 667-2539

Boston University

Dietetic Internship Prgm
Sargent Coll Grad Nutri Div
635 Commonwealth Ave
Boston, MA 02215-1605
Prgm Dir: Joan Salge Blake, MS RD
Tel: 617 353-2710

Brigham and Women's Hospital

Dietetic Internship Prgm
75 Francis St
Boston, MA 02115-6195
Prgm Dir: Alice McCarley, MS RD
Tel: 617 732-7493

Massachusetts General Hospital

Dietetic Internship Prgm
Dept of Dietetics
Boston, MA 02114
Prgm Dir: Kathleen E Creedon, MHPE RD
Tel: 617 726-2589

New England Med Ctr/Frances Stern Nutri Ctr

Dietetic Internship Prgm
Tufts University Box 783
750 Washington St
Boston, MA 02111-1533
Prgm Dir: Johanna T Dwyer, DSc RD
Tel: 617 636-5273

Simmons College

Dietetics-Didactic Prgm
Dept of Nutrition
300 The Fenway
Boston, MA 02115-5898
Prgm Dir: Margery J Gann, MS MBA RD FADA
Tel: 617 521-2713

Simmons College

Dietetic Internship Prgm
Dept of Nutrition
300 The Fenway
Boston, MA 02115
Prgm Dir: Nancie Harvey Herbold, EdD RD
Tel: 617 521-2711

Mt Auburn Hospital

Dietetic Internship Prgm
330 Mount Auburn St
Cambridge, MA 02238
Prgm Dir: Susan Tiller, MBA RD
Tel: 617 499-5665

Framingham State College

Dietetic Internship Prgm
Family and Consumer Sciences
PO Box 2000
Framingham, MA 01701
Prgm Dir: Patricia Plummer, PhD RD
Tel: 508 626-4760

Framingham State College

Dietetics-Didactic Prgm
Family and Consumer Science
100 State St
Framingham, MA 01701-9101
Prgm Dir: Patricia Luoto, EdD RD
Tel: 508 626-4759

Framingham State College

Dietetics-Coordinated Prgm
Family and Consumer Sciences
100 State St
Framingham, MA 01701-9101
Prgm Dir: Suzanne Neubauer, PhD RD
Tel: 508 626-4754

St Luke's Hospital/Marriott Corporation

Preprofessional Practice Prgm
101 Page St
New Bedford, MA 02740-3464
Prgm Dir: Elizabeth F Winthrop, MS RD
Tel: 508 997-1525

Sodexho USA

Preprofessional Practice Prgm
153 Second Ave
Waltham, MA 02254-3730
Prgm Dir: Barbara Woodland, MS RD
Tel: 800 926-7429, Ext 483

Michigan

University of Michigan Hospitals

Preprofessional Practice Prgm
Public Health
C333 Med Inn Bldg
Box 0832
1500 E Medical Ctr Dr
Ann Arbor, MI 48109-2029
Prgm Dir: Andrea Lasichak, MS RD
Tel: 313 764-3277

University of Michigan

Dietetics-Didactic Prgm
Public Hlth Human Nutrition Prgm
1420 Washington Heights
Ann Arbor, MI 48109-2029
Prgm Dir: Deborah A Lown, MS RD CNSD
Tel: 313 764-3277

University of Michigan Hospitals

Dietetic Internship Prgm
UH2C227/0056
1500 E Medical Ctr Dr
Ann Arbor, MI 48109-0056
Prgm Dir: Joyce Kerestes-Smith, MS RD
Tel: 313 936-5199

Andrews University

Dietetics-Didactic Prgm
Dept of Nutrition
Berrien Springs, MI 49104-0210
Prgm Dir: William R Proulx, MS RD
Tel: 616 471-3370

Andrews University

Preprofessional Practice Prgm
Dept of Nutrition
Berrien Springs, MI 49104-0210
Prgm Dir: Winston Craig, PhD RD
Tel: 616 471-3370

Detroit Health Department

Dietetic Internship Prgm
Nutrition Div
1151 Taylor St
Detroit, MI 48202-1732
Prgm Dir: Willie Louise Lee, MS RD
Tel: 313 876-4090

Harper Hospital

Dietetic Internship Prgm
Food & Nutrition Services
3990 John R St
Detroit, MI 48201-2018
Prgm Dir: Diane L Trippett, MS RD
Tel: 313 745-2037

Henry Ford Hospital

Dietetic Internship Prgm
Dept of Dietetics
2799 W Grand Blvd
Detroit, MI 48202-2689
Prgm Dir: Hildreth A Macy, MA RD FADA
Tel: 313 876-1071

Marygrove College

Dietetics-Didactic Prgm
Human Ecology Dept
8425 W McNichols Rd
Detroit, MI 48221-2546
Prgm Dir: Karen Kirmis, MS RD
Tel: 313 862-8000

Wayne State University

Dietetics-Coordinated Prgm
Nutrition & Food Science
3009 Science Hall
Detroit, MI 48202
Prgm Dir: Tonia Reinhard, MS RD
Tel: 313 577-2500

Michigan State University

Dietetics-Didactic Prgm
Food Sci & Human Nutrition
236 G Malcolm Trout
East Lansing, MI 48824-1030
Prgm Dir: Stella Cash, MS RD
Tel: 517 355-6483

Hurley Medical Center

Dietetic Internship Prgm
Nutrition Service Dept
One Hurley Plaza
Flint, MI 48503-5993
Prgm Dir: Constance M Hagelshaw, MS RD
Tel: 810 257-9772

Western Michigan University

Dietetics-Didactic Prgm
Consumer Resources & Tech
3025 Kohrman Hall
Kalamazoo, MI 49008
Prgm Dir: Maija Petersons, PhD RD
Tel: 616 387-3710

Western Michigan University

Dietetic Internship Prgm
Family and Consumer Sciences
3025 Kohrman Hall
Kalamazoo, MI 49008-5067
Prgm Dir: Maija Peterson, PhD RD
Tel: 616 387-3710

Madonna University

Dietetics-Didactic Prgm
Family & Consumer Resources
36600 Schoolcraft Rd
Livonia, MI 48150-1173
Prgm Dir: Karen Schmitz, PhD RD
Tel: 313 432-5534

Northern Michigan University

Dietetics-Didactic Prgm
HPER
Marquette, MI 49855
Prgm Dir: Mohey Mowafy, PhD RD
Tel: 906 227-2366

Central Michigan University

Dietetics-Didactic Prgm
Human Environmental Studies
205 Wightman Hall
Mt Pleasant, MI 48859
Prgm Dir: Robert D Lee, DrPH RD
Tel: 517 774-5604

Oakland County Health Division

Preprofessional Practice Prgm
Dept 432
1200 N Telegraph Rd
Pontiac, MI 48341-0432
Prgm Dir: Linda H Eaton, MS RD CHES
Tel: 810 858-1832

Central Michigan University

Dietetic Internship Prgm
3037 Davenport Ave
Saginaw, MI 48602-3652
Prgm Dir: Robert D Lee, DrPH RD
Tel: 517 774-5604

Eastern Michigan University

Dietetics-Coordinated Prgm
Human Environ/Cons Resources
200-K Roosevelt Hall
Ypsilanti, MI 48197
Prgm Dir: Deborah W Silverman, MS RD LD
Tel: 313 487-2491

Minnesota

College of St Scholastica

Dietetics-Didactic Prgm
Dept of Dietetics
1200 Kenwood Ave
Duluth, MN 55811
Prgm Dir: Susan Kumsha Bodin, MS RD
Tel: 218 723-6101

Mankato State University

Dietetics-Didactic Prgm
Home Economics Dept
MSU Box 44/PO Box 8400
Mankato, MN 56002-8400
Prgm Dir: Beth C Zimmer, MS RD
Tel: 507 389-6016

Minneapolis Veterans Affairs Medical Ctr

Dietetic Internship Prgm
Nutrition & Food Service
One Veterans Dr
Minneapolis, MN 55417
Prgm Dir: Heidi Hoover, MS RD
Tel: 612 725-2004

Univ of Minnesota Hosp and Clinic

Dietetic Internship Prgm
Nutrition Dept PO Box 84
Harvard St at E River Rd
Minneapolis, MN 55455
Prgm Dir: Mary C McFadden, MS RD
Tel: 612 626-3661

Concordia College - Moorhead

Dietetics-Didactic Prgm
Family & Nutrition Sciences
Moorhead, MN 56562
Prgm Dir: Betty J Larson, EdD LRD
Tel: 218 299-3748

St Marys Hospital/Mayo Medical Center

Dietetic Internship Prgm
1216 2nd St SW
Rochester, MN 55902-1906
Prgm Dir: Karen E Moxness, MS RD
Tel: 507 255-5221

College of St Benedict/St John's Univ

Dietetics-Coordinated Prgm
Nutrition Dept
37 S College Ave
St Joseph, MN 56374-2099
Prgm Dir: Amy C Olson, PhD RD
Tel: 320 363-5057

College of St Catherine

Dietetics-Didactic Prgm
Family Consumer & Nutri Sci
2004 Randolph Ave
St Paul, MN 55105-1750
Prgm Dir: Patricia J Ode, MA RD
Tel: 612 690-6204

St Paul Ramsey Medical Center

Dietetic Internship Prgm
640 Jackson St
St Paul, MN 55101-2502
Prgm Dir: Elizabeth L Orchard, MA RD
Tel: 612 221-2712

University of Minnesota - St Paul

Dietetics-Coordinated Prgm
269 Food Science & Nutrition
1334 Eckles Ave
St Paul, MN 55108-6099
Prgm Dir: Madge N Hanson, MS RD
Tel: 612 624-9278

University of Minnesota - Twin Cities

Dietetic Internship Prgm
Food Science & Nutrition
1334 Eckles Ave
St Paul, MN 55108-6099
Prgm Dir: Louise M Mullan, MS RD
Tel: 612 624-3255

University of Minnesota - Twin Cities

Dietetics-Didactic Prgm
Food Science & Nutrition
1334 Eckles Ave
St Paul, MN 55108-1040
Prgm Dir: Louise M Mullan, MS RD
Tel: 612 624-3255

Mississippi

University of Southern Mississippi

Preprofessional Practice Prgm
Southern Station
PO Box 5035
Hattiesburg, MS 39406-5035
Prgm Dir: Ruth Ann Broome, MS RD
Tel: 601 924-9769

University of Southern Mississippi

Dietetics-Didactic Prgm
School of Home Economics
PO Box 5035
Hattiesburg, MS 39406-5035
Prgm Dir: Wayne E Billon, PhD RD
Tel: 601 266-4679

University of Southern Mississippi

Dietetics-Coordinated Prgm
Nutrition and Dietetics
Southern Station Box 5035
Hattiesburg, MS 39406-5035
Prgm Dir: Mary Frances Nettles, PhD RD
Tel: 601 266-4679

St Dominic-Jackson Memorial Hospital

Dietetic Internship Prgm
969 Lakeland Dr
Jackson, MS 39216-4699
Prgm Dir: Stella Pierce, MHS RD LD
Tel: 601 364-6935

Programs

Alcorn State University
Dietetics-Didactic Prgm
Family and Consumer Sciences
1000 ASU Dr #839
Lorman, MS 39096-9402
Prgm Dir: Ivis T Forrester, PhD RD
Tel: 601 877-6252

Mississippi State University
Dietetic Internship Prgm
School of Human Sciences
Box 9745
Mississippi State, MS 39762
Prgm Dir: Sylvia H Byrd, PhD RD
Tel: 601 325-0919

Mississippi State University
Dietetics-Didactic Prgm
Dept of Home Economics
PO Box 9745
Mississippi State, MS 39762-9745
Prgm Dir: Carolyn Malone, MS RD
Tel: 601 325-3820

University of Mississippi
Dietetics-Didactic Prgm
Family and Consumer Sciences
Meek Hall
University, MS 38677
Prgm Dir: Kathy B Knight, PhD RD
Tel: 601 232-7371

Missouri

Southeast Missouri State University
Dietetics-Didactic Prgm
Human Environmental Studies
Cape Girardeau, MO 63701-4799
Prgm Dir: Marcia L Nahikian-Nelms, PhD RD
Tel: 573 651-2994

University of Missouri - Columbia
Dietetics-Coordinated Prgm
Dietetic Education
318 Clark Hall
Columbia, MO 65211
Prgm Dir: Candace S Kohnke, PhD RD
Tel: 573 882-4136

Missouri Dept of Mental Health
Dietetic Internship Prgm
Office of Administration
1706 E Elm St/PO Box 687
Jefferson City, MO 65102
Prgm Dir: Annette J Terry, MS RD
Tel: 573 751-8145

ARAMARK Healthcare Support Services SW
Preprofessional Practice Prgm
St Joseph Health System
1000 Carondelet Dr
Kansas City, MO 64114-4802
Prgm Dir: Beth F Harrell, MS RD
Tel: 816 943-2146

Northwest Missouri State University
Dietetics-Didactic Prgm
Coll of Educ & Human Services
Rm 309 Admin Bldg
Maryville, MO 64468-6001
Prgm Dir: Jenell Ciak, PhD RD
Tel: 816 562-1168

College of the Ozarks
Dietetics-Didactic Prgm
Dietetics & Nutrition Educ
Point Lookout, MO 65726
Prgm Dir: Suzanne Martin, PhD RD
Tel: 417 334-6411

Southwest Missouri State University
Dietetics-Didactic Prgm
Dept of Biomedical Sciences
Springfield, MO 65804
Prgm Dir: Helen Reid, PhD RD
Tel: 417 836-5321

Barnes-Jewish Hospital
Dietetic Internship Prgm
One Barnes Hospital Plaza
St Louis, MO 63110
Prgm Dir: Margaret Foy Shields, MEd RD
Tel: 314 362-5284

Fontbonne College
Dietetics-Didactic Prgm
Human Environmental Sciences
6800 Wydown Blvd
St Louis, MO 63105-3098
Prgm Dir: Linda L Kendrick, MA RD
Tel: 314 889-1415

St Louis University Health Sciences Ctr
Dietetic Internship Prgm
School of Allied Health Profs
1504 S Grand Blvd
St Louis, MO 63104-1304
Prgm Dir: Mildred Mattfeldt-Beman, PhD RD
Tel: 314 577-8523

Veterans Affairs Medical Center
Dietetic Internship Prgm
Nutri & Food Services (120/JB)
1 Jefferson Barracks Dr
St Louis, MO 63125
Prgm Dir: Martha R Kratzer, MS RD
Tel: 314 894-6631

Central Missouri State University
Dietetics-Didactic Prgm
Human Environmental Sciences
Grinstead 235
Warrensburg, MO 64093
Prgm Dir: Mary Anne Drake, PhD RD LD
Tel: 816 543-4217

Montana

Montana State University
Dietetics-Didactic Prgm
Health & Human Development
201 Romney
Bozeman, MT 59717
Prgm Dir: Pamela Harris, MS RD
Tel: 406 994-6338

Nebraska

University of Nebraska at Kearney
Dietetics-Didactic Prgm
Family & Consumer Science
Otto Olsen Bldg Rm 205B
Kearney, NE 68849-2130
Prgm Dir: Sharon L Davis, MS RD
Tel: 308 865-8230

University of Nebraska-Lincoln
Dietetic Internship Prgm
Nutri Science & Dietetics
202 Ruth Leverton Hall
Lincoln, NE 68583-0806
Prgm Dir: Linda O Young, MS RD
Tel: 402 472-2925

University of Nebraska-Lincoln
Dietetics-Didactic Prgm
Nutri Science & Dietetics
202 Ruth Leverton Hall
Lincoln, NE 68583-0806
Prgm Dir: Linda O Young, MS RD
Tel: 402 472-2925

University of Nebraska Medical Center
Dietetic Internship Prgm
600 S 42nd St
Box 981200
Omaha, NE 68198-1200
Prgm Dir: Glenda R Woscyna, MS RD CN
Tel: 402 559-5317

Nevada

University of Nevada - Reno
Dietetic Internship Prgm
Dept of Nutrition
Mail Stop 142
Reno, NV 89557-0132
Prgm Dir: David S Wilson, PhD RD
Tel: 702 784-6440

University of Nevada - Reno
Dietetics-Didactic Prgm
Dept of Nutrition
Mail Stop 142
Reno, NV 89557
Prgm Dir: Marsha H Read, PhD RD
Tel: 702 784-6446

New Hampshire

University of New Hampshire
Dietetic Internship Prgm
Nutrition Ctr
Colovos Rd
Durham, NH 03824
Prgm Dir: Caroline Giles, MA RD
Tel: 603 862-2811

University of New Hampshire
Dietetics-Didactic Prgm
Animal & Nutrition Science
Human Nutri Ctr Colovos Rd
Durham, NH 03824
Prgm Dir: Colette Janson-Sand, PhD RD
Tel: 603 862-1723

Keene State College
Dietetics-Didactic Prgm
Home Econ/Human Services
Joslin House/Rm 207
Keene, NH 03435-2903
Prgm Dir: Patsy Beffa-Negrini, PhD RD
Tel: 603 358-2859

New Jersey

College of St Elizabeth
Dietetics-Didactic Prgm
Dept of Foods and Nutrition
2 Convent Rd
Morristown, NJ 07960-6989
Prgm Dir: Dorothy A Addario, MS RD
Tel: 201 605-7045

College of St Elizabeth
Dietetic Internship Prgm
Dept of Foods and Nutrition
2 Convent Rd
Morristown, NJ 07960-6989
Prgm Dir: Monica Luby, MS RD
Tel: 201 605-7125

Rutgers SUNJ New Brunswick Campus
Dietetics-Didactic Prgm
Nutri Sci/Davison Hall
26 Nichol Ave
New Brunswick, NJ 08903-0270
Prgm Dir: Bernadette G Janas, PhD RD
Tel: 908 932-6568

Univ of Med & Dent of New Jersey
Dietetic Internship Prgm
Schl of Health Related Profs
1776 Raritan Rd
Scotch Plains, NJ 07076
Prgm Dir: Kay Stearns Bruening, MA RD
Tel: 908 889-2488

Marriott Health Care/Helene Fuld Med Ctr
Preprofessional Practice Prgm
750 Brunswick Ave
Trenton, NJ 08638-4143
Prgm Dir: Cheryl Margetin, MS RD
Tel: 609 394-6344

Montclair State University
Dietetics-Didactic Prgm
Dept of Human Ecology
Upper Montclair, NJ 07043
Prgm Dir: Kathleen D Bauer, PhD RD
Tel: 201 655-4171

Montclair State University
Preprofessional Practice Prgm
Dept of Home Ecology
Upper Montclair, NJ 07043
Prgm Dir: Shahla Wunderlich, PhD RD
Tel: 201 655-4373

New Mexico

University of New Mexico
Dietetic Internship Prgm
Hlth Promo Phys Ed & Leisure
Johnson Ctr 1150
Albuquerque, NM 87131-1251
Prgm Dir: Wendy M Sandoval, PhD RD
Tel: 505 277-4322

University of New Mexico
Dietetics-Didactic Prgm
Dept of Health Promo
Phys Ed & Leisure Prgms
Albuquerque, NM 87131-1251
Prgm Dir: Karen Heller, PhD RD LD
Tel: 505 277-0937

New Mexico State University
Dietetics-Didactic Prgm
Dept of Home Economics
Dept 3470/PO Box 30003
Las Cruces, NM 88003-8003
Prgm Dir: Margaret Ann Bock, PhD RD LD
Tel: 505 646-1178

New York

CUNY Herbert H Lehman College
Dietetics-Didactic Prgm
Dept of Health Services
Bedford Park Blvd W
Bronx, NY 10468-1589
Prgm Dir: Alice Tobias, EdD RD
Tel: 718 960-8775

CUNY Herbert H Lehman College
Preprofessional Practice Prgm
Dept of Health Services
Bedford Park Blvd W
Bronx, NY 10468-1589
Prgm Dir: Andrea P Boyar, PhD RD
Tel: 718 960-8487

Veterans Affairs Medical Center
Dietetic Internship Prgm
130 W Kingsbridge Rd
Bronx, NY 10468-3904
Prgm Dir: Barbara Isaacs, MS RD
Tel: 718 579-1640

ARAMARK Healthcare Support Services
Preprofessional Practice Prgm
Kingsbrook Jewish Med Ctr
585 Schenectady Ave
Brooklyn, NY 11203
Prgm Dir: Renu Sethi, MA RD
Tel: 718 604-5757

CUNY Brooklyn College
Dietetics-Didactic Prgm
Health and Nutrition Sciences
2900 Bedford Ave
Brooklyn, NY 11210-2889
Prgm Dir: Roseanne Schnoll, MS RD
Tel: 718 951-5900

CUNY Brooklyn College
Preprofessional Practice Prgm
Health and Nutrition Science
2900 Bedford Ave
Brooklyn, NY 11210-2889
Prgm Dir: Roseanne Schnoll, MS RD
Tel: 718 951-5909

Long Island College Hospital
Preprofessional Practice Prgm
Nutrition & Food Service
Atlantic Ave & Hicks St
Brooklyn, NY 11201
Prgm Dir: Elisa Zimmer, MS RD CNSD CDE
Tel: 718 780-2836

Long Island Univ - C W Post Campus
Dietetics-Didactic Prgm
Health Science Dept
Brookville, NY 11548
Prgm Dir: Clifford Rouder, MS RD
Tel: 516 299-3046

Long Island Univ - C W Post Campus
Dietetic Internship Prgm
Health Sciences Dept
Brookville, NY 11548
Prgm Dir: Alice Fornari, MS RD
Tel: 516 299-3224

D'Youville College
Dietetics-Coordinated Prgm
320 Porter Ave
Buffalo, NY 14201-1084
Prgm Dir: Edward H Weiss, PhD RD
Tel: 716 881-3200

SUNY College at Buffalo
Dietetics-Coordinated Prgm
Nutrition Hosp & Fashion Dept
1300 Elmwood Ave
Buffalo, NY 14222-1095
Prgm Dir: Donna M Hayes, MS RD
Tel: 716 878-5634

SUNY College at Buffalo
Dietetics-Didactic Prgm
Nutri Hospitality & Fashion
1300 Elmwood Ave
Buffalo, NY 14222-1095
Prgm Dir: Tejaswini Rao, PhD RD
Tel: 716 878-4333

CUNY Queens College
Dietetic Internship Prgm
Family Nutri and Exercise Sciences
Remsen Hall 306
Flushing, NY 11367-1597
Prgm Dir: Susan P Braverman, MS RD
Tel: 718 997-4150

CUNY Queens College
Dietetics-Didactic Prgm
Family Nutri and Exercise Sciences
65-30 Kissena Blvd
Flushing, NY 11367-1597
Prgm Dir: Marcia C Miller, EdD RD
Tel: 718 997-4152

Cornell University
Dietetic Internship Prgm
366 MVR Hall
Ithaca, NY 14853-4401
Prgm Dir: Gertrude Armbruster, PhD RD
Tel: 607 255-2642

Cornell University
Dietetics-Didactic Prgm
Div of Nutritional Sciences
366 Martha Van Rensselaer
Ithaca, NY 14853-4401
Prgm Dir: Gertrude Armbruster, PhD RD
Tel: 607 255-2642

Cornell University
Dietetics-Didactic Prgm
School of Hotel Admin
W209 Statler Hall
Ithaca, NY 14853
Prgm Dir: Mary H Tabacchi, PhD RD
Tel: 607 255-3458

Programs

United Health Services Hospital
Dietetic Internship Prgm
Wilson Memorial Regl Med Ctr
33-57 Harrison St
Johnson City, NY 13790-2143
Prgm Dir: Susan R Smith, MS RD
Tel: 607 763-6600

Ulster Cnty Residential Healthcare Fac
Preprofessional Practice Prgm
99 Golden Hill Dr
Kingston, NY 12401
Prgm Dir: Sheree Perez Cross, MPA RD LDN
Tel: 914 339-4540

CUNY Hunter College
Preprofessional Practice Prgm
School of Health Sciences
425 E 25th St
New York, NY 10010-2590
Prgm Dir: Karen O'Brien, MS RD
Tel: 212 481-5127

CUNY Hunter College
Dietetics-Didactic Prgm
Brookdale Hlth Science Ctr
425 E 25th St
New York, NY 10010-2590
Prgm Dir: Karen O'Brien, MS RD
Tel: 212 481-7563

New York Hospital
Dietetic Internship Prgm
525 E 68th St AN-833
New York, NY 10021-4873
Prgm Dir: Elaine Rosenthal, MS RD
Tel: 212 746-0830

New York University
Dietetics-Didactic Prgm
Nutrition and Food Studies
35 W 4th St 10th Fl
New York, NY 10012-1172
Prgm Dir: Judith A Gilbride, PhD RD
Tel: 212 998-5580

New York University
Preprofessional Practice Prgm
Nutrition and Food Studies
35 W 4th St 10th Fl
New York, NY 10012-1172
Prgm Dir: Judith A Gilbride, PhD RD
Tel: 212 998-5580

Teachers College Columbia University
Preprofessional Practice Prgm
Health & Nutrition Education
525 W 120th St Box 137
New York, NY 10027-6625
Prgm Dir: Lillian Yung, EdD RD
Tel: 212 678-3950

Marriott/Metro New York AP4 Programs
Preprofessional Practice Prgm
South Nassau Communities Hosp
2445 Oceanside Rd
Oceanside, NY 11572-1548
Prgm Dir: Judith Creeron, MS RD
Tel: 516 763-3903

New York Institute of Technology
Dietetic Internship Prgm
NYCOM-II-Rm 363-Clinical Nutrition
PO Box 8000
Old Westbury, NY 11568-8000
Prgm Dir: Therese Ann Franzese, MS RD
Tel: 516 626-7417

SUNY College at Oneonta
Dietetics-Didactic Prgm
Dept of Human Ecology
Oneonta, NY 13820-4015
Prgm Dir: Carolyn J Haessig, PhD RD
Tel: 607 436-2705

SUNY College at Plattsburgh
Dietetics-Didactic Prgm
Nursing Food and Nutrition
101 Broad St
Plattsburgh, NY 12901
Prgm Dir: Jean Coates, PhD RD
Tel: 518 564-4222

Rochester Institute of Technology
Dietetics-Coordinated Prgm
Food Hotel and Travel Mgmt
14 Lomb Memorial Dr
Rochester, NY 14623-5604
Prgm Dir: Elizabeth A Kmiecinski, MS RD
Tel: 716 475-2357

Rochester Institute of Technology
Dietetics-Didactic Prgm
Food Hotel & Tour Mgmt
14 Lomb Memorial Dr
Rochester, NY 14623-5604
Prgm Dir: Barbara Cerio, MS RD
Tel: 716 475-2352

Syracuse University Main Campus
Dietetic Internship Prgm
Nutrition & Foodservice Mgmt
034 Slocum Hall
Syracuse, NY 13244-1250
Prgm Dir: Debra Connolly, MA RD
Tel: 315 443-2386

Syracuse University Main Campus
Dietetics-Coordinated Prgm
Nutrition Foodservice Mgmt
034 Slocum Hall
Syracuse, NY 13244-1250
Prgm Dir: Lois A Schroeder, PhD RD
Tel: 315 443-2063

Syracuse University Main Campus
Dietetics-Didactic Prgm
Nutrition & Foodservice Mgmt
034 Slocum Hall
Syracuse, NY 13244-1250
Prgm Dir: Kim Dittus, PhD RD
Tel: 315 443-2386

Marymount College
Dietetics-Didactic Prgm
Dept of Human Ecology
Marian Hall
Tarrytown, NY 10591
Prgm Dir: Paula VanAken, MS RD
Tel: 914 332-6559

Russell Sage College
Dietetics-Didactic Prgm
Nutrition Science Dept
Ackerman Hall
Troy, NY 12180-4115
Prgm Dir: Ann Rogan, PhD RD
Tel: 518 270-2048

Sage Graduate School
Dietetic Internship Prgm
45 Ferry St
Troy, NY 12180-4115
Prgm Dir: Melodie Bell-Cavallino, MS RD
Tel: 518 270-2075

Westchester County Medical Center
Dietetic Internship Prgm
Food Services Div
Grasslands Rd
Valhalla, NY 10595-1689
Prgm Dir: Irene Gatto, MS RD
Tel: 914 285-7276

North Carolina

Appalachian State University
Dietetic Internship Prgm
Family and Consumer Sciences
Boone, NC 28608
Prgm Dir: Mary Etta Reeves, PhD RD
Tel: 704 262-3120

Appalachian State University
Dietetics-Didactic Prgm
Family and Consumer Sciences
Boone, NC 28608-2630
Prgm Dir: Lawrence Forman, PhD RD
Tel: 704 262-2630

Univ of North Carolina at Chapel Hill
Dietetics-Coordinated Prgm
McGavran-Greenburg Hall
Dept of Nutrition CB 7400
Chapel Hill, NC 27599-7400
Prgm Dir: Carolyn Barrett, MS MPH RD
Tel: 919 966-7214

Univ of North Carolina at Chapel Hill
Dietetics-Didactic Prgm
McGraven-Greenburg Hall
Dept of Nutrition CB 7400
Chapel Hill, NC 27599-7400
Prgm Dir: Carolyn J H Barrett, MS MPH RD
Tel: 919 966-7214

Western Carolina University
Dietetics-Didactic Prgm
Dept of Health Sciences
Cullowhee, NC 28723
Prgm Dir: Kathryn W Hosig, PhD RD
Tel: 704 227-7114

Western Carolina University
Preprofessional Practice Prgm
Nutrition/Dietetics
Dept of Health Sciences
Cullowhee, NC 28723
Prgm Dir: Barbara A Cosper, PhD RD
Tel: 704 227-7114

North Carolina Central University
Dietetic Internship Prgm
Dept of Home Economics
PO Box 19615
Durham, NC 27707-0099
Prgm Dir: Esther Okeiyi, PhD RD
Tel: 919 560-6476

North Carolina Central University
Dietetics-Didactic Prgm
Dept of Human Sciences
PO Box 19615
Durham, NC 27707-0099
Prgm Dir: Esther C Okeiyi, PhD RD LDN
Tel: 919 560-6476

Bennett College
Dietetics-Didactic Prgm
Home Economics Dept
900 E Washington St
Greensboro, NC 27401-3239
Prgm Dir: Beth P Jones, MS RD
Tel: 910 370-8795

North Carolina A & T State University
Dietetics-Didactic Prgm
Dept of Home Economics
Benbow Hall 102
Greensboro, NC 27411-1064
Prgm Dir: Wilda F Wade, PhD RD LDN
Tel: 910 334-7850

Univ of North Carolina at Greensboro
Dietetic Internship Prgm
Food, Nutrition, and Foodservice
318 Stone Bldg
Greensboro, NC 27412-5001
Prgm Dir: Martha L Taylor, PhD RD
Tel: 910 334-5313

Univ of North Carolina at Greensboro
Dietetics-Didactic Prgm
Human Environmental Sciences
318 Stone/1000 Spring Garden
Greensboro, NC 27412-5001
Prgm Dir: Cheryl A Lovelady, PhD RD LDN
Tel: 910 334-5313

East Carolina University
Dietetic Internship Prgm
Home Environmental Sciences
Nutrition & Hospitality Mgmt
Greenville, NC 27858-4353
Prgm Dir: Janet D Bryan, MSHE RD LDN
Tel: 919 328-1352

East Carolina University
Dietetics-Didactic Prgm
Nutri and Hospitality Mgmt
Greenville, NC 27858-4353
Prgm Dir: Janet D Bryan, MSHE RD LDN
Tel: 919 328-1352

Meredith College
Dietetic Internship Prgm
Human Environmental Sciences
3800 Hillsborough St
Raleigh, NC 27607-5298
Prgm Dir: William Landis, PhD RD
Tel: 919 829-8568

Meredith College
Dietetics-Didactic Prgm
Human Environmental Sciences
3800 Hillsborough St
Raleigh, NC 27607-5298
Prgm Dir: Lauree P Holliday, MS RD LDN
Tel: 919 829-2355

North Dakota

North Dakota State University
Dietetics-Coordinated Prgm
Dept of Food and Nutrition
EML Hall 351
Fargo, ND 58105-5057
Prgm Dir: Kathleen Reichert, MS LRD
Tel: 701 231-7474

North Dakota State University
Dietetics-Didactic Prgm
Dept of Food & Nutrition
Fargo, ND 58105
Prgm Dir: Vel Rae Burkholder, MS LRD
Tel: 701 231-7480

North Dakota State University
Preprofessional Practice Prgm
EML Hall 351H
PO Box 5057
Fargo, ND 58105-5057
Prgm Dir: Barbara B North, MS LRD
Tel: 701 231-7479

Univ of No Dakota Sch of Med and Hlth Sci
Dietetics-Coordinated Prgm
Nutrition and Dietetics
Univ Station/PO Box 8237
Grand Forks, ND 58202-8273
Prgm Dir: Judith Hall, MS LRD
Tel: 701 777-3752

Ohio

University of Akron
Dietetics-Coordinated Prgm
Home Econ and Family Ecology
215 Schrank Hall S
Akron, OH 44325-6103
Prgm Dir: Sue A Rasor-Greenhalgh, MS RD
Tel: 330 972-6046

University of Akron
Dietetics-Didactic Prgm
Home Econ and Family Ecology
215 Schrank Hall S
Akron, OH 44325-6103
Prgm Dir: Roberta S Hurley, PhD RD LD
Tel: 330 972-7856

Ohio University Main Campus
Dietetics-Didactic Prgm
Human and Consumer Sciences
101 A Tupper Hall
Athens, OH 45701-2979
Prgm Dir: Marjorie Hagerman, MS RD LD
Tel: 614 593-2874

Bluffton College
Dietetics-Didactic Prgm
Family & Consumer Sciences
280 W College Ave Box 896
Bluffton, OH 45817-1196
Prgm Dir: Kay Soltesz, PhD RD LD
Tel: 419 358-3233

Bowling Green State University
Preprofessional Practice Prgm
Family and Consumer Sciences
Bowling Green, OH 43403
Prgm Dir: Martha Sue Houston, PhD RD LD
Tel: 419 372-2026

Bowling Green State University
Dietetics-Didactic Prgm
Family and Consumer Sciences
206 Johnston Hall
Bowling Green, OH 43403-0254
Prgm Dir: Younghee Kim, PhD RD LD
Tel: 419 372-7859

Christ Hospital
Dietetic Internship Prgm
Food & Nutrition Services
2139 Auburn Ave
Cincinnati, OH 45219-2906
Prgm Dir: Patricia C Cooper, MS RD LD
Tel: 513 369-2396

Good Samaritan Hospital
Dietetic Internship Prgm
Nutrition Dept
375 Dixmyth Ave
Cincinnati, OH 45220-2489
Prgm Dir: Jackene M Laverty, MEd RD LD
Tel: 513 872-1983

Univ Affl Cincinnati for Devel Disorders
Dietetic Internship Prgm
Children's Hospital Med Ctr
Elland & Bethesda Aves
Cincinnati, OH 45229-2899
Prgm Dir: Shirley M Ekvall, PhD RD LD
Tel: 513 559-4614

Univ of Cincinnati
Dietetics-Didactic Prgm
Dietetics and Nutri Education
PO 210022/504 Dyer Hall
Cincinnati, OH 45221
Prgm Dir: Bonnie J Brehm, PhD RD LD
Tel: 513 556-3853

University of Cincinnati Hospital
Dietetic Internship Prgm
234 Goodman St
Cincinnati, OH 45267-0716
Prgm Dir: Ray Anne Best, MS RD LD
Tel: 513 558-4543

Case-Western Reserve University
Dietetics-Didactic Prgm
Dept of Nutrition
Cleveland, OH 44106-4906
Prgm Dir: Janice N Neville, DSc RD LD MPH
Tel: 216 368-3231

Case-Western Reserve University
Dietetic Internship Prgm
Dept of Nutrition-201
10900 Euclid Ave
Cleveland, OH 44106-1712
Prgm Dir: Isabel M Parraga, PhD RD LD
Tel: 216 368-2440

Cleveland Clinic Foundation
Dietetic Internship Prgm
Nutrition Services M17
9500 Euclid Ave
Cleveland, OH 44195-5146
Prgm Dir: Sue Kent, MS RD LD
Tel: 216 444-6487

Cleveland Veterans Affairs Med Ctr
Dietetic Internship Prgm
10701 E Blvd
Cleveland, OH 44106-1702
Prgm Dir: Anne Raguso, PhD RD
Tel: 216 421-3028

MetroHealth Medical Center
Dietetic Internship Prgm
2500 MetroHealth Dr
Cleveland, OH 44109-1998
Prgm Dir: Sharon C Borg-Madura, MS
Tel: 216 778-5316

University Hospitals of Cleveland
Dietetic Internship Prgm
11000 Euclid Ave
Cleveland, OH 44106-2602
Prgm Dir: Bonnie Rigutto, MEd RD LD CNSD
Tel: 216 844-3323

Mt Carmel College of Nursing
Dietetic Internship Prgm
127 S Davis Ave
Columbus, OH 43222-1504
Prgm Dir: Kathleen M Blanchard, MS RD LD
Tel: 614 234-5800

Ohio State University
Preprofessional Practice Prgm
Human Nutri & Food Mgmt
1787 Neil Ave
Columbus, OH 43210-1295
Prgm Dir: Alma M Saddam, PhD RD LD
Tel: 614 292-5512

Ohio State University
Dietetics-Coordinated Prgm
Sch of Allied Medical Profs
1583 Perry St
Columbus, OH 43210-1234
Prgm Dir: M Rosita Schiller, PhD RD
Tel: 614 292-0635

Ohio State University
Dietetic Internship Prgm
Schl of Allied Medical Profs
Med Dietetics/1583 Perry St
Columbus, OH 43210-1234
Prgm Dir: M Rosita Schiller, PhD RD LD
Tel: 614 292-0635

Ohio State University
Dietetics-Didactic Prgm
Human Nutrition & Food Mgmt
1787 Neil Ave
Columbus, OH 43210-1220
Prgm Dir: Mary C Mitchell, PhD RD
Tel: 614 292-8189

Riverside Methodist Hospitals
Dietetic Internship Prgm
3535 Olentangy River Rd
Columbus, OH 43214-3925
Prgm Dir: Patricia A Lubas, MS RD LD
Tel: 614 566-5346

Miami Valley Hospital
Dietetic Internship Prgm
1 Wyoming St
Dayton, OH 45409-2793
Prgm Dir: Rebecca M Lee, MS RD LD
Tel: 513 208-2448

University of Dayton
Dietetics-Didactic Prgm
Food & Nutrition Prgm
300 College Park Ave
Dayton, OH 45469-2335
Prgm Dir: Julie Palmert, MS RD LD
Tel: 513 229-2711

Kent State University
Dietetics-Didactic Prgm
Family and Consumer Studies
Nixon Hall/Nutri & Dietetics
Kent, OH 44242
Prgm Dir: Karen Lowry Gordon, PhD RD LD
Tel: 216 672-2248

Miami University
Dietetics-Didactic Prgm
Phys Ed Hlth & Sports Studies
18 Phillips Hall
Oxford, OH 45056
Prgm Dir: Susan J Rudge, PhD RD LD
Tel: 513 529-5036

Notre Dame College
Dietetics-Didactic Prgm
4545 College Rd
South Euclid, OH 44121-4293
Prgm Dir: Annette Pedersen, MS RD LD CDE
Tel: 216 381-1680

Youngstown State University
Dietetics-Didactic Prgm
Human Ecology Dept
410 Wick Ave
Youngstown, OH 44555-0001
Prgm Dir: Raj N Varma, PhD RD LD
Tel: 330 742-3346

Youngstown State University
Dietetics-Coordinated Prgm
410 Wick Ave
Youngstown, OH 44555-0001
Prgm Dir: Jean Hassell, MS RD LD
Tel: 330 742-1822

Oklahoma

University of Central Oklahoma
Dietetic Internship Prgm
Human Environmental Sciences
Edmond, OK 73034
Prgm Dir: Valerie B Knotts, EdD RD LD
Tel: 405 341-2980

University of Central Oklahoma
Dietetics-Didactic Prgm
College of Education
Human Environmental Sciences
Edmond, OK 73034
Prgm Dir: Valerie B Knotts, EdD RD LD
Tel: 405 341-2980

Langston University
Dietetics-Didactic Prgm
Dept of Home Ecology
308/304 Jones Hall
Langston, OK 73050
Prgm Dir: Saigeetha Sangiah, PhD RD LD
Tel: 405 466-3340

Univ of Oklahoma Health Sciences Center
Dietetics-Coordinated Prgm
Dept of Nutritional Sciences
PO Box 26901
Oklahoma City, OK 73190
Prgm Dir: Rachel S Barkley, MS RD LD
Tel: 405 271-2113

Univ of Oklahoma Health Sciences Center
Dietetics-Didactic Prgm
Nutritional Sci POB 26901
801 NE 13th St Rm 465
Oklahoma City, OK 73190-5005
Prgm Dir: Rachel S Barkely, MS RD LD
Tel: 405 271-2113

Univ of Oklahoma Health Sciences Center
Dietetic Internship Prgm
Dept of Nurtitional Sciences
PO Box 26901 CHB
Oklahoma City, OK 73190
Prgm Dir: Kathy Onley, PhD RD LD
Tel: 405 271-2113

Oklahoma State University Main Campus
Dietetic Internship Prgm
Dept of Nutritional Sciences
HES 425
Stillwater, OK 74078-0337
Prgm Dir: Lea L Ebro, PhD RD LD
Tel: 405 744-8294

Oklahoma State University Main Campus
Dietetics-Didactic Prgm
Nutritional Sciences Dept
425 HES
Stillwater, OK 74078-6141
Prgm Dir: Barbara J Stoecker, PhD RD LD
Tel: 405 744-5041

Northeastern State University
Dietetics-Didactic Prgm
Coll of Business & Industry
Tahlequah, OK 74464-2399
Prgm Dir: M Susie Williams, MS RD LD
Tel: 918 456-5511

Oregon

Oregon State University
Dietetics-Didactic Prgm
Nutrition and Food Mgmt
Milam Hall 108
Corvallis, OR 97331-5103
Prgm Dir: Mary Cluskey, PhD RD
Tel: 503 737-0960

Oregon Health Sciences University

Dietetic Internship Prgm
VAMC EJH-10
3181 SW Sam Jackson Park Rd
Portland, OR 97201-1034
Prgm Dir: Dorothy W Hagan, PhD RD
Tel: 503 494-7596

Mid Willamette Vlly Dietetec Internship

Dietetic Internship Prgm
Capital Manor Retirement Comm
1955 Dallas Hwy NW/Ste 1200
Salem, OR 97304
Prgm Dir: Nancy Dunton, PhD RD
Tel: 503 362-4101

Pennsylvania

Cedar Crest College

Dietetics-Didactic Prgm
The Allen Center for Nutrition
100 College Dr
Allentown, PA 18104-6132
Prgm Dir: Patricia Wenner, MS RD
Tel: 610 437-4471

The Wood Company

Preprofessional Practice Prgm
PO Box 3501
6081 Hamilton Blvd
Allentown, PA 18106-0501
Prgm Dir: Monica F Pyzia, MS RD
Tel: 610 395-3800

Geisinger Medical Center

Dietetic Internship Prgm
100 N Academy Ave
Danville, PA 17822-0123
Prgm Dir: Cynthia M Brylinsky, MS RD CNSD
Tel: 717 271-6237

Edinboro University of Pennsylvania

Dietetics-Coordinated Prgm
Biology and Health Services
Edinboro, PA 16444
Prgm Dir: Sally J Lanz, MS RD
Tel: 814 732-2447

Gannon University

Dietetics-Coordinated Prgm
Sciences Engineering and Hlth Science
109 University Square
Erie, PA 16541-0001
Prgm Dir: Dawna T Mughal, PhD RD
Tel: 814 871-5452

Mercyhurst College

Dietetics-Coordinated Prgm
Dept of Human Ecology
Glenwood Hills
Erie, PA 16546
Prgm Dir: Charlene Glispy, MS RD
Tel: 814 824-2462

Messiah College

Dietetics-Didactic Prgm
Dept of Natural Sciences
Grantham, PA 17027
Prgm Dir: Mary Ann Mihok, MS RD
Tel: 717 766-2511

Seton Hill College

Dietetics-Coordinated Prgm
Family and Consumer Sciences
Greensburg, PA 15601-1599
Prgm Dir: Janice G Sandrick, PhD RD
Tel: 412 830-1045

Immaculata College

Dietetics-Didactic Prgm
Fashion Foods & Nutrition
Box 722
Immaculata, PA 19345-0722
Prgm Dir: Marion Jeanne Bell, MS RD
Tel: 610 647-4400

Immaculata College

Dietetic Internship Prgm
Nutrition Educ
Graduate Div
Immaculata, PA 19345
Prgm Dir: Susan Johnston, MS RD
Tel: 610 647-4400

Indiana University of Pennsylvania

Dietetic Internship Prgm
Dept of Food & Nutrition
10 Ackerman Hall
Indiana, PA 15705-1087
Prgm Dir: Joanne B Steiner, PhD RD
Tel: 412 357-4440

Indiana University of Pennsylvania

Dietetics-Didactic Prgm
Dept of Food & Nutrition
10 Ackerman Hall
Indiana, PA 15705-1087
Prgm Dir: Joanne B Steiner, PhD RD
Tel: 412 357-4440

Johnstown Area/Lee Hospital

Dietetic Internship Prgm
320 Main St
Johnstown, PA 15901-1601
Prgm Dir: Cynthia M Risinger, MS RD
Tel: 814 533-0776

Mansfield University

Dietetics-Didactic Prgm
Simon B Elliott Hall
Dept of Health Sciences
Mansfield, PA 16933
Prgm Dir: Kathy Wright, MS RD
Tel: 717 662-4628

Drexel University

Dietetics-Didactic Prgm
Nutrition and Food Sciences
32nd and Chestnut Sts
Philadelphia, PA 19104-2875
Prgm Dir: Shortie McKinney, PhD RD FADA
Tel: 215 895-2417

Family Health Council Inc

Dietetic Internship Prgm
625 Stanwix St
Pittsburgh, PA 15222-1417
Prgm Dir: Karen A Virostek, MS RD
Tel: 412 288-2130

Marriott Health Care Svcs/St Francis Med Ctr

Preprofessional Practice Prgm
Nutrition Service Dept
45th and Penn Aves
Pittsburgh, PA 15201
Prgm Dir: Sheila B Kelly, MS RD
Tel: 412 622-4173

Shadyside Hospital

Dietetic Internship Prgm
5230 Centre Ave
Pittsburgh, PA 15232-1304
Prgm Dir: Joyce M Scott-Smith, MS RD
Tel: 412 623-2114

University of Pittsburgh

Dietetics-Coordinated Prgm
Health and Rehab Sciences
Forbes Tower Rm 4052
Pittsburgh, PA 15260-1802
Prgm Dir: Regina M Onda, PhD RD
Tel: 412 647-1201

University of Pittsburgh

Dietetics-Didactic Prgm
Health and Rehab Science
Forbes Tower/Rm 4052
Pittsburgh, PA 15260-1802
Prgm Dir: Regina M Onda, PhD RD
Tel: 412 647-1201

Marywood College

Dietetics-Coordinated Prgm
Dept of Nutrition and Dietetics
2300 Adams Ave
Scranton, PA 18509-1598
Prgm Dir: Marianne E Borja, EdD RD FADA
Tel: 717 348-6277

Marywood College

Dietetics-Didactic Prgm
Dept of Nutrition and Dietetics
2300 Adams Ave
Scranton, PA 18509-1514
Prgm Dir: Gina Sylvester, MS RD
Tel: 717 348-6211, Ext 2632

Marywood College

Dietetic Internship Prgm
Dept of Nutrition and Dietetics
Scranton, PA 18509
Prgm Dir: Lee Harrison, PhD RD FADA
Tel: 717 348-6211

Penn State University - Main Campus

Dietetics-Didactic Prgm
Nutrition Dept
Coll of Hlth & Human Devel
University Park, PA 16802-6500
Prgm Dir: Penny Kris-Etherton, PhD RD
Tel: 814 863-2923

Puerto Rico

Puerto Rico Department of Health

Dietetic Internship Prgm
PO Box 70184
San Juan, PR 00936
Prgm Dir: Ana E Rivera, MS RD
Tel: 787 274-6831

Programs

University of Puerto Rico
Dietetic Internship Prgm
College of Hlth Related Profs
Med Sci Campus PO Box 365067
San Juan, PR 00936-5067
Prgm Dir: Rita L Delgado, ME RD
Tel: 787 758-2525

University of Puerto Rico
Dietetics-Didactic Prgm
Box 23347 UPR Station
Rio Piedras Campus
San Juan, PR 00931-3347
Prgm Dir: Carmen Alcaraz, MS RD
Tel: 787 763-6599

Veterans Affairs Medical Center
Dietetic Internship Prgm
One Veterans Plaza
San Juan, PR 00927-5800
Prgm Dir: Carmen L De Balado, MS RD
Tel: 787 758-7575

Rhode Island

University of Rhode Island
Dietetics-Didactic Prgm
Food Science & Nutrition
17 Woodward Hall
Kingston, RI 02881-0804
Prgm Dir: Catherine English, PhD RD LDN
Tel: 401 874-5869

University of Rhode Island
Preprofessional Practice Prgm
Food Science & Nutrition
Kingston, RI 02881
Prgm Dir: Geoffrey W Greene, PhD RD
Tel: 401 792-2466

South Carolina

Medical University of South Carolina
Dietetic Internship Prgm
308 Wachovia Bank Bldg
171 Ashley Ave
Charleston, SC 29425
Prgm Dir: Joanne Milkereit, MHSA RD
Tel: 803 792-1454

Clemson University
Dietetics-Didactic Prgm
Box 340371
Clemson, SC 29634-0371
Prgm Dir: M Elizabeth Kunkel, PhD RD
Tel: 864 656-5690

So Carolina Hlth & Environmental Control
Dietetic Internship Prgm
Mills Complex
PO Box 101106
Columbia, SC 29211-0106
Prgm Dir: Phyllis Allen, MPHN RD
Tel: 803 737-3954

South Carolina State University
Dietetics-Didactic Prgm
Staley Hall PO Box 7084
300 College Ave
Orangeburg, SC 29117-0001
Prgm Dir: Juanita Bowens, PhD RD
Tel: 803 536-8620

Winthrop University
Dietetics-Didactic Prgm
Dept of Human Nutrition
Rock Hill, SC 29733
Prgm Dir: Sarah F Stallings, PhD RD
Tel: 803 323-2101

Winthrop University
Dietetic Internship Prgm
Dept of Human Nutrition
Rock Hill, SC 29733
Prgm Dir: Patricia Giblin Wolman, EdD RD
Tel: 803 323-2101

South Dakota

South Dakota State University
Dietetics-Didactic Prgm
Family and Consumer Sciences
PO Box 2275A
Brookings, SD 57007-0497
Prgm Dir: Madeleine S Rose, PhD RD
Tel: 605 688-4041

University of South Dakota
Preprofessional Practice Prgm
School of Medicine
414 E Clark St
Vermillion, SD 57069-2390
Prgm Dir: Gail Johannsen, MS RD
Tel: 605 677-5311

Mt Marty College
Dietetics-Didactic Prgm
Nutrition & Food Science
1105 W 8th St
Yankton, SD 57078-3724
Prgm Dir: Thecla Holzbauer, MS RD
Tel: 605 668-1520

Tennessee

University of Tennessee at Chattanooga
Dietetics-Didactic Prgm
Dept of Human Ecology
202 Hunter Hall
Chattanooga, TN 37403
Prgm Dir: Patricia M Garrett, MS RD LDN
Tel: 423 755-4792

Tennessee Technological University
Dietetics-Didactic Prgm
School of Home Economics
Box 5035
Cookeville, TN 38505
Prgm Dir: Cathy Hix Cunningham, PhD RD LDN
Tel: 615 372-3376

Carson-Newman College
Dietetics-Didactic Prgm
PO Box 71881
Jefferson City, TN 37760-7001
Prgm Dir: Kitty R Coffey, PhD RD LDN CFCS
Tel: 423 471-3295

East Tennessee State University
Dietetics-Didactic Prgm
Applied Human Sciences
PO Box 70671
Johnson City, TN 37614-0671
Prgm Dir: Kenneth D James, PhD RD LD
Tel: 423 439-4411

East Tennessee State University
Dietetic Internship Prgm
Applied Human Sciences
PO Box 70671
Johnson City, TN 37614-0671
Prgm Dir: Martha A Raidl, PhD RD
Tel: 423 439-4409

University of Tennessee - Knoxville
Dietetics-Didactic Prgm
Dept of Nutrition
1215 Cumberland Ave Rm 229
Knoxville, TN 37996-1900
Prgm Dir: Jean Skinner, PhD RD
Tel: 615 974-5445

University of Tennessee - Knoxville
Dietetic Internship Prgm
Human Ecology/Dept of Nutri
1215 Cumberland Ave
Knoxville, TN 37996-1900
Prgm Dir: Karen A Balnicki, MS RD LDN
Tel: 423 974-5445

University of Tennessee at Martin
Dietetics-Didactic Prgm
Human Environmental Sciences
Rm 340 Gooch Hall
Martin, TN 38238-5045
Prgm Dir: Anne L Cook, PhD RD LDN CHE
Tel: 901 587-7100

University of Tennessee at Martin
Dietetic Internship Prgm
Human Environmental Sciences
Rm 340 Gooch Hall
Martin, TN 38238-5045
Prgm Dir: Mary E Mohs, PhD RD
Tel: 901 587-7100

University of Memphis
Dietetic Internship Prgm
Consumer Science and Education
Manning Hall
Memphis, TN 38152
Prgm Dir: Mary Ann Smith, PhD RD LDN
Tel: 901 678-2301

University of Memphis
Dietetics-Didactic Prgm
Consumer Science and Education
Memphis, TN 38152
Prgm Dir: Robin Roach, EdD RD
Tel: 901 678-3110

Middle Tennessee State University
Dietetics-Didactic Prgm
Dept of Human Sciences
PO Box 86
Murfreesboro, TN 37133-0086
Prgm Dir: Dellmar Walker, PhD RD LDN
Tel: 615 898-2091

National HealthCare LP
Dietetic Internship Prgm
PO Box 1398
Murfreesboro, TN 37133-1398
Prgm Dir: Patty T Poe, MEd RD LDN
Tel: 615 890-2020

David Lipscomb University

Dietetics-Didactic Prgm
Family & Consumer Sciences
3901 Granny White Pike
Nashville, TN 37204-3951
Prgm Dir: Nancy Hunt, MS MEd RD
Tel: 615 269-1000

Tennessee State University

Dietetics-Didactic Prgm
Family and Consumer Sciences/PO Box 9535
3500 John A Merritt Blvd
Nashville, TN 37209-1561
Prgm Dir: Sandria L Godwin, PhD RD LD
Tel: 615 963-5619

Vanderbilt University Medical Center

Dietetic Internship Prgm
B-802TVC
1301 22nd Ave S
Nashville, TN 37232-5510
Prgm Dir: Cynthia B Broadhurst, MS RD
Tel: 615 322-0062

Texas

Abilene Christian University

Dietetics-Didactic Prgm
Family & Consumer Sciences
ACU Box 8155
Abilene, TX 79699
Prgm Dir: Christine Crowson, MS RD
Tel: 915 674-2089

University of Texas at Austin

Dietetics-Didactic Prgm
Dept of Human Ecology
GEA 117
Austin, TX 78712
Prgm Dir: Jane F Tillman, MS RD
Tel: 512 471-7639

University of Texas at Austin

Dietetics-Coordinated Prgm
Dept of Human Ecology
A2700
Austin, TX 78712-1097
Prgm Dir: Beth Gillham, PhD RD LD
Tel: 512 471-4934

Lamar Univ Institute of Tech - Beaumont

Preprofessional Practice Prgm
Family and Consumer Sciences
PO Box 10035
Beaumont, TX 77710-0035
Prgm Dir: Amy Pemberton, PhD RD LD
Tel: 409 880-8663

Lamar Univ Institute of Tech - Beaumont

Dietetics-Didactic Prgm
Family and Consumer Sciences
PO Box 10035
Beaumont, TX 77710-0035
Prgm Dir: Connie Elliff, MS RD
Tel: 409 880-8663

Texas A & M University

Dietetic Internship Prgm
Dept of Animal Science
Human Nutrition Section
College Station, TX 77843-2471
Prgm Dir: Carolyn Bailey, MS RD LD
Tel: 409 845-2142

Texas A & M University

Dietetics-Didactic Prgm
Human Nutrition Section
Dept of Animal Science
College Station, TX 77843-2471
Prgm Dir: Karen S Kubena, PhD RD LD
Tel: 409 845-2142

Baylor University Medical Center

Dietetic Internship Prgm
3500 Gaston Ave
Dallas, TX 75246-2045
Prgm Dir: Linda S Blue, MS RD LD FADA
Tel: 214 820-4019

Presbyterian Hospital of Dallas

Dietetic Internship Prgm
8200 Walnut Hill Ln
Dallas, TX 75231-4402
Prgm Dir: Barbara Taylor, MA RD LD
Tel: 214 345-7558

Univ of Tx Southwestern Med Ctr - Dallas

Dietetics-Coordinated Prgm
Dept of Clinical Nutrition
5323 Harry Hines Blvd
Dallas, TX 75235-8877
Prgm Dir: Jo Ann S Carson, MS RD LD
Tel: 214 648-1520

Texas Woman's University

Dietetics-Didactic Prgm
Nutrition & Food Sciences
TWU Station 425888
Denton, TX 76204-3888
Prgm Dir: Betty Alford, PhD RD LD
Tel: 817 898-2636

Texas Woman's University

Dietetic Internship Prgm
Nutrition & Food Sciences
PO Box 425888
Denton, TX 76204-3888
Prgm Dir: Martha L Rew, MS RD LD
Tel: 817 898-2636

Univ of Texas - Pan American

Dietetics-Coordinated Prgm
1201 W University Dr
Edinburg, TX 78539-2999
Prgm Dir: Alexander O Edionwe, PhD RD
Tel: 210 381-2294

Brooke Army Medical Center

Dietetic Internship Prgm
Nutrition Care Div
3851 Roger Brooke Dr
Ft Sam Houston, TX 78234-6306
Prgm Dir: Lt Col Robin Tefft, DrPH RD
Tel: 210 916-3372

Texas Christian University

Dietetics-Coordinated Prgm
Dept of Nutrition & Dietetics
TCU Box 298600
Ft Worth, TX 76129
Prgm Dir: Mary Anne Gorman, PhD RD LD
Tel: 817 921-7309

Texas Christian University

Dietetics-Didactic Prgm
Dept of Nutrition & Dietetics
Box 298600
Ft Worth, TX 76129
Prgm Dir: Anne VanBeber, PhD RD LD
Tel: 817 921-7309

Texas Southern University

Dietetics-Didactic Prgm
Human Svcs and Consumer Sci
3100 Cleburne Ave
Houston, TX 77004-4575
Prgm Dir: Oddis C Turner, DrPH RD LD CHE
Tel: 713 313-7699

Texas Woman's University

Dietetic Internship Prgm
1130 M D Anderson Blvd
Houston, TX 77030-2897
Prgm Dir: Rose M Bush, MS RD
Tel: 713 794-2376

Univ of Texas Hlth Sci Ctr at Houston

Dietetic Internship Prgm
Sch of Public Hlth/E619 RAS Bldg
1200 Herman Pressler Dr
Houston, TX 77030
Prgm Dir: Jeanne Martin, PhD RD LD
Tel: 713 500-9347

University of Houston

Dietetic Internship Prgm
Human Devel and Consumer Sci
4800 Calhoun
Houston, TX 77204-6861
Prgm Dir: Clint Stevens, MSc RD
Tel: 713 743-4110

University of Houston

Dietetics-Didactic Prgm
Human Devel and Consumer Sci
4800 Calhoun Rd
Houston, TX 77204-0096
Prgm Dir: Jenna DeBaun Anding, PhD RD LD
Tel: 713 743-4120

Veterans Affairs Medical Center

Dietetic Internship Prgm
2002 Holcombe Blvd
Houston, TX 77030-4298
Prgm Dir: Sydney R Morrow, PhD RD
Tel: 713 794-7120

Sam Houston State University

Dietetics-Didactic Prgm
Food Science & Nutrition
Huntsville, TX 77341
Prgm Dir: Zaheer Kirmani, PhD RD LD
Tel: 409 294-1242

Texas A & M University - Kingsville

Dietetics-Didactic Prgm
Dept of Human Sciences
Campus Box 168
Kingsville, TX 78363
Prgm Dir: Gloria Fernandez-Van Zante, MS RD LD
Tel: 512 595-2211

Texas A & M University - Kingsville
Dietetic Internship Prgm
Dept of Human Sciences
Campus Box 168
Kingsville, TX 78363
Prgm Dir: Sandra D Simons, PhD RD LD
Tel: 512 595-2211

Texas Tech Univ Hlth Sci Ctr
Dietetics-Didactic Prgm
Educ Nutri & Rest Hotel Mgmt
PO Box 41162
Lubbock, TX 79409-1162
Prgm Dir: Mallory Boylan, PhD RD LD
Tel: 806 742-3068

Texas Tech Univ Hlth Sci Ctr
Dietetic Internship Prgm
College of Human Sciences
PO Box 41162
Lubbock, TX 79409-1162
Prgm Dir: Elizabeth A Fox, PhD RD LD
Tel: 806 742-3068

Stephen F Austin State University
Dietetics-Didactic Prgm
Dept of Human Sciences
PO Box 13014 SFA Station
Nacogdoches, TX 75962-3014
Prgm Dir: Suzy Weems, PhD RD LD
Tel: 409 468-2060

Stephen F Austin State University
Preprofessional Practice Prgm
SFA Station 13014
Nacogdoches, TX 75962-3014
Prgm Dir: Donna-Jean Hunt, MS RD
Tel: 409 468-4502

Prairie View A & M University
Dietetic Internship Prgm
Box 4329
Prairie View, TX 77446
Prgm Dir: Sharon McWhinney, PhD RD LD
Tel: 409 857-4417

Prairie View A & M University
Dietetics-Didactic Prgm
Dept of Human Sciences
PO Box 4329
Prairie View, TX 77446-4329
Prgm Dir: Sharon McWhinney, PhD RD LD
Tel: 409 857-4417

University of the Incarnate Word
Dietetics-Didactic Prgm
4301 Broadway St
San Antonio, TX 78209-6318
Prgm Dir: Mary Kaye Sawyer-Morse, MS RD
Tel: 210 829-3167

University of the Incarnate Word
Dietetic Internship Prgm
4301 Broadway T-2
San Antonio, TX 78209
Prgm Dir: Joseph C Bonilla, PhD RD
Tel: 210 829-3908

Southwest Texas State University
Dietetics-Didactic Prgm
Family & Consumer Sciences
San Marcos, TX 78666-4616
Prgm Dir: G Sue Thompson, PhD RD LD
Tel: 512 245-2483

Southwest Texas State University
Dietetic Internship Prgm
Family and Consumer Sciences
601 University Dr
San Marcos, TX 78666-4616
Prgm Dir: B J Friedman, PhD RD LD
Tel: 512 245-2155

Tarleton State University
Dietetics-Didactic Prgm
Dept of Human Sciences
Mailstop TO380
Stephenville, TX 76402
Prgm Dir: Janet Miles-Maestas, MA RD LD
Tel: 817 968-9196

Baylor University
Dietetics-Didactic Prgm
Family and Consumer Sciences
BU Box 97346
Waco, TX 76798-7346
Prgm Dir: LuAnn Soliah, PhD RD LD
Tel: 817 755-3626

Utah

Utah State University
Dietetics-Coordinated Prgm
Nutrition and Food Science
Logan, UT 84322-8700
Prgm Dir: Noreen B Schvaneveldt, MS RD CD
Tel: 801 797-2105

Brigham Young University
Dietetics-Didactic Prgm
Food Science and Nutrition
2218 SFLC
Provo, UT 84602-1041
Prgm Dir: Nora Nyland, PhD RD CD
Tel: 801 378-3912

Brigham Young University
Dietetics-Coordinated Prgm
Food Science and Nutrition
2218 SFLC
Provo, UT 84602-6799
Prgm Dir: Nora Nyland, PhD RD CD
Tel: 801 378-3912

University of Utah
Dietetics-Coordinated Prgm
College of Health
Foods & Nutrition 239N-HPR
Salt Lake City, UT 84112
Prgm Dir: Laurie J Moyer-Mileur, PhD RD CD
Tel: 801 581-6730

Veterans Affairs Medical Center (120D)
Dietetic Internship Prgm
500 Foothill Blvd
Salt Lake City, UT 84148-0001
Prgm Dir: Ann Martin Mildenhall, MS RD CD
Tel: 801 582-1565

Vermont

Fletcher Allen Health Care
Dietetic Internship Prgm
MCHV Campus Nutrition Svcs
111 Colchester Ave
Burlington, VT 05401
Prgm Dir: Michael Kanfer, MBA RD
Tel: 802 656-3640

University of Vermont
Dietetics-Didactic Prgm
Dept of Nutritional Sciences
Terrill Hall
Burlington, VT 05405
Prgm Dir: Jane K Ross, PhD RD
Tel: 802 656-0539

Virginia

Virginia Polytechnic Inst & State Univ
Dietetic Internship Prgm
338 Wallace Hall
Blacksburg, VA 24061-0430
Prgm Dir: Carol Papillon, MPH RD
Tel: 540 231-5549

Virginia Polytechnic Inst & State Univ
Dietetics-Didactic Prgm
Human Nutrition & Foods
College Human Resources
Blacksburg, VA 24061-0430
Prgm Dir: Eleanor D Schlenker, PhD RD
Tel: 540 231-4672

Univ of Virginia Health Sciences Center
Dietetic Internship Prgm
Dietetic Education
Box 273-59
Charlottesville, VA 22908
Prgm Dir: Ana Abad Sinden, MS RD CNSD
Tel: 804 924-2286

Hampton University
Preprofessional Practice Prgm
Dept of Human Ecology
Hampton, VA 23668
Prgm Dir: Henri E Pate, PhD RD
Tel: 804 727-5273

Hampton University
Dietetics-Didactic Prgm
Dept of Human Ecology
Hampton, VA 23668
Prgm Dir: Henri E Pate, PhD RD CHE
Tel: 804 727-5273

James Madison University
Dietetics-Didactic Prgm
Dept of Health Sciences
Moody Hall 102
Harrisonburg, VA 22807
Prgm Dir: Patricia B Brevard, PhD RD
Tel: 540 568-6510

James Madison University
Dietetic Internship Prgm
Dept of Health Sciences
Harrisonburg, VA 22807
Prgm Dir: Janet W Gloeckner, PhD RD
Tel: 540 568-7084

Norfolk State University
Dietetics-Didactic Prgm
Food Sci & Nutri Chem/Physics
2401 Corprew Ave
Norfolk, VA 23504-3907
Prgm Dir: Mary Linda Allen, MS RD
Tel: 757 683-9532

Virginia State University
Dietetic Internship Prgm
PO Box 9211
Petersburg, VA 23806
Prgm Dir: Gloria Young, EdD MS RD
Tel: 804 524-5502

Virginia State University
Dietetics-Didactic Prgm
Dept of Human Ecology
Box 9211
Petersburg, VA 23806
Prgm Dir: Gloria Young, EdD RD
Tel: 804 524-5761

Radford University
Dietetics-Didactic Prgm
Dept of Health Services
PO Box 6962
Radford, VA 24142-5826
Prgm Dir: Barbara McChrisley, PhD RD MT
Tel: 540 831-5542

Med Coll of VA/Virginia Commonwealth U
Dietetic Internship Prgm
PO Box 980294
Richmond, VA 23298-0294
Prgm Dir: Ann E Robbins, MS RD
Tel: 804 828-9108

Virginia Department of Health
Preprofessional Practice Prgm
Div of Public Hlth Nutrition
1500 E Main St Rm 132
Richmond, VA 23219
Prgm Dir: Margaret Tate, MS RD
Tel: 804 371-6298

Washington

Bastyr University
Dietetics-Didactic Prgm
14500 Juanita Dr NE
Bothell, WA 98011
Prgm Dir: Suzzanne N Myer, MS RD
Tel: 206 823-1300

Bastyr University
Dietetic Internship Prgm
Nutrition Program
14500 Juanita Dr NE
Bothell, WA 98011
Prgm Dir: Suzzanne Nelson Myer, MS RD
Tel: 206 523-9585

Central Washington University
Dietetic Internship Prgm
Family and Consumer Sciences
400 E 8th Ave
Ellensburg, WA 98929-7565
Prgm Dir: Ethan Bergman, PhD RD CD
Tel: 509 963-2366

Central Washington University
Dietetics-Didactic Prgm
Family and Consumer Sciences
Ellensburg, WA 98926-7566
Prgm Dir: Ethan A Bergman, PhD RD
Tel: 509 963-2366

Washington State University
Dietetics-Coordinated Prgm
FSHN Bldg 108
Pullman, WA 99164-6376
Prgm Dir: Dorothy Pond-Smith, PhD RD
Tel: 509 335-1395

Washington State University
Dietetics-Didactic Prgm
Food Sci & Human Nutrition
Pullman, WA 99164-6376
Prgm Dir: Cindy Heiss, PhD RD
Tel: 509 335-8448

Sea Mar Community Health Center
Dietetic Internship Prgm
8720 14th Ave S
Seattle, WA 98108-4807
Prgm Dir: Janet Leader, MPH RD
Tel: 206 762-3730

Seattle Pacific University
Dietetics-Didactic Prgm
Human Environmental Sciences
3307 3rd Ave W
Seattle, WA 98119-1997
Prgm Dir: Evette M Hackman, PhD RD
Tel: 206 281-2708

University of Washington
Dietetics-Didactic Prgm (Master's Only)
305 Raitt Hall
Box 353410
Seattle, WA 98195-3410
Prgm Dir: Joan M Karkeck, MS RD CD
Tel: 206 543-1730

University of Washington
Dietetic Internship Prgm
DL-10
Seattle, WA 98195
Prgm Dir: Joan M Karkeck, MS MA RD
Tel: 206 543-9191

Washington State University
Dietetic Internship Prgm
Food Sci & Human Nutrition
601 W First Ave
Spokane, WA 99204-0399
Prgm Dir: Alice A Opryszek, MS RD
Tel: 509 358-7621

West Virginia

West Virginia Wesleyan College
Dietetics-Didactic Prgm
Dept of Human Ecology
Haymond Hall 215E/PO Box 15
Buckhannon, WV 26201-0015
Prgm Dir: Lillian S Halverson, PhD RD
Tel: 304 473-8379

Marshall University
Dietetics-Didactic Prgm
Family and Consumer Science
Huntington, WV 25755-2460
Prgm Dir: Jane U Edwards, PhD RD
Tel: 304 696-2507

Marshall University
Dietetic Internship Prgm
Corbly Hall 203 Home Econ
400 Hal Greer Blvd
Huntington, WV 25755
Prgm Dir: Susan C Linnenkohl, PhD RD
Tel: 304 696-6641

West Virginia University
Dietetic Internship Prgm
Coll of Agriculture and Forestry
PO Box 6124
Morgantown, WV 26506-6124
Prgm Dir: Betty J Forbes, MA RD
Tel: 304 293-3402

West Virginia University
Dietetics-Didactic Prgm
Coll of Agriculture and Forestry
Allen Hall PO Box 6124
Morgantown, WV 26506-6124
Prgm Dir: Betty J Forbes, MA RD
Tel: 304 293-3402

West Virginia University Hospitals, Inc
Dietetic Internship Prgm
Dept 8016
Nutrition & Dietetics
Morgantown, WV 26506-8016
Prgm Dir: Susan J Arnold, MS RD
Tel: 304 598-4105

Wisconsin

University of Wisconsin - Green Bay
Dietetics-Didactic Prgm
Human Biology Dept
2420 Nicolet Dr
Green Bay, WI 54311-7001
Prgm Dir: Andrea Wang, PhD RD
Tel: 414 465-2681

University of Wisconsin - Green Bay
Preprofessional Practice Prgm
2420 Nicolet Dr
Green Bay, WI 54311-7001
Prgm Dir: Karen Lacey
Tel: 414 465-2681

Viterbo College
Dietetic Internship Prgm
Nutrition and Dietetics Dept
815 S 9th St
La Crosse, WI 54601-4797
Prgm Dir: Lorraine C Lewis, MS RD
Tel: 608 796-3660

Viterbo College
Dietetics-Coordinated Prgm
Nutrition and Dietetics Dept
815 S 9th St
La Crosse, WI 54601-4797
Prgm Dir: Lorraine C Lewis, MS RD
Tel: 608 796-3660

University of Wisconsin - Madison

Dietetics-Didactic Prgm
Dept of Nutritional Sciences
1415 Linden Dr
Madison, WI 53706-1571
Prgm Dir: Denise M Ney, PhD RD
Tel: 608 262-4386

University of Wisconsin - Madison

Dietetics-Coordinated Prgm
Dept of Nutritional Sciences
1415 Linden Dr
Madison, WI 53706-1571
Prgm Dir: Lynette M Karls, MS RD
Tel: 608 262-5847

University of Wisconsin Hosp & Clinics

Preprofessional Practice Prgm
Food and Nutrition Services
F4/120 600 Highland Ave
Madison, WI 53792-0001
Prgm Dir: Marjorie U Morgan, MS RD
Tel: 608 263-8237

University of Wisconsin Hosp & Clinics

Dietetic Internship Prgm
Food and Nutrition Services F4/120
600 Highland Ave
Madison, WI 53792-0001
Prgm Dir: Marjorie Morgan, MS RD
Tel: 608 263-8237

University of Wisconsin - Stout

Dietetic Internship Prgm
220 Home Economics Bldg
Dept of Food & Nutrition
Menomonie, WI 54751
Prgm Dir: Barbara L Knous, PhD RD
Tel: 715 232-1994

University of Wisconsin - Stout

Dietetics-Didactic Prgm
School of Home Economics
Menomonie, WI 54751
Prgm Dir: Joy A Jocelyn, PhD RD
Tel: 715 232-1175

Mt Mary College

Preprofessional Practice Prgm
Graduate Program in Dietetics
2900 N Menomonee River Pkwy
Milwaukee, WI 53222-4597
Prgm Dir: Lisa Stark, MS RD
Tel: 414 256-1216

Mt Mary College

Dietetics-Coordinated Prgm
Dept of Dietetics
2900 N Menomonee River Pkwy
Milwaukee, WI 53222-4597
Prgm Dir: Janet Rank Fischer, MS RD
Tel: 414 256-1216

University of Wisconsin - Stevens Point

Preprofessional Practice Prgm
College of Professional Studies
Stevens Point, WI 54481
Prgm Dir: Judie M Pfiffner, MS RD
Tel: 715 346-2437

University of Wisconsin - Stevens Point

Dietetics-Didactic Prgm
College of Professional Studies
Stevens Point, WI 54481
Prgm Dir: Laura C Rall, PhD RD
Tel: 715 346-4087

Wyoming

University of Wyoming

Dietetics-Didactic Prgm
Dept of Home Economics
PO Box 3354
Laramie, WY 82071-3354
Prgm Dir: Rhoda Schantz, PhD RD
Tel: 307 766-4145

Dietetic Technician-Associate Degree

Arizona

Central Arizona College

Dietetic Technician-AD Prgm
8470 N Overfield Rd
Coolidge, AZ 85228
Prgm Dir: Glenna McCollum, MPH RD
Tel: 520 426-4497   *Fax:* 520 426-4476
E-mail: glennam@cactus.cac.cc.az.us

Arkansas

Black River Technical College

Dietetic Technician-AD Prgm
PO Box 468
Pocahontas, AR 72455
Prgm Dir: Angela C Caldwell, MS RD LD
Tel: 501 892-4565, Ext 261   *Fax:* 501 892-3546

California

Orange Coast College

Dietetic Technician-AD Prgm
2701 Fairview Rd
Costa Mesa, CA 92628-0120
Prgm Dir: Eleanor B Huang, MS RD
Tel: 714 432-5835, Ext 26   *Fax:* 714 432-5609

Grossmont College

Dietetic Technician-AD Prgm
8800 Grossmont College Dr
El Cajon, CA 92020-1799
Prgm Dir: Mary Hubbard, PhD RD
Tel: 619 465-1700, Ext 348   *Fax:* 619 461-3396

Loma Linda University

Dietetic Technician-AD Prgm
Nutrition and Dietetics
School of Allied Hlth Profs
Loma Linda, CA 92350
Prgm Dir: Georgia Hodgkin, EdD RD
Tel: 909 824-4593   *Fax:* 909 824-4291
E-mail: ghodgkin@ccmail.llu.edu

Long Beach City College

Dietetic Technician-AD Prgm
Fam and Consumer Studies Div
Liberal Arts Campus/4901 E Carson St
Long Beach, CA 90808
Prgm Dir: Linda Allen Huy, EdD RD
Tel: 310 420-4550   *Fax:* 310 420-4118

Los Angeles City College

Dietetic Technician-AD Prgm
Family and Consumer Studies
855 N Vermont Ave
Los Angeles, CA 90029-3590
Prgm Dir: Janice Johnson Young, MS RD
Tel: 213 953-4259   *Fax:* 213 953-4294

Chaffey Community College
Dietetic Technician-AD Prgm
Food Service Management
5885 Haven Ave
Rancho Cucamonga, CA 91737-3002
Prgm Dir: Suzanne Johnson, MA RD
Tel: 909 941-2711   *Fax:* 909 466-2831

San Bernardino Valley College
Dietetic Technician-AD Prgm
Family and Consumer Science
701 S Mount Vernon
San Bernardino, CA 92410
Prgm Dir: Jill Ross, MS RD
Tel: 909 888-6511, Ext 1503

Colorado

Front Range Comm College - Westminster
Dietetic Technician-AD Prgm
3645 W 112th Ave
Westminster, CO 80030
Prgm Dir: Lou Ann Dixon, MEd RD
Tel: 303 466-8811, Ext 5260   *Fax:* 303 469-9615
E-mail: louann@csn.org

Connecticut

Gateway Community - Technical College
Dietetic Technician-AD Prgm
88 Bassett Rd
New Haven, CT 06473
Prgm Dir: Nina Tiglio Ruckes, MPH RD
Tel: 203 234-3309   *Fax:* 203 234-3353
E-mail: Ruckes@gnhvax.commnet.edu

Briarwood College
Dietetic Technician-AD Prgm
2279 Mount Vernon Rd
Southington, CT 06489
Prgm Dir: Paula D Kellogg Leibovitz, MS RD CDN
Tel: 860 628-4751   *Fax:* 860 628-6444

Florida

Florida Community College - Jacksonville
Dietetic Technician-AD Prgm
North Campus
4501 Capper Rd
Jacksonville, FL 32218
Prgm Dir: Margaret Wolson, MS RD
Tel: 904 766-6743   *Fax:* 904 766-6654

Palm Beach Community College
Dietetic Technician-AD Prgm
4200 Congress Ave
Lake Worth, FL 33461-4796
Prgm Dir: Ethel M Fowler, MS RD
Tel: 407 439-8126   *Fax:* 407 439-8202

Miami-Dade Community College
Dietetic Technician-AD Prgm
New World Ctr Campus
300 NE 2nd Ave
Miami, FL 33132-2297
Prgm Dir: Bonnie Landsea, MS RD FADA
Tel: 305 237-3160   *Fax:* 305 237-7429

Pensacola Junior College
Dietetic Technician-AD Prgm
1000 College Blvd
Pensacola, FL 32504-8998
Prgm Dir: Janet Ball Levins, MPH RD LD
Tel: 904 484-2531   *Fax:* 904 484-1826

Idaho

Ricks College
Dietetic Technician-AD Prgm
Dept of Home Economics
Rexburg, ID 83460-0615
Prgm Dir: Janel D Smith, MS RD
Tel: 208 356-1370   *Fax:* 208 356-1366
E-mail: smithjd@ricks.edu

Illinois

Malcolm X College
Dietetic Technician-AD Prgm
1900 W Van Buren
Chicago, IL 60612-3145
Prgm Dir: Perla M Kushida, EdD RD RN
Tel: 312 850-7383   *Fax:* 312 942-2470
E-mail: kushida@aol.com

William Rainey Harper College
Dietetic Technician-AD Prgm
1200 W Algonquin Rd
Palatine, IL 60067-7398
Prgm Dir: Jane Allendorph, MS RD LD
Tel: 847 925-6537   *Fax:* 847 925-6047

Indiana

Purdue University-Calumet
Dietetic Technician-AD Prgm
Behavioral Sciences Dept
Hammond, IN 46323-2094
Prgm Dir: Margaret B West, MS RD
Tel: 219 989-2716   *Fax:* 219 989-2008

Ball State University
Dietetic Technician-AD Prgm
Dept of Home Economics
150 Practical Arts
Muncie, IN 47306
Prgm Dir: Corine M Carr, MS RD
Tel: 317 285-2255   *Fax:* 317 285-2314
E-mail: cmcarr777@aol.com

Louisiana

Delgado Community College
Dietetic Technician-AD Prgm
450 S Clairborne Ave
New Orleans, LA 70112-1310
Prgm Dir: Donna Pace, MBA RD LDN
Tel: 504 568-6994   *Fax:* 504 568-5494
E-mail: dmpace@pop3.dcc.edu

Maine

Southern Maine Technical College
Dietetic Technician-AD Prgm
Fort Rd
South Portland, ME 04106
Prgm Dir: Linda Gabrielson, MS RD
Tel: 207 767-9606   *Fax:* 207 767-2731
E-mail: gabriel@server.seis.com

Maryland

Baltimore City Community College
Dietetic Technician-AD Prgm
Dept of Allied Health
2901 Liberty Heights Ave
Baltimore, MD 21215-7893
Prgm Dir: Jolene R Campbell, MEd RD LD
Tel: 410 462-7724

Massachusetts

Laboure College
Dietetic Technician-AD Prgm
2120 Dorchester Ave
Boston, MA 02124-5698
Prgm Dir: Anne S Manion, MBA RD
Tel: 617 296-8300, Ext 4042   *Fax:* 617 296-7947

Essex Agriculture and Tech Institute
Dietetic Technician-AD Prgm
562 Maple St
Hathorne, MA 01937
Prgm Dir: Bernadette S Lucas, MS RD
Tel: 508 774-0050, Ext 63   *Fax:* 508 774-6530

Michigan

Wayne County Community College
Dietetic Technician-AD Prgm
Vocational and Career Educ
1001 W Fort St
Detroit, MI 48226
Prgm Dir: Ethel M Nettles, PhD RD
Tel: 313 943-4482   *Fax:* 313 943-4025

Minnesota

Normandale Community College
Dietetic Technician-AD Prgm
9700 France Ave S
Bloomington, MN 55431
Prgm Dir: Vicki Erdmann, MS RD
Tel: 612 832-6481   *Fax:* 612 832-6571
E-mail: verdmann@nr.cc.mn.us

University of Minnesota - Crookston
Dietetic Technician-AD Prgm
Hospitality and Home Econ
Crookston, MN 56716
Prgm Dir: Sharon Stewart, MS RD
Tel: 218 281-6510   *Fax:* 218 281-8050
E-mail: sstewart@mail.crk.umn.edu

Programs

Missouri

St Louis Comm Coll at Florissant Valley
Dietetic Technician-AD Prgm
3400 Pershall Rd
St Louis, MO 63135-1499
Prgm Dir: Susan S Appelbaum, MEd RD
Tel: 314 595-4426   *Fax:* 314 595-4544

Nebraska

Southeast Community College
Dietetic Technician-AD Prgm
8800 O St
Lincoln, NE 68520-1227
Prgm Dir: Bernadine J Taylor, MA RD
Tel: 402 437-2465   *Fax:* 402 437-2404

New Hampshire

University of New Hampshire
Dietetic Technician-AD Prgm
Thompson Schl of Applied Sci
Cole Hall
Durham, NH 03824
Prgm Dir: Nancy Johnson, MEd RD
Tel: 603 862-1050   *Fax:* 603 862-2915

New Jersey

Camden County College
Dietetic Technician-AD Prgm
PO Box 200
Blackwood, NJ 08012
Prgm Dir: Betty Brown Joynes, MA RD
Tel: 609 227-7200, Ext 324   *Fax:* 609 374-4856

Middlesex County College
Dietetic Technician-AD Prgm
155 Mill Rd
PO Box 3050
Edison, NJ 08818-3050
Prgm Dir: Corey J Wu Jung, MS RD
Tel: 908 906-2538   *Fax:* 908 494-8244

New York

LaGuardia Community College
Dietetic Technician-AD Prgm
City University of New York
31-10 Thomson Ave
Long Island City, NY 11101
Prgm Dir: Rosann T Ippolito, MS RD
Tel: 718 482-5758   *Fax:* 718 482-5599

SUNY Agric & Tech College at Morrisville
Dietetic Technician-AD Prgm
Bailey Annex
Morrisville, NY 13408
Prgm Dir: Marie Louise Smith, MEd MS RD
Tel: 315 684-6288   *Fax:* 315 684-6592
E-mail: snymorva.cs.syymor.edu

Dutchess Community College
Dietetic Technician-AD Prgm
53 Pendell Rd
Poughkeepsie, NY 12601-1595
Prgm Dir: Marilyn C Holsipple, EdD RD
Tel: 914 431-8323   *Fax:* 914 431-8991
E-mail: holsippl@sunydutchess.edu

Suffolk County Community College
Dietetic Technician-AD Prgm
Eastern Campus
2 Speonk-Riverhead Rd
Riverhead, NY 11901-3499
Prgm Dir: Jodie E Newman, MS RD
Tel: 516 548-2590   *Fax:* 516 548-2617

Rockland Community College
Dietetic Technician-AD Prgm
145 College Rd
Suffern, NY 10901-3699
Prgm Dir: Janice Shaer, MA RD
Tel: 914 574-4130   *Fax:* 914 574-4498

Westchester Community College
Dietetic Technician-AD Prgm
75 Grasslands Rd
Valhalla, NY 10595-1698
Prgm Dir: Juliana Snyder, MS RD
Tel: 914 785-6750   *Fax:* 914 785-6423

Erie Community College - North Campus
Dietetic Technician-AD Prgm
6205 Main St
Williamsville, NY 14221-7095
Prgm Dir: Margaret Garfoot, MS RD
Tel: 716 851-1598

Ohio

Cincinnati State Tech and Comm College
Dietetic Technician-AD Prgm
Health Technologies Div
3520 Central Pkwy
Cincinnati, OH 45223-2690
Prgm Dir: Sharman Willmore, MS RD LD
Tel: 513 569-1685   *Fax:* 513 569-1659

Cuyahoga Community College
Dietetic Technician-AD Prgm
2900 Community College Ave
Cleveland, OH 44115
Prgm Dir: Barbara Mikuszewski, MS RD LD
Tel: 216 987-4497   *Fax:* 216 987-4386
E-mail: barbmikuszewski@tri-c.cc.oh.us

Columbus State Community College
Dietetic Technician-AD Prgm
550 E Spring St
PO Box 1609
Columbus, OH 43216-1609
Prgm Dir: Louise G Conway, MS RD
Tel: 614 227-2580   *Fax:* 614 227-5146
E-mail: lconway%cscc@cougar.colstate.cc.oh.us

Sinclair Community College
Dietetic Technician-AD Prgm
444 W Third St
Dayton, OH 45402-1460
Prgm Dir: Beatriz Dykes, MEd RD
Tel: 513 226-2756   *Fax:* 513 449-4592
E-mail: bdykes@Sinclair.edu

Lima Technical College
Dietetic Technician-AD Prgm
4240 Campus Dr
Lima, OH 45804-3597
Prgm Dir: Marilyn Gilroy, MS RD LD
Tel: 419 221-1112, Ext 328   *Fax:* 419 221-0450
E-mail: gilroym@ltc.tec.oh.us

Hocking Technical College
Dietetic Technician-AD Prgm
3301 Hocking Pkwy
Nelsonville, OH 45764-9704
Prgm Dir: Deborah Murray, MS RD LD
Tel: 614 753-3591

Owens Community College
Dietetic Technician-AD Prgm
PO Box 10000
Toledo, OH 43699-1947
Prgm Dir: Martha Johnson, MEd RD LD
Tel: 419 661-7214   *Fax:* 419 661-7665
E-mail: mjohnson@owens.cc.oh.us

Youngstown State University
Dietetic Technician-AD Prgm
Dept of Human Ecology
One University Plaza
Youngstown, OH 44555-3344
Prgm Dir: David H Holben, PhD RD LD
Tel: 330 742-3344   *Fax:* 330 742-2309
E-mail: dholben@cc.ysu.edu

Muskingum Area Technical College
Dietetic Technician-AD Prgm
Hlth Pub Svcs and Gen Studies
1555 Newark Rd
Zanesville, OH 43701
Prgm Dir: Tracy Smith-Hall, MS RD LD
Tel: 614 454-2501, Ext 219   *Fax:* 614 454-0035

Oklahoma

Oklahoma State University - Okmulgee
Dietetic Technician-AD Prgm
1801 E 4th St
Okmulgee, OK 74447-3901
Prgm Dir: Alexandria Miller, PhD RD LD
Tel: 918 756-6211, Ext 220   *Fax:* 918 756-1315

Oregon

Portland Community College
Dietetic Technician-AD Prgm
12000 SW 49th
PO Box 19000
Portland, OR 97280-0990
Prgm Dir: Marie Banfe, MS RD LD
Tel: 503 977-4030   *Fax:* 503 977-4869

Pennsylvania

Community College of Philadelphia
Dietetic Technician-AD Prgm
1700 Spring Garden St
Philadelphia, PA 19130-3991
Prgm Dir: Dorothy R Koteski, MS RD
Tel: 215 751-8427   *Fax:* 215 751-8937

Comm Coll of Allegheny Cnty-Alleg Campus
Dietetic Technician-AD Prgm
808 Ridge Ave
Pittsburgh, PA 15212-6097
Prgm Dir: Elizabeth C Vargo, MS RD
Tel: 412 237-2640

Penn State University - Main Campus
Dietetic Technician-AD Prgm
Coll of Health & Human Devel
Hotel Rest & Recreation Mgmt
University Park, PA 16802-1307
Prgm Dir: Ellen P Barbrow, MEd RD
Tel: 814 863-2676   *Fax:* 814 863-4257
E-mail: epbi@psu.edu

Westmoreland County Community College
Dietetic Technician-AD Prgm
Youngwood, PA 15697-1895
Prgm Dir: Marlene C Scatena, MA RD
Tel: 412 925-4165   *Fax:* 412 925-4293

South Carolina

Greenville Technical College
Dietetic Technician-AD Prgm
Hospitality Education
PO Box 5616
Greenville, SC 29606-5616
Prgm Dir: Margaret D Condrasky, EdD RD CCE
Tel: 864 250-8404   *Fax:* 864 250-8455
E-mail: condrmde@gvltec.edu

Tennessee

Shelby State Community College
Dietetic Technician-AD Prgm
PO Box 40568
Memphis, TN 38174-0568
Prgm Dir: Cleo Long, MS RD LDN
Tel: 901 544-5051   *Fax:* 901 544-5057

Texas

Tarrant County Junior Coll - South
Dietetic Technician-AD Prgm
2100 TCJC Pkwy
Arlington, TX 76018
Prgm Dir: Anne Marie Richmond, PhD RD LD
Tel: 817 515-3609   *Fax:* 817 515-3186

El Paso Community College
Dietetic Technician-AD Prgm
9570 Gateway Blvd N
El Paso, TX 79924
Prgm Dir: Marsha Cummings, MEd RD LD
Tel: 915 757-5016   *Fax:* 915 757-5122

Houston Community College Central
Dietetic Technician-AD Prgm
1300 Holman
Houston, TX 77004
Prgm Dir: Dalia M Lima, MPH RD
Tel: 713 718-6801   *Fax:* 713 520-0896

San Jacinto College Central Campus
Dietetic Technician-AD Prgm
8060 Spencer Hwy
PO Box 2007
Pasadena, TX 77505-2007
Prgm Dir: Annette E Betz, MS RD LD
Tel: 713 476-1501, Ext 1498   *Fax:* 713 478-2790

St Philip's College
Dietetic Technician-AD Prgm
1801 Martin Luther King
San Antonio, TX 78203-2098
Prgm Dir: Mary A Kunz, MS RD LD
Tel: 210 531-3315   *Fax:* 210 531-3445
E-mail: mkunz@accd.edu

Virginia

Northern Virginia Community College
Dietetic Technician-AD Prgm
HRI/DIT CF208
8333 Little River Trnpk
Annandale, VA 22003-3796
Prgm Dir: Janet Sass, MS RD
Tel: 703 323-3458   *Fax:* 703 323-3215

J Sargeant Reynolds Community College
Dietetic Technician-AD Prgm
PO Box 85622
Richmond, VA 23285-5622
Prgm Dir: B Lynn Farmer, MA RD
Tel: 804 367-8880   *Fax:* 804 367-2703

Tidewater Community College
Dietetic Technician-AD Prgm
1700 College Crescent
Virginia Beach, VA 23456
Prgm Dir: Christine Medlin, PhD RD
Tel: 804 427-7336   *Fax:* 804 427-1338
E-mail: tcmedlc%vccsent.bitnet@vtbit.cc.ut.edu

Washington

Shoreline Community College
Dietetic Technician-AD Prgm
16101 Greenwood Ave N
Seattle, WA 98133
Prgm Dir: Venus Gomez Deming, MS RD
Tel: 206 546-4673   *Fax:* 206 546-5869
E-mail: vdeming@cte.edu

Spokane Community College
Dietetic Technician-AD Prgm
N 1810 Greene St
MS 2090
Spokane, WA 99207-5399
Prgm Dir: Erin Clason, MPH RD CDE
Tel: 509 533-7314   *Fax:* 509 533-8621

Wisconsin

Madison Area Technical College
Dietetic Technician-AD Prgm
3550 Anderson St
Madison, WI 53704-2599
Prgm Dir: Barbara A Hundt, EdS RD
Tel: 608 246-6319   *Fax:* 608 246-6880

Milwaukee Area Technical College
Dietetic Technician-AD Prgm
700 W State St
Milwaukee, WI 53233
Prgm Dir: Jean Dueling, MS RD
Tel: 414 297-6876   *Fax:* 414 297-7733
E-mail: duelingj@milwaukee.tec.wi.us.edu

Programs

Electroneurodiagnostic Technologist

History

The American Medical Association's (AMA) involvement in the evaluation and accreditation of educational programs in electro-encephalographic (EEG) technology began in 1972 with the recognition of EEG technology as an allied health profession by the AMA Council on Health Manpower. Subsequently, AMA staff worked with representatives of the professional organizations representing this clinical discipline to develop a draft of the *Standards (Essentials) of an Accredited Educational Program for the Electroencephalographic Technologist*.

In 1973, representatives of the American EEG Society, the American Medical EEG Association, and the American Society of Electroneurodiagnostic Technologists (then the American Society of EEG Technologists) presented statements supporting the *Standards*. These organizations and the AMA House of Delegates then considered and adopted the *Standards* for entry-level educational programs for the electroencephalographic technologist.

The Joint Review Committee on Education in Electroencephalographic Technology was established and held its initial meeting in September 1973. In 1988, the name of the committee was changed to the Joint Review Committee on Education in Electroneurodiagnostic Technology.

This review body is composed of six members—four members appointed by the American Society of Electroneurodiagnostic Technologists and two members appointed by the American Electroencephalographic Society. Meetings are held twice annually. The committee develops recommendations on accreditation status of programs, which are subsequently forwarded to the Commission on Accreditation of Allied Health Education Programs for final action. The *Standards* were revised in 1980, 1987, and 1995. In 1987, evoked potential (EP) techniques were included in *Standards* for programs desiring recognition in both EEG and EP techniques. In 1995, polysomnography (PSG) techniques were included for programs desiring recognition in EEG, EP, and PSG techniques.

Occupational Description

Electroneurodiagnostic technology is the scientific field devoted to recording and studying the electrical activity of the brain and nervous system. Electroneurodiagnostic technologists possess the knowledge, attributes, and skills to obtain interpretable recordings of patients' nervous system function. They work in collaboration with the electroencephalographer.

Job Description

The electroneurodiagnostic technologist is skilled in the following functions: communicating with patients, family, and other health care personnel; taking and abstracting histories; applying adequate recording electrodes and using EEG, EP, and PSG techniques; documenting the clinical condition of patients; and understanding and employing the optimal use of EEG, EP, and PSG equipment. Among other duties, the electroneurodiagnostic technologist also understands the interface between EEG, EP, and PSG equipment and other electrophysiological devices; recognizes and understands EEG and EP and sleep activity displayed; manages medical emergencies in the laboratory; and prepares a descriptive report of recorded activity for the electroencephalographer. The responsibilities of the technologist may also include laboratory management and the supervision of EEG technicians.

Employment Characteristics

Although electroneurodiagnostic personnel work primarily in the neurology departments of hospitals, many work in private offices of neurologists and neurosurgeons. Growth in employment in the profession is expected to be greater than the average for all occupations owing to the increased use of EEG and EP techniques in surgery, in diagnosing and monitoring patients with epilepsy, and in diagnosing sleep disorders. Technologists generally work a 40-hour week. According to the American Society of Electroneurodiagnostic Technologists, 1995 entry-level salaries average $25,000.

Educational Programs

Length. Programs may be 12 months or more and may be integrated into a college-sponsored program leading to a degree.

Prerequisites. High school diploma or equivalent.

Curriculum. The curriculum includes anatomy, physiology, and neuroanatomy (with major emphasis on the brain), as well as electronics, instrumentation, and personal and patient safety.

Standards. *Standards* are minimum educational standards that have been adopted by the following organizations collaborating with the AMA as well as by the AMA itself: the American Electroencephalographic Society, American Medical Electroencephalographic Association, and American Society of Electroneurodiagnostic Technologists. Each new program is assessed in accordance with the *Standards*, and accredited programs are periodically reviewed to determine whether they remain in substantial compliance. The *Standards* are available on written request to the Committee on Accreditation in Electroneurodiagnostic Technology.

Inquiries

Accreditation

Requests for information on program accreditation, including *Standards*, preparing the self-study report, and arranging a site visit, should be submitted to

Joint Review Committee in Electroneurodiagnostic Technology
Rte 1 Box 62A
Genoa, WI 54632
608 689-2058

Careers

Inquiries regarding careers and curriculum should be addressed to

American Society of Electroneurodiagnostic Technologists
204 W Seventh St
Carroll, IA 51401-2135
712 792-2978

Certification/Registration

Inquiries regarding certification may be addressed to

Executive Director
American Board of Registration of Electroencephalographic and Evoked Potential Technologists
PO Box 916633
Longwood, FL 32791-6633

Electroneuro-diagnostic Technologist

California

Orange Coast College

Electroneurodiagnostic Tech Prgm
2701 Fairview Rd
Costa Mesa, CA 92626
Prgm Dir: Walter Banoczi, R EEG/EP T CNIM
Tel: 714 432-5591 *Fax:* 714 432-5534
Med Dir: Hugh McIntyre, MD
Class Cap: 25 *Begins:* Aug
Length: 22 mos *Award:* Cert, AA
Tuition per yr: $462 res, $3,626 non-res
Evening or weekend classes available

Florida

David G Erwin Technical Center

Electroneurodiagnostic Tech Prgm
2010 E Hillsborough Ave
Tampa, FL 33610
Prgm Dir: Henry Coet III, R EEG T
Tel: 813 231-1800 *Fax:* 813 231-1820
Med Dir: David Dillenbeck, MD
Class Cap: 18 *Begins:* Aug
Length: 12 mos *Award:* Dipl
Tuition per yr: $550 res, $4,070 non-res
Evening or weekend classes available

Illinois

St John's Hospital

Electroneurodiagnostic Tech Prgm
800 E Carpenter
Springfield, IL 62769
Prgm Dir: Janice Walbert, R EEG EPT
Tel: 217 544-6464, Ext 4704 *Fax:* 217 535-3695
Med Dir: Wesley Betsill, MD
Class Cap: 6 *Begins:* Jul
Length: 12 mos *Award:* Dipl
Tuition per yr: $3,140

Iowa

Scott Community College

Electroneurodiagnostic Tech Prgm
500 Belmont Rd
Bettendorf, IA 52722
Prgm Dir: Deborah K Hahn, R EEG EPT
Tel: 319 359-7531
Med Dir: M Sanguino, MD
Class Cap: 12 *Begins:* Aug Sep
Length: 22 mos *Award:* AAS
Tuition per yr: $2,660 res, $3,300 non-res
Evening or weekend classes available

Kirkwood Community College

Electroneurodiagnostic Tech Prgm
6301 Kirkwood Blvd SW
PO Box 2068
Cedar Rapids, IA 52406-9973
Prgm Dir: Margaret Gordon, R EEG T
Tel: 319 356-8768
Med Dir: Thoru Yamada, MD
Class Cap: 12 *Begins:* Sep
Length: 21 mos *Award:* AAS
Tuition per yr: $3,684 res, $7,367 non-res
Evening or weekend classes available

Maryland

Naval School of Health Sciences - MD

Electroneurodiagnostic Tech Prgm
8901 Wisonsin Ave
Bethesda, MD 20889-5611
Prgm Dir: Sherry M Burton, R EEGT HM2 USN
  R EE
Tel: 301 295-0124 *Fax:* 301 295-0621
E-mail: sburton@nsh20.med.naymil
Med Dir: Jean Panagakos, MD EEG CAPT MC
Class Cap: 10 *Begins:* Varies
Length: 6 mos *Award:* Cert

Massachusetts

Children's Hospital

Electroneurodiagnostic Tech Prgm
300 Longwood Ave
Boston, MA 02115
Prgm Dir: Lewis L Kull, R EEG/EPT
Tel: 617 355-7970
Med Dir: Gregory L Holmes, MD
Class Cap: 7 *Begins:* Sep
Length: 12 mos *Award:* Cert
Tuition per yr: $2,000

Laboure College

Electroneurodiagnostic Tech Prgm
2120 Dorchester Ave
Boston, MA 02124
Prgm Dir: Jean Wilkins Farley, MA R EEG T
Tel: 617 296-8300, Ext 4043 *Fax:* 617 296-7947
Med Dir: Sanford Auerbach, MD
Class Cap: 8 *Begins:* Sep
Length: 20 mos *Award:* Cert, AS
Tuition per yr: $12,360
Evening or weekend classes available

New York

Niagara County Community College

Electroneurodiagnostic Tech Prgm
3111 Saunders Settlement Rd
Sanborn, NY 14132
Prgm Dir: Nicholas J T Lo Cascio, PhD
Tel: 716 731-3271 *Fax:* 716 731-4053
Med Dir: Michael Kohrman, MD
Class Cap: 22 *Begins:* Sep
Length: 20 mos *Award:* AAS
Tuition per yr: $2,454 res, $3,629 non-res
Evening or weekend classes available

Pennsylvania

Crozer-Chester Med Ctr/Delaware Co CC

Electroneurodiagnostic Tech Prgm
One Medical Ctr Blvd
Upland, PA 19013
Prgm Dir: Kellee W Tirce, REEG/EPT, RPSGT
Tel: 610 447-2688 *Fax:* 610 447-2696
Med Dir: Lawrence Green, MD
Class Cap: 12 *Begins:* Sep
Length: 15 mos *Award:* Cert
Tuition per yr: $2,500 res, $2,500 non-res

Wisconsin

Western Wisconsin Technical College

Electroneurodiagnostic Tech Prgm
304 No 6th St
PO Box 908
La Crosse, WI 54601
Prgm Dir: Clayton Pollert, R EEG T
Tel: 608 785-9253
Med Dir: Gregory Fischer, MD
Class Cap: 14 *Begins:* Jun
Length: 24 mos *Award:* AAS
Tuition per yr: $2,159 res, $12,693 non-res

Programs

Emergency Medical Technician-Paramedic

History

The emergency medical technician-paramedic (EMT-paramedic) was first recognized as an allied health occupation in 1975 by the American Medical Association (AMA) for the purpose of accrediting entry-level educational programs in the profession. Beginning in 1976, a concerted effort by many organizations was begun to develop the educational *Standards (Essentials)* that would be used to evaluate EMT-paramedic programs seeking accreditation. Following several drafts of the proposed *Standards*, with wide distribution to the appropriate communities of interest, the *Standards* were adopted in 1978. Adoption was by the AMA Council on Medical Education (CME) on behalf of the AMA and by the organizations collaborating with the AMA in this accreditation process and sponsoring the newly formed Joint Review Committee on Educational Programs for the EMT-Paramedic (JRC/EMT-P): the American College of Emergency Physicians, American College of Surgeons, American Psychiatric Association, American Society of Anesthesiologists, National Association of Emergency Medical Technicians, and National Registry of Emergency Medical Technicians. Today, the AMA's role of adopting *Standards* is now the responsibility of the Commission on Accreditation of Allied Health Education Programs and the collaborating agencies.

The JRC/EMT-P is currently sponsored by the American Academy of Pediatrics, American College of Cardiology, American College of Emergency Physicians, American College of Surgeons, American Society of Anesthesiologists, National Association of Emergency Medical Technicians, National Council of State Emergency Medical Services Training Coordinators, and National Registry of Emergency Medical Technicians.

Occupational Description

Emergency medical technician-paramedics, working under the direction of a physician (often through radio communication), recognize, assess, and manage medical emergencies of acutely ill or injured patients in prehospital care settings. EMT-paramedics work principally in advanced life-support units and ambulance services under medical supervision and direction.

Job Description

To fulfill the role of the EMT-paramedic, an individual must be able to

1. Recognize a medical emergency; assess the situation; manage emergency care and, if needed, extricate the patient; coordinate efforts with those of other agencies that may be involved in the care and transportation of the patient; and establish rapport with the patient and significant others to decrease their state of anxiety.
2. Assign priorities to emergency treatment data for the designated medical command authority or assign priorities of emergency treatment.
3. Record and communicate pertinent data to the designated medical command authority.
4. Initiate and continue emergency medical care under medical control, including the recognition of presenting conditions and initiation of appropriate treatments—for example, traumatic and medical emergencies, airway and ventilation problems, cardiac dysrhythmias, cardiac standstill, and psychological crises—and assess the response of the patient to that treatment, modifying medical therapy as directed.
5. Exercise personal judgment and provide such emergency care as has been specifically authorized in advance in cases where medical direction is interrupted by communication failure or in cases of immediate life-threatening conditions.
6. Direct and coordinate the transport of the patient by selecting the best available method(s) in conjunction with medical command authority.
7. Record in writing or dictate the details related to the patient's emergency care and the incident.
8. Direct the maintenance and preparation of emergency care equipment and supplies.

Employment Characteristics

Variations in geographic, sociologic, and economic factors have an impact on emergency medical services and subsequently on the type of practice engaged in by EMT-paramedics. Some EMT-paramedics are employed by community fire and police departments and have related responsibilities in those fields; some serve as community volunteers. Not only are these individuals being employed in the prehospital phase of acute care provided by fire departments, police departments, public services, and private purveyors, but there is also an increased demand for their skills in hospital emergency departments and private industry.

According to the 1992 CAHEA Annual Supplemental Survey, entry-level salaries averaged $21,672.

Educational Programs

Length. Some programs are designed as a part-time study model, whereas others are organized as full-time collegiate curricula. Instruction dealing specifically with emergency medical care requires anywhere from 600 to 1,000 hours of instruction, the variation largely owing to the availability of actual emergency care incidents through which the student may acquire supervised clinical practice experience.

Prerequisites. Successful completion of a course of training for EMT-ambulance and evidence of certification as an EMT-ambulance are the principal prerequisites for entrance into the EMT-paramedic program. In addition, a prospective student is expected to be a high school graduate or the equivalent. In those programs offering a combination of EMT-ambulance and EMT-paramedic training, the clinical, didactic, and supervised practice portions of both programs must be completed before the EMT-paramedic student begins the required field internship. In addition, students are expected to be able to meet the physical and mental demands of the occupation. Individuals who have acquired the equivalent of basic EMT training in the military services within the past 12 months and whose work experience is approved by a recognized state agency may be considered qualified to matriculate in an EMT-paramedic program.

Curriculum. The accreditation standards require that a course of instruction be composed of three components: didactic clinical instruction, in-hospital clinical practice, and a supervised field internship in an advanced life-support unit that functions under an emergency medical services command authority. The courses of instruction are expected to be competency-based and supported by performance assessments. Instruction should provide the student with knowledge of acute and critical changes in physiology and psychological and clinical symptoms as they pertain to the prehospital emergency medical care of individuals of all ages. The curriculum also should provide students with an understanding of the ethical and legal responsibilities that they assume as students and that they are being prepared to assume as graduates.

Standards. *Standards* are minimum educational standards adopted by the American College of Emergency Physicians, American College of Surgeons, American Society of Anesthesiologists, National Association of Emergency Medical Technicians, National Registry of Emergency Medical Technicians, and AMA CME. Each new program is assessed in accordance with the *Standards*, and accredited programs are periodically reviewed to determine whether they remain in substantial compliance. The *Standards and Guidelines* are available on written request from the Joint Review Committee in Educational Programs for the EMT-Paramedic.

Inquiries

Accreditation

Requests for information on program accreditation, including *Standards*, preparing the self-study report, and arranging a site visit, should be submitted to

Joint Review Committee on Educational Programs
    for the EMT-Paramedic
7108-C S Alton Way/Ste 150
Englewood, CO 80112-2106
303 694-6191
303 741-3655 Fax

Careers

Inquiries regarding careers should be addressed to

National Association of Emergency Medical Technicians
102 W Leake St
Clinton, MS 39056
601 924-7744

Certification/Licensure

Inquiries regarding certification may be addressed to

National Registry of Emergency Medical Technicians
Rocco V Morando Bldg
Box 29233/6610 Busch Blvd
Columbus, OH 43229-0233
614 888-4484

Emergency Medical Technician-Paramedic

Alabama

University of Alabama at Birmingham
Emergency Med Tech-Paramedic Prgm
Sch of Hlth Related Professions
912 S 18th St
Birmingham, AL 35205
Prgm Dir: Marie S Gospodareck, BS EMT-P
Tel: 205 934-3611
Med Dir: Alan R Dimick, MD
Class Cap: 135 *Begins:* Sep Mar Jan Jun
Length: 15 mos *Award:* Cert
Tuition per yr: $1,900 res, $1,900 non-res

George C Wallace State Comm College
Emergency Med Tech-Paramedic Prgm
Dept of Emergency Medicine
Rt 6, Box 62
Dothan, AL 36303
Prgm Dir: Earl Shaw, AAS NREMT-P
Tel: 334 983-3521 *Fax:* 334 983-4255
Med Dir: James M Jones, DO
Class Cap: 10 *Begins:* Mar Sep
Length: 9 mos *Award:* Cert, AAS
Tuition per yr: $1,190 res, $1,828 non-res

Gadsden State Community College
Emergency Med Tech-Paramedic Prgm
1001 George Wallace Dr
PO Box 227
Gadsden, AL 35902-0227
Prgm Dir: John E Blue II, EMT-P
Tel: 205 235-5674 *Fax:* 205 235-5600
Med Dir: Howard E McVeigh, MD
Class Cap: 220 *Begins:* Sep Jan Mar Jun
Length: 18 mos, 24 mos *Award:* Cert, AAS
Tuition per yr: $1,490 res, $2,740 non-res
Evening or weekend classes available

Wallace State College
Emergency Med Tech-Paramedic Prgm
301 Main St NW
PO Box 2000
Hanceville, AL 35077-2000
Prgm Dir: Daryl R Eustace, AS NREMT-P
Tel: 205 352-8000 *Fax:* 205 352-8228
Med Dir: Lynn A Jetton, MD
Class Cap: 20 *Begins:* Sep
Length: 9 mos *Award:* Cert, AAS
Tuition per yr: $935 res, $1,870 non-res
Evening or weekend classes available

Programs

University of Alabama at Huntsville

Emergency Med Tech-Paramedic Prgm
School of Primary Medical Care
Clinical Science Ctr/Rm 109
109 Governors Dr SW
Huntsville, AL 35801
Prgm Dir: Richard K Beck, NREMT-P
Tel: 205 551-4416   *Fax:* 205 551-4451
E-mail: beckr@email.uah.edu
Med Dir: David James Garvey, MD PhD
Class Cap: 40   *Begins:* Sep Jan Mar Jun
Length: 22 mos   *Award:* Cert, BS
Tuition per yr: $3,330 res, $5,000 non-res
Evening or weekend classes available

University of South Alabama

Emergency Med Tech-Paramedic Prgm
2002 Old Bay Front Dr
Mobile, AL 36615-1427
Prgm Dir: Edward J Carlson, MEd NREMT-P
Tel: 334 431-6418   *Fax:* 334 431-6525
E-mail: ecarlson@usouthal.campus.mci.net
Med Dir: Frank S Petty John, MD
Class Cap: 800   *Begins:* Quarterly
Length: 6 mos   *Award:* Cert
Tuition per yr: $1,936 res, $2,482 non-res
Evening or weekend classes available

H Councill Trenholm State Technical College

Emergency Med Tech-Paramedic Prgm
1225 Air Base Blvd
Montgomery, AL 36108
Prgm Dir: Gail Taylor
Tel: 334 240-9674   *Fax:* 334 832-9777
Med Dir: Richard M Sobel, MD
Class Cap: 20   *Begins:* Mar Sep
Length: 15 mos   *Award:* Cert, AAT
Tuition per yr: $1,500 res, $2,250 non-res
Evening or weekend classes available

Shelton St Comm Coll/Alabama Fire Coll

Emergency Med Tech-Paramedic Prgm
2015 McFarland Blvd E
Tuscaloosa, AL 35404-1399
Prgm Dir: Phillip K Bobo, MD
Tel: 205 391-3754
Med Dir: Steve R Lovelady, MD
Class Cap: 40   *Begins:* Jun Aug Jan
Length: 18 mos   *Award:* Cert
Tuition per yr: $525 res, $600 non-res

California

Daniel Freeman Memorial Hospital

Emergency Med Tech-Paramedic Prgm
333 N Prairie Ave
Inglewood, CA 90301
Prgm Dir: Carol L Gallagher, MPA BSN
Tel: 310 674-7050   *Fax:* 310 419-8256
Med Dir: Walter S Graf, MD
Class Cap: 35
Length: 6 mo , 9 mos   *Award:* Cert
Tuition per yr: $1,216 res, $3,650 non-res
Evening or weekend classes available

Crafton Hills College

Emergency Med Tech-Paramedic Prgm
11711 Sand Canyon Rd
Yucaipa, CA 92399
Prgm Dir: James R Holbrook, EMTP MA
Tel: 909 389-3251   *Fax:* 909 389-3256
Med Dir: Doug Grudz, MD FACEP
Class Cap: 35   *Begins:* Sep Feb
Length: 12 mos, 9 mos   *Award:* Dipl,Cert, AAS
Tuition per yr: $100 res, $3,400 non-res

Colorado

Provenant - St Anthony Hospitals/Central

Emergency Med Tech-Paramedic Prgm
4231 W 16th Ave
Denver, CO 80204
Prgm Dir: Tracy Lynn Collins, RN BSN
Tel: 303 629-3911
Med Dir: W Peter Vellman, MD
Class Cap: 20   *Begins:* Jan Sep
Length: 10 mos   *Award:* Cert
Tuition per yr: $2,400

Swedish Medical Center

Emergency Med Tech-Paramedic Prgm
Columbia Colorado Division
300 E Hampden Ave #100m
Englewood, CO 80110
Prgm Dir: Patricia Tritt, RN MA
Tel: 303 788-6302   *Fax:* 303 788-7656
Med Dir: Michael Hunt, MD
Class Cap: 20   *Begins:* Jan Jul
Length: 6 mos   *Award:* Cert
Tuition per yr: $2,400 res, $2,400 non-res

Colorado Assn of Paramedical Educ, Inc

Emergency Med Tech-Paramedic Prgm
9191 Grant St
Thornton, CO 80229
Prgm Dir: Carol Hurdelbrink, RN
Tel: 303 450-4436   *Fax:* 303 450-4458
Med Dir: Donald Massey, DO
Class Cap: 30   *Begins:* Sep
Length: 10 mos   *Award:* Cert
Tuition per yr: $2,450
Evening or weekend classes available

Connecticut

CCTC/St Francis Hosp & Med Ctr

Emergency Med Tech-Paramedic Prgm
North Suburban Med Ctr
61 Woodland St
Hartford, CT 06105-2354
Prgm Dir: Terry DeVito, MEd EMT-P CEN
Tel: 203 520-7872   *Fax:* 860 520-7906
E-mail: devito@commnet.edu
Med Dir: Alison Lane-Reticker, MD
Class Cap: 30   *Begins:* Aug
Length: 10 mos   *Award:* Cert
Tuition per yr: $1,560 res, $4,680 non-res

Delaware

Kent General Hosp

Emergency Med Tech-Paramedic Prgm
640 S State St
Dover, DE 19901
Prgm Dir: Bruce W Tuitt, NREMT-P
Tel: 302 674-7200   *Fax:* 302 674-7984
E-mail: banepon@aol.com
Med Dir: John Sewell, MD
Begins: Sep Feb
Length: 12 mos   *Award:* Cert

Medical Center of Delaware

Emergency Med Tech-Paramedic Prgm
501 W 14th St/PO Box 1668
Wilmington, DE 19899
Prgm Dir: Paula K Riley, RN BSN CCRN CEN
Tel: 302 428-2913   *Fax:* 302 428-2797
Med Dir: Ross Megargel, DO FACEP
Begins: Sep
Length: 12 mos   *Award:* Cert

Florida

Manatee Area Vocational-Technical Center

Emergency Med Tech-Paramedic Prgm
5603 34th St W
Bradenton, FL 34210
Prgm Dir: John M Beyer, BS EMT
Tel: 941 751-7977   *Fax:* 941 751-7927
Med Dir: Steve C Watsky, MD
Class Cap: 20   *Begins:* Aug
Length: 10 mos   *Award:* Cert
Tuition per yr: $259 res, $518 non-res

Brevard Community College

Emergency Med Tech-Paramedic Prgm
1519 Clearlake Rd
Cocoa, FL 32922
Prgm Dir: Melissa B Robinson, RN BSH EMT-P
Tel: 407 632-1111, Ext 4550   *Fax:* 407 634-3731
Med Dir: John McPherson, MD
Class Cap: 21   *Begins:* Aug
Length: 11 mos, 24 mos   *Award:* Cert, AS
Tuition per yr: $1,369
Evening or weekend classes available

Daytona Beach Community College

Emergency Med Tech-Paramedic Prgm
1200 International Speedway Blvd
PO Box 2811
Daytona Beach, FL 32120-2811
Prgm Dir: Adam W Lebowitz, MPH EMT-P
Tel: 904 255-8131   *Fax:* 904 254-4491
E-mail: lebowia@dbcc.cc.fl.us
Med Dir: John Steven Bohannon, MD
Class Cap: 168   *Begins:* May
Length: 12 mos, 24 mos   *Award:* Cert, AS
Tuition per yr: $1,145 res, $4,295 non-res
Evening or weekend classes available

Lake County Vocational Technical Center
Emergency Med Tech-Paramedic Prgm
2001 Kurt St
Eustis, FL 32726
Prgm Dir: Thomas C Lackey, BS EMT-P
Tel: 352 383-2555 *Fax:* 352 735-3013
Med Dir: John Geeslin, MD
Class Cap: 32 *Begins:* Aug Jan
Length: 11 mos *Award:* Cert
Tuition per yr: $561
Evening or weekend classes available

Broward Community College
Emergency Med Tech-Paramedic Prgm
3501 SW Davie Rd
Davie, FL 33314
Prgm Dir: Elizabeth Jordan, MN REMT-P
Tel: 954 475-6776 *Fax:* 954 473-9037
Med Dir: Barry R Weiss, MD
Class Cap: 160 *Begins:* Aug Jan May
Length: 12 mos *Award:* Cert
Tuition per yr: $1,249 res, $4,044 non-res
Evening or weekend classes available

Edison Community College
Emergency Med Tech-Paramedic Prgm
8099 College Pkwy SW
Ft Myers, FL 33906-6210
Prgm Dir: Nancy A Jerz, BPS
Tel: 941 489-9114 *Fax:* 941 489-9331
Med Dir: Daniel Booth, MD
Class Cap: 110 *Begins:* Jan May Aug
Length: 12 mos *Award:* Cert, AS
Tuition per yr: $1,033 res, $3,192 non-res

Indian River Community College
Emergency Med Tech-Paramedic Prgm
3209 Virginia Ave
Ft Pierce, FL 34981-5599
Prgm Dir: Marjorie Bowers, EdD
Tel: 561 462-4471
Med Dir: James Robelli, MD
Class Cap: 30 *Begins:* Aug
Length: 10 mos, 24 mos *Award:* Cert, AS
Tuition per yr: $1,545 res, $6,180 non-res

Santa Fe Community College
Emergency Med Tech-Paramedic Prgm
3000 NW 83rd St
W-201-I
Gainesville, FL 32606-6200
Prgm Dir: Gail A Stewart, BS EMT-P
Tel: 352 395-5755 *Fax:* 352 395-5711
E-mail: gail.stewart@santafe.cc.fl.us
Med Dir: Carl W Peters, MD
Class Cap: 16 *Begins:* Aug
Length: 12 mos, 22 mos *Award:* Cert, AS
Tuition per yr: $1,400 res, $5,410 non-res

Florida Community College - Jacksonville
Emergency Med Tech-Paramedic Prgm
4501 Capper Rd/A234
Jacksonville, FL 32218
Prgm Dir: Marjorie Fisher, BS EMT-P
Tel: 904 766-6513 *Fax:* 904 766-6654
Med Dir: Jeffrey S Smowton, MD
Class Cap: 24 *Begins:* Jan May
Length: 12 mos, 24 mos *Award:* Dipl,Cert, AS
Tuition per yr: $1,375 res, $5,191 non-res
Evening or weekend classes available

Lake City Community College
Emergency Med Tech-Paramedic Prgm
Rte 19/PO Box 1030
Lake City, FL 32025-8703
Prgm Dir: Bruce Willms, EdS NREMT-P
Tel: 904 752-1822 *Fax:* 904 758-9959
Med Dir: Carlos Castellon, MD
Class Cap: 20 *Begins:* Jun
Length: 12 mos *Award:* Cert, AS
Tuition per yr: $1,144 res, $4,167 non-res
Evening or weekend classes available

Palm Beach Community College
Emergency Med Tech-Paramedic Prgm
4200 S Congress Ave
Lake Worth, FL 33461
Prgm Dir: Albert L Howe, NREMT-P
Tel: 561 439-8260 *Fax:* 561 439-8202
E-mail: alshusband@msn.com
Med Dir: William L Davis, DO
Class Cap: 60 *Begins:* Jun
Length: 11 mos *Award:* Cert, AS
Tuition per yr: $1,148 res, $4,271 non-res
Evening or weekend classes available

Miami-Dade Community College
Emergency Med Tech-Paramedic Prgm
Medical Ctr Campus
950 NW 20th St
Miami, FL 33127
Prgm Dir: Karen Mattox, MS
Tel: 305 237-4030 *Fax:* 305 237-4278
Med Dir: Armando Santelices, MD
Class Cap: 76 *Begins:* Aug Jan
Length: 12 mos *Award:* Cert, AS
Tuition per yr: $1,567 res, $5,510 non-res

Pasco-Hernando Community College
Emergency Med Tech-Paramedic Prgm
10230 Ridge Rd
New Port Richey, FL 34654-5199
Prgm Dir: Toni Vineyard, REMT-P MA
Tel: 813 847-2727 *Fax:* 813 816-3300
Med Dir: Charles Boothby, DO
Class Cap: 30 *Begins:* Aug
Length: 11 mos *Award:* Cert, AS
Tuition per yr: $1,283 res, $4,782 non-res
Evening or weekend classes available

Central Florida Community College
Emergency Med Tech-Paramedic Prgm
3001 SW College Rd
PO Box 1388
Ocala, FL 34478
Prgm Dir: Michael McMurrer, MA EMT
Tel: 352 237-2111
Med Dir: Arthur Osberg, MD
Class Cap: 22 *Begins:* Aug
Length: 10 mos *Award:* Cert, AS
Tuition per yr: $1,461 res, $5,232 non-res

Valencia Community College
Emergency Med Tech-Paramedic Prgm
1800 S Kirkman Rd
PO Box 3028
Orlando, FL 32811
Prgm Dir: Raymond V Taylor
Tel: 407 299-5000 *Fax:* 407 293-8839
Med Dir: Mark Trach, MD
Class Cap: 75 *Begins:* Aug
Length: 12 mos, 24 mos *Award:* Cert, AS
Tuition per yr: $1,911 res, $6,734 non-res
Evening or weekend classes available

Gulf Coast Community College
Emergency Med Tech-Paramedic Prgm
5230 W Hwy 98
Panama City, FL 32401-9978
Prgm Dir: Daniel Finley, PhD NREMPT
Tel: 904 769-1551 *Fax:* 904 747-3246
E-mail: dfinley@ccmail.gc.cc.fl.us
Med Dir: Fred Epstein, MD
Class Cap: 20 *Begins:* Aug
Length: 10 mos *Award:* Cert, AS
Tuition per yr: $1,197 res, $4,788 non-res
Evening or weekend classes available

Pensacola Junior College
Emergency Med Tech-Paramedic Prgm
Warrington Campus
5555 W Hwy 98
Pensacola, FL 32505-1097
Prgm Dir: Vicki Garlock, RN BSN
Tel: 904 484-2215 *Fax:* 904 484-2365
Med Dir: John Hybart, MD
Class Cap: 20 *Begins:* Jan
Length: 16 mos, 24 mos *Award:* Cert, AS
Tuition per yr: $1,775 res, $9,315 non-res

St Petersburg Junior College
Emergency Med Tech-Paramedic Prgm
Health Education Ctr
PO Box 13489
St Petersburg, FL 33733
Prgm Dir: Nerina Stepanovsky, MSN RN EMT-P
Tel: 813 341-3680
Med Dir: Laurie Romig, MD
Class Cap: 50 *Begins:* Aug Jan
Length: 11 mos, 24 mos *Award:* Cert, AS
Tuition per yr: $1,350 res, $4,650 non-res

Seminole Community College
Emergency Med Tech-Paramedic Prgm
100 Weldon Blvd
Sanford, FL 32773
Prgm Dir: Sandra W Fraser, RN EMT-P
Tel: 407 328-2198 *Fax:* 407 328-2139
Med Dir: Ronald D Brown, MD
Class Cap: 30 *Begins:* Jan
Length: 16 mos, 31 mos *Award:* Cert, AS
Tuition per yr: $1,250
Evening or weekend classes available

Sarasota County Technical Institute
Emergency Med Tech-Paramedic Prgm
4748 Beneva Rd
Sarasota, FL 34233-1756
Prgm Dir: Deborah Metheny
Tel: 813 924-1365
Med Dir: Steven R Newman, MD
Class Cap: 20 *Begins:* Jul
Length: 11 mos *Award:* Cert
Tuition per yr: $806 res, $4,830 non-res

St Augustine Technical Center
Emergency Med Tech-Paramedic Prgm
2980 Collins Ave
St Augustine, FL 32095-9970
Prgm Dir: Dick Talbert, BA MEd
Tel: 904 829-1080 *Fax:* 904 824-6750
Med Dir: Luis Rios, MD
Class Cap: 30 *Begins:* Sep
Length: 10 mos *Award:* Cert
Tuition per yr: $782 res, $3,136 non-res

Tallahassee Community College

Emergency Med Tech-Paramedic Prgm
444 Appleyard Dr
Tallahassee, FL 32304-2895
Prgm Dir: Brian P Dunmyer, BA RP
Tel: 904 922-8156   *Fax:* 904 921-5722
E-mail: dunmyerbWmail.tallahassee.cc.fl.us
Med Dir: Thomas G Lareau, MD
Class Cap: 15   *Begins:* Aug
Length: 11 mos, 23 mos   *Award:* Cert, AS
Tuition per yr: $992 res, $3,659 non-res
Evening or weekend classes available

Hillsborough Community College

Emergency Med Tech-Paramedic Prgm
PO Box 30030
Tampa, FL 33630
Prgm Dir: Michael L Moats, EMT-P MEd
Tel: 813 253-7420
Med Dir: I Charles Sand, MD
Class Cap: 72   *Begins:* Aug Jan
Length: 10 mos, 22 mos   *Award:* Cert, AS
Tuition per yr: $1,660 res, $5,600 non-res

Polk Community College

Emergency Med Tech-Paramedic Prgm
999 Ave H NE
Winter Haven, FL 33881-4299
Prgm Dir: Craig N Story, NREMT-P
Tel: 941 297-1000   *Fax:* 941 297-1010
E-mail: cstory@mail.polk.cc.fl.us
Med Dir: David Brooke, MD
Class Cap: 15   *Begins:* Aug
Length: 12 mos   *Award:* Cert
Tuition per yr: $1,127 res, $3,151 non-res

Illinois

Loyola University Med Ctr

Emergency Med Tech-Paramedic Prgm
2160 S First Ave
Maywood, IL 60153
Prgm Dir: Brian E Sobeck, NREMT-P
Tel: 708 327-2544   *Fax:* 708 327-2548
Med Dir: Ron Lee, MD MBA
Class Cap: 25   *Begins:* Jan
Length: 12 mos   *Award:* Cert
Tuition per yr: $1,400

Trinity Medical Center

Emergency Med Tech-Paramedic Prgm
501 10th Ave
Moline, IL 61265
Prgm Dir: Jo Chambers, RN REMT-P
Tel: 309 757-3168   *Fax:* 309 757-3138
Med Dir: Walter J Bradley, MD MBA FACEP
Class Cap: 25   *Begins:* Aug
Length: 13 mos   *Award:* Cert
Tuition per yr: $1,997
Evening or weekend classes available

Indiana

Ivy Tech/Evansville Adv Life Support Consort

Emergency Med Tech-Paramedic Prgm
3501 First Ave
Evansville, IN 47711
Prgm Dir: Mary E Ostrye, MEd
Tel: 812 479-4191
Med Dir: Samuel Fitzsimmons, MD
Class Cap: 24   *Begins:* Aug
Length: 18 mos   *Award:* Cert
Tuition per yr: $2,000 res, $3,500 non-res

Methodist Hospital of Indiana, Inc

Emergency Med Tech-Paramedic Prgm
Ball State Univ
1701 N Senate Blvd
Indianapolis, IN 46206
Prgm Dir: Shirley Jones, MSEd MHA EMT-P
Tel: 317 929-3785
Med Dir: Michael L Olinger, MD
Class Cap: 20   *Begins:* Aug
Length: 12 mos, 24 mos   *Award:* Cert, AS
Tuition per yr: $2,100

Iowa

Mercy School of Health Sciences

Emergency Med Tech-Paramedic Prgm
928 6th Ave
Des Moines, IA 50309-1234
Prgm Dir: Christopher S Perrin, BA EMT-P
Tel: 515 247-4097   *Fax:* 515 246-1278
E-mail: mercy@mchs.edu
Med Dir: David G Stilley, MD
Class Cap: 30   *Begins:* Aug
Length: 6 mo , 9 mos   *Award:* Cert
Tuition per yr: $2,400 res, $4,495 non-res

Kansas

Johnson County Community College

Emergency Med Tech-Paramedic Prgm
12345 College Blvd & Quivira Rd
Overland Park, KS 66210-1299
Prgm Dir: Denny Kurogi, EMS
Tel: 913 469-8500   *Fax:* 913 469-2315
E-mail: dkurogi@johnco.cc.ks.us
Med Dir: Mark Holcomb, MD FACEP
Class Cap: 20   *Begins:* Jan
Length: 12 mos   *Award:* Cert, AS
Tuition per yr: $2,162 res, $5,734 non-res

Kentucky

Eastern Kentucky University

Emergency Med Tech-Paramedic Prgm
Dizney 225, EKU
Richmond, KY 40475-3135
Prgm Dir: Nancy Davis, RN MSN
Tel: 606 622-1028   *Fax:* 606 622-1140
Med Dir: S Delbert Fritz, MD
Class Cap: 90   *Begins:* Aug
Length: 13 mos, 16 mos   *Award:* Cert, AS
Tuition per yr: $4,428 res, $12,258 non-res
Evening or weekend classes available

Louisiana

University of Southwestern Louisiana

Emergency Med Tech-Paramedic Prgm
PO Box 42732
Lafayette, LA 70504-2732
Prgm Dir: Sheryl M Gonsoulin, MN
Tel: 318 482-5603   *Fax:* 318 482-5649
E-mail: smg3846@usl.edu
Med Dir: Leslie Greco, DO
Class Cap: 140   *Begins:* Jan Jun Aug
Length: 21 mos   *Award:* AD
Tuition per yr: $1,885 res, $4,585 non-res

Maryland

University of Maryland Baltimore County

Emergency Med Tech-Paramedic Prgm
5401 Wilkens Ave
Academic IV/Rm 316
Baltimore, MD 21228-5398
Prgm Dir: Dwight A Polk, BA NREMT-P
Tel: 410 455-3223   *Fax:* 410 455-3045
E-mail: polk@umbc.edu
Med Dir: Kevin Seaman, MD
Class Cap: 15   *Begins:* Sep
Length: 48 mos   *Award:* BS, MS
Tuition per yr: $4,136 res, $8,928 non-res

Michigan

Lansing Community College

Emergency Med Tech-Paramedic Prgm
3400 Human Health & Public Svcs Dept
PO Box 40010
Lansing, MI 48901-7210
Prgm Dir: Rexine A Finn, BSN EMT
Tel: 517 483-1410
Med Dir: Robert K Orr, DO
Class Cap: 60   *Begins:* Aug Jan
Length: 9 mos   *Award:* Cert, AD
Tuition per yr: $1,901 res, $2,974 non-res
Evening or weekend classes available

Minnesota

Northwest Technical Coll - E Grand Forks

Emergency Med Tech-Paramedic Prgm
PO Box 111 Hwy 220 N
East Grand Forks, MN 56721
Prgm Dir: Daniel L Sponsler, NREMT-P BS
Tel: 218 773-3441   *Fax:* 218 773-4502
E-mail: sponsler@adm.egf.tec.mn.us
Med Dir: James Fasbender, MD
Class Cap: 30   *Begins:* Aug
Length: 21 mos   *Award:* AAS
Tuition per yr: $3,955 res, $7,909 non-res

Century Community and Technical College

Emergency Med Tech-Paramedic Prgm
3300 Century Ave N
White Bear Lake, MN 55110
Prgm Dir: Diana Van Wormer, RN
Tel: 612 779-5794   *Fax:* 612 779-5779
Med Dir: Brent Saetrum, MD
Class Cap: 26   *Begins:* Varies
Length: 12 mos, 24 mos   *Award:* Dipl, AAS
Tuition per yr: $3,078 res, $6,156 non-res

Mississippi

Jones County Junior College
Emergency Med Tech-Paramedic Prgm
900 S Court St
Ellisville, MS 39437
Prgm Dir: Gregory M. Cole, AA NREMT-P
Tel: 601 477-4074 *Fax:* 601 477-4152
Med Dir: Roger Meadows, DO
Class Cap: 25 *Begins:* Aug
Length: 12 mos, 21 mos *Award:* Cert, AAS
Tuition per yr: $1,152 res, $2,485 non-res

Itawamba Community College
Emergency Med Tech-Paramedic Prgm
602 W Hill St
Fulton, MS 38843
Prgm Dir: Deborah Roebuck, RM REMT-P
Tel: 601 682-3101 *Fax:* 601 862-4614
Med Dir: James M Kirksey, MD
Class Cap: 15 *Begins:* Varies
Length: 5 mo , 10 mos *Award:* Cert, AAS
Tuition per yr: $1,275 res, $1,290 non-res
Evening or weekend classes available

Forrest General Hospital
Emergency Med Tech-Paramedic Prgm
6051 US Hwy 49 N
Hattiesburg, MS 39404-6389
Prgm Dir: Joe Jones, REMT-P
Tel: 601 288-2655
Med Dir: Mark Mitchell, DO
Class Cap: 25 *Begins:* Sep
Length: 12 mos *Award:* Cert
Tuition per yr: $1,200

University of Mississippi Medical Center
Emergency Med Tech-Paramedic Prgm
2500 N State St
Jackson, MS 39216-4505
Prgm Dir: Clyde Deschamp, MEd REMT-P
Tel: 601 984-5585 *Fax:* 601 984-6768
Med Dir: Frederick B Carlton, Jr, MD
Class Cap: 25 *Begins:* Aug
Length: 12 mos *Award:* Cert
Tuition per yr: $500 res, $976 non-res
Evening or weekend classes available

Mississippi Gulf Coast Community College
Emergency Med Tech-Paramedic Prgm
PO Box 67
Parkinston, MS 39573
Prgm Dir: Gary Shirley, EMT-P
Tel: 601 928-5211 *Fax:* 601 896-2520
Med Dir: William Bradford, MD
Begins: Aug
Length: 12 mos, 24 mos *Award:* Cert, AS
Tuition per yr: $1,352

Southwest Mississippi Regl Medical Ctr
Emergency Med Tech-Paramedic Prgm
215 Marion Ave
PO Box 1307
McComb, MS 39648
Prgm Dir: Sandra Stinson, NREMT-P
Tel: 601 684-5163
Med Dir: C Foster Lowe, MD
Class Cap: 20 *Begins:* Jun *Award:* Cert

Missouri

IHM Health Studies Ctr/St Louis University Med Ctr/Barnes Hosp
Emergency Med Tech-Paramedic Prgm
2500 Abbott Pl
St Louis, MO 63143
Prgm Dir: Tina J Stumpf, RN EMT-P
Tel: 314 768-1234 *Fax:* 314 768-1595
Med Dir: Lawrence Lewis, MD
Class Cap: 50 *Begins:* Jan
Length: 18 mos *Award:* Cert
Tuition per yr: $2,300
Evening or weekend classes available

Nebraska

Creighton University
Pre-Hosp Educ & Training Prgm
2514 Cuming St
Omaha, NE 68131-1632
Prgm Dir: Judy Janing, RN MA EMT-P
Tel: 402 280-1280 *Fax:* 402 280-1288
E-mail: jjaning@creighton.edu
Med Dir: Richard Walker, MD
Class Cap: 60 *Begins:* Aug Jan
Length: 12 mos, 18 mos *Award:* Cert, AD, BS
Tuition per yr: $4,850

New Hampshire

New Hampshire Technical Institute
Emergency Med Tech-Paramedic Prgm
11 Institute Dr
Concord, NH 03301-7412
Prgm Dir: Nancy L Brubaker, MEd EMT-P
Tel: 603 225-1836 *Fax:* 603 225-1895
Med Dir: David J Connor, MD
Class Cap: 27 *Begins:* Aug
Length: 21 mos *Award:* AS
Tuition per yr: $3,747 res, $4,865 non-res

New Mexico

Univ of New Mexico School of Medicine
Emergency Med Tech-Paramedic Prgm
2700 Yale Blvd SE
Albuquerque, NM 87106
Prgm Dir: Larry Hatfield, MEd REMT-P
Tel: 505 277-5757 *Fax:* 505 244-1505
Med Dir: David Johnson, MD
Class Cap: 24 *Begins:* Aug
Length: 11 mos *Award:* Cert
Tuition per yr: $2,315 res, $7,015 non-res

Dona Ana Community College
Emergency Med Tech-Paramedic Prgm
Box 30001/Dept 3DA
Las Cruces, NM 88003-0001
Prgm Dir: Ann Bellows, RN NREMT-P MA
Tel: 505 527-7529 *Fax:* 505 527-7515
E-mail: mmakris@nmsu.edu
Med Dir: Benjamin Diven, MD
Class Cap: 25 *Begins:* Jul
Length: 13 mos, 24 mos *Award:* Cert, AAS
Tuition per yr: $1,116 res, $2,952 non-res
Evening or weekend classes available

Eastern New Mexico University-Roswell
Emergency Med Tech-Paramedic Prgm
PO Box 6000
Roswell, NM 88202-6000
Prgm Dir: Mike Buldra, R EMT-P
Tel: 505 624-7239 *Fax:* 505 624-7100
E-mail: buldran@hib.enmuros.cc.nm.us
Med Dir: Don R Clark, MD
Class Cap: 16 *Begins:* Jun
Length: 14 mos, 24 mos *Award:* Cert, AS
Tuition per yr: $1,100 res, $2,800 non-res
Evening or weekend classes available

New York

Borough of Manhattan Community Coll of CUNY/New York Downtown Hosp
Emergency Med Tech-Paramedic Prgm
199 Chambers St
Dept of Allied Hlth Sciences
New York, NY 10007
Prgm Dir: Richard Lanzara, RRT MPH PhD
Tel: 212 346-8730
Med Dir: Diane Sixsmith, MPH MD
Begins: Sep
Length: 12 mos, 24 mos *Award:* Cert, AAS
Tuition per yr: $2,600 res, $4,200 non-res

North Carolina

Western Carolina University
Emergency Med Tech-Paramedic Prgm
Dept of Health Sciences
Cullowhee, NC 28723
Prgm Dir: Barbara K Lovin, EdD
Tel: 704 227-7113 *Fax:* 704 227-7446
E-mail: lovinb@wcuvax1.wcu.edu
Med Dir: David C Trigg, MD
Class Cap: 20 *Begins:* Aug
Length: 48 mos *Award:* BS
Tuition per yr: $874 res, $8,028 non-res

Catawba Valley Community College
Emergency Med Tech-Paramedic Prgm
2550 Hwy 70 SE
Hickory, NC 28602-9699
Prgm Dir: Martha McCrea, RN PA-C
Tel: 704 327-7000 *Fax:* 704 327-7276
Med Dir: Frank Donatelli, MD
Class Cap: 25 *Begins:* Sep
Length: 24 mos *Award:* Dipl, AD
Tuition per yr: $766 res, $6,044 non-res

Ohio

Akron General Medical Center
Emergency Med Tech-Paramedic Prgm
400 Wabash Ave
Akron, OH 44307
Prgm Dir: Scott W Martin, BS REMT-P
Tel: 330 384-6655 *Fax:* 330 996-2300
Med Dir: Thomas J Elson, MD FACEP
Class Cap: 45 *Begins:* Sep
Length: 10 mos *Award:* Dipl,Cert
Tuition per yr: $1,500
Evening or weekend classes available

University of Cincinnati Hospital
Emergency Med Tech-Paramedic Prgm
231 Bethesda Ave
Cincinnati, OH 45267-0769
Prgm Dir: Alan Mistler, RN
Tel: 513 558-4995   *Fax:* 513 558-5719
Med Dir: Michael Sayre, MD
Begins: Sep
Length: 10 mos   *Award:* Cert
Tuition per yr: $1,500
Evening or weekend classes available

Columbus State Community College
Emergency Med Tech-Paramedic Prgm
550 E Spring St
Columbus, OH 43215
Prgm Dir: Arthur K Ghiloni, EMT-P AS
Tel: 614 227-2510   *Fax:* 614 227-5144
Med Dir: Douglas Rund, MD
Class Cap: 22   *Begins:* Jun Jan
Length: 12 mos   *Award:* Cert
Tuition per yr: $1,938 res, $4,125 non-res
Evening or weekend classes available

Parma Community General Hospital
Emergency Med Tech-Paramedic Prgm
7300 State Rd
Parma, OH 44134
Prgm Dir: Mary Jane Pavlick, RN CEN REMT-P
Tel: 216 886-7323   *Fax:* 216 886-1295
Med Dir: J Michael Lonergan, MD
Class Cap: 50   *Begins:* Jan
Length: 11 mos   *Award:* Cert
Tuition per yr: $2,200 res, $2,200 non-res

Youngstown State University
Emergency Med Tech-Paramedic Prgm
410 Wick Ave
Youngstown, OH 44555
Prgm Dir: Randall W Benner, MEd NREMT-P
Tel: 330 742-3327   *Fax:* 330 742-2921
E-mail: rwbenner@cc.ysu.edu
Med Dir: Craig A Soltis, MD FACEP
Class Cap: 40   *Begins:* Sep
Length: 11 mos, 21 mos   *Award:* Cert, AAS
Tuition per yr: $4,260 res, $9,100 non-res
Evening or weekend classes available

Oregon

Oregon Health Sciences University
Emergency Med Tech-Paramedic Prgm
Dept of Emer Med-UHN/52
3181 SW Sam Jackson Pk Rd
Portland, OR 97201-3098
Prgm Dir: John Saito, EMT-P MPH
Tel: 503 494-7250
Med Dir: James Bryan, MD
Class Cap: 24   *Begins:* Sep
Length: 12 mos   *Award:* Cert
Tuition per yr: $4,000

Pennsylvania

Harrisburg Area Community College
Emergency Med Tech-Paramedic Prgm
One HACC Dr
Harrisburg, PA 17110-2999
Prgm Dir: Craig Davis, MEd EMT-P
Tel: 717 780-2564   *Fax:* 717 780-2551
E-mail: cadavis@hacc01b.hacc.edu
Med Dir: Jesse A Weigel, MD FACEP
Class Cap: 30   *Begins:* Aug
Length: 12 mos   *Award:* Dipl,Cert, AA
Tuition per yr: $1,145 res, $3,435 non-res
Evening or weekend classes available

St Joseph Hospital
Emergency Med Tech-Paramedic Prgm
250 College Ave
Lancaster, PA 17604-3509
Prgm Dir: Charles Bortle
Tel: 717 291-8224   *Fax:* 717 291-8516
Med Dir: Harris Baderak, DO
Class Cap: 48   *Begins:* Sep
Length: 12 mos   *Award:* Cert
Tuition per yr: $4,500
Evening or weekend classes available

Ctr for Emer Med of Western Pennsylvania
Emergency Med Tech-Paramedic Prgm
230 McKee Pl/Ste 500
Pittsburgh, PA 15213
Prgm Dir: Gregg Margolis, MS NREMT-P
Tel: 412 578-3200   *Fax:* 412 578-3241
Med Dir: Ronald N Roth, MD FACEP
Class Cap: 50   *Begins:* Jan Sep Apr
Length: 12 mos, 15 mos   *Award:* Cert
Tuition per yr: $1,950 res, $3,950 non-res
Evening or weekend classes available

Williamsport Hospital
Emergency Med Tech-Paramedic Prgm
777 Rural Ave
Williamsport, PA 17701
Prgm Dir: Charles G Stutzman, REMT-P
Tel: 717 321-2387   *Fax:* 717 321-2263
E-mail: twhmcpti@csrlink.net
Med Dir: Earl R Miller, MD
Class Cap: 42   *Begins:* Nov
Length: 15 mos   *Award:* Cert
Tuition per yr: $5,200

South Carolina

Greenville Technical College
Emergency Med Tech-Paramedic Prgm
PO Box 5616 Station B
Greenville, SC 29606-5616
Prgm Dir: Christopher K Cothran, MS NREMT-P
Tel: 864 250-8218   *Fax:* 864 250-8462
E-mail: cothrack@gvltec.edu
Med Dir: Stephen E Parks, MD
Class Cap: 30   *Begins:* Aug
Length: 21 mos   *Award:* AD
Tuition per yr: $1,500 res, $1,620 non-res
Evening or weekend classes available

Tennessee

Northeast State Technical Comm College
Emergency Med Tech-Paramedic Prgm
2425 Hwy 75
PO Box 246
Blountville, TN 37617-0246
Prgm Dir: Donald S Coleman, MEd EMT-P
Tel: 423 323-3191   *Fax:* 423 323-3083
E-mail: dscoleman@nstcc.cc.tn.us
Med Dir: Joseph D Barker, MD
Class Cap: 25   *Begins:* Aug
Length: 12 mos   *Award:* Cert
Tuition per yr: $1,200 res, $2,500 non-res
Evening or weekend classes available

Volunteer State Community College
Emergency Med Tech-Paramedic Prgm
Nashville Pike
Gallatin, TN 37066
Prgm Dir: Richard A Collier, BSN CEN EMT-P
Tel: 615 452-8600   *Fax:* 615 230-3344
E-mail: rcollier@uscc.cc.tn.us
Med Dir: John Nixon, MD ACEP
Class Cap: 30   *Begins:* Jun Aug
Length: 15 mos, 24 mos   *Award:* Cert, AAS
Tuition per yr: $1,525 res, $3,772 non-res
Evening or weekend classes available

Roane State Community College
Emergency Med Tech-Paramedic Prgm
8393 Kingston Pike
Knoxville, TN 37919
Prgm Dir: Kirk Harris, AS BS EMT-P
Tel: 423 539-6905
Med Dir: Bert Toney, MD
Class Cap: 60   *Begins:* Aug
Length: 12 mos   *Award:* Cert
Tuition per yr: $1,234 res, $4,554 non-res

Jackson State Community College
Emergency Med Tech-Paramedic Prgm
2406 N Parkway St
Jackson, TN 38301-3797
Prgm Dir: Thomas H Coley, BEd EMT-P
Tel: 901 424-3520   *Fax:* 901 425-2647
E-mail: tcoley@jscc.cc.tn.us
Med Dir: Doug Phillips, MD
Class Cap: 35   *Begins:* Sep
Length: 12 mos   *Award:* Dipl,Cert, AAS
Tuition per yr: $1,491 res, $5,880 non-res
Evening or weekend classes available

Shelby State Community College
Emergency Med Tech-Paramedic Prgm
H Bldg
PO Box 40568
Memphis, TN 38174-0568
Prgm Dir: Gerald Foon, EMT-P MS
Tel: 901 544-5400   *Fax:* 901 544-5391
E-mail: foon@sscc.cc.tn.us
Med Dir: Loren Crown, MD
Begins: Sep
Length: 12 mos   *Award:* Cert, AAS
Tuition per yr: $1,536 res, $6,144 non-res

Texas

Austin Community College

Emergency Med Tech-Paramedic Prgm
1020 Grove Blvd
Austin, TX 78741
Prgm Dir: Jeffrey Hayes, BS NREMT-P
Tel: 512 389-4112 *Fax:* 512 369-6700
E-mail: jhayes@flash.net
Med Dir: B Duke Kimbrough, MD
Class Cap: 35 *Begins:* Jan Sep
Length: 18 mos, 12 mos *Award:* AAS
Tuition per yr: $1,035 res, $1,980 non-res
Evening or weekend classes available

Lee College

Emergency Med Tech-Paramedic Prgm
PO Box 818
Baytown, TX 77522-0818
Prgm Dir: Ernest K Whitener, MS EMT-P
Tel: 713 425-6836
Med Dir: David Hall, MD
Class Cap: 20 *Begins:* Sep Jan
Length: 12 mos *Award:* Cert, AAS
Tuition per yr: $600 res, $800 non-res

Univ of Tx Southwestern Med Ctr/El Centro College

Emergency Med Tech-Paramedic Prgm
5323 Harry Hines Blvd
Dallas, TX 75235-8890
Prgm Dir: Debra Cason, RN MS EMT-P
Tel: 214 648-3131 *Fax:* 214 648-7580
E-mail: dcason@mednet.sswmed.edu
Med Dir: James M Atkins, MD
Class Cap: 129 *Begins:* Sep Jan May
Length: 5 mos *Award:* Cert
Tuition per yr: $1,375

Houston Community College System

Emergency Med Tech-Paramedic Prgm
22 Waugh Dr
Houston, TX 77007
Prgm Dir: Josiah W Tyson III, EMT-P, AA
Tel: 713 237-1040 *Fax:* 713 641-9653
Med Dir: Arlo F Weltge, MD
Class Cap: 120 *Begins:* Sep
Length: 5 mo , 12 mos *Award:* Cert
Tuition per yr: $660 res, $1,144 non-res

Texas Tech Univ Hlth Sci Ctr

Emergency Med Tech-Paramedic Prgm
3601 Fourth St
Lubbock, TX 79430
Prgm Dir: Neil B Coker, BS EMT-P
Tel: 806 743-3218 *Fax:* 806 743-1315
E-mail: alhubc@ttuhsc.edu
Med Dir: CRF Baker, Jr, MD
Class Cap: 60 *Begins:* Aug
Length: 11 mos *Award:* Cert
Tuition per yr: $1,250 res, $1,250 non-res
Evening or weekend classes available

Univ of Texas Hlth Sci Ctr at San Antonio

Emergency Med Tech-Paramedic Prgm
4201 Medical Dr/Ste 250
San Antonio, TX 77229-5631
Prgm Dir: Charles E Garoni, BA EMT-P
Tel: 210 567-7860 *Fax:* 210 567-7887
E-mail: garoni@uthscsa.edu
Med Dir: Donald J Gordon, MD
Begins: Varies
Length: 5 mo , 14 mos *Award:* Cert
Tuition per yr: $1,600

College of the Mainland

Emergency Med Tech-Paramedic Prgm
1200 Amburn Rd
Texas City, TX 77591
Prgm Dir: Nancy Ann Eubanks, RN RMT-P EMSC
Tel: 409 938-1211, Ext 255 *Fax:* 409 938-1211
E-mail: neubanks@campus.mainland.cc.tx.us
Med Dir: Robert Fromm, MD
Class Cap: 200 *Begins:* Aug Jan
Length: 10 mos *Award:* Cert, AAS
Tuition per yr: $152 res, $275 non-res
Evening or weekend classes available

Utah

Weber State University

Emergency Med Tech-Paramedic Prgm
3800 Harrison Blvd
Ogden, UT 84408-3902
Prgm Dir: Valory Poncelet-Quick, RN MS
Tel: 801 626-6521 *Fax:* 801 626-6610
E-mail: vquick\@weber.edu
Med Dir: Joan Balcombe, MD
Begins: Sep
Length: 8 mo , 16 mos *Award:* Cert, AA
Tuition per yr: $1,854 res, $5,541 non-res

Virginia

Northern Virginia Community College

Emergency Med Tech-Paramedic Prgm
8333 Little River Trnpk
Annandale, VA 22003
Prgm Dir: Pamela B doCarmo, PhD EMT-P
Tel: 703 323-3037 *Fax:* 703 323-4576
Med Dir: James F Vafier, MD
Class Cap: 32 *Begins:* Aug Jan
Length: 8 mo , 24 mos *Award:* Cert, AAS
Tuition per yr: $1,344
Evening or weekend classes available

Comm Hosp of Roanoke Valley/College of Health Sciences

Emergency Med Tech-Paramedic Prgm
PO Box 13186
Roanoke, VA 24031-3186
Prgm Dir: Glen Mayhew, BA REMT-P
Tel: 540 985-8398 *Fax:* 540 985-9773
Med Dir: Michael Donato, DO
Class Cap: 30 *Begins:* Aug
Length: 0 mo , 18 mos *Award:* AD
Tuition per yr: $6,400
Evening or weekend classes available

Washington

Central Washington University

Emergency Med Tech-Paramedic Prgm
Ellensburg, WA 98926
Prgm Dir: Dorothy M Purser, MEd
Tel: 509 963-1451
Med Dir: Jackson Horsley, MD
Class Cap: 24 *Begins:* Sep
Length: 9 mo , 12 mos *Award:* Dipl,Cert, BS
Tuition per yr: $1,317 res, $4,584 non-res

Univ of Washington/Harborview Med Ctr

Emergency Med Tech-Paramedic Prgm
325 Ninth Ave
Mailstop 2A-40
Seattle, WA 98104
Prgm Dir: Martha Taylor
Tel: 206 223-3489 *Fax:* 206 731-8554
E-mail: rwaugh@u.washington.edu
Med Dir: Leonard A Cobb, MD
Class Cap: 18 *Begins:* Oct
Length: 10 mos *Award:* Cert
Tuition per yr: $10,000

Spokane Community College

Emergency Med Tech-Paramedic Prgm
N 1810 Greene St
Spokane, WA 99207-5399
Prgm Dir: Mary Pat Sesso, RN MSN ARNP
Tel: 509 533-7299 *Fax:* 509 533-8621
E-mail: msesso@clc.ctc.edu
Med Dir: Gary Gularte, MD
Class Cap: 18 *Begins:* Jan
Length: 10 mos *Award:* Cert
Tuition per yr: $588

Tacoma Community College

Emergency Med Tech-Paramedic Prgm
5900 S 12th St
Tacoma, WA 98465
Prgm Dir: Lisa Evenbly, RN BSN
Tel: 206 566-5162 *Fax:* 206 566-5273
Med Dir: Patricia Hastings, DO
Class Cap: 24 *Begins:* Jun
Length: 12 mos, 21 mos *Award:* Cert, AAS
Tuition per yr: $2,870 res, $7,350 non-res
Evening or weekend classes available

Health Information Management

History

Standards for educational programs for medical record administrators (formerly librarians) were established in 1935 by the American Medical Record Association (now the American Health Information Management Association [AHIMA]) through its committee on training. The first four programs for medical record administrators were accredited in that year, three of which were hospital-based and one of which was a college-based program. In 1942, the AHIMA invited the American Medical Association (AMA) to serve as the official accrediting agency for educational programs for medical record administrators. This responsibility was accepted by the AMA House of Delegates. *Standards (Essentials)* for educational programs for medical record administrators were initially developed and adopted in 1943 and were subsequently revised in 1952, 1960, 1967, 1974, 1981, 1988, and 1994.

In 1953, the first *Standards* for educational programs for medical record technicians were established and approved by both the AHIMA and the AMA. The first educational programs for medical record technicians were hospital-based. Over the years there has been a gradual transition from hospital-based educational programs for medical record administrators and medical record technicians to college- and university-based programs. In 1965, 1976, 1983, 1988, and 1994, the AHIMA—in collaboration with the AMA Council on Medical Education (CME)—revised and adopted the *Standards and Guidelines for Accredited Programs for the Health Information Technician and the Health Information Administrator*. Today, the *Standards* are adopted by the Commission on Accreditation of Allied Health Education Programs (CAAHEP) in collaboration with AHIMA.

Definition of the Profession

Health information management is the profession that focuses on health care data and the management of health care information resources. The profession addresses the nature, structure, and translation of data into usable forms of information for the advancement of health and health care of individuals and populations.

Health information management professionals collect, integrate, and analyze primary and secondary health care data; disseminate information; and manage information resources related to the research, planning, provision, and evaluation of health care services.

Health Information Administrator

Occupational Description

Health information administrators manage health information systems consistent with the medical, administrative, ethical, and legal requirements of the health care delivery system. Although these administrators are not often directly involved in patient contact, their work with the medical and hospital administrative staff is of critical importance to patient care. Because they deal with patient records and information, they should not be confused with medical librarians, who work chiefly with books, periodicals, and other medical publications.

Job Description

The health information administrator is the professional responsible for the management of health information systems consistent with professional standards and the medical, administrative, ethical, and legal requirements of the health care delivery system. The administrator possesses the administrative knowledge and skills necessary to plan and develop health information systems that meet standards of accrediting and regulating agencies; to design health information systems appropriate for various sizes and types of health care facilities; to manage the human, financial, and physical resources of a health information service; to participate in medical staff and institutional activities, including utilization management, risk management, and quality assessment; to collect and analyze patient and facility data for reimbursement, facility planning, marketing, risk management, utilization management, quality assessment, and research; to serve as an advocate for privacy and confidentiality of health information; and to plan and offer in-service educational programs for health care personnel.

Employment Characteristics

The demand for health information administrators is greatest in hospitals. Other growing areas of employment are ambulatory and long-term care facilities, state health departments, peer review organizations, government agencies, and private industry. Health information administrators interested in teaching may accept faculty appointments in academic programs for health information administration.

According to the AHIMA, entry-level salaries average between $25,000 and $30,000.

Educational Programs

Length. Baccalaureate degree programs are 4 years. Postbaccalaureate and other certificate programs are generally 1 year.
Prerequisites. Applicants for the 4-year baccalaureate degree program should have a high school diploma or equivalent. Applicants for the 1-year postbaccalaureate certificate program should have a baccalaureate degree that includes coursework in science and statistics, as specified.
Curriculum. The preprofessional curriculum should include studies in humanities, behavioral and biological sciences, mathematics, and data processing. The professional curriculum requires medical sciences, including language of medicine, structure and function of the human body, and disease process; organization of the health care industry; systems and processes for collecting, maintaining, and disseminating health-related information; computer concepts and microcomputer applications; computer applications in health care; laws, regulations, ethics, and standards affecting the management of health information; management theory, principles and practices, classifications, nomenclatures, and reimbursement systems; data analysis and presentation; systems analysis and design and project management concepts; health care financial management; clinical quality assessment and improvement; and statistics, research and evaluation methods, and supervised practice in health information departments of facilities and agencies.
Standards. *Standards* are minimum educational standards developed by the AHIMA in collaboration with the Commission on Accreditation of Allied Health Education Programs (CAAHEP). Each new program is assessed in accordance with the *Standards*, and accredited programs are reviewed periodically to determine whether they remain in compliance. The *Standards* are available on written request from the AHIMA

Health Information Technician

Occupational Description

The medical record is a permanent document prepared for each person treated in a healthcare facility. It contains the "who, what, why, where, when, and how" details of patient care during diagnosis and treatment, as well as information of medical, scientific, and legal value. Health information technicians are important members of the healthcare team. Traditionally, health information technicians have been employed in the medical records department of hospitals. With the increasing expansion of healthcare needs, opportunities for employment are also available in ambulatory healthcare facilities, industrial clinics, state and federal health agencies, long-term care facilities, and a number of other areas.

Job Description

The health information technician is the professional responsible for maintaining components of health information systems in a manner consistent with the medical, administrative, ethical, legal, accreditation, and regulatory requirements of the healthcare delivery system. In all types of facilities, and in various locations within a facility, the technician possesses the technical knowledge and skills necessary to process, maintain, compile, and report patient data for reimbursement, facility planning, marketing, risk management, utilization management, quality assessment, and research; to abstract and code clinical data using appropriate classification systems; and to analyze health records according to standards. The health information technician may be responsible for functional supervision of the various components of the health information system.

Employment Characteristics

Although the demand for health information technicians is greatest in hospitals, other growing areas of employment may include long-term care facilities, ambulatory care centers, rehabilitation centers, state and local health departments, and large group medical practices.

According to the AHIMA, entry-level salaries average $22,000.

Educational Programs

Length. Programs are generally 2 years, offering an associate degree.

Prerequisites. High school diploma or equivalent.

Curriculum. In addition to general education courses, the professional component of the technician program requires medical sciences, including language of medicine, structure and function of the human body, and disease process; organization of the health care industry; systems and processes for collecting, maintaining, and disseminating health-related information; computer concepts and microcomputer applications; computer applications in health care; laws, regulations, ethics, and standards affecting management of health information; supervisory principles and practices, classifications, nomenclatures, and reimbursement systems; data analysis and presentation; clinical quality assessment and improvement; and supervised practice in health information departments of health care facilities and agencies.

Standards. *Standards* are minimum educational standards developed by the AHIMA in collaboration with the Commission on Accreditation of Allied Health Education Programs. Each new program is assessed in accordance with the *Standards*, and accredited programs are reviewed periodically to determine whether they remain in compliance. The *Standards* are available on written request from the AHIMA.

Inquiries

Accreditation

Requests for information on program accreditation, including *Standards*, preparing the self-study report, and arranging a site visit, should be submitted to

American Health Information Management Association
Education & Accreditation Division
919 N Michigan Ave/Ste 1400
Chicago, IL 60611-1683
312 787-2672 ext 403

Careers and Credentialing

Inquiries regarding careers and credentialing should be addressed to

American Health Information Management Association
919 N Michigan Ave/Ste 1400
Chicago, IL 60611-1683
312 787-2672 ext 207

Health Information Administrator

Alabama

University of Alabama at Birmingham
Health Information Admin Prgm
University Station
Birmingham, AL 35294
Prgm Dir: Sara S Grostick, RRA
Tel: 205 934-3509   *Fax:* 205 975-6608
E-mail: him0004@uabdpo.dpo.uab.edu
Class Cap: 25   *Begins:* Sep
Length: 12 mos   *Award:* BS
Tuition per yr: $2,100 res, $4,200 non-res
Evening or weekend classes available

Arkansas

Arkansas Tech University
Health Information Admin Prgm
Wilson 105
Russellville, AR 72801
Prgm Dir: Melinda Heaton, MEd RRA
Tel: 501 968-0441   *Fax:* 501 964-0504
E-mail: pimh@atuvm.atu.edu
Class Cap: 20   *Begins:* Aug
Length: 37 mos   *Award:* BS
Tuition per yr: $902 res, $3,804 non-res

California

Loma Linda University
Health Information Admin Prgm
Office of the Dean
Loma Linda, CA 92350
Prgm Dir: Marilyn R Davidian, RRA
Tel: 909 824-4976   *Fax:* 909 824-4291
E-mail: mdavidian@ccmail.llu.edu
Class Cap: 25   *Begins:* Sep
Length: 18 mos   *Award:* Cert, BS
Tuition per yr: $13,510 res, $13,510 non-res

Colorado

Regis University
Health Information Admin Prgm
3333 Regis Blvd
Denver, CO 80221-1099
Prgm Dir: Debra L Bennett-Woods, MA ART
Tel: 303 458-4157   *Fax:* 308 964-5533
Class Cap: 20   *Begins:* Jan Aug
Length: 24 mos, 30 mos   *Award:* Cert, BS
Tuition per yr: $5,096 res, $5,096 non-res
Evening or weekend classes available

Florida

Florida International University
Health Information Admin Prgm
N Miami Campus
ACI-Rm 394C
Miami, FL 33181
Prgm Dir: Maha Yunis, RRA
Tel: 305 940-5631   *Fax:* 305 919-5507
E-mail: yunism@fiu.edu
Class Cap: 95   *Begins:* Aug
Length: 20 mos   *Award:* BSHIM
Tuition per yr: $1,892 res, $6,579 non-res

University of Central Florida
Health Information Admin Prgm
PO Box 25000
Orlando, FL 32816
Prgm Dir: Carol J Barr, RRA
Tel: 407 823-2353   *Fax:* 407 823-2353
E-mail: harr@pegasus.cc.ucf.edu
Class Cap: 30   *Begins:* Aug
Length: 24 mos   *Award:* BS
Tuition per yr: $2,095 res, $7,978 non-res
Evening or weekend classes available

Florida A & M University
Health Information Admin Prgm
Tallahassee, FL 32307
Prgm Dir: Barbara W Mosley, PhD RRA
Tel: 904 599-3822   *Fax:* 904 561-2457
Class Cap: 20   *Begins:* Aug
Length: 24 mos   *Award:* BS
Tuition per yr: $1,650 res, $6,652 non-res

Georgia

Clark Atlanta University
Health Information Admin Prgm
James P Brawley Dr at Fair St SW
Atlanta, GA 30314
Prgm Dir: Barbara Brice, PhD RRA
Tel: 404 880-8115   *Fax:* 404 880-6165
Class Cap: 20   *Begins:* Sep
Length: 13 mos, 36 mos   *Award:* Cert, BS
Tuition per yr: $5,711 res, $4,000 non-res

Medical College of Georgia
Health Information Admin Prgm
AL-122
Augusta, GA 30912-0400
Prgm Dir: Charlotte A Johnston, PhD RRA
Tel: 706 721-3436   *Fax:* 706 721-6067
E-mail: chjohnstamail.mcg.edu
Class Cap: 40   *Begins:* Sep
Length: 18 mos, 33 mos   *Award:* Dipl, BS
Tuition per yr: $2,148 res, $6,435 non-res
Evening or weekend classes available

Illinois

Chicago State University
Health Information Admin Prgm
9501 S King Dr
BHS 610
Chicago, IL 60628-1598
Prgm Dir: Leona M Thomas, MHS RRA
Tel: 312 995-2552   *Fax:* 312 995-4484
Class Cap: 25   *Begins:* Aug
Length: 48 mos   *Award:* BS
Tuition per yr: $2,420 res, $6,464 non-res
Evening or weekend classes available

Univ of Illinois at Chicago
Health Information Admin Prgm
1919 W Taylor, Rm 811
M/C520
Chicago, IL 60612
Prgm Dir: Karen Patena, MBA RRA
Tel: 312 996-3530   *Fax:* 312 413-0205
E-mail: patena@uic.edu
Class Cap: 50   *Begins:* Aug
Length: 24 mos   *Award:* Dipl, BS
Tuition per yr: $4,124 res, $9,864 non-res

Illinois State University
Health Information Admin Prgm
Moulton Hall 103
Normal, IL 61761
Prgm Dir: Francis L Waterstraat, Jr, MBA RRA
Tel: 309 438-8329
Begins: Aug
Length: 24 mos   *Award:* BS
Tuition per yr: $3,712 res, $9,402 non-res

Indiana

Indiana University Northwest
Health Information Admin Prgm
3400 Broadway
Gary, IN 46408
Prgm Dir: Margaret A Skurka, MS RRA
Tel: 219 980-6654   *Fax:* 219 980-6649
E-mail: mskurk@iunhaw1.iun.indiana.edu
Class Cap: 15   *Begins:* Aug
Length: 24 mos   *Award:* BS
Tuition per yr: $2,449 res, $6,480 non-res
Evening or weekend classes available

Indiana University School of Medicine
Health Information Admin Prgm
1140 W Michigan St
CF 322
Indianapolis, IN 46202-5119
Prgm Dir: Janatha R Ashton, MS RRA
Tel: 317 274-7317   *Fax:* 317 278-1820
E-mail: jashton@iupui.edu
Class Cap: 20   *Begins:* Aug
Length: 9 mos   *Award:* BS
Tuition per yr: $4,086 res, $12,540 non-res

Kansas

University of Kansas Medical Center
Health Information Admin Prgm
3901 Rainbow Blvd
Kansas City, KS 66160-7607
Prgm Dir: Alice Junghans
Tel: 913 588-2422 *Fax:* 913 588-2428
E-mail: ajunghan@kumc.edu
Class Cap: 30 *Begins:* Jun
Length: 12 mos *Award:* Dipl, BS
Tuition per yr: $2,908 res, $12,190 non-res

Kentucky

Eastern Kentucky University
Health Information Admin Prgm
Dizney 117
Richmond, KY 40475-3135
Prgm Dir: Frances A Hindsman, MBA RRA
Tel: 606 622-1915 *Fax:* 606 622-1140
E-mail: hrshinds@acs.eku.edu
Class Cap: 32 *Begins:* Aug Jan
Length: 18 mos, 36 mos *Award:* Cert, BS
Tuition per yr: $1,970 res, $5,450 non-res
Evening or weekend classes available

Louisiana

University of Southwestern Louisiana
Health Information Admin Prgm
PO Box 41007
Lafayette, LA 70504
Prgm Dir: Carol A Venable, MPH RRA
Tel: 318 482-6629 *Fax:* 318 482-5902
E-mail: venable@usl.edu
Class Cap: 35 *Begins:* Aug
Length: 48 mos *Award:* BS
Tuition per yr: $1,893 res, $5,492 non-res

Louisiana Tech University
Health Information Admin Prgm
PO Box 3171
Ruston, LA 71272
Prgm Dir: Lou H Davison, DBA RRA
Tel: 318 257-2854 *Fax:* 318 257-4896
E-mail: 1105993@vm.cc.latech.edu
Class Cap: 35 *Begins:* Aug Nov Feb May
Length: 39 mos *Award:* BS
Tuition per yr: $2,352 res, $4,347 non-res

Massachusetts

Northeastern University
Health Information Admin Prgm
269 Ryder Hall
Boston, MA 02115
Prgm Dir: Annalee Collins, MEd.,RRA
Tel: 617 373-2525 *Fax:* 607 373-2325
E-mail: ancollin@lynx.neu.edu
Class Cap: 64 *Begins:* Jan Apr Sep
Length: 18 mos, 36 mos *Award:* Cert, BS
Tuition per yr: $5,600
Evening or weekend classes available

Michigan

Ferris State University
Health Information Admin Prgm
Coll of Allied Hlth Sciences
200 Ferris Dr/VFS402
Big Rapids, MI 49307-2740
Prgm Dir: Ellen J Haneline, MEd RRA
Tel: 616 592-2313 *Fax:* 616 592-3788
Begins: Aug
Length: 38 mos *Award:* Dipl, BS
Tuition per yr: $3,630 res, $7,364 non-res
Evening or weekend classes available

Baker College
Health Information Admin Prgm
1050 W Bristol Rd
Flint, MI 48507
Prgm Dir: Brenda Brown
Tel: 810 766-4195
Class Cap: 35 *Begins:* Sep
Length: 48 mos *Award:* BA
Tuition per yr: $1,344 res, $1,344 non-res

Minnesota

College of St Scholastica
Health Information Admin Prgm
1200 Kenwood Ave
Duluth, MN 55811
Prgm Dir: Kathleen M LaTour, MA RRA
Tel: 218 723-6011 *Fax:* 219 723-6290
E-mail: klatour@fac1.css.edu
Class Cap: 40 *Begins:* Sep
Length: 18 mos, 27 mos *Award:* Cert, BA
Tuition per yr: $13,056

Mississippi

University of Mississippi Medical Center
Health Information Admin Prgm
2500 N State St
Jackson, MS 39216
Prgm Dir: Rebecca J Yates, MEd RRA
Tel: 601 984-6305 *Fax:* 601 984-6344
E-mail: yates@shrp.umsmed.edu
Begins: Aug
Length: 18 mos *Award:* Dipl, BS
Tuition per yr: $2,071 res, $4,530 non-res

Missouri

Stephens College
Health Information Admin Prgm
Campus Box 2083
Columbia, MO 65215
Prgm Dir: Joan T Rines, PhD RRA
Tel: 573 876-7283 *Fax:* 573 876-7248
E-mail: joanr@wc.stephens.edu
Class Cap: 125 *Begins:* Varies *Award:* Cert, BS
Tuition per yr: $1,950 res, $1,950 non-res
Evening or weekend classes available

St Louis University Health Sciences Ctr
Health Information Admin Prgm
Dept of Hlth Info Management
3525 Caroline
St Louis, MO 63104
Prgm Dir: Karen Jody Smith, MSM RRA
Tel: 314 577-8516 *Fax:* 314 268-5135
E-mail: smit2kj@sluvca.edu
Class Cap: 25 *Begins:* Aug
Length: 48 mos *Award:* Dipl, BS
Tuition per yr: $11,690

Montana

Carroll College
Health Information Admin Prgm
Faculty Box 90
Helena, MT 59625
Prgm Dir: David Westlake, RRA
Tel: 406 447-4365
E-mail: dwestlak@carroll.edu
Class Cap: 45 *Begins:* Aug
Length: 36 mos *Award:* BA
Tuition per yr: $8,650

Nebraska

College of St Mary
Health Information Admin Prgm
1901 S 72nd St
Omaha, NE 68124
Prgm Dir: Ellen B Jacobs, MEd RRA
Tel: 402 399-2611 *Fax:* 402 399-2657
Begins: Aug Jan
Length: 24 mos *Award:* BS
Tuition per yr: $10,994
Evening or weekend classes available

New Jersey

Kean College of New Jersey
Health Information Admin Prgm
Morris Ave
Union, NJ 07083
Prgm Dir: Natalie Sartori, MEd
Tel: 908 527-3010
Class Cap: 20 *Begins:* Sep
Length: 24 mos, 48 mos *Award:* Cert, BS
Tuition per yr: $3,367 res, $4,685 non-res
Evening or weekend classes available

New York

SUNY Health Science Center - Brooklyn
Health Information Admin Prgm
450 Clarkson Ave
PO Box 105
Brooklyn, NY 11203
Prgm Dir: Isaac Topor, EdD RRA
Tel: 718 270-7770 *Fax:* 718 270-7751
Class Cap: 20 *Begins:* Sep
Length: 24 mos *Award:* Cert, BS
Tuition per yr: $1,808 res, $4,258 non-res
Evening or weekend classes available

Programs

Long Island Univ - C W Post Campus

Health Information Admin Prgm
Northern Blvd
Greenvale, NY 11548
Prgm Dir: Nancy E Katz-Johnson, MHS RRA
Tel: 516 299-2485
Begins: Sep Jan May Jun Jul
Length: 48 mos   *Award:* Dipl,Cert, BS
Tuition per yr: $12,430

Ithaca College

Health Information Admin Prgm
953 Danby Rd
Ithaca, NY 14850-7182
Prgm Dir: Christine H Pogorzala, MS RRA
Tel: 607 274-3355   *Fax:* 607 274-1137
E-mail: pogorzal@ithaca.edu
Class Cap: 40   *Begins:* Aug Jan
Length: 18 mos   *Award:* Dipl, BS
Tuition per yr: $16,130

SUNY Institute of Tech - Utica/Rome

Health Information Admin Prgm
PO Box 3050
Utica, NY 13504-3050
Prgm Dir: Donna L Silsbee, MS RRA
Tel: 315 792-7391   *Fax:* 315 792-7138
E-mail: fdls1@sunyit.edu
Class Cap: 20   *Begins:* Sep
Length: 18 mos   *Award:* BS, BPS
Tuition per yr: $3,400 res, $4,150 non-res
Evening or weekend classes available

North Carolina

Western Carolina University

Health Information Admin Prgm
139 Moore Hall
Cullowhee, NC 28723
Prgm Dir: Walter R Floreani, RRA
Tel: 704 227-7113   *Fax:* 704 227-7446
E-mail: floreani@wpoff.ecu.edu
Class Cap: 17   *Begins:* Aug
Length: 18 mos   *Award:* BS
Tuition per yr: $1,732 res, $8,574 non-res

East Carolina University

Health Information Admin Prgm
Sch Allied Hlth Science
Greenville, NC 27858
Prgm Dir: Elizabeth J Layman, PhD RRA
Tel: 919 328-4444   *Fax:* 919 328-4470
E-mail: hrlayman@ecuvm.cis.ecu.edu
Class Cap: 20   *Begins:* Aug
Length: 18 mos   *Award:* BS
Tuition per yr: $1,200 res, $5,000 non-res

Ohio

Ohio State University

Health Information Admin Prgm
1583 Perry St
Columbus, OH 43210
Prgm Dir: Melanie Brodnik, PhD RRA
Tel: 614 292-0567   *Fax:* 614 292-0210
E-mail: brodnik.2@osu.edu
Class Cap: 20   *Begins:* Sep
Length: 18 mos   *Award:* Cert, BS
Tuition per yr: $3,273 res, $9,813 non-res

Oklahoma

East Central University

Health Information Admin Prgm
Ada, OK 74820
Prgm Dir: Sandra A Dixon, MEd MCE RRA
Tel: 405 332-8000   *Fax:* 405 332-1623
E-mail: sdixon@mailclerk.ecok.edu
Class Cap: 16   *Begins:* Aug
Length: 24 mos   *Award:* BS
Tuition per yr: $1,834 res, $4,523 non-res

Southwestern Oklahoma State University

Health Information Admin Prgm
100 Campus Dr
Weatherford, OK 73096
Prgm Dir: Marion Prichard, RRA
Tel: 405 774-3287   *Fax:* 405 774-3795
E-mail: pricham@swasd.edu
Class Cap: 16   *Begins:* Aug
Length: 24 mos   *Award:* BS
Tuition per yr: $1,712 res, $4,320 non-res

Pennsylvania

Gwynedd-Mercy College

Health Information Admin Prgm
Gwynedd Valley, PA 19437
Prgm Dir: Jennifer Hornung, RRA CPHQ CCS
Tel: 610 646-7300
Class Cap: 15   *Begins:* Aug
Length: 24 mos   *Award:* Cert, BS
Tuition per yr: $12,300

Temple University

Health Information Admin Prgm
College of Allied Health Professions
3307 N Broad St
Philadelphia, PA 19140
Prgm Dir: L B Harman, PhD, RRA
Tel: 215 221-4811   *Fax:* 215 707-7819
E-mail: lharman@vm.temple.edu
Class Cap: 36   *Begins:* Sep
Length: 9 mos   *Award:* BS
Tuition per yr: $6,408 res, $11,340 non-res

Duquesne University

Health Information Admin Prgm
Chair Dept of Health Mgmt Systems
323 Rangos Sch of Hlth Sciences
Pittsburgh, PA 15282-0001
Prgm Dir: Joan M Kiel, PhD
Tel: 412 396-4772   *Fax:* 412 396-5554
Class Cap: 30   *Begins:* Aug
Length: 48 mos, 60 mos   *Award:* MHMS , MBA
Tuition per yr: $13,696 res, $14,486 non-res
Evening or weekend classes available

University of Pittsburgh

Health Information Admin Prgm
6051 Forbes Tower
Pittsburgh, PA 15260
Prgm Dir: Mervat Abdelhak, PhD RRA
Tel: 412 647-1190   *Fax:* 412 647-1199
E-mail: madelhakt@pitt.edu
Class Cap: 36   *Begins:* Sep
Length: 18 mos, 24 mos   *Award:* Cert, BS, MS
Tuition per yr: $8,036 res, $12,274 non-res
Evening or weekend classes available

York College of Pennsylvania

Health Information Admin Prgm
Country Club Rd
York, PA 17405
Prgm Dir: Jean A Fultz, RRA
Tel: 717 816-1616, Ext 1295   *Fax:* 717 849-1619
Class Cap: 20   *Begins:* Sep
Length: 36 mos   *Award:* BS
Tuition per yr: $5,525
Evening or weekend classes available

Puerto Rico

University of Puerto Rico

Health Information Admin Prgm
GPO Box 365067
San Juan, PR 00936-5067
Prgm Dir: Anna Orabona-Ocasio, RRA CCS
Tel: 787 764-3609   *Fax:* 787 759-3645
Class Cap: 14   *Begins:* Aug
Length: 22 mos   *Award:* MS
Tuition per yr: $2,250 res, $3,500 non-res

South Carolina

Medical University of South Carolina

Health Information Admin Prgm
Coll of Hlth Professions
171 Ashley Ave
Charleston, SC 29425
Prgm Dir: Karen A Wager, RRA
Tel: 803 792-4491   *Fax:* 803 792-3327
E-mail: wagerka@musc.edu
Class Cap: 20   *Begins:* Aug Jan May
Length: 18 mos, 26 mos   *Award:* , MHS
Tuition per yr: $4,401 res, $12,822 non-res
Evening or weekend classes available

South Dakota

Dakota State University

Health Information Admin Prgm
C B Kennedy Ctr #151
Madison, SD 57042-1799
Prgm Dir: Dorine Bennett, MBA RA
Tel: 605 256-5137   *Fax:* 605 256-5316
E-mail: bennettd@columbia.dsu.edu
Class Cap: 45   *Begins:* Sep
Length: 18 mos, 36 mos   *Award:* BS
Tuition per yr: $2,813 res, $6,006 non-res

Tennessee

University of Tennessee Memphis

Health Information Admin Prgm
822 Beale St
Memphis, TN 38163
Prgm Dir: Mary C McCain, MPA RRA
Tel: 901 448-6486   *Fax:* 901 448-7545
Begins: Sep
Length: 12 mos   *Award:* Dipl, BS
Tuition per yr: $1,952 res, $4,336 non-res

Tennessee State University

Health Information Admin Prgm
3500 John A Merritt Blvd
Nashville, TN 37209-1561
Prgm Dir: Elizabeth I Kunnu, MEd RRA
Tel: 615 963-7441   *Fax:* 615 963-7498
E-mail: in%"kunne@harpo.tnstate.edu
Class Cap: 35   *Begins:* Aug Jan
Length: 36 mos   *Award:* BS
Tuition per yr: $1,950 res, $6,280 non-res
Evening or weekend classes available

Texas

University of Texas Medical Branch

Health Information Admin Prgm
301 University Blvd
Galveston, TX 77555-1028
Prgm Dir: Tella-Marie Williams, BA RRA
Tel: 409 772-3051   *Fax:* 409 747-1613
E-mail: twilliam%sahs@mhost.utmb.edu
Class Cap: 26   *Begins:* Aug
Length: 24 mos   *Award:* BS
Tuition per yr: $1,212 res, $5,500 non-res

Texas Southern University

Health Information Admin Prgm
3100 Cleburne St
Houston, TX 77004
Prgm Dir: Debra J Butts, RRA
Tel: 713 527-7265   *Fax:* 713 313-1094
Class Cap: 15   *Begins:* Sep
Length: 49 mos   *Award:* Dipl, BS
Tuition per yr: $1,577 res, $5,128 non-res
Evening or weekend classes available

Southwest Texas State University

Health Information Admin Prgm
San Marcos, TX 78666
Prgm Dir: Sue E Biedermann, RRA
Tel: 512 245-8242   *Fax:* 512 245-3791
E-mail: sb5220@samson.health.swt.edu
Class Cap: 30   *Begins:* Aug
Length: 24 mos   *Award:* BS
Tuition per yr: $2,385 res, $8,800 non-res
Evening or weekend classes available

Virginia

Norfolk State University

Health Information Admin Prgm
2401 Corprew Ave
Norfolk, VA 23504
Prgm Dir: Joyce B Harvey, PhD RRA
Tel: 757 683-8209   *Fax:* 757 683-9114
Begins: Aug Jan
Length: 48 mos   *Award:* BS
Tuition per yr: $3,024 res, $6,600 non-res

Washington

University of Washington

Health Information Admin Prgm
1107 NE 45th
Ste 355 JD-02
Seattle, WA 98105
Prgm Dir: Mary Alice Hanken, PhD RRA
Tel: 206 543-8810   *Fax:* 206 685-4719
E-mail: mahanken@u.washington.edu
Class Cap: 20   *Begins:* Sep
Length: 9 mos   *Award:* Cert
Tuition per yr: $10,000 res, $10,000 non-res
Evening or weekend classes available

Wisconsin

University of Wisconsin - Milwaukee

Health Information Admin Prgm
PO Box 413
Milwaukee, WI 53201
Prgm Dir: John J Lynch, PhD RRA
Tel: 414 229-5615   *Fax:* 414 229-5100
E-mail: johnjl@csd.uwm.edu
Class Cap: 20   *Begins:* Sep
Length: 24 mos   *Award:* BS
Tuition per yr: $3,102 res, $9,964 non-res
Evening or weekend classes available

Health Information Technician

Alabama

Wallace State College

Health Information Tech Prgm
Beville Health Education Bldg
Hanceville, AL 35077-9080
Prgm Dir: Donna S Stanley, EdS RRA
Tel: 205 352-8327   *Fax:* 205 352-8228
Class Cap: 45   *Begins:* Sep
Length: 21 mos   *Award:* Dipl, AAS
Tuition per yr: $1,100 res, $3,025 non-res
Evening or weekend classes available

Bishop State Community College

Health Information Tech Prgm
351 N Broad St
Mobile, AL 36603-5898
Prgm Dir: Anna Sharp
Tel: 334 690-6413   *Fax:* 334 405-4505
Class Cap: 20   *Begins:* Sep
Length: 21 mos   *Award:* AAS
Tuition per yr: $1,188 res, $2,079 non-res
Evening or weekend classes available

Alaska

University of Alaska Southeast

Health Information Tech Prgm
UAS Sitka Campus
1332 Seward Ave
Sitka, AK 99835-9498
Prgm Dir: Carol Petrie Liberty, RRA MS
Tel: 907 747-7718   *Fax:* 907 747-3552
E-mail: tfcpl@aca01.alaska.edu
Class Cap: 20   *Begins:* Aug Jan
Length: 24 mos, 36 mos   *Award:* AAS
Tuition per yr: $1,690 res, $5,002 non-res

Arizona

Phoenix College

Health Information Tech Prgm
1202 W Thomas Rd
Phoenix, AZ 85013
Prgm Dir: Deborah S Dennis, RRA
Tel: 602 285-7148   *Fax:* 602 285-7700
E-mail: dennis@pc.maricopa
Class Cap: 35   *Begins:* Aug
Length: 9 mo , 18 mos   *Award:* Cert, AAS
Tuition per yr: $1,088 res, $5,088 non-res
Evening or weekend classes available

Programs

Arkansas

Garland County Community College
Health Information Tech Prgm
101 College Dr
Hot Springs, AR 71913-9174
Prgm Dir: Susan Wallace, MEd RRA
Tel: 501 767-9371 *Fax:* 501 767-6896
E-mail: swallace@jill.gccc.cc.ar.us
Class Cap: 18 *Begins:* Aug
Length: 45 mos *Award:* AAS
Tuition per yr: $888 res, $1,124 non-res
Evening or weekend classes available

California

Cypress College
Health Information Tech Prgm
9200 Valley View St
Cypress, CA 90630
Prgm Dir: Rosalie Majid, RRA
Tel: 714 826-2220 *Fax:* 714 527-2175
E-mail: majidr@nocccd.cc.ca.us
Class Cap: 100 *Begins:* Aug Jan
Length: 18 mos *Award:* Cert, AS
Tuition per yr: $390 res, $3,420 non-res
Evening or weekend classes available

Fresno City College
Health Information Tech Prgm
1101 E University Ave
Fresno, CA 93741
Prgm Dir: Mary Ann Woods, PhD
Tel: 209 442-4600
Class Cap: 50 *Begins:* Aug Jan
Length: 24 mos *Award:* AS

Chabot College
Health Information Tech Prgm
25555 Hesperian Blvd
Hayward, CA 94545-5001
Prgm Dir: Diane Premean, RRA ART
Tel: 510 786-6904 *Fax:* 510 782-9315
E-mail: Premeau@aol.com
Class Cap: 24 *Begins:* Aug
Length: 18 mos, 36 mos *Award:* Dipl, AS
Tuition per yr: $325 res, $2,500 non-res
Evening or weekend classes available

Charles R Drew Univ of Med & Science
Health Information Tech Prgm
1621 E 120th St
Los Angeles, CA 90059
Prgm Dir: Barbara J Penn, MS RRA
Tel: 213 563-5888 *Fax:* 213 563-4923
Class Cap: 30 *Begins:* Sep
Length: 24 mos *Award:* Cert, AS
Tuition per yr: $10,400 res, $10,400 non-res
Evening or weekend classes available

East Los Angeles College
Health Information Tech Prgm
1301 Avenida Cesar Chavez
Monterey Park, CA 91754
Prgm Dir: Lea T Davidson, MPH RRA
Tel: 213 265-8884 *Fax:* 213 265-8631
Class Cap: 180 *Begins:* Aug Jan
Length: 21 mos *Award:* AS
Tuition per yr: $429 res, $4,983 non-res
Evening or weekend classes available

Cosumnes River College
Health Information Tech Prgm
8401 Center Pkwy
Sacramento, CA 95823
Prgm Dir: Colleen Pearson, ART
Tel: 916 688-7226 *Fax:* 916 688-7443
Class Cap: 30 *Begins:* Aug
Length: 24 mos *Award:* AA
Tuition per yr: $390 res, $4,140 non-res

San Diego Mesa College
Health Information Tech Prgm
7250 Mesa College Dr
San Diego, CA 92111
Prgm Dir: Teddy L Scribner, MS RRA
Tel: 619 627-2606 *Fax:* 619 279-5668
Class Cap: 25 *Begins:* Aug
Length: 24 mos *Award:* Dipl, AS
Tuition per yr: $390 res, $1,500 non-res
Evening or weekend classes available

City College of San Francisco
Health Information Tech Prgm
John Adams Campus
1860 Hayes St
San Francisco, CA 94117
Prgm Dir: Marie T Conde, BS ART
Tel: 415 561-1818
Class Cap: 40 *Begins:* Jan Aug
Length: 24 mos *Award:* Cert, AS
Tuition per yr: $300

Colorado

Arapahoe Community College
Health Information Tech Prgm
5900 S Santa Fe Dr
Littleton, CO 80120
Prgm Dir: Annette Bigalk, RRA
Tel: 303 797-5795 *Fax:* 303 797-5935
Class Cap: 20 *Begins:* Aug
Length: 24 mos *Award:* AAS
Tuition per yr: $1,336 res, $4,948 non-res
Evening or weekend classes available

Pueblo Community College
Health Information Tech Prgm
900 W Orman Ave
Pueblo, CO 81004
Prgm Dir: Jill Sell-Kruse, RRA
Tel: 719 549-3143 *Fax:* 719 549-3108
E-mail: sell_kruse@pcc.cccoes.edu
Class Cap: 20 *Begins:* Sept
Length: 21 mos *Award:* AAS
Tuition per yr: $3,762 res, $16,830 non-res
Evening or weekend classes available

Connecticut

Briarwood College
Health Information Tech Prgm
2279 Mt Vernon Rd
Southington, CT 06489
Prgm Dir: A H Lenne Klopfer, MS RRA
Tel: 203 628-4751
Class Cap: 30 *Begins:* Aug
Length: 24 mos, 12 mos *Award:* Dipl, AAS
Tuition per yr: $9,212

Florida

Broward Community College
Health Information Tech Prgm
Ctr for Hlth Science Educ
1000 Coconut Creek Pkwy
Coconut Creek, FL 33066
Prgm Dir: Mary Spivey, MLIS RRA
Tel: 954 969-2084 *Fax:* 954 973-2348
E-mail: maryspivey@aol.com
Class Cap: 20 *Begins:* Aug
Length: 24 mos *Award:* AS
Tuition per yr: $1,100 res, $4,200 non-res

Daytona Beach Community College
Health Information Tech Prgm
PO Box 2811
Daytona Beach, FL 32120-2811
Prgm Dir: Nancy Thomas, EdD RRA
Tel: 904 255-8131 *Fax:* 904 254-4491
E-mail: thomasn@dbcc.cc.fl.edu
Class Cap: 20 *Begins:* Aug
Length: 21 mos *Award:* AS
Tuition per yr: $1,253 res, $4,698 non-res
Evening or weekend classes available

Indian River Community College
Health Information Tech Prgm
3209 Virginia Ave
Fort Pierce, FL 34981-5599
Prgm Dir: Claudia Keating, MEd RRA
Tel: 407 462-4265
Class Cap: 50 *Begins:* Aug
Length: 24 mos *Award:* AS
Tuition per yr: $528 res, $2,112 non-res

Florida Community College - Jacksonville
Health Information Tech Prgm
601 W State St
Jacksonville, FL 32202
Prgm Dir: Eudelia S Thomas, MS RRA
Tel: 904 632-5065 *Fax:* 904 632-5053
E-mail: www.fccj.fl.us/~urc/hlth.mgmt.html
Class Cap: 24 *Begins:* Aug
Length: 30 mos *Award:* AS
Tuition per yr: $1,181 res, $4,429 non-res
Evening or weekend classes available

Miami-Dade Community College
Health Information Tech Prgm
Medical Ctr Campus
950 NW 20th St
Miami, FL 33127
Prgm Dir: Josephine M Gordon, RRA
Tel: 305 237-4104
Class Cap: 40 *Begins:* Aug May
Length: 24 mos *Award:* AS
Tuition per yr: $1,476 res, $5,160 non-res

International College
Health Information Tech Prgm
2654 E Tamiami Trail
Naples, FL 33962
Prgm Dir: Janice Madden, ART
Tel: 941 774-4700
Med Dir: Janice Madden, ART
Class Cap: 30 *Begins:* Jan May Sep
Length: 24 mos *Award:* AS
Tuition per yr: $5,000

Pensacola Junior College

Health Information Tech Prgm
Dept of Allied Health
1000 College Blvd
Pensacola, FL 32504
Prgm Dir: Barbara H Edwards, MEd RRA
Tel: 904 484-2213 *Fax:* 904 484-2375
Class Cap: 30 *Begins:* Aug
Length: 20 mos *Award:* AS
Tuition per yr: $1,200 res, $4,320 non-res
Evening or weekend classes available

St Petersburg Junior College

Health Information Tech Prgm
PO Box 13489
St Petersburg, FL 33733
Prgm Dir: Sheila Newberry, MEd., RRT
Tel: 813 341-3623 *Fax:* 813 341-3744
E-mail: newberrys@email.spjc.cc.fl.us
Class Cap: 25 *Begins:* Aug
Length: 21 mos, 60 mos *Award:* AS
Tuition per yr: $1,343 res, $4,796 non-res
Evening or weekend classes available

Georgia

Darton College

Health Information Tech Prgm
2400 Gillionville Rd
Albany, GA 31707
Prgm Dir: Ruth B Shingleton, MBA DDA
Tel: 912 430-6894 *Fax:* 912 430-6910
Class Cap: 30 *Begins:* Sep
Length: 21 mos *Award:* AS
Tuition per yr: $1,080 res, $2,904 non-res
Evening or weekend classes available

Medical College of Georgia

Health Information Tech Prgm
AL-122
Augusta, GA 30912-0400
Prgm Dir: Charlotte A Johnston, PhD RRA
Tel: 706 721-3436 *Fax:* 706 721-6067
E-mail: chjohnst@mail.mcg.edu
Class Cap: 5 *Begins:* Sep
Length: 12 mos *Award:* Dipl, AS
Tuition per yr: $2,864 res, $8,580 non-res
Evening or weekend classes available

Idaho

Boise State University

Health Information Tech Prgm
College of Health Science
Boise State University
Boise, ID 83725
Prgm Dir: Patricia Elison, RRA
Tel: 208 385-1130 *Fax:* 208 385-3469
E-mail: pelison@bsu.ibsu.edu
Class Cap: 40 *Begins:* Aug Jan
Length: 24 mos *Award:* AS
Tuition per yr: $1,964 res, $7,310 non-res
Evening or weekend classes available

Idaho State University

Health Information Tech Prgm
Campus Box 8380
Pocatello, ID 83209-8380
Prgm Dir: Suzanne Griffin, MEd RRA
Tel: 208 236-4169 *Fax:* 208 236-4641
E-mail: fs/gnfsuza@isu.edu
Class Cap: 20 *Begins:* Jan
Length: 22 mos *Award:* AAS
Tuition per yr: $3,204 res, $5,216 non-res
Evening or weekend classes available

Illinois

Belleville Area College

Health Information Tech Prgm
2500 Carlyle Ave
Belleville, IL 62221
Prgm Dir: Wendy Holder, RRA
Tel: 618 235-2700 *Fax:* 618 235-1578
Class Cap: 20 *Begins:* Aug
Length: 22 mos *Award:* AAS
Tuition per yr: $1,445 res, $3,094 non-res
Evening or weekend classes available

Truman College

Health Information Tech Prgm
1145 W Wilson Ave
Chicago, IL 60640
Prgm Dir: Daphine D Lenton, MS, RRA
Tel: 312 907-4781 *Fax:* 312 907-4781
Class Cap: 80 *Begins:* Aug Jan
Length: 24 mos *Award:* Dipl, AAS
Tuition per yr: $1,125 res, $3,007 non-res

Oakton Community College

Health Information Tech Prgm
1600 E Golf Rd
Des Plaines, IL 60016
Prgm Dir: Cynthia L DeBerg, MA RRA
Tel: 708 635-1957 *Fax:* 847 635-1764
E-mail: cindyd@oakton.edu
Class Cap: 20 *Begins:* Aug
Length: 21 mos, 16 mos *Award:* Dipl,Cert, AAS
Tuition per yr: $1,050 res, $3,750 non-res
Evening or weekend classes available

College of DuPage

Health Information Tech Prgm
22nd St and Lambert Rd
Glen Ellyn, IL 60137-6599
Prgm Dir: Kim D Pack, RRA
Tel: 630 942-2532 *Fax:* 630 858-5409
Class Cap: 20 *Begins:* Sep
Length: 21 mos *Award:* AAS
Tuition per yr: $1,392 res, $5,664 non-res
Evening or weekend classes available

College of Lake County

Health Information Tech Prgm
19351 W Washington St
Grayslake, IL 60030-1198
Prgm Dir: Denise Anastasio, MPA RRA
Tel: 847 223-6601 *Fax:* 847 223-1357
E-mail: danastasio@clc.cc.il.us
Class Cap: 30 *Begins:* Aug
Length: 18 mos *Award:* AAS
Tuition per yr: $1,581 res, $6,045 non-res
Evening or weekend classes available

Southern Illinois Collegiate Common Mkt

Health Information Tech Prgm
3213 S Park Ave
Herrin, IL 62948
Prgm Dir: Mary J Sullivan, MS RRA
Tel: 618 985-2898 *Fax:* 618 942-6658
E-mail: siccm@midwest.net
Class Cap: 24 *Begins:* Aug
Length: 18 mos *Award:* AS
Tuition per yr: $2,112 res, $5,887 non-res
Evening or weekend classes available

Robert Morris College

Health Information Tech Prgm
43 Orland Square Dr
Orland Park, IL 60462
Prgm Dir: Andrea Bunker, MS ART
Tel: 708 349-5108 *Fax:* 708 349-5119
Med Dir: Elaine Carroll, MD
Class Cap: 55 *Begins:* April
Length: 15 mos *Award:* AAS
Tuition per yr: $9,750 res, $9,750 non-res
Evening or weekend classes available

Moraine Valley Community College

Health Information Tech Prgm
10900 S 88th Ave
Palos Hills, IL 60465
Prgm Dir: Charlotte Razor, MHA
Tel: 708 974-5315 *Fax:* 708 974-1184
Class Cap: 23 *Begins:* Aug
Length: 10 mos *Award:* AAS
Tuition per yr: $1,209 res, $4,557 non-res

Indiana

Indiana Univ/Purdue Univ Ft Wayne

Health Information Tech Prgm
2101 Coliseum Blvd E
Ft Wayne, IN 46805
Prgm Dir: Barbara A Ellison, BS RRA
Tel: 219 481-6168 *Fax:* 219 481-6083
E-mail: ellison@smtplink.ipfw.indiana.edu
Class Cap: 15 *Begins:* Aug
Length: 24 mos, 5 mos *Award:* AS
Tuition per yr: $3,407 res, $7,854 non-res
Evening or weekend classes available

Indiana University Northwest

Health Information Tech Prgm
3400 Broadway
Gary, IN 46408
Prgm Dir: Margaret A Skurka, MS RRA
Tel: 219 980-6654 *Fax:* 219 980-6649
E-mail: mskurk@iunhaw1.iun.indiana.edu
Class Cap: 26 *Begins:* Aug
Length: 21 mos *Award:* AS
Tuition per yr: $2,700 res, $6,500 non-res
Evening or weekend classes available

Vincennes University

Health Information Tech Prgm
1002 N First St
Vincennes, IN 47591-9986
Prgm Dir: Darrel W King, MS RRA
Tel: 812 888-4437 *Fax:* 812 888-4550
E-mail: dking@vunet.vinu.edu
Class Cap: 24 *Begins:* Aug
Length: 19 mos *Award:* AS
Tuition per yr: $2,797 res, $4,158 non-res

Programs

Iowa

Northeast Iowa Community College
Health Information Tech Prgm
Box 400
Calmar, IA 52132
Prgm Dir: Rhonda Seibert, BS ART
Tel: 319 562-3263
Class Cap: 30 *Begins:* Aug
Length: 9 mo , 18 mos *Award:* Dipl, AAS
Tuition per yr: $2,232 res, $3,125 non-res
Evening or weekend classes available

Kirkwood Community College
Health Information Tech Prgm
6301 Kirkwood Blvd SW
PO Box 2068
Cedar Rapids, IA 52406-9973
Prgm Dir: Joanne Becker, ART
Tel: 319 398-4923 *Fax:* 319 398-1293
E-mail: jbecker@kirkwood.cc.ia.us
Class Cap: 30 *Begins:* Aug
Length: 18 mos *Award:* AAS
Tuition per yr: $1,759 res, $3,519 non-res
Evening or weekend classes available

Indian Hills Community College
Health Information Tech Prgm
Ottumwa Campus
Ottumwa, IA 52501
Prgm Dir: Heidi Clayton, BS RRA
Tel: 515 683-5164 *Fax:* 515 683-5184
Class Cap: 40 *Begins:* Aug
Length: 18 mos *Award:* AAS
Tuition per yr: $2,376 res, $3,564 non-res

Kansas

Dodge City Community College
Health Information Tech Prgm
2501 N 14th Ave
Dodge City, KS 67801
Prgm Dir: Barbara Rubin, MEd RRA
Tel: 316 225-1321 *Fax:* 316 227-9319
Class Cap: 9 *Begins:* Aug
Length: 24 mos *Award:* AD
Tuition per yr: $1,080 res, $1,620 non-res

Hutchinson Community College
Health Information Tech Prgm
1300 N Plum
Hutchinson, KS 67501
Prgm Dir: Loretta A Horton, RRA
Tel: 316 665-4955 *Fax:* 316 662-6647
E-mail: hortonl@hutchcc.edu
Class Cap: 16 *Begins:* Aug
Length: 22 mos *Award:* AAS
Tuition per yr: $1,200 res, $2,910 non-res
Evening or weekend classes available

Washburn University of Topeka
Health Information Tech Prgm
1700 College Ave SW
Topeka, KS 66621
Prgm Dir: Michelle Shipley, RRA CCS
Tel: 913 231-1010
E-mail: zzship@sace.wuacc.edu
Class Cap: 20 *Begins:* Aug
Length: 24 mos *Award:* Cert, AS
Tuition per yr: $3,813 res, $7,831 non-res
Evening or weekend classes available

Kentucky

Western Kentucky University
Health Information Tech Prgm
207 Academic Complex
Bowling Green, KY 42101
Prgm Dir: Karen C Sansom, RRA
Tel: 502 745-3815 *Fax:* 502 745-6869
E-mail: karen.sansom@wku.edu
Class Cap: 22 *Begins:* Aug
Length: 21 mos *Award:* AS
Tuition per yr: $2,066 res, $2,942 non-res

Eastern Kentucky University
Health Information Tech Prgm
Dizney 117
Richmond, KY 40475-3135
Prgm Dir: Frances A Hindsman, MBA RRA
Tel: 606 622-1915 *Fax:* 606 622-1140
E-mail: hrshinds@acs.eku.edu
Class Cap: 32 *Begins:* Aug Jan
Length: 18 mos *Award:* AS
Tuition per yr: $1,970 res, $5,450 non-res
Evening or weekend classes available

Louisiana

Delgado Community College
Health Information Tech Prgm
615 City Park Ave
New Orleans, LA 70119-4399
Prgm Dir: Melissa LaCour, RRA
Tel: 504 483-4429 *Fax:* 504 483-4609
Class Cap: 20 *Begins:* Aug
Length: 22 mos *Award:* AS
Tuition per yr: $1,674 res, $4,284 non-res
Evening or weekend classes available

Louisiana Tech University
Health Information Tech Prgm
PO Box 3171
Ruston, LA 71272
Prgm Dir: Helen D Baxter, MA RRA
Tel: 318 257-2854 *Fax:* 318 257-4896
E-mail: iflil2c@vm.cc.latech.edu
Class Cap: 35 *Begins:* Aug Nov Feb May
Length: 21 mos *Award:* ASMRT
Tuition per yr: $2,328 res, $4,323 non-res
Evening or weekend classes available

Southern Univ at Shreveport - Bossier City
Health Information Tech Prgm
610 Texas St 328A
Shreveport, LA 71101
Prgm Dir: Ann E Marohn, MS RRA
Tel: 318 674-3487 *Fax:* 318 674-3460
Class Cap: 15 *Begins:* Aug
Length: 24 mos *Award:* AAS
Tuition per yr: $1,403 res, $2,809 non-res
Evening or weekend classes available

Maine

University of Maine - Bangor
Health Information Tech Prgm
Univ. College of Bangor UMA
128 Texas Ave
Bangor, ME 04401
Prgm Dir: Susan M Benson, MPA MS RRA
Tel: 207 581-6144 *Fax:* 207 581-6066
E-mail: sbenson@maine.maine.edu
Class Cap: 25 *Begins:* Sep Jan
Length: 16 mos *Award:* AS
Tuition per yr: $2,880 res, $7,040 non-res
Evening or weekend classes available

Kennebec Valley Technical College
Health Information Tech Prgm
92 Western Ave
Fairfield, ME 04937
Prgm Dir: Joan M Frisina, BS RRA
Tel: 207 453-5156 *Fax:* 207 453-5194
E-mail: kjfrisin@krtc.mtcs.tac.me.us
Class Cap: 24 *Begins:* Aug
Length: 18 mos *Award:* AAS
Tuition per yr: $2,992 res, $4,653 non-res
Evening or weekend classes available

Maryland

Baltimore City Community College
Health Information Tech Prgm
2901 Liberty Heights Ave
Baltimore, MD 21215-7893
Prgm Dir: Betty Neely Mitchell, RRA
Tel: 410 462-7729 *Fax:* 410 462-7785
Begins: Sep
Length: 9 mos *Award:* AA
Tuition per yr: $1,322 res, $5,775 non-res

Hagerstown Business College
Health Information Tech Prgm
18616 Crestwood Dr
Hagerstown, MD 21742
Prgm Dir: M Beth Shanholtzer, RRA
Tel: 301 739-2670 *Fax:* 301 791-7661
Begins: Sep
Length: 20 mos *Award:* AS
Tuition per yr: $5,940 res, $5,940 non-res
Evening or weekend classes available

Prince George's Community College
Health Information Tech Prgm
301 Largo Rd
Largo, MD 20772
Prgm Dir: Muriel Adams, RRA CCS
Tel: 301 322-0735 *Fax:* 301 808-0418
Class Cap: 25 *Begins:* Sep
Length: 21 mos *Award:* AAS
Tuition per yr: $2,346 res, $4,488 non-res
Evening or weekend classes available

Montgomery College
Health Information Tech Prgm
7600 Takoma Ave
Takoma Park, MD 20912
Prgm Dir: Shirley Suzanne Meiskey, MSA RRA
Tel: 301 650-1337 *Fax:* 301 650-1335
Class Cap: 22 *Begins:* Sep
Length: 21 mos *Award:* AAS
Tuition per yr: $1,834 res, $3,504 non-res

Massachusetts

Fisher College

Health Information Tech Prgm
118 Beacon St
Boston, MA 02116
Prgm Dir: Nancy L Allen-Tuch, MBA RRA
Tel: 617 236-8800   *Fax:* 617 236-8858
Class Cap: 20   *Begins:* Sep Jan
Length: 24 mos   *Award:* AS
Tuition per yr: $17,750
Evening or weekend classes available

Laboure College

Health Information Tech Prgm
2120 Dorchester Ave
Boston, MA 02124
Prgm Dir: Eileen C Perry, MBA RRA
Tel: 617 296-8300   *Fax:* 617 296-7947
Class Cap: 40   *Begins:* Aug
Length: 24 mos   *Award:* Cert, AS
Tuition per yr: $5,000
Evening or weekend classes available

Hennepin Technical College

Health Information Tech Prgm
777 Elsbree St
Fall River, MA 02777
Prgm Dir: Edward J Dobbs, BBA RRA
Tel: 508 678-2811, Ext 2329   *Fax:* 508 676-7146
E-mail: edobbs@bristol.mass.edu
Class Cap: 20   *Begins:* Sep
Length: 21 mos   *Award:* AS
Tuition per yr: $2,870 res, $8,050 non-res

Northern Essex Community College

Health Information Tech Prgm
Elliot Way
Haverhill, MA 01830
Prgm Dir: Patricia E Taglianetti, RRA
Tel: 508 374-5826   *Fax:* 508 374-3729
E-mail: ptaglianetti@necc.mass.edu
Class Cap: 25   *Begins:* Sep
Length: 24 mos   *Award:* AS
Tuition per yr: $1,600 res, $3,990 non-res
Evening or weekend classes available

Holyoke Community College

Health Information Tech Prgm
303 Homestead Ave
Holyoke, MA 01040
Prgm Dir: Marylou Theilman, MEd
Tel: 413 538-7000
Med Dir: Mary Delong, ART
Class Cap: 35   *Begins:* Sep
Length: 24 mos   *Award:* Cert, AS
Tuition per yr: $1,008 res, $4,680 non-res

Michigan

Ferris State University

Health Information Tech Prgm
Coll of Allied Hlth Sciences
200 Ferris Dr/VFS 402
Big Rapids, MI 49307-2740
Prgm Dir: Ellen J Haneline, MEd RRA
Tel: 616 592-2313   *Fax:* 616 592-3788
Class Cap: 30   *Begins:* Aug
Length: 18 mos   *Award:* Dipl, AAS
Tuition per yr: $3,630 res, $7,364 non-res
Evening or weekend classes available

Henry Ford Community College

Health Information Tech Prgm
22586 Ann Arbor Trail
Dearborn Heights, MI 48127
Prgm Dir: M Marsha C Steele, RRA
Tel: 313 730-5975   *Fax:* 313 730-5965
Class Cap: 25   *Begins:* Aug
Length: 24 mos   *Award:* AS
Tuition per yr: $1,710 res, $2,490 non-res
Evening or weekend classes available

Baker College

Health Information Tech Prgm
G 1050 W Bristol Rd
Flint, MI 48507
Prgm Dir: Cheryl J Foster, BS RRA
Tel: 810 766-4147
Class Cap: 150   *Begins:* Sep
Length: 18 mos   *Award:* AS
Tuition per yr: $4,080

Schoolcraft College

Health Information Tech Prgm
1751 Radcliff
Garden City, MI 48135
Prgm Dir: Patricia A Rubio, MSA RRA
Tel: 313 462-4770   *Fax:* 313 462-4775
Class Cap: 30   *Begins:* Aug
Length: 24 mos   *Award:* AAS
Tuition per yr: $2,274 res, $3,171 non-res
Evening or weekend classes available

Gogebic Community College

Health Information Tech Prgm
E4946 Jackson Rd
Ironwood, MI 49938
Prgm Dir: Carla J Pogliano, MA RRA
Tel: 906 932-4231   *Fax:* 906 932-0868
Class Cap: 20   *Begins:* Aug
Length: 18 mos   *Award:* AS
Tuition per yr: $1,260 res, $1,750 non-res
Evening or weekend classes available

Davenport College - Kalamazoo

Health Information Tech Prgm
4123 W Main St
Kalamazoo, MI 49006
Prgm Dir: Cecilia McDermott, RRA
Tel: 616 382-2835
Class Cap: 77   *Begins:* Sep Jun
Length: 18 mos   *Award:* AS
Tuition per yr: $6,400

Baker College of Muskegon

Health Information Tech Prgm
Baker College System
123 Apple Ave
Muskegon, MI 49442
Prgm Dir: Cheryl J Foster, BS RRA
Tel: 616 726-4904   Fax: 616 728-1417
E-mail: foster_c@muskegon.baker.edu
Class Cap: 30   *Begins:* Sep
Length: 18 mos   *Award:* AAS
Tuition per yr: $6,000

Minnesota

Anoka-Hennepin Technical College

Health Information Tech Prgm
1335 W Hwy 10
Anoka, MN 55303
Prgm Dir: Gwen J Enzler, RRA
Tel: 612 427-1880
Class Cap: 35   *Begins:* Sep
Length: 20 mos   *Award:* AAS
Tuition per yr: $1,301 res, $2,602 non-res

College of St Catherine

Health Information Tech Prgm
601 25th Ave S
Minneapolis, MN 55454
Prgm Dir: Joanne Odegaard Valerius, RRA
Tel: 612 690-7756   *Fax:* 612 690-6849
Class Cap: 20   *Begins:* Sep Jan
Length: 30 mos, 18 mos   *Award:* Dipl, AAS
Tuition per yr: $10,168

Northwest Technical Coll - Moorhead

Health Information Tech Prgm
1900 28th Ave S
Moorhead, MN 56560
Prgm Dir: Carolyn Linnell, RRA ART
Tel: 218 235-6277   *Fax:* 218 236-0342
Begins: Sep
Length: 20 mos   *Award:* Dipl, AAS
Tuition per yr: $1,862 res, $3,724 non-res

Rasmussen Colleges

Health Information Tech Prgm
245 N 37th Ave
St Cloud, MN 56303-3091
Prgm Dir: Margaret A Johnson, RRA
Tel: 320 251-5600   *Fax:* 320 251-3702
Class Cap: 75   *Begins:* Sep Oct
Length: 18 mos   *Award:* AAS
Tuition per yr: $8,760 res, $8,760 non-res
Evening or weekend classes available

Ridgewater College - Willmar Campus

Health Information Tech Prgm
2101 15th Ave NW
PO Box 1097
Willmar, MN 56201
Prgm Dir: Pete Fisk, RRA
Tel: 320 231-2947   *Fax:* 320 231-7677
Class Cap: 20   *Begins:* Sep
Length: 21 mos   *Award:* AAS

Mississippi

Hinds Community College District

Health Information Tech Prgm
1750 Chadwick Dr
Jackson, MS 39204
Prgm Dir: Judith E Moore, MHS RRA
Tel: 601 372-6507   *Fax:* 601 371-3703
E-mail: jmoore@its.state.ms.us
Class Cap: 15   *Begins:* Aug
Length: 24 mos   *Award:* AAS
Tuition per yr: $1,120 res, $3,576 non-res
Evening or weekend classes available

Programs

Meridian Community College

Health Information Tech Prgm
910 Hwy 19 N
Meridian, MS 39307
Prgm Dir: Robin Allen Jones, BS MRA RRA
Tel: 601 484-8759 *Fax:* 601 482-3936
Class Cap: 15 *Begins:* Aug
Length: 18 mos *Award:* AA
Tuition per yr: $960 res, $2,000 non-res

Missouri

Penn Valley Community College

Health Information Tech Prgm
3201 SW Trafficway
Kansas City, MO 64111
Prgm Dir: Tracy Rockwell, RRA
Tel: 816 759-4245 *Fax:* 816 759-4553
Class Cap: 32 *Begins:* Aug
Length: 24 mos *Award:* AAS
Tuition per yr: $1,558 res, $2,563 non-res

Ozarks Technical Community College

Health Information Tech Prgm
PO Box 5958
Springfield, MO 65801
Prgm Dir: Beth Climer, RRA
Tel: 417 895-7062 *Fax:* 417 895-7085
Class Cap: 24 *Begins:* Aug
Length: 21 mos *Award:* Cert, AAS
Tuition per yr: $1,221 res, $1,881 non-res
Evening or weekend classes available

Missouri Western State College

Health Information Tech Prgm
4525 Downs Dr
St Joseph, MO 64507
Prgm Dir: David Heizer, RRA
Tel: 816 271-4404 *Fax:* 816 271-5849
Class Cap: 30 *Begins:* Sep
Length: 24 mos *Award:* AS
Tuition per yr: $1,976 res, $3,738 non-res

St Charles County Community College

Health Information Tech Prgm
4601 Mid Rivers Mall Dr
St Peters, MO 63376
Prgm Dir: Candace E Neu, RRA CCS
Tel: 314 922-8000 *Fax:* 314 922-8352
E-mail: cneu@chuck.stchas.edu
Class Cap: 30 *Begins:* Aug
Length: 21 mos *Award:* AS
Tuition per yr: $1,505 res, $2,205 non-res
Evening or weekend classes available

Montana

Montana State Univ Coll of Technology

Health Information Tech Prgm
2100 16th Ave S
Great Falls, MT 59405
Prgm Dir: Irene L Mueller, MLS RRA
Tel: 406 771-4358 *Fax:* 406 771-4317
E-mail: zgf6013@maia.oscs.montana.edu
Class Cap: 15 *Begins:* Sep
Length: 24 mos *Award:* AAS
Tuition per yr: $1,743 res, $4,112 non-res
Evening or weekend classes available

Salish Kootenai College

Health Information Tech Prgm
PO Box 117
Pablo, MT 59855
Prgm Dir: Roberta Yankovich, ART
Tel: 406 675-4800 *Fax:* 406 675-4801
E-mail: roberta_yankovich@skc.edu
Class Cap: 25 *Begins:* Sep
Length: 24 mos *Award:* AS
Tuition per yr: $1,635 res, $2,139 non-res

Nebraska

College of St Mary

Health Information Tech Prgm
1901 S 72nd St
Omaha, NE 68124
Prgm Dir: Ellen B Jacobs, MEd RRA
Tel: 402 399-2611 *Fax:* 402 399-2657
Class Cap: 20 *Begins:* Aug
Length: 24 mos, 36 mos *Award:* AS
Tuition per yr: $10,994
Evening or weekend classes available

Nevada

Community College of Southern Nevada

Health Information Tech Prgm
3200 E Cheyenne Ave
N Las Vegas, NV 89030
Prgm Dir: Hyla Winters, MHCA RRA
Tel: 702 651-5742 *Fax:* 702 651-5738
E-mail: winters@pioneer.nevada.edu
Class Cap: 15 *Begins:* Sep
Length: 18 mos *Award:* Cert, AS
Tuition per yr: $1,241 res, $3,100 non-res

New Jersey

Hudson County Community College

Health Information Tech Prgm
2039 Kennedy Blvd
Science 330
Jersey City, NJ 07305
Prgm Dir: Jacqueline Gibbons, MS RRA
Tel: 201 200-3320
Med Dir: Lloyd M Kahn, DPM
Class Cap: 25 *Begins:* Sep Jan
Length: 18 mos *Award:* AAS
Tuition per yr: $1,380 res, $2,512 non-res

Burlington County College

Health Information Tech Prgm
Pemberton-Brown Mills Rd
Pemberton, NJ 08068-1599
Prgm Dir: Suzanne K Davis, RRA
Tel: 609 894-9311 *Fax:* 609 726-1781
Class Cap: 20 *Begins:* Sep
Length: 21 mos, 45 mos *Award:* AAS
Tuition per yr: $1,584 res, $1,764 non-res
Evening or weekend classes available

New Mexico

University of New Mexico - Gallup/IHS

Health Information Tech Prgm
200 College Rd
Gallup, NM 87301
Prgm Dir: Carol Fleming, RRA CCS
Tel: 505 863-7659
Class Cap: 20 *Begins:* Aug
Length: 20 mos *Award:* AS
Tuition per yr: $624 res, $1,536 non-res

New York

SUNY College of Technology at Alfred

Health Information Tech Prgm
Allied Health Bldg
Rm 114
Alfred, NY 14802
Prgm Dir: Janette B Thomas, MPS RRA
Tel: 607 587-3661 *Fax:* 607 587-3684
E-mail: thomasj@alfredtech.edu
Class Cap: 25 *Begins:* Aug
Length: 20 mos, 30 mos *Award:* AAS
Tuition per yr: $3,200 res, $8,300 non-res

Broome Community College

Health Information Tech Prgm
Business Bldg
PO Box 1017
Binghamton, NY 13902
Prgm Dir: Mary L Rosato, MA
Tel: 607 778-5051 *Fax:* 607 778-5345
E-mail: rosato_m@sunybroome.edu
Class Cap: 24 *Begins:* Aug
Length: 18 mos *Award:* AAS
Tuition per yr: $2,040 res, $4,080 non-res
Evening or weekend classes available

Trocaire College

Health Information Tech Prgm
110 Red Jacket Pkwy
Buffalo, NY 14220
Prgm Dir: Deborah Shelvay, BA ART
Tel: 716 826-1200 *Fax:* 716 826-0059
Class Cap: 24 *Begins:* Sep
Length: 19 mos *Award:* AAS
Tuition per yr: res, $5,300 non-res
Evening or weekend classes available

CUNY Borough of Manhattan Community Coll

Health Information Tech Prgm
199 Chambers St
Rm 747
New York, NY 10007
Prgm Dir: Camille V Layne, RRA
Tel: 212 346-8739 *Fax:* 212 346-8730
Class Cap: 100 *Begins:* Sep
Length: 24 mos, 36 mos *Award:* AAS
Tuition per yr: $2,500 res, $3,076 non-res
Evening or weekend classes available

Adirondack Community College

Health Information Tech Prgm
634 Bay Rd
Queensbury, NY 12804-1498
Prgm Dir: Lisa Potocar, RRA BPS ART AAS
Tel: 518 743-2286 *Fax:* 518 745-1433
Med Dir: Susan Letuak, PhD MSN RN
Begins: Sep
Length: 24 mos *Award:* AAS
Tuition per yr: $1,900 res, $3,800 non-res

Monroe Community College

Health Information Tech Prgm
1000 E Henrietta Rd
Rochester, NY 14623
Prgm Dir: Sharon L Insero, RRA
Tel: 716 292-2375   *Fax:* 716 427-2749
Class Cap: 30   *Begins:* Sep
Length: 18 mos   *Award:* Dipl, AAS
Tuition per yr: $2,410 res, $4,820 non-res

Molloy College

Health Information Tech Prgm
1000 Hempstead Ave
PO Box 5002
Rockville Centre, NY 11571-5002
Prgm Dir: Ellen Spector Haigney
Tel: 516 678-5000   *Fax:* 516 256-2252
Class Cap: 20   *Begins:* Sep Jan
Length: 20 mos   *Award:* AAS
Tuition per yr: $9,502

Rockland Community College

Health Information Tech Prgm
145 College Rd
Suffern, NY 10901
Prgm Dir: Isabelle Janzen, RRA
Tel: 914 574-4000   *Fax:* 914 574-4498
Class Cap: 25   *Begins:* Sep
Length: 12 mos, 12 mos   *Award:* AAS
Tuition per yr: $2,200 res, $4,500 non-res

Onondaga Community College

Health Information Tech Prgm
Rte 173
Syracuse, NY 13215
Prgm Dir: Judith Chrisman, MS RRA
Tel: 315 469-2102
Class Cap: 40   *Begins:* Aug Jan
Length: 24 mos   *Award:* AAS
Tuition per yr: $1,225 res, $2,450 non-res
Evening or weekend classes available

Mohawk Valley Community College

Health Information Tech Prgm
1101 Sherman Dr
Utica, NY 13501
Prgm Dir: Sue Ellen Bice, MS RRA
Tel: 315 792-5513   *Fax:* 315 792-5666
E-mail: sbice@mucc.edu
Class Cap: 32   *Begins:* Aug
Length: 19 mos   *Award:* AAS
Tuition per yr: $2,500 res, $5,000 non-res
Evening or weekend classes available

Erie Community College - City Campus

Health Information Tech Prgm
6205 Main St
Williamsville, NY 14221-7095
Prgm Dir: Gail M Lauritsen, EdM RRA
Tel: 716 851-1513   *Fax:* 716 851-1429
E-mail: lauritsen@nstaff.sunyerie.edu
Class Cap: 32   *Begins:* Sep
Length: 22 mos   *Award:* AAS
Tuition per yr: $2,500 res, $5,000 non-res
Evening or weekend classes available

North Carolina

Central Piedmont Community College

Health Information Tech Prgm
PO Box 35009
Charlotte, NC 28235
Prgm Dir: Susan C McDermott, RRA
Tel: 704 330-6452   *Fax:* 704 330-5930
Class Cap: 20   *Begins:* Sep
Length: 21 mos   *Award:* AAS
Tuition per yr: $742 res, $6,020 non-res
Evening or weekend classes available

Pitt Community College

Health Information Tech Prgm
PO Drawer 7007
Greenville, NC 27835-7007
Prgm Dir: Kay Gooding, MPH MA Ed RRA
Tel: 919 321-4361   *Fax:* 919 231-4451
E-mail: kgooding@pcc.pitt.cc.nc.us
Class Cap: 18   *Begins:* Sep
Length: 24 mos   *Award:* AD
Tuition per yr: $742 res, $6,020 non-res

Catawba Valley Community College

Health Information Tech Prgm
2550 Hwy 70 SE
Hickory, NC 28602
Prgm Dir: Debra W Cook, MAEd RRA
Tel: 704 327-7000   *Fax:* 704 327-7276
Class Cap: 18   *Begins:* Sep
Length: 18 mos   *Award:* AS, AAS
Tuition per yr: $557 res, $4,515 non-res
Evening or weekend classes available

Davidson County Community College

Health Information Tech Prgm
PO Box 1287
Lexington, NC 27293-1287
Prgm Dir: Mary Daniel Wilson, RRA BS
Tel: 910 249-8186   *Fax:* 910 249-9060
Class Cap: 20   *Begins:* Aug
Length: 21 mos   *Award:* AAS
Tuition per yr: $742 res, $6,020 non-res

Southeastern Regl Allied Hlth Consortium

Health Information Tech Prgm
PO Box 30
Supply, NC 28462
Prgm Dir: Kathleen Howard, RRA
Tel: 910 754-6900   *Fax:* 910 754-7805
Class Cap: 25   *Begins:* Sep
Length: 21 mos   *Award:* AAS
Tuition per yr: $742 res, $6,020 non-res

Edgecombe Community College

Health Information Tech Prgm
2009 W Wilson St
Tarboro, NC 27886
Prgm Dir: Christy W McBryde
Tel: 919 446-0436
Class Cap: 15   *Begins:* Sep
Length: 21 mos   *Award:* AAS
Tuition per yr: $111 res, $981 non-res

North Dakota

United Tribes Technical College

Health Information Tech Prgm
3315 University Dr
Bismarck, ND 58504
Prgm Dir: James C Steen, BBA BS RRA
Tel: 701 255-3285, Ext 245   *Fax:* 701 255-1844
Class Cap: 30   *Begins:* Aug
Length: 24 mos   *Award:* AAS
Tuition per yr: $2,000 res, $2,000 non-res

North Dakota State College of Science

Health Information Tech Prgm
800 N Sixth St
Wahpeton, ND 58076
Prgm Dir: Brian H Gaarder, RRA
Tel: 701 671-2297   *Fax:* 701 671-3587
Class Cap: 25   *Begins:* Aug
Length: 18 mos   *Award:* AAS
Tuition per yr: $1,701 res, $4,293 non-res
Evening or weekend classes available

Ohio

Stark State College of Technology

Health Information Tech Prgm
6200 Frank Ave NW
Canton, OH 44720
Prgm Dir: Darlene S Horn, RRA
Tel: 330 494-6170
Class Cap: 20   *Begins:* Aug
Length: 18 mos   *Award:* Dipl, AAS
Tuition per yr: $2,822 res, $3,842 non-res
Evening or weekend classes available

Cincinnati State Tech and Comm College

Health Information Tech Prgm
3520 Central Pkwy
Cincinnati, OH 45223
Prgm Dir: Gail I Smith, MA RRA
Tel: 513 569-1678   *Fax:* 513 569-1659
Class Cap: 30   *Begins:* Sep Nov
Length: 24 mos   *Award:* Dipl, AAS
Tuition per yr: $2,935 res, $5,665 non-res
Evening or weekend classes available

Cuyahoga Community College

Health Information Tech Prgm
Metro Campus
700 Carnegie Ave
Cleveland, OH 44115
Prgm Dir: Nancy N Donahue, RRA
Tel: 216 987-4456   *Fax:* 216 987-4386
Class Cap: 20   *Begins:* Sep
Length: 12 mos, 9 mos   *Award:* AAS
Tuition per yr: $2,200 res, $5,700 non-res

Columbus State Community College

Health Information Tech Prgm
550 E Spring St
Columbus, OH 43215
Prgm Dir: Lisa A Cerrato, BS RRA
Tel: 614 227-2541   *Fax:* 614 227-5144
E-mail: lcerrato@netexp.net
Med Dir: Jay H Benedict, MS
Class Cap: 40   *Begins:* Sep
Length: 18 mos   *Award:* Cert, AAS
Tuition per yr: $1,656 res, $3,600 non-res
Evening or weekend classes available

Sinclair Community College

Health Information Tech Prgm
444 W Third St
Dayton, OH 45402
Prgm Dir: Catharine A Huber, RRA
Tel: 513 226-2973 *Fax:* 513 226-7960
E-mail: chuber@sinclair.edu
Class Cap: 25 *Begins:* Sep
Length: 22 mos *Award:* AAS
Tuition per yr: $1,953 res, $3,087 non-res
Evening or weekend classes available

Bowling Green State University

Health Information Tech Prgm
901 Rye Beach Rd
Huron, OH 44839
Prgm Dir: Mona M Burke, MA RRA
Tel: 419 433-5560 *Fax:* 419 433-9696
Class Cap: 15 *Begins:* Aug
Length: 18 mos *Award:* AS
Tuition per yr: $3,166 res, $7,906 non-res
Evening or weekend classes available

Hocking Technical College

Health Information Tech Prgm
3301 Hocking Pkwy
Nelsonville, OH 45764
Prgm Dir: Karen Lewis, MHSA RRA ART
Tel: 614 753-3591 *Fax:* 614 753-5105
Class Cap: 65 *Begins:* Sep
Length: 18 mos *Award:* AS
Tuition per yr: $2,088 res, $4,176 non-res
Evening or weekend classes available

Oklahoma

Rose State College

Health Information Tech Prgm
6420 SE 15th St
Midwest City, OK 73110
Prgm Dir: Cecil D Brooks, RRA
Tel: 405 733-7578 *Fax:* 405 736-0338
E-mail: cbrooks@ms.rose.cc.ok.us
Class Cap: 20 *Begins:* Aug
Length: 24 mos *Award:* AAS
Tuition per yr: $1,287 res, $3,267 non-res
Evening or weekend classes available

Tulsa Community College

Health Information Tech Prgm
Allied Health Div Metro Campus
909 S Boston Ave
Tulsa, OK 74119-2095
Prgm Dir: Sandra S Smith, BS MEd/RRA
Tel: 918 595-7201 *Fax:* 918 595-7298
E-mail: ssmith@vin.tulsa.cc.ok.us
Class Cap: 18 *Begins:* Aug
Length: 24 mos *Award:* AAS
Tuition per yr: $1,167 res, $3,120 non-res
Evening or weekend classes available

Oregon

Central Oregon Community College

Health Information Tech Prgm
NW College Way
Bend, OR 97701
Prgm Dir: Gloria M Ahern, RRA
Tel: 541 383-7736 *Fax:* 541 383-7535
E-mail: gahern@cocc.edu
Class Cap: 25 *Begins:* Sep
Length: 9 mo , 18 mos *Award:* Dipl,Cert, AAS
Tuition per yr: $1,728 res, $2,256 non-res
Evening or weekend classes available

Portland Community College

Health Information Tech Prgm
12000 SW 49th Ave
Portland, OR 97219
Prgm Dir: Susan Williams, RRA
Tel: 503 978-5665 *Fax:* 503 978-5257
E-mail: slwillia@pcc.edu
Class Cap: 30 *Begins:* Sep
Length: 18 mos *Award:* AAS
Tuition per yr: $3,255 res, $11,625 non-res
Evening or weekend classes available

Pennsylvania

Gwynedd-Mercy College

Health Information Tech Prgm
Sumneytown Pike
Gwynedd Valley, PA 19437
Prgm Dir: Jennifer Hornung, RRA CPHQ CCS
Tel: 610 646-7300
Class Cap: 25 *Begins:* Aug
Length: 24 mos *Award:* AS
Tuition per yr: $12,300

Community College of Philadelphia

Health Information Tech Prgm
1700 Spring Garden St
Philadelphia, PA 19130
Prgm Dir: Joyce Garozzo, MS RRA
Tel: 215 751-8946 *Fax:* 215 751-8937
Class Cap: 36 *Begins:* Sep
Length: 16 mos *Award:* AAS
Tuition per yr: $1,830 res, $3,660 non-res
Evening or weekend classes available

Comm Coll of Allegheny Cnty-Alleg Campus

Health Information Tech Prgm
808 Ridge Ave
Pittsburgh, PA 15212
Prgm Dir: JoAnn Avoli, RRA
Tel: 412 237-2614 *Fax:* 412 237-4521
E-mail: javoli@ccac.edu
Class Cap: 25 *Begins:* Aug
Length: 18 mos *Award:* AS
Tuition per yr: $2,040 res, $4,080 non-res
Evening or weekend classes available

Sawyer School

Health Information Tech Prgm
717 Liberty Ave
Pittsburgh, PA 15222
Prgm Dir: Susan Nidere, RN
Tel: 412 261-5701 *Fax:* 412 281-7269
Med Dir: Edgar Cordero, MD
Class Cap: 72 *Begins:* Varies
Length: 16 mos *Award:* AS
Tuition per yr: $7,140

Lehigh Carbon Community College

Health Information Tech Prgm
4525 Education Park Dr
Schnecksville, PA 18078-2598
Prgm Dir: George Peters
Tel: 610 799-1596 *Fax:* 610 799-1527
Med Dir: Paul H Schenck, MD
Class Cap: 60 *Begins:* Aug
Length: 24 mos *Award:* AAS
Tuition per yr: $1,612 res, $3,410 non-res

South Hills Business School

Health Information Tech Prgm
480 Waupelani Dr
State College, PA 16801
Prgm Dir: Dan Christopher, MBA RRA
Tel: 814 234-7755 *Fax:* 814 234-0926
Class Cap: 25 *Begins:* Aug
Length: 20 mos *Award:* ASB
Tuition per yr: $7,080

Puerto Rico

Huertas Junior College

Health Information Tech Prgm
PO Box 8429
Caguas, PR 00726
Prgm Dir: Nelida Anderson, RRA
Tel: 809 743-1242 *Fax:* 809 743-0203
Class Cap: 200 *Begins:* Sep
Length: 24 mos *Award:* AS
Tuition per yr: $900 res, $900 non-res

Colegio Universitario Del Este

Health Information Tech Prgm
PO Box 2010
Carolina, PR 00984-2010
Prgm Dir: Evelyn Rosario-Ortiz, RRA
Tel: 787 257-7373
Class Cap: 40 *Begins:* Sep
Length: 20 mos *Award:* Dipl, AS
Tuition per yr: $3,000

Universidad Adventista de las Antillas

Health Information Tech Prgm
PO Box 118
Mayaguez, PR 00681-0118
Prgm Dir: Zilma Santiago de Sepulveda, RRA
  CMSC
Tel: 787 834-9595 *Fax:* 787 834-9597
Class Cap: 20 *Begins:* Aug Jan
Length: 21 mos *Award:* AS
Tuition per yr: $3,500

Interamerican University - San German

Health Information Tech Prgm
Call Box 5100
San German, PR 00683
Prgm Dir: Magda Lopez, MS
Tel: 787 264-1912 *Fax:* 787 892-6350
E-mail: maglopez@ns.inter.edu
Class Cap: 25 *Begins:* Aug
Length: 24 mos *Award:* AD
Tuition per yr: $3,000
Evening or weekend classes available

South Carolina

Midlands Technical College

Health Information Tech Prgm
PO Box 2408
Columbia, SC 29202
Prgm Dir: Jill L Dority, RRA CTR
Tel: 803 822-3072 *Fax:* 803 822-3619
Class Cap: 18 *Begins:* Aug
Length: 21 mos *Award:* AD
Tuition per yr: $1,857 res, $2,970 non-res
Evening or weekend classes available

Florence-Darlington Technical College

Health Information Tech Prgm
PO Box 100548
Florence, SC 29501-0548
Prgm Dir: Mattie G Wilson, MA RRA
Tel: 803 661-8146
Class Cap: 20 *Begins:* Aug
Length: 19 mos *Award:* AD
Tuition per yr: $1,000 res, $1,150 non-res

South Dakota

Dakota State University

Health Information Tech Prgm
CB Kennedy Ctr #151
Madison, SD 57042
Prgm Dir: Dorine Bennett, MBA RRA
Tel: 605 256-5137 *Fax:* 605 256-5316
E-mail: bennett@columbia.dsu.edu
Class Cap: 35 *Begins:* Sep
Length: 18 mos *Award:* AS
Tuition per yr: $2,813 res, $6,006 non-res

National College

Health Information Tech Prgm
PO Box 1780
Rapid City, SD 57709-1780
Prgm Dir: Marilyn Holmgren, MS RRA
Tel: 605 394-4839 *Fax:* 605 394-4871
E-mail: mholmgr@server1.natcol-rcy.edu
Class Cap: 20 *Begins:* Sep
Length: 20 mos *Award:* AS
Tuition per yr: $9,240 res, $9,240 non-res

Tennessee

Chattanooga State Technical Comm College

Health Information Tech Prgm
4501 Amnicola Hwy
Chattanooga, TN 37406-1097
Prgm Dir: Kathryn L McMillan, MEd RRA
Tel: 423 697-4450 *Fax:* 423 634-3071
E-mail: kmcmillan@cstcc.cc.tn.us
Class Cap: 20 *Begins:* Aug
Length: 18 mos *Award:* AAS
Tuition per yr: $994 res, $3,920 non-res
Evening or weekend classes available

Volunteer State Community College

Health Information Tech Prgm
1480 Nashville Pike
Gallatin, TN 37066-3188
Prgm Dir: Lois Anne Knobeloch, RRA
Tel: 615 452-8600 *Fax:* 615 230-3317
E-mail: lknobeloch@uscc.cc.tn.us
Class Cap: 40 *Begins:* Sep
Length: 21 mos *Award:* AAS
Tuition per yr: $1,536 res, $6,144 non-res
Evening or weekend classes available

Roane State Community College

Health Information Tech Prgm
276 Patton Ln
Harriman, TN 37748-5011
Prgm Dir: Alice A Moore, RRA CCS
Tel: 423 882-4624 *Fax:* 423 882-4549
E-mail: moore_a@ai.rscc.cc.tn.us
Class Cap: 17 *Begins:* Aug
Length: 21 mos *Award:* AAS
Tuition per yr: $1,066 res, $4,138 non-res
Evening or weekend classes available

Texas

Lee College

Health Information Tech Prgm
511 S Whiting St
Baytown, TX 77520-0818
Prgm Dir: Ann Marice Ivey, MS RRA CMT
Tel: 713 425-6569 *Fax:* 713 425-6520
Begins: Jun Aug Jan
Length: 12 mos, 24 mos *Award:* Cert, AAS
Tuition per yr: $749 res, $1,337 non-res
Evening or weekend classes available

El Paso Community College

Health Information Tech Prgm
PO Box 20500
El Paso, TX 79998
Prgm Dir: Jean A Garrison, RRA
Tel: 915 534-4074 *Fax:* 915 534-4114
Class Cap: 12 *Begins:* Aug
Length: 5 mo , 22 mos *Award:* Cert, AAS
Tuition per yr: $990 res, $2,960 non-res
Evening or weekend classes available

North Central Texas College

Health Information Tech Prgm
1525 W California St
Gainesville, TX 76240
Prgm Dir: Linda Jones, BS RRA
Tel: 817 668-7731 *Fax:* 972 436-6214
Class Cap: 40 *Begins:* Aug Jan Jun
Length: 12 mos, 24 mos *Award:* Cert, AAS
Tuition per yr: $350 res, $555 non-res
Evening or weekend classes available

Texas State Technical College

Health Information Tech Prgm
2424 Boxwood
Harlingen, TX 78551-3697
Prgm Dir: Gayla J Holmes, MS RRA
Tel: 210 425-0763 *Fax:* 210 425-0630
Class Cap: 24 *Begins:* Sep
Length: 18 mos *Award:* AAS
Tuition per yr: $1,256 res, $4,424 non-res

Houston Community College Central

Health Information Tech Prgm
Health Careers Education Div
3100 Shenandoah
Houston, TX 77021
Prgm Dir: Carla Tyson, MHA RRA
Tel: 713 746-5337
E-mail: tyson_c@hccs.cc.tx.us
Class Cap: 25 *Begins:* Aug
Length: 24 mos *Award:* Cert, AAS
Tuition per yr: $1,008 res, $1,500 non-res
Evening or weekend classes available

Tarrant Junior College

Health Information Tech Prgm
828 Harwood Rd
Hurst, TX 76054
Prgm Dir: Delores J McDonald, RRA CCS
Tel: 817 788-6544 *Fax:* 817 788-6601
Class Cap: 21 *Begins:* Aug
Length: 24 mos *Award:* AAS
Tuition per yr: $680 res, $1,020 non-res

South Plains College

Health Information Tech Prgm
1302 Main St
Lubbock, TX 79401
Prgm Dir: Bette J Green, MPA RRA
Tel: 806 747-0576, Ext 4644 *Fax:* 806 765-2775
E-mail: dwiggins@mail.spc.cc.tx.us
Class Cap: 32 *Begins:* Aug
Length: 9 mo , 18 mos *Award:* Dipl,Cert, AAS
Tuition per yr: $1,698 res, $1,918 non-res

Howard College

Health Information Tech Prgm
3197 Executive Dr
San Angelo, TX 76904
Prgm Dir: Nancy L Rendon, RRA
Tel: 915 944-9585
Class Cap: 18 *Begins:* Aug
Length: 21 mos *Award:* AAS
Tuition per yr: $1,276 res, $1,458 non-res

St Philip's College

Health Information Tech Prgm
1801 Martin Luther King Dr.
San Antonio, TX 78203
Prgm Dir: Elizabeth Bernasconi, RRA
Tel: 512 531-3416
Class Cap: 30 *Begins:* Aug
Length: 9 mo , 20 mos *Award:* Cert, AAS
Tuition per yr: $500 res, $1,600 non-res
Evening or weekend classes available

Tyler Junior College

Health Information Tech Prgm
PO Box 9020
Tyler, TX 75711
Prgm Dir: Charlotte Creason, BS RRA
Tel: 903 510-2669 *Fax:* 903 510-2592
Class Cap: 25 *Begins:* Aug
Length: 24 mos *Award:* AAS
Tuition per yr: $842 res, $1,322 non-res
Evening or weekend classes available

Programs

Wharton County Junior College

Health Information Tech Prgm
911 Boling Hwy
Wharton, TX 77488
Prgm Dir: Mary W King, MS RRA
Tel: 409 532-6363   *Fax:* 409 532-6545
Class Cap: 30   *Begins:* Aug Sep
Length: 20 mos   *Award:* AAS
Tuition per yr: $1,161 res, $1,978 non-res
Evening or weekend classes available

Utah

Weber State University

Health Information Tech Prgm
3911 University Circle
Odgen, UT 84408-3911
Prgm Dir: Christ R Elliott, RRA
Tel: 801 626-7242   *Fax:* 801 626-7683
E-mail: celliott@weber.edu
Begins: Sep
Length: 18 mos   *Award:* AAS
Tuition per yr: $1,743 res, $5,514 non-res
Evening or weekend classes available

Virginia

Northern Virginia Community College

Health Information Tech Prgm
8333 Little River Trnpk
Annandale, VA 22003
Prgm Dir: Sandra Bailey, RRA
Tel: 703 323-3413   *Fax:* 703 323-4576
E-mail: nubails@nv.cc.va.us
Class Cap: 25   *Begins:* Aug
Length: 18 mos   *Award:* AAS
Tuition per yr: $1,682 res, $5,507 non-res
Evening or weekend classes available

College of Health Sciences

Health Information Tech Prgm
PO Box 13186
Roanoke, VA 24031-3186
Prgm Dir: Mildred P St Leger, BA RRA
Tel: 540 985-4020   *Fax:* 540 985-9773
Class Cap: 15   *Begins:* Aug
Length: 18 mos   *Award:* Dipl, AS
Tuition per yr: $4,200
Evening or weekend classes available

Tidewater Community College

Health Information Tech Prgm
1700 College Crescent
Virginia Beach, VA 23456
Prgm Dir: Gussie L Hammond, MS BS RRA
Tel: 804 427-7262   *Fax:* 804 427-1338
Class Cap: 40   *Begins:* Aug
Length: 21 mos   *Award:* AAS
Tuition per yr: $1,612 res, $5,002 non-res
Evening or weekend classes available

Washington

Shoreline Community College

Health Information Tech Prgm
16101 Greenwood Ave N
Seattle, WA 98133
Prgm Dir: Donna J Wilde, MPA RRA
Tel: 206 543-4757   *Fax:* 206 543-4604
E-mail: dwilde@ctc.edu
Class Cap: 355   *Begins:* Sep
Length: 18 mos   *Award:* AAS
Tuition per yr: $1,390 res, $5,500 non-res
Evening or weekend classes available

Spokane Community College

Health Information Tech Prgm
N 1810 Greene St
MS 2090
Spokane, WA 99207
Prgm Dir: Shirley Higgin, MEd RRA
Tel: 509 536-8032   *Fax:* 509 533-8621
E-mail: shiggin@ctc.edu
Class Cap: 25   *Begins:* Sep
Length: 18 mos   *Award:* AAS
Tuition per yr: $1,350 res, $5,298 non-res
Evening or weekend classes available

Tacoma Community College

Health Information Tech Prgm
6501 S 19th St
Tacoma, WA 98466
Prgm Dir: Ingrid Bentzen, RRA
Tel: 206 566-5163   *Fax:* 206 566-5273
Class Cap: 30   *Begins:* Sep
Length: 18 mos   *Award:* Cert, AAS
Tuition per yr: $1,401 res, $5,511 non-res
Evening or weekend classes available

West Virginia

Fairmont State College

Health Information Tech Prgm
Locust Ave
Fairmont, WV 26554
Prgm Dir: Sr Marie Horvath, RRA
Tel: 304 367-4764   *Fax:* 304 366-4870
Class Cap: 25   *Begins:* Aug
Length: 18 mos   *Award:* AAS
Tuition per yr: $1,918 res, $4,428 non-res

Marshall University

Health Information Tech Prgm
Huntington, WV 25755
Prgm Dir: Jane Barker, RRA
Tel: 304 696-6796   *Fax:* 304 696-3013
E-mail: barker@marshall.edu
Class Cap: 25   *Begins:* Aug
Length: 21 mos   *Award:* AAS
Tuition per yr: $1,058 res, $1,974 non-res
Evening or weekend classes available

Wisconsin

Chippewa Valley Technical College

Health Information Tech Prgm
620 W Clairemont Ave
Eau Claire, WI 54701
Prgm Dir: Carol Ryan, RRA
Tel: 715 833-6423   *Fax:* 715 833-6470
E-mail: chippewa.tech.wi.us
Class Cap: 20   *Begins:* Jan
Length: 16 mos   *Award:* AS
Tuition per yr: $1,997 res, $15,405 non-res

Northeast Wisconsin Technical College

Health Information Tech Prgm
2740 W Mason St
PO Box 19042
Green Bay, WI 54307-9042
Prgm Dir: Marilyn Toninato, BS RRA
Tel: 414 498-5577   *Fax:* 414 498-5673
Class Cap: 16   *Begins:* Jun
Length: 20 mos   *Award:* AAS
Tuition per yr: $1,832 res, $14,007 non-res

Western Wisconsin Technical College

Health Information Tech Prgm
304 N Sixth St
PO Box 908
La Crosse, WI 54602-0908
Prgm Dir: Tamra R Brown, ME RRA
Tel: 608 785-9549   *Fax:* 608 785-9497
E-mail: brown@a1.western.tec.wi.us
Class Cap: 16   *Begins:* Aug
Length: 20 mos   *Award:* AS
Tuition per yr: $2,090 res, $13,047 non-res

Gateway Technical College

Health Information Tech Prgm
1001 S Main St
Racine, WI 53403
Prgm Dir: Cynthia Fickenscher, BS RRA
Tel: 414 631-7307   *Fax:* 414 631-1044
Class Cap: 22   *Begins:* Aug
Length: 20 mos   *Award:* AAS
Tuition per yr: $1,800

Moraine Park Technical College

Health Information Tech Prgm
2151 N Main St
West Bend, WI 53095
Prgm Dir: Lucia Francis, RRA
Tel: 414 334-3413   *Fax:* 414 335-5708
Class Cap: 30   *Begins:* Aug
Length: 18 mos   *Award:* AAS
Tuition per yr: $2,741

Medical Assistant

History

Since its founding in 1956, the American Association of Medical Assistants (AAMA) has been the only professional association devoted exclusively to the profession of medical assisting. The AAMA holds an important role in improving the educational preparation and continuing education opportunities for the medical assistant.

The first certification examination was administered in 1963, preceding the establishment of the accreditation program. In 1966, the AAMA began work on formal curriculum standards in collaboration with the AMA. A task force of physicians and medical assistants surveyed existing medical assistant programs and drew up tentative standards, which were adopted in 1969. Approximately 3 years were spent in laying a solid groundwork for a 2-year associate degree program. In 1971, after 2 years of actual accreditation activity, the initial standards were revised to allow for the accreditation of 1-year educational programs.

Occupational Description

Medical assisting is a multiskilled allied health profession; practitioners work primarily in ambulatory settings such as medical offices and clinics. Medical assistants function as members of the health care delivery team and perform administrative and clinical procedures.

Job Description

Medical assistants are allied health professionals who assist physicians in their offices or other medical settings. In accordance with respective state laws, they perform a broad range of administrative and clinical duties, as indicated by the AAMA's recent role delineation study.

Administrative duties include scheduling and receiving patients, preparing and maintaining medical records, performing basic secretarial skills and medical transcription, handling telephone calls and writing correspondence, serving as a liaison between the physician and other individuals, and managing practice finances.

Clinical duties include asepsis and infection control, taking patient histories and vital signs, performing first aid and CPR, preparing patients for procedures, assisting the physician with examinations and treatments, collecting and processing specimens, performing selected diagnostic tests, and preparing and administering medications as directed by the physician.

Both administrative and clinical duties involve maintenance of equipment and supplies for the practice. A medical assistant who is sufficiently qualified by education and/or experience may be responsible for supervising personnel, developing and conducting public outreach programs to market the physician's professional services, and participating in the negotiation of leases and of equipment and supply contracts.

Employment Characteristics

More medical assistants are employed by practicing physicians than any other type of allied health personnel. Medical assistants are usually employed in physicians' offices, where they perform a variety of administrative and clinical tasks to facilitate the work of the physician. The responsibilities of medical assistants vary, depending on whether they work in a clinic, hospital, large group practice, or small private office. With a demand from more than 200,000 physicians, there are, and will probably continue to be, almost unlimited opportunities for formally educated medical assistants.

According to the AAMA, the average entry-level salary in 1995 was $18,000.

Educational Programs

Length. Programs are either 2 years, resulting in an associate degree, or 1 year, resulting in a certificate or diploma.
Prerequisites. High school diploma or equivalent.
Curriculum. The curricula of accredited programs must ensure achievement of the *Entry-Level Competencies for the Medical Assistant*. The curriculum must include anatomy and physiology, medical terminology, medical law and ethics, psychology, communications (oral and written), medical assisting administrative procedures, and medical assisting clinical procedures. Programs must include an externship that provides practical experience in qualified physicians' offices, accredited hospitals, or other health care facilities.
Standards. *Standards (Essentials)* are minimum standards developed by the Curriculum Board of the AAMA's Endowment. Each new program is assessed in accordance with the *Standards*, and accredited programs are reviewed periodically to determine whether they remain in substantial compliance. The *Standards and Guidelines* are available on written request from the American Association of Medical Assistants' Endowment.

Inquiries

Accreditation

Requests for information on program accreditation, including *Standards*, preparing the self-study report, and arranging for a site visit, should be submitted to

American Association of Medical Assistants' Endowment
Department of Accreditation
20 N Wacker Dr/Ste 1575
Chicago, IL 60606-2903
800 228-2262

Careers

Inquiries regarding careers or accredited programs should be addressed to

American Association of Medical Assistants
20 N Wacker Dr/Ste 1575
Chicago, IL 60606-2903
800 228-2262

Certification/Registration

Inquiries regarding certification may be addressed to

Director of Certification
American Association of Medical Assistants
20 N Wacker Dr/Ste 1575
Chicago, IL 60606-2903
312 424-3100

Programs

Medical Assistant

Alabama

George C Wallace State Comm College
Medical Assistant Prgm
Napier Field Rd
Rt 6 Box 62
Dothan, AL 36303
Prgm Dir: Jane Ann Shannon, MT(ASCP) CMA-C
Tel: 334 983-3521 *Fax:* 334 983-3600
Med Dir: William Lupinacci, MD
Class Cap: 96 *Begins:* Jan Mar Jun Sep
Length: 12 mos, 18 mos *Award:* Dipl,Cert, AAS
Tuition per yr: $2,410 res, $4,385 non-res
Evening or weekend classes available

Wallace State College
Medical Assistant Prgm
PO Box 2000
Hanceville, AL 35077-2000
Prgm Dir: Tracie Fuqua, AAS CMA
Tel: 205 352-2090, Ext 235 *Fax:* 205 352-6400
Med Dir: James Thomason, MD FAAP
Class Cap: 35 *Begins:* Sep
Length: 24 mos *Award:* AAS
Tuition per yr: $1,474 res, $2,580 non-res
Evening or weekend classes available

Draughons Junior College
Medical Assistant Prgm
122 Commerce St
Montgomery, AL 36104
Prgm Dir: Sadie Sky
Tel: 334 263-1013 *Fax:* 334 262-7326
Class Cap: 100 *Begins:* Jan Apr Jun Oct
Length: 18 mos, 24 mos *Award:* Cert, AS
Tuition per yr: $7,580
Evening or weekend classes available

H Councill Trenholm State Technical College
Medical Assistant Prgm
1225 Air Base Blvd
PO Box 9000
Montgomery, AL 36108
Prgm Dir: Sylvia Nobles, MSN RN CMA
Tel: 334 832-9000 *Fax:* 334 832-9777
Med Dir: J W Strickland Jr, MD
Class Cap: 40 *Begins:* Sep
Length: 12 mos, 18 mos *Award:* Cert, AAT
Tuition per yr: $2,800
Evening or weekend classes available

Alaska

University of Alaska Anchorage
Medical Assistant Prgm
3211 Providence Dr
Anchorage, AK 99508
Prgm Dir: Robin Wahto, BSN RN CMA
Tel: 907 786-1547 *Fax:* 907 786-1244
E-mail: AFRJW@ALAS
Med Dir: Judith Whitcomb, MD
Class Cap: 30 *Begins:* Sep Jan May
Length: 10 mos, 24 mos *Award:* Cert, AAS
Tuition per yr: $2,870 res, $8,610 non-res
Evening or weekend classes available

Arizona

The Bryman School
Medical Assistant Prgm
4343 N 16th St
Phoenix, AZ 85016
Prgm Dir: Valoria A Bradford, CMA
Tel: 602 274-4300 *Fax:* 602 230-9942
Med Dir: Alfonso Puyana, MD
Class Cap: 240 *Begins:* Monthly
Length: 7 mos *Award:* Dipl
Tuition per yr: $5,950
Evening or weekend classes available

Arkansas

Arkansas Tech University
Medical Assistant Prgm
Russellville, AR 72801
Prgm Dir: Tom Palko, MT(ASCP)MCS
Tel: 501 968-0328 *Fax:* 501 964-0504
Med Dir: Stanley Bradley, MD
Class Cap: 20 *Begins:* Aug Jan
Length: 19 mos *Award:* AS
Tuition per yr: $1,902 res, $3,804 non-res
Evening or weekend classes available

California

ConCorde Career Institute
Medical Assistant Prgm
1717 S Brookhurst St
Anaheim, CA 92804
Prgm Dir: Tonya Hallock
Tel: 714 635-3450 *Fax:* 714 535-3168
Med Dir: Benny Hall, MD
Begins: Monthly
Length: 8 mos *Award:* Dipl
Tuition per yr: $6,500

Orange Coast College
Medical Assistant Prgm
2701 Fairview Rd
Costa Mesa, CA 92628-5005
Prgm Dir: Margie Willis, CMA-AC
Tel: 714 432-0202 *Fax:* 714 432-5532
Med Dir: Jeffrey Barke, MD
Class Cap: 36 *Begins:* Jan
Length: 18 mos *Award:* Cert
Tuition per yr: $351 res, $3,429 non-res

De Anza College
Medical Assistant Prgm
21250 Stevens Creek Blvd
Cupertino, CA 95014
Prgm Dir: Patricia L Hassel, RN CMA-AC
Tel: 408 864-8789 *Fax:* 408 864-5444
Med Dir: Stanley Markowski, MD
Class Cap: 70 *Begins:* Sep Jan Apr Jul
Length: 12 mos, 24 mos *Award:* Dipl,Cert
Tuition per yr: $3,980 res, $5,460 non-res
Evening or weekend classes available

Chabot College
Medical Assistant Prgm
25555 Hesperian Blvd
Hayward, CA 94545-5001
Prgm Dir: Jane Vallely, BS RN CMA
Tel: 510 786-6901 *Fax:* 510 782-9315
Med Dir: Jeffrey Mandel, MD
Class Cap: 40 *Begins:* Aug
Length: 9 mo , 18 mos *Award:* Cert, AA
Tuition per yr: $380 res, $122 non-res
Evening or weekend classes available

Modesto Junior College
Medical Assistant Prgm
435 College Ave
Modesto, CA 95350-9977
Prgm Dir: Shirley Buzbee, CMA
Tel: 209 575-6377
Med Dir: Roland C Nyegaard
Class Cap: 25 *Begins:* Aug
Length: 9 mos *Award:* Cert, AS
Tuition per yr: $512 res, $3,977 non-res

CSi Bryman College
Medical Assistant Prgm
1120 W La Veta/Ste 100
Orange, CA 92668
Prgm Dir: Donna Kucharski, CMA
Tel: 714 953-6500 *Fax:* 714 953-4163
Med Dir: Daniel Jimenez, MD
Class Cap: 616 *Begins:* Monthly
Length: 8 mos *Award:* Dipl
Tuition per yr: $6,175 res, $6,175 non-res
Evening or weekend classes available

Pasadena City College
Medical Assistant Prgm
1570 E Colorado Blvd
Pasadena, CA 91106
Prgm Dir: Joyce Y Nakano, CMA-A
Tel: 818 585-7431
Med Dir: Richard Shapiro, MD
Class Cap: 24 *Begins:* Aug
Length: 9 mos *Award:* Cert
Tuition per yr: $416 res, $3,515 non-res
Evening or weekend classes available

National Education Ctr - Bryman Campus
Medical Assistant Prgm
3505 N Hart Ave
Rosemead, CA 91770
Prgm Dir: Debra R Hrisoulas, CMA
Tel: 818 573-5470 *Fax:* 818 280-4011
Med Dir: Sami Juma, MD
Begins: Jan Dec
Length: 8 mos *Award:* Dipl
Tuition per yr: $5,520
Evening or weekend classes available

Cosumnes River College
Medical Assistant Prgm
8401 Center Pkwy
Sacramento, CA 95823
Prgm Dir: Patricia Goshorn, RN CMA-AC
Tel: 916 688-7296 *Fax:* 916 688-7443
Med Dir: Daniel J Fields, MD
Class Cap: 30 *Begins:* Sep Feb
Length: 24 mos *Award:* Cert, AA
Tuition per yr: $120 res, $3,200 non-res

Western Career College

Medical Assistant Prgm
8909 Folsom Blvd
Sacramento, CA 95826
Prgm Dir: Terry Wade, CMA
Tel: 916 361-1660 *Fax:* 916 361-6666
Med Dir: Martha Miller, MD
Class Cap: 288 *Begins:* Monthly
Length: 9 mos *Award:* Cert, AS
Tuition per yr: $7,270 res, $7,270 non-res
Evening or weekend classes available

ConCorde Career Institute

Medical Assistant Prgm
570 W Fourth St
San Bernardino, CA 92401
Prgm Dir: Vicki Prater, CMA-C
Tel: 909 884-8891 *Fax:* 909 384-1768
Med Dir: Benny Hau, MD
Class Cap: 365 *Begins:* Varies
Length: 9 mos *Award:* Dipl
Tuition per yr: $6,795
Evening or weekend classes available

National Education Ctr - Skadron Campus

Medical Assistant Prgm
825 E Hospitality Ln
San Bernardino, CA 92408
Prgm Dir: Ruth Darton, CMA
Tel: 909 885-3893 *Fax:* 909 885-2396
Begins: Monthly
Length: 8 mos *Award:* Dipl
Tuition per yr: $5,459 res, $5,459 non-res

San Diego Mesa College

Medical Assistant Prgm
7250 Mesa College Dr
San Diego, CA 92111
Prgm Dir: Temma Al-Mukhtar, CMA MBChB
Tel: 619 627-2949
Med Dir: Donald Weiss, MD
Class Cap: 35 *Begins:* Aug
Length: 9 mo , 24 mos *Award:* Dipl,Cert, AS
Tuition per yr: $403 res, $3,913 non-res
Evening or weekend classes available

City College of San Francisco

Medical Assistant Prgm
1860 Hayes St
San Francisco, CA 94117
Prgm Dir: Margaret Guichard
Tel: 415 561-1826 *Fax:* 415 561-1861
Med Dir: Francis J Charlton, MD
Class Cap: 125 *Begins:* Aug Jan
Length: 12 mos, 24 mos *Award:* Cert, AS
Tuition per yr: $416 res, $4,388 non-res
Evening or weekend classes available

National Education Ctr - Bryman Campus

Medical Assistant Prgm
731 Market St
San Francisco, CA 94103
Prgm Dir: Linda Albertson, CMA
Tel: 415 777-2500 *Fax:* 415 495-3457
Med Dir: Pedro Pinto, MD
Begins: Monthly
Length: 8 mos *Award:* Dipl
Tuition per yr: $6,140 res, $6,140 non-res

National Education Ctr - Bryman Campus

Medical Assistant Prgm
2015 Naglee Ave
San Jose, CA 95128
Prgm Dir: Haig Movsesian, RMA
Tel: 408 275-8800 *Fax:* 408 275-0662
Med Dir: Robert Roth, MD
Begins: Monthly
Length: 8 mos *Award:* Dipl
Tuition per yr: $6,050 res, $6,050 non-res

Western Career College of San Leandro

Medical Assistant Prgm
170 Bayfair Mall
San Leandro, CA 94578
Prgm Dir: Cris McTighe, RMA
Tel: 510 276-3888 *Fax:* 510 276-3653
Med Dir: Martha Miller, MD
Class Cap: 24 *Begins:* Monthly
Length: 9 mos *Award:* Dipl
Tuition per yr: $6,395 res, $6,395 non-res

Coastal Valley College

Medical Assistant Prgm
731 S Lincoln St
Santa Maria, CA 93454
Prgm Dir: Stella P Martin, CMA BS
Tel: 805 925-1478 *Fax:* 805 925-4189
Med Dir: Randy Johnson, MD
Class Cap: 12
Length: 8 mos *Award:* Dipl
Tuition per yr: $5,000

West Valley Community College District

Medical Assistant Prgm
14000 Fruitvale Ave
Saratoga, CA 95070
Prgm Dir: Diane Herschfelt, CMA-A
Tel: 408 741-2139
Med Dir: William Hamilton, MD
Class Cap: 25 *Begins:* Sep Jan
Length: 11 mos, 22 mos *Award:* Cert, AS

National Education Ctr - Bryman Campus

Medical Assistant Prgm
4212 W Artesia Blvd
Torrance, CA 90504
Prgm Dir: Jacqueline Hornsby, CMA
Tel: 310 542-6951 *Fax:* 310 542-3294
Med Dir: Pramod Multani, MD
Class Cap: 275 *Begins:* Monthly
Length: 8 mos *Award:* Dipl
Tuition per yr: $5,820 res, $5,820 non-res

Golden State Business College Inc

Medical Assistant Prgm
3356 S Fairway
Visalia, CA 93277
Prgm Dir: Linda Sanchez
Tel: 209 733-4040 *Fax:* 209 733-7831
Med Dir: Alex C Torres, MD FAAFP
Class Cap: 80 *Begins:* Monthly
Length: 8 mos *Award:* Cert
Tuition per yr: $5,845 res, $5,845 non-res

Colorado

T H Pickens Technical Center

Medical Assistant Prgm
500 Airport Blvd
Aurora, CO 80011
Prgm Dir: Pamela Wiebelhaus, BS RN CMA
Tel: 303 344-4910 *Fax:* 303 340-1898
Med Dir: Michael Dennington, MD
Class Cap: 15 *Begins:* Aug Jan
Length: 10 mos *Award:* Cert
Tuition per yr: $1,620 res, $3,240 non-res
Evening or weekend classes available

Front Range Comm College - Westminster

Medical Assistant Prgm
6600 Arapahoe
Boulder, CO 80303
Prgm Dir: Sandra L Love, MBA RN CMA
Tel: 303 447-5588 *Fax:* 303 447-5258
Med Dir: John Hudson, MD
Class Cap: 16 *Begins:* Aug Jan
Length: 9 mos *Award:* Cert
Tuition per yr: $2,880 res, $12,318 non-res
Evening or weekend classes available

Blair Junior College

Medical Assistant Prgm
828 Wooten Rd
Colorado Springs, CO 80915
Prgm Dir: Pat Vidic, CMA
Tel: 719 574-1082 *Fax:* 719 574-4493
Med Dir: Joyce Michael, DO
Class Cap: 80 *Begins:* Jan Apr Jul Oct
Length: 24 mos *Award:* AAS
Tuition per yr: $12,413
Evening or weekend classes available

Community College of Denver

Medical Assistant Prgm
3532 Franklin St
Denver, CO 80205
Prgm Dir: Priscilla E Lindsey, RN BSN
Tel: 303 293-8737
Med Dir: Jeannette Brake, MD
Class Cap: 90 *Begins:* Varies
Length: 10 mos *Award:* Cert
Tuition per yr: $3,898 res, $12,675 non-res

Denver Institute of Technology

Medical Assistant Prgm
Health Careers Division
7350 N Broadway
Denver, CO 80221
Prgm Dir: Loretta Mitchel
Tel: 303 650-5050
Class Cap: 80 *Begins:* Jan Apr Jul Oct
Length: 18 mos *Award:* AA
Tuition per yr: $10,995

Emily Griffith Opportunity School

Medical Assistant Prgm
1250 Welton St
Denver, CO 80204
Prgm Dir: Jeanne L Avery, CMA
Tel: 303 575-4737 *Fax:* 303 575-4840
Med Dir: Alan Burgess, MD
Class Cap: 20 *Begins:* Sep Jan
Length: 9 mos *Award:* Cert
Tuition per yr: $1,500 res, $5,100 non-res

Parks College

Medical Assistant Prgm
9065 Grant St
Denver, CO 80229
Prgm Dir: Rogene D Lowe, MT(ASCP)CMA
Tel: 303 457-2757 *Fax:* 303 457-4030
Med Dir: Zachary Shpall, MD
Class Cap: 25 *Begins:* Jan Apr Jul Oct
Length: 24 mos *Award:* AAS
Tuition per yr: $13,525
Evening or weekend classes available

Connecticut

Branford Hall Career Institute

Medical Assistant Prgm
One Summit Pl
Branford, CT 06405
Prgm Dir: Carol R Quale, RN
Tel: 203 488-2525 *Fax:* 203 488-5233
E-mail: branford@micro-net.com
Class Cap: 50 *Begins:* Sep Nov Feb Apr
Length: 12 mos *Award:* Dipl
Tuition per yr: $9,950 res, $9,950 non-res

Quinebaug Valley Comm - Tech College

Medical Assistant Prgm
742 Upper Maple St
Danielson, CT 06239
Prgm Dir: Lorraine Fleming, BA MT(ASCP)
Tel: 860 774-1160 *Fax:* 860 774-7768
E-mail: qr_markos_76@apollo.columnet.edu
Med Dir: Philip Raiford, MD
Class Cap: 50 *Begins:* Aug Jan
Length: 18 mos *Award:* AS
Tuition per yr: $1,520 res, $4,440 non-res
Evening or weekend classes available

Data Institute Business School

Medical Assistant Prgm
745 Burnside Ave
East Hartford, CT 06108
Prgm Dir: Nancy Peacos, RN
Tel: 860 528-4111 *Fax:* 860 291-9550
Med Dir: Dominick Roto, DO RP BS
Class Cap: 60 *Begins:* Jan Mar May Jul Sep
Length: 12 mos *Award:* Dipl
Tuition per yr: $7,900 res, $7,900 non-res

Porter and Chester Institute - Enfield

Medical Assistant Prgm
138 Weymouth Rd
Enfield, CT 06082
Prgm Dir: Christine A Jette, LPN
Tel: 203 741-2561 *Fax:* 203 741-0234
Med Dir: Paul D Nitti, MD
Class Cap: 30 *Begins:* Oct Jan Apr Jul
Length: 1 mos *Award:* Dipl
Tuition per yr: $9,400 res, $9,400 non-res

Stone Academy

Medical Assistant Prgm
1315 Dixwell Ave
Hamden, CT 06514
Prgm Dir: Holly E Mulrenan, BSN RN
Tel: 203 288-7474 *Fax:* 203 288-8869
Med Dir: Leonard Fasano, MD
Class Cap: 250 *Begins:* Feb Apr Jul Sep
Length: 12 mos, 24 mos *Award:* Dipl
Tuition per yr: $10,025
Evening or weekend classes available

Morse School of Business

Medical Assistant Prgm
275 Asylum St
Hartford, CT 06103
Prgm Dir: Carol Boardman, MA
Tel: 203 522-2261
Med Dir: Richard Stone, MD
Class Cap: 75 *Begins:* Feb May Sep Nov
Length: 15 mos, 18 mos *Award:* Dipl,Cert
Tuition per yr: $11,160

Porter and Chester Institute - Stratford

Medical Assistant Prgm
670 Lordship Blvd
Stratford, CT 06497
Prgm Dir: Carl Ottowell, EMT-P
Tel: 203 375-4463 *Fax:* 203 375-5285
Med Dir: Bruce Wainer, MD
Class Cap: 30 *Begins:* Oct Jan Apr Jul
Length: 1 mos *Award:* Dipl
Tuition per yr: $9,400 res, $9,400 non-res

Porter and Chester Institute - Watertown

Medical Assistant Prgm
320 Sylvan Lake Rd
Watertown, CT 06779
Prgm Dir: Gail Martinelli, LPN AS
Tel: 203 274-9294 *Fax:* 203 274-3075
Med Dir: Paul Kraus, MD
Class Cap: 30 *Begins:* Oct Jan Apr Jul
Length: 1 mos *Award:* Dipl
Tuition per yr: $9,400 res, $9,400 non-res

Fox Institute of Business

Medical Assistant Prgm
99 South St
West Hartford, CT 06110-1922
Prgm Dir: Linda K Navitsky, BA MA
Tel: 860 947-2299 *Fax:* 860 947-2290
E-mail: patrickfox@aol.com
Med Dir: Steven Meltzer, DMD
Class Cap: 96 *Begins:* Oct Feb Jun
Length: 15 mos, 24 mos *Award:* Dipl,Cert
Tuition per yr: $6,400 res, $6,400 non-res
Evening or weekend classes available

Porter and Chester Institute

Medical Assistant Prgm
125 Silas Deane Hwy
Wethersfield, CT 06109
Prgm Dir: Susan Perrerira
Tel: 203 529-2519 *Fax:* 203 563-2595
Med Dir: Larry E Blitstein, MD
Class Cap: 30 *Begins:* Oct Jan Apr Jul
Length: 14 mos, 21 mos *Award:* Dipl
Tuition per yr: $9,400 res, $9,400 non-res

Northwestern Connecticut Comm College

Medical Assistant Prgm
Park Place E
Winsted, CT 06098
Prgm Dir: Barbara C Berger, RN CMA
Tel: 203 738-6378 *Fax:* 860 738-6439
E-mail: nw_berger
Med Dir: Clifford Rosenberg, MD
Class Cap: 60 *Begins:* Sep
Length: 16 mos *Award:* AS
Tuition per yr: $1,722
Evening or weekend classes available

Florida

Broward Community College

Medical Assistant Prgm
3501 SW Davie Rd
Ft Lauderdale, FL 33301
Prgm Dir: Adelaida DeLaGuardia, AS CMA
Tel: 954 475-6906 *Fax:* 954 473-9037
Med Dir: Glen Motlan, MD
Class Cap: 30 *Begins:* Aug
Length: 10 mos *Award:* Cert
Tuition per yr: $1,500 res, $3,600 non-res

Keiser College of Technology

Medical Assistant Prgm
1500 NW 49th St
Ft Lauderdale, FL 33309
Prgm Dir: Diane M Klieger, RMA CMA MBA
Tel: 954 776-4456 *Fax:* 954 771-4894
Med Dir: Gohar Khan, MD
Begins: Varies
Length: 24 mos *Award:* AS
Tuition per yr: $6,560 res, $6,560 non-res

Minnesota Riverland Tech Coll-Faribault

Medical Assistant Prgm
2401 N Harbor City Blvd
Melbourne, FL 32935
Prgm Dir: Jahangir Moini, MD MPH
Tel: 407 253-2929 *Fax:* 407 255-2017
Class Cap: 200 *Begins:* Jan Apr Jul Oct
Length: 24 mos *Award:* AS
Tuition per yr: $4,500 res, $4,500 non-res
Evening or weekend classes available

Orlando College-Melbourne Campus

Medical Assistant Prgm
2401 N Harbor City Blvd
Melbourne, FL 32935
Prgm Dir: Jahangir Moini, MD
Tel: 407 254-6459 *Fax:* 407 255-2017
Class Cap: 50 *Begins:* Jan Apr Jul Oct
Length: 24 mos *Award:* AAS
Tuition per yr: $4,500 res, $4,500 non-res
Evening or weekend classes available

Pensacola Junior College

Medical Assistant Prgm
Warrington Campus
5555 W Hwy 98
Pensacola, FL 32507
Prgm Dir: Carmen Schlaffer, MS RN
Tel: 904 484-2223 *Fax:* 904 454-2365
Med Dir: William Nass, MD
Class Cap: 30 *Begins:* Aug
Length: 12 mos *Award:* Cert
Tuition per yr: $1,200 res, $2,161 non-res

Sarasota County Technical Institute

Medical Assistant Prgm
4748 Beneva Rd
Sarasota, FL 34233
Prgm Dir: Linda W Swisher, RN EdD
Tel: 941 924-1365 *Fax:* 941 361-6886
Med Dir: Anthony M Muniz, MD
Class Cap: 25 *Begins:* Mar July Nov
Length: 13 mos *Award:* Cert
Tuition per yr: $1,265 res, $7,121 non-res

Pinellas Tech Educ Ctr - St Petersburg

Medical Assistant Prgm
901 34th St S
St Petersburg, FL 33711
Prgm Dir: Diane M Klieger, RN MBA CMA
Tel: 813 893-2500   *Fax:* 813 893-2776
Med Dir: Edgar Buren, MD
Class Cap: 50   *Begins:* Varies
Length: 12 mos, 18 mos   *Award:* Dipl
Tuition per yr: $675 res, $5,063 non-res
Evening or weekend classes available

David G Erwin Technical Center

Medical Assistant Prgm
2010 E Hillsborough Ave
Tampa, FL 33610-8299
Prgm Dir: Elaine Waldbart, RN
Tel: 813 231-1800   *Fax:* 813 231-1820
Med Dir: Alan Iezzi, MD
Class Cap: 43   *Begins:* Varies
Length: 14 mos   *Award:* Dipl
Tuition per yr: $660 res, $4,884 non-res
Evening or weekend classes available

New England Institute of Tech at Palm Beach

Medical Assistant Prgm
1126 53rd Ct
West Palm Beach, FL 33407
Prgm Dir: Amy Rae, RN BSN
Tel: 561 842-8324   *Fax:* 561 842-9503
Class Cap: 20   *Begins:* Jan Apr Jul Oct
Length: 18 mos   *Award:* AS
Tuition per yr: $4,800 res, $4,800 non-res
Evening or weekend classes available

South College

Medical Assistant Prgm
1760 N Congress Ave
West Palm Beach, FL 33409
Prgm Dir: Carmen Carpenter, RN BSN CMA
Tel: 561 697-9200
Med Dir: Stephen Shavitz, MD
Class Cap: 100   *Begins:* Jan Apr Jun Sep
Length: 18 mos, 24 mos   *Award:* Cert, AS
Tuition per yr: $1,300

Winter Park Adult Vocational Center

Medical Assistant Prgm
901 Webster Ave
Winter Park, FL 32789
Prgm Dir: Barbara Matthews, LPN CMA
Tel: 407 647-6366   *Fax:* 407 647-6366
E-mail: mattheb@ocps.k12.fl.us
Med Dir: Lon Dawson, MD
Class Cap: 100   *Begins:* Monthly
Length: 12 mos   *Award:* Dipl,Cert
Tuition per yr: $725 res, $5,551 non-res

Georgia

Atlanta Area Technical School

Medical Assistant Prgm
1560 Stewart Ave SW
Atlanta, GA 30310
Prgm Dir: Katrina Green
Tel: 404 756-3779   *Fax:* 404 756-0932
Med Dir: Muhammed A Muhammed, MD
Class Cap: 20   *Begins:* Mar Oct
Length: 15 mos   *Award:* Dipl
Tuition per yr: $1,480

Augusta Technical Institute

Medical Assistant Prgm
3116 Deans Bridge Rd
Augusta, GA 30906
Prgm Dir: Lisa Nagle, CMA
Tel: 706 771-4189   *Fax:* 706 771-4181
E-mail: lnagle@augusta.tec.ga.us
Med Dir: Paul Fischer, MD
Class Cap: 50   *Begins:* Sep Mar
Length: 12 mos   *Award:* Dipl
Tuition per yr: $1,096 res, $1,096 non-res
Evening or weekend classes available

Columbus Technical Institute

Medical Assistant Prgm
928 Forty Fifth St
Columbus, GA 31904-6572
Prgm Dir: Edith M Thompson, RN PhD CMA
Tel: 706 649-1499   *Fax:* 706 649-1937
Med Dir: Antonio R Rodriguez, MD
Class Cap: 25   *Begins:* Sep
Length: 12 mos   *Award:* Dipl
Tuition per yr: $1,008
Evening or weekend classes available

Heart of Georgia Technical Institute

Medical Assistant Prgm
560 Pinehill Rd
Dublin, GA 31021
Prgm Dir: Gwendolyn Upshaw, BSN NCMA
Tel: 912 274-7885   *Fax:* 912 275-6642
Med Dir: Monty Shuman, MD
Class Cap: 20   *Begins:* Jan
Length: 12 mos   *Award:* Dipl
Tuition per yr: $1,638

Medix School

Medical Assistant Prgm
2480 Windy Hill Rd
Marietta, GA 30067
Prgm Dir: Vicki Schaller, CMA CPT
Tel: 770 980-0002   *Fax:* 770 980-0811
Med Dir: Gerald D Kumin, MD PC
Class Cap: 550   *Begins:* Monthly
Length: 9 mos   *Award:* Dipl
Tuition per yr: $6,150 res, $6,150 non-res

Savannah Technical Institute

Medical Assistant Prgm
5717 White Bluff Rd
Savannah, GA 31405-5594
Prgm Dir: Marcia P Jones, MEd CMA
Tel: 912 351-4562   *Fax:* 912 352-4362
Med Dir: Ester McAlpine, MD
Class Cap: 20   *Begins:* Oct
Length: 12 mos   *Award:* Dipl
Tuition per yr: $1,104 res, $2,112 non-res
Evening or weekend classes available

South College

Medical Assistant Prgm
709 Mall Blvd
Savannah, GA 31406
Prgm Dir: Cecilia Miller, RN BSN CMA
Tel: 912 651-8100   *Fax:* 912 356-1409
E-mail: southcollege@sava.gulfnet.com
Med Dir: Gustave Kreh, MD
Class Cap: 30   *Begins:* Sep Jan Mar Jun
Length: 12 mos, 24 mos   *Award:* Cert, AS
Tuition per yr: $6,000
Evening or weekend classes available

Swainsboro Technical Institute

Medical Assistant Prgm
346 Kite Rd
Swainsboro, GA 30401
Prgm Dir: Eugenia M Fulcher, RN BSN MEd
Tel: 912 237-6465   *Fax:* 912 237-4043
E-mail: gtulcher@admin1.swainsborn.ti.ga.us
Med Dir: James L Ray, MD
Class Cap: 30   *Begins:* Sep Jan Mar Jul
Length: 12 mos   *Award:* Dipl
Tuition per yr: res, $1,008 non-res
Evening or weekend classes available

Thomas Technical Institute

Medical Assistant Prgm
15689 US Hwy 19 N
Thomasville, GA 31792
Prgm Dir: Glenda Hatcher, BSN RN CMA
Tel: 912 225-4096   *Fax:* 912 225-4330
E-mail: glenda@ttin1.thomas.tec.ga.us
Med Dir: Charles Sanders, MD
Class Cap: 24   *Begins:* Sep
Length: 12 mos   *Award:* Dipl
Tuition per yr: $1,008 res, $2,016 non-res
Evening or weekend classes available

Valdosta Technical Institute

Medical Assistant Prgm
4089 Valtec Rd
PO Box 928
Valdosta, GA 31603-0928
Prgm Dir: Cecelia Bruce, RN
Tel: 912 333-2100   *Fax:* 912 333-2129
Med Dir: James R Wilhoite
Class Cap: 20   *Begins:* Sep Mar
Length: 12 mos   *Award:* Dipl
Tuition per yr: $1,192 res, $2,000 non-res
Evening or weekend classes available

Hawaii

Kapiolani Community College

Medical Assistant Prgm
4303 Diamond Head Rd
Honolulu, HI 96816
Prgm Dir: Joan A Young, BEd RN CMA-AC
Tel: 808 734-9349   *Fax:* 808 734-9126
Med Dir: Franklin Young, MD
Class Cap: 50   *Begins:* Jan Aug
Length: 13 mos, 18 mos   *Award:* Cert, AS
Tuition per yr: $788 res, $5,132 non-res
Evening or weekend classes available

Idaho

College of Southern Idaho

Medical Assistant Prgm
PO Box 1238
Twin Falls, ID 83303-1238
Prgm Dir: Penny Glenn, MEd
Tel: 208 733-9554   *Fax:* 208 736-4743
E-mail: pglenn@aspent.csi.cc.id.us
Med Dir: Kurt Seppi, MD
Class Cap: 12   *Begins:* Aug
Length: 12 mos, 24 mos   *Award:* Cert, AAS
Tuition per yr: $1,100 res, $2,500 non-res
Evening or weekend classes available

Illinois

Belleville Area College

Medical Assistant Prgm
2500 Carlyle Rd
Belleville, IL 62221
Prgm Dir: Rose M Hall, BS RN CMA-AC
Tel: 618 235-2700   *Fax:* 618 235-1578
Med Dir: R Attala, MD
Class Cap: 36   *Begins:* Aug Jan
Length: 12 mos   *Award:* Cert
Tuition per yr: $1,178 res, $2,000 non-res

Northwestern Business College

Medical Assistant Prgm
4829 N Lipps Ave
Chicago, IL 60630
Prgm Dir: Catherine M Gierman, BA/RN CMA
Tel: 312 777-4220
Med Dir: Renee Schickler, MD
Class Cap: 150   *Begins:* Sep Dec Mar Jun
Length: 18 mos   *Award:* AAS
Tuition per yr: $6,670

Robert Morris College

Medical Assistant Prgm
180 N LaSalle St
Chicago, IL 60601
Prgm Dir: Elba Soto, RRA
Tel: 312 836-4888
Med Dir: Elaine Carroll, MD
Class Cap: 500   *Begins:* Sep Feb May
Length: 10 mos, 15 mos   *Award:* Dipl, AAS
Tuition per yr: $9,300

Northwestern Business College

Medical Assistant Prgm
Southwest Campus
8020 W 87th St
Hickory Hills, IL 60457
Prgm Dir: Catherine M Gierman, RN BA CMA
Tel: 312 777-4220   *Fax:* 312 777-2861
Med Dir: Renee Schickler, MD
Class Cap: 48   *Begins:* Sep Dec Mar Jun
Length: 18 mos   *Award:* AAS
Tuition per yr: $6,250 res, $6,250 non-res

Robert Morris College

Medical Assistant Prgm
43 Orland Square
Orland Park, IL 60462
Prgm Dir: Lora Stotler, MPH CMA
Tel: 708 349-5122   *Fax:* 708 349-5119
Med Dir: Elaine Carroll, MD
Class Cap: 40   *Begins:* Feb May Jul Sep Dec
Length: 10 mos, 15 mos   *Award:* Dipl, AAS
Tuition per yr: $9,750 res, $9,750 non-res

William Rainey Harper College

Medical Assistant Prgm
1200 W Algonquin Rd
Palatine, IL 60067
Prgm Dir: Vera Davis, RN CMA
Tel: 847 925-6444   *Fax:* 847 925-6047
Med Dir: Thomas Cronin, MD
Class Cap: 30   *Begins:* Aug Jan Jun
Length: 24 mos, 18 mos   *Award:* Cert, AAS
Tuition per yr: $2,560 res, $12,190 non-res
Evening or weekend classes available

Midstate College

Medical Assistant Prgm
224 SW Jefferson St
Peoria, IL 61602
Prgm Dir: Judith S Bell, BA RT CMA-C
Tel: 309 673-6365   *Fax:* 309 673-5814
Med Dir: M Kim Rodine, MD
Class Cap: 80   *Begins:* Dec Mar June Sep
Length: 18 mos   *Award:* AAS
Tuition per yr: $5,700 res, $5,700 non-res
Evening or weekend classes available

Rockford Business College

Medical Assistant Prgm
730 N Church
Rockford, IL 61103
Prgm Dir: Catherine Rogers, RN BSN MBA CMA
Tel: 815 965-8616   *Fax:* 815 965-0360
Med Dir: Phillip DuPont, MD PC
Class Cap: 62   *Begins:* Jun Sep Nov Mar
Length: 24 mos   *Award:* AAS
Tuition per yr: $4,080 res, $4,080 non-res

Indiana

Ivy Tech State Coll - Columbus

Medical Assistant Prgm
4475 Central Ave
Columbus, IN 47203
Prgm Dir: Marilyn Ryser, RN CMA
Tel: 812 372-9925   *Fax:* 812 372-0311
Med Dir: Robert W Petry, MD
Class Cap: 25   *Begins:* Aug Jan May
Length: 12 mos, 18 mos   *Award:* Cert, AAS
Tuition per yr: $2,713 res, $5,018 non-res

Ivy Tech State Coll SW - Evansville

Medical Assistant Prgm
3501 First Ave
Evansville, IN 47710
Prgm Dir: Patricia A Bailey, RN BS CMA
Tel: 812 429-1381   *Fax:* 812 429-1483
Med Dir: William Blume, MD
Begins: Aug
Length: 16 mos, 21 mos   *Award:* Cert, AAS
Tuition per yr: $3,007 res, $5,477 non-res
Evening or weekend classes available

International Business Coll - Ft Wayne

Medical Assistant Prgm
3811 Old Illinois Rd
Ft Wayne, IN 46804-1298
Prgm Dir: Pamela L Neu, AS CMA
Tel: 219 432-8702   *Fax:* 219 436-1896
Med Dir: Gordon Franke, MD
Class Cap: 40   *Begins:* Jul Mar Sep
Length: 10 mos   *Award:* Dipl
Tuition per yr: $8,790

Ivy Tech State Coll NE - Ft Wayne

Medical Assistant Prgm
3800 N Anthony Blvd
Ft Wayne, IN 46805
Prgm Dir: Margaret Frazier, BS RN CMA
Tel: 219 480-4273   *Fax:* 219 480-4149
Med Dir: Kathryn Einhaus, MD
Begins: Aug Jan May
Length: 24 mos, 18 mos   *Award:* Dipl,Cert, AAS
Tuition per yr: $2,318 res, $4,222 non-res
Evening or weekend classes available

Michiana College

Medical Assistant Prgm
4807 Illinois Rd
Ft Wayne, IN 46804
Prgm Dir: Cheryl Beaman, CMA
Tel: 219 237-0774   *Fax:* 219 237-3585
Med Dir: William Carter, MD
Class Cap: 50   *Begins:* Various
Length: 14 mos   *Award:* AAS
Tuition per yr: $8,784 res, $8,784 non-res

Indiana Business College

Medical Assistant Prgm
5460 Victory Dr/Ste 100
Indianapolis, IN 46203
Prgm Dir: Linda Foster, NSG
Tel: 317 783-5100   *Fax:* 317 783-4898
Med Dir: Kim Hoefgen, NSG
Length: 12 mos, 15 mos   *Award:* Dipl, AS
Tuition per yr: $0 res, $6,200 non-res

International Business Coll - Indianapolis

Medical Assistant Prgm
7205 Shadeland Station
Indianapolis, IN 46256
Prgm Dir: Melissa Stieneker, CMA
Tel: 317 841-6400   *Fax:* 317 841-6419
Med Dir: Edwin Campbell, MD
Class Cap: 30   *Begins:* Sep
Length: 10 mos   *Award:* Dipl
Tuition per yr: $9,375 res, $9,375 non-res

Ivy Tech State Coll - Indianapolis

Medical Assistant Prgm
Central Indiana Region
One W 26th St/PO Box 1763
Indianapolis, IN 46206-1763
Prgm Dir: Linda Reed, MA RN CMA
Tel: 317 921-4450   *Fax:* 317 921-4511
E-mail: lreed@ivy.tec.in.us
Med Dir: Tom Moran, MD
Class Cap: 46   *Begins:* Aug Jan May
Length: 12 mos, 24 mos   *Award:* Dipl,Cert, TC, AAS
Tuition per yr: $2,418 res, $4,901 non-res
Evening or weekend classes available

Professional Careers Institute

Medical Assistant Prgm
2611 Waterfront Pkwy E Dr
Indianapolis, IN 46214
Prgm Dir: Cathy Below, CMA
Tel: 317 299-6001   *Fax:* 317 298-6842
Med Dir: Norman Glanzman, MD
Class Cap: 240   *Begins:* Quarterly
Length: 8 mo , 14 mos   *Award:* Dipl, AAS
Tuition per yr: $5,950 res, $5,950 non-res
Evening or weekend classes available

Ivy Tech State Coll - Kokomo

Medical Assistant Prgm
1815 E Morgan St
Kokomo, IN 46901
Prgm Dir: Connie Morgan, BSN RN CMA
Tel: 317 459-0561   *Fax:* 317 454-5111
Med Dir: Don Wagoner, MD
Begins: Aug
Length: 18 mos, 24 mos   *Award:* Cert, AAS
Tuition per yr: $2,263 res, $6,500 non-res
Evening or weekend classes available

Ivy Tech State Coll - Lafayette
Medical Assistant Prgm
3101 S Creasy Ln
PO Box 6299
Lafayette, IN 47903
Prgm Dir: Cindy Abel, BS CMA
Tel: 317 772-9206 *Fax:* 317 772-9214
Med Dir: Dennis Richmond, MD
Class Cap: 30 *Begins:* Aug Sep
Length: 12 mos, 24 mos *Award:* Cert, AAS
Tuition per yr: $3,007 res, $5,477 non-res

Ivy Tech State Coll SE - Madison
Medical Assistant Prgm
Health & Human Services Div
590 IVY Tech Dr
Madison, IN 47250
Prgm Dir: Annabet Garner, CMA AAS
Tel: 812 265-2580
Med Dir: Thomas Eckert, MD
Begins: Jan May Aug
Length: 12 mos, 18 mos *Award:* Cert, TC
Tuition per yr: $2,820 res, $5,135 non-res

Ivy Tech State Coll EC - Muncie
Medical Assistant Prgm
4301 Cowan Rd
Muncie, IN 47307
Prgm Dir: Jeff Turner, CMA
Tel: 317 289-2291 *Fax:* 317 289-2291
Med Dir: Dr Charles Dinwiddie, MD
Class Cap: 50 *Begins:* Aug Jan
Length: 12 mos, 18 mos *Award:* Cert, AAS
Tuition per yr: $3,007
Evening or weekend classes available

Ivy Tech State Coll - Richmond
Medical Assistant Prgm
2325 Chester Blvd
Richmond, IN 47374
Prgm Dir: Idris Bond, BSN CMA
Tel: 317 966-2656, Ext 372 *Fax:* 317 962-8741
E-mail: ibond@ivytech.in.us
Med Dir: David DeSantis, MD
Class Cap: 50 *Begins:* Jan May Aug
Length: 24 mos *Award:* AAS
Tuition per yr: $3,946 res, $7,188 non-res
Evening or weekend classes available

Ivy Tech State Coll SC - Sellersburg
Medical Assistant Prgm
8204 Hwy 311
Sellersburg, IN 47172
Prgm Dir: Deborah D Rawles, PA
Tel: 812 246-3301 *Fax:* 812 246-9905
Med Dir: Richard E Riehl, MD
Begins: Aug Jan May
Length: 12 mos, 18 mos *Award:* Cert, AAS
Tuition per yr: $2,418 res, $4,401 non-res
Evening or weekend classes available

Ivy Tech State Coll NC - South Bend
Medical Assistant Prgm
1534 W Sample St
South Bend, IN 46619
Prgm Dir: Martha C Garrels, BS CMA MT(ASCP)
Tel: 219 289-7001 *Fax:* 219 236-7172
E-mail: mgarrels@ivy.tec.in.us
Med Dir: Lynn D Day, MD FAAFP
Class Cap: 44 *Begins:* Aug Jan May
Length: 12 mos, 20 mos *Award:* Cert, AAS
Tuition per yr: $2,900 res, $4,300 non-res

Michiana College
Medical Assistant Prgm
1030 E Jefferson Blvd
South Bend, IN 46617
Prgm Dir: Karen Stewart, CMA
Tel: 219 436-2738 *Fax:* 219 436-2958
Med Dir: William Carter, MD
Class Cap: 50 *Begins:* Varies
Length: 14 mos *Award:* AAS
Tuition per yr: $8,784 res, $8,784 non-res

Ivy Tech State Coll - Terre Haute
Medical Assistant Prgm
7999 US Hwy 41
Terre Haute, IN 47802-4898
Prgm Dir: Joretta J Roloff, RN CMA
Tel: 812 299-1121 *Fax:* 812 299-5723
Med Dir: Harold Loveall, MD
Class Cap: 30 *Begins:* Sep
Length: 12 mos, 18 mos *Award:* Cert, AAS
Tuition per yr: $3,947 res, $7,188 non-res

Ivy Tech State Coll - Valparaiso
Medical Assistant Prgm
2401 Valley Dr
Valparaiso, IN 46383
Prgm Dir: Ethel Morikis, BSN RNC
Tel: 219 464-8514 *Fax:* 219 464-9751
Med Dir: J Timothy Ames, MD
Begins: Aug
Length: 10 mos *Award:* Cert
Tuition per yr: $4,200 res, $6,300 non-res
Evening or weekend classes available

Iowa

Des Moines Area Community College
Medical Assistant Prgm
2006 Ankeny Blvd
Ankeny, IA 50021
Prgm Dir: Diane M VanderPloeg, MS CMA
Tel: 515 964-6457 *Fax:* 515 964-6440
Med Dir: Joellen Heims, MD
Class Cap: 36 *Begins:* Aug
Length: 11 mos *Award:* Dipl
Tuition per yr: $2,666 res, $4,908 non-res
Evening or weekend classes available

Kirkwood Community College
Medical Assistant Prgm
6301 Kirkwood Blvd SW
PO Box 2068
Cedar Rapids, IA 52406-9973
Prgm Dir: Judith A Cowan, BS RN CMA
Tel: 319 398-5564 *Fax:* 319 398-1293
Med Dir: Donald A F Nelson, MD
Class Cap: 39 *Begins:* Jan Sep
Length: 12 mos *Award:* Dipl
Tuition per yr: $2,420 res, $4,840 non-res
Evening or weekend classes available

Iowa Western Community College
Medical Assistant Prgm
2700 College Rd
PO Box 4-C
Council Bluffs, IA 51502-3004
Prgm Dir: Colleen Getsfred, CMA
Tel: 712 325-3348 *Fax:* 712 325-3717
Med Dir: Gary Leitch, MD
Class Cap: 20 *Begins:* Aug
Length: 10 mos *Award:* Dipl
Tuition per yr: $2,680 res, $4,020 non-res

American Institute of Commerce
Medical Assistant Prgm
1801 E Kimberly Rd
Davenport, IA 52807
Prgm Dir: Grace Keys, BSN CMA
Tel: 319 355-3500
Med Dir: C L Peterson, MD
Begins: Quarterly
Length: 15 mos, 18 mos *Award:* Dipl, AAS
Tuition per yr: $8,250 res, $8,250 non-res

Hamilton College
Medical Assistant Prgm
2300 Euclid Ave
Des Moines, IA 50310
Prgm Dir: Theodore Along
Tel: 515 279-0253 *Fax:* 515 279-2054
Med Dir: Bernard Munro, MD
Class Cap: 12 *Begins:* Quarterly
Length: 15 mos, 18 mos *Award:* Dipl, AAS
Tuition per yr: $9,410
Evening or weekend classes available

Iowa Central Community College
Medical Assistant Prgm
330 Ave M
Ft Dodge, IA 50501
Prgm Dir: Barbara Kolesar, RN CMA
Tel: 515 576-7201 *Fax:* 515 576-7206
Med Dir: Mark Marner, MD
Class Cap: 28 *Begins:* Sep
Length: 11 mos *Award:* Cert
Tuition per yr: $2,530 res, $3,333 non-res

Iowa Lakes Community College
Medical Assistant Prgm
217 W Fifth St
Spencer, IA 51301
Prgm Dir: Carol Hartig, RN
Tel: 712 262-8428
Med Dir: David Robinson, DO
Class Cap: 25 *Begins:* Sep
Length: 15 mos *Award:* Dipl
Tuition per yr: $8,875

Southeastern Community College
Medical Assistant Prgm
1015 S Gear Ave
Drawer F
West Burlington, IA 52655
Prgm Dir: Anita M Stineman, MSN
Tel: 319 752-2731 *Fax:* 319 752-4957
Med Dir: Carl Hays, MD
Class Cap: 30 *Begins:* Aug
Length: 11 mos *Award:* Dipl
Tuition per yr: $1,721 res, $2,581 non-res

Kansas

Wichita Area Technical College
Medical Assistant Prgm
324 N Emporia
Wichita, KS 67202
Prgm Dir: Beth Buchholz, CMA
Tel: 316 833-4370
Med Dir: Paul Davis, MD
Class Cap: 20 *Begins:* Aug
Length: 9 mos, 24 mos *Award:* Dipl, AAS
Tuition per yr: $976 res, $6,480 non-res

Programs

Kentucky

Fugazzi College

Medical Assistant Prgm
406 Lafayette Ave
Lexington, KY 40502
Prgm Dir: Earlane Cox, MA
Tel: 606 266-0401 *Fax:* 606 268-2118
Med Dir: J W Hammons, MD
Class Cap: 3540 *Begins:* Jan Apr Jul Sep
Length: 18 mos, 24 mos *Award:* AA
Tuition per yr: $4,700 res, $4,700 non-res
Evening or weekend classes available

Kentucky Tech Central Campus

Medical Assistant Prgm
104 Vo-Tech Rd
Lexington, KY 40510-1020
Prgm Dir: Joyce Combs, AAS CMA
Tel: 606 246-2400, Ext 254 *Fax:* 606 246-2417
Med Dir: Michael Carr, MD
Class Cap: 15 *Begins:* April
Length: 12 mos *Award:* Dipl
Tuition per yr: $750 res, $1,500 non-res
Evening or weekend classes available

Kentucky College of Business

Medical Assistant Prgm
3950 Dixie Hwy
Louisville, KY 40216-4147
Prgm Dir: Barbara Bishop, CMA
Tel: 502 447-7634 Fax: 502 447-7665
Med Dir: Melissa Bushnell, EMT MLT AMT
Class Cap: 70 *Begins:* Monthly
Length: 24 mos *Award:* AS
Tuition per yr: $5,232

Kentucky Tech/Jefferson State Campus

Medical Assistant Prgm
800 W Chestnut St
Louisville, KY 40203
Prgm Dir: Jannie Washington, BS CMA-C
Tel: 502 595-4275 *Fax:* 502 595-2387
Med Dir: Robert Hammer
Class Cap: 1 *Begins:* Oct Apr
Length: 12 mos, 15 mos *Award:* Dipl
Tuition per yr: $750 res, $1,500 non-res
Evening or weekend classes available

Spencerian College

Medical Assistant Prgm
4627 Dixie Hwy
Louisville, KY 40216
Prgm Dir: Kim Wilson, MT(AMT)
Tel: 502 447-1000 *Fax:* 502 447-4574
Med Dir: Kathy Nieder, MD
Class Cap: 40 *Begins:* Jan Mar Jun Sep
Length: 12 mos *Award:* Dipl
Tuition per yr: $9,840
Evening or weekend classes available

West Kentucky Tech

Medical Assistant Prgm
Blandville Rd
PO Box 7408
Paducah, KY 42002-7408
Prgm Dir: Vicki Barclay, MS CMA
Tel: 502 554-4991 *Fax:* 502 554-2695
Med Dir: Ronald Wilson, MD
Class Cap: 12 *Begins:* Aug
Length: 11 mos *Award:* Dipl
Tuition per yr: $600 res, $1,200 non-res
Evening or weekend classes available

Eastern Kentucky University

Medical Assistant Prgm
Dizney 225
Richmond, KY 40475-3135
Prgm Dir: Joy Renfro, MA RRA CMA
Tel: 606 622-1028 *Fax:* 606 622-1140
E-mail: mas renfr@asc.eku.edu
Med Dir: Joseph Bark, MD
Class Cap: 60 *Begins:* Aug Jan
Length: 22 mos *Award:* AS
Tuition per yr: $1,970 res, $5,450 non-res
Evening or weekend classes available

Kentucky College of Business

Medical Assistant Prgm
139 Killarney Ln
Richmond, KY 40475
Prgm Dir: Penny VanDierendonck, AS CMA
Tel: 606 623-8956 *Fax:* 606 624-5544
Class Cap: 43 *Begins:* Jan Apr Jun Sep
Length: 24 mos *Award:* AS
Tuition per yr: $5,496 res, $5,496 non-res

Maine

Beal College

Medical Assistant Prgm
629 Main St
Bangor, ME 04401
Prgm Dir: Theresa C Morrow, MT(ASCP)CMA
Tel: 207 947-4591 *Fax:* 207 947-0208
Med Dir: Kenneth Simone, DO
Class Cap: 20 *Begins:* Bimonthly
Length: 24 mos *Award:* AS
Tuition per yr: $3,840 res, $3,840 non-res
Evening or weekend classes available

Husson College

Medical Assistant Prgm
One College Circle
Bangor, ME 04401
Prgm Dir: Theresa F Perry, MS
Tel: 207 941-7169 *Fax:* 207 941-7988
E-mail: perry@husson.husson.edu
Med Dir: James A Raczek, MD
Class Cap: 0 *Begins:* Sep Jan
Length: 18 mos *Award:* AS
Tuition per yr: $8,960
Evening or weekend classes available

Maryland

Medix School

Medical Assistant Prgm
1017 York Rd
Towson, MD 21204
Prgm Dir: Rona E Goldman, CCVT CMA-AC
Tel: 410 337-5155 *Fax:* 410 337-5104
Med Dir: John D Griswold, MD
Class Cap: 0 *Begins:* Monthly
Length: 9 mos *Award:* Cert
Tuition per yr: $6,150

Massachusetts

Porter and Chester Institute - Chicopee

Medical Assistant Prgm
134 Dulong Circle
Chicopee, MA 01022
Prgm Dir: Dale Miller, RN
Tel: 413 593-3339 *Fax:* 413 593-6439
Med Dir: Paul D Nitti, MD
Class Cap: 30 *Begins:* Oct Jan Apr Jul
Length: 1 mos *Award:* Dipl
Tuition per yr: $9,400 res, $9,400 non-res

Northern Essex Community College

Medical Assistant Prgm
100 Elliott Way
Haverhill, MA 01830
Prgm Dir: Joan Hagopian, MEd CMA
Tel: 508 374-3884
Med Dir: James Brackbill, MD
Class Cap: 20 *Begins:* Sep
Length: 9 mos *Award:* Cert
Tuition per yr: $2,001 res, $6,612 non-res

Aquinas College at Milton

Medical Assistant Prgm
303 Adams St
Milton, MA 02186
Prgm Dir: Marie F Newman, MEd
Tel: 617 696-3100 *Fax:* 617 696-8706
Med Dir: Barbara Ann Payne, MD
Begins: Sep
Length: 18 mos *Award:* AS
Tuition per yr: $8,150

Southeastern Technical Institute

Medical Assistant Prgm
250 Foundry St
S Easton, MA 02375
Prgm Dir: Faith A Ward, BS CMA
Tel: 508 238-1860 *Fax:* 508 278-7266
Med Dir: William Lawrence, MD
Class Cap: 24 *Begins:* Sep
Length: 10 mos *Award:* Dipl
Tuition per yr: $1,000 res, $2,300 non-res

Springfield Technical Community College

Medical Assistant Prgm
One Amory Square
Springfield, MA 01105
Prgm Dir: Noreen Sullivan, RN MEd
Tel: 413 781-7822 *Fax:* 413 781-5805
Med Dir: Paul Farkas, MD
Class Cap: 50 *Begins:* Sep
Length: 18 mos *Award:* AS
Tuition per yr: $1,296 res, $4,680 non-res
Evening or weekend classes available

Worcester Technical Institute

Medical Assistant Prgm
251 Belmont St
Worcester, MA 01605
Prgm Dir: Jacqueline J Walsh, MED BA LPN CMA
Tel: 508 799-1945 *Fax:* 508 799-1932
Med Dir: Dean Morrell, MD
Class Cap: 24 *Begins:* Aug
Length: 9 mos *Award:* Cert
Tuition per yr: $1,600 res, $3,000 non-res

Michigan

Great Lakes Junior College - Bay City
Medical Assistant Prgm
3930 Traxler Court
Bay City, MI 48706
Prgm Dir: Meredith Livingston, LPN CMA
Tel: 517 673-5857 *Fax:* 517 673-7543
Med Dir: Larry L Carr, DO
Begins: Sep
Length: 36 mos *Award:* AS
Tuition per yr: $2,148

Great Lakes Junior College - Caro
Medical Assistant Prgm
1231 Cleaver Rd
Caro, MI 48723
Prgm Dir: Meredith Livingston, LPN CMA
Tel: 517 673-5857 *Fax:* 517 673-7543
Med Dir: Larry L Carr, DO
Begins: Sep
Length: 36 mos *Award:* AS
Tuition per yr: $2,148

Macomb Community College
Medical Assistant Prgm
Business Health & Human Serv
44575 Garfield Rd
Clinton Township, MI 48038-1139
Prgm Dir: M Janisse, RN BS
Tel: 810 286-2097 *Fax:* 810 286-2098
Med Dir: Albert Przyblski, DO
Class Cap: 64 *Begins:* Aug
Length: 9 mo , 18 mos *Award:* Cert, AAS
Tuition per yr : $1,746 res, $2,646 non-res

Henry Ford Community College
Medical Assistant Prgm
22586 Ann Arbor Trail
Dearborn Heights, MI 48127
Prgm Dir: Catherine McCartney, MA RN CMA
Tel: 313 730-5974 *Fax:* 313 730-5965
Med Dir: John M Battle, MD
Class Cap: 30 *Begins:* Aug Jan
Length: 10 mos *Award:* Cert
Tuition per yr: $1,827 res, $2,685 non-res
Evening or weekend classes available

Baker College
Medical Assistant Prgm
G 1050 W Bristol Rd
Flint, MI 48507
Prgm Dir: Marsh A L Beneduct, MSA CMA A
Tel: 810 766-4133 *Fax:* 810 766-4049
E-mail: Benedi_m@acaofl.baker.edu
Med Dir: Richard Antell, MD
Class Cap: 34 *Begins:* Jan Mar Jun Sep
Length: 24 mos *Award:* AAS
Tuition per yr: $6,500 res, $6,500 non-res
Evening or weekend classes available

Davenport College
Medical Assistant Prgm
415 E Fulton St
Grand Rapids, MI 49503
Prgm Dir: Patricia Allen, CMA
Tel: 616 451-3511 *Fax:* 616 732-1142
Med Dir: Timothy Tobolic, MD
Class Cap: 90 *Begins:* Sep Jan Mar
Length: 18 mos *Award:* AAS
Tuition per yr: $8,010
Evening or weekend classes available

Jackson Community College
Medical Assistant Prgm
2111 Emmons Rd
Jackson, MI 49201
Prgm Dir: Jean Tannis Dennerll, BS CMA
Tel: 517 787-0800
Med Dir: Brian Adamczyk, MD
Class Cap: 40 *Begins:* qtrly
Length: 20 mos, 16 mos *Award:* Cert, AS
Tuition per yr: res, $2,901 non-res
Evening or weekend classes available

Kalamazoo Valley Community College
Medical Assistant Prgm
Kalamazoo Valley Com College TX Township
PO Box 4070 6767 West O Ave.
Kalamazoo, MI 49003
Prgm Dir: Carol K Merrill
Tel: 616 372-5324 *Fax:* 616 372-5458
Med Dir: Kim J. Gloystein, MD
Class Cap: 48 *Begins:* Aug Jan
Length: 10 mos, 24 mos *Award:* AAS
Tuition per yr: $1,440 res, $2,680 non-res
Evening or weekend classes available

Great Lakes Junior College - Midland
Medical Assistant Prgm
3555 E Patrick Rd
Midland, MI 48642
Prgm Dir: Meredith Livingston, LPN CMA
Tel: 517 673-5857 *Fax:* 517 673-7543
Med Dir: Larry L Carr, DO
Begins: Sep
Length: 36 mos *Award:* AS
Tuition per yr: $2,148

Baker College of Muskegon
Medical Assistant Prgm
123 Apple Ave
Muskegon, MI 49442
Prgm Dir: Gertrude A Kenny, BSN RN CMA
Tel: 616 726-4904 *Fax:* 616 728-1417
E-mail: kenny_t@moskegon.baker.edu
Med Dir: J Max Busard, MD
Class Cap: 36 *Begins:* Sep Jan Mar
Length: 18 mos *Award:* AAS
Tuition per yr: $6,240
Evening or weekend classes available

Baker College of Owosso
Medical Assistant Prgm
1020 S Washington St
Owosso, MI 48867
Prgm Dir: Kimberly S Poag, CMA
Tel: 517 723-5251 *Fax:* 517 723-3355
Med Dir: Harry Atoynatan, MD
Class Cap: 32 *Begins:* Sep Jan Apr
Length: 24 mos *Award:* AAS
Tuition per yr: $6,500 res, $6,500 non-res
Evening or weekend classes available

Great Lakes Junior College - Saginaw
Medical Assistant Prgm
310 S Washington Ave
Saginaw, MI 48607
Prgm Dir: Meredith Livingston, LPN CMA
Tel: 517 673-5857 *Fax:* 517 673-7543
Med Dir: Larry L Carr, DO
Begins: Sep
Length: 36 mos *Award:* AS
Tuition per yr: $2,148

Carnegie Institute
Medical Assistant Prgm
550 Stephenson Hwy/Ste 100
Troy, MI 48083
Prgm Dir: Bonnie Normile, RN CMA CCVT
Tel: 313 589-1078 *Fax:* 810 589-1631
E-mail: carnegie47@aol.com
Med Dir: William E Rizzo, MD
Class Cap: 225 *Begins:* Jan Mar Jun Sep
Length: 12 mos, 24 mos *Award:* Dipl
Tuition per yr: $6,450

Oakland Community College - Waterford
Medical Assistant Prgm
7350 Cooley Lake Rd
Waterford, MI 48327
Prgm Dir: Karen A Kittle, CMA CPT
Tel: 810 360-3094 *Fax:* 810 360-3203
Med Dir: C Kohler Champion, MD
Begins: Sep Jan May
Length: 10 mos, 20 mos *Award:* Cert, AAS
Tuition per yr: $1,932 res, $3,276 non-res
Evening or weekend classes available

Minnesota

Anoka-Hennepin Technical College
Medical Assistant Prgm
1355 W Hwy 10
Anoka, MN 55303
Prgm Dir: Anita Johnson, RN
Tel: 612 427-1880 *Fax:* 612 576-4715
Med Dir: Mark Brakke, MD
Class Cap: 35 *Begins:* Sep
Length: 12 mos *Award:* Dipl
Tuition per yr: $3,334 res, $6,667 non-res

Medical Institute of Minnesota
Medical Assistant Prgm
5503 Green Valley Dr
Bloomington, MN 55437
Prgm Dir: Vicki Scott, BA CMA
Tel: 612 844-0064 *Fax:* 612 844-0671
Med Dir: George Cembrowski, MD
Class Cap: 20 *Begins:* Oct Jan Apr Jul
Length: 17 mos *Award:* AAS
Tuition per yr: $7,275
Evening or weekend classes available

Duluth Business Univ/MN Sch of Business
Medical Assistant Prgm
412 W Superior St
Duluth, MN 55802
Prgm Dir: Dee Leskey, CMA
Tel: 218 722-3361 *Fax:* 218 722-8376
Med Dir: John J Vukelich, MD
Begins: Jan Apr Jul Oct
Length: 14 mos *Award:* Dipl
Tuition per yr: $8,200
Evening or weekend classes available

Northwest Technical Coll - E Grand Forks
Medical Assistant Prgm
Hwy 220 N
East Grand Forks, MN 56721
Prgm Dir: Elizabeth McMahon, BSN RN CMA
Tel: 218 773-3441
Med Dir: Keith W Millette, MD
Class Cap: 28 *Begins:* Sep Dec Mar
Length: 12 mos *Award:* Dipl
Tuition per yr: $2,689 res, $3,359 non-res

Lakeland Medical Dental Academy

Medical Assistant Prgm
1402 W Lake St
Minneapolis, MN 55408
Prgm Dir: Virginia Johnson
Tel: 612 827-5656
Class Cap: 220   *Begins:* Jan Mar Jun Sep
Length: 11 mos, 20 mos   *Award:* Dipl, AAS
Tuition per yr: $5,850
Evening or weekend classes available

Minnesota School of Business - Richfield

Medical Assistant Prgm
1401 W 76t St/Ste 500
Richfield, MN 55423
Prgm Dir: John P Cody, BS MBA CMA
Tel: 612 798-3726   *Fax:* 612 861-5548
Med Dir: John Vukelich, MD
Begins: Jan Apr Jul Oct
Length: 14 mos, 20 mos   *Award:* Dipl, AAS
Tuition per yr: $11,055 res, $11,055 non-res
Evening or weekend classes available

Rochester Community and Technical College

Medical Assistant Prgm
851 30th Ave SE
Rochester, MN 55904-4999
Prgm Dir: Marjorie R Reif, PA-C CMA
Tel: 507 285-7117   *Fax:* 507 285-7496
E-mail: marj.reif@roch.edu
Med Dir: Thomas W Miller, MD
Class Cap: 20   *Begins:* Sep
Length: 11 mos, 24 mos   *Award:* Cert, AA
Tuition per yr: $2,911 res, $5,490 non-res

Dakota County Technical College

Medical Assistant Prgm
1300 E 145th St
Rosemount, MN 55068-2999
Prgm Dir: Dianne Tempel, RN CMA BSc
Tel: 612 423-8375   *Fax:* 612 423-7028
Med Dir: Leslie Atwood, MD
Class Cap: 30   *Begins:* Sep
Length: 12 mos   *Award:* Dipl
Tuition per yr: $2,551 res, $5,053 non-res
Evening or weekend classes available

Minneapolis Business College

Medical Assistant Prgm
1711 W County Rd B
Roseville, MN 55113
Prgm Dir: Susan Ende, CMA
Tel: 612 636-7406
Med Dir: Paul L Olson, MD
Class Cap: 56   *Begins:* Sep
Length: 10 mos   *Award:* Dipl
Tuition per yr: $8,930

Globe College of Business

Medical Assistant Prgm
175 Fifth St E Ste 201
Galtier Plaza Box 60
St Paul, MN 55101-2901
Prgm Dir: John P Cody, MBA CMA
Tel: 612 798-3726   *Fax:* 612 861-5548
Med Dir: John J Vukelich, BA MD
Class Cap: 125   *Begins:* Jan Apr Jul Oct
Length: 14 mos, 20 mos   *Award:* Dipl, AAS
Tuition per yr: $11,055 res, $11,055 non-res
Evening or weekend classes available

Century College

Medical Assistant Prgm
3300 Century Ave N
White Bear Lake, MN 55110
Prgm Dir: Mary Braun
Tel: 612 773-1731
Med Dir: Mary Ann Leukuma, MD
Class Cap: 5060   *Begins:* Quarterly
Length: 15 mos   *Award:* Dipl
Tuition per yr: $3,604 res, $6,555 non-res

Ridgewater College - Willmar Campus

Medical Assistant Prgm
2101 15th Ave VW
PO Box 1097
Willmar, MN 56201
Prgm Dir: Julene Bredeson, RN BSN CMA
Tel: 320 231-2947   *Fax:* 320 231-7677
Med Dir: Mary Bretzman, MD
Class Cap: 30   *Begins:* Sep
Length: 14 mos   *Award:* Dipl
Tuition per yr: $3,380 res, $5,994 non-res

Mississippi

Northeast Mississippi Community College

Medical Assistant Prgm
Cunningham Blvd
Booneville, MS 38829
Prgm Dir: Kaye Roberson, BA CMA
Tel: 601 720-7393   *Fax:* 601 728-1165
Med Dir: Horton G Taylor, MD
Class Cap: 15   *Begins:* Aug
Length: 18 mos   *Award:* AAS
Tuition per yr: $950 res, $2,050 non-res
Evening or weekend classes available

Hinds Community College District

Medical Assistant Prgm
3805 Hwy 80 E
Pearl, MS 39208
Prgm Dir: Christine M King, CMA
Tel: 601 932-5582   *Fax:* 601 936-5569
Med Dir: Donald C Faucett, MD
Class Cap: 16   *Begins:* Aug
Length: 18 mos   *Award:* AAS
Tuition per yr: $1,070 res, $3,276 non-res
Evening or weekend classes available

Missouri

Springfield College

Medical Assistant Prgm
1010 W Sunshine St
Springfield, MO 65807-2446
Prgm Dir: Steve Marshall
Tel: 417 864-7220   *Fax:* 417 864-5697
Med Dir: Kit Murphy
Class Cap: 75   *Begins:* Jan Apr July Oct
Length: 24 mos   *Award:* AAS
Tuition per yr: $5,198

Nebraska

Spencer School of Business

Medical Assistant Prgm
410 W Second St
Grand Island, NE 68801
Prgm Dir: Diane Samuelson
Tel: 308 382-8044   *Fax:* 308 382-5072
Med Dir: Richard E Goble, MD
Begins: Jan Apr Jul Sep
Length: 12 mos, 15 mos   *Award:* Dipl, AS
Tuition per yr: $4,937 res, $4,687 non-res

Central Community College

Medical Assistant Prgm
Hastings Campus
PO Box 1024
Hastings, NE 68902-1024
Prgm Dir: Joann Wieland, MS MEd RN
Tel: 402 461-2473   *Fax:* 402 461-2473
E-mail: wiehmea@ccadm.gi.cccneb.edu
Med Dir: Fred Catlett, DDS
Begins: Varies
Length: 18 mos   *Award:* AAS
Tuition per yr: $1,295 res, $1,903 non-res
Evening or weekend classes available

Southeast Community College

Medical Assistant Prgm
8800 O St
Lincoln, NE 68520
Prgm Dir: Jeanette Goodwin, BS BSN RN
Tel: 402 437-2756
Med Dir: Patrick Bertoline, MD
Class Cap: 50   *Begins:* Mar Sep
Length: 12 mos   *Award:* Dipl
Tuition per yr: $1,871 res, $2,228 non-res

Gateway Electronics Institute

Medical Assistant Prgm
808 S 74th Plaza/Ste 100
Omaha, NE 68114
Prgm Dir: Julie Johnette, RN CMA
Tel: 402 398-0900
Med Dir: Jay Matzke, MD
Class Cap: 24   *Begins:* Every 8 wks
Length: 12 mos   *Award:* Cert
Tuition per yr: $7,320

Omaha College of Health Careers

Medical Assistant Prgm
10845 Harney St
Omaha, NE 68154-2655
Prgm Dir: Deborah K Romaire, RN CMA
Tel: 402 333-1400   *Fax:* 402 333-4598
Med Dir: Stephen H Williams, MD
Class Cap: 15   *Begins:* Monthly
Length: 9 mo , 16 mos   *Award:* Dipl
Tuition per yr: $6,772
Evening or weekend classes available

New Hampshire

New Hampshire Community Technical College

Medical Assistant Prgm
One College Dr
Claremont, NH 03743
Prgm Dir: Arlene C Hadsted
Tel: 603 542-7744 *Fax:* 603 543-1844
E-mail: a_halste@tec.nh.us
Class Cap: 24 *Begins:* Aug
Length: 11 mos *Award:* Dipl
Tuition per yr: $3,286 res, $7,564 non-res

Northeast Career Schools

Medical Assistant Prgm
749 E Industrial Park Dr
Manchester, NH 03109
Prgm Dir: Joanna Bligh, RT MEd
Tel: 603 669-1151, Ext 533 *Fax:* 603 622-2866
Med Dir: Bill Windler, MD
Class Cap: 216 *Begins:* Varies
Length: 9 mos *Award:* Cert
Evening or weekend classes available

New Jersey

Hudson County Community College

Medical Assistant Prgm
2039 Kennedy Blvd
Science 330
Jersey City, NJ 07305
Prgm Dir: Judith Bender, MA CMA
Tel: 201 200-3320 *Fax:* 201 332-5546
Med Dir: Edgar Braunstein, MD
Class Cap: 200 *Begins:* Sep Jan
Length: 12 mos, 24 mos *Award:* Cert, AAS
Tuition per yr: $2,250 res, $4,500 non-res
Evening or weekend classes available

Bergen Community College

Medical Assistant Prgm
400 Paramus Rd
Paramus, NJ 07652
Prgm Dir: John E Clement, CMA-AC
Tel: 201 447-7178 *Fax:* 201 612-8225
Med Dir: Hugh McGee, Jr, MD
Begins: Sep
Length: 18 mos *Award:* Dipl, AAS
Tuition per yr: $2,828 res, $5,294 non-res

Technical Institute of Camden County

Medical Assistant Prgm
Cross Keys Rd
PO Box 566
Sicklerville, NJ 08081
Prgm Dir: Eldora Wright, CMA
Tel: 609 767-7000 *Fax:* 609 767-6625
Med Dir: Sloon A Robinson, MD
Class Cap: 24 *Begins:* Sep
Length: 10 mos *Award:* Cert
Tuition per yr: $700

Berdan Institute

Medical Assistant Prgm
265 Rt 46 W
Totowa, NJ 07512
Prgm Dir: Irene Figliolina, CMA
Tel: 201 256-3444 *Fax:* 201 256-0816
Med Dir: Giovanni Lima, MD
Begins: Varies
Length: 9 mo , 12 mos *Award:* Dipl
Tuition per yr: $7,100
Evening or weekend classes available

New York

Broome Community College

Medical Assistant Prgm
Business Bldg
PO Box 1017
Binghamton, NY 13902
Prgm Dir: Bonnie Lou Deister, BSN RN CMA-C
Tel: 607 778-5088 *Fax:* 607 778-5345
Med Dir: Bruce T Bowling, MD
Class Cap: 35 *Begins:* Aug
Length: 18 mos *Award:* AAS
Tuition per yr: $2,168 res, $4,336 non-res
Evening or weekend classes available

Ridley-Lowell Business & Technical Institute

Medical Assistant Prgm
116 Front St
Binghamton, NY 13905
Prgm Dir: Lynn Augenstern, CMA MS
Tel: 607 724-2941 *Fax:* 607 724-0799
Med Dir: Louis P Mateya Jr, MD
Class Cap: 10 *Begins:* Jan Apr Sep
Length: 12 mos *Award:* Dipl
Tuition per yr: $6,000 res, $6,000 non-res

Suffolk Community College

Medical Assistant Prgm
Crooked Hill Rd
Brentwood, NY 11717
Prgm Dir: Jean Riddell, MA CMA
Tel: 516 851-6739 *Fax:* 516 851-6532
Med Dir: Clive D Caplan, MD
Class Cap: 36 *Begins:* Sep
Length: 24 mos *Award:* AAS
Tuition per yr: $2,100 res, $4,200 non-res

Byrant & Stratton Business Institute

Medical Assistant Prgm
1028 Main St
Buffalo, NY 14202
Prgm Dir: Carolyn M Merlino, BSN CMA
Tel: 716 884-9120
Med Dir: Gambino Baloy, MD PC
Class Cap: 80 *Begins:* Jan Apr Jul Oct
Length: 18 mos *Award:* AOS
Tuition per yr: $4,480

Wood-Tobe Coburn School

Medical Assistant Prgm
8 E 40th St
New York, NY 10016
Prgm Dir: Lynn Mc Manus, LPN
Tel: 212 686-9040 *Fax:* 212 686-9171
Med Dir: Richard Belli, DPM
Class Cap: 30 *Begins:* Sep
Length: 10 mos *Award:* Dipl
Tuition per yr: $10,800 res, $10,800 non-res

Bryant & Stratton Business Institute

Medical Assistant Prgm
82 St Paul St
Rochester, NY 14604
Prgm Dir: Anne Marie Kuder, RN BS
Tel: 716 325-6010 *Fax:* 716 325-6805
Med Dir: Carol J Peterson, MD
Begins: Jan Apr Jul Sep
Length: 18 mos *Award:* AOS
Tuition per yr: $6,192
Evening or weekend classes available

Bryant & Stratton Business Institute

Medical Assistant Prgm
Henrietta Campus
1225 Jefferson Rd
Rochester, NY 14623-3136
Prgm Dir: Barbara L Stein, MS MT(ASCP) SH
CMA
Tel: 716 292-5627 *Fax:* 716 292-6015
Med Dir: Carole Peterson, MD
Class Cap: 200 *Begins:* Jan Apr Jul Oct
Length: 18 mos *Award:* AOS
Tuition per yr: $6,720
Evening or weekend classes available

Bryant & Stratton Business Institute

Medical Assistant Prgm
953 James St
Syracuse, NY 13202
Prgm Dir: Susan Schilling, BS CMA
Tel: 315 472-6603 *Fax:* 315 474-4383
Med Dir: Leonard Levy, MD
Class Cap: 150 *Begins:* Jan Apr Jul Sep
Length: 18 mos *Award:* AOS
Tuition per yr: $8,965
Evening or weekend classes available

Erie Community College - City Campus

Medical Assistant Prgm
North Campus
6205 Main St
Williamsville, NY 14221-7095
Prgm Dir: Myrtle M Green, MT(ASCP)MSCMA
Tel: 716 851-1553 *Fax:* 716 851-1429
Med Dir: William Scheuler, MD
Class Cap: 60 *Begins:* Sep
Length: 18 mos *Award:* AAS
Tuition per yr: $2,500 res, $5,000 non-res
Evening or weekend classes available

North Carolina

Central Piedmont Community College

Medical Assistant Prgm
PO Box 35009
Charlotte, NC 28235
Prgm Dir: Janice F Mayhew, BS RN CMA
Tel: 704 330-6965 *Fax:* 704 330-5930
E-mail: http://www.cpcc.cc.nc.us
Class Cap: 120 *Begins:* Sep Nov Mar Jun
Length: 12 mos *Award:* Dipl
Tuition per yr: $762 res, $6,040 non-res
Evening or weekend classes available

Programs

King's College

Medical Assistant Prgm
322 Lamar Ave
Charlotte, NC 28204
Prgm Dir: Linda Ramge, MT CMA
Tel: 704 372-0266 *Fax:* 704 348-2029
Med Dir: Maureen L Beurskens, MD
Class Cap: 130 *Begins:* Mar Sep
Length: 10 mos *Award:* Dipl
Tuition per yr: $9,225 res, $9,225 non-res

Haywood Community College

Medical Assistant Prgm
Freelander Dr
Clyde, NC 28721-9454
Prgm Dir: Barbara Ensley, RN CMA-C
Tel: 704 627-4533 *Fax:* 704 627-4525
Med Dir: George Brown, MD
Class Cap: 35 *Begins:* Sep
Length: 21 mos *Award:* AAS
Tuition per yr: $742 res, $6,020 non-res

Gaston College

Medical Assistant Prgm
201 Hwy 321 S
Dallas, NC 28034-1499
Prgm Dir: Betty Jones, MA RN CMA
Tel: 704 922-6377 *Fax:* 704 922-6484
Med Dir: Lee Barro, MD
Class Cap: 40 *Begins:* Sep
Length: 18 mos *Award:* AAS
Tuition per yr: $742 res, $6,020 non-res

Pitt Community College

Medical Assistant Prgm
Hwy 11 S
PO Drawer 7007
Greenville, NC 27835-7007
Prgm Dir: Marsha Hemby, BA RN CMA
Tel: 919 355-4284 *Fax:* 919 321-4451
E-mail: mhemby@pcc.pitt.cc.nc.us
Med Dir: Leo Wavers, MD
Class Cap: 36 *Begins:* Sep Dec
Length: 21 mos *Award:* Cert, AAS
Tuition per yr: $742 res, $6,020 non-res
Evening or weekend classes available

Guilford Technical Community College

Medical Assistant Prgm
PO Box 309
Jamestown, NC 27282
Prgm Dir: Kimberly G Cannon, BS CMA
Tel: 910 334-4822 *Fax:* 910 454-2510
Med Dir: E B Mabry, MD
Class Cap: 35 *Begins:* Sep
Length: 21 mos *Award:* AAS
Tuition per yr: $742 res, $6,020 non-res
Evening or weekend classes available

James Sprunt Community College

Medical Assistant Prgm
JSCC PO Box 398
Hwy 11 South
Kenansville, NC 28349
Prgm Dir: Angelia Williams, AAS/CMA
Tel: 910 296-2565 *Fax:* 910 296-1636
Med Dir: Roland Draughn, MD
Class Cap: 20 *Begins:* Sep
Length: 21 mos *Award:* AAS
Tuition per yr: $771 res, $6,052 non-res
Evening or weekend classes available

Mitchell Community College

Medical Assistant Prgm
219 N Academy St
Mooresville, NC 28115
Prgm Dir: Priscilla Stanley, BS RN CMA
Tel: 704 663-1923 *Fax:* 704 663-5239
Med Dir: Stephen Ferguson, MD
Class Cap: 30 *Begins:* Sep
Length: 12 mos *Award:* Dipl
Tuition per yr: $742 res, $6,020 non-res
Evening or weekend classes available

Carteret Community College

Medical Assistant Prgm
3505 Arendell St
Morehead City, NC 28557
Prgm Dir: Julie Hosley, RN CMA
Tel: 919 247-3097 *Fax:* 919 247-2514
Med Dir: Darryl Falls, MD
Class Cap: 20 *Begins:* Sep
Length: 12 mos *Award:* Dipl
Tuition per yr: $775 res, $6,040 non-res

Western Piedmont Community College

Medical Assistant Prgm
1001 Burkemont Ave
Morganton, NC 28655
Prgm Dir: Ann Giles, MHS CMA
Tel: 704 438-6129 *Fax:* 704 438-6015
Med Dir: W L Sims, MD
Class Cap: 23 *Begins:* Sep
Length: 12 mos, 21 mos *Award:* Dipl, AAS
Tuition per yr: $728 res, $6,000 non-res
Evening or weekend classes available

Wake Technical Community College

Medical Assistant Prgm
9101 Fayetteville Rd
Raleigh, NC 27603-5676
Prgm Dir: Wanda J Orsett, CMA
Tel: 919 231-4500
Med Dir: Robert S Watkins, MD
Class Cap: 25 *Begins:* Sep
Length: 12 mos *Award:* Dipl
Tuition per yr: $742 res, $6,020 non-res

Miller-Motte Business College

Medical Assistant Prgm
606 S College Rd
Wilmington, NC 28403
Prgm Dir: Glenn Grady, MEd BSMT(ASCP)CMA
Tel: 910 392-4660 *Fax:* 910 799-6224
Med Dir: James J Pence, Jr, MD
Class Cap: 135 *Begins:* Sep Dec Mar Jun
Length: 18 mos *Award:* Dipl, AAS
Tuition per yr: res, $3,150 non-res
Evening or weekend classes available

Wingate College

Medical Assistant Prgm
PO Box 3024
Wingate, NC 28174
Prgm Dir: Pat V Thompson, MA HT(ASCP)CMA
Tel: 704 233-8104
Med Dir: Alex Snyder, MD
Class Cap: 25 *Begins:* Sep
Length: 18 mos *Award:* AAS , BSAH
Tuition per yr: $6,270

Ohio

Southern Ohio College - NE

Medical Assistant Prgm
2791 Mogadore Rd
Akron, OH 44312
Prgm Dir: Judith L Julagay, BSN RN
Tel: 330 733-8766 *Fax:* 330 733-5853
Med Dir: Leslie Parchment, DO
Class Cap: 175 *Begins:* Jan Apr Jun Oct
Length: 24 mos *Award:* AAS
Tuition per yr: $6,240

University of Akron

Medical Assistant Prgm
Akron, OH 44325-3702
Prgm Dir: Rebecca Gibson, MS CMA
Tel: 330 972-6515 *Fax:* 330 972-6952
Med Dir: Glenda Wickstram, MD
Class Cap: 75 *Begins:* Sep Jan
Length: 24 mos *Award:* AAS
Tuition per yr: $3,486 res, $8,686 non-res
Evening or weekend classes available

Ashland County-West Holmes Career Center

Medical Assistant Prgm
1783 State Rte 60
Ashland, OH 44805
Prgm Dir: Carol L Hale, RN CMA
Tel: 419 289-3313 *Fax:* 419 289-3729
Med Dir: J Stephen Torski, MD
Class Cap: 25 *Begins:* Sep Dec
Length: 9 mos *Award:* Cert
Tuition per yr: $3,200

Stark State College of Technology

Medical Assistant Prgm
6200 Frank Ave NW
Canton, OH 44720
Prgm Dir: Jennie L Self, MSTE RN CMA
Tel: 330 494-6170 *Fax:* 330 966-6586
Med Dir: Lawrence Ronning, MD
Class Cap: 32 *Begins:* Aug
Length: 20 mos *Award:* AAS
Tuition per yr: $2,988 res, $4,068 non-res
Evening or weekend classes available

Fairfield Career Center (EVSD)

Medical Assistant Prgm
4000 Columbus-Lancaster Rd
Carroll, OH 43112
Prgm Dir: Stephen Winegardner, MEd
Tel: 614 756-9245 *Fax:* 614 837-9447
Med Dir: Stephen Kock, MD
Class Cap: 25 *Begins:* Sep
Length: 9 mos *Award:* Cert
Tuition per yr: $2,970

Cincinnati State Tech and Comm College

Medical Assistant Prgm
3520 Central Pkwy
Cincinnati, OH 45223
Prgm Dir: Olivia Watts, BSN RN
Tel: 513 569-1676 *Fax:* 513 569-1659
E-mail: owatts@cinstate.cc.oh
Med Dir: Greg Ebner, DO
Class Cap: 30 *Begins:* Sep
Length: 12 mos, 10 mos *Award:* Cert, AAS
Tuition per yr: $4,189 res, $8,370 non-res
Evening or weekend classes available

Southern Ohio College - Woodlawn

Medical Assistant Prgm
1011 Glendale-Milford Rd
Cincinnati, OH 45215-1107
Prgm Dir: Rachael C Allstatter, LPN BSEd MEd
 CMA
Tel: 513 771-2424   *Fax:* 513 771-3413
Med Dir: Theodore Cole, OD
Class Cap: 200   *Begins:* Mar Jun Sep Jan
Length: 18 mos   *Award:* AS
Tuition per yr: $7,200
Evening or weekend classes available

Cuyahoga Community College

Medical Assistant Prgm
Metro Campus
700 Carnegie Ave
Cleveland, OH 44115
Prgm Dir: Barbara Freeman, BS MEd MT(ASCP)
Tel: 216 987-4438   *Fax:* 216 987-4438
Med Dir: Carl F Asseff, MD
Class Cap: 24   *Begins:* Sep
Length: 12 mos, 21 mos   *Award:* Dipl,Cert, AAS
Tuition per yr: $1,326 res, $3,133 non-res
Evening or weekend classes available

MTI Business College

Medical Assistant Prgm
1140 Euclid Ave/2nd Flr
Cleveland, OH 44115-1603
Prgm Dir: Martha Weidenbach, CMA LPN
Tel: 216 621-8228   *Fax:* 216 621-6488
Med Dir: Lonnie Marsh II, MD
Class Cap: 120   *Begins:* Quarterly
Length: 12 mos   *Award:* Dipl

Bradford School

Medical Assistant Prgm
6170 Busch Blvd
Columbus, OH 43229
Prgm Dir: Kay E Biggs, CMA
Tel: 614 846-9410   *Fax:* 614 846-9656
Med Dir: Jack Stevens, MD
Begins: Sep
Length: 10 mos   *Award:* Dipl
Tuition per yr: $7,320

Akron Medical-Dental Institute

Medical Assistant Prgm
1625 Portage Trail
Cuyahoga Falls, OH 44223-2122
Prgm Dir: Christine Fessler, CMA
Tel: 330 928-3400   *Fax:* 330 928-1906
Med Dir: William B Rogers, MD
Class Cap: 400   *Begins:* Sep Jan Mar Jun
Length: 11 mos, 17 mos   *Award:* Dipl
Tuition per yr: $7,400
Evening or weekend classes available

Miami-Jacobs College

Medical Assistant Prgm
400 E Second St
PO Box 1433
Dayton, OH 45401
Prgm Dir: Christina Dosland, BS
Tel: 513 461-5174
Med Dir: Kosi Auotn, MD
Class Cap: 25   *Begins:* Sep Jan Mar Jun
Length: 18 mos   *Award:* AD
Tuition per yr: $5,510

Ohio Institute of Photography and Technology

Medical Assistant Prgm
Division of Allied Health
2029 Edgefield Rd
Dayton, OH 45439
Prgm Dir: Karen R Seagraves, CMA AS
Tel: 513 294-6155   *Fax:* 513 294-2259
Med Dir: Kevin Hornbeck, DO
Class Cap: 30   *Begins:* Quarterly
Length: 14 mos, 18 mos   *Award:* Dipl, AS
Tuition per yr: $5,850 res, $11,700 non-res

Sinclair Community College

Medical Assistant Prgm
444 W Third St
Dayton, OH 45402
Prgm Dir: Jennifer L Barr, MEd MS CMA
Tel: 513 449-5163   *Fax:* 513 226-7960
Med Dir: Daniel L Whitmer, MD
Class Cap: 40   *Begins:* Sep
Length: 21 mos   *Award:* AAS
Tuition per yr: $1,457 res, $2,303 non-res
Evening or weekend classes available

Ohio Valley Business College

Medical Assistant Prgm
500 Maryland St
PO Box 7000
East Liverpool, OH 43920
Prgm Dir: Lynnette Burnett, MT CMA
Tel: 330 330-1070   *Fax:* 330 385-4606
Med Dir: J Fraser Jackson, MD
Class Cap: 35   *Begins:* Aug Jan
Length: 18 mos   *Award:* AD
Tuition per yr: $3,500 res, $3,500 non-res

Southern State Community College

Medical Assistant Prgm
200 Hobart Dr
Hillsboro, OH 45133
Prgm Dir: Saundra Stevens, MEd
Tel: 513 393-3431   *Fax:* 513 393-9370
Med Dir: Michael Kenner, DO
Class Cap: 60   *Begins:* Sep
Length: 18 mos   *Award:* AAS
Tuition per yr: $2,572 res, $4,736 non-res
Evening or weekend classes available

Medina County Career Center

Medical Assistant Prgm
1101 W Liberty St
Medina, OH 44256-9969
Prgm Dir: Lori Bamrick, RN CMA
Tel: 216 725-8461
Med Dir: John Funk, MD
Class Cap: 24   *Begins:* Sep
Length: 9 mos   *Award:* Cert
Tuition per yr: $3,385

Knox County Career Center

Medical Assistant Prgm
306 Martinsburg Rd
Mt Vernon, OH 43050
Prgm Dir: B Waynette Bridwell, BSN RN
Tel: 614 397-5820   *Fax:* 614 397-7040
Med Dir: Robert L Westerheide, MD
Begins: Aug
Length: 11 mos   *Award:* Cert
Tuition per yr: $3,050

Hocking Technical College

Medical Assistant Prgm
3301 Hocking Pkwy
Nelsonville, OH 45764-9704
Prgm Dir: Kathy West, MEd CMA-C
Tel: 614 753-3591
Med Dir: Rose Labrador, MD
Class Cap: 50   *Begins:* Sep
Length: 18 mos   *Award:* AAS
Tuition per yr: $2,082 res, $2,082 non-res
Evening or weekend classes available

Belmont Technical College

Medical Assistant Prgm
120 Fox-Shannon Pl
St Clairsville, OH 43950
Prgm Dir: Sally Hindman, BS RN CMA
Tel: 614 695-9500   *Fax:* 614 695-2247
Med Dir: Joseph Gabis, MD
Class Cap: 70   *Begins:* Sep
Length: 18 mos   *Award:* AAS
Tuition per yr: $2,379 res, $2,958 non-res
Evening or weekend classes available

Jefferson Community College

Medical Assistant Prgm
4000 Sunset Blvd
Steubenville, OH 43952
Prgm Dir: Robin S Flohr, MBA BSN RN CMA
Tel: 614 264-5591
Med Dir: John D Kuruc, MD
Class Cap: 25   *Begins:* Aug
Length: 11 mos, 18 mos   *Award:* Cert, AD
Tuition per yr: $2,294 res, $2,600 non-res
Evening or weekend classes available

Davis Junior College of Business

Medical Assistant Prgm
4747 Monroe St
Toledo, OH 43623
Prgm Dir: Laurie Schofield
Tel: 419 473-2700
Med Dir: Philip Lepkowski, MD
Class Cap: 120   *Begins:* Varies
Length: 18 mos   *Award:* Dipl,Cert, AD
Tuition per yr: $5,532

University of Toledo

Medical Assistant Prgm
Community and Technical Coll
2801 W Bancroft St
Toledo, OH 43606
Prgm Dir: Mary Ellen Wedding, CMA
Tel: 419 530-3149   *Fax:* 419 530-3096
Med Dir: Douglas Lyons, DO
Class Cap: 200   *Begins:* Sep Jan Mar Jun
Length: 18 mos   *Award:* AD
Tuition per yr: $2,997 res, $8,282 non-res
Evening or weekend classes available

Youngstown State University

Medical Assistant Prgm
Dept of Allied Health
410 Wick Ave
Youngstown, OH 44555
Prgm Dir: Kathylynn Feld, MS RN CMA
Tel: 330 742-1760   *Fax:* 330 742-2309
Med Dir: Thomas N Detesco, MD
Class Cap: 30   *Begins:* Sep Jan Mar
Length: 21 mos   *Award:* AAS
Tuition per yr: $970 res, $1,642 non-res

Muskingum Area Technical College

Medical Assistant Prgm
1555 Newark Rd
Zanesville, OH 43701
Prgm Dir: Tim Berger, RN CMA
Tel: 614 454-2501   *Fax:* 614 454-0035
Med Dir: Krist Sandland, MD
Class Cap: 50   *Begins:* Sep
Length: 21 mos   *Award:* Cert, AAS
Tuition per yr: $2,940 res, $4,740 non-res

Oklahoma

Canadian Valley Area Vocational Tech Sch

Medical Assistant Prgm
1401 Michigan Ave
Chickasha, OK 73018
Prgm Dir: Bernadette Burns, RN MPH MEd
Tel: 405 224-7220   *Fax:* 405 222-3839
Med Dir: Pilar Escobar, MD
Class Cap: 18   *Begins:* Monthly
Length: 16 mos   *Award:* Dipl
Tuition per yr: $675 res, $4,212 non-res

Tulsa Community College

Medical Assistant Prgm
909 S Boston Ave
Tulsa, OK 74119
Prgm Dir: Jeanette Girkin, EdD CMA
Tel: 918 595-7006
Med Dir: Walter Kempe, MD
Class Cap: 35   *Begins:* Jan Aug
Length: 10 mos, 24 mos   *Award:* Cert, AAS
Tuition per yr: $1,332 res, $3,598 non-res

Oregon

Mt Hood Community College

Medical Assistant Prgm
26000 SE Stark St
Gresham, OR 97030
Prgm Dir: Sue Boulden, RN
Tel: 503 667-7136   *Fax:* 503 667-7618
E-mail: bouldens@mhcc.cc.or.us
Med Dir: Robert Sayson, MD
Class Cap: 100   *Begins:* Sep Jan Mar Jun
Length: 18 mos   *Award:* AAS
Tuition per yr: $1,500 res, $4,950 non-res
Evening or weekend classes available

Portland Community College

Medical Assistant Prgm
12000 SW 49th Ave
Portland, OR 97219
Prgm Dir: Denise A Rigsbee, LPN CMA
Tel: 503 978-5665   *Fax:* 503 978-5257
E-mail: drigsbee@pcc.edu
Med Dir: Susan Williams, RRA
Class Cap: 24   *Begins:* Sep
Length: 9 mos   *Award:* Cert
Tuition per yr: $1,540 res, $5,500 non-res
Evening or weekend classes available

Chemeketa Community College

Medical Assistant Prgm
PO Box 14007
Salem, OR 97309
Prgm Dir: Elizabeth A Bode, PhD RN CMA
Tel: 503 399-3994
E-mail: bettyb@chemk.cc.or.us
Med Dir: Julie A Kurian, MD
Class Cap: 28   *Begins:* Sep
Length: 10 mos   *Award:* Cert
Tuition per yr: $1,530 res, $1,530 non-res

Pennsylvania

Butler County Community College

Medical Assistant Prgm
PO Box 1203
Butler, PA 16003-1203
Prgm Dir: Deborah B Kennedy, RN BS MS
Tel: 412 287-8711, Ext 373   *Fax:* 412 285-6047
Med Dir: Stephen E Sargent, MD
Class Cap: 35   *Begins:* Aug
Length: 16 mos   *Award:* AAS
Tuition per yr: $850 res, $1,700 non-res
Evening or weekend classes available

Mt Aloysius College

Medical Assistant Prgm
7373 Admiral Peary Hwy
Cresson, PA 16630-1999
Prgm Dir: Pauline Leventry, RN CMA
Tel: 814 886-4131   *Fax:* 814 886-2978
Med Dir: William P Hirsch, MD
Begins: Aug
Length: 18 mos   *Award:* AS
Tuition per yr: $8,780

Delaware County Community College

Medical Assistant Prgm
Rte 252 and Media Line Rd
Media, PA 19063
Prgm Dir: Marian D Edmiston, MSN RN CMA
Tel: 610 359-5274   *Fax:* 610 359-7350
Med Dir: Leonard Rosen, MD
Class Cap: 24   *Begins:* Sep
Length: 12 mos, 15 mos   *Award:* Cert, AAS
Tuition per yr: $2,428 res, $5,389 non-res
Evening or weekend classes available

Career Training Academy, Inc

Medical Assistant Prgm
ExpoMart
105 Mall Blvd/Ste 301-W
Monroeville, PA 15146
Prgm Dir: Deborah Jordan, CMA
Tel: 412 372-3900   *Fax:* 412 373-4262
Class Cap: 150   *Begins:* Monthly
Length: 9 mos   *Award:* Dipl
Tuition per yr: $4,095 res, $4,095 non-res

Career Training Academy, Inc

Medical Assistant Prgm
703 Fifth Ave
New Kensington, PA 15068
Prgm Dir: Deborah Vernon, CMA
Tel: 412 337-1000   *Fax:* 412 335-7140
Med Dir: Bernard L Rottschaeffer, MD
Class Cap: 120   *Begins:* Monthly
Length: 9 mo , 16 mos   *Award:* Dipl, AST
Tuition per yr: $4,095

Community College of Philadelphia

Medical Assistant Prgm
1700 Spring Garden St
Philadelphia, PA 19130
Prgm Dir: Deborah L Donaldson, MA CMA
Tel: 215 751-8947   *Fax:* 215 751-8937
Med Dir: Philip Ingaglio, MD
Class Cap: 30   *Begins:* Sep
Length: 18 mos   *Award:* AAS
Tuition per yr: $2,277 res, $4,554 non-res

Thompson Learning Corporation

Medical Assistant Prgm
Thompson Institute
3440 Market St/2nd Fl
Philadelphia, PA 19104
Prgm Dir: William Thorn, CMA NRMA ARMA
Tel: 215 387-1530   *Fax:* 215 387-0106
E-mail: wthorn1@mail.idt.nett
Med Dir: David Kountz, MD
Class Cap: 300   *Begins:* Monthly, Quartely
Length: 8 mo , 18 mos   *Award:* Dipl, AST
Tuition per yr: $5,450 res, $5,450 non-res
Evening or weekend classes available

Bradford School-Pittsburgh

Medical Assistant Prgm
Gulf Tower
707 Grant St
Pittsburgh, PA 15219
Prgm Dir: Linda N DeFalle, CMA
Tel: 412 391-6366
Med Dir: Kimberly A Parks, CMA
Class Cap: 150   *Begins:* Feb Sep Jul
Length: 10 mos   *Award:* Dipl
Tuition per yr: $9,575

Comm Coll of Allegheny Cnty-Alleg Campus

Medical Assistant Prgm
808 Ridge Ave
Pittsburgh, PA 15212
Prgm Dir: Grace J Cammarata, CMA
Tel: 412 237-2614   *Fax:* 412 237-4521
E-mail: gcammara@ccac.edu
Class Cap: 25   *Begins:* Aug
Length: 18 mos   *Award:* AS
Tuition per yr: $2,040 res, $4,080 non-res
Evening or weekend classes available

Duffs Business Institute

Medical Assistant Prgm
110 Ninth St
Pittsburgh, PA 15222
Prgm Dir: Lynn Slack, CMA
Tel: 412 261-4530   *Fax:* 412 261-4546
Med Dir: Jesse Mitchell, MD
Class Cap: 79   *Begins:* Jan Apr Jul Oct
Length: 9 mos   *Award:* Dipl
Tuition per yr: $5,850

ICM School of Business and Medical Careers
Medical Assistant Prgm
10 Wood St
Pittsburgh, PA 15222
Prgm Dir: Susan K Baker-Schutz
Tel: 412 261-2647 *Fax:* 412 261-6491
Med Dir: Michael Wald, MD
Class Cap: 225 *Begins:* Oct Jan Apr Jul
Length: 8 mo , 15 mos *Award:* Dipl,Cert
Tuition per yr: $7,776

Median School of Allied Health Careers
Medical Assistant Prgm
125 Seventh St
Pittsburgh, PA 15222
Prgm Dir: Kimberly Rubesne, CMA-ME
Tel: 412 391-0422 *Fax:* 412 232-4348
Med Dir: Marc Schneiderman, MD
Class Cap: 100 *Begins:* Sep Jan Apr Jun
Length: 10 mos, 15.5 mos *Award:* Dipl, AST
Tuition per yr: $6,300

Sawyer School
Medical Assistant Prgm
717 Liberty Ave
Pittsburgh, PA 15222
Prgm Dir: Susan Nibert, RN
Tel: 412 261-5700 *Fax:* 412 281-7269
Med Dir: Edgar Cordero, MDPC
Class Cap: 100 *Begins:* Varies
Length: 12 mos, 16 mos *Award:* Dipl, ASB
Tuition per yr: $6,730 res, $7,140 non-res

Lehigh Carbon Community College
Medical Assistant Prgm
4525 Education Park Dr
Schnecksville, PA 18078-2598
Prgm Dir: Judith K Ehninger, BS RN CMA
Tel: 610 799-1516 *Fax:* 610 799-1527
Med Dir: Paul H Schenck, MD
Begins: Aug
Length: 21 mos *Award:* AAS
Tuition per yr: $2,015 res, $4,030 non-res
Evening or weekend classes available

Central Pennsylvania Business School
Medical Assistant Prgm
Campus on College Hill
Summerdale, PA 17093
Prgm Dir: Crystal Wilson, CMA
Tel: 717 732-0702 *Fax:* 717 732-5254
Med Dir: Charles E Darowish, DO
Class Cap: 40 *Begins:* July Oct Jan
Length: 20 mos *Award:* ASB
Tuition per yr: $9,980

Berks Technical Institute
Medical Assistant Prgm
2205 Ridgewood Rd
Wyomissing, PA 19610
Prgm Dir: John Buynak, RN
Tel: 610 372-1722 *Fax:* 610 376-4684
Med Dir: Timothy Jameson, DO
Class Cap: 50 *Begins:* Feb May Jul Sep
Length: 7 mo , 18 mos *Award:* Dipl, AS
Tuition per yr: $6,272
Evening or weekend classes available

South Carolina

Forrest Junior College
Medical Assistant Prgm
601 E River St
Anderson, SC 29624
Prgm Dir: Carol Bagwell, MA
Tel: 864 225-7653 *Fax:* 864 261-7471
Med Dir: Stephen Worsham, MD
Class Cap: 100 *Begins:* May
Length: 12 mos *Award:* Dipl
Tuition per yr: $4,826
Evening or weekend classes available

Trident Technical College
Medical Assistant Prgm
PO Box 118067
Charleston, SC 29423-8067
Prgm Dir: Deborah White, BHS CMA
Tel: 803 572-6103
Med Dir: William M Lyman, MD
Class Cap: 30 *Begins:* Aug
Length: 12 mos *Award:* Dipl
Tuition per yr: $1,536 res, $1,776 non-res
Evening or weekend classes available

Midlands Technical College
Medical Assistant Prgm
PO Box 2408
Columbia, SC 29202
Prgm Dir: Marie D Robertson, CMA-AC
Tel: 803 822-3398 *Fax:* 803 822-3619
Class Cap: 22 *Begins:* Jan
Length: 12 mos *Award:* Cert
Tuition per yr: $1,500

Orangeburg Calhoun Technical College
Medical Assistant Prgm
3250 St Matthews Rd
Orangeburg, SC 29118
Prgm Dir: Precious F Mayer, MS
Tel: 803 535-1346 *Fax:* 803 535-1388
Med Dir: Willie B Louis, MD
Class Cap: 24 *Begins:* Aug
Length: 12 mos *Award:* Dipl
Tuition per yr: $1,155 res, $1,444 non-res
Evening or weekend classes available

South Dakota

National College
Medical Assistant Prgm
321 Kansas City St
Rapid City, SD 57709
Prgm Dir: Rita Landrus, CMA
Tel: 605 394-4839 *Fax:* 605 394-4871
Med Dir: Ray D Strand, MD
Class Cap: 20 *Begins:* Sep
Length: 19 mos *Award:* AAS
Tuition per yr: $8,415
Evening or weekend classes available

Lake Area Technical Institute
Medical Assistant Prgm
230 11th St NE
Watertown, SD 57201
Prgm Dir: Audrey Rausch, RN
Tel: 605 882-5284 *Fax:* 605 882-6299
E-mail: latiinfo@lati.tec.sd.us
Med Dir: Kevin Bjordahl, MD
Class Cap: 30 *Begins:* Sep Jan
Length: 14 mos, 18 mos *Award:* Dipl, AAS
Tuition per yr: $2,864
Evening or weekend classes available

Tennessee

Miller-Motte Business College
Medical Assistant Prgm
1820 Business Park Dr
Clarksville, TN 37040
Prgm Dir: Carolyn Duplessis, MT(ASCP) CMA
Tel: 615 553-0071 *Fax:* 615 552-2916
Med Dir: Danny W Futrell, MD
Class Cap: 180 *Begins:* Varies
Length: 24 mos *Award:* AAS
Tuition per yr: $5,400
Evening or weekend classes available

East Tennessee State University
Medical Assistant Prgm
1000 West E St
ETSU Nave Center
Elizabethton, TN 37643
Prgm Dir: Brenda M Foster, CMA
Tel: 423 547-4905 *Fax:* 423 547-4921
Med Dir: Tedford S Taylor, MD
Class Cap: 15 *Begins:* Aug
Length: 22 mos *Award:* AAS
Tuition per yr: $2,892 res, $9,396 non-res
Evening or weekend classes available

Tennessee Technology Center - Livingston
Medical Assistant Prgm
PO Box 219
740 High Tech Dr
Livingston, TN 38570
Prgm Dir: Patrice S Gilliam, BSN RN CMA MA
Tel: 615 823-5525 *Fax:* 615 823-7484
Med Dir: Albert E Hensel III, MD
Class Cap: 20 *Begins:* Jul
Length: 12 mos *Award:* Cert
Tuition per yr: $448 res, $448 non-res

Shelby State Community College
Medical Assistant Prgm
PO Box 40568
Memphis, TN 38174-0568
Prgm Dir: Darius Y. Wilson, MAT,MT(ASCP)
Tel: 901 544-5390 *Fax:* 901 544-5391
Med Dir: Hettie S Gibbs, MD
Class Cap: 15 *Begins:* Jun
Length: 24 mos *Award:* AAS
Tuition per yr: $1,536 res, $6,144 non-res
Evening or weekend classes available

Texas

Cisco Junior College
Medical Assistant Prgm
Box 3 Rt 3
Cisco, TX 76437
Prgm Dir: Mary Franklin, CMA
Tel: 915 673-4567 *Fax:* 915 673-4575
Med Dir: Austin King, MD
Class Cap: 35 *Begins:* Sep Jan Jun Jul
Length: 12 mos, 24 mos *Award:* Cert, AD
Tuition per yr: $500 res, $700 non-res

El Paso Community College
Medical Assistant Prgm
PO Box 20500
El Paso, TX 79998
Prgm Dir: Jeanne Howard, CMA AAS
Tel: 915 534-4139
Med Dir: Leonard Duran, MD
Class Cap: 20 *Begins:* Aug
Length: 12 mos, 20 mos *Award:* Cert, AAS
Tuition per yr: $1,495 res, $4,078 non-res

Western Technical Institute
Medical Assistant Prgm
4710 Alabama St
El Paso, TX 79930
Prgm Dir: Andreas Fester, CMA
Tel: 915 566-9621
Med Dir: Albert Unger, MD
Class Cap: 90 *Begins:* Monthly
Length: 7 mo , 12 mos *Award:* Cert
Tuition per yr: $5,109

Bradford School
Medical Assistant Prgm
4669 SW Frwy #300
Houston, TX 77027
Prgm Dir: Betty Burgan, CMA
Tel: 713 629-1500 *Fax:* 713 629-0059
Med Dir: Tom Salek, MD FAAFP ABFP
Class Cap: 28 *Begins:* Feb Apr Jul Sep Nov
Length: 8 mos *Award:* Dipl
Tuition per yr: $8,240

San Antonio College
Medical Assistant Prgm
1300 San Pedro Ave
San Antonio, TX 78284
Prgm Dir: Sunnee A Rakowitz
Tel: 210 733-2437 *Fax:* 210 733-2907
Med Dir: George Richmond, MD
Class Cap: 50 *Begins:* Sep Jan Jun
Length: 12 mos, 18 mos *Award:* Cert, AAS
Tuition per yr: $1,200 res, $2,845 non-res
Evening or weekend classes available

Utah

American Inst of Med/Dental Tech
Medical Assistant Prgm
1675 N Freedom Blvd/Bldg 9A
Provo, UT 84604
Prgm Dir: Carol A Lee, RN
Tel: 801 377-2900 *Fax:* 801 375-3077
Med Dir: Roger Lewis, MD
Class Cap: 100 *Begins:* Varies
Length: 8 mos *Award:* Dipl
Tuition per yr: $4,095 res, $4,095 non-res
Evening or weekend classes available

Bryman School
Medical Assistant Prgm
1144 W 3300 S
Salt Lake City, UT 84119
Prgm Dir: Tina Landskroener, CMA-C(BSBAM)
Tel: 801 975-7000 *Fax:* 801 975-7872
Med Dir: Peter Hasby, MD
Class Cap: 384 *Begins:* Monthly
Length: 8 mo , 18 mos *Award:* Cert, AAS
Tuition per yr: $7,500 res, $11,880 non-res
Evening or weekend classes available

Latter Day Saints Business College
Medical Assistant Prgm
411 E South Temple
Salt Lake City, UT 84111
Prgm Dir: Edith Hamelin, BSN RN CMA
Tel: 801 524-8131 *Fax:* 801 524-1900
Med Dir: Don Stromquist, MD
Class Cap: 100 *Begins:* Sep Jan Mar Jun
Length: 12 mos, 24 mos *Award:* Cert, AAS
Tuition per yr: $2,500
Evening or weekend classes available

Salt Lake Community College
Medical Assistant Prgm
4600 S Redwood Rd
PO Box 30808
Salt Lake City, UT 84130
Prgm Dir: Jana Tucker, CMA LPRT
Tel: 801 957-4090 *Fax:* 801 957-4612
Med Dir: Raymond Middleton, MD
Class Cap: 80 *Begins:* Jan Mar Jun Sep
Length: 12 mos *Award:* Cert
Tuition per yr: $1,784 res, $5,004 non-res
Evening or weekend classes available

Virginia

Commonwealth College - Hampton College
Medical Assistant Prgm
1120 W Mercury Blvd
Hampton, VA 23666-3309
Prgm Dir: Terry Raynor, BA RN CMA EMT
Tel: 804 838-2122 *Fax:* 804 745-6884
Med Dir: Kamal Luoka, MD
Class Cap: 50 *Begins:* Jan Apr Jul Oct
Length: 18 mos *Award:* AAS
Tuition per yr: $5,952 res, $5,952 non-res

Dominion Business School of Harrisonburg
Medical Assistant Prgm
933 Reservoir St
Harrisonburg, VA 22801
Prgm Dir: Judy Hobbie, RN
Tel: 540 433-6977 *Fax:* 540 433-3726
Class Cap: 120 *Begins:* Monthly
Length: 15 mos *Award:* Dipl

Commonwealth College - Richmond Campus
Medical Assistant Prgm
8141 Hull Street Rd
Richmond, VA 23235-6411
Prgm Dir: Nina Blodgett, BA RN CMA EMT
Tel: 804 745-2444 *Fax:* 804 745-6884
Med Dir: Kevin Harvey, MD
Class Cap: 50 *Begins:* Jan Apr Jul Oct
Length: 18 mos *Award:* AAS
Tuition per yr: $5,952 res, $5,952 non-res

Dominion Business School of Roanoke
Medical Assistant Prgm
4142 Melrose Ave NW/Ste 1
Roanoke, VA 24017
Prgm Dir: Kelly Pike
Tel: 540 362-7738 *Fax:* 540 563-0512
Class Cap: 50 *Begins:* Jan Apr Jul Oct
Length: 15 mos *Award:* Dipl
Tuition per yr: $8,500 res, $8,500 non-res
Evening or weekend classes available

National Business College
Medical Assistant Prgm
PO Box 6400
Roanoke, VA 24017-0400
Prgm Dir: Karen Wright-Ellis, CMA AS RTT
Tel: 540 986-1800 *Fax:* 540 986-1344
Med Dir: K Le Gree Hallman, MD
Class Cap: 40 *Begins:* Sep Jan Apr Jun
Length: 24 mos *Award:* AS
Tuition per yr: $6,000
Evening or weekend classes available

Dominion Business School of Staunton
Medical Assistant Prgm
825 Richmond Rd
Staunton, VA 24401
Prgm Dir: Judy Arline, CMA
Tel: 703 886-3596 *Fax:* 703 885-8647
Class Cap: 75 *Begins:* Quarterly
Length: 15 mos *Award:* Dipl
Tuition per yr: $7,200 res, $7,200 non-res

Commonwealth College - Virginia Beach Campus
Medical Assistant Prgm
4160 Virginia Beach Blvd
Virginia Beach, VA 23452-0222
Prgm Dir: Cornelia Mutts, BA RN CMA EMT
Tel: 804 499-7900 *Fax:* 804 745-6884
Med Dir: C O Barclay, MD
Class Cap: 18 *Begins:* Jan Apr Jul Oct
Length: 18 mos *Award:* AAS
Tuition per yr: $5,952 res, $5,952 non-res

Washington

Highline Community College
Medical Assistant Prgm
PO Box 98000
Des Moines, WA 98198-9800
Prgm Dir: Carol D Tamparo, CMA-A PhD
Tel: 206 878-3710 *Fax:* 206 870-3780
E-mail: ctamparo@hcc.etc.c
Med Dir: T J Huchala, MD
Class Cap: 50 *Begins:* Sep
Length: 18 mos *Award:* AAS
Tuition per yr: $1,484 res, $5,511 non-res
Evening or weekend classes available

Everett Community College
Medical Assistant Prgm
801 Wetmore
Everett, WA 98201
Prgm Dir: Debra Tri
Tel: 206 388-9362 *Fax:* 206 388-9129
Med Dir: Earl Beegle, MD
Class Cap: 60 *Begins:* Sep Jan Apr Jun
Length: 18 mos *Award:* Cert
Tuition per yr: $2,206 res, $7,386 non-res
Evening or weekend classes available

South Puget Sound Community College

Medical Assistant Prgm
2011 Mottman Rd SW
Olympia, WA 98502-6218
Prgm Dir: Margaret Fowler-Floyd, RN BS CMA
Tel: 206 754-7711, Ext 256   *Fax:* 206 664-0780
Med Dir: Lowell R Dightman, MD
Class Cap: 20   *Begins:* Sep Jan Apr
Length: 18 mos   *Award:* ATA
Tuition per yr: $999 res, $3,939 non-res
Evening or weekend classes available

North Seattle Community College

Medical Assistant Prgm
9600 College Way N
Seattle, WA 98103
Prgm Dir: Deborah J Bedford, AAS
Tel: 206 525-4561   *Fax:* 206 527-3784
Med Dir: Roger Higgs, MD
Class Cap: 30   *Begins:* Sep
Length: 12 mos   *Award:* Cert, AAS
Tuition per yr: $1,838 res, $7,316 non-res
Evening or weekend classes available

Wisconsin

Lakeshore Technical College

Medical Assistant Prgm
1290 North Ave
Cleveland, WI 53015
Prgm Dir: Barbara I Dodge, RN
Tel: 414 458-4183
Med Dir: Robert A Gahl, MD
Class Cap: 30   *Begins:* Aug Jan
Length: 9 mos   *Award:* Dipl
Tuition per yr: $3,230 res, $10,745 non-res

Northeast Wisconsin Technical College

Medical Assistant Prgm
2740 W Mason St
PO Box 19042
Green Bay, WI 54307-9042
Prgm Dir: Mary M Rahr, MS RN CMA-C
Tel: 414 498-5523   *Fax:* 414 498-5673
Med Dir: Bertram Milson, MD
Class Cap: 36   *Begins:* Aug
Length: 10 mos   *Award:* Dipl
Tuition per yr: $1,587 res, $10,657 non-res
Evening or weekend classes available

Blackhawk Technical College

Medical Assistant Prgm
6004 Prairie Rd
PO Box 53547
Janesville, WI 53547
Prgm Dir: Stephanie Richardson, RN BSN
Tel: 608 757-7608
Med Dir: K Eugene Bostian, MD
Class Cap: 30   *Begins:* Aug
Length: 9 mos   *Award:* Dipl
Tuition per yr: $1,740 res, $1,740 non-res
Evening or weekend classes available

Western Wisconsin Technical College

Medical Assistant Prgm
304 N Sixth St
PO Box 908
La Crosse, WI 54602-0908
Prgm Dir: Margaret Napoli, BS RN
Tel: 608 785-9922   *Fax:* 608 785-9407
E-mail: napoli@a1.western.tec.wi.us
Med Dir: Laura Krister, MD
Class Cap: 24   *Begins:* Aug
Length: 9 mos   *Award:* Dipl
Tuition per yr: $1,716 res, $11,342 non-res

Madison Area Technical College

Medical Assistant Prgm
3550 Anderson St
Madison, WI 53791-9674
Prgm Dir: Susan Buboltz, RN CMA
Tel: 608 246-6110   *Fax:* 608 246-6013
E-mail: swb4913@madison.tec.wi.us
Med Dir: Kay Heggestad, MD
Class Cap: 68   *Begins:* Jan Aug
Length: 9 mo , 13 mos   *Award:* Dipl
Tuition per yr: $1,638 res, $1,638 non-res

Mid-State Technical College

Medical Assistant Prgm
2600 W Fifth St
Marshfield, WI 54449
Prgm Dir: Barbara Lato, RN CMA
Tel: 715 387-2538   *Fax:* 715 389-2864
Med Dir: Richard Leer, MD
Class Cap: 36   *Begins:* Aug Jan
Length: 9 mos   *Award:* Dipl
Tuition per yr: $2,000
Evening or weekend classes available

Concordia University Wisconsin

Medical Assistant Prgm
12800 N Lake Shore Dr
Mequon, WI 53097
Prgm Dir: Sharon L Cooper, MT MS
Tel: 414 243-4362   *Fax:* 414 243-4351
Class Cap: 30   *Begins:* Aug
Length: 9 mos   *Award:* Cert
Tuition per yr: $4,000

Milwaukee Area Technical College

Medical Assistant Prgm
700 W State St
Milwaukee, WI 53233
Prgm Dir: Patricia Suminski, RN CMA
Tel: 414 297-6934   *Fax:* 414 297-6851
Med Dir: Ken Redlin, MD
Class Cap: 32   *Begins:* Sep
Length: 9 mos   *Award:* Dipl
Tuition per yr: $2,500 res, $10,789 non-res

Stratton College

Medical Assistant Prgm
1300 N Jackson St
Milwaukee, WI 53202
Prgm Dir: Paula Nordwig, BS CMA
Tel: 414 276-5200   *Fax:* 414 276-3930
Med Dir: Margaret Leonhardt, MD
Class Cap: 200   *Begins:* Varies
Length: 18 mos   *Award:* AS
Tuition per yr: $6,160

Wisconsin Indianhead Technical College

Medical Assistant Prgm
1019 S Knowles Ave
New Richmond, WI 54017
Prgm Dir: Lynette Waschke, RN CMA-C
Tel: 715 246-6561   *Fax:* 715 246-2777
Med Dir: James Craig, MD
Class Cap: 30   *Begins:* Sep Jan
Length: 9 mos   *Award:* Dipl
Tuition per yr: $1,690
Evening or weekend classes available

Waukesha County Technical College

Medical Assistant Prgm
800 Main St
Pewaukee, WI 53072
Prgm Dir: Kay Braaten, MS RN
Tel: 414 691-5563   *Fax:* 414 691-5451
E-mail: kbraaten@waukesha.tec.wi.us
Med Dir: David Brockway, DO
Class Cap: 30   *Begins:* Aug Jan
Length: 9 mos   *Award:* Dipl
Tuition per yr: $1,740
Evening or weekend classes available

Gateway Technical College

Medical Assistant Prgm
1001 S Main St
Racine, WI 53403
Prgm Dir: Ann Zion
Tel: 414 631-7353   *Fax:* 414 631-1044
Med Dir: Kevin Benson, MD
Class Cap: 30   *Begins:* Aug Jan
Length: 10 mos   *Award:* Dipl
Tuition per yr: $1,380 res, $9,880 non-res
Evening or weekend classes available

Programs

Medical Illustrator

History

Formal educational programs for the medical illustrator date back to the early 1900s, with Max Broedel's school at Johns Hopkins University. The Association of Medical Illustrators (AMI) was established in 1945. Under the auspices of the AMI, standards were developed by which the organization has accredited medical illustration programs in this country since 1967.

In 1986, the AMI expressed a desire to have educational programs for the medical illustrator accredited by the Committee on Allied Health Education and Accreditation (CAHEA) of the American Medical Association (AMA). This desire stemmed from the recognition that professional medical illustrator programs were more closely related to allied health than to the visual arts.

An ad hoc committee on outside accreditation of the AMI worked with staff of the AMA Division of Allied Health Education and Accreditation to modify the existing standards to comply with the format recommended by the CAHEA. The resulting *Essentials and Guidelines of an Accredited Educational Program for the Medical Illustrator* were adopted by the AMI and the AMA Council on Medical Education (CME) in 1987. Revised standards were adopted by the AMI and the AMA in 1992. Today, the standards are adopted by the Commission on Accreditation of Allied Health Education Programs (CAAHEP) in collaboration with the AMI.

Occupational Description

The term "medical illustrator" applies to competent professionals in the discipline of medical illustration. Medical illustrators create visual material designed to facilitate the recording and dissemination of medical, biological, and related knowledge. The medical illustration profession not only embraces production of such material but also functions in an administrative, consultative, and advisory capacity. Medical illustration employs a variety of artistic techniques, ranging from drawing, painting, sculpting, layout, design, and typography to computer graphics and electronic imaging.

With a strong foundation in biological sciences, anatomy, physiology, pathology, and general medical knowledge, combined with a high degree of proficiency in the visual arts, medical illustrators are able to depict subjects with extreme accuracy and realism or to interpret and reduce a complex idea to a simple explanatory diagram or schematic concept.

Job Description

Through the medical graphics they create, medical illustrators are communicators and teachers. Although some medical illustrators specialize in a single art medium or confine their interest to one of the medical specialties, the majority handle an ever-changing variety of assignments. They work with many different media to produce the highly accurate and authentic illustrations used in the publication of medical books, journals, films, videotapes, exhibits, posters, wall charts, and computer programs. Materials prepared by medical illustrators also may be used for projection in the classroom or for professional group presentations.

A medical illustrator also may work as a member of a research team to provide illustrations or to participate directly in the research problem. Some specialize in preparing prosthetics or in preparing models for instructional purposes.

In addition to the production of graphics and three-dimensional works, medical illustrators may serve as producers/directors or designers in the development of instructional programs. They also may organize and administer biomedical communication centers or illustration services at major teaching hospitals, health science centers, or elsewhere.

Employment Characteristics

The majority of medical illustrators are employed by medical schools and large medical centers that conduct teaching and research programs. Others are in private, state, and federal hospitals, clinics, and dental and veterinary schools. Many work independently on a freelance basis for medical publishers, pharmaceutical houses, and advertising agencies, in commercial settings, or for lawyers. Medical illustrators with appropriate background and professional experience are qualified to direct an illustration service unit or a biomedical communication center.

Entry level salaries for graduates of medical illustration schools range from $27,000 to $35,000. Experienced medical illustrators can earn an average of anywhere from $35,000 to $100,000.

Educational Programs

Length. Programs are generally 2 years, resulting in a master's degree.

Prerequisites. All current medical illustrator programs are at an advanced level and are based on a master's model. Generally, 4 years of undergraduate study are necessary to gain the required foundation. All programs culminating in a graduate degree require a baccalaureate degree and a good academic record. A preparatory program for the professional or graduate level of study should include a balance of art, premedical biology, and the humanities. Applicants for the advanced professional level programs must submit a portfolio of artwork.

Curriculum. Although the area of major emphasis may vary from school to school, programs of study usually include most of the following courses: human gross anatomy (with detailed dissection); histology; physiology; embryology; neuroanatomy; pathology; illustration techniques; anatomical illustration; surgical illustration; three-dimensional modeling; prosthetics; design for charts, graphs, and statistical data; exhibit design and construction; medical photography; television and multimedia production; computer graphics; business management; instructional design; and production technology.

Standards. *Standards* are national standards developed by the AMI in collaboration with the AMA. Each new program is assessed in accordance with the *Standards*, and accredited programs are reviewed periodically to determine whether they remain in substantial compliance. The *Standards and Guidelines* are available on written request from the AMI.

Inquiries

Accreditation

Direct requests for information on program accreditation, including *Standards*, preparing the self-study report, and arranging a site visit, should be submitted to

Accreditation Review Committee for the Medical Illustrator
CAAHEP
35 E Wacker Dr/Ste 1970
Chicago, IL 60601-2208
312 553-9355

Careers

Inquiries regarding careers and curriculum should be addressed to

Association of Medical Illustrators
1819 Peachtree St NE/Ste 560
Atlanta, GA 30309

Medical Illustrator

Georgia

Medical College of Georgia

Medical Illustrator Prgm
Allied Hlth and Grad Studies
1120 15th St
Augusta, GA 30912-0300
Prgm Dir: Steven J Harrison, MS
Tel: 706 721-3266   *Fax:* 706 721-7855
E-mail: curtice@mail.mcg.edu
Class Cap: 8   *Begins:* Aug
Length: 21 mos   *Award:* MS
Tuition per yr: $2,960 res, $7,252 non-res

Illinois

Univ of Illinois at Chicago

Medical Illustrator Prgm
Biomed Visualiz (MC-527)
School of Biomedical and Health Information
  Sciences
Coll of Assoc Hlth Professions
Chicago, IL 60612-7249
Prgm Dir: Alice A Katz, PhD
Tel: 312 996-7337   *Fax:* 312 996-8342
E-mail: aakatz@uic.edu
Class Cap: 12   *Begins:* Aug
Length: 21 mos   *Award:* MA, MS
Tuition per yr: $5,686 res, $13,163 non-res

Maryland

Johns Hopkins School of Medicine

Medical Illustrator Prgm
Dept of Art Applied to Med
1830 E Monument St Ste 7000
Baltimore, MD 21205
Prgm Dir: Gary P Lees, MS
Tel: 410 955-3213   *Fax:* 410 955-1085
E-mail: glees@welchlink.welch.jhu.edu
Class Cap: 6   *Begins:* Aug
Length: 21 mos   *Award:* MA
Tuition per yr: $20,740

Michigan

University of Michigan Medical Center

Medical Illustrator Prgm
Sch of Art
2000 Bonisteel Blvd/Rm 1075
Ann Arbor, MI 48109
Prgm Dir: Denis C Lee, MC
Tel: 313 998-6270   *Fax:* 313 936-0469
E-mail: stdenis@umich.edu
Med Dir: Edward West, MFA Assoc Dean
Class Cap: 8   *Begins:* Sep
Length: 19 mos   *Award:* MFA
Tuition per yr: $13,200 res, $27,000 non-res

Texas

Univ of Tx Southwestern Med Ctr - Dallas

Medical Illustrator Prgm
Biomed Comm/Illust Grad Prgm
5323 Harry Hines Blvd/Ex Park
Dallas, TX 75235-8881
Prgm Dir: Lewis E Calver, MS
Tel: 214 648-4699   *Fax:* 214 648-5353
E-mail: calver@utsw.swmed.edu
Class Cap: 6   *Begins:* May
Length: 24 mos   *Award:* Dipl, MA
Tuition per yr: $952 res, $5,814 non-res

Programs

Music Therapist

Job Description

Music therapy is a health profession in which music is used within a therapeutic relationship to address individuals' physical, psychological, cognitive, and social needs. After assessing the strengths and needs of each client, the qualified music therapist provides the indicated treatment, including creating, singing, moving to, and/or listening to music. Through musical involvement in the therapeutic context, patients' abilities are strengthened and transferred to other areas of their lives. Music therapy also provides avenues for communication that can be helpful to those who find it difficult to express themselves in words. Research in music therapy supports the effectiveness of music therapy in many areas, such as facilitating movement and overall physical rehabilitation, motivating people to cope with treatment, providing emotional support for clients and their families, and providing an outlet for expressing feelings.

Music therapists must have an interest in people and desire to help others empower themselves. The essence of music therapy practice involves establishing caring and professional relationships with people of all ages and abilities. Empathy, patience, creativity, imagination, receptivity to new ideas, and self-understanding are also important attributes. Because music therapists are musicians as well as therapists, a background in and love of music are also essential. Individuals considering a career in music therapy are advised to gain experience through volunteer opportunities or summer work in nursing homes, camps for children with disabilities, and other settings that serve the needs of people with disabilities.

Employment Characteristics

Music therapists are employed in many different settings, including general and psychiatric hospitals, mental health agencies, rehabilitation centers, day care facilities, nursing homes, schools, and private practices. Other emerging areas of health care delivery where music therapy is used include hospice care, substance abuse programs, oncology treatment centers, pain/stress management clinics, and correctional settings. Music therapists provide services for adults and children with psychiatric disorders, mental retardation and developmental disabilities, speech and hearing impairments, physical disabilities, and neurological impairments, among others. Music therapists are usually members of an interdisciplinary team that supports patients' goals within the context of the music therapy setting.

According to the NAMT, the average reported salary for music therapists is $30,000.

Educational Programs

Length. Undergraduate students in music therapy undertake a 4-year baccalaureate program of 127 semester hours. Successful completion of a 1,040-hour supervised clinical internship is also required. The master's degree in music therapy requires at least 30 semester hours for completion.

Prerequisites. For entry into undergraduate programs, a high school degree is required, along with demonstration of musicianship. Candidates for the master's degree must hold a baccalaureate degree or equivalency in music therapy (see "Board Certification," below) or be working concurrently toward fulfilling degree equivalency requirements.

Curriculum. The core curriculum for the baccalaureate degree includes coursework in music therapy; psychology; music; biological, social, and behavioral sciences; disabling conditions; and general studies. This curriculum is followed by a 6-month clinical internship in an approved mental health, special education, or health care facility, where students learn to assess clients' needs, develop and implement treatment plans, and evaluate and document clinical changes.

Graduate programs examine, with greater breadth and depth, issues relevant to the clinical, professional, and academic preparation of music therapists, usually in combination with established methods of research inquiry.

Standards. The National Association of Schools of Music publishes a biannual handbook that specifies the standards and guidelines required of educational programs in music therapy. Each new program is assessed in accordance with these standards, and approved programs are periodically reviewed to ensure that they remain in substantial compliance.

Certification

Each student who has completed academic and clinical training at the baccalaureate level is eligible to sit for the examination administered by the Certification Board for Music Therapists, leading to the credential Music Therapist - Board Certified (MT-BC).

Individuals who have an earned baccalaureate degree in music may elect to complete the degree equivalency program in music therapy offered by most NAMT-approved universities. Under this program, the student completes only the coursework required for Board certification without necessarily earning a second baccalaureate degree.

Inquiries

Accreditation

Requests for information on accreditation should be directed to

National Association of Schools of Music
11250 Roger Bacon Dr/Ste 21
Reston, VA 22090
703 437-0700
703 437-6312 Fax
E-mail: kpmnasm@aol.com

Education and Careers

Requests for information on education and careers should be directed to

National Association for Music Therapy
8455 Colesville Rd/Ste 1000
Silver Spring, MD 20910
301 589-3300
301 589-5175 Fax
Internet: http://www.namt.com/namt/
E-mail: career@namt.com

Certification

Requests for information on Board certification should be directed to

Certification Board for Music Therapists
589 Southlake Blvd
Richmond, VA 23236
800 765-CBMT or 804 379-9497
804 379-9354 Fax

Note: As of January 1, 1998, the National Association for Music Therapy will merge with the American Association for Music Therapy to form the American Music Therapy Association (AMTA).

Music Therapist

Alabama

University of Alabama

Music Therapist Prgm
School of Music
PO Box 870366
Tuscaloosa, AL 35487-0366
Prgm Dir: Carol A Prickett, PhD RMT
Tel: 205 348-1432
E-mail: cpricket@wolfgang.music.ua
Award: BA

Arizona

Arizona State University

Music Therapist Prgm
School of Music
Box 870405
Tempe, AZ 85287-0405
Prgm Dir: Barbara Crowe, MM RMT-BC
Tel: 602 965-7413
E-mail: barbaraj.crowe@asu.edu
Award: BA

California

California State University - Northridge

Music Therapist Prgm
18111 Nordhoff St
Northridge, CA 91330
Prgm Dir: Ronald Borczon, MM RMT-BC
Tel: 818 677-3174
E-mail: rborczon@csun.edu
Award: BA

Chapman University

Music Therapist Prgm
School of Music
333 N Glassell St
Orange, CA 92666
Prgm Dir: Kay Roskam, PhD RMT-BC
Tel: 714 532-6032
Award: BA

University of the Pacific

Music Therapist Prgm
Conservatory of Music
Dept of Music Therapy
Stockton, CA 95211
Prgm Dir: David Wolfe, PhD RMT
Tel: 209 946-3194
E-mail: dwolfe@uop.edu
Award: BA, MA

Colorado

Colorado State University

Music Therapist Prgm
Dept of Music, Theatre and Dance
Fort Collins, CO 80523
Prgm Dir: William Davis, PhD RMT
Tel: 970 491-5888
E-mail: davis@lamar.colostate.edu
Award: BA, MA

District of Columbia

Howard University

Music Therapist Prgm
College of Fine Arts/Music Dept
6th and Fairmont St NW
Washington, DC 20059
Prgm Dir: Donna Washington, MCAT RMT-BC
Tel: 202 806-7136
Award: BA

Florida

University of Miami

Music Therapist Prgm
School of Music
PO Box 248165
Coral Gables, FL 33124
Prgm Dir: Cathy McKinney, PhD RMT-BC
Tel: 305 284-3943
E-mail: cmckinne@umiami.miami.edu
Award: BA, MA

Florida State University

Music Therapist Prgm
School of Music
Tallahassee, FL 32306-2098
Prgm Dir: Jayne M Standley, PhD RMT
Tel: 904 644-4565
E-mail: standl-j@cmr.fsu.edu
Award: BA, MA

Georgia

University of Georgia

Music Therapist Prgm
School of Music
Fine Arts Bldg
Athens, GA 30602-3153
Prgm Dir: Roy Grant, PhD RMT
Tel: 706 542-3737
E-mail: rgrant@uga.cc.uga.edu
Award: BA, MA

Georgia College and State University

Music Therapist Prgm
Dept of Music and Theatre CPO 66
Milledgeville, GA 31061
Prgm Dir: Sandra L Curtis, PhD RMT-BC
Tel: 912 454-2645
E-mail: scurtis@mail.gac.peachnet.edu
Award: BA

Illinois

Western Illinois University

Music Therapist Prgm
Music Dept
Macomb, IL 61455
Prgm Dir: Bruce A Prueter, MS RMT-BC
Tel: 309 298-1187
Award: BA

Illinois State University

Music Therapist Prgm
Music Dept 5660
Normal, IL 61790-5660
Prgm Dir: Marie Di Giammarino, EdD RMT-BC
Tel: 309 438-8198
E-mail: mdigiam@oratmail.cfa.ilstu.edu
Award: BA, MA

Indiana

University of Evansville

Music Therapist Prgm
Dept of Music
1800 Lincoln Ave
Evansville, IN 47722
Prgm Dir: Alan Solomon, PhD RMT
Tel: 812 479-2754
E-mail: as7@evansville.edu
Award: BA

Indiana Univ/Purdue Univ Ft Wayne

Music Therapist Prgm
2101 Coliseum Blvd E
Fort Wayne, IN 46805-1499
Prgm Dir: Linda M Wright-Bower, MS RMT-BC
Tel: 219 481-6714
Award: BA

Iowa

University of Iowa

Music Therapist Prgm
School of Music
1006 Voxman Music Bldg
Iowa City, IA 52242
Prgm Dir: Kate Gfeller, PhD RMT
Tel: 319 335-1657
E-mail: kay-gfeller@uiowa.edu
Award: BA

Wartburg College

Music Therapist Prgm
School of Music
222 9th St
Waverly, IA 50677
Prgm Dir: Carol Culton-Hoine, MME RMT-BC
Tel: 319 352-8401
Award: BA

Kansas

University of Kansas

Music Therapist Prgm
Art, Music Ed and Music Therapy
311 Bailey Hall
Lawrence, KS 66045
Prgm Dir: Alicia Clair, PhD RMT-BC
Tel: 913 864-4784
E-mail: elmer@falcon.cc.ukans.edu
Award: BA, MA

Programs

Louisiana

Loyola University New Orleans
Music Therapist Prgm
College of Music
6363 St Charles Ave
New Orleans, LA 70118
Prgm Dir: Darlene Brooks, MMT RMT-BC
Tel: 504 865-2142
E-mail: brooks@bcta.loyno.edu
Award: BA, MA

Massachusetts

Berklee College of Music
Music Therapist Prgm
Chair Music Therapy Dept
1140 Boylston St
Boston, MA 02215-3693
Prgm Dir: Suzanne B Hanser, EdD RMT-BC
Tel: 617 266-1400, Ext 639
E-mail: shanser@it.berklee.edu
Award: BA

Anna Maria College
Music Therapist Prgm
Dept of Music/Box 45
Paxton, MA 01612-1198
Prgm Dir: Lisa Summer, MCAT RMT-BC
Tel: 508 849-3454
E-mail: summer@anna-maria.edu
Award: BA

Michigan

Michigan State University
Music Therapist Prgm
School of Music
East Lansing, MI 48824-1043
Prgm Dir: Roger Smeltekop, MM RMT-BC
Tel: 517 355-6753
Award: BA, MA

Western Michigan University
Music Therapist Prgm
School of Music
Kalamazoo, MI 49008-3834
Prgm Dir: Brian Wilson, MM RMT-BC
Tel: 616 387-4679
E-mail: brian.wilson@wmich.edu
Award: BA, MA

Eastern Michigan University
Music Therapist Prgm
Dept of Music
Ypsilanti, MI 48197
Prgm Dir: Michael McGuire, MM RMT-BC
Tel: 313 487-0292
Award: BA

Minnesota

Augsburg College
Music Therapist Prgm
731 21st Ave
Minneapolis, MN 55454
Prgm Dir: Roberta Kagin Metzler, MME RMT-BC
Tel: 612 330-1273
Award: BA

University of Minnesota - Twin Cities
Music Therapist Prgm
School of Music
2106 4th St S
Minneapolis, MN 55455
Prgm Dir: Charles Furman, PhD RMT
Tel: 612 624-7512
E-mail: furma001@maroon.tc.umn.edu
Award: BA

Mississippi

William Carey College
Music Therapist Prgm
498 Tuscan Ave
Hattiesburg, MS 39401
Prgm Dir: Paul D Cotton, PhD RMT
Tel: 601 582-5051
Award: BA

Missouri

University of Missouri - Kansas City
Music Therapist Prgm
Conservatory of Music
4949 Cherry
Kansas City, MO 64110-2229
Prgm Dir: George Petrie III, PhD RMT
Tel: 816 235-2912
E-mail: petrie@cctr.umkc.edu
Award: BA

Maryville University
Music Therapist Prgm
Dept of Music
13550 Conway Rd
St Louis, MO 63141
Prgm Dir: Joseph Moreno, PhD RMT-BC
Tel: 314 529-9441
Award: BA

New Jersey

Montclair State University
Music Therapist Prgm
Music Dept
Upper Montclair, NJ 07043
Prgm Dir: Barbara Wheeler, PhD RMT-BC
Tel: 201 655-7613
E-mail: wheelerb@alpha.montclair.edu
Award: BA

New York

SUNY College at Fredonia
Music Therapist Prgm
School of Music
Mason Hall
Fredonia, NY 14063
Prgm Dir: Constance E Willeford, MM RMT-BC
Tel: 716 673-3401
Award: BA

SUNY College at New Paltz
Music Therapist Prgm
Music Dept
New Paltz, NY 12561
Prgm Dir: Robert Krout, EdD RMT-BC
Tel: 914 257-2708
E-mail: rkroutmtbc@aol.com
Award: BA

Nazareth College of Rochester
Music Therapist Prgm
4245 East Ave
Rochester, NY 14618
Prgm Dir: Bryan C Hunter, PhD RMT-BC
Tel: 716 389-2702
Award: BA

North Carolina

Queens College
Music Therapist Prgm
Music Dept
1900 Selwyn Ave
Charlotte, NC 28274-0001
Prgm Dir: Frances J McClain, PhD RMT-BC
Tel: 704 337-2301
Award: BA

East Carolina University
Music Therapist Prgm
Fletcher Music Center
Greenville, NC 27858
Prgm Dir: Barbara Cobb Memory, PhD RMT-BC
Tel: 919 328-6331
Award: BA

Ohio

Ohio University Main Campus
Music Therapist Prgm
School of Music
440 Music Bldg
Athens, OH 45701
Prgm Dir: Peggy Codding, PhD RMT
Tel: 614 593-4248
E-mail: codding@ouvaxa.cats.ohiou.edu
Award: BA, MA

Baldwin-Wallace College
Music Therapist Prgm
Cleveland Consortium
275 Eastland Rd
Berea, OH 44017
Prgm Dir: Lalene DyShere Kay, MM RMT-BC
Tel: 216 826-2171
Award: BA

College of Mount St Joseph
Music Therapist Prgm
5701 Delhi Rd
Cincinnati, OH 45233-1670
Prgm Dir: Nancy A Nornhold, RMT
Tel: 513 244-4435
Award: BA

University of Dayton
Music Therapist Prgm
Music Dept
300 College Park
Dayton, OH 45469-0290
Prgm Dir: Marilyn J Sandness, MM RMT-BC
Tel: 937 229-3908
E-mail: sandess@yar.udayton.edu
Award: BA

Oklahoma

Phillips University
Music Therapist Prgm
100 S University Ave
Enid, OK 73701
Prgm Dir: Maria Hossenlopp, RMT-BC
Tel: 405 548-2358
Award: BA

Southwestern Oklahoma State University
Music Therapist Prgm
100 Campus Dr
Weatherford, OK 73096
Prgm Dir: Michael D Cassity, PhD RMT-BC
Tel: 405 774-3218
Award: BA

Oregon

Willamette University
Music Therapist Prgm
900 State St
Salem, OR 97301
Prgm Dir: Myra Staum, PhD RMT-BC
Tel: 503 370-6450
E-mail: mstaum@williamette.edu
Award: BA

Pennsylvania

Elizabethtown College
Music Therapist Prgm
Dept of Fine and Performing Arts
One Alpha Dr
Elizabethtown, PA 17022-2298
Prgm Dir: James L Haines, PhD RMT
Tel: 717 361-1212
E-mail: hainesjl@acad.etown.edu
Award: BA

Mansfield University
Music Therapist Prgm
Dept of Music
Mansfield, PA 16933
Prgm Dir: Elizabeth Eidenier, RMT-BC
Tel: 717 662-4710
Award: BA

Allegheny University of the Health Sciences
Music Therapist Prgm
Broad and Vine Sts/MS 905
Philadelphia, PA 19102-1192
Prgm Dir: Paul Nolan, MCAT RMT-BC
Tel: 215 762-6927
E-mail: nolan@hal.hahnemann.edu
Award: BA

Temple University
Music Therapist Prgm
College of Music 012-00
Philadelphia, PA 19122
Prgm Dir: Kenneth Bruscia, PhD ACMT-BC
Tel: 215 204-8310
Award: BA, MA

Duquesne University
Music Therapist Prgm
School of Music
Forbes Ave
Pittsburgh, PA 15282
Prgm Dir: Donna Marie Beck, PhD RMT-BC
Tel: 412 396-6086
Award: BA

Marywood College
Music Therapist Prgm
2300 Adams Ave
Scranton, PA 18509
Prgm Dir: Mariam Pfeifer, MA RMT-BC
Tel: 717 348-6211, Ext 2527
E-mail: pfeifer@ac.marywood.edu
Award: BA

Slippery Rock University
Music Therapist Prgm
SRU Dept of Music
Slippery Rock, PA 16057
Prgm Dir: Sue Shuttleworth, MM RMT-BC
Tel: 412 738-2447
E-mail: sue.shuttleworth@sru.edu
Award: BA

South Carolina

Charleston Southern University
Music Therapist Prgm
9200 University Blvd
PO Box 118087
Charleston, SC 29423-8087
Prgm Dir: Myra J Jordan, MME RMT
Tel: 803 863-7969
E-mail: mjjordan@aol.com
Award: BA

Tennessee

Tennessee Technological University
Music Therapist Prgm
Dept of Music and Art
Box 5045
Cookeville, TN 38505
Prgm Dir: Michael Clark, MME RMT-BC
Tel: 615 372-3065
E-mail: mec2197@tntech.edu
Award: BA

Texas

West Texas A & M University
Music Therapist Prgm
Dept of Music and Dance
WTA&M Box 879
Canyon, TX 79016-0001
Prgm Dir: Martha Estes, MA RMT
Tel: 806 656-2822
Award: BA

Southern Methodist University
Music Therapist Prgm
Meadows School of the Arts
Div of Music Therapy/Music
Dallas, TX 75275
Prgm Dir: Kaja Jensen, PhD MT-BC
Tel: 214 768-3175
E-mail: kjensen@mail.smu.edu
Award: BA, MA

Texas Woman's University
Music Therapist Prgm
PO Box 425768
TWU Station
Denton, TX 76204
Prgm Dir: Nancy Hadsell, PhD RMT-BC
Tel: 817 898-2514
E-mail: f_hasdell@twu.edu
Award: BA, MA

Sam Houston State University
Music Therapist Prgm
Dept of Music SHSU
Huntsville, TX 77341
Prgm Dir: Mary Ann Nolteriek, PhD RMT
Tel: 409 294-1376
Award: BA

Utah

Utah State University
Music Therapist Prgm
USU Music Dept
Logan, UT 84322-4015
Prgm Dir: Bruce Saperston, PhD RMT-BC
Tel: 801 797-3036
E-mail: bsaperston@wpo.hass.usu.edu
Award: BA

Virginia

Radford University
Music Therapist Prgm
Dept of Music
Radford, VA 24142
Prgm Dir: James E Borling, MM RMT-BC
Tel: 540 831-5177
E-mail: jborling@runet.edu
Award: BA, MA

Shenandoah University
Music Therapist Prgm
1460 University Dr
Winchester, VA 22601-5195
Prgm Dir: Michael J Rohrbacher, PhD RMT-BC
Tel: 540 665-4560
E-mail: mrohrbac@su.ed
Award: BA

Programs

Wisconsin

University of Wisconsin - Eau Claire

Music Therapist Prgm
Dept of Allied Health Professions
Sch of Human Sciences and Services
Eau Claire, WI 54702-4004
Prgm Dir: Dale B Taylor, PhD RMT-BC
Tel: 715 836-2628
E-mail: taylordb@uwec.edu
Award: BA

Alverno College

Music Therapist Prgm
3401 S 39th St
PO Box 3439222
Milwaukee, WI 53234-3922
Prgm Dir: Diane Knight, MS RMT-BC
Tel: 414 382-6135
Award: BA

University of Wisconsin - Oshkosh

Music Therapist Prgm
Dept of Music
800 Algoma Blvd
Oshkosh, WI 54901-8636
Prgm Dir: Nancy M Lloyd, MME RMT
Tel: 414 424-4224
Award: BA

Nuclear Medicine Technologist

History

The Joint Review Committee on Educational Programs in Nuclear Medicine Technology was formed by the Society of Nuclear Medicine, Society of Nuclear Medical Technologists, American College of Radiology, American Society of Clinical Pathologists, American Society for Medical Technology, and American Society of Radiologic Technologists. The first meeting of the Joint Review Committee was held in January 1970.

The Society of Nuclear Medical Technologists, one of the original sponsors, terminated its corporate status as a professional organization in 1975. The American Society for Medical Technology and the American Society of Clinical Pathologists relinquished sponsorship in 1994. Current representation of collaborating sponsors on the review committee includes two public members and three members appointed from each of the following organizations: the American College of Radiology, American Society of Radiologic Technologists, Society of Nuclear Medicine, and Society of Nuclear Medicine-Technologist Section. The current sponsorship maintains a balance between physicians and technologists.

The responsibilities of the Joint Review Committee include coordinating the preparation and revision of educational standards for adoption by collaborating organizations and conducting program reviews. The committee meets twice annually to review educational programs and determine accreditation status.

The first *Essentials of an Accredited Educational Program for the Nuclear Medicine Technologist* were adopted by the collaborating organizations in 1969. The *Essentials* were substantially revised in 1976, 1984, and 1991.

Occupational Description

Nuclear medicine is the medical specialty that uses the nuclear properties of radioactive and stable nuclides to make diagnostic evaluations of the anatomic or physiologic conditions of the body and to provide therapy with unsealed radioactive sources. The skills of the nuclear medicine technologist complement those of the nuclear medicine physician and of other professionals in the field.

Job Description

Nuclear medicine technologists perform a number of tasks in the areas of patient care, technical skills, and administration. When caring for patients, they acquire adequate knowledge of the patients' medical histories to understand and relate to their illnesses and pending diagnostic procedures for therapy, instruct patients before and during procedures, evaluate the satisfactory preparation of patients before commencing a procedure, and recognize emergency patient conditions and initiate life-saving first aid when appropriate.

Nuclear medicine technologists apply their knowledge of radiation physics and safety regulations to limit radiation exposure, prepare and administer radiopharmaceuticals, use radiation detection devices and other kinds of laboratory equipment that measure the quantity and distribution of radionuclides deposited in the patient or in a patient specimen, perform in vivo and in vitro diagnostic procedures, use quality control techniques as part of a quality assurance program covering all procedures and products in the laboratory, and participate in research activities.

Administrative functions may include supervising other nuclear medicine technologists, students, laboratory assistants, and other personnel; participating in procuring supplies and equipment; documenting laboratory operations; participating in departmental inspections conducted by various licensing, regulatory, and accrediting agencies; and participating in scheduling patient examinations.

Employment Characteristics

The employment outlook in nuclear medicine technology is good. Opportunities may be found in major medical centers, smaller hospitals, and independent imaging centers. Opportunities also are available for obtaining positions in clinical research, education, and administration. Salaries vary depending on the employer and geographic location.

According to a 1994 survey of 1,514 nuclear medicine technologists by the Society of Nuclear Medicine, 32% earned between $31,000 and $40,000 per year, 27% earned between $40,000 and $49,000, and 26% earned $50,000 or more.

Educational Programs

Length. The professional portion of the programs is 1 year. Institutions offering accredited programs may provide an integrated educational sequence leading to an associate or baccalaureate degree over a period of 2 or 4 years.

Prerequisites. Applicants for admission must have graduated from high school or the equivalent and have acquired postsecondary competencies in human anatomy and physiology, physics, mathematics, medical terminology, oral and written communications, chemistry, and medical ethics.

Curriculum. The curriculum includes patient care, nuclear physics, instrumentation and statistics, health physics, biochemistry, immunology, radiopharmacology, administration, radiation biology, clinical nuclear medicine, radionuclide therapy, and introduction to computer application.

Standards. *Essentials* are minimum educational standards adopted by the collaborating organizations. Each new program is assessed in accordance with the *Essentials*, and accredited programs are periodically reviewed to determine whether they remain in substantial compliance. The *Essentials and Guidelines* are available on written request from the Division of Allied Health Education and Accreditation.

Inquiries

Accreditation

Requests for information on program accreditation, including the *Essentials*, preparing the self-study report, and arranging a site visit, should be submitted to

Executive Director
Joint Review Committee on Educational Programs in
    Nuclear Medicine Technology
350 South 400 East/Ste 200
Salt Lake City, UT 84111-2938
801 364-4310
801 364-9234 Fax

Careers

Inquiries regarding careers and curriculum should be addressed to

American Society of Radiologic Technologists
15000 Central Ave SE
Albuquerque, NM 87123

Society of Nuclear Medicine–Technologist Section
1850 Samuel Morse Dr
Reston, VA 22090-5316
703 708-9000

Certification/Registration

Inquiries regarding certification may be addressed to

Nuclear Medicine Technology Certification Board
2970 Clairmont Rd NE/Ste 610
Atlanta, GA 30329-1634
404 315-1739

American Registry of Radiologic Technologists
1255 Northland Dr
Mendota Heights, MN 55120

Nuclear Medicine Technologist

Canada

British Columbia Institute of Technology

Nuclear Medicine Tech Prgm
3700 Willingdon Ave
Burnaby, BC V5G 3H2
Prgm Dir: Lawrence Parisotto, BSc RTNM
Tel: 604 432-8303   *Fax:* 604 436-9590
E-mail: lparisot@bcit.bc.ca
Med Dir: P Cohen, MD
Class Cap: 18   *Begins:* Sep
Length: 24 mos   *Award:* Dipl, AS
Tuition per yr: $2,300 res, $5,000 non-res

Alabama

University of Alabama at Birmingham

Nuclear Medicine Tech Prgm
Sch of Hlth Related Profs
Birmingham, AL 35294-1270
Prgm Dir: Ann M Steves, MS CNMT
Tel: 205 934-2004   *Fax:* 205 934-7387
E-mail: stevesa@admin.shrp.uab.edu
Med Dir: Eva V Dubovsky, MD PhD
Class Cap: 15   *Begins:* Sep
Length: 15 mos   *Award:* Cert, BS
Tuition per yr: $4,800 res, $9,600 non-res
Evening or weekend classes available

Arkansas

Baptist Medical System

Nuclear Medicine Tech Prgm
11900 Colonel Glenn Rd
Ste 1000
Little Rock, AR 72210-2820
Prgm Dir: Arthur G Maune, BS CNMT
Tel: 501 223-7447   *Fax:* 501 223-7406
Med Dir: Charles Boyd, MD
Class Cap: 6   *Begins:* Jul
Length: 12 mos   *Award:* Cert
Tuition per yr: $2,350

St Vincent Infirmary Medical Center

Nuclear Medicine Tech Prgm
Two St Vincent Circle
Little Rock, AR 72205-5499
Prgm Dir: Rick Bearden, BS MT CNMT
Tel: 501 660-2195   *Fax:* 501 671-4075
E-mail: rbearden@aristotle
Med Dir: Jerry L Prather, MD
Class Cap: 15   *Begins:* Aug
Length: 12 mos   *Award:* BS

Univ of Ark for Med Sci/St Vincent Infirmary

Nuclear Medicine Tech Prgm
4301 W Markham
Little Rock, AR 72205
Prgm Dir: Martha W Pickett, MHSA CNMT
Tel: 501 686-6848   *Fax:* 501 686-6513
E-mail: mwpickett@chrp.uams.edu
Med Dir: Gary Purnell, MD
Class Cap: 15   *Begins:* Aug
Length: 12 mos   *Award:* BS
Tuition per yr: $2,625 res, $6,562 non-res
Evening or weekend classes available

Univ of Arkansas for Medical Sciences

Nuclear Medicine Tech Prgm
4301 W Markham
Slot 714
Little Rock, AR 72205
Prgm Dir: Martha W Pickett, MHSA CNMT
Tel: 501 686-6848   *Fax:* 501 686-6073
E-mail: mwpickett@chrp.uams.edu
Med Dir: Gary Purnell, MD
Class Cap: 15   *Begins:* Aug
Length: 12 mos   *Award:* BS
Tuition per yr: $2,625 res, $6,562 non-res
Evening or weekend classes available

California

California State Univ-Dominguez Hills

Nuclear Medicine Tech Prgm
1000 E Victoria St
Carson, CA 90747
Prgm Dir: Kathleen McEnerney, DA
   MT(ASCP)CNMT
Tel: 310 243-3979   *Fax:* 310 516-3865
E-mail: kmenerney@dhvx20.csudh.edu
Med Dir: Fred S Mishkin, MD
Class Cap: 12   *Begins:* Jul
Length: 12 mos   *Award:* Dipl, BS
Tuition per yr: $1,791 res, $8,679 non-res

Loma Linda University

Nuclear Medicine Tech Prgm
Office of the Dean
Loma Linda, CA 92350
Prgm Dir: Arthur W Kroetz, MA RT
Tel: 909 824-4931
Med Dir: Gerald M Kirk, MD
Class Cap: 9   *Begins:* Sep
Length: 12 mos   *Award:* Cert
Tuition per yr: $2,480

Charles R Drew Univ of Med & Science

Nuclear Medicine Tech Prgm
Coll Allied Hlth Med Imaging Tech
1621 E 120th St
Los Angeles, CA 90059
Prgm Dir: Will Wade, CNMT
Tel: 213 563-5835
Med Dir: Panukorn Vasinrapee, MD
Class Cap: 5   *Begins:* Aug
Length: 12 mos   *Award:* Cert
Tuition per yr: $3,000

Los Angeles County - USC Medical Center

Nuclear Medicine Tech Prgm
1200 N State St
PO Box 2082/Rm 4516
Los Angeles, CA 90033
Prgm Dir: Lawrence J Szpila
Tel: 213 226-7266   *Fax:* 213 226-8064
Med Dir: Michael Siegel, MD
Class Cap: 6   *Begins:* Sep
Length: 12 mos   *Award:* Cert

Veterans Affairs Med Ctr W Los Angeles

Nuclear Medicine Tech Prgm
Wilshire and Sawtelle Blvds
Los Angeles, CA 90073
Prgm Dir: George L Colouris, CNMT
Tel: 310 268-3547   *Fax:* 310 268-4916
Med Dir: William H Blahd, MD
Class Cap: 11   *Begins:* Jul
Length: 12 mos   *Award:* Cert

Univ of California San Diego Med Ctr

Nuclear Medicine Tech Prgm
200 W Arbor Dr
San Diego, CA 92103-8758
Prgm Dir: Sara G Neff, CNMT RT(N)
Tel: 619 543-6682   *Fax:* 619 543-1975
E-mail: sneff@vcsd.edu
Med Dir: David Young, MD
Class Cap: 5   *Begins:* Oct
Length: 12 mos   *Award:* Cert
Tuition per yr: $2,500

University of California - San Francisco

Nuclear Medicine Tech Prgm
505 Parnassus Ave
San Francisco, CA 94143
Prgm Dir: Sylvia W Corpuz, BA CNMT
Tel: 415 476-1521
Med Dir: David C Price, MD
Class Cap: 9   *Begins:* Sep
Length: 12 mos   *Award:* Cert

Cancer Foundation of Santa Barbara

Nuclear Medicine Tech Prgm
300 W Pueblo St
PO Box 837
Santa Barbara, CA 93105
Prgm Dir: Lynette Robbins, CNMT
Tel: 805 682-7300   *Fax:* 805 569-7389
Med Dir: Pawan Gupta, MD
Class Cap: 4   *Begins:* Sep
Length: 12 mos   *Award:* Cert
Tuition per yr: $2,000

Colorado

Community Coll of Denver - Auraria Campus

Nuclear Medicine Tech Prgm
PO Box 173363
Campus Box 950
Denver, CO 80217-3363
Prgm Dir: Christine Yamasaki, BA CNMT
Tel: 303 556-2472   *Fax:* 303 556-8555
E-mail: col_christine@cccs.cccoes.edu
Med Dir: William Klingensmith, MD
Class Cap: 15   *Begins:* May Aug
Length: 12 mos, 15 mos   *Award:* Dipl,Cert, AAS
Tuition per yr: $2,214 res, $6,933 non-res

Connecticut

St Vincent's Medical Center
Nuclear Medicine Tech Prgm
2800 Main St
Bridgeport, CT 06606
Prgm Dir: Mary E Campbell, RT(N)CNMT
Tel: 203 576-5083   *Fax:* 203 576-5531
Med Dir: Norman R Vincent, MD
Class Cap: 4   *Begins:* Sep
Length: 12 mos   *Award:* Cert
Tuition per yr: $1,800

Middlesex Community - Technical College
Nuclear Medicine Tech Prgm
100 Training Hill Rd
Middletown, CT 06457
Prgm Dir: Elaine Lisitano, RT(R)
Tel: 860 344-6505
Med Dir: Ravi Jain, MD PhD
Class Cap: 3   *Begins:* Jun
Length: 15 mos   *Award:* Cert
Tuition per yr: $1,130 res, $2,920 non-res

Gateway Community - Technical College
Nuclear Medicine Tech Prgm
88 Bassett Rd
North Haven, CT 06473
Prgm Dir: Kathleen Murphy, BS CNMT ARRT(N)
Tel: 203 234-3314   *Fax:* 203 234-3353
E-mail: murphy5@gnhvax.commnet.edu
Med Dir: John Seibyl, MD
Class Cap: 13   *Begins:* Sep
Length: 24 mos   *Award:* AS
Tuition per yr: $1,560 res, $4,680 non-res
Evening or weekend classes available

Delaware

Delaware Tech & Comm Coll - Wilmington
Nuclear Medicine Tech Prgm
333 Shipley St
Wilmington, DE 19801
Prgm Dir: LaRay A Fox, BS CNMT
Tel: 302 428-6876   *Fax:* 302 428-2691
E-mail: fox.l@mcd.gen.de.us
Med Dir: Vidya V Sagar, MD
Class Cap: 11   *Begins:* Jun
Length: 24 mos   *Award:* AAS
Tuition per yr: $1,850 res, $4,725 non-res
Evening or weekend classes available

District of Columbia

George Washington University
Nuclear Medicine Tech Prgm
2300 I St NW
Rm 703
Washington, DC 20037
Prgm Dir: Miriam K Miller, MA CNMT
Tel: 202 994-3718   *Fax:* 202 994-3718
E-mail: mkmiller@gwis2.circ.gwu.edu
Med Dir: Vijay Varma, MD
Class Cap: 10   *Begins:* Sep
Length: 12 mos, 42 mos   *Award:* Cert, BS
Tuition per yr: $12,825

Florida

Broward Community College
Nuclear Medicine Tech Prgm
Ctr for Hlth Sciences Educ Bldg #8
3501 SW Davie Rd
Davie, FL 33314
Prgm Dir: Lorenzo Harrison, MBA CNMT
Tel: 954 475-6907
Med Dir: Maureen Sullivan, MD
Class Cap: 25   *Begins:* Aug
Length: 16 mos, 24 mos   *Award:* Cert, AS
Tuition per yr: $1,300 res, $4,800 non-res

Halifax Medical Center
Nuclear Medicine Tech Prgm
303 N Clyde Morris Blvd
Daytona Beach, FL 32120
Prgm Dir: Ronald S Smith, BS CNMT (N)ARRT
Tel: 904 254-4043   *Fax:* 904 254-4231
Med Dir: Thomas J Yuschok, MD
Class Cap: 4   *Begins:* Sep
Length: 15 mos   *Award:* Cert

Santa Fe Community College
Nuclear Medicine Tech Prgm
3000 NW 83rd St
Gainesville, FL 32606-6200
Prgm Dir: Edwin J Dice, MS CNMT
Tel: 352 395-5702   *Fax:* 352 395-5700
E-mail: ed.dice@santafe.cc.fl.us
Med Dir: Edward V Staab, MD
Class Cap: 12   *Begins:* Aug
Length: 22 mos   *Award:* AS
Tuition per yr: $1,271 res, $1,271 non-res
Evening or weekend classes available

Univ of Miami/Jackson Memorial Hosp
Nuclear Medicine Tech Prgm
1611 NW 12th Ave
Miami, FL 33136
Prgm Dir: Sharon S Halula, BS CNMT
Tel: 305 585-6345   *Fax:* 305 585-2620
Med Dir: George Sfakianakis, MD
Class Cap: 9   *Begins:* Jul
Length: 15 mos   *Award:* Cert
Tuition per yr: $1,500 res, $1,800 non-res

Mt Sinai Medical Center of Greater Miami
Nuclear Medicine Tech Prgm
4300 Alton Rd
Miami Beach, FL 33140
Prgm Dir: Douglas C Fuller, MS CNMT
Tel: 305 674-2980   *Fax:* 305 674-2692
Med Dir: William Smoak, MD
Class Cap: 2   *Begins:* Jan
Length: 12 mos   *Award:* Cert
Tuition per yr: $1,000

Valencia Community College
Nuclear Medicine Tech Prgm
1800 S Kirkman Rd
Orlando, FL 32811
Prgm Dir: Karen L Blondeau, MEd CNMT
Tel: 407 841-5111, Ext 8922   *Fax:* 407 423-3204
E-mail: kblondea@pegasus.cc.ucf.edu
Med Dir: Richard Lovas, MD
Class Cap: 7   *Begins:* Aug
Length: 22 mos   *Award:* AS
Tuition per yr: $1,359 res, $4,791 non-res
Evening or weekend classes available

Hillsborough Community College
Nuclear Medicine Tech Prgm
PO Box 30030
Tampa, FL 33630
Prgm Dir: Max Lombardi, ABSNM
Tel: 813 253-7418   *Fax:* 813 253-7400
Med Dir: Ian Tyson, MD
Class Cap: 18   *Begins:* Aug
Length: 24 mos   *Award:* Dipl, AS
Tuition per yr: $1,461 res, $5,444 non-res

Georgia

Medical College of Georgia
Nuclear Medicine Tech Prgm
Medical College of Georgia
Augusta, GA 30912
Prgm Dir: Wanda M Mundy, EdD
Tel: 706 721-3691   *Fax:* 706 721-8293
E-mail: wmundy@mail.mcg.edu
Med Dir: George Burke, MD
Class Cap: 14   *Begins:* Sep
Length: 12 mos, 24 mos   *Award:* Cert, AS, BS
Tuition per yr: $3,820 res, $6,908 non-res
Evening or weekend classes available

Illinois

College of DuPage
Nuclear Medicine Tech Prgm
22nd St and Lambert Rd
Glen Ellyn, IL 60137-6599
Prgm Dir: Joanne M Metler, MS CNMT
Tel: 630 942-3065   *Fax:* 630 858-5409
E-mail: metler@cdnet.cod.edu
Med Dir: Constance Wojtowicz, MD
Class Cap: 15   *Begins:* Sep
Length: 15 mos   *Award:* Cert
Tuition per yr: $1,800

Edward Hines Jr VA Hospital
Nuclear Medicine Tech Prgm
Fifth Ave and Roosevelt Rd
115 F
Hines, IL 60141
Prgm Dir: Nancy McDonald, BS CNMT
Tel: 708 343-7200   *Fax:* 708 216-2390
Med Dir: Parvez Shirazi, MD
Class Cap: 7   *Begins:* Jan Jul
Length: 12 mos   *Award:* Cert, BS

St Francis Medical Center
Nuclear Medicine Tech Prgm
530 NE Glen Oak Ave
Peoria, IL 61637
Prgm Dir: Tim Claxton, BS RT
Tel: 309 655-2005
Med Dir: Gordon Campbell, MD
Class Cap: 6   *Begins:* Aug
Length: 14 mos   *Award:* Dipl
Tuition per yr: $500

Programs

Triton College
Nuclear Medicine Tech Prgm
2000 Fifth Ave
River Grove, IL 60171
Prgm Dir: Charles Burchett, MA MT(ASCP)
Tel: 708 456-0300   *Fax:* 708 583-3121
E-mail: cchett@triton.cc.il.us
Med Dir: Robert Henkin, MD
Begins: Sep
Length: 22 mos   *Award:* AAS
Tuition per yr: $1,548 res, $4,563 non-res

Indiana

Ball State University
Nuclear Medicine Tech Prgm
c/o Methodist Hosp of Ind
1701 N Senate Blvd
Indianapolis, IN 46202
Prgm Dir: James J Wirrell, MEd CNMT
Tel: 317 929-8088   *Fax:* 317 929-2102
Med Dir: Larry L Heck, MD
Class Cap: 12   *Begins:* May
Length: 26 mos   *Award:* AS
Tuition per yr: $3,200

Indiana University School of Medicine
Nuclear Medicine Tech Prgm
541 Clinical Dr
CL 120
Indianapolis, IN 46202
Prgm Dir: Emily Hernandez, MS RT
Tel: 317 274-3801   *Fax:* 317 274-4074
E-mail: ehernande@xray.indyrad.iupui.edu
Med Dir: Robert Burt, MD
Class Cap: 7   *Begins:* Jun
Length: 22 mos   *Award:* BS
Tuition per yr: $3,541 res, $10,329 non-res
Evening or weekend classes available

Iowa

University of Iowa
Nuclear Medicine Tech Prgm
Dept of Radiology
Iowa City, IA 52242-1009
Prgm Dir: Anthony W Knight, MBA CNMT
Tel: 319 356-1911   *Fax:* 319 356-2220
E-mail: anthony-knight@uiowa.edu
Med Dir: Peter T Kirchner, MD
Class Cap: 10   *Begins:* Aug
Length: 12 mos   *Award:* Cert, BS
Tuition per yr: $3,088 res, $10,189 non-res

Kansas

University of Kansas Medical Center
Nuclear Medicine Tech Prgm
3901 Rainbow Blvd
Kansas City, KS 66160
Prgm Dir: Tina R Crain, MS CNMT RT(R)(N
Tel: 913 588-6858   *Fax:* 913 588-7899
E-mail: tcrain@kumc.edu
Med Dir: David F Preston, MD
Class Cap: 6   *Begins:* Sep
Length: 12 mos   *Award:* Cert
Tuition per yr: $2,000 res, $2,000 non-res

Kentucky

Lexington Community College
Nuclear Medicine Tech Prgm
Cooper Dr
330A Oswald Bldg
Lexington, KY 40506-0235
Prgm Dir: Charles H Coulston, MSEd CNMT
RT(N)
Tel: 606 257-4056   *Fax:* 606 257-4339
E-mail: chcoul01@ukec.uky.edu
Med Dir: Edward B Moody, MD MSE
Class Cap: 6   *Begins:* Aug
Length: 24 mos   *Award:* AAS
Tuition per yr: $2,942 res, $8,122 non-res
Evening or weekend classes available

University of Louisville
Nuclear Medicine Tech Prgm
Health Sciences Ctr
Louisville, KY 40292
Prgm Dir: Mark H Crosthwaite, MEd CNMT RT
Tel: 502 852-5624
Med Dir: Nolan Sa Kow, MD
Class Cap: 24   *Begins:* Aug
Length: 21 mos   *Award:* BSH
Tuition per yr: $3,585 res, $10,125 non-res

Louisiana

Alton Ochsner Medical Foundation
Nuclear Medicine Tech Prgm
1516 Jefferson Hwy
New Orleans, LA 70121
Prgm Dir: Evelyn R Merritt, CNMT(NMTCB)
Tel: 504 842-3267   *Fax:* 504 842-9129
Med Dir: Stanton E Shuler, MD
Begins: Jul
Length: 12 mos   *Award:* Cert

Delgado Community College
Nuclear Medicine Tech Prgm
501 City Park Ave
New Orleans, LA 70119
Prgm Dir: Ellen Thomas, BS RT(N) CNMT
Tel: 504 483-4015   *Fax:* 504 483-4609
Med Dir: Richard J Campeau, MD
Class Cap: 12   *Begins:* Jan
Length: 12 mos   *Award:* Cert
Tuition per yr: $1,526 res, $3,816 non-res
Evening or weekend classes available

Overton Brooks VA Medical Center
Nuclear Medicine Tech Prgm
510 E Stoner Ave
Shreveport, LA 71101-4295
Prgm Dir: Shirley H Ledbetter, BS CNMT
Tel: 318 424-6060   *Fax:* 318 424-6156
Med Dir: Frederick E Reinke, MD
Class Cap: 7   *Begins:* Jul
Length: 12 mos   *Award:* Cert

Maryland

Johns Hopkins Hospital
Nuclear Medicine Tech Prgm
600 N Wolfe St
Radiology Admin B179
Baltimore, MD 21287
Prgm Dir: Jay K Rhine, CNMT
Tel: 410 955-8422   *Fax:* 410 955-0059
E-mail: jkrhine@rad.jhu.edu
Med Dir: A Cahid Civelek, MD
Class Cap: 15   *Begins:* Jul
Length: 13 mos   *Award:* Cert
Tuition per yr: $4,100 res, $4,100 non-res
Evening or weekend classes available

Naval School of Health Sciences - MD
Nuclear Medicine Tech Prgm
Bethesda, MD 20889-5611
Prgm Dir: Daniel L Matangga, RT(N)
Tel: 301 295-5477   *Fax:* 301 295-0621
E-mail: matangga@nsh20.med.navy.mil
Med Dir: Capt E D Silverman, MD USNR
Class Cap: 30   *Begins:* Jan Jul
Length: 12 mos   *Award:* Cert

Prince George's Community College
Nuclear Medicine Tech Prgm
301 Largo Rd
Largo, MD 20772
Prgm Dir: Joseph R Hawkins, BS CNMT
Tel: 301 322-0733   *Fax:* 301 386-7504
Med Dir: Andrew M Keenan, MD
Class Cap: 15   *Begins:* Sep June
Length: 21 mos, 13 mos   *Award:* Cert, AAS
Tuition per yr: $2,800 res, $4,700 non-res
Evening or weekend classes available

Massachusetts

Bunker Hill Community College
Nuclear Medicine Tech Prgm
New Rutherford Ave
Boston, MA 02129
Prgm Dir: Susan W C Allen, CNMT RT(N)
Tel: 617 228-2418   *Fax:* 617 228-2082
Med Dir: Belton A Burrows, MD
Class Cap: 17   *Begins:* Sep
Length: 24 mos   *Award:* AS
Tuition per yr: $1,800 res, $5,622 non-res

Mass Coll of Pharmacy & Allied Hlth Sci
Nuclear Medicine Tech Prgm
179 Longwood Ave
Boston, MA 02215
Prgm Dir: George Matelli, EdD
Tel: 617 735-2933   *Fax:* 617 732-2801
Med Dir: S Ted Treves, MD
Class Cap: 20   *Begins:* Sep
Length: 24 mos, 42 mos   *Award:* AS, BS
Tuition per yr: $12,360 res, $12,360 non-res
Evening or weekend classes available

Salem State College

Nuclear Medicine Tech Prgm
352 Lafayette St
Salem, MA 01970
Prgm Dir: John W Metcalfe, PhD
Tel: 508 741-6236   *Fax:* 508 741-6176
Med Dir: Robert E Belliveau, MD
Class Cap: 14   *Begins:* Sep
Length: 38 mos   *Award:* Dipl, BS
Tuition per yr: $1,408 res, $5,726 non-res
Evening or weekend classes available

Springfield Technical Community College

Nuclear Medicine Tech Prgm
One Armory Square
Springfield, MA 01105
Prgm Dir: Richard T Serino, MEd CNMT
Tel: 413 781-7822
Med Dir: Said Zu'bi, MD
Class Cap: 15   *Begins:* Sep
Length: 24 mos   *Award:* AS
Tuition per yr: $1,733 res, $6,469 non-res

Univ Mass Med Ctr/Worcester State Coll

Nuclear Medicine Tech Prgm
U of Massachusetts Med Ctr
55 Lake Ave N
Worcester, MA 01655
Prgm Dir: Lewis E Braverman, MD
Tel: 508 856-3115   *Fax:* 508 856-6867
Class Cap: 7   *Begins:* Jun
Length: 48 mos, 12 mos   *Award:* Dipl,Cert, BS
Tuition per yr: $2,978 res, $6,692 non-res
Evening or weekend classes available

Michigan

Ferris State University

Nuclear Medicine Tech Prgm
200 Ferris Dr
VFS 411
Big Rapids, MI 49307
Prgm Dir: Sheila Squicciarini, CNMT
Tel: 616 592-2319   *Fax:* 616 592-3788
Med Dir: Anthony Keller, MD
Class Cap: 36   *Begins:* Aug
Length: 21 mos, 39 mos   *Award:* AAS , BS
Tuition per yr: $3,565 res, $7,186 non-res
Evening or weekend classes available

William Beaumont Hospital

Nuclear Medicine Tech Prgm
3601 W 13 Mile Rd
Royal Oak, MI 48073-6769
Prgm Dir: Mary L Premo, BA CNMT ARRT(N)
Tel: 810 551-4125   *Fax:* 810 551-0768
E-mail: mpremo@beaumont.edu
Med Dir: Howard Dworkin, MD
Class Cap: 10   *Begins:* Aug
Length: 14 mos   *Award:* Cert
Tuition per yr: $500

Minnesota

Mayo Clinic/Mayo Foundation

Nuclear Medicine Tech Prgm
School/Hlth Related Sciences
200 First St SW
Rochester, MN 55905
Prgm Dir: Nancy Hockert, NMT(ASCP)
Tel: 507 284-3245   *Fax:* 507 284-0656
E-mail: hockert.nancy@mayo.edu
Med Dir: Brian P Mullan, MD
Class Cap: 10   *Begins:* Sep
Length: 12 mos   *Award:* Cert
Tuition per yr: $2,150

St Mary's University of Minnesota

Nuclear Medicine Tech Prgm
700 Terrace Hts #10
Winona, MN 55987-1399
Prgm Dir: Donald J Alsum, PhD
Tel: 507 457-1546   *Fax:* 507 457-1633
E-mail: dalsum@smu.edu
Med Dir: Jeanette V Moulthrop, MD
Class Cap: 6   *Begins:* Sep
Length: 39 mos, 48 mos   *Award:* Cert, BA
Tuition per yr: $12,045 res, $12,045 non-res

Mississippi

University of Mississippi Medical Center

Nuclear Medicine Tech Prgm
2500 N State St
Jackson, MS 39216
Prgm Dir: John Vanderslice Jr, BS CNMT
Tel: 601 984-2585   *Fax:* 601 984-2502
E-mail: juandus@fiona.umsmed.edu
Med Dir: Bharti R Patel, MD
Class Cap: 8   *Begins:* Jul
Length: 12 mos   *Award:* Cert

Missouri

University of Missouri - Columbia

Nuclear Medicine Tech Prgm
One Hospital Dr
Columbia, MO 65211
Prgm Dir: Kimberly G Hoffman, CNMT
Tel: 573 443-2511   *Fax:* 573 882-1663
E-mail: hoggmank@ext.missouri.edu
Med Dir: Bennett S Greenspan, MD
Class Cap: 7   *Begins:* Aug
Length: 12 mos   *Award:* Cert, BS
Tuition per yr: $4,580 res, $13,486 non-res

Research Medical Center

Nuclear Medicine Tech Prgm
2316 E Meyer Blvd
Kansas City, MO 64132
Prgm Dir: Charlotte Ament, BS MA CNMT
Tel: 816 276-4235   *Fax:* 816 276-3138
Med Dir: Barry Gubin, MD
Class Cap: 8   *Begins:* Sep
Length: 12 mos   *Award:* Cert
Tuition per yr: $800 res, $800 non-res

St Louis University Health Sciences Ctr

Nuclear Medicine Tech Prgm
1504 S Grand Blvd
St Louis, MO 63104
Prgm Dir: Sheila D Rosenfeld, MA CNMT
Tel: 314 289-7054   *Fax:* 314 289-6533
E-mail: rosenfeld@nucmed.slu.edu
Med Dir: James Fletcher, MD
Class Cap: 14   *Begins:* Sep
Length: 12 mos, 39 mos   *Award:* Cert, BS
Tuition per yr: $11,690

Nebraska

University of Nebraska Medical Center

Nuclear Medicine Tech Prgm
600 S 42nd St
Omaha, NE 68198-1045
Prgm Dir: Carol L Dworak, CNMT
Tel: 402 559-7224   *Fax:* 402 559-1011
E-mail: cldworak@unmc.edu
Med Dir: Lisa Gobar, MD
Class Cap: 6   *Begins:* Aug
Length: 12 mos, 24 mos   *Award:* BS
Tuition per yr: $3,150 res, $8,364 non-res
Evening or weekend classes available

Nevada

University of Nevada Las Vegas

Nuclear Medicine Tech Prgm
4505 Maryland Pkwy
Las Vegas, NV 89154
Prgm Dir: Kenneth M Winch, ARRT(R)(N)
Tel: 702 895-3136   *Fax:* 702 895-3872
Med Dir: Paul Bandt, MD
Class Cap: 13   *Begins:* Aug
Length: 48 mos   *Award:* BS
Tuition per yr: $1,856 res, $6,606 non-res

New Jersey

Univ of Med & Dent of New Jersey

Nuclear Medicine Tech Prgm
Schl Hlth Related Professions
150 Bergen St Rm H41
Newark, NJ 07103
Prgm Dir: Timothy J Lynch, RT(N)
Tel: 201 982-6021   *Fax:* 201 982-6954
E-mail: lynchtj@umdnj.edu
Med Dir: Gerard W Moskowitz, MD
Class Cap: 10   *Begins:* Sep
Length: 15 mos   *Award:* Cert
Tuition per yr: $5,000 res, $6,500 non-res

Riverview Medical Center

Nuclear Medicine Tech Prgm
One Riverview Plaza
Red Bank, NJ 07701
Prgm Dir: Virginia Chiafullo, BS CNMT
Tel: 908 530-2407
Med Dir: John A Parrella, MD
Class Cap: 7   *Begins:* Jul
Length: 12 mos   *Award:* Cert
Tuition per yr: $5,000

Gloucester County College
Nuclear Medicine Tech Prgm
1400 Tanyard Rd
Sewell, NJ 08080
Prgm Dir: Laura J Sharkey, CNMT
Tel: 609 468-5000 *Fax:* 609 464-8463
Med Dir: Howard P Rothenberg, MD MS
Class Cap: 22 *Begins:* Sep
Length: 20 mos *Award:* AAS
Tuition per yr: $1,944 res, $1,980 non-res

New York

CUNY Bronx Community College
Nuclear Medicine Tech Prgm
Univ Ave and W 181st St
Bronx, NY 10453
Prgm Dir: Jack Prince, PhD
Tel: 718 289-5400 *Fax:* 718 289-6373
Med Dir: M Donald Blaufox, MD, PhD
Class Cap: 60 *Begins:* Sep Jan
Length: 30 mos *Award:* AAS
Tuition per yr: $2,100 res, $2,676 non-res
Evening or weekend classes available

SUNY at Buffalo
Nuclear Medicine Tech Prgm
105 Parker Hall
Buffalo, NY 14226
Prgm Dir: Elpida S Crawford, MS CNMT
Tel: 716 892-2141 *Fax:* 716 838-4918
E-mail: elpida@nucmed.buffalo.edu
Med Dir: Hani Nabi, MD
Class Cap: 15 *Begins:* Sep
Length: 18 mos *Award:* Dipl, BS
Tuition per yr: $3,400 res, $8,300 non-res
Evening or weekend classes available

Institute of Allied Medical Professions
Nuclear Medicine Tech Prgm
405 Park Ave/Ste 501
New York, NY 10022-4405
Prgm Dir: John W Hart, CNMT RT(N)
Tel: 212 758-1410 *Fax:* 212 758-1424
Med Dir: Josef Machac, MD
Class Cap: 24 *Begins:* Jun Dec
Length: 12 mos *Award:* Cert
Tuition per yr: $8,900
Evening or weekend classes available

New York University Medical Center
Nuclear Medicine Tech Prgm
550 First Ave
New York, NY 10016
Prgm Dir: Raymond Lopez, MPA RT CNMT
Tel: 212 263-7410 *Fax:* 212 263-7519
E-mail: lopez@nucmed
Med Dir: Joseph J Sanger, MD
Class Cap: 12 *Begins:* Sep
Length: 12 mos *Award:* Cert
Tuition per yr: $7,200 res, $7,200 non-res

St Vincent's Hosp & Med Ctr of New York
Nuclear Medicine Tech Prgm
153 W 11th St
New York, NY 10011
Prgm Dir: Raul Rapun, PhD
Tel: 212 604-8716 *Fax:* 212 604-3889
Med Dir: Hussein Abdel-Dayem, MD
Class Cap: 9 *Begins:* Sep
Length: 15 mos *Award:* Cert
Tuition per yr: $6,500

Northport VA Medical Center #632C
Nuclear Medicine Tech Prgm
79 Middleville Rd
Northport, NY 11768
Prgm Dir: Lillian J Gucciardi, BS CNMT RT(N)
Tel: 516 261-4400
Med Dir: Mohammed A Antar, MD
Class Cap: 7 *Begins:* Jul
Length: 24 mos *Award:* Cert
Tuition per yr: $500

Manhattan College
Nuclear Medicine Tech Prgm
Manhattan College Pkwy
Riverdale, NY 10471
Prgm Dir: Lawrence W Hough, MA CNMT
Tel: 718 862-7370 *Fax:* 718 862-7816
E-mail: lhough@manhattan.edu
Med Dir: Donald Margouleff, MD
Class Cap: 30 *Begins:* Sep Jan
Length: 15 mos, 48 mos *Award:* Cert, BS
Tuition per yr: $13,800

Rochester Institute of Technology
Nuclear Medicine Tech Prgm
Dept of Allied Health Sciences
Rochester, NY 14623
Prgm Dir: Kristin Waterstram-Rich, CNMT
Tel: 716 475-5117 *Fax:* 716 475-5766
E-mail: kmw4088@rit.edu
Med Dir: Robert E O'Mara, MD
Class Cap: 18 *Begins:* Jun Sep
Length: 12 mos, 37 mos *Award:* Cert, BS
Tuition per yr: $14,670
Evening or weekend classes available

Molloy College
Nuclear Medicine Tech Prgm
1000 Hempstead Ave
Rockville Centre, NY 11570
Prgm Dir: Marc Fischer, BS CNMT ARRT MDA
Tel: 516 678-5000, Ext 166 *Fax:* 516 256-2252
Med Dir: Joseph J Macy, MD ABR
Class Cap: 12 *Begins:* Sep
Length: 24 mos *Award:* AAS
Tuition per yr: $9,600
Evening or weekend classes available

St Vincent's Medical Center of Richmond
Nuclear Medicine Tech Prgm
355 Bard Ave
Staten Island, NY 10310
Prgm Dir: Kathleen A Quince, MPA BS CNMT
Tel: 718 876-2010 *Fax:* 718 876-2006
Med Dir: Orlando L Manfredi, MD/ABR ABNM
Class Cap: 4 *Begins:* July
Length: 48 mos *Award:* Cert, BS
Tuition per yr: $2,550 res, $5,050 non-res

SUNY Health Science Center at Syracuse
Nuclear Medicine Tech Prgm
750 E Adams St
Syracuse, NY 13210
Prgm Dir: Bradford J Hellwig, BS CNMT
Tel: 315 464-7031 *Fax:* 315 464-7068
E-mail: hellwihb@vax.cs.hscsyr.edu
Med Dir: F Deaver Thomas
Class Cap: 5 *Begins:* Apr Sep
Length: 12 mos *Award:* Cert
Tuition per yr: $6,500

North Carolina

University of North Carolina Hospitals
Nuclear Medicine Tech Prgm
101 Manning Dr
CB 7600(NL) Radiology-Nuclear Medcine
Chapel Hill, NC 27514
Prgm Dir: Marilyn W Parrish, RT(N) CNMT
Tel: 919 966-5233 *Fax:* 919 966-7898
E-mail: mparrish.rad1@mail.unch.unc.edu
Med Dir: William H McCartney, MD
Class Cap: 7 *Begins:* Aug
Length: 12 mos *Award:* Cert
Tuition per yr: $700

Pitt Community College
Nuclear Medicine Tech Prgm
PO Drawer 7007
Greenville, NC 27835-7007
Prgm Dir: Merritt W Clark III, BS ARRT (N)(R)
Tel: 919 321-4453
Med Dir: Julian R Vainright Jr, MD
Class Cap: 5 *Begins:* Sep
Length: 12 mos *Award:* Dipl, AAS
Tuition per yr: $758 res, $6,022 non-res

Caldwell Comm College & Tech Institute
Nuclear Medicine Tech Prgm
1000 Hickory Blvd
Hudson, NC 28638
Prgm Dir: Jimmy L Council, RT(N) CNMT
Tel: 704 726-2322 *Fax:* 704 726-2216
Med Dir: Richard Curtis, MD
Class Cap: 15 *Begins:* Sep
Length: 24 mos *Award:* AAS
Tuition per yr: $742 res, $6,020 non-res
Evening or weekend classes available

Forsyth Technical Community College
Nuclear Medicine Tech Prgm
2100 Silas Creek Pkwy
Winston-Salem, NC 27103
Prgm Dir: Donald G Harkness, MEd CNMT
Tel: 910 723-0371 *Fax:* 910 748-9395
Med Dir: Robert J Cowan, MD
Class Cap: 10 *Begins:* Sep
Length: 24 mos *Award:* AAS
Tuition per yr: $742 res, $6,020 non-res

Ohio

Aultman Hospital
Nuclear Medicine Tech Prgm
2600 Sixth St SW
Canton, OH 44710
Prgm Dir: Joseph G Markley, BS RTN
Tel: 330 438-6204 *Fax:* 330 438-9811
Med Dir: Laurence G Hanelin, MD
Class Cap: 6 *Begins:* Jul
Length: 12 mos *Award:* Cert
Tuition per yr: $2,500

University of Cincinnati Medical Center
Nuclear Medicine Tech Prgm
234 Goodman St
Cincinnati, OH 45267
Prgm Dir: Alan Vespie, MEd CNMT
Tel: 513 558-9081 *Fax:* 513 558-7690
E-mail: vespieaw@email.uc.edu
Med Dir: Mariano Fernandez-Ulloa, MD
Class Cap: 13 *Begins:* Sep
Length: 21 mos, 39 mos *Award:* AS, BS
Tuition per yr: $3,471 res, $8,745 non-res
Evening or weekend classes available

Ohio State University Hospitals
Nuclear Medicine Tech Prgm
203F E Doan Hall
Columbus, OH 43210
Prgm Dir: Robert Reid, MS CNMT
Tel: 614 293-8433 *Fax:* 614 293-4366
Med Dir: John Olsen, MD
Class Cap: 7 *Begins:* Jun
Length: 13 mos *Award:* Cert
Tuition per yr: $1,000 res, $1,000 non-res

The University of Findlay
Nuclear Medicine Tech Prgm
1000 N Main St
Findlay, OH 45840
Prgm Dir: Elaine M Markon, MS CNMT
Tel: 419 424-4708 *Fax:* 419 424-4822
Med Dir: Daniel Singer, MD
Class Cap: 70 *Begins:* Aug Jan
Length: 12 mos, 48 mos *Award:* Cert, BS
Tuition per yr: $7,700 res, $7,700 non-res
Evening or weekend classes available

St Elizabeth Health Center
Nuclear Medicine Tech Prgm
1044 Belmont Ave
Youngstown, OH 44501
Prgm Dir: Richard M Blanco, RT CNMT
Tel: 330 746-7211
Med Dir: Jae J Lee, MD
Class Cap: 5 *Begins:* Jul
Length: 24 mos *Award:* Cert
Tuition per yr: $1,000 res, $1,000 non-res

Oklahoma

Univ of Oklahoma Health Sciences Center
Nuclear Medicine Tech Prgm
PO Box 26901
Oklahoma City, OK 73190
Prgm Dir: Jan Winn, MEd RT(N)(ARRT)
Tel: 405 271-6477 *Fax:* 405 271-1424
E-mail: jan-winn@uokhsc.edu
Med Dir: Carl Bogardus, MD
Class Cap: 12 *Begins:* Aug
Length: 48 mos *Award:* BS
Tuition per yr: $3,117 res, $8,076 non-res
Evening or weekend classes available

Pennsylvania

Cedar Crest College
Nuclear Medicine Tech Prgm
100 College Dr
Allentown, PA 18104-6196
Prgm Dir: Brian S Misanko, PhD
Tel: 610 437-4471 *Fax:* 610 606-4616
E-mail: bsmisnko@cedarcrest.edu
Med Dir: Stuart Jones, MD
Class Cap: 8 *Begins:* Jun
Length: 12 mos, 48 mos *Award:* Cert, BS
Tuition per yr: $7,605
Evening or weekend classes available

Lancaster Institute for Health Education
Nuclear Medicine Tech Prgm
PO Box 3555
Lancaster, PA 17604-3555
Prgm Dir: Penni L Aten, BS CNMT
Tel: 717 290-5668 *Fax:* 717 290-5970
Med Dir: Robert Basarab, MD
Class Cap: 12 *Begins:* Jun
Length: 12 mos *Award:* Cert
Tuition per yr: $4,000 res, $4,000 non-res

Comm Coll of Allegheny Cnty-Alleg Campus
Nuclear Medicine Tech Prgm
808 Ridge Ave
Pittsburgh, PA 15212
Prgm Dir: Carl Mazzetti, CNMT
Tel: 412 237-2751 *Fax:* 412 237-4521
E-mail: cmazzett@cacc.edu
Med Dir: Mustafa Adatepe, MD
Class Cap: 30 *Begins:* Sep
Length: 24 mos, 12 mos *Award:* Dipl,Cert, AS
Tuition per yr: $2,040 res, $4,080 non-res
Evening or weekend classes available

Wyoming Valley Health Care System Inc
Nuclear Medicine Tech Prgm
N River and Auburn Sts
Wilkes Barre, PA 18764
Prgm Dir: Cindy Turchin, CNMT
Tel: 717 552-2075 *Fax:* 717 552-2080
E-mail: turch@epix.net
Med Dir: E Joan Graham, DO
Class Cap: 5 *Begins:* Sep
Length: 12 mos *Award:* Cert
Tuition per yr: $2,000

Puerto Rico

University of Puerto Rico
Nuclear Medicine Tech Prgm
GPO Box 5067
San Juan, PR 00936
Prgm Dir: Miriam Espada, CNMT
Tel: 787 751-4434 *Fax:* 787 764-1760
Med Dir: Frieda Silva, MD
Class Cap: 10 *Begins:* Aug
Length: 12 mos *Award:* BS
Tuition per yr: $1,080

Rhode Island

Rhode Island Hospital
Nuclear Medicine Tech Prgm
593 Eddy St
Providence, RI 02902
Prgm Dir: Pamela C Maisano, ARRT CNMT
Tel: 401 444-8621
Med Dir: Richard B Noto, MD
Class Cap: 9 *Begins:* Jul
Length: 12 mos *Award:* Cert
Tuition per yr: $3,500

South Carolina

Midlands Technical College
Nuclear Medicine Tech Prgm
PO Box 2408
Columbia, SC 29202
Prgm Dir: Miriam E Hunt, BHS CNMT ARRT
Tel: 803 434-6343 *Fax:* 803 434-4500
Med Dir: Samuel Friedman, MD
Class Cap: 8 *Begins:* Aug
Length: 12 mos *Award:* Cert
Tuition per yr: $1,620 res, $2,016 non-res
Evening or weekend classes available

South Dakota

Southeast Technical Institute
Nuclear Medicine Tech Prgm
2301 Career Pl
Sioux Falls, SD 57107
Prgm Dir: Carole South-Winter, RT(R) CNMT BS
Tel: 605 338-8459
Med Dir: W.A. Boade, MD
Class Cap: 26 *Begins:* Sep
Length: 27 mos *Award:* AAS
Tuition per yr: $4,955
Evening or weekend classes available

Tennessee

Chattanooga State Technical Comm College
Nuclear Medicine Tech Prgm
4501 Amnicola Hwy
Chattanooga, TN 37406
Prgm Dir: Sandra Dobbs, RT(R)(N) CNMT
Tel: 423 634-7711 *Fax:* 423 634-7711
Med Dir: Alan D Hughes, MD
Class Cap: 25 *Begins:* August
Length: 12 mos *Award:* Cert
Tuition per yr: $1,253 res, $5,000 non-res

Univ of Tennessee Med Ctr at Knoxville
Nuclear Medicine Tech Prgm
1924 Alcoa Hwy
Knoxville, TN 37920
Prgm Dir: Glen Hathaway, CNMT
Tel: 423 544-9726 *Fax:* 423 544-9074
E-mail: ghathawa@scanner.hosp.utk.edu
Med Dir: Karl F Hubner, MD
Class Cap: 7 *Begins:* Aug
Length: 12 mos *Award:* Cert, BS
Tuition per yr: $2,300 res, $2,300 non-res

Programs

Baptist Memorial Health Care Systems
Nuclear Medicine Tech Prgm
1003 Monroe Ave
Memphis, TN 38104
Prgm Dir: Kathy Thompson, BS CNMT
Tel: 901 227-3042 *Fax:* 901 227-4310
Med Dir: M Moinuddin, MD
Class Cap: 10 *Begins:* Sep
Length: 12 mos *Award:* Cert
Tuition per yr: $2,500 res, $2,500 non-res

Methodist Hospitals of Memphis
Nuclear Medicine Tech Prgm
1265 Union Ave
Memphis, TN 38104
Prgm Dir: Pamela J Simmons, CNMT RT(R)(N)
Tel: 901 726-7363 *Fax:* 901 726-7390
Med Dir: Alvin J Weber, MD
Class Cap: 4 *Begins:* Sep
Length: 12 mos *Award:* Cert

Vanderbilt University Medical Center
Nuclear Medicine Tech Prgm
Rad Dept 21st and Garland
CCC-1124 MCN
Nashville, TN 37232-2675
Prgm Dir: James A Patton, PhD
Tel: 615 322-0508 *Fax:* 615 322-3764
E-mail: jim.patton@mcmail.vanderbilt.edu
Med Dir: Martin P Sandler, MD
Class Cap: 8 *Begins:* Aug
Length: 12 mos *Award:* BS
Tuition per yr: $1,900

Texas

Amarillo College
Nuclear Medicine Tech Prgm
PO Box 447
Amarillo, TX 79178
Prgm Dir: Howard Bacon, AAS BAAS RTR(N)
Tel: 806 354-6071
Med Dir: Antonio C Gonzalez, MD
Class Cap: 10 *Begins:* Aug
Length: 24 mos *Award:* AAS
Tuition per yr: $600 res, $950 non-res

Galveston College-University of Texas
Nuclear Medicine Tech Prgm
4015 Ave Q
Galveston, TX 77550
Prgm Dir: Bobby R Brown, BS CNMT
Tel: 409 772-3042 *Fax:* 409 772-3014
E-mail: bobrown%sahs@mhost.utmb.edu
Med Dir: Martin L Nusynowitz, MD
Class Cap: 5 *Begins:* Sep
Length: 23 mos *Award:* Dipl,Cert, AAS
Tuition per yr: $1,146 res, $1,146 non-res

Baylor College of Medicine
Nuclear Medicine Tech Prgm
1200 Moursund Ave
Houston, TX 77030
Prgm Dir: Paul H Murphy, PhD
Tel: 713 791-3141 *Fax:* 713 791-3141
E-mail: pmurphy@bcm.tmc.edu
Med Dir: Warren H Moore, MD
Class Cap: 12 *Begins:* Sep
Length: 12 mos *Award:* Cert
Tuition per yr: $1,800

Houston Community College Central
Nuclear Medicine Tech Prgm
3100 Shenandoah
Houston, TX 77021-1042
Prgm Dir: Glenn X Smith, BS CNMT
Tel: 713 718-7354 *Fax:* 713 718-7401
Med Dir: Donald A Podoloff, MD
Class Cap: 31 *Begins:* Aug
Length: 24 mos, 18 mos *Award:* Cert, AAS
Tuition per yr: $1,092 res, $1,833 non-res
Evening or weekend classes available

University of the Incarnate Word
Nuclear Medicine Tech Prgm
4301 Broadway
San Antonio, TX 78209
Prgm Dir: Pamela King, CNMT
Tel: 210 829-3149 *Fax:* 210 829-3153
Med Dir: Angelita Ramos-Gabatin, MD FACD
Class Cap: 12 *Begins:* Aug Jan
Length: 18 mos *Award:* BS
Tuition per yr: $6,000
Evening or weekend classes available

Utah

Univ of Utah Health Sciences Center
Nuclear Medicine Tech Prgm
50 N Medical Dr
Salt Lake City, UT 84132
Prgm Dir: Paul E Christian, BS CNMT
Tel: 801 581-2716 *Fax:* 801 585-2403
Med Dir: Wayne Adams, MD
Class Cap: 5 *Begins:* Jul
Length: 12 mos *Award:* Cert
Tuition per yr: $700 res, $700 non-res

Vermont

University of Vermont
Nuclear Medicine Tech Prgm
302 Rowell Bldg
Burlington, VT 05405
Prgm Dir: Louis M Izzo, CNMT MS
Tel: 802 656-3455 *Fax:* 802 656-8876
E-mail: louis.izzo@uvm.edu
Med Dir: Jonathan Fairbank, MD
Class Cap: 8 *Begins:* Aug
Length: 24 mos *Award:* AS
Tuition per yr: $6,732 res, $16,824 non-res

Virginia

Univ of Virginia Health Sciences Center
Nuclear Medicine Tech Prgm
Jefferson Park Ave
Box 486
Charlottesville, VA 22908
Prgm Dir: Christopher Puckett, BS CNMT
Tel: 804 924-5201
Med Dir: Charles D Teates, MD
Class Cap: 7 *Begins:* Aug
Length: 15 mos *Award:* Cert
Tuition per yr: $1,000

Old Dominion University
Nuclear Medicine Tech Prgm
Norfolk, VA 23529-0287
Prgm Dir: Scott R Sechrist, MS CNMT ARRT(N)
Tel: 757 683-3589 *Fax:* 757 683-5028
E-mail: srs100f@cianium.hs.
Med Dir: David Weaver, PhD MD
Class Cap: 10 *Begins:* Aug
Length: 22 mos *Award:* BS
Tuition per yr: $4,389 res, $11,385 non-res
Evening or weekend classes available

Med Coll of VA/Virginia Commonwealth U
Nuclear Medicine Tech Prgm
Dept of Radiation Sciences
PO Box 9804595 MCV Campus
Richmond, VA 23298-0495
Prgm Dir: Joanne S Greathouse, EdS FASRT
  RT(R)
Tel: 804 828-9104 *Fax:* 804 828-9104
E-mail: jgreathouse@gems.vcu.edu
Med Dir: James L Tatum, MD
Class Cap: 8 *Begins:* Aug
Length: 21 mos *Award:* BS
Tuition per yr: $5,841 res, $17,396 non-res
Evening or weekend classes available

Carilion Health System/Carilion Roanoke Mem Hosp
Nuclear Medicine Tech Prgm
Roanake Memorial Hospitals
Belleview at Jefferson St
Roanoke, VA 24033
Prgm Dir: Norma F Arthur, MSEd RTR
Tel: 540 981-7731
Med Dir: Marshall A Wakat, MD PhD
Class Cap: 3 *Begins:* Sep
Length: 12 mos *Award:* Cert
Tuition per yr: $1,000

Washington

Bellevue Community College
Nuclear Medicine Tech Prgm
Box 900
Seattle, WA 98111
Prgm Dir: Jennifer L Prekeges, MS CNMT
Tel: 206 223-6951 *Fax:* 206 625-7295
Med Dir: Marie E Lee, MD
Class Cap: 5 *Begins:* Sep
Length: 12 mos *Award:* Cert
Tuition per yr: $3,000 res, $3,000 non-res

West Virginia

West Virginia State College
Nuclear Medicine Tech Prgm
PO Box 1000
Campus Box 183
Institute, WV 25112-1000
Prgm Dir: James D Wilson, CNMT MS
Tel: 304 766-3118
Med Dir: Steven A Artz, MD
Class Cap: 11 *Begins:* Aug
Length: 24 mos *Award:* AAS
Tuition per yr: $2,783 res, $4,304 non-res
Evening or weekend classes available

West Virginia University Hospitals, Inc

Nuclear Medicine Tech Prgm
Medical Ctr Dr
PO Box 6401
Morgantown, WV 26506
Prgm Dir: Connie Y Felton, CNMT
Tel: 304 598-4260 *Fax:* 304 598-4348
Med Dir: Naresh C Gupta, MD
Class Cap: 4 *Begins:* Jul
Length: 12 mos *Award:* Cert
Tuition per yr: $800

Wheeling Jesuit University

Nuclear Medicine Tech Prgm
316 Washington Ave
Wheeling, WV 26003
Prgm Dir: Angela R Macci, RT BS MPM
Tel: 304 243-2387
Class Cap: 88 *Begins:* Aug
Length: 48 mos *Award:* Dipl, BS
Tuition per yr: $12,000

Wisconsin

Gundersen Med Found/La Crosse Lutheran

Nuclear Medicine Tech Prgm
1836 South Ave
La Crosse, WI 54601
Prgm Dir: Beverly A Lewis, BS CNMT
Tel: 608 782-7300 *Fax:* 608 791-6642
E-mail: blewis@gc.gundluth.org
Med Dir: Sue Beier-Hanratty, MD
Class Cap: 2 *Begins:* Sep
Length: 12 mos *Award:* Cert
Tuition per yr: $1,200

St Joseph's Hospital

Nuclear Medicine Tech Prgm
611 St Joseph Ave
Marshfield, WI 54449
Prgm Dir: Jesse R Johnson, BS CNMT
Tel: 715 387-7787
E-mail: johnsoj@mfldclin.edu
Med Dir: G John Weir, MD
Class Cap: 6 *Begins:* Aug
Length: 12 mos *Award:* Cert, BS
Tuition per yr: $3,000 res, $5,000 non-res
Evening or weekend classes available

Froedtert Memorial Lutheran Hospital

Nuclear Medicine Tech Prgm
9200 W Wisconsin Ave
PO Box 26099
Milwaukee, WI 53226
Prgm Dir: Frank G Steffel, BS CNMT
Tel: 414 259-2071 *Fax:* 414 771-3460
Med Dir: Arthur Z Krasnow, MD
Class Cap: 8 *Begins:* Sep
Length: 12 mos *Award:* Cert
Tuition per yr: $1,000 res, $1,000 non-res

St Luke's Medical Center

Nuclear Medicine Tech Prgm
2900 W Oklahoma Ave
Milwaukee, WI 53215
Prgm Dir: Lannice Meyer, CNMT
Tel: 414 649-6418 *Fax:* 414 649-2118
Med Dir: A Michael Kistler, MD
Class Cap: 6 *Begins:* Jun
Length: 12 mos *Award:* Cert
Tuition per yr: $1,000

Occupational Therapy

History

The National Society for the Promotion of Occupational Therapy was founded in 1917 and incorporated under the laws of the District of Columbia.

The objective of the association as set forth in its Constitution "shall be to study and advance curative occupations for invalids and convalescents; to gather news of progress in occupational therapy and to use such knowledge to the common good; to encourage original research, [and] to promote cooperation among occupational therapy societies and with other agencies of rehabilitation."

About 3 years after its incorporation, the association was urged by several leading physicians and authorities on hospital administration to establish a national register or directory of occupational therapists "for the protection of hospitals and institutions from unqualified persons posing as occupational therapists."

After careful consideration and on the advice of other national organizations in the field of medicine, the Association decided that the first step toward the establishment of a national register or directory was the establishment of minimum standards of training for occupational therapists.

In 1921, the name of the Association was changed to the American Occupational Therapy Association (AOTA). In 1923, accreditation of educational programs became a stated function of the American Occupational Therapy Association, and basic educational standards were developed.

AOTA approached the Council on Medical Education of the American Medical Association in 1933 to request cooperation in the development and improvement of educational programs for occupational therapists.

The *Essentials of an Acceptable School of Occupational Therapy* were adopted the AMA House of Delegates in 1935. This action represented the first cooperative accreditation activity by the AMA.

In 1958, AOTA assumed responsibility for approval of educational programs for the occupational therapy assistant. The standards on which accreditation was based were modeled after the *Essentials* established for baccalaureate programs.

In 1964, the AOTA/AMA collaborative relationship in accreditation was officially recognized by the National Commission on Accrediting (NCA). The NCA was a private agency serving as a coordinating agency for accrediting activities in higher education. Although it had no legal authority, it had great influence on educational accreditation through the listing of accrediting agencies it recommended to its members. The NCA continued its activities in merger with the Federation of Regional Accrediting Commissions of Higher Education since January 1975. The new organization was the Council on Postsecondary Accreditation (COPA).

In 1990, AOTA petitioned the Committee on Allied Health Education and Accreditation (CAHEA) to include the accreditation of the occupational therapy assistant programs in the CAHEA system. Following approval of the change by the AMA Council on Medical Education, CAHEA petitioned both COPA and the US Department of Education (ED) for recognition as the accrediting body for occupational therapy assistant education.

In 1991, occupational therapy assistant programs with approval status from the AOTA Accreditation Committee became accredited by CAHEA/AMA in collaboration with the AOTA Accreditation Committee.

On January 1, 1994, the AOTA Accreditation Committee changed its name to the AOTA Accreditation Council for Occupational Therapy Education (ACOTE) and became operational as an accrediting agency independent of CAHEA/AMA.

During 1994, the ACOTE became listed by the ED as a nationally recognized accrediting agency for professional programs in the field of occupational therapy. The ACOTE was also granted initial recognition by the Commission on Recognition of Postsecondary Accreditation (CORPA). CORPA is the nongovernmental recognition agency for accrediting bodies that was formed when the Council on Postsecondary Accreditation (COPA) dissolved in 1994.

On March 1, 1994, 197 previously accredited/approved and developing occupational therapy and occupational therapy assistant educational programs were transferred into the ACOTE accreditation system.

In a ballot election concluded October 31, 1994, the AOTA membership approved the proposed AOTA Bylaws Amendment that reflected the creation of AOTAs new accrediting body and establishment of the ACOTE as a standing committee of the AOTA Executive Board.

Occupational Therapist

Occupational Description

Occupational therapy is the use of purposeful activity and interventions to achieve functional outcomes to maximize the independence and the maintenance of health of any individual who is limited by a physical injury or illness, a cognitive impairment, a psychosocial dysfunction, a mental illness, a developmental or learning disability, or an adverse environmental condition.

Job Description

Occupational therapy services are based on assessment methods, including the use of skilled observation or the administration and interpretation of standardized or nonstandardized tests and measurements to identify areas for occupational therapy services.

Occupational therapy services include, but are not limited to, the assessment, treatment, and education of, or consultation with, the individual, family, or other persons; interventions directed toward developing daily living skills, work readiness or work performance, play skills or leisure capacities, or enhancing educational performances skills; or providing for the development of sensory-motor, perceptual or neuromuscular functioning, or range of motion, or emotional, motivational, cognitive, or psychosocial components of performance.

Occupational therapy services may require assessment of the need for and use of interventions such as the design, development, adaptation, application, or training in the use of assistive technology devices; the design, fabrication, or application of rehabilitative technology such as selected orthotic devices; training in the use of assistive technology and orthotic or prosthetic devices; the application of physical agent modalities as an adjunct to or in preparation for purposeful activity; the use of ergonomic principles; the adaptation of environments and processes to enhance functional performance; or the promotion of health and wellness.

Employment Characteristics

The wide population served by occupational therapists is located in a variety of settings, such as hospitals, clinics, rehabilitation facilities, long-term care facilities, extended care facilities, schools, camps, and the patients' own homes. Occupational therapists both receive referrals from and make referrals to the appropriate health, educational, or medical specialists.

AOTA studies indicate that the average entry-level salary in 1995 for occupational therapists was $38,300.

Educational Programs

Length. Programs at the baccalaureate level entail 4 years of college or university preparation. Postbaccalaureate programs leading to a certificate or master's degree are generally 2 years. Following completion of all educational requirements, individuals take a national certification examination. Many states also regulate the practice of occupational therapy.

Prerequisites. Applicants to baccalaureate programs should have a high school diploma or equivalent. A baccalaureate degree is a prerequisite for postbaccalaureate occupational therapy programs.

Curriculum. Curricula of accredited programs are required to include basic human sciences, the human development process, specific life tasks and activities, health and illness, and occupational therapy theory and practice, which includes a minimum of 6 months of supervised field experiences. The education of the occupational therapist is broadly based in human anatomy and physiology, behavioral sciences such as psychology and sociology, humanities and the arts, specialized professional subjects, and field work experience.

Standards. *Essentials*, revised in 1991 and updated in 1995, are the minimum educational standards adopted by AOTA's ACOTE. Each new program is assessed in accordance with the *Essentials*, and accredited programs are periodically reviewed to determine whether they remain in substantial compliance. The *Essentials and Guidelines* are available on written request from the AOTA Accreditation Department (address below).

Occupational Therapy Assistant

Occupational Description

Under the direction of an occupational therapist, the occupational therapy assistant directs an individual's participation in selected tasks to restore, reinforce, and enhance performance; to facilitate learning of those skills and functions essential for adaptation and productivity; to diminish or correct pathology; and to promote and maintain health. The occupational orientation of the assistant is that of guiding the individual's goal-directed use of time, energy, interest, and attention. A fundamental concern is the development and maintenance of the capacity throughout the life span to perform with satisfaction to self and others those tasks and roles essential to productive living and to the mastery of self and the environment.

Under the therapist's direction, the assistant participates in the development of adaptive skills and performance capacity and is concerned with factors that promote, influence, or enhance performance, as well as those that serve as barriers or impediments to the individual's ability to function. The occupational therapy assistant provides service to those individuals whose abilities to cope with tasks of living are threatened or impaired by developmental deficits, the aging process, poverty and cultural differences, physical injury or illness, or psychological and social disability.

Job Description

Entry-level occupational therapy assistant technical education prepares the individual to:
1. Collaborate in providing occupational therapy services with appropriate supervision to prevent deficits and to maintain or improve functions in the activities of daily living, work, and play/leisure and in the underlying components, including sensorimotor, cognitive, and psychosocial.
2. Participate in managing occupational therapy service.
3. Direct activity programs.
4. Incorporate values and attitudes congruent with the profession's standards and ethics.

Employment Characteristics

COTAs assist in the planning and implementation of treatment of a diverse population in a variety of settings such as nursing homes, hospitals and clinics, rehabilitation facilities, long-term care facilities, extended care facilities, sheltered workshops, schools and camps, private homes, and community agencies. AOTA studies indicate that the average entry-level salary in 1995 for certified occupational therapy assistants was $27,400.

Educational Programs

Length. Education may be acquired in either a 2-year associate degree program or a 1-year certificate program. These technical-level education programs are located in 2-year and 4-year colleges and universities, medical schools, and postsecondary vocational/technical schools and institutions and include academic and field work components, as do the professional level programs. Following completion of all educational requirements, individuals take a national certification examination. Many states also regulate the practice of occupational therapy.

Prerequisites. High school diploma or equivalent. A foundation of liberal arts, sciences, and technical education, as well as biological, behavioral, and health sciences, may be prerequisite to, or concurrent with, the technical education of the program curriculum.

Curriculum. Curricula of accredited programs are required to include normal and abnormal conditions across the life span, occupational therapy principles and practice skills, the occupational therapy process, treatment planning, implementation of skills and knowledge, documentation of services, management assistive services, direction of program activity, and field work education (Levels I and II).

Standards. *Essentials*, revised in 1991 and updated in 1995, are the minimum educational standards adopted by AOTA's ACOTE. Each new program is assessed in accordance with the *Essentials*, and accredited programs are periodically reviewed to determine whether they remain in substantial compliance. The *Essentials and Guidelines* are available on written request from the AOTA Accreditation Department (address below).

Inquiries

Accreditation

Requests for information on program accreditation, including the *Essentials*, preparing the self-study report, and arranging a site visit, should be submitted to

Director, Accreditation Department
American Occupational Therapy Association
4720 Montgomery Ln
PO Box 31220
Bethesda, MD 20824-1220
301 652-2682

Careers

Inquiries regarding careers should be addressed to

Public Relations Department
American Occupational Therapy Association
4720 Montgomery Ln
PO Box 31220
Bethesda, MD 20824-1220
301 652-2682

Certification

Inquiries regarding certification may be addressed to

National Board for Certification in Occupational Therapy (NBCOT)
800 S Frederick Ave/Ste 200
Gaithersburg, MD 20877-4150
301 990-7979
E-mail: NatBdCrtOT@AOL.COM

Occupational Therapist

Alabama

University of Alabama at Birmingham

Occupational Therapist Prgm
1714 Ninth Ave S/Rm 237
Birmingham, AL 35294-1270
Prgm Dir: Carroline F Amari, MA OTR/L FAOTA
Tel: 205 934-3568   *Fax:* 205 975-7302
E-mail: amaric@admin.shrp.uab.edu
Class Cap: 30   *Begins:* Sep
Length: 24 mos   *Award:* Cert, BS
Tuition per yr: $3,840 res, $6,160 non-res
Evening or weekend classes available

University of South Alabama

Occupational Therapist Prgm
Springhill Academic Campus/Rm 5108
1504 Springhill Ave
Mobile, AL 36604
Prgm Dir: Marjorie E Scaffa, PhD OTR
Tel: 334 434-3939   *Fax:* 334 434-3934
E-mail: mscaffa@jaguar1.usouthal.edu
Class Cap: 30   *Begins:* Jun
Length: 20 mos   *Award:* BS
Tuition per yr: $5,579 res, $7,679 non-res

Tuskegee University

Occupational Therapist Prgm
School of Nursing
Dept of Allied Health
Tuskegee, AL 36088-1696
Prgm Dir: Marie Moore Lyles, MS OTR/L FAOTA
Tel: 334 727-8696   *Fax:* 334 727-5461
Class Cap: 20   *Begins:* Jun Sep
Length: 24 mos   *Award:* BS
Tuition per yr: $9,876 res, $9,876 non-res

Arkansas

University of Central Arkansas

Occupational Therapist Prgm
201 Donaghey Ave HSC Ste 300
Box 5001
Conway, AR 72035-0001
Prgm Dir: Linda D Shalik, PhD OTR/L
Tel: 501 450-3192   *Fax:* 501 450-5503
E-mail: lindas@cci.uca.edu
Class Cap: 48   *Begins:* Jun
Length: 25 mos   *Award:* BS
Tuition per yr: $2,392 res, $4,364 non-res

California

Loma Linda University

Occupational Therapist Prgm
Sch of Allied Hlth Prof
Nichol Hall, Rm 903
Loma Linda, CA 92350-0001
Prgm Dir: Lynn M Arrateig, MA OTR
Tel: 909 824-4628   *Fax:* 909 824-4291
E-mail: arrateig@ccmail.llu.edu
Begins: June
Length: 24 mos   *Award:* BS
Tuition per yr: $15,330 res, $15,330 non-res

University of Southern California

Occupational Therapist Prgm
1540 Alcazar/CHP 133
Los Angeles, CA 90033-1091
Prgm Dir: Florence A Clark, PhD OTR FAOTA
Tel: 213 342-2850   *Fax:* 213 342-1540
E-mail: otdept@usc.edu
Class Cap: 120   *Begins:* Jun Sep
Length: 17 mos, 30 mos   *Award:* BS, MA
Tuition per yr: $19,140 res, $19,140 non-res

Samuel Merritt College

Occupational Therapist Prgm
370 Hawthorne Ave
Oakland, CA 94609-3108
Prgm Dir: Guy L McCormack, MS OTR
Tel: 510 869-8023   *Fax:* 510 869-6282
Med Dir: Thomas P Forde, MD
Class Cap: 44   *Begins:* Sep
Length: 27 mos   *Award:* MOT
Tuition per yr: $19,200 res, $19,200 non-res

San Jose State University

Occupational Therapist Prgm
Coll of Applied Sciences and Arts
One Washington Square
San Jose, CA 95192-0059
Prgm Dir: Kay Schwartz, EdD OTR FAOTA
Tel: 408 924-3070   *Fax:* 408 924-3088
E-mail: kschwart@sjsuvm1.sjsu.edu
Begins: Aug Jan
Length: 54 mos   *Award:* BS
Tuition per yr: $1,632 res, $9,504 non-res

Colorado

Colorado State University

Occupational Therapist Prgm
228 Occupational Therapy Bldg
Ft Collins, CO 80523
Prgm Dir: Elnora M Gilfoyle, OTR FAOTA
Tel: 970 491-6253   *Fax:* 970 491-6290
E-mail: gilfoyle@cahs.colostate.edu
Class Cap: 90   *Begins:* Aug Jan
Length: 42 mos, 24 mos   *Award:* BS, MS
Tuition per yr: $2,855 res, $9,791 non-res
Evening or weekend classes available

Connecticut

Quinnipiac College

Occupational Therapist Prgm
Sch of Health Sciences
Hamden, CT 06518
Prgm Dir: Kimberly D Hartmann, MHS OTR/L
   FAOTA
Tel: 203 281-8679   *Fax:* 203 281-8706
E-mail: hartmann@quinnipiac.edu
Class Cap: 400   *Begins:* Sep
Length: 44 mos   *Award:* Cert, BS
Tuition per yr: $12,800
Evening or weekend classes available

University of Hartford

Occupational Therapist Prgm
College of Educ, Nursing, & Health
200 Bloomfield Ave
Dana Hall Rm 232
West Hartford, CT 06117-1599
Prgm Dir: Betsey C Smith, MS OTR/L
Tel: 860 768-4831   *Fax:* 860 768-5244
E-mail: bsmith@uhavax.hartford.edu
Class Cap: 40   *Begins:* Sep
Length: 24 mos   *Award:* BS
Tuition per yr: $15,600
Evening or weekend classes available

District of Columbia

Howard University

Occupational Therapist Prgm
College of Allied Health Science
Sixth and Bryant Sts NW
Washington, DC 20059-0001
Prgm Dir: Shirley Jackson, MS OTR/L
Tel: 202 806-7614   *Fax:* 202 806-7918
Class Cap: 35   *Begins:* Aug
Length: 21 mos   *Award:* BS
Tuition per yr: $10,000

Florida

Nova Southeastern University

Occupational Therapist Prgm
Health Profs Div/Coll of Allied Health
3200 S University Dr
Ft Lauderdale, FL 33328
Prgm Dir: Reba L Anderson, PhD OTR FAOTA
Tel: 954 423-1242   *Fax:* 954 916-2290
E-mail: reba@hpd.acast.nova.edu
Class Cap: 100   *Begins:* Jun
Length: 30 mos   *Award:* MOT
Tuition per yr: $15,500 res, $17,500 non-res

University of Florida

Occupational Therapist Prgm
PO Box 100164 JHMHC
Gainesville, FL 32610-0164
Prgm Dir: Julia Van Deusen, PhD OTR
Tel: 352 392-2617   *Fax:* 352 846-1042
Med Dir: David R Challoner, MD
Class Cap: 60   *Begins:* Aug
Length: 24 mos   *Award:* Dipl, BHS
Tuition per yr: $1,793 res, $4,995 non-res

Florida International University

Occupational Therapist Prgm
University Park Campus
CH101
Miami, FL 33199
Prgm Dir: Pamela K Shaffner, MS OTR/L
Tel: 305 348-3105   *Fax:* 305 348-1240
E-mail: shaffner@fiu.edu
Class Cap: 50   *Begins:* Aug Jun
Length: 25 mos, 36 mos   *Award:* Cert, BS
Tuition per yr: $1,898 res, $7,496 non-res

Barry University

Occupational Therapist Prgm
11300 NE 2nd Ave
Miami Shores, FL 33161-6695
Prgm Dir: Douglas Mitchell, MS OTR/L
Tel: 305 899-3213   *Fax:* 305 899-2958
Class Cap: 35   *Begins:* Aug
Length: 36 mos   *Award:* BS
Tuition per yr: $8,100
Evening or weekend classes available

Florida A & M University

Occupational Therapist Prgm
Div of Occupational Therapy
223 Ware-Rhaney Bldg
Tallahassee, FL 32307
Prgm Dir: Brian Gibbs, PhD OTR/L
Tel: 904 561-2014   *Fax:* 904 561-2457
E-mail: jbeck@nsi.famu.edu
Class Cap: 34   *Begins:* Aug
Length: 48 mos   *Award:* BS
Tuition per yr: $2,180 res, $8,226 non-res

Georgia

Medical College of Georgia

Occupational Therapist Prgm
Sch of Allied Health
EF 102
Augusta, GA 30912-0700
Prgm Dir: Ricardo C Carrasco, PhD OTR/L FAOTA
Tel: 706 721-3641   *Fax:* 706 721-9718
E-mail: roarrasc@mail.mcg.edu
Begins: Sep
Length: 24 mos   *Award:* Dipl, BS
Tuition per yr: $2,780

Illinois

Chicago State University

Occupational Therapist Prgm
9501 S King Dr
Chicago, IL 60628-1598
Prgm Dir: Kuzhilethu K Kshepakaran, MEd OTR
Tel: 773 995-2366   *Fax:* 773 995-2839
Class Cap: 30   *Begins:* Jun
Length: 24 mos, 36 mos   *Award:* BS
Tuition per yr: $2,972 res, $7,859 non-res
Evening or weekend classes available

Rush University

Occupational Therapist Prgm
1653 W Harrison St
Chicago, IL 60612-3833
Prgm Dir: Marlene Morgan, MOT OTR/L
Tel: 312 942-7138   *Fax:* 312 942-6989
E-mail: mmorgan@rpslm.edu
Class Cap: 25   *Begins:* Jun
Length: 27 mos   *Award:* MS
Tuition per yr: $15,288 res, $15,288 non-res

Univ of Illinois at Chicago

Occupational Therapist Prgm
Coll of Associated Health Profs
1919 W Taylor St M/C 811
Chicago, IL 60612
Prgm Dir: Gary Kielhofner, DrPH OTR/L FAOTA
Tel: 312 996-6901   *Fax:* 312 413-0256
E-mail: Kielhfnr@uic.edu
Class Cap: 56   *Begins:* Aug
Length: 22 mos, 28 mos   *Award:* BS, MS
Tuition per yr: $5,124 res, $12,300 non-res

Indiana

University of Southern Indiana

Occupational Therapist Prgm
8600 University Blvd
Evansville, IN 47712-3534
Prgm Dir: Aimee J Luebben, MS OTR FAOTA
Tel: 812 465-1179   *Fax:* 812 465-7092
E-mail: aluebben.ucs@smtp.usi.edu
Class Cap: 30   *Begins:* Jul
Length: 22 mos   *Award:* BS
Tuition per yr: $2,424
Evening or weekend classes available

Indiana University School of Medicine

Occupational Therapist Prgm
1140 W Michigan St
Coleman Hall 311
Indianapolis, IN 46202-5119
Prgm Dir: Celestine Hamant, MS OTR FAOTA
Tel: 317 274-8006   *Fax:* 317 274-2150
E-mail: chamant@indyunix.iupui.edu
Class Cap: 50   *Begins:* Aug
Length: 20 mos   *Award:* BS, MS
Tuition per yr: $3,030 res, $9,300 non-res

University of Indianapolis

Occupational Therapist Prgm
1400 E Hanna Ave
Indianapolis, IN 46227-3697
Prgm Dir: Penelope A Moyers, EdD OTR CHT
Tel: 317 788-3432   *Fax:* 317 788-3480
E-mail: moyers@gandlf.uindy.edu
Class Cap: 52   *Begins:* Aug
Length: 30 mos   *Award:* MS
Tuition per yr: $15,000 res, $15,000 non-res
Evening or weekend classes available

Iowa

St Ambrose University

Occupational Therapist Prgm
518 W Locust
Davenport, IA 52803
Prgm Dir: Theresa Lyn Schlabach, MA OTR/L
    BCPOT
Tel: 319 333-6279   *Fax:* 319 333-6243
E-mail: tschlabh@saunix.sau.edu
Class Cap: 50   *Begins:* Jun
Length: 26 mos   *Award:* Dipl, BSOT
Tuition per yr: $11,180

Kansas

University of Kansas Medical Center

Occupational Therapist Prgm
3033 Robinson
3901 Rainbow Blvd
Kansas City, KS 66160-7602
Prgm Dir: Winnie Dunn, PhD OTR FAOTA
Tel: 913 588-7195   *Fax:* 913 588-4568
E-mail: wdunn@kumc.edu
Class Cap: 48   *Begins:* Jun
Length: 33 mos, 45 mos   *Award:* BS, MS
Evening or weekend classes available

Kansas Newman College

Occupational Therapist Prgm
3100 McCormick Ave
Wichita, KS 67213-2097
Prgm Dir: Diane Overstreet, MOT OTR
Tel: 316 942-4291   *Fax:* 316 942-4483
E-mail: overstreet@ksnewman.edu
Class Cap: 30   *Begins:* Aug
Length: 30 mos   *Award:* BS
Tuition per yr: $8,500

Kentucky

Eastern Kentucky University

Occupational Therapist Prgm
Dizney 103
Richmond, KY 40475-3135
Prgm Dir: Linda Martin, MS
Tel: 606 622-3300   *Fax:* 606 622-1140
E-mail: otsmarti@acs.eku.edu
Begins: Jan Aug July
Length: 24 mos, 36 mos   *Award:* Cert, BS, MS
Tuition per yr: $1,970 res, $5,450 non-res
Evening or weekend classes available

Louisiana

Northeast Louisiana University

Occupational Therapist Prgm
Monroe, LA 71209-0430
Prgm Dir: Kathryn H Davis, MA L/OTR
Tel: 318 342-1610   *Fax:* 318 342-1687
Class Cap: 30   *Begins:* Aug
Length: 46 mos   *Award:* Dipl, BS
Tuition per yr: $1,925 res, $4,326 non-res
Evening or weekend classes available

Louisiana State Univ Med Ctr - New Orleans
Occupational Therapist Prgm
Sch of Allied Health Professions
1900 Gravier St
New Orleans, LA 70112-2223
Prgm Dir: M Suzanne Poulton, MHS L/OTR
Tel: 504 568-4301   *Fax:* 504 568-4249
E-mail: spoult@lsumc.edu
Begins: Jun
Length: 26 mos   *Award:* BS
Tuition per yr: $3,359 res, $6,484 non-res

Maine

University of New England
Occupational Therapist Prgm
College of Arts and Sciences
Biddeford, ME 04005-9599
Prgm Dir: Judith G Kimball, PhD OTR/L FAOTA
Tel: 207 283-0171   *Fax:* 207 282-6379
E-mail: jgk@mailbox.une.edu
Class Cap: 52   *Begins:* Sep
Length: 48 mos   *Award:* BS
Tuition per yr: $13,050

University of Southern Maine
Occupational Therapist Prgm
Lewiston-Auburn College
51 Westminster St
Lewiston, ME 04240-3534
Prgm Dir: Yvette Hatchel, JD MEd OTR/L
Tel: 207 753-6584   *Fax:* 207 754-6555
E-mail: hachtel@maine.maine.edu
Class Cap: 24   *Begins:* Sep
Length: 27 mos   *Award:* MOT
Tuition per yr: $5,486 res, $15,525 non-res

Maryland

Towson State University
Occupational Therapist Prgm
Towson, MD 21252-7097
Prgm Dir: Charlotte E Exner, PhD OTR/L FAOTA
Tel: 410 830-2762   *Fax:* 410 830-2322
E-mail: exner-c@midget,towson.edu
Begins: Sep Jan
Length: 34 mos, 38 mos   *Award:* BS, MS

Massachusetts

Boston University
Occupational Therapist Prgm
Sargent Coll Allied Hlth & Rehab Profs
635 Commonwealth Ave
Boston, MA 02215
Prgm Dir: Elsie R Vergara, ScD OTR FAOTA
Tel: 617 353-2727   *Fax:* 617 353-7500
E-mail: evergara@bu.edu
Med Dir: Richard H Egdahl, MD PhD
Class Cap: 45   *Begins:* Sep
Length: 30 mos, 54 mos   *Award:* BS, MS
Tuition per yr: $20,570 res, $20,570 non-res
Evening or weekend classes available

Tufts University
Occupational Therapist Prgm
26 Winthrop St
Medford, MA 02155-7084
Prgm Dir: Sharan L Schwartzberg, EdD OTR
   FAOTA
Tel: 617 627-3720   *Fax:* 617 627-3722
E-mail: sschwart@pearl.tufts.edu
Class Cap: 60   *Begins:* Sep
Length: 18 mos   *Award:* MA, MS
Tuition per yr: $16,427

Springfield College
Occupational Therapist Prgm
263 Alden St
Springfield, MA 01109-3797
Prgm Dir: Katherine M Post, MS OTR/L FAOTA
Tel: 413 748-3762   *Fax:* 413 748-3796
Class Cap: 45   *Begins:* Sep
Length: 23 mos, 28 mos   *Award:* MEd , MS
Tuition per yr: $17,056
Evening or weekend classes available

Worcester State College
Occupational Therapist Prgm
486 Chandler St
Worcester, MA 01602-2597
Prgm Dir: Donna M Joss, EdD OTR/L
Tel: 508 793-8119   *Fax:* 508 793-8192
E-mail: djoss@worc.mass.edu
Class Cap: 60   *Begins:* Sep Jan
Length: 22 mos, 38 mos   *Award:* BS
Tuition per yr: $1,408 res, $5,542 non-res
Evening or weekend classes available

Michigan

Wayne State University
Occupational Therapist Prgm
Coll of Pharmacy and Allied Hlth Profs
Detroit, MI 48202-3489
Prgm Dir: Susan A Esdaile, PhD SROT
Tel: 313 577-5877   *Fax:* 313 577-5822
E-mail: sesdail@cms.cc.wayne.edu
Class Cap: 45   *Begins:* May
Length: 32 mos, 54 mos   *Award:* Cert, BS
Tuition per yr: $3,245 res, $6,685 non-res

Baker College
Occupational Therapist Prgm
G 1050 W Bristol Rd
Flint, MI 48507-5508
Prgm Dir: Darrell Hagen, MA OTR
Tel: 810 766-4192   *Fax:* 810 766-4049
E-mail: hagen_d@flint.baker.edu
Class Cap: 47   *Begins:* Apr
Length: 50 mos   *Award:* BOT
Tuition per yr: $6,630 res, $6,630 non-res
Evening or weekend classes available

Western Michigan University
Occupational Therapist Prgm
Kalamazoo, MI 49008-5051
Prgm Dir: Susan K Meyers, EdD OTR
Tel: 616 387-3850   *Fax:* 616 387-3845
E-mail: susan.meyers@wmich.edu
Class Cap: 64   *Begins:* Sep Jan
Length: 28 mos   *Award:* Dipl, BS
Tuition per yr: $3,622 res, $8,317 non-res

Saginaw Valley State University
Occupational Therapist Prgm
Ryder Ctr W Rm 105
7400 Bay Rd
University Center, MI 48710-0001
Prgm Dir: Alfred G Bracciano, EdD OTR
Tel: 517 791-7355   *Fax:* 517 790-0545
E-mail: bracc@tardis.svsu.edu
Class Cap: 38   *Begins:* Apr
Length: 48 mos   *Award:* BSOT
Tuition per yr: $3,242 res, $23,882 non-res

Eastern Michigan University
Occupational Therapist Prgm
Dept of Assoiciated Health Professions
328 King Hall
Ypsilanti, MI 48197-2239
Prgm Dir: Virginia A Dickie, PhD OTR FAOTA
Tel: 313 487-0461   Fax: 313 487-4095
E-mail: virginia.dickie@emich.edu
Class Cap: 250   *Begins:* Jan Sep
Length: 30 mos   *Award:* BS
Tuition per yr: $2,295 res, $5,880 non-res

Minnesota

College of St Scholastica
Occupational Therapist Prgm
1200 Kenwood Ave
Duluth, MN 55811
Prgm Dir: Thomas H Dillon, MA OTR
Tel: 218 723-6698   *Fax:* 218 723-6472
E-mail: tdillon@fac1.css.edu
Class Cap: 30   *Begins:* Sep
Length: 28 mos   *Award:* , MA
Tuition per yr: $14,016
Evening or weekend classes available

Univ of Minnesota Hosp and Clinic
Occupational Therapist Prgm
Box 388 UMHC
420 Delaware St SE
Minneapolis, MN 55455-0392
Prgm Dir: Judith Reisman, PhD OTR FAOTA
Tel: 612 626-4358   *Fax:* 612 625-7192
E-mail: reism001@maroon.tc.umn.edu
Med Dir: Dennis Dykstra, MD PhD
Class Cap: 35   *Begins:* Sep
Length: 39 mos   *Award:* BS
Tuition per yr: $4,992 res, $13,457 non-res

College of St Catherine
Occupational Therapist Prgm
2004 Randolph Ave
St Paul, MN 55105-1794
Prgm Dir: Julie Bass Haugen, PhD OTR
Tel: 612 690-6602   *Fax:* 612 690-6024
E-mail: jobhaugen@alex.stkate.edu
Begins: Sep
Length: 27 mos   *Award:* Cert, BA
Tuition per yr: $12,224
Evening or weekend classes available

Mississippi

University of Mississippi Medical Center

Occupational Therapist Prgm
School of Health Related Profs
2500 N State St
Jackson, MS 39216-4505
Prgm Dir: Bette A Groat, MA OTR/L
Tel: 601 984-6350 *Fax:* 601 984-6344
E-mail: groat@shrp.umsmed.edu
Class Cap: 28 *Begins:* Jun
Length: 24 mos *Award:* BS
Tuition per yr: $2,935 res, $5,730 non-res

Missouri

University of Missouri - Columbia

Occupational Therapist Prgm
School of Health Related Profs
126 Lewis Hall
Columbia, MO 65211
Prgm Dir: Diana J Baldwin, MA OTR/L FAOTA
Tel: 573 882-3988 Fax: 573 884-8369
E-mail: baldwind@ext.missouri.edu
Class Cap: 80 *Begins:* Jun
Length: 30 mos *Award:* BHS
Tuition per yr: $4,329 res, $12,940 non-res

Rockhurst College

Occupational Therapist Prgm
College of Arts and Sciences
1100 Rockhurst Rd
Kansas City, MO 64110-2561
Prgm Dir: Jane P Rues, EdD OTR
Tel: 816 501-4635 *Fax:* 816 501-4169
E-mail: rues@vaxl.rockhurst.edu
Class Cap: 36 *Begins:* Aug
Length: 36 mos, 48 mos *Award:* Dipl, MOT
Tuition per yr: $6,175

St Louis University Health Sciences Ctr

Occupational Therapist Prgm
1755 S Grand Blvd Rm 427
St Louis, MO 63104-1395
Prgm Dir: Shirley K Behr, PhD OTR
Tel: 314 577-8514 *Fax:* 314 268-5414
E-mail: behrsk@sluvca.slu.edu
Class Cap: 40 *Begins:* Aug
Length: 30 mos, 40 mos *Award:* BS
Tuition per yr: $13,900
Evening or weekend classes available

Washington University

Occupational Therapist Prgm
4444 Forest Park Ave
St Louis, MO 63108
Prgm Dir: M Carolyn Baum, PhD OTR/C FAOTA
Tel: 314 286-1600 Fax: 314 286-1601
Class Cap: 200 *Begins:* Aug
Length: 28 mos *Award:* BSOT , MSOT
Tuition per yr: $17,500

Nebraska

Creighton University

Occupational Therapist Prgm
Sch of Pharmacy and Allied Health
2500 California Plaza
Omaha, NE 68178-0259
Prgm Dir: Claudia Peyton, MS OTR/L
Tel: 402 280-1856 *Fax:* 402 280-5692
E-mail: crunyon@creighton.edu
Class Cap: 60 *Begins:* Aug Jan May
Length: 24 mos, 20 mos *Award:* Dipl, BS
Tuition per yr: $18,000
Evening or weekend classes available

New Hampshire

University of New Hampshire

Occupational Therapist Prgm
Sch of Health and Human Services
Hewitt Hall/4 Library Way
Durham, NH 03824-3563
Prgm Dir: Alice Seidel, EdD OTR/L
Tel: 603 862-2167 *Fax:* 603 862-0778
E-mail: acseidel@christa.unh.edu
Class Cap: 55 *Begins:* Sep
Length: 18 mos, 36 mos *Award:* Cert, BS
Tuition per yr: $3,870 res, $12,540 non-res

New Jersey

Kean College of New Jersey

Occupational Therapist Prgm
Willis 311 Morris Ave
Union, NJ 07083-9982
Prgm Dir: Karen Stern, EdD OTR
Tel: 908 527-2590 *Fax:* 908 354-2746
E-mail: kstern@turbo.kean.edu
Class Cap: 30 *Begins:* Sep
Length: 30 mos *Award:* Cert, BS
Tuition per yr: $3,089 res, $4,288 non-res
Evening or weekend classes available

New Mexico

University of New Mexico

Occupational Therapist Prgm
Sch of Medicine
Hlth Sci & Serv Bldg Rm 215
Albuquerque, NM 87131-5641
Prgm Dir: Terry K Crowe, PhD OTR/L
Tel: 505 277-1753 *Fax:* 505 277-7011
E-mail: tkcrowe@unm.edu
Class Cap: 24 *Begins:* Jun
Length: 30 mos *Award:* Dipl, BS
Tuition per yr: $2,475 res, $8,291 non-res

New York

SUNY Health Science Center - Brooklyn

Occupational Therapist Prgm
450 Clarkson Ave Box 81
Brooklyn, NY 11203-2098
Prgm Dir: Patricia B Trossman, EdD OTR FAOTA
Tel: 718 270-7731 *Fax:* 718 270-7751
E-mail: ptrossman@netmail.hscbklyn.edu
Class Cap: 33 *Begins:* May
Length: 33 mos, 45 mos *Award:* BS
Tuition per yr: $3,490 res, $3,490 non-res

D'Youville College

Occupational Therapist Prgm
320 Porter Ave
Buffalo, NY 14201-1084
Prgm Dir: Onda Bennett, MS OTR
Tel: 716 881-7624 *Fax:* 716 881-7790
Class Cap: 70 *Begins:* Sep Jan
Length: 60 mos *Award:* Comb BS/MS
Tuition per yr: $9,690
Evening or weekend classes available

SUNY at Buffalo

Occupational Therapist Prgm
515 Stockton Kimball Tower
3435 Main St
Buffalo, NY 14214-3079
Prgm Dir: William C Mann, PhD OTR
Tel: 716 829-3141 *Fax:* 716 829-3217
E-mail: wmann@acsu.buffalo.edu
Class Cap: 50 *Begins:* Jun
Length: 24 mos *Award:* BS
Tuition per yr: $3,400 res, $8,300 non-res
Evening or weekend classes available

Touro College

Occupational Therapist Prgm
135 Carman Rd/Bldg 10
Dix Hills, NY 11746-5641
Prgm Dir: Anthony Hollander, PhD OTR/L
Tel: 516 673-3200, Ext 231 *Fax:* 516 425-9249
Class Cap: 120 *Begins:* Aug
Length: 34 mos *Award:* BS, MA
Tuition per yr: $16,100

Mercy College

Occupational Therapist Prgm
555 Broadway
Dobbs Ferry, NY 10522-1189
Prgm Dir: Joan Toglia, MA OTR/L
Tel: 914 674-9331, Ext 600 *Fax:* 914 674-9457
E-mail: jtoglia@eagle.liunet.edu
Class Cap: 30 *Begins:* Sep
Length: 26 mos *Award:* Dipl, BS, MS
Tuition per yr: $11,850 res, $11,850 non-res
Evening or weekend classes available

CUNY York College

Occupational Therapist Prgm
94-20 Guy R Brewer Blvd
Jamaica, NY 11451-9902
Prgm Dir: Ruth Kraiem, MS OTR
Tel: 718 262-2720 *Fax:* 718 262-2027
Class Cap: 40 *Begins:* Sep
Length: 32 mos *Award:* BS
Tuition per yr: $2,200 res, $4,800 non-res
Evening or weekend classes available

Keuka College

Occupational Therapist Prgm
Keuka Park, NY 14478-0098
Prgm Dir: Peter M Talty, MS OTR
Tel: 315 536-5255 *Fax:* 315 536-5216
E-mail: ptalty@mail.keuka.edu
Class Cap: 60 *Begins:* Sep
Length: 42 mos *Award:* BS
Tuition per yr: $10,490 res, $10,490 non-res
Evening or weekend classes available

Columbia University

Occupational Therapist Prgm
Neurological Institute 8th Fl
710 W 168th St
New York, NY 10032
Prgm Dir: Cynthia Hughes Harris, PhD OTR
  FAOTA
Tel: 212 305-3781 *Fax:* 212 305-4569
E-mail: harryc@cudept.cis.columbia.edu
Class Cap: 49 *Begins:* Sep
Length: 24 mos *Award:* MS
Tuition per yr: $17,970

New York University

Occupational Therapist Prgm
School of Education
35 W 4th St 11th Fl
New York, NY 10012-1172
Prgm Dir: Deborah R Labovitz, PhD OTR/L
  FAOTA
Tel: 212 998-5825 *Fax:* 212 995-4044
E-mail: labovitz@is2.nyu.edu
Class Cap: 75 *Begins:* Sep
Length: 48 mos, 30 mos *Award:* BS, MA
Evening or weekend classes available

Dominican College

Occupational Therapist Prgm
10 Western Hwy
Orangeburg, NY 10962-1299
Prgm Dir: Rita P Cottrell, MA OTR
Tel: 914 359-6449 *Fax:* 914 359-2313
Class Cap: 60 *Begins:* Sep Jan
Length: 22 mos *Award:* Dipl, BS
Tuition per yr: $8,775
Evening or weekend classes available

SUNY Health Science Ctr at Stony Brook

Occupational Therapist Prgm
Sch of Health Technology and Mgmt/L2-031
Div of Rehabilitation Sciences
Stony Brook, NY 11794-8201
Prgm Dir: Roger Fleming, MPA MA OTR/L
Tel: 516 444-8160 *Fax:* 516 444-7621
Class Cap: 25 *Begins:* Jul
Length: 20 mos *Award:* BS
Tuition per yr: $3,400 res, $8,300 non-res

The Sage Colleges

Occupational Therapist Prgm
45 Ferry St
Troy, NY 12180-4115
Prgm Dir: Martha M Frank, MS OTR
Tel: 518 270-2266 *Fax:* 518 271-4545
E-mail: frankm@sage.edu
Class Cap: 40 *Begins:* Sep
Length: 36 mos *Award:* BS, MS
Tuition per yr: $17,000 res, $12,000 non-res

Utica College of Syracuse University

Occupational Therapist Prgm
Div of Health Sciences
1600 Burrstone Rd
Utica, NY 13502-4892
Prgm Dir: Nancy Hollins, MS OTR/L
Tel: 315 792-3059 Fax: 315 792-3292
E-mail: nlh@uc1.ucsu.edu
Class Cap: 60 *Begins:* Aug Sep
Length: 48 mos *Award:* BS
Tuition per yr: $14,116
Evening or weekend classes available

North Carolina

Univ of North Carolina at Chapel Hill

Occupational Therapist Prgm
Medical School Wing E, CB 7120
Chapel Hill, NC 27599-7120
Prgm Dir: Ruth Humphry, PhD OTR/L
Tel: 919 966-2451 Fax: 919 966-3678
E-mail: rhumphry@css.unc.edu
Class Cap: 24 *Begins:* Jun
Length: 26 mos *Award:* MS
Tuition per yr: $2,150 res, $10,682 non-res
Evening or weekend classes available

East Carolina University

Occupational Therapist Prgm
School of Allied Hlth Sciences
Greenville, NC 27858-4353
Prgm Dir: Anne Dickerson, PhD OTR/L
Tel: 919 328-4441 *Fax:* 919 328-4470
E-mail: otdicker@ecuvm.cls.ecu.edu
Class Cap: 36 *Begins:* May
Length: 27 mos *Award:* BS
Tuition per yr: $2,594 res, $7,648 non-res
Evening or weekend classes available

Lenoir-Rhyne College

Occupational Therapist Prgm
Box 7547
Hickory, NC 28603
Prgm Dir: Susan Stallings-Sahler, PhD OTR/L
  BCP
Tel: 704 328-7367 *Fax:* 704 328-7364
E-mail: sssahler@aol.com
Class Cap: 16 *Begins:* Aug
Length: 18 mos *Award:* BS
Tuition per yr: $7,480 res, $5,443 non-res

North Dakota

Univ of No Dakota Sch of Med and Hlth Sci

Occupational Therapist Prgm
Box 7126 University Station
Grand Forks, ND 58202-7126
Prgm Dir: Sue McIntyre, MS OTR/L
Tel: 701 777-2209 *Fax:* 701 777-2212
E-mail: smcintyr@mail.med.und.nodak.edu
Class Cap: 138 *Begins:* Aug
Length: 42 mos *Award:* BS
Tuition per yr: $2,428 res, $5,952 non-res

Ohio

Xavier University

Occupational Therapist Prgm
3800 Victory Pkwy
Cincinnati, OH 45207-7341
Prgm Dir: Judith S Bloomer, PhD OTR/L
Tel: 513 745-3150 *Fax:* 513 745-3261
E-mail: bloomer@xavier.xu.edu
Class Cap: 32 *Begins:* Aug
Length: 33 mos *Award:* Cert, BS
Tuition per yr: $12,000 res, $12,000 non-res
Evening or weekend classes available

Cleveland State University

Occupational Therapist Prgm
Euclid Ave at E 24th St
Fenn Tower 705
Cleveland, OH 44115-2440
Prgm Dir: John J Bazyk, MS OTR/L
Tel: 216 687-2379 *Fax:* 216 687-9316
E-mail: j.bazyk@csuohio.edu
Class Cap: 39 *Begins:* Jun
Length: 24 mos, 48 mos *Award:* Cert, BS
Tuition per yr: $4,308 res, $8,616 non-res

Ohio State University

Occupational Therapist Prgm
School of Allied Medical Profs
1583 Perry St
Columbus, OH 43210-1234
Prgm Dir: H Kay Grant, PhD OTR/L FAOTA
Tel: 614 292-5824 *Fax:* 614 292-0210
E-mail: grant.2@osu.edu
Class Cap: 60 *Begins:* Sep
Length: 26 mos *Award:* Cert, BS
Tuition per yr: $3,273 res, $9,813 non-res

The University of Findlay

Occupational Therapist Prgm
1000 N Main St
Findlay, OH 45840-3695
Prgm Dir: Peggy Owens, MA OTR/L FAOTA
Tel: 419 424-4863 *Fax:* 419 424-4822
E-mail: owens@lucy.findlay.edu
Class Cap: 32 *Begins:* Apr
Length: 23 mos *Award:* BS
Tuition per yr: $9,951 res, $9,951 non-res

Shawnee State University

Occupational Therapist Prgm
940 Second St
Portsmouth, OH 45662-4303
Prgm Dir: Catherine O Perry, MEd OTR/L
Tel: 614 355-2272 *Fax:* 614 355-2354
E-mail: cperry@shawnee.edu
Class Cap: 15 *Begins:* Jan
Length: 27 mos *Award:* BS
Tuition per yr: $2,976 res, $5,151 non-res
Evening or weekend classes available

Medical College of Ohio

Occupational Therapist Prgm
School of Allied Health
PO Box 10008
Toledo, OH 43699-0008
Prgm Dir: Julie J Thomas, PhD OTR/L
Tel: 419 381-4429 *Fax:* 419 381-3051
E-mail: jjthomas@opus.mco.edu
Class Cap: 20 *Begins:* Sep
Length: 27 mos *Award:* MOT
Tuition per yr: $5,280 res, $9,256 non-res
Evening or weekend classes available

Oklahoma

Univ of Oklahoma Health Sciences Center
Occupational Therapist Prgm
College of Allied Health
801 NE 13th St
Oklahoma City, OK 73190-1090
Prgm Dir: Toby B Hamilton, MPH OTR
Tel: 405 271-2411, Ext 151 *Fax:* 405 271-2432
E-mail: toby_hamilton@uokhsc.edu
Class Cap: 32 *Begins:* Aug
Length: 23 mos *Award:* BS
Tuition per yr: $2,822 res, $8,113 non-res

Oregon

Pacific University
Occupational Therapist Prgm
2043 College Way
Forest Grove, OR 97116-1797
Prgm Dir: Molly McEwen, MHS OTR/L
Tel: 503 359-2203 *Fax:* 503 359-2980
E-mail: mcewenm@pacificu.edu
Class Cap: 26 *Begins:* Sep
Length: 24 mos *Award:* Dipl, BS
Tuition per yr: $14,120

Pennsylvania

College Misericordia
Occupational Therapist Prgm
Division of Health Sciences
301 Lake St
Dallas, PA 18612-1098
Prgm Dir: Christine L Hischmann, MS OTR/L
Tel: 717 674-6413 *Fax:* 717 675-2441
E-mail: miser16@epix.net
Class Cap: 100 *Begins:* Aug
Length: 30 mos, 60 mos *Award:* BS, MS
Tuition per yr: $10,500

Elizabethtown College
Occupational Therapist Prgm
One Alpha Dr
Elizabethtown, PA 17022-2298
Prgm Dir: Jacqueline L Jones, PhD OTR/L
Tel: 717 361-1172 *Fax:* 717 361-1207
E-mail: jonesjl@acad.etown.edu
Class Cap: 40 *Begins:* Aug
Length: 44 mos *Award:* BS
Tuition per yr: $14,190

Gannon University
Occupational Therapist Prgm
University Square
Erie, PA 16541-0001
Prgm Dir: Linda M DiJoseph, MS OTR FAOTA
Tel: 814 871-7653 *Fax:* 814 871-5662
E-mail: dijoseph@cluster.gannon.edu
Class Cap: 40 *Begins:* Aug
Length: 38 mos *Award:* BSOT
Tuition per yr: $12,100 res, $12,100 non-res

Temple University
Occupational Therapist Prgm
College of Allied Hlth Profs
3307 N Broad St
Philadelphia, PA 19140
Prgm Dir: Judith M Perinchief, MS OTR/L
Tel: 215 707-4843 *Fax:* 215 707-7656
E-mail: judiep@um.temple.edu
Class Cap: 32 *Begins:* Jul
Length: 25 mos, 22 mos *Award:* Cert, BS, MS
Tuition per yr: $6,408 res, $11,340 non-res
Evening or weekend classes available

Thomas Jefferson University
Occupational Therapist Prgm
Rm 820 Edison Bldg
130 S Ninth St
Philadelphia, PA 19107-5233
Prgm Dir: Roseann C Schaaf, MEd OTR/L FAOTA
Tel: 215 503-9606 *Fax:* 215 923-2475
Class Cap: 74 *Begins:* Sep
Length: 23 mos, 28 mos *Award:* Dipl,Cert, BS, MS
Tuition per yr: $14,350 res, $14,350 non-res
Evening or weekend classes available

Chatham College
Occupational Therapist Prgm
Woodland Rd
Pittsburgh, PA 15232-2826
Prgm Dir: Eileen Henry, EdD OTR/L
Tel: 412 365-1183 Fax: 412 365-1502
E-mail: henry@chatham.edu
Class Cap: 40 *Begins:* Sep
Length: 22 mos *Award:* MOT
Tuition per yr: $6,900

Duquesne University
Occupational Therapist Prgm
Rangos Sch of Hlth Sciences
Health Sciences Bldg/Rm 227
Pittsburgh, PA 15282-0001
Prgm Dir: Patricia Crist, PhD OTR/L FAOTA
Tel: 412 396-5945 *Fax:* 412 396-5554
E-mail: crist@duq2.cc.duq.edu
Class Cap: 40 *Begins:* Aug
Length: 56 mos *Award:* MOT
Tuition per yr: $15,428 res, $15,428 non-res
Evening or weekend classes available

University of Pittsburgh
Occupational Therapist Prgm
Sch of Health and Rehab Sciences
5012 Forbes Tower
Pittsburgh, PA 15260
Prgm Dir: Jennifer Angelo, PhD OTR/L FAOTA
Tel: 412 647-1183 *Fax:* 412 647-1255
E-mail: octangel+@pitt.edu
Class Cap: 40 *Begins:* Jun
Length: 22 mos *Award:* Dipl, BS
Tuition per yr: $9,824 res, $21,048 non-res

Puerto Rico

University of Puerto Rico
Occupational Therapist Prgm
Med Sci Bldg/PT & OT Dept
PO Box 365067
San Juan, PR 00936-5067
Prgm Dir: Migdalia Morales-Berrios, MS OTR
Tel: 787 758-2525 *Fax:* 787 759-3645
Class Cap: 35 *Begins:* Aug
Length: 35 mos *Award:* BS
Tuition per yr: $1,894 res, $2,400 non-res

South Carolina

Medical University of South Carolina
Occupational Therapist Prgm
Coll of Health Profs
171 Ashley Ave/Rm 123-CHP
Charleston, SC 29425-2701
Prgm Dir: Becki A Trickey, PhD OTR/L
Tel: 803 792-2961 *Fax:* 803 492-0710
E-mail: trickeyb@musc.edu
Class Cap: 35 *Begins:* Jun
Length: 24 mos *Award:* BS
Tuition per yr: $4,401 res, $11,822 non-res

South Dakota

University of South Dakota
Occupational Therapist Prgm
414 E Clark St
Vermillion, SD 57069-2390
Prgm Dir: Dorothy Anne Elsberry, PhD OTR/L FAOTA
Tel: 605 677-5600 *Fax:* 605 677-6581
Class Cap: 26 *Begins:* Aug
Length: 28 mos *Award:* MS
Tuition per yr: $2,632 res, $7,763 non-res

Tennessee

University of Tennessee Memphis
Occupational Therapist Prgm
822 Beale St/Rm 338
Memphis, TN 38163
Prgm Dir: Ann Nolen, PsyD OTR
Tel: 901 448-8393 *Fax:* 901 448-7545
E-mail: anolen@utmem1.utmem.edu
Class Cap: 26 *Begins:* Sep
Length: 24 mos *Award:* BSOT
Tuition per yr: $2,380 res, $7,816 non-res

Tennessee State University
Occupational Therapist Prgm
Sch of Allied Hlth Profs
3500 John A Merritt Blvd
Nashville, TN 37209-1561
Prgm Dir: Rachelle D Hyman, MEd OTR
Tel: 615 963-5953 *Fax:* 615 963-5926
E-mail: hymanr@harpo.tnstate.edu
Class Cap: 35 *Begins:* May
Length: 24 mos *Award:* BS
Tuition per yr: $2,823 res, $9,054 non-res

Programs

Texas

Texas Woman's University
Occupational Therapist Prgm
Box 425648 TWU Station
Denton, TX 76204-5648
Prgm Dir: Janette Schkade, PhD OTR
Tel: 817 898-2803 *Fax:* 817 898-2486
E-mail: a_schkade@venus.twu.edu
Med Dir: Martin Grabois, MD
Class Cap: 200 *Begins:* Aug Jan Jun Jul
Length: 24 mos, 57 mos *Award:* Cert, BSMOT
Tuition per yr: $1,667 res, $6,759 non-res

University of Texas Medical Branch
Occupational Therapist Prgm
J-28/301 University Blvd
Galveston, TX 77555-1028
Prgm Dir: Jaclyn Low, PhD OTR
Tel: 409 772-3060 *Fax:* 409 747-1615
E-mail: jlow%sahs@mhost.utmb.edu
Class Cap: 40 *Begins:* Jun
Length: 24 mos *Award:* BS
Tuition per yr: $988 res, $6,156 non-res

Texas Tech Univ Hlth Sci Ctr
Occupational Therapist Prgm
School of Allied Health
3601 4th St
Lubbock, TX 79430
Prgm Dir: Kayla Cotkin, MS OTR
Tel: 806 743-3240 *Fax:* 806 743-2515
E-mail: alhkc@ttuhsc.edu
Class Cap: 60 *Begins:* Jun
Length: 27 mos *Award:* BS
Tuition per yr: $904 res, $5,904 non-res
Evening or weekend classes available

Univ of Texas Hlth Sci Ctr at San Antonio
Occupational Therapist Prgm
7703 Floyd Curl Dr
San Antonio, TX 78284-7770
Prgm Dir: Gale S Haradon, PhD OTR
Tel: 210 567-3111 *Fax:* 210 567-3114
E-mail: haradon@uthscsa.edu
Med Dir: Nicolas E Walsh, MD
Class Cap: 120 *Begins:* Jun
Length: 33 mos *Award:* BS
Tuition per yr: $1,260 res, $8,442 non-res

Virginia

Med Coll of VA/Virginia Commonwealth U
Occupational Therapist Prgm
PO Box 980008
Richmond, VA 23298-0008
Prgm Dir: Shelly J Lane, PhD OTR/L FAOTA
Tel: 804 828-2219 *Fax:* 804 828-0782
Class Cap: 32 *Begins:* Aug Jun
Length: 24 mos, 25 mos *Award:* BS, MSOT
Tuition per yr: $4,018 res, $11,633 non-res

Shenandoah University
Occupational Therapist Prgm
333 W Cork St
Winchester, VA 22601
Prgm Dir: Gretchen V M Stone, PhD OTR
Tel: 540 665-5543 *Fax:* 540 665-5564
E-mail: gstone@su.edu
Class Cap: 40 *Begins:* Aug
Length: 25 mos *Award:* Dipl, MS
Tuition per yr: $13,000
Evening or weekend classes available

Washington

University of Washington
Occupational Therapist Prgm
Dept of Rehab Medicine
Box 356490
Seattle, WA 98195
Prgm Dir: Elizabeth M Kanny, PhD OTR/L FAOTA
Tel: 206 685-7412 *Fax:* 206 685-3244
E-mail: ekanny@u.washington.edu
Class Cap: 25 *Begins:* Sep
Length: 27 mos *Award:* BS
Tuition per yr: $3,138 res, $9,753 non-res

University of Puget Sound
Occupational Therapist Prgm
School of Occupational Therapy
1500 N Warner
Tacoma, WA 98416-0510
Prgm Dir: Katherine B Stewart, MS OTR/L
Tel: 206 756-3281 *Fax:* 206 756-8309
E-mail: kbstewart@ups.edu
Class Cap: 55 *Begins:* Aug
Length: 24 mos *Award:* BS, MOT
Tuition per yr: $18,030

Wisconsin

University of Wisconsin - Madison
Occupational Therapist Prgm
1300 University Ave (2110/MSC)
Madison, WI 53706-1532
Prgm Dir: Mary L Schneider, PhD OTR
Tel: 608 262-1639 *Fax:* 608 263-6434
E-mail: schneider@soemadison.wisc.edu
Class Cap: 45 *Begins:* Sep
Length: 30 mos *Award:* Dipl, BS
Tuition per yr: $3,032 res, $10,150 non-res

Concordia University Wisconsin
Occupational Therapist Prgm
12800 N Lake Shore Dr
Mequon, WI 53097-2402
Prgm Dir: Suzanne L Floyd, MS OTR
Tel: 414 243-4278 *Fax:* 414 243-4506
E-mail: sfloyd@bach.cuw.edu
Class Cap: 24 *Begins:* Aug Jan
Length: 24 mos *Award:* BS
Tuition per yr: $5,325 res, $5,325 non-res

Mt Mary College
Occupational Therapist Prgm
2900 N Menomonee River Pkwy
Milwaukee, WI 53222-4597
Prgm Dir: Diana S Bartels, MS OTR
Tel: 414 256-1246, Ext 411 *Fax:* 414 256-1224
E-mail: bartelsd@mtmary.edu
Class Cap: 65 *Begins:* Aug
Length: 20 mos, 36 mos *Award:* BS, MS
Tuition per yr: $10,230 res, $10,230 non-res
Evening or weekend classes available

University of Wisconsin - Milwaukee
Occupational Therapist Prgm
School of Allied Health Professions
PO Box 413
Milwaukee, WI 53201-0413
Prgm Dir: Judith A Falconer, PhD OTR
Tel: 414 229-6160 *Fax:* 414 229-5100
E-mail: falconer@csd.uwm.edu
Class Cap: 125 *Begins:* Sep
Length: 20 mos *Award:* BS
Tuition per yr: $2,947 res, $9,398 non-res

Wyoming

Casper College
Occupational Therapist Prgm
125 College Dr
Casper, WY 82601
Prgm Dir: Sue McIntyre, MS OTR/L
Tel: 701 777-2209
Class Cap: 48 *Begins:* May
Length: 42 mos *Award:* BS

Occupational Therapy Assistant

Alabama

Jefferson State Community College

Occupational Therapy Asst Prgm
Pinson Valley Parkway
2601 Carson Rd
Birmingham, AL 35215-3098
Prgm Dir: Barbara Veigl, OTR/L
Tel: 205 856-6043 *Fax:* 205 856-7725
E-mail: health@jscc.ol.us
Class Cap: 16 *Begins:* Jan
Length: 24 mos *Award:* AAS
Tuition per yr: $943 res, $1,528 non-res

Wallace State College

Occupational Therapy Asst Prgm
PO Box 2000
Hanceville, AL 35077-2000
Prgm Dir: Lynn M Hazard, MA OTR/L
Tel: 205 352-8333 *Fax:* 205 352-8228
E-mail: hazard@bham.mindspring.com
Class Cap: 45 *Begins:* Sep
Length: 24 mos *Award:* AAS
Tuition per yr: $1,232 res, $2,156 non-res
Evening or weekend classes available

Arizona

Apollo College

Occupational Therapy Asst Prgm
2701 W Bethany Home Rd
Phoenix, AZ 85017-1705
Prgm Dir: Christine Merchant, OTR/L
Tel: 602 433-1333 *Fax:* 602 433-1414
Class Cap: 75 *Begins:* varies
Length: 15 mos *Award:* AAS
Tuition per yr: $6,890 res, $6,890 non-res
Evening or weekend classes available

California

Grossmont College

Occupational Therapy Asst Prgm
8800 Grossmont College Dr
El Cajon, CA 92020-1799
Prgm Dir: Marianne Maynard, PhD OTR FAOTA
Tel: 619 465-1700, Ext 304 *Fax:* 619 461-3396
Class Cap: 30 *Begins:* Jun
Length: 18 mos *Award:* AS

Loma Linda University

Occupational Therapy Asst Prgm
Sch of Allied Hlth Professions
SAHP-Nichol Hall/Rm A912
Loma Linda, CA 92350-0001
Prgm Dir: Liane Hewitt, MPH OTR
Tel: 909 824-4948 *Fax:* 909 478-4239
E-mail: lhewitt@sahp.llu.edu
Class Cap: 60 *Begins:* Sep
Length: 15 mos *Award:* AA
Tuition per yr: $10,224

Mt St Mary's College

Occupational Therapy Asst Prgm
Doheny Campus
10 Chester Pl
Los Angeles, CA 90007-2598
Prgm Dir: Elizabeth Snow, MA OTR
Tel: 213 746-0450, Ext 2221 *Fax:* 213 744-0833
Class Cap: 30 *Begins:* Sep Mar
Length: 24 mos *Award:* AA
Tuition per yr: $12,420

Sacramento City College

Occupational Therapy Asst Prgm
Allied Health Dept
3835 Freeport Blvd
Sacramento, CA 95822-1386
Prgm Dir: Susan M Hussey, MS OTR
Tel: 916 558-2297 *Fax:* 916 558-2392
E-mail: husseys@mail.scc.losrios.cc.ca.us
Class Cap: 30 *Begins:* Jan
Length: 24 mos *Award:* Dipl, AS
Tuition per yr: $117 res, $1,080 non-res
Evening or weekend classes available

Maric College of Medical Careers

Occupational Therapy Asst Prgm
(Educational Medical Inc)
3666 Kearny Villa Rd
San Diego, CA 92123
Prgm Dir: Gale Seefeld, MA OTR
Tel: 619 654-3650 *Fax:* 619 279-1620
Class Cap: 35 *Begins:* Mar Aug
Length: 12 mos *Award:* AS
Tuition per yr: $12,723 res, $12,723 non-res

Colorado

Denver Institute of Technology

Occupational Therapy Asst Prgm
7350 N Broadway
Denver, CO 80221-3653
Prgm Dir: Kelley McBride, OTR EMT
Tel: 303 650-5050, Ext 330 *Fax:* 303 426-1832
Class Cap: 60 *Begins:* Jan Apr Jul Oct
Length: 18 mos *Award:* AS
Tuition per yr: $10,995

Morgan Community College

Occupational Therapy Asst Prgm
17800 Rd 20
Ft Morgan, CO 80701-4399
Prgm Dir: Alessandra F Zapiecki, OTR
Tel: 970 867-3081 *Fax:* 970 867-6608
E-mail: s_zapiecki%mcc@cccs.cccoes.edu
Class Cap: 20 *Begins:* Jan
Length: 24 mos *Award:* AAS
Tuition per yr: $1,720 res, $7,000 non-res

Arapahoe Community College

Occupational Therapy Asst Prgm
2500 W College Dr
PO Box 9002
Littleton, CO 80160-9002
Prgm Dir: Wanda Figueroa Rosario, MS OTR
Tel: 303 797-5939 *Fax:* 303 797-5935
Class Cap: 20 *Begins:* Aug Jan
Length: 18 mos *Award:* Dipl, AAS
Tuition per yr: $1,583 res, $5,757 non-res
Evening or weekend classes available

Pueblo Community College

Occupational Therapy Asst Prgm
900 W Orman Ave
Pueblo, CO 81004-1499
Prgm Dir: Terry R Hawkins, MPH OTR FAOTA
Tel: 719 549-3268 *Fax:* 714 549-3136
E-mail: hawkins@pcc.colorado.edu
Class Cap: 30 *Begins:* Sep
Length: 21 mos *Award:* AAS
Tuition per yr: $2,081 res, $10,822 non-res
Evening or weekend classes available

Connecticut

Manchester Community - Technical College

Occupational Therapy Asst Prgm
60 Bidwell St/MS 19
PO Box 1046
Manchester, CT 06045-1046
Prgm Dir: Brenda Smaga, MS OTR/L
Tel: 860 647-6183 Fax: 860 647-6370
E-mail: ma_smaga@comnet.edu
Class Cap: 26 *Begins:* Sep Jan
Length: 24 mos *Award:* AS
Tuition per yr: $1,646 res, $4,622 non-res

Delaware

Delaware Tech & Comm Coll - Owens Campus

Occupational Therapy Asst Prgm
Owens Campus
PO Box 610
Georgetown, DE 19947-0610
Prgm Dir: Anne M Lawton, OTR/L
Tel: 302 856-5400 *Fax:* 302 856-5773
E-mail: alawton@outland.dtcc.edu
Class Cap: 36 *Begins:* Aug
Length: 24 mos *Award:* AAS
Tuition per yr: $1,146 res, $2,865 non-res
Evening or weekend classes available

Florida

Daytona Beach Community College

Occupational Therapy Asst Prgm
1200 International Spdwy Blvd
Daytona Beach, FL 32114
Prgm Dir: Alice L Godbey, MS OTR/L
Tel: 904 255-8131, Ext 3751 *Fax:* 904 254-4492
Class Cap: 25 *Begins:* Aug
Length: 22 mos *Award:* AS
Tuition per yr: $2,700 res, $9,787 non-res
Evening or weekend classes available

Palm Beach Community College

Occupational Therapy Asst Prgm
4200 S Congress Ave
Lake Worth, FL 33461-4796
Prgm Dir: Sophia Munro, MS OTR
Tel: 561 439-8094 *Fax:* 561 439-8202
Med Dir: Patrick Haney, DDS MS
Class Cap: 26 *Begins:* Aug
Length: 21 mos *Award:* AS
Tuition per yr: $1,340 res, $4,983 non-res
Evening or weekend classes available

Programs

Central Florida Community College

Occupational Therapy Asst Prgm
3001 SW College Rd
Ocala, FL 34474
Prgm Dir: Dorothy J Grabowski, OTR/L
Tel: 352 237-2111, Ext 327 *Fax:* 352 237-0510
E-mail: hypw87a@prodigy
Class Cap: 24 *Begins:* Jan
Length: 17 mos *Award:* AS
Tuition per yr: $2,768 res, $9,914 non-res
Evening or weekend classes available

Hillsborough Community College

Occupational Therapy Asst Prgm
PO Box 30030
Tampa, FL 33630-3030
Prgm Dir: Susan Adams, BHS OTR/L
Tel: 813 253-7431 *Fax:* 813 253-7506
Class Cap: 20 *Begins:* Aug
Length: 22 mos *Award:* AS
Tuition per yr: $1,096 res, $4,208 non-res
Evening or weekend classes available

Georgia

Medical College of Georgia

Occupational Therapy Asst Prgm
School of Allied Health Sciences
EF-102
Augusta, GA 30912-0700
Prgm Dir: Ricardo C Carrasco, PhD OTR/L
Tel: 706 721-3641 *Fax:* 706 721-9718
E-mail: rcarrasc@mail.mcg.edu
Begins: Sep
Length: 10 mos *Award:* AA
Tuition per yr: $2,085 res, $5,790 non-res

Middle Georgia College

Occupational Therapy Asst Prgm
1100 Second St SE
Cochran, GA 31014-1599
Prgm Dir: Heather Copan, OTR/L
Tel: 912 934-3402 *Fax:* 912 934-3199
E-mail: hcopan@warrior.mgc.peachnet.edu
Class Cap: 20 *Begins:* Sep
Length: 24 mos *Award:* AS
Tuition per yr: $420 res, $1,230 non-res

Hawaii

Kapiolani Community College

Occupational Therapy Asst Prgm
Health Sciences Dept
4303 Diamond Head Rd/Kavila 210
Honolulu, HI 96816
Prgm Dir: Ann Kadoguchi, OTR
Tel: 808 734-9229 *Fax:* 808 734-9126
Begins: Aug
Length: 20 mos *Award:* AS
Tuition per yr: $435 res, $2,595 non-res

Idaho

American Institute of Health Technology

Occupational Therapy Asst Prgm
6600 Emerald
Boise, ID 83704-8738
Prgm Dir: Carrie L Mori, MS OTR/L
Tel: 208 377-8080 Fax: 208 322-7658
E-mail: moric@micron.net
Class Cap: 24 *Begins:* May Sep
Length: 20 mos *Award:* AAS
Tuition per yr: $6,000

Illinois

Parkland College

Occupational Therapy Asst Prgm
2400 W Bradley Ave
Champaign, IL 61821-1899
Prgm Dir: Rebecca R Bahnke, OTR/L
Tel: 217 351-2394 *Fax:* 217 373-3830
E-mail: rbahnke@parkland.cc.il.usa
Class Cap: 20 *Begins:* Aug
Length: 24 mos *Award:* AAS
Tuition per yr: $1,440 res, $4,676 non-res
Evening or weekend classes available

Wilbur Wright College

Occupational Therapy Asst Prgm
4300 N Narragansett Ave
Chicago, IL 60634-1591
Prgm Dir: Joyce Wandel, MS OTR/L
Tel: 773 481-8875 *Fax:* 773 481-8892
E-mail: jwandel@ccc.ec
Class Cap: 28 *Begins:* Sep
Length: 26 mos *Award:* AAS
Tuition per yr: $2,025
Evening or weekend classes available

College of DuPage

Occupational Therapy Asst Prgm
Occupational and Vocational Education
425 22nd St
Glen Ellyn, IL 60137-6599
Prgm Dir: Kathleen Mital, MS MOT OTR
Tel: 630 942-2419 *Fax:* 630 858-5409
Class Cap: 30 *Begins:* Jan
Length: 24 mos *Award:* AAS
Tuition per yr: $1,450 res, $4,600 non-res
Evening or weekend classes available

Southern Illinois Collegiate Common Mkt

Occupational Therapy Asst Prgm
3213 S Park Ave
Carterville, IL 62918
Prgm Dir: Sharon J Benshoff, MEd OTR/L
Tel: 618 942-6902 *Fax:* 618 942-6658
E-mail: benshoff@midwest.net
Class Cap: 20 *Begins:* Aug
Length: 20 mos *Award:* AAS
Tuition per yr: $1,015
Evening or weekend classes available

Illinois Central College

Occupational Therapy Asst Prgm
201 SW Adams
Peoria, IL 61635-0001
Prgm Dir: Janet Bishop, MS OTR/L
Tel: 309 999-4674 *Fax:* 309 673-9626
Class Cap: 16 *Begins:* Aug
Length: 18 mos *Award:* AAS
Tuition per yr: $1,512 res, $4,680 non-res

South Suburban College of Cook County

Occupational Therapy Asst Prgm
15800 S State St
South Holland, IL 60473-1262
Prgm Dir: Jennifer Myler, OTR/L
Tel: 708 596-2000, Ext 264 *Fax:* 708 210-5758
E-mail: ssclib@cedar.cic.net
Class Cap: 40 *Begins:* Aug
Length: 20 mos *Award:* Dipl, AAS
Tuition per yr: $1,815 res, $5,025 non-res
Evening or weekend classes available

Indiana

Ivy Tech State Coll - Indianapolis

Occupational Therapy Asst Prgm
Central Indiana Region
One W 26th St
Indianapolis, IN 46206-1763
Prgm Dir: Christy A Troxell, MA OTR
Tel: 317 921-4325 *Fax:* 317 921-4511
E-mail: ctroxell@ivy.tec.in.us
Class Cap: 20 *Begins:* Aug Jan
Length: 24 mos *Award:* AS
Tuition per yr: $2,088 res, $3,780 non-res
Evening or weekend classes available

Iowa

Kirkwood Community College

Occupational Therapy Asst Prgm
6301 Kirkwood Blvd SW
PO Box 2068
Cedar Rapids, IA 52406-9973
Prgm Dir: Mary Ellen Dunford, OTR/L
Tel: 319 398-4941 *Fax:* 319 398-1293
E-mail: mdunfor@kirkwood.c.ia.us
Class Cap: 40 *Begins:* Aug
Length: 22 mos *Award:* AAS
Tuition per yr: $954 res, $1,908 non-res
Evening or weekend classes available

Western Iowa Tech Community College

Occupational Therapy Asst Prgm
4647 Stone Ave/PO Box 265
Sioux City, IA 51102-0265
Prgm Dir: Linda Tronvold, OTR/L
Tel: 712 274-8733, Ext 1339 *Fax:* 712 274-6412
Class Cap: 24 *Begins:* Jan
Length: 24 mos *Award:* AAS
Tuition per yr: $3,724 res, $7,448 non-res
Evening or weekend classes available

Kansas

Barton County Community College

Occupational Therapy Asst Prgm
RR 3 Box 136Z
Great Bend, KS 67530-9283
Prgm Dir: Lee Frye, MS OTR
Tel: 316 792-9368 *Fax:* 316 792-3056
E-mail: fryel@cougar.barton.cc.ks.us
Class Cap: 40 *Begins:* Aug
Length: 21 mos, 16 mos *Award:* AAS
Tuition per yr: $732 res, $4,523 non-res
Evening or weekend classes available

Louisiana

Northeast Louisiana University
Occupational Therapy Asst Prgm
Coll of Pharmacy and Hlth Sci
Sch Allied Hlth Sciences
Monroe, LA 71209-0430
Prgm Dir: Kathryn H Davis, MA L/OTR
Tel: 318 342-1610   *Fax:* 318 342-1687
Class Cap: 35   *Begins:* Aug
Length: 25 mos, 28 mos   *Award:* AS
Tuition per yr: $1,925 res, $4,326 non-res
Evening or weekend classes available

Maine

Kennebec Valley Technical College
Occupational Therapy Asst Prgm
92 Western Ave
Fairfield, ME 04937-1367
Prgm Dir: Diane Sauter-Davis, OTR/L
Tel: 207 453-5172   *Fax:* 207 453-5010
E-mail: kdsauter@kvtc.mtcs.tec.me.us
Class Cap: 24   *Begins:* Sep
Length: 18 mos   *Award:* Dipl, AAS
Tuition per yr: $2,368 res, $5,217 non-res
Evening or weekend classes available

Maryland

Catonsville Community College
Occupational Therapy Asst Prgm
800 S Rolling Rd
Catonsville, MD 21228-9987
Prgm Dir: Judy Blum, MS OTR/L
Tel: 410 455-4482   *Fax:* 410 455-4998
Class Cap: 20   *Begins:* Feb Jun
Length: 18 mos   *Award:* Dipl, AAS
Tuition per yr: $1,440 res, $1,440 non-res
Evening or weekend classes available

Allegany College of Maryland
Occupational Therapy Asst Prgm
12401 Willowbrook Rd SE
Cumberland, MD 21502-2596
Prgm Dir: Jeffrey Hopkins, MS OTR/L
Tel: 301 724-7700, Ext 536   Fax: 301 724-6892
Class Cap: 16   *Begins:* Aug
Length: 20 mos   *Award:* AAS
Tuition per yr: $5,046 res, $6,646 non-res

Massachusetts

Bay State College
Occupational Therapy Asst Prgm
31 St James Ave
Boston, MA 02116
Prgm Dir: Susan Gelfman, MS OTR/L
Tel: 617 375-0195   *Fax:* 617 375-0197
Class Cap: 30   *Begins:* Sep
Length: 24 mos   *Award:* AS
Tuition per yr: $9,800

North Shore Community College
Occupational Therapy Asst Prgm
PO Box 3340
1 Ferncroft Rd
Danvers, MA 01923-0840
Prgm Dir: Maureen S Nardella, BS, OTR/L
Tel: 508 762-4164   *Fax:* 508 762-4022
Class Cap: 60   *Begins:* Sep
Length: 21 mos, 12 mos   *Award:* AS
Tuition per yr: $1,976 res, $5,784 non-res
Evening or weekend classes available

Bristol Community College
Occupational Therapy Asst Prgm
777 Elsbree St
Fall River, MA 02720-9960
Prgm Dir: Johanna Duponte, MS OTR/L
Tel: 508 678-2811, Ext 2325   *Fax:* 508 676-7146
E-mail: jduponte@bristol.mass.edu
Class Cap: 20   *Begins:* Sep
Length: 24 mos   *Award:* AS
Tuition per yr: $2,788 res, $7,820 non-res
Evening or weekend classes available

Greenfield Community College
Occupational Therapy Asst Prgm
270 Main St
Greenfield, MA 01301
Prgm Dir: Marilyn Micka-Pickunka, MA OTR/L
Tel: 413 774-3131, Ext 317   *Fax:* 413 774-2285
E-mail: nursing@gcc.mass.edu
Class Cap: 25   *Begins:* Sep
Length: 18 mos   *Award:* AS
Tuition per yr: $1,638 res, $6,768 non-res

Bay Path College
Occupational Therapy Asst Prgm
588 Longmeadow St
Longmeadow, MA 01106
Prgm Dir: Irene L Herden, MBA OTR/L FAOTA
Tel: 413 567-0621, Ext 450   *Fax:* 413 567-9324
Class Cap: 22   *Begins:* Sep
Length: 16 mos   *Award:* AS
Tuition per yr: $20,400

Mt Ida College
Occupational Therapy Asst Prgm
Junior College Div
777 Dedham St
Newton Centre, MA 02159-3310
Prgm Dir: Jeraldine C Perron, MS OTR/L FAOTA
Tel: 617 928-4770   *Fax:* 617 244-7532
E-mail: jerrie@aol.com
Begins: Sep
Length: 18 mos   *Award:* AS
Tuition per yr: $10,320
Evening or weekend classes available

Springfield Technical Community College
Occupational Therapy Asst Prgm
One Armory Square
Springfield, MA 01101
Prgm Dir: Marianne Joyce, OTR/L
Tel: 413 781-7822   *Fax:* 413 781-5805
Begins: Sep
Length: 18 mos   *Award:* AS
Tuition per yr: $5,880 non-res

Massachusetts Bay Community College
Occupational Therapy Asst Prgm
Wellesley Hills Campus
50 Oakland St
Wellesley Hills, MA 02181-5399
Prgm Dir: Iris G Leigh, MS OTR/L
Tel: 617 239-2240   *Fax:* 617 239-1047
E-mail: leighiri@mbcc.mass.edu
Begins: Sep
Length: 21 mos   *Award:* AS
Tuition per yr: $4,850 res, $12,850 non-res

Becker College
Occupational Therapy Asst Prgm
61 Sever St Box 15071
Worcester, MA 01615-0071
Prgm Dir: Edith C Fenton, MS OTR/L
Tel: 508 791-9241   *Fax:* 508 890-1500
Class Cap: 50   *Begins:* Sep Jan
Length: 18 mos   *Award:* AS
Tuition per yr: $8,790
Evening or weekend classes available

Quinsigamond Community College
Occupational Therapy Asst Prgm
670 W Boylston St
Worcester, MA 01606
Prgm Dir: Elaine Fallon, MS OTR FAOTA
Tel: 508 854-4254   *Fax:* 508 852-6943
Class Cap: 35   *Begins:* Sep Feb
Length: 20 mos   *Award:* Dipl, AS
Tuition per yr: $2,120 res, $5,936 non-res

Michigan

Wayne County Community College
Occupational Therapy Asst Prgm
1001 W Fort St
Detroit, MI 48226-9975
Prgm Dir: Jean Whicker, MS OTR
Tel: 313 496-2692   Fax: 313 962-5097
Class Cap: 36   *Begins:* June
Length: 18 mos, 21 mos   *Award:* AAS
Tuition per yr: $1,296 res, $1,680 non-res
Evening or weekend classes available

Charles Stewart Mott Community College
Occupational Therapy Asst Prgm
Southern Lakes Campus
2100 W Thompson Rd
Fenton, MI 48430
Prgm Dir: Wendy Blair Early, MS OTR
Tel: 810 750-8550   *Fax:* 810 750-8588
Class Cap: 15   *Begins:* Sep
Length: 24 mos   *Award:* Dipl, AAS
Tuition per yr: $4,250 res, $7,735 non-res
Evening or weekend classes available

Schoolcraft College
Occupational Therapy Asst Prgm
1751 Radcliff St
Garden City, MI 48135-1197
Prgm Dir: Nancy M Vandewiele-Milligan, MS OTR
Tel: 313 462-4770, Ext 6002   *Fax:* 313 462-4775
Class Cap: 30   *Begins:* Aug Jan
Length: 27 mos   *Award:* AAS
Tuition per yr: $1,550 res, $2,263 non-res
Evening or weekend classes available

Programs

Grand Rapids Community College

Occupational Therapy Asst Prgm
143 Bostwick NE
Grand Rapids, MI 49503-3295
Prgm Dir: Alice A Donahue, MA OTR
Tel: 616 771-4236 *Fax:* 616 771-3741
E-mail: adonahue@post.grcc.cc.mi.us
Class Cap: 34 *Begins:* Aug
Length: 22 mos *Award:* AAAS
Tuition per yr: $2,028 res, $3,003 non-res
Evening or weekend classes available

Baker College of Muskegon

Occupational Therapy Asst Prgm
123 Apple Ave
Muskegon, MI 49442-9982
Prgm Dir: Lenee Gabris, MS OTR
Tel: 616 726-4904, Ext 339 *Fax:* 616 728-1417
E-mail: gabris_l@muskegon.baker.edu
Class Cap: 30 *Begins:* Sep Jan
Length: 22 mos, 28 mos *Award:* AAS
Tuition per yr: $7,375 res, $7,375 non-res
Evening or weekend classes available

Lake Michigan College

Occupational Therapy Asst Prgm
South Campus
111 Spruce St
Niles, MI 49120
Prgm Dir: Martha Branson-Banks, OTR
Tel: 616 684-5850 *Fax:* 616 684-3270
E-mail: branson@raptor.lmc.cc.mi.us
Class Cap: 21 *Begins:* Aug
Length: 24 mos *Award:* AAS
Tuition per yr: $1,440 res, $2,145 non-res

Minnesota

Anoka-Hennepin Technical College

Occupational Therapy Asst Prgm
1355 W Hwy 10
Anoka, MN 55303-1590
Prgm Dir: Marietta Cosky Saxon, OTR
Tel: 612 576-4935 *Fax:* 612 576-4715
E-mail: msaxon@ank.tec.mn.us
Class Cap: 40 *Begins:* Sep
Length: 18 mos *Award:* AAS
Tuition per yr: $2,646
Evening or weekend classes available

Riverland Community College

Occupational Therapy Asst Prgm
1900 8TH Ave NW
Austin, MN 55912-1407
Prgm Dir: Carol Davis, OTR
Tel: 507 433-0567 *Fax:* 507 433-0515
E-mail: Davisca@au.cc.mn.us
Class Cap: 25 *Begins:* Sep
Length: 22 mos *Award:* AS
Tuition per yr: $2,105 res, $4,102 non-res
Evening or weekend classes available

Lake Superior College

Occupational Therapy Asst Prgm
2101 Trinity Rd
Duluth, MN 55811-3399
Prgm Dir: Janna M Dreher, MS OTR
Tel: 218 722-2801, Ext 332 *Fax:* 218 722-2899
E-mail: j.dreher@lsc.cc.mn.us
Class Cap: 26 *Begins:* Sep Mar
Length: 18 mos *Award:* AAS
Tuition per yr: $1,872 res, $3,744 non-res
Evening or weekend classes available

Northwest Technical Coll - E Grand Forks

Occupational Therapy Asst Prgm
Hwy 220 N
East Grand Forks, MN 56721
Prgm Dir: Cassie Hilts, OTR/L
Tel: 218 773-3441 *Fax:* 218 773-4502
E-mail: hilts@adm.egf.tec.mn.us
Class Cap: 24 *Begins:* Aug
Length: 27 mos *Award:* AAS
Tuition per yr: $1,955 res, $3,910 non-res
Evening or weekend classes available

College of St Catherine-Minneapolis

Occupational Therapy Asst Prgm
601 25th Ave S
Minneapolis, MN 55454-1494
Prgm Dir: Marianne F Christiansen, MA OTR
Tel: 612 690-7772 *Fax:* 612 690-7849
E-mail: mfchristians@alex.state.edu
Class Cap: 50 *Begins:* Sep
Length: 18 mos *Award:* AAS
Tuition per yr: $11,152 res, $11,152 non-res
Evening or weekend classes available

Missouri

Sanford Brown College Hazelwood Campus

Occupational Therapy Asst Prgm
368 Brookes Dr
Hazelwood, MO 63042
Tel: 314 731-3995 *Fax:* 314 731-7044
Class Cap: 36 *Begins:* Varies
Length: 21 mos *Award:* AAS
Tuition per yr: $16,340

Penn Valley Community College

Occupational Therapy Asst Prgm
3201 SW Trafficway
Kansas City, MO 64111-2764
Prgm Dir: Sandy McIlnay, MEd OTR
Tel: 816 759-4235 *Fax:* 816 759-4553
E-mail: mcilnay@pennvalley.cc.mo.us
Class Cap: 36 *Begins:* Aug
Length: 22 mos *Award:* AAS
Tuition per yr: $1,643 res, $2,738 non-res
Evening or weekend classes available

St Louis Community College at Meramec

Occupational Therapy Asst Prgm
11333 Big Bend Blvd
St Louis, MO 63122
Prgm Dir: Nancy M Klein, MS OTR
Tel: 314 984-7364 *Fax:* 314 984-7250
Class Cap: 32 *Begins:* Aug
Length: 21 mos *Award:* AAS
Tuition per yr: $1,528 res, $1,924 non-res

Montana

Montana State Univ Coll of Technology

Occupational Therapy Asst Prgm
Allied Health Dept
2100 16th Ave S
Great Falls, MT 59405-4998
Prgm Dir: Helen Quarles, MS OTR/L
Tel: 406 771-4364 *Fax:* 406 771-4317
E-mail: zgf6018@maia.oscs.montana.edu
Class Cap: 20 *Begins:* Jan
Length: 24 mos *Award:* AAS
Tuition per yr: $1,743 res, $4,112 non-res
Evening or weekend classes available

Nebraska

Clarkson College

Occupational Therapy Asst Prgm
101 S 42nd St
Omaha, NE 68131-2739
Prgm Dir: Yvonne Parde, MS OTR/L
Tel: 402 552-6139 *Fax:* 402 552-6019
E-mail: parde@clrkcol.chrsnet.edu
Class Cap: 16 *Begins:* Sept
Length: 24 mos *Award:* AS
Tuition per yr: $8,400 res, $8,400 non-res

New Hampshire

New Hampshire Community Technical College

Occupational Therapy Asst Prgm
One College Dr
Claremont, NH 03743-9707
Prgm Dir: Joan Holcombe Larsen, MEd OTR/L
   RTC
Tel: 603 542-7744 *Fax:* 603 542-1844
E-mail: j_larsen@tec.nh.us
Class Cap: 30 *Begins:* Aug Jan
Length: 20 mos *Award:* AAS
Tuition per yr: $3,286 res, $4,929 non-res
Evening or weekend classes available

New Jersey

Atlantic Community College

Occupational Therapy Asst Prgm
Allied Health Division
5100 Black Horse Pike
Mays Landing, NJ 08330-9888
Prgm Dir: Angela J Busillo, MEd OTR
Tel: 609 343-5044 *Fax:* 609 343-5122
E-mail: busillo@nsvm.atlantic.edu
Class Cap: 16 *Begins:* Sep
Length: 22 mos *Award:* AAS
Tuition per yr: $2,500
Evening or weekend classes available

Union County College

Occupational Therapy Asst Prgm
232 E Second St
Plainfield, NJ 07060
Prgm Dir: Carol Keating, MA OTR
Tel: 908 412-3587 *Fax:* 908 754-2798
E-mail: keatin@hawk.ucc.edu
Class Cap: 24 *Begins:* Sep
Length: 24 mos *Award:* AAS
Tuition per yr: $2,046 res, $4,092 non-res

New Mexico

Eastern New Mexico University-Roswell
Occupational Therapy Asst Prgm
Div of Health
52 Univ Blvd/PO Box 6000
Roswell, NM 88202-6000
Prgm Dir: Patsy Herrera, OTR/L
Tel: 505 624-7267 *Fax:* 505 624-7100
E-mail: herrerap@lib.enmuros.cc.nm.us
Class Cap: 25 *Begins:* Aug
Length: 18 mos *Award:* AS
Tuition per yr: $1,018 res, $2,794 non-res

Western New Mexico University
Occupational Therapy Asst Prgm
PO Box 680
Silver City, NM 88062-0680
Prgm Dir: Gwen Cassel, MOT OTR/L
Tel: 505 538-6293 *Fax:* 505 538-6178
E-mail: casselg@silver.wnmu.edu
Class Cap: 25 *Begins:* Aug
Length: 24 mos *Award:* AS
Tuition per yr: $1,516

New York

Maria College
Occupational Therapy Asst Prgm
700 New Scotland Ave
Albany, NY 12208-1798
Prgm Dir: Sandra C Jung, OTR
Tel: 518 489-7436 *Fax:* 518 438-7170
Class Cap: 46 *Begins:* Sep
Length: 18 mos *Award:* AAS
Tuition per yr: $5,200 res, $5,200 non-res
Evening or weekend classes available

Genesee Community College
Occupational Therapy Asst Prgm
One College Rd
Batavia, NY 14020-9704
Prgm Dir: Mary K Hartman, MS OTR/L
Tel: 716 345-6838 *Fax:* 716 343-0433
Class Cap: 32 *Begins:* Aug Jan
Length: 18 mos *Award:* AAS
Tuition per yr: $1,150 res, $1,275 non-res
Evening or weekend classes available

Erie Community College - City Campus
Occupational Therapy Asst Prgm
6205 Main St
Williamsville, NY 14221-7095
Prgm Dir: Betsy Jones, ORT/L
Tel: 716 851-1320 *Fax:* 716 851-1429
E-mail: jones@nstaff.sunyerie.edu
Class Cap: 55 *Begins:* Sep
Length: 20 mos, 30 mos *Award:* AAS
Tuition per yr: $2,270 res, $4,540 non-res
Evening or weekend classes available

Herkimer County Community College
Occupational Therapy Asst Prgm
Reservoir Rd
Herkimer, NY 13350-1598
Prgm Dir: Brice R Kistler, OTR/L
Tel: 315 866-0300, Ext 237 *Fax:* 315 866-7253
Class Cap: 45 *Begins:* Aug
Length: 20 mos *Award:* AAS
Tuition per yr: $2,250 res, $3,600 non-res
Evening or weekend classes available

LaGuardia Community College
Occupational Therapy Asst Prgm
31-10 Thomson Ave
Long Island City, NY 11101-3083
Prgm Dir: Naomi S Greenberg, PhD MPH OTR FAOTA
Tel: 718 482-5777 *Fax:* 718 482-5599
Class Cap: 250 *Begins:* Sep Mar
Length: 24 mos, 36 mos *Award:* AS
Tuition per yr: $2,204 res, $2,676 non-res

Orange County Community College
Occupational Therapy Asst Prgm
115 South St
Middletown, NY 10940-6404
Prgm Dir: Mary Sands, MSEd OTR FAOTA
Tel: 914 341-4323 *Fax:* 914 343-1228
E-mail: msands@mail.sunyorange.edu
Class Cap: 24 *Begins:* Sep
Length: 18 mos *Award:* AAS
Tuition per yr: $2,100 res, $4,200 non-res
Evening or weekend classes available

Rockland Community College
Occupational Therapy Asst Prgm
145 College Rd
Suffern, NY 10901-3699
Prgm Dir: Ellen Spergel, MS OTR
Tel: 914 574-4312 *Fax:* 914 574-4399
Class Cap: 60 *Begins:* Sep Feb
Length: 19 mos *Award:* AAS
Tuition per yr: $1,025 res, $1,025 non-res
Evening or weekend classes available

North Carolina

Stanly Community College
Occupational Therapy Asst Prgm
141 College Dr
Albemarle, NC 28001-9402
Prgm Dir: Karen Babcock Smith, OTR/L
Tel: 704 982-0121, Ext 209 *Fax:* 704 982-0819
E-mail: babcocks@stanly.cc.nc.us
Class Cap: 24 *Begins:* Aug
Length: 24 mos *Award:* AAS
Tuition per yr: $853 res, $6,588 non-res
Evening or weekend classes available

Durham Technical Community College
Occupational Therapy Asst Prgm
1637 Lawson St
Durham, NC 27703-5023
Prgm Dir: Teepa Snow, MS OTR/L FAOTA
Tel: 919 686-3459 *Fax:* 919 686-3601
E-mail: teepas@nando.net
Class Cap: 36 *Begins:* Sep
Length: 21 mos *Award:* Dipl, AAS
Tuition per yr: $812 res, $6,072 non-res
Evening or weekend classes available

Pitt Community College
Occupational Therapy Asst Prgm
PO Drawer 7007
Hwy 11 S
Greenville, NC 27835-7007
Prgm Dir: Roselyn V Armstrong, MA OTR/L
Tel: 919 321-4458 *Fax:* 919 321-4451
E-mail: rarmstro@pcc.pitt.nc.us
Class Cap: 25 *Begins:* Aug
Length: 24 mos *Award:* AAS
Tuition per yr: $742 res, $6,020 non-res
Evening or weekend classes available

Caldwell Comm College & Tech Institute
Occupational Therapy Asst Prgm
2855 Hickory Blvd
Hudson, NC 28638-1399
Prgm Dir: Rebecca L Withers, MPH OTR/L
Tel: 704 726-2344 *Fax:* 704 726-2216
Class Cap: 25 *Begins:* Sep
Length: 21 mos *Award:* AAS
Tuition per yr: $556 res, $4,515 non-res

Southwestern Community College
Occupational Therapy Asst Prgm
275 Webster Rd
Sylva, NC 28779
Prgm Dir: Helen Nodzak, MOT OTR/L
Tel: 704 586-4091, Ext 272 *Fax:* 704 586-3129
E-mail: helenn@southwest.cc.nc.us
Class Cap: 20 *Begins:* Sep
Length: 21 mos *Award:* AAS
Tuition per yr: $742 res, $6,020 non-res
Evening or weekend classes available

North Dakota

North Dakota State College of Science
Occupational Therapy Asst Prgm
Hektner Hall
Wahpeton, ND 58076-0002
Prgm Dir: Sr Carolita Mauer, MA OTR/L
Tel: 701 671-2982 *Fax:* 701 671-2587
E-mail: mauer@plains.nodak.edu
Class Cap: 50 *Begins:* Aug
Length: 18 mos *Award:* AS
Tuition per yr: $1,751 res, $2,139 non-res

Ohio

Stark State College of Technology
Occupational Therapy Asst Prgm
6200 Frank Ave NW
Canton, OH 44720-7299
Prgm Dir: Doris Huston, OTR
Tel: 330 966-5458, Ext 200 *Fax:* 330 966-6586
E-mail: dhuston@stark.cc.oh.us
Class Cap: 12 *Begins:* Aug Jan
Length: 20 mos *Award:* AAS
Tuition per yr: $2,800 res, $3,800 non-res
Evening or weekend classes available

Cincinnati State Tech and Comm College
Occupational Therapy Asst Prgm
3520 Central Pkwy
Cincinnati, OH 45223-2690
Prgm Dir: Anne Zobay, ORT/L
Tel: 513 569-1598 *Fax:* 513 569-1659
Class Cap: 25 *Begins:* Sep
Length: 24 mos *Award:* AAS
Tuition per yr: $4,020 res, $8,040 non-res

Cuyahoga Community College
Occupational Therapy Asst Prgm
2900 Community College Ave
Cleveland, OH 44115-3196
Prgm Dir: Hector L Merced, OTR/L
Tel: 216 987-4498 *Fax:* 216 987-4386
E-mail: hector.merced@tri-c.cc.oh.us
Class Cap: 25 *Begins:* Sep
Length: 18 mos *Award:* AAS
Tuition per yr: $1,417 res, $1,878 non-res

Sinclair Community College

Occupational Therapy Asst Prgm
444 W Third St
Dayton, OH 45402-1460
Prgm Dir: S Kay Ashworth, MAT OTR/L
Tel: 513 449-5178 *Fax:* 513 449-5192
E-mail: kashwort@sinclair.edu
Class Cap: 30 *Begins:* Sep
Length: 21 mos *Award:* AAS
Tuition per yr: $1,885 res, $3,835 non-res

Kent State University

Occupational Therapy Asst Prgm
East Liverpool Campus
400 E Fourth St
East Liverpool, OH 43920-3497
Prgm Dir: Elizabeth Fowler, OTR/L
Tel: 330 385-4272 *Fax:* 330 385-6348
E-mail: bfowler@el2.kenteliv.kent.edu
Class Cap: 26 *Begins:* Sep
Length: 21 mos *Award:* AAS
Evening or weekend classes available

Shawnee State University

Occupational Therapy Asst Prgm
Dept of Occupational Therapy
940 Second St
Portsmouth, OH 45662-4303
Prgm Dir: Catherine O Perry, MEd OTR/L
Tel: 614 355-2272 *Fax:* 614 355-2354
E-mail: cperry@shawnee.edu
Class Cap: 18 *Begins:* Sep
Length: 21 mos *Award:* AAS
Tuition per yr: $2,976 res, $5,151 non-res
Evening or weekend classes available

Lourdes College

Occupational Therapy Asst Prgm
6832 Convent Blvd
Sylvania, OH 43560-2898
Prgm Dir: Cynthia L Goodwin, MS OTR/L
Tel: 419 885-3211, Ext 222 *Fax:* 419 882-3786
Class Cap: 20 *Begins:* Aug
Length: 22 mos *Award:* Dipl, AAS
Tuition per yr: $8,296
Evening or weekend classes available

Muskingum Area Technical College

Occupational Therapy Asst Prgm
1555 Newark Rd
Zanesville, OH 43701-2694
Prgm Dir: Mary Arnold, MA OTR/L
Tel: 614 454-2501, Ext 194 *Fax:* 614 454-0035
E-mail: marnold@matc.tec.oh.us
Begins: Sep
Length: 21 mos *Award:* Dipl, AAS
Tuition per yr: $2,880 res, $4,800 non-res
Evening or weekend classes available

Oklahoma

Oklahoma City Community College

Occupational Therapy Asst Prgm
Hlth, Soc Sci and Human Svcs Div
7777 S May Ave
Oklahoma City, OK 73159-4444
Prgm Dir: Phyllis Baker, OTR/L
Tel: 405 682-7506 *Fax:* 405 682-1611
E-mail: phbaker@okc.cc.ok.us
Class Cap: 20 *Begins:* Aug Jan
Length: 24 mos *Award:* AAS
Tuition per yr: $1,431 res, $3,471 non-res
Evening or weekend classes available

Tulsa Community College

Occupational Therapy Asst Prgm
Allied Health Services Div
909 S Boston Ave
Tulsa, OK 74119-2095
Prgm Dir: Gary Braswell, OTR/L
Tel: 918 595-7319 *Fax:* 918 595-7298
Class Cap: 15 *Begins:* Jun
Length: 24 mos, 36 mos *Award:* AAS
Tuition per yr: $1,200 res, $2,190 non-res

Oregon

Mt Hood Community College

Occupational Therapy Asst Prgm
26000 SE Stark St
Gresham, OR 97030-3300
Prgm Dir: Chris Hencinski, MS OTR/L
Tel: 503 667-7129 *Fax:* 503 492-6047
E-mail: hencinsc@mhee.cc.or.us
Class Cap: 20 *Begins:* Sep
Length: 9 mos *Award:* AAS
Tuition per yr: $1,620 res, $6,069 non-res

Pennsylvania

Harcum College

Occupational Therapy Asst Prgm
Bryn Mawr, PA 19010-3476
Prgm Dir: Kerstin Potter, MS OTR
Tel: 610 526-6115 *Fax:* 610 526-6086
Class Cap: 54 *Begins:* Sep
Length: 24 mos *Award:* Dipl, AS
Tuition per yr: $8,840
Evening or weekend classes available

Mt Aloysius College

Occupational Therapy Asst Prgm
Cresson, PA 16630
Prgm Dir: E Nelson Clark, MS OTR/L
Tel: 814 886-6328 Fax: 814 886-2978
Class Cap: 60 *Begins:* Aug
Length: 24 mos *Award:* AS
Tuition per yr: $9,800

Comm Coll of Allegheny Cnty-Boyce Campus

Occupational Therapy Asst Prgm
595 Beatty Rd
Monroeville, PA 15146-1395
Prgm Dir: Lillian Briola, MOT OTR/L
Tel: 412 325-6751 *Fax:* 412 325-6799
E-mail: lbriola@ccac.edu
Class Cap: 51 *Begins:* Aug
Length: 25 mos *Award:* AS
Tuition per yr: $2,040 res, $4,080 non-res
Evening or weekend classes available

Penn State University

Occupational Therapy Asst Prgm
Mont Alto Campus
Campus Dr
Mont Alto, PA 17237-9703
Prgm Dir: Janet DeLany, MS OTR/L
Tel: 717 749-6218 *Fax:* 717 749-6069
E-mail: jud102@psu.edu
Begins: Aug
Length: 16 mos *Award:* AS
Tuition per yr: $5,024 res, $7,808 non-res

Lehigh Carbon Community College

Occupational Therapy Asst Prgm
4525 Education Park Dr
Schnecksville, PA 18078-2598
Prgm Dir: Cindy J Rifenburg, OTR/L
Tel: 610 799-1548 *Fax:* 610 799-1527
Class Cap: 40 *Begins:* Aug
Length: 24 mos, 36 mos *Award:* AAS
Tuition per yr: $2,040 res, $4,080 non-res
Evening or weekend classes available

Pennsylvania College of Technology

Occupational Therapy Asst Prgm
One College Ave
Williamsport, PA 17701-5799
Prgm Dir: Barbara J Natell, MSEd OTR/L
Tel: 717 326-3761, Ext 7600 *Fax:* 717 327-4529
E-mail: bnatell@pct.edu
Class Cap: 32 *Begins:* Aug
Length: 22 mos *Award:* AAS
Tuition per yr: $5,740 res, $8,700 non-res
Evening or weekend classes available

Puerto Rico

Humacao University College

Occupational Therapy Asst Prgm
University of Puerto Rico
CUH Postal Station
Humacao, PR 00791-9998
Prgm Dir: Milagros Marrero, MPH OTR/L
Tel: 787 850-9390 *Fax:* 787 850-9461
Class Cap: 35 *Begins:* Aug
Length: 22 mos *Award:* Dipl, AAS
Tuition per yr: $1,125 res, $1,400 non-res

South Carolina

Trident Technical College

Occupational Therapy Asst Prgm
PO Box 118067
Charleston, SC 29423-8067
Prgm Dir: Susan D Stockmaster, MHS OTR/L
Tel: 803 572-6254 *Fax:* 803 569-6585
E-mail: zpstockmasters@trident.tec.sc.us
Class Cap: 22 *Begins:* May Jun
Length: 21 mos *Award:* AS
Tuition per yr: $1,536 res, $1,776 non-res
Evening or weekend classes available

Tennessee

Roane State Community College

Occupational Therapy Asst Prgm
276 Patton Ln
Harriman, TN 37748-5011
Prgm Dir: Susan Sain, MS OTR/L
Tel: 423 481-3496 *Fax:* 423 483-0441
E-mail: sain_s@rscc.tn.us
Class Cap: 20 *Begins:* Aug
Length: 24 mos *Award:* AAS
Tuition per yr: $1,024 res, $2,926 non-res

Nashville State Technical Institute

Occupational Therapy Asst Prgm
120 White Bridge Rd
PO Box 90285
Nashville, TN 37209-4515
Prgm Dir: Linda Twelves, MS OTR CDRS
Tel: 615 353-3383 *Fax:* 615 353-3376
E-mail: twelves_p@nsti.tec.tn.us
Class Cap: 24 *Begins:* Aug
Length: 20 mos *Award:* AAS
Tuition per yr: $950 res, $2,926 non-res

Texas

Amarillo College

Occupational Therapy Asst Prgm
PO Box 447
Amarillo, TX 79178-0001
Prgm Dir: Virginia R Gass, MEd OTR
Tel: 806 354-6079 *Fax:* 806 354-6076
E-mail: vrgass@actx.edu
Class Cap: 25 *Begins:* Jan
Length: 22 mos *Award:* AAS
Tuition per yr: $753 res, $2,516 non-res
Evening or weekend classes available

Austin Community College

Occupational Therapy Asst Prgm
7748 Hwy 290 W
Austin, TX 78736-3290
Prgm Dir: Martha Sue Carrell, OTR
Tel: 512 223-8079 *Fax:* 512 288-8185
Class Cap: 20 *Begins:* Aug
Length: 24 mos *Award:* AAS
Tuition per yr: $690 res, $1,320 non-res
Evening or weekend classes available

Navarro College

Occupational Therapy Asst Prgm
3200 W 7th Ave
Corsicana, TX 75110-4818
Prgm Dir: Anita Lane, MEd OTR
Tel: 903 874-6501, Ext 367 *Fax:* 903 874-4636
E-mail: alane@nav.cc.tx.us
Class Cap: 30 *Begins:* Aug
Length: 24 mos *Award:* AAS
Tuition per yr: $1,200 res, $1,800 non-res

North Central Texas College

Occupational Therapy Asst Prgm
601 E Hickory St/Ste B
Denton, TX 76201-4305
Prgm Dir: Carolyn Mohair, OTR
Tel: 817 381-1142 *Fax:* 817 380-0274
Class Cap: 40 *Begins:* Aug
Length: 24 mos *Award:* AAS
Tuition per yr: $776 res, $776 non-res
Evening or weekend classes available

Army Medical Dept Center and School

Occupational Therapy Asst Prgm
Dept of Med Sci
Attn: MCCS-HMO Ltc Rice
Ft Sam Houston, TX 78234-6131
Prgm Dir: LTC Valerie J Rice, PhD OTR/L CPE
Tel: 210 221-3694 *Fax:* 210 221-4447
E-mail: ltc_valerie_rice@
  medcom1.smtplink.amedd.army.mil
Class Cap: 90 *Begins:* Jan April Aug
Length: 7 mos *Award:* Cert

Houston Community College Central

Occupational Therapy Asst Prgm
Health Careers Division
3100 Shenandoah
Houston, TX 77021-1098
Prgm Dir: Linda Williams, MA OTR/L
Tel: 713 718-7392 *Fax:* 713 718-7401
Begins: Aug
Length: 12 mos *Award:* Cert
Tuition per yr: $1,130 res, $3,480 non-res

San Jacinto College South

Occupational Therapy Asst Prgm
13735 Beamer Rd
Houston, TX 77089
Prgm Dir: Jane F Moes, MOT OTR
Tel: 713 484-1900 *Fax:* 713 922-3487
E-mail: jmoes@south.sjcd.cc.tx.us
Class Cap: 26 *Begins:* Aug
Length: 21 mos *Award:* AAS
Tuition per yr: $852 res, $3,195 non-res
Evening or weekend classes available

St Philip's College

Occupational Therapy Asst Prgm
1801 Martin Luther King St
San Antonio, TX 78203-2098
Prgm Dir: Edward E Beaty, Jr, MSIS OTR
Tel: 210 531-3416 *Fax:* 210 531-3459
E-mail: ebeaty@accdvm.accd.edu
Class Cap: 36 *Begins:* Aug
Length: 20 mos *Award:* AAS
Tuition per yr: $690 res, $1,234 non-res

Utah

Salt Lake Community College

Occupational Therapy Asst Prgm
4600 S Redwood Rd
PO Box 30808
Salt Lake City, UT 84130-0808
Prgm Dir: Anne A England, MEd OTR/L
Tel: 801 957-4314 *Fax:* 801 957-4444
E-mail: englanan@slcc.edu
Class Cap: 24 *Begins:* Sep
Length: 12 mos *Award:* AAS
Tuition per yr: $1,455 res, $4,710 non-res
Evening or weekend classes available

Virginia

J Sargeant Reynolds Community College

Occupational Therapy Asst Prgm
PO Box 85622
Richmond, VA 23285-5622
Prgm Dir: Kathryn Mason, OTR
Tel: 804 786-3484 *Fax:* 804 786-5298
E-mail: srmasok@jsr.cc.va.us
Class Cap: 35 *Begins:* Aug
Length: 22 mos *Award:* Dipl, AAS
Tuition per yr: $2,172
Evening or weekend classes available

College of Health Sciences

Occupational Therapy Asst Prgm
Comm Hosp of Roanoke Valley
920 S Jefferson St
Roanoke, VA 24016
Prgm Dir: Ave Mitta, OTR
Tel: 540 985-4097 *Fax:* 540 985-9773
E-mail: ave@health.chs.edu
Class Cap: 30 *Begins:* Aug
Length: 18 mos *Award:* AS
Tuition per yr: $6,400
Evening or weekend classes available

Washington

Green River Community College

Occupational Therapy Asst Prgm
12401 SE 320th St
Auburn, WA 98002-3699
Prgm Dir: Barbara J Rom, MS OTR/L
Tel: 206 833-9111, Ext 4319 *Fax:* 206 288-3479
E-mail: brom@grcc.ctc.edu
Class Cap: 32 *Begins:* Sep Mar
Length: 18 mos *Award:* AAS
Tuition per yr: $1,350 res, $5,298 non-res

Yakima Valley Community College

Occupational Therapy Asst Prgm
16th Ave and Nob Hill Blvd
PO Box 1647
Yakima, WA 98907-1647
Prgm Dir: Peg Bryant, OTR/L
Tel: 509 574-4951 *Fax:* 509 574-4734
E-mail: pbryant@ctc.edu
Class Cap: 27 *Begins:* Sep
Length: 18 mos *Award:* ATA
Tuition per yr: $1,431 res, $5,541 non-res
Evening or weekend classes available

Wisconsin

Fox Valley Technical College

Occupational Therapy Asst Prgm
1825 N Bluemound Dr
PO Box 2277
Appleton, WI 54913-2277
Prgm Dir: Patricia Holz, OTR
Tel: 414 735-4843   *Fax:* 414 735-2582
E-mail: holz@foxvalley.tec.wi.us
Class Cap: 28   *Begins:* Sep Jan
Length: 18 mos   *Award:* AA
Tuition per yr: $2,455

Madison Area Technical College

Occupational Therapy Asst Prgm
211 N Carroll St
Madison, WI 53703-2285
Prgm Dir: Toni Walski, MS OTR
Tel: 608 258-2314   *Fax:* 608 258-2480
Class Cap: 90   *Begins:* Aug Jan
Length: 20 mos   *Award:* AA
Tuition per yr: $2,004

Milwaukee Area Technical College

Occupational Therapy Asst Prgm
700 W State St
Milwaukee, WI 53233-1443
Prgm Dir: Elaine Strachota, MS OTR
Tel: 414 297-7160   *Fax:* 414 297-6851
E-mail: strachoe@milwaukee.tec.wi.us
Begins: Aug Jan
Length: 18 mos   *Award:* AAS
Tuition per yr: $1,639 res, $10,957 non-res
Evening or weekend classes available

Ophthalmic Medical Technician/Technologist

History

Established in 1969 as the Joint Commission on Allied Health Personnel in Ophthalmology (JCAHPO) represents all segments of ophthalmology, including representatives of the American Academy of Ophthalmology, the Association of University Professors in Ophthalmology, the Contact Lens Association of Ophthalmologists, the Society of Military Ophthalmologists, the Canadian Ophthalmological Society, the American Ophthalmological Society, the Association of Technical Personnel in Ophthalmology (ATPO, formerly AACA-HPO), the American Orthoptic Council, the American Society of Ophthalmic Registered Nurses, the American Association of Certified Orthoptists, the Association of Veterans Affairs Ophthalmologists, and the Canadian Orthoptic Society. JCAHPO and ATPO are the agencies jointly designated to collaborate with the Commission on Accreditation of Allied Health Education Programs (CAAHEP) in the accrediting of educational programs.

In February 1974, the AMA Council on Health Manpower approved the concept of the ophthalmic medical assistant and agreed that a need for a single category of ophthalmic assistant had been demonstrated. To develop educational *Standards (Essentials)*, the AMA Council on Medical Education (CME) worked with representatives of the American Association of Certified Allied Health Personnel in Ophthalmology (AACAHPO), the American Association of Medical Assistants (AAMA), the American Association of Ophthalmology (AAO), the American Academy of Ophthalmology and Otolaryngology (AAOO), the Association of University Professors in Ophthalmology (AUPO), the Contact Lens Association of Ophthalmologists (CLAO), the COA-OMP, and the Society of Military Ophthalmologists (SMO).

It was agreed that in the establishment of *Standards* and the accreditation of educational programs for the ophthalmic medical assistant, the interests of ophthalmological medicine would be represented by COA-OMP and the interests of the allied health occupations by AACAHPO and AAMA. These three organizations developed and adopted the *Standards and Guidelines of an Accredited Educational Program for the Ophthalmic Medical Assistant*, which were then adopted by the AMA House of Delegates at its June 1975 meeting. The Joint Review Committee for the Ophthalmic Medical Assistant changed its name to the Joint Review Committee for Ophthalmic Medical Personnel in 1988, then to the Committee on Accreditation for Ophthalmic Medical Personnel (CoA-OMP) in 1995. The AACAHPO also changed its name in 1988 to Association of Technical Personnel in Ophthalmology. Under the *Standards* approved in 1988, "ophthalmic medical assistant" was omitted and no longer accredited by the Committee on Allied Health Education and Accreditation (CAHEA). The *Standards* now include two levels of programs, ophthalmic medical technician and ophthalmic medical technologist, that are accredited by CAAHEP.

Occupational Description

Ophthalmic medical technicians and technologists are skilled persons qualified by academic and clinical training to perform ophthalmic procedures under the direction or supervision of the ophthalmologist.

Job Description

Ophthalmic medical technicians and technologists assist ophthalmologists by performing tasks delegated to them, such as collecting data and administering treatment ordered by ophthalmologists. They are qualified to take a medical history, administer diagnostic tests, take anatomical and functional ocular measurements, test ocular functions (including visual acuity, visual fields, and sensori-motor functions), administer topical ophthalmic and oral medications, and instruct the patient (as in home care and in use of contact lenses). Duties include caring for and maintaining ophthalmic instruments, sterilizing surgical instruments, assisting in ophthalmic surgery in the office or hospital, taking optical measurements, assisting in the fitting of contact lenses, and adjusting and making minor repairs on spectacles. Ophthalmic medical technicians and technologists may also maintain ophthalmic and surgical instruments as well as office equipment.

Ophthalmic medical technologists perform all duties performed by technicians but are expected to do so at a higher level of expertise and to exercise considerable technical clinical judgment. Additionally, technologists may be expected to perform ophthalmic clinical photography and fluorescence angiography, ocular motility and binocular function tests, and electrophysiological and microbiological procedures, as well as to provide instruction to and supervision of other ophthalmic personnel and patients. (Ophthalmic medical technologist programs are designated with an asterisk in the program listing.)

Employment Characteristics

Ophthalmic medical technicians and technologists render supportive services to the ophthalmologist. They are employed primarily by ophthalmologists but may be employed by medical institutions, clinics, or physician groups and assigned to an ophthalmologist who is responsible for their direction. They may be involved with patients of an ophthalmologist in any setting for which the ophthalmologist is responsible. Salaries vary depending on employer and geographic location.

Educational Programs

Length. Programs are generally 1 year for technicians and 2 years for technologists.

Prerequisites. High school diploma or equivalent for technicians and two years of undergraduate study for technologists.

Curriculum. Instruction should follow a planned outline, which includes courses in anatomy and physiology, medical terminology, medical laws and ethics, psychology, ocular anatomy and physiology, ophthalmic optics, microbiology, ophthalmic pharmacology and toxicology, ocular motility, and diseases of the eye. The curriculum also includes diagnostic and treatment procedures, including visual field testing, contact lenses, ophthalmic surgery, and the care and maintenance of ophthalmic instruments and equipment. Students also must have supervised clinical experience, during which they have opportunities to apply theory to practice through correlated and supervised instruction in clinical practice areas.

Standards. *Standards* are minimum educational standards adopted by the organizations listed above. Each new program is assessed in accordance with the *Standards*, and accredited programs are periodically reviewed to determine whether they remain in substantial compliance. The *Standards* are available on written request from the Committee on Accreditation for Ophthalmic Medical Personnel.

Inquiries

Accreditation

Requests for information on program accreditation, including the *Standards*, preparing the self-study report, and arranging a site visit, should be submitted to

Joint Commission on Allied Health Personnel in Ophthalmology
2025 Woodlane Dr
St Paul, MN 55125-2995
612 731-2944 or 800 284-3937

Careers and Certification

Inquiries regarding careers, continuing education, and certification criteria should be addressed to

Joint Commission on Allied Health Personnel in Ophthalmology
2025 Woodlane Dr
St Paul, MN 55125-2995
612 731-2944 or 800 284-3937

Ophthalmic Medical Technician/ Technologist

District of Columbia

Georgetown University Medical Center
Ophthalmic Med Technologist Prgm*
Center for Sight
3800 Reservoir Rd NW
Washington, DC 20007
Prgm Dir: Phyllis L Fineberg, BA COMT
Tel: 202 687-4862 *Fax:* 202 687-4978
Med Dir: Peter Y Evans, MD
Class Cap: 9 *Begins:* Jul
Length: 23 mos *Award:* Cert
Tuition per yr: $3,700

Florida

University of Florida
Ophthalmic Med Technologist Prgm*
PO Box 100284 JHMHC
Gainesville, FL 32610
Prgm Dir: Diana J Shamis, MHSE CO COMT
Tel: 352 392-3111 *Fax:* 352 392-4201
E-mail: dshamis@eye1.eye.ufi.edu
Med Dir: Melvin Rubin, MD
Begins: Jul
Length: 24 mos *Award:* Cert
Tuition per yr: $2,000

Illinois

Triton College
Ophthalmic Med Technician Prgm
2000 N Fifth Ave
River Grove, IL 60171
Prgm Dir: Debra Baker, COMT
Tel: 708 456-0300 *Fax:* 708 583-3121
Med Dir: Mary Dougal, MD
Class Cap: 30 *Begins:* Aug
Length: 24 mos *Award:* Dipl, AAS
Tuition per yr: $1,200

Louisiana

Louisiana State Univ Med Ctr - New Orleans
Ophthalmic Med Technologist Prgm*
2020 Gravier St/Ste #B
New Orleans, LA 70112
Prgm Dir: Robin Cooper, COMT
Tel: 504 568-6700 *Fax:* 504 568-4470
Med Dir: Herbert E Kaufman, MD
Class Cap: 4 *Begins:* May
Length: 24 mos *Award:* BS
Tuition per yr: $2,359 res, $5,359 non-res

*Designates Ophthalmic Medical Technologist program

Michigan

Detroit Institute of Ophthalmology
Ophthalmic Med Technologist Prgm*
15415 E Jefferson Ave
Grosse Pointe Pk, MI 48230
Prgm Dir: Deanna Presnell, COMT CST
Tel: 313 824-4710 *Fax:* 313 822-4233
Med Dir: Philip C Hessburg, MD
Class Cap: 2 *Begins:* Aug
Length: 22 mos, 20 mos *Award:* Cert
Tuition per yr: $3,120 res, $3,120 non-res
Evening or weekend classes available

Minnesota

St Paul Ramsey Medical Center
Ophthalmic Med Technologist Prgm*
640 Jackson St
St Paul, MN 55101
Prgm Dir: Dianna E Graves, BS COMT
Tel: 612 221-3000 *Fax:* 612 221-2256
Med Dir: Leslie Kopietz, MD
Class Cap: 6 *Begins:* Sep
Length: 21 mos *Award:* Cert
Tuition per yr: $3,400 res, $3,400 non-res

New York

New York Eye and Ear Infirmary
Ophthalmic Med Technologist Prgm*
310 E 14th St
New York, NY 10003
Prgm Dir: Sara Shippman, CO
Tel: 212 979-4375 *Fax:* 212 979-4564
Med Dir: Alan C Weseley, MD
Class Cap: 3 *Begins:* Sep
Length: 22 mos *Award:* Cert
Tuition per yr: $1,500

North Carolina

Duke University Medical Center
Ophthalmic Med Technician Prgm
Eye Ctr PO Box 3802
Durham, NC 27710
Prgm Dir: Judy Seaber, PhD
Tel: 919 684-2038 *Fax:* 919 684-6096
Med Dir: Banks Anderson, MD
Class Cap: 6 *Begins:* Jul
Length: 12 mos *Award:* Cert
Tuition per yr: $2,800

Oregon

Portland Community College
Ophthalmic Med Technician Prgm
PO Box 19000
Portland, OR 97280-0990
Prgm Dir: Joanne M Harris, COT
Tel: 503 978-5666 *Fax:* 503 978-5257
E-mail: jmharris@pcc.edu
Med Dir: James K Tsujimura, MD
Class Cap: 29 *Begins:* Sep
Length: 21 mos *Award:* AAS
Tuition per yr: $1,584 res, $5,520 non-res
Evening or weekend classes available

Virginia

Old Dominion University
Ophthalmic Med Technologist Prgm*
Sight and Hearing Ctr
600 Gresham Dr
Norfolk, VA 23507
Prgm Dir: Kelley J Fleming, CO COMT
Tel: 757 628-2100 *Fax:* 757 668-2109
Med Dir: Ira R Lederman, MD
Class Cap: 3 *Begins:* Sep
Length: 22 mos *Award:* Cert, BS
Tuition per yr: $3,100
Evening or weekend classes available

Ophthalmic-related Occupations

Accreditation History

The Commission on Opticianry Accreditation was formed in 1979 with the sole purpose of accrediting ophthalmic dispensing and ophthalmic laboratory technician educational programs, formerly a function of the National Academy of Opticianry. In 1985, the US Department of Education recognized the commission as the accrediting body for 2-year ophthalmic dispensing and 1-year ophthalmic laboratory technology programs.

Ophthalmic Dispensing Optician

Occupational Description

Ophthalmic dispensing opticians adapt and fit corrective eyewear, including eyeglasses and in some cases contact lenses, as prescribed by an ophthalmologist or optometrist. They help customers select appropriate and attractive frames, then prepare work orders for ophthalmic laboratory technicians, who grind and insert lenses into frames. The dispensing optician then adjusts the finished eyewear to fit customer needs.

Job Description

The ophthalmic dispensing optician combines an understanding of the human eye and vision with customer service skills to order the production of corrective eyewear, aid the patient/customer in selecting appropriate, aesthetically pleasing frames, and adjust the frames to fit the customer's face.

Chief duties of the dispensing optician include

- identifying eye structure, function, and pathology, and determining facial and eye measurements
- assisting the customer in selecting frames and lenses that match the customer's physical features and aesthetic desires
- using an ophthalmologist's or optometrist's prescription to prepare work orders for the ophthalmic laboratory technician
- delivering prescription eyewear/vision aids and instructing customers in use and care
- maintaining patient/customer records and address complaints
- providing follow-up services, including eyewear adjustment, repair, and replacement
- operating and maintaining equipment and demonstrating proficiency in lens finishing techniques
- adapting, dispensing, and fitting contact lenses
- assisting in various business duties, including frame and lens inventory, supply and equipment maintenance, and patient insurance/claim forms submission and record keeping.

Employment Characteristics

Most dispensing opticians work 40-hour weeks in retail stores, some of which may offer one-stop eye examinations, frames, and on-the-spot lens grinding and fitting.

Employment Outlook

As the percentage of middle-aged and elderly people increases, so will these individuals' need for corrective eyewear. Eyewear as fashion—more and more people today now own two or more pairs of eyeglasses for different occasions—also translates into strong future demand for ophthalmic dispensing opticians, as do the many new vision products, such as photochromic lenses (glasses that turn into sunglasses outdoors), now available in plastic and glass; tinted lenses; and bifocal, extended-wear, and disposable contact lenses.

Educational Programs

Length. Ophthalmic dispensing optician programs are 2 years.
Prerequisites. Although no formal requirements exist, ophthalmic dispensing optician students should be familiar with the principles of physics, basic anatomy, algebra, geometry, and mechanical drawing.
Curriculum. Ophthalmic dispensing opticianry educational programs include instruction in optical mathematics, optical physics, and the use of precision measuring instruments and other machinery and tools.
Standards. Each new ophthalmic dispensing opticianry educational program is assessed in accordance with standards published by the Commission on Opticianry Accreditation, and accredited programs are periodically reviewed to ensure that they remain in substantial compliance.

Ophthalmic Laboratory Technician

Occupational Description

Ophthalmic laboratory technicians cut, grind, edge, and finish lenses and fabricate eyewear. Duties include transcribing prescriptions, selecting appropriate lens forms, and processing the materials to meet the prescription.

Job Description

Working from a prescription written by an ophthalmologist or optometrist, the ophthalmic laboratory technician uses various types of equipment and machines, including grinders, polishers, and lensometers, to ensure that the finished lenses match the specifications. The technician also assembles the lens and frame parts into a finished set of eyeglasses.

Chief duties of the ophthalmic laboratory technician include

- safely and effectively operating and maintaining equipment needed to produce lenses and make eyewear
- performing basic mathematical and algebraic operations required on the job
- tinting and coating lenses and performing minor frame repair
- performing impact resistance treatment and testing
- working with ophthalmic dispensing opticians to address and rectify customer/patient complaints
- providing follow-up services, including eyewear adjustment, repair, and replacement
- discussing prescription eyewear/vision aids and consumer/patient-related information with the prescriber
- assisting in various business duties, including frame and lens inventory, supply and equipment maintenance, and record keeping.

Employment Characteristics

Most ophthalmic laboratory technicians work 40-hour weeks, either in retail stores that make and sell prescription glasses or for optical laboratories. Some technicians work for optometrists or ophthalmologists. Depending on the size of the business, the technician may either handle every phase of lenses and frame production or work with other technicians, assembly-line style.

Employment Outlook

As the percentage of middle-aged and elderly people increases, so will these individuals' need for corrective eyewear. Much of the growth in this profession will occur in retail optical chain stores that make prescription eyewear on the premises and offer quick turnaround time.

Educational Programs

Length. Ophthalmic laboratory technician programs are 1 year.
Prerequisites. Although no formal requirements exist, ophthalmic laboratory technician students should have a broad knowledge of science and mathemathics and a high level of manual dexterity.
Curriculum. Ophthalmic laboratory technician educational programs include instruction in optical theory, surfacing and lens finishing, and reading and applying prescriptions.
Standards. Each new ophthalmic laboratory technician educational program is assessed in accordance with standards published by the Commission on Opticianry Accreditation, and accredited programs are periodically reviewed to ensure that they remain in substantial compliance.

Inquiries

Accreditation

Inquiries regarding accreditation should be directed to

Floyd H Holmgrain, Jr, EdD, Executive Director
Commission on Opticianry Accreditation
10111 Martin Luther King Jr Hwy/Ste 100
Bowie, MD 20720-4200
301 459-8075
301 577-3880 Fax

Careers

Inquiries regarding careers should be directed to

Contact Lens Society of America
441 Carlisle Dr
Reston, VA 22070
703 437-5100

National Academy of Opticianry
National Federation of Opticianry Schools
10111 Martin Luther King Jr Hwy/#112
Bowie, MD 20720-4299
301 577-4828

Optical Laboratories Association
PO Box 2000
Merrifield, VA 22116-2000
703 849-8550

Optical Manufacturers Association
6055-A Arlington Blvd
Falls Church, VA 22044
703 237-8433

Opticians Association of America
10341 Democracy Ln
Fairfax, VA 22030-2521
703 691-8355

Ophthalmic Dispensing Optician

Connecticut

Middlesex Community - Technical College
Ophthalmic Dispenser Prgm
Ophthalmic Design and Dispensing
100 Training Hill Rd
Middletown, CT 06457
Prgm Dir: Raymond P Dennis
Tel: 860 343-5845

Florida

Miami-Dade Community College
Ophthalmic Dispenser Prgm
Vision Care Technology/Opticianry
950 NW 20th St
Miami, FL 33127
Prgm Dir: Jerry Brown
Tel: 305 237-4267

Hillsborough Community College
Ophthalmic Dispenser Prgm
PO Box 30030
Tampa, FL 33630
Prgm Dir: William Underwood
Tel: 813 253-7433

Georgia

De Kalb Technical Institute
Ophthalmic Dispenser Prgm
495 Indian Creek Dr
Clarkston, GA 30021
Prgm Dir: Thomas Schulz
Tel: 404 297-9522, Ext 207 *Fax:* 404 294-4234
E-mail: tschulz@atlcom.net
Class Cap: 26 *Begins:* Sep
Length: 18 mos *Award:* Dipl, AAT
Tuition per yr: $882 res, $882 non-res
Evening or weekend classes available

Massachusetts

Mt Ida College
Ophthalmic Dispenser Prgm
Opticianry
777 Dedham St
Newton Centre, MA 02159
Prgm Dir: Maynard Rosen
Tel: 617 969-7000, Ext 324
Class Cap: 30 *Begins:* Sep
Length: 24 mos *Award:* AAS
Tuition per yr: $11,000

Worcester Technical Institute
Ophthalmic Dispenser Prgm
251 Belmont St
Worcester, MA 01605
Prgm Dir: Charles Walsh
Tel: 508 799-1945
Class Cap: 16 *Begins:* Aug
Length: 18 mos *Award:* Dipl, AAS
Tuition per yr: $1,600 res, $3,000 non-res

Michigan

Ferris State University
Ophthalmic Dispenser Prgm
Opticianry
VFS 424
Big Rapids, MI 49307
Prgm Dir: Russell B Hess
Tel: 616 592-2224 *Fax:* 616 592-2394
Class Cap: 32 *Begins:* Aug
Length: 22 mos *Award:* AAS
Tuition per yr: $3,665 res, $3,665 non-res

Minnesota

Anoka-Hennepin Technical College
Ophthalmic Dispenser Prgm
1355 W Main St
Anoka, MN 55303
Prgm Dir: Myron Moe
Tel: 612 427-1880, Ext 267 *Fax:* 612 576-4715
E-mail: mmoe@ank.tec.mn.us
Class Cap: 24 *Begins:* Sep
Length: 9 mo , 18 mos *Award:* Cert, AAS
Tuition per yr: $1,400 res, $1,400 non-res
Evening or weekend classes available

New Hampshire

New Hampshire Tech College - Nashua
Ophthalmic Dispenser Prgm
Opticianry
505 Amherst St
Nashua, NH 03061-2052
Prgm Dir: Michael A Szczerbiak
Tel: 603 882-6923, Ext 66

New Jersey

Camden County College
Ophthalmic Dispenser Prgm
Ophthalmic Science
PO Box 200
Blackwood, NJ 08012
Prgm Dir: Raymond J DiDonato
Tel: 609 227-7200, Ext 322

Essex County College
Ophthalmic Dispenser Prgm
303 University Ave
Newark, NJ 07102
Prgm Dir: Russell Elmo Jr
Tel: 201 877-3367

Raritan Valley Community College
Ophthalmic Dispenser Prgm
Ophthalmic Science
PO Box 3300
Somerville, NJ 08876
Prgm Dir: Brian Thomas
Tel: 908 526-1200, Ext 8277

New Mexico

Southwestern Indian Polytechnic Institute
Ophthalmic Dispenser Prgm
Optical Technology-Dispensing
9169 Coors Rd NW
Albuquerque, NM 87184
Prgm Dir: Samuel Henderson
Tel: 505 897-5359

New York

CUNY New York City Technical College
Ophthalmic Dispenser Prgm
300 Jay St
Brooklyn, NY 11201
Prgm Dir: Edward C August
Tel: 718 260-5298

Interboro Institute
Ophthalmic Dispenser Prgm
450 W 56th St
New York, NY 10019
Prgm Dir: Jayne H Weinberger
Tel: 212 399-0091

Mater Dei College
Ophthalmic Dispenser Prgm
Opticianry
5428 State Hwy 37
Ogdensburg, NY 13669
Prgm Dir: Debra White
Tel: 315 393-5930 *Fax:* 315 393-5056
Class Cap: 30 *Begins:* Sep Jan
Length: 24 mos *Award:* AAS
Tuition per yr: $6,350
Evening or weekend classes available

Erie Community College - North Campus
Ophthalmic Dispenser Prgm
6205 Main St
Williamsville, NY 14221-7095
Prgm Dir: Paul E Will
Tel: 716 634-0800, Ext 400

North Carolina

Durham Technical Community College
Ophthalmic Dispenser Prgm
1637 Lawson St
Durham, NC 27703
Prgm Dir: Ellen Stoner
Tel: 919 686-3485 *Fax:* 919 317-1317
E-mail: ellen@nccu.campus.mci.net
Class Cap: 30 *Begins:* Sept Aug
Length: 21 mos *Award:* AAS
Tuition per yr: $800 res, $4,500 non-res

Tennessee

Roane State Community College
Ophthalmic Dispenser Prgm
Opticianry
Patton Ln
Harriman, TN 37748
Prgm Dir: Michael Goggin
Tel: 423 882-4594 *Fax:* 423 882-4549
E-mail: goggin_mt@a1.rscc.cc.tn.us
Med Dir: John B Cousar, MD
Class Cap: 20 *Begins:* Aug
Length: 24 mos *Award:* AAS
Tuition per yr: $0 res, $1,463 non-res

Texas

El Paso Community College
Ophthalmic Dispenser Prgm
Ophthalmic Technology
PO Box 20500
El Paso, TX 79998
Prgm Dir: Jose Baca, BS FNAO
Tel: 915 594-2000 *Fax:* 915 534-4114
Class Cap: 15 *Begins:* Aug Jan
Length: 12 mos, 24 mos *Award:* Cert, AAS
Tuition per yr: $1,267 res, $4,160 non-res
Evening or weekend classes available

Virginia

J Sargeant Reynolds Community College
Ophthalmic Dispenser Prgm
Opticianry
PO Box 85622
Richmond, VA 23285-5622
Prgm Dir: Joel Adler
Tel: 804 786-3494

Tri-Service Optician Schools (TOPS)
Ophthalmic Dispenser Prgm
Naval Ophthalmic Support & Trng Activity
NWS PO Box 350
Yorktown, VA 23691-0350
Prgm Dir: HMC William J Dufort, USN
Tel: 757 887-7148 *Fax:* 757 887-4511
E-mail: dufort@nos5.med.navy.mil
Class Cap: 130 *Begins:* Quarterly
Length: 6 mos *Award:* Cert

Washington

Seattle Central Community College
Ophthalmic Dispenser Prgm
1701 Broadway
Seattle, WA 98122
Prgm Dir: Gary Clayton
Tel: 206 344-4321

Programs

Ophthalmic Laboratory Technician

New Mexico

Southwestern Indian Polytechnic Institute
Ophthalmic Laboratory Technician Prgm
Optical Technology
9169 Coors Rd NW
Albuquerque, NM 87184
Prgm Dir: Samuel Henderson
Tel: 505 897-5359

New York

Nat'l Tech Inst for Deaf/Rochester Inst Tech
Ophthalmic Laboratory Technician Prgm
Optical Finishing Technology
52 Lomb Memorial Dr/Bldg LBJ
Rochester, NY 14623-0887
Prgm Dir: Douglas Wachter
Tel: 716 475-6585
Class Cap: 16   *Begins:* Sep
Length: 27 mos   *Award:* AAS , AOS
Tuition per yr: $5,211 res, $5,211 non-res

Virginia

Tri-Service Optician Schools (TOPS)
Ophthalmic Laboratory Technician Prgm
Naval Ophthalmic Support & Trng Activity
NWS PO Box 350
Yorktown, VA 23691-0350
Prgm Dir: HMC William J Dufort, USN
Tel: 757 887-7148

Orthotist and Prosthetist

History

The Educational Accreditation Commission (EAC) was created in August 1972 by the American Board of Certification in Orthotics and Prosthetics, Inc (ABC) to meet the orthotics and prosthetics profession's need for an institutional accreditation program. That same year the EAC set out to establish criteria to assess and compare orthotics and prosthetics curricula. These criteria *Standards (Essentials)* were developed and revised to meet the profession's needs in training orthotists and prosthetists.

In 1991, the EAC was reorganized and renamed the National Commission on Orthotic and Prosthetic Education (NCOPE). NCOPE's primary mission and obligation is to ensure that educational programs meet the minimum standards of quality to prepare individuals to enter the orthotics and prosthetics profession.

During 1992, the NCOPE and its collaborating organizations, the American Orthotic and Prosthetic Association (AOPA) and the American Academy of Orthotists and Prosthetists (AAOP), applied to the American Medical Association (AMA) Council of Medical Education (CME) for recognition of orthotics and prosthetics as an allied health profession. Recognition was granted in August 1992.

In February 1993, the NCOPE reformatted its existing *Standards* to meet the requirements of the Committee on Allied Health Education and Accreditation (CAHEA) Recommended Format for *Standards and Guidelines*. The *Standards* were adopted by AOPA in April 1993. The AMA CME adopted the *Standards* in August 1993, and the AAOP adopted the *Standards* in September 1993.

Occupational Description

Orthotics and prosthetics are applied physical disciplines that address neuromuscular and structural skeletal problems in the human body with a treatment process that includes evaluation and transfer of forces using orthoses and protheses to achieve optimum function, prevent further disability, and provide cosmesis.

The orthotist and prosthetist work directly with the physician and representatives of other allied health professions in the rehabilitation of the physically challenged. The orthotist designs and fits devices, known as orthoses, to provide care to patients who have disabling conditions of the limbs and spine. The prosthetist designs and fits devices, known as prostheses, for patients who have partial or total absence of a limb.

Job Description

In 1990 and 1991, a role delineation study was conducted by the profession to study the primary tasks performed by the entry-level orthotist and prosthetist. It focused on which tasks are performed on the job, how important each task is, how frequently the task is performed, and how critical the task is. The study concluded that the role of the orthotist and prosthetist includes, but may not be limited to, five major domains: clinical assessment, patient management, technical implementation, practice management, and professional responsibility.

Employment Characteristics

Orthotists and prosthetists typically provide their services in one or more of the following settings: private facilities, hospitals and clinics, colleges and universities, and medical schools.

According to the NCOPE, the salary for board-certified orthotists and prosthetists averaged between $36,000 and $59,000 in 1995.

Educational Programs

Length. Orthotic and/or prosthetic education occurs in two forms: baccalaureate degree and certificate programs. Degree programs are based on a standard 4-year curriculum, and certificate courses range from 6 months to 1 year for one discipline to 18 months to 2 years for both disciplines.

Prerequisites. Applicants for the 4-year baccalaureate degree programs should have a high school diploma or equivalent and meet institutional entrance requirements. Applicants for post-baccalaureate programs should have a baccalaureate degree that includes appropriate course work in biology, chemistry, physics, psychology, computer science, algebra, human anatomy, and physiology, as well as any other specified by the institution.

Curriculum. The professional curriculum includes formal instruction in biomechanics gait analysis/pathomechanics, kinesiology, pathology, materials science, research methods, diagnostic imaging techniques, measurement, impression taking, model rectification, diagnostic fitting, definitive fitting, postoperative management, external power, static and dynamic alignment of sockets related to various amputation levels, and fitting and alignment of orthoses for lower limb, upper limb, and spine with various systems to be included. The curriculum also includes a clinical experience.

Standards. *Standards* are the minimum educational standards developed by NCOPE, AOPA, AAOP, and the AMA. Each new program is assessed in accordance with the *Standards and Guidelines for an Accredited Educational Program for the Orthotist and Prosthetist*, and accredited programs are reviewed periodically to determine whether they remain in compliance.

Inquiries

Accreditation

Requests for information on program accreditation, including *Standards*, preparing the self-study report, and arranging a site visit, should be submitted to

National Commission on Orthotic and Prosthetic Education
1650 King St/Ste 500
Alexandria, VA 22314
703 836-7114   703 836-0838 Fax
E-mail: opncope@aol.com

Careers

Inquiries regarding careers should be addressed to

National Commission on Orthotic and Prosthetic Education
1650 King St/Ste 500
Alexandria, VA 22314
703 836-7114   703 836-0838 Fax
E-mail: opncope@aol.com

American Academy of Orthotists and Prosthetists
1650 King St/Ste 500
Alexandria, VA 22314
703 836-7118   703 836-0838 Fax

American Orthotic & Prosthetic Association
1650 King St/Ste 500
Alexandria, VA 22314
703 836-7116
E-mail: www.theaopa.org

Certification

Inquiries regarding certification may be addressed to

American Board for Certification in Orthotics & Prosthetics, Inc
1650 King St/Ste 500
Alexandria, VA 22314
703 836-7114   703 836-0838 Fax
E-mail: lanceabc@aol.com

Orthotist/Prosthetist

California

California State Univ-Dominguez Hills
Orthotist/Prosthetist Prgm
1000 E Victoria Blvd/ERC A505
Carson, CA 90747
Prgm Dir: Scott Hornbeak, MBA CPO
Tel: 310 516-4170   *Fax:* 310 516-3846
Class Cap: 28   *Begins:* Jul
Length: 9 mos   *Award:* Cert
Tuition per yr: $10,000 res, $10,000 non-res

Connecticut

Connecticut Children's Medical Center
Orthotist/Prosthetist Prgm
Newington Certificate Prgm
181 E Cedar St
Newington, CT 06111
Prgm Dir: Robert S Lin, CPO
Tel: 860 667-5360   *Fax:* 860 667-1719
Med Dir: Joseph Smey, EdD
Class Cap: 40   *Begins:* Sep
Length: 9 mos   *Award:* Cert
Tuition per yr: $12,500
Evening or weekend classes available

Programs

Perfusionist

History

The field of cardiovascular perfusion emerged in the mid-1960s, with most of its practitioners trained on the job until the mid-1970s. Trainees often come from other disciplines: nursing, respiratory therapy, biomedical engineering, surgical technology, monitoring technicians, and the laboratory sciences.

In 1972, the American Society of Extra-Corporeal Technologists (AmSECT) began a program of certification for perfusionists. In 1975, this program was turned over to a new agency established to conduct certification as an independent activity: the American Board of Cardiovascular Perfusion (ABCP). The ABCP also adopted minimum standards for training programs as developed by AmSECT and began evaluation and accreditation activities. AmSECT, with the cosponsorship of the American Association of Thoracic Surgeons (AATS) and the Society of Thoracic Surgeons (STS), petitioned the American Medical Association (AMA) for recognition of the occupation in January 1975. The petition was amended on several occasions, and in December 1976 the Committee on Emerging Health Manpower recommended approval; the AMA Council on Medical Education (CME) granted recognition in that same month.

In 1977, four collaborating organizations sponsored the formation of the Joint Review Committee for Perfusion Education (JRC-PE)—the AATS, ABCP, AmSECT, and STS. From 1978 to 1979, the JRC-PE and others developed the *Standards (Essentials) and Guidelines for an Accredited Educational Program for the Perfusionist*. The *Standards* were adopted in 1980 and accreditation of programs began in 1981. The *Standards* were revised in 1984 and 1989. In 1984, the Perfusion Program Directors Council became an additional sponsor, as did the Society of Cardiovascular Anesthesiologists in 1989. In 1991, the review committee became known as the Accreditation Committee for Perfusion Education (AC-PE). In 1996, the American Academy of Cardiovascular Perfusion became an additional sponsor of the review committee.

Occupational Description

A perfusionist is a skilled person, qualified by academic and clinical education, who operates extracorporeal circulation and autotransfusion equipment during any medical situation where it is necessary to support or temporarily replace the patient's circulatory or respiratory function. The perfusionist is knowledgeable concerning the variety of equipment available to perform extracorporeal circulation functions and is responsible, in consultation with the physician, for selecting the appropriate equipment and techniques to be used.

Job Description

Perfusionists conduct extracorporeal circulation and ensure the safe management of physiologic functions by monitoring the necessary variables. Perfusion (extracorporeal circulation) procedures involve specialized instrumentation and/or advanced life-support techniques and may include a variety of related functions. The perfusionist provides consultation to the physician in the selection of the appropriate equipment and techniques to be used during extracorporeal circulation.

During cardiopulmonary bypass, the perfusionist may administer blood products, anesthetic agents, or drugs through the extracorporeal circuit on prescription and/or appropriate protocol. The perfusionist is responsible for the monitoring of blood gases and the adequate anticoagulation of the patient, induction of hypothermia, hemodilution, and other duties, when prescribed. Perfusionists may be administratively responsible for purchasing supplies and equip-

ment, as well as for personnel and departmental management. Final medical responsibility for extracorporeal perfusion rests with the surgeon-in-charge.

Employment Characteristics

Perfusionists may be employed in hospitals, by surgeons, and as employees of a group practice. They typically work during the week and are frequently on call for emergency procedures on weekends and nights. They also may work in an on-call system, depending on the number of perfusionists employed by the institution.

According to the AmSECT, the average base salary for a recently graduated perfusionist is $40,000; for a certified perfusionist with 2 to 5 years experience, $55,000 to $60,000; 5 to 10 years experience, $60,000 to $100,000; and chief perfusionist, $100,000 and higher.

Educational Programs

Length. Programs are generally 1 to 4 years in length, depending on the program design, objectives, prerequisites, and student qualifications.

Prerequisites. Prerequisites vary depending on the length and design of the program. Most programs require college-level science and mathematics. A background in medical technology, respiratory therapy, or nursing is suggested for some programs.

Curriculum. Curricula of accredited programs include courses covering heart-lung bypass for adult, pediatric, and infant patients undergoing heart surgery; long-term supportive extracorporeal circulation; monitoring of the patient undergoing extracorporeal circulation; autotransfusion; and special applications of the technology. Curricula include clinical experience that incorporates and requires performance of an adequate number and variety of circulation procedures.

Standards. *Standards* are minimum educational standards adopted by the American Academy of Cardiovascular Perfusion, American Association for Thoracic Surgery, American Board of Cardiovascular Perfusion, American Medical Association, American Society of Extra-Corporeal Technology, Commission on Accreditation of Allied Health Education Programs, the Perfusion Program Directors Council, the Society of Cardiovascular Anesthesiologists, and the Society of Thoracic Surgeons. Each new program is assessed in accordance with the *Standards*, and accredited programs are periodically reviewed to determine whether they remain in substantial compliance. The *Standards and Guidelines* are available on written request from the Accreditation Committee for Perfusion Education.

Inquiries

Accreditation

Requests for information on program accreditation, including *Standards*, preparing the self-study report, and arranging a site visit, should be submitted to

Accreditation Committee for Perfusion Education
7108-C S Alton Way/Ste 150
Englewood, CO 80112
303 741-3598
303 741-3655 Fax

Careers

Inquiries regarding careers and curriculum should be addressed to

AmSECT National Office
11480 Sunset Hills Rd/Ste 200E
Reston, VA 22090-9955
703 435-8556

American Academy of Cardiovascular Perfusion
PO Box 468
Pell City, AL 35125
205 338-6355
E-mail: OfficeAACP@aol.com
Internet: http://users.aol.com/OfficeAACP

Certification

Inquiries regarding certification may be addressed to

American Board of Cardiovascular Perfusion
207 N 25th Ave
Hattiesburg, MS 39401
601 582-3309

Perfusionist

Arizona

University of Arizona
Perfusionist Prgrm
1501 N Campbell Ave
Tucson, AZ 85724
Prgm Dir: Douglas L Larson, PhD CCP
Tel: 520 626-6339   *Fax:* 520 626-4042
E-mail: dlarson@ccit.arizona.edu
Med Dir: Gulshan Sethi, MD
Class Cap: 3   *Begins:* Aug
Length: 20 mos   *Award:* Cert, MS
Tuition per yr: $1,950 res, $7,978 non-res

Connecticut

Quinnipiac College
Perfusionist Prgm
275 Mt Carmel Ave
Hamden, CT 06518
Prgm Dir: Michael J Smith, PhD RRT CCP
Tel: 203 288-5251   *Fax:* 203 281-8706
E-mail: msmith@quinnipiac
Med Dir: Charles G Newton, MD
Class Cap: 10   *Begins:* Sep
Length: 16 mos   *Award:* Cert, BS
Tuition per yr: $13,685

District of Columbia

Walter Reed Army Medical Center
Perfusionist Prgm
Washington, DC 20307-5001
Prgm Dir: James M Ogletree, MMS PA-C CCP
Tel: 202 782-6438   *Fax:* 202 782-8253
Med Dir: Christopher A Danby, Maj MC
Class Cap: 10   *Begins:* Jan Jul
Length: 18 mos   *Award:* Cert

Florida

Barry University
Perfusionist Prgm
11300 NE 2nd Ave
Miami Shores, FL 33161
Prgm Dir: Jason L Freed, MS CCP
Tel: 305 899-3214   *Fax:* 305 899-3845
E-mail: jfreed@buaxpi.barry.edu
Med Dir: Richard A Perryman, MD
Class Cap: 22   *Begins:* Aug
Length: 21 mos   *Award:* Dipl, BS
Tuition per yr: $19,285

Programs

Illinois

Rush University
Perfusionist Prgm
1653 W Harrison St
Chicago, IL 60612
Prgm Dir: Michael Djuric, BA MA CCP
Tel: 312 942-2305 *Fax:* 312 942-6989
Med Dir: William M Piccione, BS MD
Class Cap: 6 *Begins:* Sep
Length: 21 mos *Award:* BS
Tuition per yr: $15,200

Iowa

University of Iowa Hospitals and Clinics
Perfusionist Prgm
Dept of Surgery
Iowa City, IA 52242
Prgm Dir: Robin Sutton, MS CCP
Tel: 319 356-8496 *Fax:* 319 353-7174
E-mail: robin-sutton@uiowa.edu
Med Dir: Wayne E Richenbacher, MD
Class Cap: 6 *Begins:* Aug
Length: 21 mos *Award:* Cert
Tuition per yr: $3,705 res, $13,602 non-res

Kansas

Via Christi Regional Med Ctr/St Joseph Campus
Perfusionist Prgm
3600 E Harry
Wichita, KS 67218
Prgm Dir: Linda Cantu, RN CCP
Tel: 316 689-6017 *Fax:* 316 689-5297
Med Dir: Daniel Tatpati, MD
Class Cap: 3 *Begins:* Aug
Length: 12 mos *Award:* BS
Tuition per yr: $9,990

Maryland

Johns Hopkins Hospital
Perfusionist Prgm
600 N Wolfe St
Baltimore, MD 21287-4814
Prgm Dir: Adam Clark
Tel: 410 955-5168 *Fax:* 410 955-4163
Med Dir: William A Baumgartner, MD
Class Cap: 6 *Begins:* Sep
Length: 16 mos *Award:* Cert
Tuition per yr: $9,500 res, $9,500 non-res

Massachusetts

Northeastern University
Perfusionist Prgm
360 Huntington Ave
Boston, MA 02215
Prgm Dir: Patrick F Plunkett, EdD
Tel: 617 373-2407 *Fax:* 617 373-3030
E-mail: p.plunkett@nunet.neu.edu
Med Dir: Fred G Davis, MD
Class Cap: 8 *Begins:* Sep
Length: 24 mos *Award:* MS
Tuition per yr: $9,500

Minnesota

Univ of Minnesota Hosp and Clinic
Perfusionist Prgm
Health and Lung Institute
425 E River Rd
Minneapolis, MN 55455
Prgm Dir: Richard J Irmiter, AS-CCP
Tel: 612 625-7168 *Fax:* 612 625-1683
E-mail: irmit001@maroon.tc.umn.edu
Med Dir: Yoshio Sako, MD
Class Cap: 5 *Begins:* Jan
Length: 18 mos *Award:* Cert
Tuition per yr: $10,500 res, $10,500 non-res

Mississippi

Garden Park Community Hospital
Perfusionist Prgm
PO Box 299
Pelahatchie, MS 39145
Prgm Dir: Pat H Courtney Jr, CCP
Tel: 601 854-8667
Med Dir: E T Warren, MD
Class Cap: 40 *Begins:* Mar Sep
Length: 12 mos *Award:* Dipl
Tuition per yr: $5,350

Nebraska

University of Nebraska Medical Center
Perfusionist Prgm
600 S 42nd St
Omaha, NE 68198-5155
Prgm Dir: Alfred H Stammers, MSA CCP
Tel: 402 559-7227 *Fax:* 402 559-6455
E-mail: astammer@unmc.edu
Med Dir: Timothy A Galbraith, MD
Class Cap: 6 *Begins:* Aug
Length: 20 mos *Award:* Cert
Tuition per yr: $3,375 res, $8,339 non-res

New Jersey

Cooper Hospital/University Medical Ctr
Perfusionist Prgm
One Cooper Plaza/Box 217
Camden, NJ 08103
Prgm Dir: Louis Brownstein, CCP
Tel: 609 342-3277 *Fax:* 609 541-1833
Med Dir: Anthony Del Rossi, MD
Class Cap: 5 *Begins:* Sep
Length: 21 mos *Award:* Cert
Tuition per yr: $6,000

Eastern Heart Inst Gen Hosp Ctr-Passaic
Perfusionist Prgm
350 Blvd
Passaic, NJ 07053
Prgm Dir: Richard Chan, CCP
Tel: 201 365-4492 Fax: 201 916-2514
Med Dir: Kenneth N Howlitt, MD
Class Cap: 6 *Begins:* Nov
Length: 15 mos *Award:* Cert
Tuition per yr: $10,800

New York

SUNY Health Science Center at Syracuse
Perfusionist Prgm
750 E Adams St
Syracuse, NY 13210
Prgm Dir: Jeanne S Lange, RN
Tel: 315 464-6933 *Fax:* 315 464-6914
E-mail: langej@vax.cs.hscsyr.edu
Med Dir: Frederick B Parker, MD
Class Cap: 4 *Begins:* Aug
Length: 19 mos *Award:* AAS
Tuition per yr: $3,390 res, $7,836 non-res

Ohio

Christ Hospital
Perfusionist Prgm
2139 Auburn Ave
Cincinnati, OH 45219
Prgm Dir: Craig Warmuth, MEd, CCP
Tel: 513 369-1106 *Fax:* 513 629-3299
Med Dir: George M Callard, MD
Class Cap: 6 *Begins:* Sep
Length: 24 mos *Award:* Cert
Tuition per yr: $6,400 res, $12,420 non-res

Cleveland Clinic Foundation
Perfusionist Prgm
9500 Euclid Ave (G-33)
Cleveland, OH 44195-5130
Prgm Dir: Carolyn Moyers, BS CCP
Tel: 216 444-3895 *Fax:* 216 445-2725
Med Dir: Lee Wallace, MD
Class Cap: 6 *Begins:* Sep
Length: 24 mos *Award:* Cert
Tuition per yr: $4,765 res, $11,632 non-res

Ohio State University
Perfusionist Prgm
1583 Perry St
Columbus, OH 43210
Prgm Dir: Paul D Shinko, MEd CCP
Tel: 614 292-7261 *Fax:* 614 292-0210
Med Dir: Leon Camerlengo, MD
Class Cap: 8 *Begins:* Sep
Length: 21 mos *Award:* Cert, BS
Tuition per yr: $5,459 res, $14,615 non-res
Evening or weekend classes available

Oregon

Providence/St. Vincent & Medical Center
Perfusionist Prgm
9155 SW Barnes Rd Ste 230
Portland, OR 97225
Prgm Dir: Gregory A Meiling, BS PA CCP
Tel: 503 297-1419 *Fax:* 503 216-2488
Med Dir: Jeffrey Swanson, MD
Class Cap: 7 *Begins:* Sep
Length: 12 mos *Award:* Cert
Tuition per yr: $9,000

Pennsylvania

M S Hershey Med Center/Penn State Univ
Perfusionist Prgm
PO Box 850
Hershey, PA 17033
Prgm Dir: Dennis R Williams, CCP
Tel: 717 531-8550 *Fax:* 717 531-4017
E-mail: dwilliam@nursing.hmc.psu.edu
Med Dir: William S Pierce, MD
Class Cap: 3 *Begins:* Jul
Length: 24 mos *Award:* Cert
Tuition per yr: $12,500 res, $12,500 non-res

Allegheny University of the Health Sciences
Perfusionist Prgm
Broad and Vine Sts
Philadelphia, PA 19102-1192
Prgm Dir: Robert B Stroud, BS CCP
Tel: 215 762-7895 *Fax:* 215 246-5347
Med Dir: Stanley K Brockman, MD
Class Cap: 8 *Begins:* Aug
Length: 21 mos *Award:* Dipl,Cert, BS
Tuition per yr: $9,000

Episcopal Hospital
Perfusionist Prgm
Front and Lehigh Aves
Philadelphia, PA 19125
Prgm Dir: Roberta Myers, RN CCP
Tel: 215 427-7748
Med Dir: Peter Figueroa, MD
Class Cap: 8 *Begins:* Feb Aug
Length: 12 mos *Award:* Dipl
Tuition per yr: $13,000

Duquesne University
Perfusionist Prgm
Rangos Sch of Hlth Sciences
Hlth Sciences Bldg/Room 216
Pittsburgh, PA 15282
Prgm Dir: Joyce A D'Antonio, PhD
Tel: 412 396-5556 *Fax:* 412 396-5554
E-mail: dantonio@dug2.cc.dug.edu
Med Dir: Ronald V Pellegrini, MD
Class Cap: 15 *Begins:* Aug
Length: 44 mos *Award:* BS
Tuition per yr: $15,428 res, $15,428 non-res
Evening or weekend classes available

Shadyside Hospital
Perfusionist Prgm
5230 Centre Ave
Pittsburgh, PA 15232
Prgm Dir: R D Rush, CCP
Tel: 412 623-2482
Med Dir: Richard Feduska, MD
Class Cap: 12 *Begins:* Jun
Length: 15 mos *Award:* Cert, BS
Tuition per yr: $10,588

South Carolina

Medical University of South Carolina
Perfusionist Prgm
Coll Hlth Related Professions
171 Ashley Ave
Charleston, SC 29425
Prgm Dir: Jeffrey B Riley, BA CCT CCP
Tel: 803 792-2298
Med Dir: John R Handy Jr
Class Cap: 24 *Begins:* Aug
Length: 21 mos *Award:* BS
Tuition per yr: $3,520 res, $9,630 non-res

Tennessee

Vanderbilt University Medical Center
Perfusionist Prgm
The Vanderbilt Clinic/Rm 2973
Nashville, TN 37232
Prgm Dir: Walter H Merrill, MD
Tel: 615 322-0064 *Fax:* 615 343-9194
Med Dir: Harvey W Bender, Jr, MD
Class Cap: 3 *Begins:* July
Length: 18 mos *Award:* Cert
Tuition per yr: $5,000 res, $5,000 non-res

Texas

Texas Heart Institute
Perfusionist Prgm
PO Box 20345
Houston, TX 77225
Prgm Dir: Raymond J McInnis Jr, MEd CCP
Tel: 713 791-4026 *Fax:* 713 791-4993
E-mail: tstafford@biostl.thi.time.edu
Med Dir: John R Cooper, MD
Class Cap: 12 *Begins:* Jan Jul
Length: 12 mos *Award:* Cert
Tuition per yr: $4,000 res, $9,000 non-res

Wisconsin

Milwaukee School of Engineering
Perfusionist Prgm
1025 N Broadway St
Milwaukee, WI 53202-3109
Prgm Dir: Vincent R Canino, PhD PE
Tel: 414 277-7331 *Fax:* 414 277-7465
E-mail: canino@warp.msor.edu
Med Dir: Alfred J Tector, MD
Class Cap: 12 *Begins:* Sep
Length: 18 mos *Award:* MS
Tuition per yr: $5,100

Physician Assistant Practice

The concept of the physician assistant arose in the mid-1960s and early 1970s when a number of institutions and creative members of their faculty and staff began exploring new territory in American medical education. Their goal was to assist physicians in patient care. In the process, they developed curricula that taught individuals a body of clinical knowledge and skills that previously had largely been limited to the professional preserve of the physician.

In its restricted meaning, "physician assistant" is the title used since the late 1970s to identify a person prepared in the clinical knowledge and skills that are common to primary care medicine. Initially, this person was identified as an assistant to the primary care physician.

In its general meaning, "physician assistant" is used to encompass the primary care physician assistant, as described above, but it also has been applied to personnel such as surgeon assistants, anesthesiologist assistants, pathologists' assistants, radiologist assistants, urologist assistants, and others. While several of these types of physician assistants are very small in number, two occupations with listings in this *Directory* have obtained recognition from the American Medical Association: anesthesiologist assistant and physician assistant. (*Note*: For information on the occupation of anesthesiologist assistant, including program listings, see pages 15-17.)

Physician Assistant

History

The profession of physician assistant originated in the mid-1960s with leadership from Duke University, the University of Colorado, the University of Washington, and Wake Forest University. The early 1970s brought a rapid growth in the number of such educational programs, which were supported initially with $6.1 million appropriated under the authority of the Health Manpower Act of 1972. This funding also supported some of the initial organization and administration of the national program for the accreditation of educational programs in this field, specifically those designed to prepare individuals as assistants to primary care practitioners.

Interest in the development of national accreditation standards for the education of assistants to primary care physicians was first expressed by the American Society of Internal Medicine.

By 1971, standards had been developed collaboratively by a committee composed of representatives from the American Academy of Family Physicians (AAFP), the American Academy of Pediatrics (AAP), the American College of Physicians (ACP), the American Medical Association (AMA), the Association of American Medical Colleges (AAMC), the American College of Obstetrics and Gynecology (ACOG), the American Society of Internal Medicine (ASIM), the nursing profession, and educators of the physician assistant. These standards were adopted in that year by the AMA, AAFP, AAP, ACP, and ASIM. (The ASIM withdrew its sponsorship of accreditation in September 1981.)

Early in 1972, the medical specialty organizations that had adopted the new educational standards established the Joint Review Committee on Educational Programs for the Assistant to the Primary Care Physician. A principal function of the committee was to assess the extent to which applicant programs were in compliance with the *Standards (Essentials) and Guidelines for the Assistant to the Primary Care Physician* and to formulate recommendations for accreditation to the AMA Council on Medical Education (CME). This committee was composed of three representatives from each of the four sponsoring organizations. In April 1973, the committee appointed three graduate physician assistants to serve

as members-at-large for 1-year terms. By March 1974, the sponsors of the committee and the AMA had recognized the American Academy of Physician Assistants as the fifth sponsor of the review committee.

Standards for the surgeon assistant were adopted by the American College of Surgeons in 1973 and by the AMA in 1974. Originally, the American College of Surgeons Committee on Allied Health Personnel reviewed applicant programs' compliance with these standards.

As a result of discussions initiated in 1975, the review committees for the assistant to the primary care physician and surgeon assistant were brought together in 1976 into a unified accreditation review committee. On petition from the Association of Physician Assistant Programs, the collaborating sponsoring organizations of the accreditation review committee and the AMA recognized it as the seventh sponsor of the committee in 1978. The AMA became a sponsor of the review committee in 1994 following the dissolution of the Committee on Allied Health Education and Accreditation. The committee was renamed the Accreditation Review Committee on Education for the Physician Assistant in 1988.

Following a 2-year consultation with accredited educational programs, sponsors of the accreditation service, and other interested parties, revised *Standards* were adopted for the education of assistants to primary care physicians in 1978. Following a similar consultation, the revised *Standards* were adopted in 1985 as standards for the education of physician assistants. In 1990, the accreditation standards were consolidated for physician assistant and surgeon assistant education and training, to ensure that both received a comparable base of knowledge and skill in primary care medicine. The *Standards* were last revised in 1997.

Accreditation was offered from 1970 through 1975 for orthopedic and urologic physician assistants. Unlike the *Standards* for the education of the surgeon assistant and the physician assistant, the standards for education of the orthopedic and urologic assistants did not require education and training for competence in eliciting a comprehensive health history and in performing a comprehensive physical examination. Accreditation for these programs was discontinued owing to the withdrawal of support by the American Academy of Orthopaedic Surgeons and the American Urological Association.

Occupational Description

The physician assistant (PA) is academically and clinically prepared to practice medicine with the supervision of a licensed doctor of medicine or osteopathy. Within the physician/PA relationship, physician assistants exercise autonomy in medical decision-making and provide a broad range of diagnostic and therapeutic services. The clinical role of physician assistants includes primary and specialty care in medical and surgical practice settings in both urban and rural areas. Physician assistant practice is centered on patient care and may include educational, research, and administrative activities. Physician assistants are accountable for their own actions as well as being accountable to their supervising physicians. The supervising physician is ultimately responsible for the patient care rendered by the physician assistant.

The specific tasks performed by individual physician assistants cannot be delineated precisely because of the variations in practice requirements mandated by geographic, political, economic, and social factors. At a minimum, however, physician assistants are educated in areas of basic medical science, clinical disciplines, and discipline-specific problem solving.

The role of the physician assistant demands intelligence, sound judgment, intellectual honesty, appropriate interpersonal skills, and the capacity to react to emergencies in a calm and reasoned manner. An attitude of respect for oneself and others, adherence to the concepts of privilege and confidentiality in communicating with patients, and a commitment to the patient's welfare are essential attributes.

Physician assistant practice is characterized by clinical knowledge and skills in areas traditionally defined by family medicine, internal medicine, pediatrics, obstetrics, gynecology, surgery, and psychiatry/behavioral medicine. Physician assistants practice in ambulatory, emergency, inpatient, and long-term care settings. Physician assistants deliver health care services to diverse patient populations of all ages with a range of acute and chronic medical and surgical conditions. They need knowledge and skills that allow them to function effectively in a dynamic health care environment.

Services performed by physician assistants while practicing with physician supervision include but are not limited to the following:

1. *Evaluation*
   Elicit a detailed and accurate history; perform an appropriate physical examination; order, perform, and interpret appropriate diagnostic studies; delineate problems; develop management plans; and record and present data.

2. *Monitoring*
   Implement patient management plans, record progress notes, and participate in the provision of the continuity of care.

3. *Therapeutic*
   Perform therapeutic procedures and manage or assist in the management of medical and surgical conditions, which may include assisting surgeons in the conduct of operations and taking initiative in performing evaluation and therapeutic procedures in response to life-threatening situations.

4. *Patient Education*
   Counsel patients regarding issues of health care management to include compliance with prescribed therapeutic regimens, normal growth and development, family planning, and emotional problems of daily living.

5. *Referral*
   Facilitate the referral of patients to other health care providers or agencies as appropriate.

Licensure

Forty-nine states, the District of Columbia, and Guam have enacted legislation or regulations affecting physician assistants. Forty-two of these jurisdictions allow physicians to delegate prescriptive authority to the PAs they supervise.

Employment Characteristics

The *1996 Census Report of Physician Assistants*, published in 1996 by the American Academy of Physician Assistants, indicates that of the more than 29,000 practicing physician assistants, almost half are practicing in primary care. Family practice is the most common specialty for physician assistants (40%), followed by surgery and surgical subspecialties, general internal medicine, emergency medicine, orthopedics, occupational medicine, pediatrics, and subspecialties of internal medicine, such as cardiology.

The majority of physician assistants practice in ambulatory care settings. Solo and group practices employ 40% of all physician assistants. The number of physician assistants employed by hospitals is 30%, owing in part to the number of physician assistants working as house staff. The government employs almost 15% of the physician assistant workforce, primarily in the military and the Department of Veterans Affairs. The remaining members of the profession are practicing in managed care organizations, rural and urban clinics, correctional facilities, and other settings.

Physician assistants in outpatient settings work an average of 40 hours per week, while those in inpatient facilities work 43 hours.

The number of patient visits for physician assistants in outpatient settings averages 21 per day; in inpatient settings the average is 16 patient visits per day. More than one-third of physician assistants have on-call responsibilities that average 29 hours per week.

Salaries vary depending on the experience of the individual, the practice specialty, job responsibilities, and the regional cost of living. The median income for new physician assistant graduates is $51,240. Experienced physician assistants working full-time commonly earn more than $60,000, and the upper salary range exceeds $100,000. It is anticipated that the demand for PAs will continue to increase.

Educational Programs

Length. Although 25 to 27 months is most common, the length of programs varies, largely owing to differences in student selection criteria and in the educational objectives of the individual program.
Prerequisites. Although requirements differ widely, a majority of programs require 2 years of undergraduate study and some work experience in health care. A balance of study in the applied behavioral sciences and the biological sciences is advised for students who wish to qualify for admission to a physician assistant program.
Curriculum. Accreditation standards require competency-based curricula. Programs provide integrated clinical didactic and practice components that cover anatomy, pathophysiology, microbiology, and pharmacology. Additional areas of focus include development of critical thinking skills, applied behavioral science courses that deal with development of personality, mechanisms for coping with stress in daily living, development of listening and interviewing skills, and recognition of individual values relating to such dimensions of human experience as sexuality and death and dying. For programs offering an option of study to prepare as a surgeon assistant, preclinical instruction in anatomy extends to include neuroanatomy and human prosection or dissection. Four-year programs are designed to provide the student with a balance of traditional liberal arts courses and biological and applied behavioral science courses. These courses are prerequisites to clinical didactic and supervised clinical practice instruction common to both 2-year and 4-year programs.

Supervised clinical practice rotations in pediatrics, family medicine, internal medicine, obstetrics and gynecology, geriatrics, and surgery offer advanced applied content and supervised clinical work experience in dealing with commonly encountered demands for the primary health care of individuals from infancy through childhood, adolescence, and the various phases of adulthood. Students choosing a surgeon assistant program will receive greater focus on general surgery than other physician assistant students, without compromising their preparation in general medicine.
Standards. *Standards and Guidelines for an Accredited Educational Program for the Physician Assistant* are minimum acceptable standards that were adopted, as revised in 1997, by the American Academy of Family Physicians, American Academy of Pediatrics, American Academy of Physician Assistants, American College of Physicians, American College of Surgeons, American Medical Association, and Association of Physician Assistant Programs. Applicant programs that seek provisional, initial, and continuing accreditation are assessed in accordance with these standards. The *Standards and Guidelines* are available on written request from the Accreditation Review Committee on Education for the Physician Assistant.

Inquiries

Accreditation

Requests for information on curriculum and accreditation of a physician assistant and/or surgeon assistant program should be addressed to

Executive Director
Accreditation Review Committee on Education
  for the Physician Assistant
1000 N Oak Ave
Marshfield, WI 54449
715 389-3785

Careers

Inquiries regarding physician assistant careers may be addressed to

American Academy of Physician Assistants
950 N Washington St
Alexandria, VA 22314
703 836-2272

Association of Physician Assistant Programs
950 N Washington St
Alexandria, VA 22314
703 548-5538

National Certification

Inquiries regarding physician assistant certification may be addressed to

National Commission on Certification of Physician Assistants
6849-B2 Peachtree Dunwoody Rd
Atlanta, GA 30328
770 399-9971

Physician Assistant

Alabama

University of Alabama at Birmingham

Surgeon Assistant Prgm
Sch of Hlth Related Professions
222 H SHRP Bldg
Birmingham, AL 35294-1270
Prgm Dir: M.Craig Cilimberg, PA-C
Tel: 205 934-4407   *Fax:* 205 975-7302
E-mail: cilimbec@admin.shrp.uab.edu
Med Dir: Joaquin S Aldrete, MD
Class Cap: 24   *Begins:* Sep
Length: 24 mos   *Award:* Cert, BS
Tuition per yr: $3,840 res, $7,680 non-res

University of South Alabama

Physician Assistant Prgm
Dept of Physician Asst Studies
1504 Springhill Ave/Ste 1715
Mobile, AL 36604-3273
Prgm Dir: Kenneth Harbert, PA-C PhD
Tel: 334 434-3641   *Fax:* 334 434-3646
Med Dir: Allen S Craig, MD

Arizona

Kirksville Coll of Osteopathic Med-SW Center

Physician Assistant Prgm
3210 W Camelback Rd
Phoenix, AZ 85017
Prgm Dir: Richard E Davis, MS PA-C
Tel: 602 841-4077   *Fax:* 602 841-4092
Med Dir: James J Dearing, DO
Class Cap: 50   *Begins:* Sep
Length: 24 mos   *Award:*MS
Tuition per yr: $14,500 res, $14,500 non-res

California

Charles R Drew Univ of Med & Science

Physician Assistant Prgm
1621 E 120th St/MP#42
Los Angeles, CA 90059
Prgm Dir: Beverly Lassiter-Brown, MPH PA-C
Tel: 213 563-5879   *Fax:* 213 563-5950
Med Dir: Eugene Hardin, MD
Class Cap: 50   *Begins:* Aug
Length: 24 mos, 36 mos   *Award:* Cert, BS
Tuition per yr: $6,250 res, $6,250 non-res

University of Southern California

Physician Assistant Prgm
Health Sciences Campus
1975 Zonal Park/KAM-B29
Los Angeles, CA 90033
Prgm Dir: Jack Liskin, MA PA-C
Tel: 213 342-1328   *Fax:* 213 342-1260
E-mail: jliskin@usc.usc.edu
Med Dir: Allan V Abbott, MD
Class Cap: 60   *Begins:* Aug
Length: 23 mos   *Award:* Dipl, BS
Tuition per yr: $19,500

Western Univ of Health Sciences

Physician Assistant Prgm
Primary Care
College Plaza
Pomona, CA 91766-1889
Prgm Dir: Stephanie Haywood-Bowlin, MS PAC
Tel: 909 469-5390 *Fax:* 909 629-7255
Med Dir: Alan Cundari, PA DO
Class Cap: 60 *Begins:* Aug
Length: 24 mos *Award:* Cert,
Tuition per yr: $9,900 res, $9,900 non-res

University of California - Davis

Physician Assistant Prgm
2525 Stockton Blvd/Ste 1025
Sacramento, CA 95817
Prgm Dir: Janet Mentink, PhD
Tel: 916 734-3550 *Fax:* 916 452-2112
E-mail: carol.cash@ucdmc.ucdavis.edu
Med Dir: Walter Morgan, MD
Begins: Sep
Length: 24 mos *Award:* Cert,
Tuition per yr: $4,098 res, $11,799 non-res

Naval School of Hlth Sciences - San Diego

Physician Assistant Prgm
34101 Farenholt Ave
San Diego, CA 92134-5291
Prgm Dir: Lt M Chris Polkpski
Tel: 619 532-7938 *Fax:* 619 532-7796
E-mail: rlfrance@swdio.med.navy.mil
Med Dir: Joel Lees, Capt ME USN MD
Class Cap: 25 *Begins:* Sep
Length: 24 mos *Award:* Cert, BS

Stanford University School of Medicine

Physician Assistant Prgm
Primary Care Associate Prgm
703 Welch Rd Ste F-1
Palo Alto, CA 94304-1760
Prgm Dir: Virginia Fowkes, MHS
Tel: 415 723-7043
Med Dir: Dianne Higgins, MD
Class Cap: 54 *Begins:* Sep
Length: 15 mos *Award:* Dipl,Cert, AS
Tuition per yr: $6,481 res, $11,573 non-res

Colorado

University of Colorado Hlth Science Ctr

Physician Assistant Prgm
Child Hlth Assoc Prgm
4200 E Ninth Ave/PO Box C219
Denver, CO 80262
Prgm Dir: Gerald B Merenstein, MD
Tel: 303 315-7963 *Fax:* 303 315-6976
E-mail: gerald.merenstein@uchsc.edu
Med Dir: Jane Gray, MD
Class Cap: 28 *Begins:* Jun Aug
Length: 33 mos *Award:* Cert, BS, MS
Tuition per yr: $6,441 res, $22,579 non-res

Connecticut

Quinnipiac College

Physician Assistant Prgm
275 Mt Carmel Ave
Hamden, CT 06518
Prgm Dir: Dana L Sayre-Stanghope, MS PA-C
Tel: 203 281-8983 *Fax:* 203 287-5303
Med Dir: Ronald Robbins, MD
Class Cap: 30 *Begins:* May
Length: 27 mos *Award:* Cert, MHS
Tuition per yr: $15,000
Evening or weekend classes available

Yale University School of Medicine

Physician Assistant Prgm
47 College St Ste 220
New Haven, CT 06510
Prgm Dir: Elaine E Grant, PA-C MPH
Tel: 203 785-4252
E-mail: gantee@maspob.mas.yale.edu
Med Dir: Richard S K Young, MD
Class Cap: 32 *Begins:* Aug
Length: 25 mos *Award:* Cert,
Tuition per yr: $16,250 res, $16,250 non-res

District of Columbia

George Washington University

Physician Assistant Prgm
2300 I St NW
Himmelfarb 307
Washington, DC 20037
Prgm Dir: Lisa Mustone Alexander, MPH PA-C
Tel: 202 994-4034 *Fax:* 202 994-2124
E-mail: gwu_pa@gwis2.circ.gwu.edu
Med Dir: John Voss, MD
Class Cap: 55 *Begins:* Aug
Length: 24 mos, 36 mos *Award:* Cert, MS
Tuition per yr: $20,625 res, $20,625 non-res

Howard University

Physician Assistant Prgm
6th & Bryant Sts NW/Annex I
Washington, DC 20059
Prgm Dir: Brenda J Jasper, MEd PA-C
Tel: 202 806-7536 *Fax:* 202 806-4476
Med Dir: Thomas E Gaiter, MD
Class Cap: 40 *Begins:* Aug
Length: 24 mos *Award:* BS
Tuition per yr: $7,700 res, $7,700 non-res

Florida

Nova Southeastern University

Physician Assistant Prgm
3200 S University Dr
Ft Lauderdale, FL 33328
Prgm Dir: David Binsmeister, PAC MMS
Tel: 954 723-1652 *Fax:* 954 916-2285
Med Dir: Morton A Diamond, MD
Class Cap: 100 *Begins:* Jun
Length: 24 mos *Award:* BS
Tuition per yr: $15,500 res, $15,500 non-res

University of Florida

Physician Assistant Prgm
College of Medicine
PO Box 100176
Gainesville, FL 32610-0176
Prgm Dir: Wayne D Bottom, PA-C MPH
Tel: 352 395-7955 *Fax:* 352 395-7996
E-mail: ops.pap@mhs1.sth.ur.edu
Med Dir: Kerry I Edwards, MD
Class Cap: 60 *Begins:* Jun Jul
Length: 24 mos *Award:* Cert, MPAS
Tuition per yr: $4,971 res, $15,057 non-res

Georgia

Emory University

Physician Assistant Prgm
School of Medicine
1462 Clifton Rd Ste 280
Atlanta, GA 30322
Prgm Dir: Virginia H Joslin, PA-C MPH
Tel: 404 727-7825 *Fax:* 404 727-7836
E-mail: vjoslin@emory.edu
Med Dir: Allison Lauber, MD
Class Cap: 50 *Begins:* Aug
Length: 28 mos *Award:* Dipl, MMSc
Tuition per yr: $11,825 res, $11,825 non-res
Evening or weekend classes available

Medical College of Georgia

Physician Assistant Prgm
1120 15th St
AE 1032
Augusta, GA 30912
Prgm Dir: Bonnie A Dadig, MS PA-C
Tel: 706 721-3246 *Fax:* 706 721-3990
E-mail: bdadig@mail.mcg.edu
Med Dir: Rene Cormier, MD
Class Cap: 36 *Begins:* Aug
Length: 24 mos *Award:* Dipl, BS
Tuition per yr: $3,213 res, $10,121 non-res

Illinois

Cook County Hosp/Malcolm X College

Physician Assistant Prgm
1900 W Van Buren/Rm 3241
Chicago, IL 60612
Prgm Dir: Kristine M Healy, PA-C
Tel: 312 850-7268
Med Dir: Margaret M Dolan, MD
Class Cap: 26 *Begins:* Jul
Length: 25 mos *Award:* Cert, AAS
Tuition per yr: $1,800 res, $5,900 non-res
Evening or weekend classes available

Midwestern University

Physician Assistant Prgm
555 31st St
Downers Grove, IL 60515
Prgm Dir: R Scott Chavez, MPA PA-C
Tel: 630 515-6034
Med Dir: Andre Gibaldi, DO
Class Cap: 90 *Begins:* Jun
Length: 24 mos, 27 mos *Award:* Dipl, BMS , MMS
Tuition per yr: $11,500 res, $12,500 non-res

Programs

Finch U of Hlth Science/Chicago Med Sch
Physician Assistant Prgm
3333 Green Bay Rd/Bldg 51
North Chicago, IL 60064
Prgm Dir: Patrick Knott, MS PAC
Tel: 847 578-3312 *Fax:* 847 578-8690
Med Dir: Walid F Khayr, MD
Class Cap: 50 *Begins:* May
Length: 24 mos *Award:*MS
Tuition per yr: $15,450 res, $15,450 non-res

Indiana

Butler University/Clarian Health
Physician Assistant Prgm
Butler Univ Coll of Pharm and Hlth Sci
4600 Sunset Ave
Indianapolis, IN 46208-3485
Prgm Dir: Laurie Lipsig Pylitt, MHPE
Tel: 317 929-5133 *Fax:* 317 940-6172
E-mail: pylitt@butler.edu
Med Dir: Bradley M Sutter, MD
Class Cap: 30 *Begins:* Aug
Length: 21 mos *Award:*BS
Tuition per yr: $16,220 res, $16,220 non-res

Iowa

University of Osteopathic Medicine
Physician Assistant Prgm
3200 Grand Ave
Des Moines, IA 50312
Prgm Dir: Jodi L Cahalan, MS PA-C
Tel: 515 271-1415 *Fax:* 515 271-1543
E-mail: jcaholan@uomhs.edu
Med Dir: Fred Strickland, DO
Class Cap: 32 *Begins:* Jun
Length: 24 mos *Award:* Cert, BS
Tuition per yr: $10,000

University of Iowa
Physician Assistant Prgm
College of Medicine
2333 Steindler Bldg
Iowa City, IA 52242
Prgm Dir: Denis R Oliver, PhD
Tel: 319 335-8922 *Fax:* 319 335-8923
E-mail: denis-oliver@uiowa.edu
Med Dir: Daniel S Fick, MD
Class Cap: 25 *Begins:* May
Length: 25 mos *Award:* Cert, MPAS
Tuition per yr: $4,401 res, $14,178 non-res

Kansas

Wichita State University
Physician Assistant Prgm
Campus Box 43
Wichita, KS 67260
Prgm Dir: Marvis J Lary, PhD RPAC
Tel: 316 978-3011 *Fax:* 316 978-3025
E-mail: lary@chp.twsu.edu
Med Dir: Donald S. Seery, MD
Class Cap: 46 *Begins:* Aug
Length: 24 mos *Award:*BS
Tuition per yr: $4,029 res, $13,770 non-res

Kentucky

Univ of Kentucky
Physician Assistant Prgm
Dept of Health Services
121 Washington Ave Rm 118
Lexington, KY 40536-0003
Prgm Dir: Herbert Ridings, MA PA-C
Tel: 606 323-1100, Ext 292 *Fax:* 606 257-2454
Med Dir: Samuel R Scott, MD
Class Cap: 50 *Begins:* Aug
Length: 24 mos *Award:* Dipl,Cert, BHS
Tuition per yr: $2,676 res, $7,356 non-res

Louisiana

Louisiana State Univ Med Ctr - Shreveport
Physician Assistant Prgm
1501 Kings Hwy
PO Box 33932
Shreveport, LA 71130
Prgm Dir: Valgene Valgora, MSEd PA-C
Tel: 318 675-7317 *Fax:* 318 675-6937
Med Dir: Ronald B George, MD
Class Cap: 30 *Begins:* May
Length: 27 mos *Award:*BS
Tuition per yr: $3,359 res, $6,484 non-res

Maine

University of New England
Physician Assistant Prgm
Gregory Hall Annex Ste 4
11 Hills Beach Rd
Biddeford, ME 04005-9599
Prgm Dir: Carl M Toney, PA
Tel: 207 283-0171, Ext 2812 *Fax:* 207 282-6379
Med Dir: Stephen Shannon, DO MPH

Maryland

Anne Arundel Community College
Physician Assistant Prgm
101 College Prkwy
Arnold, MD 21012
Prgm Dir: Michael Olds, BS PAC
Tel: 410 315-7392 *Fax:* 410 315-7099
Med Dir: S David Krimins, MD FACP

Essex Community College
Physician Assistant Prgm
7201 Rossville Blvd
Baltimore, MD 21237
Prgm Dir: Donna Sewell, MS PA-C
Tel: 410 780-6579
Med Dir: Edwin W Whiteford, Jr, MD
Class Cap: 35 *Begins:* Sep
Length: 24 mos *Award:* Cert, AAS
Tuition per yr: $1,365 res, $4,305 non-res
Evening or weekend classes available

Massachusetts

Northeastern University
Physician Assistant Prgm
360 Huntington Ave
202 Robinson
Boston, MA 02115
Prgm Dir: Suzanne B Greenberg, MS
Tel: 617 373-3195 *Fax:* 617 373-3338
E-mail: sgreenberg@lynx.neu.edu
Med Dir: Donald Wexler, MD
Class Cap: 34 *Begins:* Sep
Length: 24 mos *Award:* Cert, MHP
Tuition per yr: $9,600 res, $9,600 non-res

Springfield College/Baystate Health Sys
Physician Assistant Prgm
263 Alden St
Springfield, MA 01109
Prgm Dir: Ira W. Gabrielson, MD
Tel: 413 746-2335 *Fax:* 413 739-5211
E-mail: spfldcol.edu
Med Dir: Carol Richardson, MD
Class Cap: 30 *Begins:* Sep Jun
Length: 24 mos, 48 mos *Award:* Cert, BS
Tuition per yr: $17,300 res, $11,900 non-res

Michigan

University of Detroit Mercy
Physician Assistant Prgm
8200 W Outer Dr
Detroit, MI 48219
Prgm Dir: Suzanne Warnimont, PA-C MPH
Tel: 313 993-6057 *Fax:* 313 993-6175
E-mail: warnismk@udmery.edu
Med Dir: Walid A Harb, MD
Class Cap: 40 *Begins:* Sep
Length: 24 mos, 36 mos *Award:* Cert, MS
Tuition per yr: $16,920 res, $16,920 non-res
Evening or weekend classes available

Wayne State University
Physician Assistant Prgm
Coll of Pharmacy and Allied Hlth Profs
217 Shapero Hall
Detroit, MI 48202
Prgm Dir: Howard James Normile, PhD
Tel: 313 577-1368 *Fax:* 313 577-2033
Med Dir: Mohamed Siddique, MD

Western Michigan University
Physician Assistant Prgm
Kalamazoo, MI 49008
Prgm Dir: Janet I Pisaneschi, PhD
Tel: 616 387-5314
Med Dir: Dan Christian
Class Cap: 80 *Begins:* Sep
Length: 24 mos *Award:* Cert, BSM
Tuition per yr: $5,867 res, $11,852 non-res

Central Michigan University
Physician Assistant Prgm
249 Foust Hall
Mt Pleasant, MI 48859
Prgm Dir: Laura W Capozzi, PA-C PhD
Tel: 517 774-7963 *Fax:* 517 774-2908
Med Dir: Daniel Radawski, PhD MD

Minnesota

Augsburg College
Physician Assistant Prgm
2211 Riverside Ave/CB 149
Minneapolis, MN 55454
Prgm Dir: Dawn B Ludwig, PA-C MS PA
Tel: 612 330-1331 *Fax:* 612 330-1757
Med Dir: Manuel E Kaplan, MD
Class Cap: 28 *Begins:* May
Length: 27 mos *Award:*BA
Tuition per yr: $18,516 res, $18,516 non-res

Missouri

St Louis University Health Sciences Ctr
Physician Assistant Prgm
1504 S Grand Blvd
St Louis, MO 63104
Prgm Dir: Laura Stuetzer, MA PA-C
Tel: 314 577-8521 *Fax:* 314 577-8503
E-mail: stuetzlj@Wsluvca.slu.edu
Med Dir: Frances L Horvath, MD
Class Cap: 30 *Begins:* May
Length: 27 mos *Award:* Cert, BMS
Tuition per yr: $15,536 res, $15,536 non-res

Montana

Rocky Mountain College
Physician Assistant Prgm
1511 Poly Dr
Billings, MT 59102
Prgm Dir: Robert L Bunnell, MS PA-C
Tel: 406 657-1190 *Fax:* 406 657-1194
Med Dir: Leonard W Etchart, MD

Nebraska

University of Nebraska Medical Center
Physician Assistant Prgm
600 S 42nd St
Omaha, NE 68198-4300
Prgm Dir: James E Somers, PhD PA-C
Tel: 402 559-7953 *Fax:* 402 559-5356
Med Dir: Gerald F Moore, MD
Class Cap: 42 *Begins:* Aug
Length: 28 mos *Award:*MPAS
Tuition per yr: $5,856 res, $14,470 non-res

New Jersey

Rutgers/Univ of Med & Dent of New Jersey
Physician Assistant Prgm
Robert Wood Johnson Med Sch
675 Hoes Ln
Piscataway, NJ 08854
Prgm Dir: Ruth Fixelle, EdM PA-C
Tel: 908 235-4444 *Fax:* 908 235-4820
Med Dir: Robert Spierer, MD
Class Cap: 50 *Begins:* Aug
Length: 36 mos, 48 mos *Award:*MS
Tuition per yr: $7,260 res, $10,890 non-res

New York

Hudson Valley Community College
Physician Assistant Prgm
Albany Medical College A-4
47 New Scotland Ave
Albany, NY 12208
Prgm Dir: S McLaughlin Bauer, MS MT
Tel: 518 262-5251 *Fax:* 518 262-6698
E-mail: bauersal@office.hvcc.edu
Med Dir: Luise Ahlers, MD
Class Cap: 36 *Begins:* Aug
Length: 24 mos *Award:* Cert, AAS
Tuition per yr: $3,225 res, $7,500 non-res

Bronx Lebanon Hospital Center
Physician Assistant Prgm
1650 Selwyn Ave/Ste 4F
Bronx, NY 10457
Prgm Dir: Jimmy Santana, BS RPA-C
Tel: 718 960-1255 *Fax:* 718 960-1329
Med Dir: Wayne Longmore, MD
Class Cap: 35 *Begins:* Sep
Length: 24 mos *Award:* Cert,
Tuition per yr: $9,000 res, $9,000 non-res

SUNY Health Science Center - Brooklyn
Physician Assistant Prgm
450 Clarkson Ave
PO Box 1222
Brooklyn, NY 11203
Prgm Dir: Dawn Morton-Rias, BS PA-C
Tel: 718 270-2324 *Fax:* 718 270-7751
Med Dir: Luther T Clark, MD
Class Cap: 30 *Begins:* Jun
Length: 27 mos *Award:*BS
Tuition per yr: $4,903 res, $8,300 non-res

The Brooklyn Hosp/Long Island Univ
Physician Assistant Prgm
121 DeKalb Ave
Brooklyn, NY 11201
Prgm Dir: Lydia Posin, MA RPAC
Tel: 718 250-8144 *Fax:* 718 797-1598
Med Dir: Meenakshi Gulrajani, MD
Class Cap: 41 *Begins:* Sep
Length: 24 mos *Award:* Cert, BS
Tuition per yr: $12,565
Evening or weekend classes available

D'Youville College
Physician Assistant Prgm
320 Porter Ave
Buffalo, NY 14201
Prgm Dir: Lynn Rivers
Tel: 716 881-7712, Ext 7713 *Fax:* 716 881-7790
Med Dir: Lovie C Tripoli, MD
Class Cap: 30 *Begins:* Aug
Length: 42 mos *Award:*BS
Tuition per yr: $9,500 res, $9,500 non-res

Touro College
Physician Assistant Prgm
Barry Z Levine Sch Hlth Sci
135 Carman Rd, Bldg 14
Dix Hills, NY 11746
Prgm Dir: Anne Marie Bozzarelli, RPAC
Tel: 516 673-3200
Med Dir: Jay P Slotkin, MD
Class Cap: 35 *Begins:* Aug
Length: 23 mos *Award:*BS
Tuition per yr: $12,500

City Univ of NY/Harlem Hosp Ctr
Physician Assistant Prgm
506 Malcolm X Blvd
WP Rm 619
New York, NY 10037
Prgm Dir: Stephen S Robinson, MD MPH
Tel: 212 939-2525 *Fax:* 212 939-2529
E-mail: ssrbh@cunyvm.cuny.edu
Med Dir: Brenda Bennett, MD
Class Cap: 35 *Begins:* Mar
Length: 28 mos *Award:* Cert, BS
Tuition per yr: $4,800 res, $10,200 non-res

Cornell University Medical College
Physician Assistant Prgm
1300 York Ave/F-1906
Physician Assistant Program
New York, NY 10021
Prgm Dir: Eva Fisher, MD
Tel: 212 746-5134 *Fax:* 212 746-8680
Class Cap: 30 *Begins:* Nov
Length: 26 mos *Award:* Cert,
Tuition per yr: $9,288

Rochester Institute of Technology
Physician Assistant Prgm
85 Lamb Memorial Drive
Rochester, NY 14623-5604
Prgm Dir: Heidi B Miller, RPA-C
Tel: 716 475-5945 *Fax:* 716 475-5766
E-mail: hbmsclevitvax.isc.rit.edu
Med Dir: Betty Rabinowitz, MD
Class Cap: 25 *Begins:* Sep
Length: 48 mos *Award:*BS
Tuition per yr: $15,375 res, $15,375 non-res

Bayley Seton Hospital
Physician Assistant Prgm
75 Vanderbilt Ave
Staten Island, NY 10304
Prgm Dir: Diane Berato Pane, PA-C HPA
Tel: 718 354-5570 *Fax:* 718 390-6146
Med Dir: James J Lamia, MD
Class Cap: 45 *Begins:* Aug
Length: 23 mos *Award:* Cert,
Tuition per yr: $8,800 res, $8,800 non-res

Wagner College
Physician Assistant Prgm
Staten Island Univ Hospital
74 Melville St
Staten Island, NY 10309
Prgm Dir: Timothy K Glennon, MBA MSN
Tel: 718 226-2453 *Fax:* 718 226-2464

SUNY Health Science Ctr at Stony Brook
Physician Assistant Prgm
SHTM-HSC/L2-052
Stony Brook, NY 11794-8202
Prgm Dir: Paul Lombardo, MPS RPAC
Tel: 516 444-3190 *Fax:* 516 444-7621
E-mail: plombardo@epo.hsc.sunysb.edu
Med Dir: Anne Robbins, MD
Class Cap: 95 *Begins:* Jul
Length: 24 mos *Award:* Dipl, BS
Tuition per yr: $4,085 res, $10,030 non-res

Le Moyne College
Physician Assistant Prgm
Dept of Biology
Syracuse, NY 13214-1399
Prgm Dir: Norbert J Henry, EdD
Tel: 315 445-4144 *Fax:* 314 445-4787
Med Dir: James Longo, MD FACC

Programs

Catholic Med Ctr of Brooklyn & Queens Inc
Physician Assistant Prgm
St Anthony's Health Professions & Nursing
   Institute
175-05 Horace Harding Expwy
Fresh Meadows, NY 11365
Prgm Dir: JoAnn A Deasy, PA-C MPH
Tel: 718 357-0500   *Fax:* 718 357-4588
Med Dir: Anthony Pesiri, MD
Class Cap: 55   *Begins:* Aug
Length: 22 mos   *Award:* Cert, BS
Tuition per yr: $12,700

North Carolina

Duke University Medical Center
Physician Assistant Prgm
PO Box 2914
Durham, NC 27710
Prgm Dir: Reginald D Carter, PhD PA-C
Tel: 919 286-8225   *Fax:* 919 286-7916
E-mail: carte00@mc.duke.edu
Med Dir: Joyce A Copeland, MD
Class Cap: 44   *Begins:* Aug
Length: 25 mos   *Award:* Cert, MHS
Tuition per yr: $17,280

Methodist College
Physician Assistant Prgm
5400 Ramsey St
Fayetteville, NC 28311
Prgm Dir: Ernest R Foster, PAC BS MA
Tel: 910 630-7495   *Fax:* 910 630-2123
Med Dir: Christopher Aul, MD

East Carolina University
Physician Assistant Prgm
School of Allied Health Sciences/Belk Bldg
Greenville, NC 27858-4353
Prgm Dir: Edward D Huechtner, MPH PA-C
Tel: 919 328-4423   *Fax:* 919 328-4470
Med Dir: C Christopher Bremer, MD

Bowman Gray School of Medicine
Physician Assistant Prgm
Medical Ctr Blvd
Winston-Salem, NC 27157-1006
Prgm Dir: Glen E Combs, MA PA-C
Tel: 910 716-4356   *Fax:* 910 716-4432
Med Dir: Venita W Morell, MD
Class Cap: 48   *Begins:* Aug
Length: 24 mos   *Award:* Cert,
Tuition per yr: $12,500

North Dakota

Univ of No Dakota Sch of Med and Hlth Sci
Physician Assistant Prgm
PO Box 9037
Grand Forks, ND 58202
Prgm Dir: Mickey Knutson, MSN FNP PA-C
Tel: 701 777-2344
E-mail: miknutso@plains.nodak.edu
Med Dir: Robert C Eelkema, MD MPH
Class Cap: 80   *Begins:* Jan
Length: 12 mos   *Award:* Cert,
Tuition per yr: $6,550 res, $7,550 non-res

Ohio

Kettering College of Medical Arts
Physician Assistant Prgm
3737 Southern Blvd
Kettering, OH 45429
Prgm Dir: A Patrick Jonas, MD ABFP
Tel: 513 296-7238   *Fax:* 513 296-4238
Med Dir: A Patrick Jonas, MD ABFP
Class Cap: 93   *Begins:* Aug
Length: 22 mos   *Award:* AAS
Tuition per yr: $10,740 res, $10,740 non-res

Cuyahoga Community College
Surgeon Assistant Prgm
11000 Pleasant Valley Rd
Parma, OH 44130
Prgm Dir: Joyce R Janicek, MA
Tel: 216 987-5123   *Fax:* 216 987-5050
E-mail: joyce.janicek@tri-c.oh.us
Med Dir: Stephen ReMine, MD FACS
Class Cap: 29   *Begins:* Sep
Length: 22 mos   *Award:* AAS
Tuition per yr: $2,965 res, $3,854 non-res

Cuyahoga Community College
Physician Assistant Prgm
11000 Pleasant Valley Rd
Parma, OH 44130
Prgm Dir: Joyce R Janicek, MA
Tel: 216 987-5123   *Fax:* 216 987-5050
E-mail: joyce.janicek@tri-c.oh.us
Med Dir: Ellen Corey, MD
Class Cap: 29   *Begins:* Sep
Length: 22 mos   *Award:* AAS
Tuition per yr: $2,965 res, $3,854 non-res

Medical College of Ohio
Physician Assistant Prgm
3000 Arlington Ave
Toledo, OH 43614
Prgm Dir: Anthony A Miller, MEd PA-C
Tel: 419 381-4637   *Fax:* 419 381-3051
Med Dir: William A Sodeman Jr, MD

Oklahoma

Univ of Oklahoma Health Sciences Center
Physician Assistant Prgm
PO Box 26901
Oklahoma City, OK 73190
Prgm Dir: Daniel L McNeill, PA PhD
Tel: 405 271-2058   *Fax:* 405 271-3621
Med Dir: Lynn Hitchell, MD MPH
Class Cap: 50   *Begins:* Jul
Length: 30 mos   *Award:* Dipl, MHS
Tuition per yr: $4,400 res, $12,800 non-res

Oregon

Oregon Health Sciences University
Physician Assistant Prgm
3181 SW Sam Jackson Park Rd
GH 219
Portland, OR 97201
Prgm Dir: Ted J Ruback, MS PA-C
Tel: 503 494-1408   *Fax:* 503 494-1409
Med Dir: Bruce W Goldberg, MD
Class Cap: 32   *Begins:* Sep
Length: 24 mos   *Award:* BS
Tuition per yr: $10,000 res, $18,000 non-res

Pennsylvania

Gannon University
Physician Assistant Prgm
109 University Square
Erie, PA 16541
Prgm Dir: Dawna Mughal, PhD
Tel: 814 871-5452   *Fax:* 814 871-5662
Med Dir: John C Jageman, MD
Class Cap: 35   *Begins:* Sep
Length: 42 mos   *Award:* BS
Tuition per yr: $13,024 res, $13,024 non-res
Evening or weekend classes available

Beaver College
Physician Assistant Prgm
450 S Easton Rd
Glenside, PA 19038
Prgm Dir: Michael Dryer, PA-C, MPH
Tel: 215 572-2082   *Fax:* 215 881-8795

St Francis College
Physician Assistant Prgm
PO Box 600
Loretto, PA 15940
Prgm Dir: Albert F Simon, MEd PA-C
Tel: 814 472-3130   *Fax:* 814 472-3137
E-mail: bsimon@sfcpa.edu
Med Dir: Lawrence Stem, MD
Class Cap: 60   *Begins:* Aug
Length: 24 mos, 48 mos   *Award:* Dipl,Cert, BS
Tuition per yr: $19,584

Allegheny University of the Health Sciences
Physician Assistant Prgm
Broad and Vine Sts MS 504
Philadelphia, PA 19102
Prgm Dir: Sherry L Stolberg, MGPGP PA-C
Tel: 215 762-7349   *Fax:* 215 762-1164
E-mail: stolbergs@allieghenny.edu
Med Dir: Ana Nonez, MD
Class Cap: 100   *Begins:* Aug
Length: 24 mos   *Award:* Dipl,Cert, , BS
Tuition per yr: $11,655 res, $11,655 non-res

Philadelphia College of Textiles and Science
Physician Assistant Prgm
School of Science and Health
School House Ln and Henry Ave
Philadelphia, PA 19144
Prgm Dir: Matt Dane Baker, PA-C MS
Tel: 215 951-2908   *Fax:* 215 951-2651
Med Dir: Joel Chinitz, MD MPH
Class Cap: 50   *Begins:* Aug
Length: 24 mos   *Award:* BS
Tuition per yr: $16,182 res, $16,182 non-res

Duquesne University

Physician Assistant Prgm
Rangos Sch of Health Sciences
123 Health Sci Bldg
Pittsburgh, PA 15282-0001
Prgm Dir: Anthony J Pinevich, MD
Tel: 412 396-5914   *Fax:* 412 396-5554
Med Dir: Michael Essig, MD
Class Cap: 35   *Begins:* Aug
Length: 60 mos   *Award:* , MPA
Tuition per yr: $15,428 res, $15,428 non-res
Evening or weekend classes available

King's College

Physician Assistant Prgm
133 N River St
Wilkes Barre, PA 18711
Prgm Dir: Eleanor Babonis, PhD PA-C
Tel: 717 826-5853   *Fax:* 717 826-5353
E-mail: erbaroni@kssoo2
Med Dir: Robert Czwalina, DO
Class Cap: 40   *Begins:* Aug
Length: 24 mos   *Award:* Cert, BS
Tuition per yr: $15,200 res, $15,200 non-res
Evening or weekend classes available

Pennsylvania College of Technology

Physician Assistant Prgm
One College Ave
Williamsport, PA 17701
Prgm Dir: Russell M Trapp Jr, BS PA-C
Tel: 717 327-4779   *Fax:* 717 321-5538
Med Dir: Michael A Gross, MD MPH

South Carolina

Medical University of South Carolina

Physician Assistant Prgm
171 Ashley Ave
Charleston, SC 29425
Prgm Dir: Arnold E Metz, MA PAC
Tel: 803 792-6490   *Fax:* 803 792-0506
E-mail: Metzae@musc.edu
Med Dir: D Glen Askins, MD
Class Cap: 30   *Begins:* Jun
Length: 27 mos   *Award:* BS
Tuition per yr: $4,260 res, $11,655 non-res

South Dakota

University of South Dakota

Physician Assistant Prgm
414 E Clark
Vermillion, SD 57069
Prgm Dir: Gloria M. Stewart, EdD PA-C ATC
Tel: 605 677-5128   *Fax:* 605 677-6569
E-mail: gstewart@sunflowr.usd.edu
Med Dir: Bruce Vogt, MD
Class Cap: 16   *Begins:* Aug
Length: 24 mos   *Award:* Dipl,Cert, BS
Tuition per yr: $6,575 res, $11,708 non-res

Tennessee

Trevecca Nazarene University

Physician Assistant Prgm
333 Murfreesboro Rd
Nashville, TN 37210-2877
Prgm Dir: David Lennon, RN PA-C MEd
Tel: 615 248-1225   *Fax:* 615 248-1622
E-mail: dlennon@trevecca.edu
Med Dir: G Michael Moredock, MD
Class Cap: 33   *Begins:* Aug
Length: 24 mos   *Award:* Cert, BS
Tuition per yr: $18,360

Texas

Univ of Tx Southwestern Med Ctr - Dallas

Physician Assistant Prgm
6011 Harry Hines Blvd/Ste V4114
Dallas, TX 75235-9090
Prgm Dir: P Eugene Jones, PhD PA-C
Tel: 214 648-1700   *Fax:* 214 648-1003
E-mail: ejones@mednet.swmed.edu
Med Dir: Patricia Cook, MD
Class Cap: 45   *Begins:* May
Length: 27 mos   *Award:* Dipl,Cert, BS
Tuition per yr: $1,728 res, $13,284 non-res
Evening or weekend classes available

Army Medical Dept Center and School

Interservice Physician Assistant Prgm
MCCS HMP (PA Br)
3151 Scott Rd/Ste 1230
Ft Sam Houston, TX 78234-6138
Prgm Dir: Donald L Parsons, SP PA-C
Tel: 210 221-6776   *Fax:* 210 221-8612
Med Dir: Chandra M Tiwary
Class Cap: 60   *Begins:* Jan May Sep
Length: 24 mos   *Award:* Cert, BS

University of Texas Medical Branch

Physician Assistant Prgm
301 University Blvd
Galveston, TX 77555-1028
Prgm Dir: Richard R Rahr, EdD PA-C
Tel: 409 772-3046   *Fax:* 409 772-9710
E-mail: rrahr%sahs@mhost.utmb.edu
Med Dir: Michael Warren, MD
Class Cap: 90   *Begins:* Jun
Length: 24 mos   *Award:* Dipl,Cert, BS
Tuition per yr: $1,700 res, $12,000 non-res

Baylor College of Medicine

Physician Assistant Prgm
One Baylor Plaza/Rm633E
Houston, TX 77030
Prgm Dir: C Emil Fasser, PA-C
Tel: 713 798-4619   *Fax:* 713 798-6128
E-mail: cfasser@bcm.tmc.edu
Med Dir: Michael P Tristan, MD MPH
Class Cap: 40   *Begins:* Jul
Length: 30 mos   *Award:* Dipl,Cert, MS
Tuition per yr: $8,200 res, $8,200 non-res

882 Training Group - US Air Force

Physician Assistant Prgm
381 TS/CSP
917 Missile Rd
Sheppard AFB, TX 76311-2246
Prgm Dir: Major Henry R Lemke, MMS PA-C
Tel: 817 676-6575
Med Dir: Major Thomas E Applegate, USAF MC
Class Cap: 25   *Begins:* Feb Jun Oct
Length: 24 mos   *Award:* Cert, BS

Utah

Univ of Utah Health Sciences Center

Physician Assistant Prgm
50 N Medical Dr/Bldg 528
Salt Lake City, UT 84132
Prgm Dir: Don M Pedersen, PA-C PhD
Tel: 801 581-7766   *Fax:* 801 581-5807
E-mail: dpedersen@upap.utah.edu
Med Dir: Stephen D Ratcliffe, MD MSPH
Class Cap: 32   *Begins:* Sep
Length: 20 mos   *Award:* Cert,
Tuition per yr: $9,868 res, $11,496 non-res

Washington

University of Washington

Physician Assistant Prgm
MEDEX Northwest
4245 Roosevelt Way NE
Seattle, WA 98105-6920
Prgm Dir: Ruth Ballweg, PA-C
Tel: 206 548-2600   *Fax:* 206 548-5195
E-mail: rballweg@u.washington.edu
Med Dir: P Jeffrey Hummel, MD MPH
Class Cap: 86   *Begins:* Sep
Length: 21 mos, 32 mos   *Award:* Cert, BCHS
Tuition per yr: $7,428 res, $7,428 non-res

West Virginia

College of West Virginia

Physician Assistant Prgm
PO Box AG
Beckley, WV 25802
Prgm Dir: Kay A Ericson, PA-C
Tel: 304 253-7351, Ext 420   *Fax:* 304 253-0789
Med Dir: Eileen Catterson, MD
Class Cap: 35   *Begins:* Aug
Length: 24 mos   *Award:* BS
Tuition per yr: $11,550 res, $11,550 non-res
Evening or weekend classes available

Alderson-Broaddus College

Physician Assistant Prgm
PO Box 578
College Hill
Philippi, WV 26416
Prgm Dir: Linda E Reed, PA MEd
Tel: 304 457-6290   *Fax:* 304 457-6308
Med Dir: Scott Dove, DO

Wisconsin

University of Wisconsin - Madison

Physician Assistant Prgm
1300 University Ave
1050 MSC
Madison, WI 53706
Prgm Dir: Jerry J Noack, PA
Tel: 608 263-5620
Med Dir: Jerry Ryan, MD
Class Cap: 60 *Begins:* Jun
Length: 24 mos *Award:* Dipl, Cert, BS
Tuition per yr: $4,049 res, $12,000 non-res

Radiologic Technology

History

In 1944, X-ray technology, the predecessor of radiologic technology, joined the health professions of occupational therapy, clinical laboratory sciences, and medical records as the fourth health occupation to establish standards of education and qualifications for accreditation. The first *Essentials of an Acceptable School for X-Ray Technicians* were the product of negotiation between the American Society of X-Ray Technicians, now the American Society of Radiologic Technologists (ASRT), and the Council on Medical Education and Hospitals of the American Medical Association (AMA). During this time, X-ray technology was limited to diagnostic imaging using radiation produced by the simple, and certainly by today's standards, primitive equipment. Very little radiation therapy was performed—the X-ray technician "did it all." Radiation therapy technology, the treating of malignant diseases with radiation, was recognized as a separate discipline from radiography in 1964. The ASRT and the American College of Radiology (ACR) adopted the first set of dedicated radiation therapy technology *Essentials* in 1968. In 1994, the discipline became known as radiation therapy, and practitioners as radiation therapists.

In 1969, the ASRT and the ACR established the Joint Review Committee on Education in Radiologic Technology (JRCERT) within the structure for allied health educational accreditation provided by the AMA Council on Medical Education (AMA CME).

The AMA CME delegated responsibility for allied health educational accreditation to a newly formed Committee on Allied Health Education and Accreditation (CAHEA) in 1976. In 1992, the Association of Educators in Radiological Sciences joined the ASRT and ACR as a participating organization in the JRCERT. That same year, the AMA announced that it had elected to dissolve CAHEA as of June 1994. In January 1994, the US Department of Education recognized the JRCERT as the national accrediting agency for radiography and radiation therapy educational programs.

Known as *Essentials* since 1944, educational standards continually evolve. In 1997, a totally new document, *Standards for an Accredited Program in Radiologic Sciences*, was implemented. The *Standards* define the requirements to achieve and maintain programmatic accreditation.

The *Standards* measure a program's compliance in areas of mission and goals, integrity, effectiveness and outcomes, curriculum, academic practices, human and learning resources, physical safety, student services, fiscal responsibility, and student outcomes. Accreditation assures that a program operates in substantial compliance with these *Standards*.

Radiation Therapist

Occupational Description

Radiation therapists deliver radiation to patients for therapeutic purposes. Radiation therapists provide for appropriate patient care and safety; apply problem-solving and critical thinking skills in the administration of prescribed treatment protocols, tumor localization, and dosimetry; and maintain pertinent records. Radiation therapists are particularly concerned with the principles of radiation protection for the patient, themselves, and others while performing these responsibilities.

Job Description

Professional competence requires that radiation therapists apply knowledge of anatomy and physiology, oncologic pathology, radiation biology, radiation oncology techniques, treatment planning procedures, and dosimetry in the performance of their duties. They must also communicate effectively with patients, health professionals, and the public.

The radiation therapist accepts responsibility for administering a radiation oncologist (physician)-prescribed course of radiation therapy, observing the patient during treatment, and maintaining pertinent records of treatment. Radiation therapists also evaluate and assess treatment delivery components, evaluate and assess the daily physiologic and psychologic responsiveness of the patient, and promote total quality care for patients undergoing radiation therapy. Additional duties may include tumor localization, dosimetry, patient follow-up, and patient education. Radiation therapists must display competence, compassion, and concern in meeting the special needs of the oncology patient.

Employment Characteristics

Radiation therapists are employed in health care facilities, including cancer centers and private offices; they are also employed in settings where their responsibilities focus on education, management, research, and sales. Salaries and benefits vary with experience and employment location, but are generally competitive with other health specialties.

Educational Programs

Programs may be 1, 2, or 4 years in length, depending on program design, objectives, and the degree or certificate awarded. The curriculum of an accredited program includes an extensive component of technical and professional courses, including an emphasis on structured, competency-based clinical education. Interested individuals should contact a particular program for information on specific courses and prerequisites.

Radiographer

Occupational Description

Radiographers use imaging equipment to provide patient services as prescribed by physicians. When providing patient services, radiographers continually strive to provide quality patient care and are particularly concerned with limiting radiation exposure to patients, themselves, and others. Radiographers utilize problem solving and critical thinking skills to perform medical imaging procedures by adapting variable technical parameters of the procedure to the condition of the patient and by initiating life support procedures as necessary during medical emergencies.

Job Description

Professional competence requires that radiographers apply knowledge of anatomy, physiology, positioning, radiographic technique, and radiation biology and protection in the performance of their responsibilities. They must be able to communicate effectively with patients, other health professionals, and the public. Additional duties may include evaluating radiologic equipment, conducting a radiographic quality assurance program, providing patient education, and managing a medical imaging department. The radiographer must display compassion, competence, and concern in meeting the special needs of the patient.

Employment Characteristics

Radiographers are employed in health care facilities—including specialized imaging centers, urgent care clinics, and private physicians' offices—and as educators or imaging department administrators. Salaries and benefits are generally competitive with other health professions, and vary according to experience and employment location.

Educational Programs

Programs are generally 2 to 4 years in length, depending on program design, objectives, and the degree or certificate awarded. The curriculum of an accredited program includes an extensive component of technical and professional courses, including an emphasis on structured competency-based clinical education. Interested individuals should contact a particular program for information on specific courses and prerequisites.

Inquiries

Accreditation/Accredited Programs

Requests for information on radiation therapy or radiography educational program accreditation, including requests for a list of accredited programs, should be submitted to

Joint Review Committee on Education in Radiologic Technology
20 N Wacker Dr/Ste 900
Chicago, IL 60606-2901
312 704-5300
312 704-5304 Fax

Careers/Curriculum

Information regarding careers and curriculum should be addressed to

American Society of Radiologic Technologists
15000 Central Ave SE
Albuquerque, NM 87123
505 298-4500

Certification/Registration

Information regarding certification should be directed to

American Registry of Radiologic Technologists
1255 Northland Dr
Mendota Heights, MN 55120

Radiation Therapist

Alabama

University of Alabama at Birmingham

Radiation Therapy Prgm
(SHRP) 354-1714 9th Ave S
Birmingham, AL 35294-1270
Prgm Dir: Shirlee E Maihoff, MEd RT(T)
Tel: 205 934-7368 *Fax:* 205 934-7387
Med Dir: Sharon Spencer, MD
Class Cap: 19 *Begins:* Sep
Length: 18 mos *Award:* BS
Evening or weekend classes available

Mobile Infirmary Medical Center

Radiation Therapy Prgm
PO Box 2144
W End Louiselle St
Mobile, AL 36652
Prgm Dir: Patricia Ann Brewer, RT(T)(R)
Tel: 334 431-3549 *Fax:* 334 431-4884
Class Cap: 8 *Begins:* Jun
Length: 12 mos *Award:* Cert
Tuition per yr: $350

Arkansas

Northwest Arkansas Community College

Radiation Therapy Prgm
PO Box 1408
Bentonville, AR 72712
Prgm Dir: Melvin C Cheney, MS RT(T)
Tel: 501 361-2585
Class Cap: 8 *Begins:* Aug
Length: 24 mos *Award:* AAS
Evening or weekend classes available

Central Arkansas Radiation Therapy Inst

Radiation Therapy Prgm
Markham at University
PO Box 55050
Little Rock, AR 72215
Prgm Dir: Linda S Wingfield, MEd
RT(R)(T)FASRT
Tel: 501 664-8573 *Fax:* 501 663-1746
Med Dir: Alvah J Nelson III, MD FACR
Class Cap: 15 *Begins:* Sep
Length: 12 mos *Award:* Cert
Tuition per yr: $500

California

City of Hope National Medical Center

Radiation Therapy Prgm
1500 E Duarte Rd
Duarte, CA 91010-0269
Prgm Dir: Christine Homan-Forell, BS RT(R)(T)
Tel: 818 301-8247
E-mail: cfarell@smtplink.ca
Med Dir: Nayana Vora, MD
Class Cap: 6 *Begins:* Oct
Length: 12 mos *Award:* Cert
Tuition per yr: $300

Loma Linda University

Radiation Therapy Prgm
Nichol Hall Rm A829
Loma Linda, CA 92350
Prgm Dir: Carol A L Davis, BA RT(T)
Tel: 909 824-4378 *Fax:* 909 478-4264
E-mail: cdavis@prolit.ccu.edu
Class Cap: 18 *Begins:* Sep
Length: 12 mos *Award:* Cert
Tuition per yr: $4,560

California State University - Long Beach

Radiation Therapy Prgm
1250 Bellflower Blvd
Long Beach, CA 90840-4902
Prgm Dir: Stephanie Eatmon, MEd RT(R)(T)
Tel: 310 985-7507
Class Cap: 18 *Begins:* Jan
Length: 48 mos *Award:* BS
Evening or weekend classes available

Foothill College

Radiation Therapy Prgm
12345 El Monte Rd
Los Altos Hills, CA 94022-4599
Prgm Dir: Michael A Pignataro, MA RT(T)
Tel: 415 949-7595 *Fax:* 415 949-7375
E-mail: pignabest.com
Med Dir: Richard Borreson, MD
Class Cap: 15 *Begins:* Jul Sep
Length: 24 mos *Award:* Cert, AS
Tuition per yr: $700 res, $7,600 non-res

Los Angeles County - USC Medical Center

Radiation Therapy Prgm
1200 N State St
Los Angeles, CA 90033
Prgm Dir: Maura A Fitzgerald, AS RT(T)
Tel: 213 226-5017
Class Cap: 5 *Begins:* Sep
Length: 12 mos *Award:* Cert

Univ of California San Diego Med Ctr

Radiation Therapy Prgm
200 W Arbor Dr
San Diego, CA 92103-8757
Prgm Dir: Elaine M Chin, BS RT(T)
Tel: 619 543-6729 *Fax:* 619 543-6723
E-mail: echin@ucsd.edu
Med Dir: Peter Johnstone, MD
Class Cap: 10 *Begins:* Sep
Length: 12 mos *Award:* Cert
Tuition per yr: $3,500 res, $3,500 non-res

City College of San Francisco

Radiation Therapy Prgm
50 Phelan Ave Box S91
San Francisco, CA 94112
Prgm Dir: Les K Yim, BS RT(T)(R)
Tel: 415 239-3458
Class Cap: 45 *Begins:* Aug
Length: 26 mos *Award:* AS

Cancer Foundation of Santa Barbara

Radiation Therapy Prgm
300 W Pueblo St
PO Box 837
Santa Barbara, CA 93105-4311
Prgm Dir: Sofiann Enrico Langhorne, RT(R)(T)
Tel: 805 682-7300 *Fax:* 805 569-7406
E-mail: school2@cfsb.org
Class Cap: 5 *Begins:* Sep
Length: 24 mos *Award:* Cert
Tuition per yr: $2,000

Connecticut

Danbury Hospital

Radiation Therapy Prgm
24 Hospital Ave
Danbury, CT 06810
Prgm Dir: Stephanie Ambra, BS RT(T)
Tel: 203 797-7190
Med Dir: John A Sperk, MD
Class Cap: 3 *Begins:* Oct
Length: 12 mos *Award:* Cert
Tuition per yr: $2,500

Hartford Hospital

Radiation Therapy Prgm
80 Seymour St
Hartford, CT 06115-0729
Prgm Dir: Nora Uricchio, MEd RT(R)(T)
Tel: 860 545-3953 *Fax:* 860 545-1500
Med Dir: Andrew L Salner, MD
Class Cap: 13 *Begins:* Jun Oct
Length: 24 mos *Award:* Cert
Tuition per yr: $2,000

Gateway Community - Technical College

Radiation Therapy Prgm
88 Bassett Rd
North Haven, CT 06473
Prgm Dir: Kathleen E Ring, BA RT(T)
Tel: 203 785-5831 *Fax:* 203 785-3023
Med Dir: Bruce Hafty, MD
Class Cap: 13 *Begins:* Sep
Length: 23 mos *Award:* AS
Tuition per yr: $1,560 res, $4,680 non-res
Evening or weekend classes available

District of Columbia

George Washington University

Radiation Therapy Prgm
2300 Eye St NW
Washington, DC 20037
Prgm Dir: Catherine L Turley, MS RT(T)
Tel: 202 994-3564 *Fax:* 202 994-1299
E-mail: turley@gwis2.circ.gwu.edu
Class Cap: 8 *Begins:* Aug
Length: 16 mos, 42 mos *Award:* Cert, BS
Tuition per yr: $12,825

Howard University

Radiation Therapy Prgm
2400 6th St NW
Washington, DC 20059
Prgm Dir: Mattie J Tabron, EdD RT(R)(T)FASRT
Tel: 202 806-7609 *Fax:* 202 806-4476
E-mail: tab@cldc.howard.edu
Begins: Aug *Award:* Cert, BS
Tuition per yr: $8,725 res, $8,725 non-res

Florida

Broward Community College

Radiation Therapy Prgm
1000 Coconut Creek Blvd
Bldg41 Rm 123
Coconut Creek, FL 33066
Prgm Dir: Maryanne Loser, BS RT(T)
Tel: 954 973-2352   *Fax:* 954 973-2348
Class Cap: 30   *Begins:* Aug
Length: 24 mos, 72 mos   *Award:* Cert, AS
Tuition per yr: $2,193 res, $7,931 non-res

Halifax Medical Center

Radiation Therapy Prgm
303 N Clyde Morris Blvd
PO Box 2830
Daytona Beach, FL 32120-2830
Prgm Dir: Belinda H Phillips, BS RT(R)(T)
Tel: 904 254-4075   *Fax:* 904 254-4231
Med Dir: Terry Bloom, MD
Class Cap: 9   *Begins:* May
Length: 12 mos   *Award:* Cert

Radiation Therapy Regional Center

Radiation Therapy Prgm
Lakes Park Office
7341 Gladiolas Dr
Ft Meyers, FL 33908
Prgm Dir: Donald E Moody, RT(R)(T)
Tel: 941 489-3420   *Fax:* 941 489-3219
Med Dir: James H Rubenstien, MD ABR
Class Cap: 18   *Begins:* Varies
Length: 14 mos   *Award:* Cert
Tuition per yr: $500 res, $1,000 non-res

St Vincent's Medical Center

Radiation Therapy Prgm
1800 Barrs St
PO Box 2982
Jacksonville, FL 32203
Prgm Dir: Todd A Blobe, BA RT(T)
Tel: 904 387-7310   *Fax:* 904 308-8737
Med Dir: Scot Ackerman, MD
Class Cap: 12   *Begins:* Sep
Length: 12 mos   *Award:* Cert
Tuition per yr: $1,500 res, $1,500 non-res

Miami-Dade Community College

Radiation Therapy Prgm
Medical Center Campus
950 NW 20th St
Miami, FL 33127
Prgm Dir: Janet G Darlington, BS RT(R)(T)
Tel: 305 585-6672   *Fax:* 305 585-7866
Class Cap: 15   *Begins:* Aug
Length: 24 mos   *Award:* Cert, AS
Tuition per yr: $1,500 res, $3,000 non-res
Evening or weekend classes available

Florida Hospital Medical Center

Radiation Therapy Prgm
College of Health Sciences
800 Lake Estelle Dr
Orlando, FL 32803
Prgm Dir: Mary Lou DeMarco, MS RT(T)
Tel: 407 895-7747   *Fax:* 407 895-7820
E-mail: mld@poboxes.com
Med Dir: Burkhard Weppelmann, MD
Class Cap: 10   *Begins:* Aug
Length: 24 mos   *Award:* Cert, AA
Tuition per yr: $4,158

Hillsborough Community College

Radiation Therapy Prgm
PO Box 30030
Tampa, FL 33630
Prgm Dir: Karen M Nelson, BA RT(R)(T)
Tel: 813 253-7372
Med Dir: Robert Miller, MD
Class Cap: 20   *Begins:* Aug May
Length: 16 mos, 24 mos   *Award:* Cert, AS
Tuition per yr: $1,100 res, $4,100 non-res

Georgia

Grady Health System

Radiation Therapy Prgm
80 Butler St SE
PO Box 26095
Atlanta, GA 30335
Prgm Dir: Deborah B Amodeo, BS RT(R)(T)
Tel: 404 616-5024   *Fax:* 404 616-3512
Med Dir: William Thomas, MD
Class Cap: 13   *Begins:* Oct
Length: 12 mos   *Award:* Cert
Tuition per yr: $2,400

Medical College of Georgia

Radiation Therapy Prgm
Bldg HK
Augusta, GA 30912-3965
Prgm Dir: Ann Marie Vann, MEd RT(R)(T)
Tel: 706 721-2971   *Fax:* 706 721-7248
Class Cap: 7   *Begins:* Sep
Length: 24 mos   *Award:* Cert, AS
Tuition per yr: $2,820 res, $6,908 non-res
Evening or weekend classes available

Armstrong Atlantic State University

Radiation Therapy Prgm
11935 Abercorn St
Savannah, GA 31419-1997
Prgm Dir: Laurie Adams, MHS RT(T)
Tel: 912 927-5360   *Fax:* 912 921-5889
E-mail: laurie_adams@mailgate.armstrong.edu
Med Dir: John Duttenhaver
Class Cap: 11   *Begins:* Sep
Length: 12 mos   *Award:* Cert
Tuition per yr: $2,448 res, $7,620 non-res

Thomas Technical Institute

Radiation Therapy Prgm
15689 US Hwy 19 N
Thomasville, GA 31792
Prgm Dir: Giles C Toole, MS RT(R)(T)
Tel: 912 225-4078   *Fax:* 912 225-5289
Med Dir: J Steven Johnson, MD
Class Cap: 11   *Begins:* Jul Sep
Length: 12 mos, 21 mos   *Award:* Dipl, AAT
Tuition per yr: $1,512 res, $2,016 non-res
Evening or weekend classes available

Illinois

Univ of Chicago Hosp/Roosevelt Univ

Radiation Therapy Prgm
5841 S Maryland Ave/MC0085
Chicago, IL 60637
Prgm Dir: Helen Schmit
Tel: 312 791-8176   *Fax:* 312 791-3499
E-mail: hschmit@rover.uchicago.edu
Med Dir: Howard Halpern, MD PhD
Class Cap: 22   *Begins:* Sep
Length: 24 mos   *Award:* BS
Tuition per yr: $7,000

St Joseph Hospital

Radiation Therapy Prgm
77 N Airlite St
Elgin, IL 60123
Prgm Dir: Heather Dam, BA RT(R)(T)
Tel: 708 695-3200   *Fax:* 847 695-3319
Class Cap: 5   *Begins:* Oct
Length: 12 mos   *Award:* Cert

National-Louis University

Radiation Therapy Prgm
2840 N Sheridan Rd
Evanston, IL 60201
Prgm Dir: Leia Levy, BA RT(T)
Tel: 847 475-1100   *Fax:* 847 256-1057
Med Dir: Krystyna Kiel, MD
Class Cap: 20   *Begins:* Sep
Length: 24 mos, 48 mos   *Award:* Dipl,Cert, BA
Tuition per yr: $12,614
Evening or weekend classes available

Edward Hines Jr VA Hospital

Radiation Therapy Prgm
Fifth Ave & Roosevelt Rd
(Dept 114B)
Hines, IL 60141
Prgm Dir: Gwendolyn Grice, BS RT(R)(T)
Tel: 708 216-2649
Class Cap: 10   *Begins:* Sep
Length: 12 mos   *Award:* Cert

Swedish American Hospital

Radiation Therapy Prgm
1400 Charles St
Rockford, IL 61104-2298
Prgm Dir: Dawna R Menke, BS RT(T)
Tel: 815 961-2030   *Fax:* 815 966-3966
Med Dir: Thornton Kline
Class Cap: 5   *Begins:* Sep
Length: 12 mos   *Award:* Cert

Indiana

Welborn Cancer Center

Radiation Therapy Prgm
401 SE Sixth St
Evansville, IN 47713
Prgm Dir: Joann Marie Murray, BS RT(R)(T)
Tel: 812 474-1110   *Fax:* 812 474-1303
Class Cap: 5   *Begins:* Jul
Length: 12 mos   *Award:* Cert
Tuition per yr: $1,000

Programs

Indiana University Northwest
Radiation Therapy Prgm
3400 Broadway
Gary, IN 46408-1197
Prgm Dir: Sandy L Piehl, MPART(R)(T)
Tel: 219 981-4204 *Fax:* 219 980-6649
E-mail: spiehl@iunhaw1.iun.indiana.edu
Class Cap: 10 *Begins:* Aug
Length: 22 mos *Award:* AS
Tuition per yr: $3,150 res, $8,150 non-res
Evening or weekend classes available

Indiana University School of Medicine
Radiation Therapy Prgm
1140 W Michigan St
Coleman Hall Rm 326
Indianapolis, IN 46202-5119
Prgm Dir: Donna Kay Dunn, MS RT(T)
Tel: 317 274-1302 *Fax:* 317 274-4723
Med Dir: Shailaja Reddy, MD
Class Cap: 16 *Begins:* Jun Aug
Length: 48 mos *Award:* BS
Tuition per yr: $4,560 res, $12,840 non-res
Evening or weekend classes available

Methodist Hospital of Indiana, Inc
Radiation Therapy Prgm
1701 N Senate Blvd
PO Box 1367
Indianapolis, IN 46206-1367
Prgm Dir: Dan R Strahan, BS RT(T)
Tel: 317 929-3377 *Fax:* 317 929-2102
Med Dir: William Rate, MD
Class Cap: 6 *Begins:* May
Length: 14 mos *Award:* Cert, AS
Tuition per yr: $3,350

Iowa

University of Iowa Hospitals and Clinics
Radiation Therapy Prgm
W189Z GH
Iowa City, IA 522421009
Prgm Dir: Pamela R Jones, BA RT(T)
Tel: 319 356-8286 *Fax:* 319 356-1530
Med Dir: David Hussey, MD
Class Cap: 8 *Begins:* Sep
Length: 12 mos *Award:* Cert
Tuition per yr: $1,000

Kansas

University of Kansas Medical Center
Radiation Therapy Prgm
3901 Rainbow Blvd
Kansas City, KS 66160-7321
Prgm Dir: Larry M Oliver, RT(T)
Tel: 913 588-3600
Class Cap: 19 *Begins:* Sep
Length: 12 mos *Award:* Cert
Tuition per yr: $3,500

Washburn University of Topeka
Radiation Therapy Prgm
1700 SW College Ave
Topeka, KS 66621
Prgm Dir: Kathryn E Frye, BS RT(R)(T)
Tel: 913 231-1010 *Fax:* 913 231-1027
E-mail: zzfrye@sace.wuacc.edu
Med Dir: Terry Walls, MD
Class Cap: 20 *Begins:* Aug
Length: 12 mos *Award:* Cert
Tuition per yr: $3,007 res, $6,541 non-res

Kentucky

Univ of Kentucky Chandler Med Ctr
Radiation Therapy Prgm
800 Rose St Rm C-39
Lexington, KY 40536-0084
Prgm Dir: Debra Mercer, BHS RT(R)(T)
Tel: 606 323-6486 *Fax:* 606 257-4931
Med Dir: P Patel, MD
Class Cap: 9 *Begins:* Jul
Length: 12 mos *Award:* Cert
Tuition per yr: $500

JG Brown Cancer Ctr/U of Louisville Hosp
Radiation Therapy Prgm
529 S Jackson St
Louisville, KY 40202
Prgm Dir: Judith M Turner, BS RT(R)(T)
Tel: 502 852-5254
Class Cap: 9 *Begins:* Sep
Length: 12 mos *Award:* Cert
Tuition per yr: $1,500

Louisiana

Alton Ochsner Medical Foundation
Radiation Therapy Prgm
Sch of Allied Health Sciences
1516 Jefferson Hwy
New Orleans, LA 70121
Prgm Dir: Robin L Wegener, BS RT(R)(T)
Tel: 504 842-3267 *Fax:* 504 842-9129
Med Dir: Robert R Kuske, MD
Class Cap: 7 *Begins:* Sep
Length: 13 mos *Award:* Cert

Maine

Southern Maine Technical College
Radiation Therapy Prgm
2 Fort Rd
South Portland, ME 04106
Prgm Dir: Dennis T Leaver, MS RT(R)(T)
Tel: 207 767-9593
Class Cap: 6 *Begins:* Aug
Length: 24 mos, 12 mos *Award:* Cert, AAS
Tuition per yr: $3,000 res, $5,400 non-res

Maryland

Essex Community College
Radiation Therapy Prgm
7201 Rossville Blvd
Baltimore, MD 21237-9987
Prgm Dir: Joseph M Digel, RT(R)(T)
Tel: 410 955-7222 *Fax:* 410 955-3691
E-mail: digeljo@welchlink.welch.jhu.edu
Med Dir: Moody D Wharam
Class Cap: 12 *Begins:* Sep
Length: 24 mos *Award:* AA
Tuition per yr: $2,400 res, $4,240 non-res

Massachusetts

Laboure College
Radiation Therapy Prgm
2120 Dorchester Ave
Boston, MA 02124-5698
Prgm Dir: Susan Beth Belinsky, MPA RT(R)(T)
Tel: 617 296-8300 *Fax:* 617 296-7947
Med Dir: Julie Shockley, MD
Class Cap: 19 *Begins:* Sep
Length: 24 mos *Award:* AS
Tuition per yr: $12,454
Evening or weekend classes available

Mass Coll of Pharmacy & Allied Hlth Sci
Radiation Therapy Prgm
179 Longwood Ave
Boston, MA 02115
Prgm Dir: Grant Guan, MD MS CMD RT(T)
Tel: 617 732-2916 *Fax:* 617 732-2801
E-mail: ghou@jcrt.harvard.edu
Med Dir: Jay Harris, MD
Class Cap: 21 *Begins:* Sep
Length: 25 mos *Award:* AS, BS
Tuition per yr: $15,759 res, $15,759 non-res
Evening or weekend classes available

Springfield Technical Community College
Radiation Therapy Prgm
One Armory Sq
Springfield, MA 01105
Prgm Dir: Julianne Kinsman, MEd RT(T)
Tel: 413 781-7822 *Fax:* 413 781-5805
E-mail: kinsman@stcc.adm.stcc.mass.edu
Med Dir: Mary Ann Lowen, MD
Class Cap: 8 *Begins:* Sep
Length: 24 mos *Award:* AS
Tuition per yr: $1,713 res, $6,745 non-res

Univ Mass Med Ctr/Worcester State Coll
Radiation Therapy Prgm
55 Lake Ave N
Worcester, MA 01655
Prgm Dir: Patricia E Webster, BS RT(T)
Tel: 508 856-5551 *Fax:* 508 856-5006
Med Dir: T J Fitzgerald, MD
Class Cap: 7 *Begins:* Oct
Length: 15 mos *Award:* Cert
Tuition per yr: $2,000

Michigan

University of Michigan Medical Center

Radiation Therapy Prgm
1500 E Medical Ctr Dr
Box 0010 Rm B2C490
Ann Arbor, MI 48109
Prgm Dir: Sue M Merkel, MSA RT(R)(T)
Tel: 313 936-9522   *Fax:* 313 936-7859
E-mail: smerkel@umich.edu
Med Dir: Howard Sandler, MD
Class Cap: 13   *Begins:* Jan Jul
Length: 12 mos   *Award:* Cert
Tuition per yr: $750

Henry Ford Hospital

Radiation Therapy Prgm
2799 W Grand Blvd
Detroit, MI 48202
Prgm Dir: Cheryl L Martin, MA RT(R)(T)
Tel: 313 876-1021   *Fax:* 313 876-3235
Med Dir: Jae Ho Kim, MD PhD
Class Cap: 8   *Begins:* Sep
Length: 12 mos   *Award:* Cert
Tuition per yr: $1,100 res, $1,100 non-res

Wayne State University

Radiation Therapy Prgm
121 Shapero Annex
Detroit, MI 48202
Prgm Dir: Diane K Chadwell, MA RT(R)(T)
Tel: 313 577-1137
Class Cap: 23   *Begins:* Sep
Length: 48 mos   *Award:* BS

Lansing Community College

Radiation Therapy Prgm
PO Box 40010/Dept 3400
Lansing, MI 48901-7210
Prgm Dir: Denise Crouch, BS RT(R)
Tel: 517 483-1428
Class Cap: 19   *Begins:* Aug
Length: 15 mos   *Award:* AS
Tuition per yr: $1,435 res, $2,345 non-res
Evening or weekend classes available

William Beaumont Hospital

Radiation Therapy Prgm
3601 W Thirteen Mile Rd
Royal Oak, MI 48073-6769
Prgm Dir: Laura L Sykes, BS RT(CT)
Tel: 810 551-7156
Class Cap: 8
Length: 18 mos   *Award:* Cert

Minnesota

Abbott Northwestern Hospital

Radiation Therapy Prgm
Virginia Piper Cancer Inst
800 E 28th St
Minneapolis, MN 55406
Prgm Dir: Mary M Durand, BS RT(R)(T)
Tel: 612 863-5386   *Fax:* 612 863-4963
E-mail: durand@allina.com
Class Cap: 5   *Begins:* Sep
Length: 12 mos   *Award:* Cert
Tuition per yr: $1,220

Univ of Minnesota Hosp and Clinic

Radiation Therapy Prgm
Harvard St at E River Rd
Box 494
Minneapolis, MN 55455
Prgm Dir: Mary Beth Hartzell, BAS RT(T)
Tel: 612 626-6404
Med Dir: Seymour H Levitt, MD
Class Cap: 7   *Begins:* Sep
Length: 12 mos   *Award:* Cert
Tuition per yr: $2,200

Mayo Clinic/Mayo Foundation

Radiation Therapy Prgm
Sch of Hlth Related Sciences
200 First St SW
Rochester, MN 55905
Prgm Dir: Leila A Bussman, BS RT(R)(T)
Tel: 507 284-4148   *Fax:* 507 284-0079
E-mail: bussmanyeakel.leila@mayo.edu
Med Dir: James A Martenson, MD
Class Cap: 12   *Begins:* Sep
Length: 5 mos   *Award:* Cert
Tuition per yr: $1,000

Missouri

St Luke's Hospital of Kansas City

Radiation Therapy Prgm
4400 Wornall Rd
Kansas City, MO 64111
Prgm Dir: Myra A Troutwine, BS RT (R)(T)
Tel: 816 932-2575   *Fax:* 816 932-2344
Class Cap: 4   *Begins:* Jan
Length: 12 mos   *Award:* Cert
Tuition per yr: $6,000

Barnes-Jewish Hospital

Radiation Therapy Prgm
One Barnes Hospital Plaza
St Louis, MO 63110
Prgm Dir: Kathleen O Kienstra, BS RT(T)
Tel: 314 362-7756   *Fax:* 314 747-1279
Med Dir: Marie E Taylor
Class Cap: 14   *Begins:* Jul
Length: 12 mos   *Award:* Cert
Tuition per yr: $2,200

Nebraska

NE Methodist Coll Nursing & Allied Hlth

Radiation Therapy Prgm
8501 W Dodge Rd
Omaha, NE 68114
Prgm Dir: Victoria Zenor, BS RT(R)(T)
Tel: 402 390-4982
Class Cap: 7   *Begins:* May
Length: 12 mos   *Award:* BS

University of Nebraska Medical Center

Radiation Therapy Prgm
600 S 42nd St
Omaha, NE 68198-1045
Prgm Dir: Cheryl K Sanders, MPA RT(R)(T)
Tel: 402 559-7604   *Fax:* 402 559-4667
E-mail: csanders@unmc.edu
Med Dir: T J Imray, MD
Class Cap: 6   *Begins:* Aug
Length: 12 mos   *Award:* BS
Tuition per yr: $2,877 res, $7,843 non-res

New Jersey

Cooper Hospital/University Medical Ctr

Radiation Therapy Prgm
One Cooper Plaza
Camden, NJ 08103
Prgm Dir: Donna Stinson, MPA RT(R)(T)
Tel: 609 342-2734   *Fax:* 609 365-8504
Begins: Sep
Length: 12 mos   *Award:* Cert
Tuition per yr: $4,000

St Barnabas Medical Center

Radiation Therapy Prgm
Old Short Hills Rd
Livingston, NJ 07039
Prgm Dir: Jennie S Lichtenberger, BS RT(T)
Tel: 201 533-5628
Med Dir: Louis J Sanfilippo, MD
Class Cap: 25   *Begins:* Sep
Length: 12 mos   *Award:* Cert
Tuition per yr: $2,500

New York

Montefiore Medical Center

Radiation Therapy Prgm
Moses Division
111 E 210th St
Bronx, NY 10467
Prgm Dir: Gerald Squillante, RT(T)
Tel: 212 920-5083   *Fax:* 718 882-6913
Class Cap: 18   *Begins:* Oct
Length: 24 mos   *Award:* Cert
Tuition per yr: $12,000

New York Methodist Hospital

Radiation Therapy Prgm
506 Sixth St/Box 159008
Brooklyn, NY 11215-9008
Prgm Dir: JoAnne Habenicht, MPA RT(R)(T)(M)
Tel: 718 780-3677   *Fax:* 718 780-3688
Med Dir: E Youssef
Class Cap: 9   *Begins:* Sep
Length: 24 mos   *Award:* Cert
Tuition per yr: $2,000

Erie Community College - City Campus

Radiation Therapy Prgm
121 Ellicott St
Buffalo, NY 14203
Prgm Dir: Peter D Blacher, EdM RT(T)
Tel: 716 851-1048
Class Cap: 17   *Begins:* Sep
Length: 24 mos   *Award:* AAS

Nassau Community College

Radiation Therapy Prgm
One Education Dr
Garden City, NY 11530
Prgm Dir: Catherine Smyth, BA RT(T)
Tel: 516 572-7551   *Fax:* 516 572-7092
Med Dir: Jay Bosworth, MD
Class Cap: 49   *Begins:* Sep
Length: 24 mos   *Award:* AAS

Programs

Memorial Sloan - Kettering Cancer Ctr

Radiation Therapy Prgm
1275 York Ave/Box 255
New York, NY 10021
Prgm Dir: Mary Reynolds, BA RT(T)
Tel: 212 639-6835 *Fax:* 121 717-3104
Med Dir: Zvi Fuks, MD
Class Cap: 12 *Begins:* Sep
Length: 24 mos *Award:* Cert
Tuition per yr: $4,000

University of Rochester Cancer Center

Radiation Therapy Prgm
601 Elmwood Ave/Box 647
Rochester, NY 14642
Prgm Dir: George M Uschold, EdD RT(T)
Tel: 716 275-5464 *Fax:* 716 275-1531
E-mail: gusch@radonc.medinfo.rochester.edu
Class Cap: 6 *Begins:* Sep
Length: 24 mos *Award:* Cert
Tuition per yr: $3,000

SUNY Health Science Ctr at Stony Brook

Radiation Therapy Prgm
School of Health Tech & Mgmt
Stony Brook, NY 11794-8200
Prgm Dir: David B LaBelle, BS RT(T)
Tel: 516 444-7761 *Fax:* 516 689-8801
E-mail: dlabelle@radonc.sunysb.edu
Med Dir: Alan G Meek, MD
Class Cap: 10 *Begins:* Sep
Length: 24 mos *Award:* Cert
Tuition per yr: $2,100 res, $7,000 non-res

SUNY Health Science Center at Syracuse

Radiation Therapy Prgm
750 E Adams St
Syracuse, NY 13210
Prgm Dir: Joan E O'Brien, MSEd RT(T)
Tel: 315 464-6937 *Fax:* 315 464-6914
E-mail: obrienj@vax.cs.hscsyr.edu
Med Dir: Robert Sagerman, PhD
Class Cap: 10 *Begins:* Aug
Length: 24 mos *Award:* AAS
Tuition per yr: $1,350 res, $3,200 non-res

North Carolina

University of North Carolina Hospitals

Radiation Therapy Prgm
101 Manning Dr
Chapel Hill, NC 27514
Prgm Dir: Robert D Adams, BS RT(T)
Tel: 919 966-1101 *Fax:* 919 966-7681
Class Cap: 9 *Begins:* Aug
Length: 12 mos *Award:* Cert
Tuition per yr: $922

Pitt Community College

Radiation Therapy Prgm
PO Drawer 7007
Greenville, NC 27835-7007
Prgm Dir: Lee Braswell, BS RT(R)(T)
Tel: 919 551-2900 *Fax:* 919 321-4451
Class Cap: 10 *Begins:* Sep
Length: 24 mos *Award:* Cert, AAS
Tuition per yr: $742 res, $6,020 non-res

Forsyth Technical Community College

Radiation Therapy Prgm
2100 Silas Creek Pkwy
Winston-Salem, NC 27103
Prgm Dir: Christina R Gibson, BS RT(R)(T)
Tel: 910 723-0371 *Fax:* 910 748-9395
Med Dir: Lisa Evans, MD
Class Cap: 20 *Begins:* Sep
Length: 24 mos, 12 mos *Award:* AAS
Tuition per yr: $742 res, $6,020 non-res
Evening or weekend classes available

Ohio

Aultman Hospital

Radiation Therapy Prgm
2600 Sixth St SW
Canton, OH 44710
Prgm Dir: Victoria L DiSabatino, BA RT(R)(T)
Tel: 330 438-6201 *Fax:* 330 438-9811
Class Cap: 5 *Begins:* Jul
Length: 12 mos *Award:* Cert
Tuition per yr: $2,500

Univ of Cincinnati

Radiation Therapy Prgm
234 Goodman Ave
ML 757
Cincinnati, OH 45267
Prgm Dir: Carolyn Hollan, MS RT(R)(T)
Tel: 513 558-9099 *Fax:* 513 558-4007
Med Dir: Bernard Aron, MD
Class Cap: 15 *Begins:* Sep
Length: 24 mos, 12 mos *Award:* Cert, AS
Tuition per yr: $3,471 res, $8,745 non-res

Cleveland Clinic Foundation

Radiation Therapy Prgm
9500 Euclid Ave (T28)
Cleveland, OH 44195
Prgm Dir: Patricia A Barrett, BS RT(R)(T)
Tel: 216 444-5484 *Fax:* 216 444-5331
E-mail: barrett@radonc.ccf.org
Med Dir: Roger Macklis, MD
Class Cap: 8 *Begins:* Jul
Length: 12 mos *Award:* Cert
Tuition per yr: $1,100 res, $1,100 non-res

University Hospitals of Cleveland

Radiation Therapy Prgm
11100 Euclid Ave
Cleveland, OH 44106
Prgm Dir: David G Ward, BS RT(R)(T)
Tel: 216 844-3103 *Fax:* 216 844-1058
Med Dir: Donald C Shine, MD
Class Cap: 7 *Begins:* Jul
Length: 12 mos *Award:* Cert
Tuition per yr: $1,000

Arthur G James Cancer Hosp & Res Inst

Radiation Therapy Prgm
300 W Tenth Ave
Columbus, OH 43210
Prgm Dir: Ruth M Hackworth, BS RT(R)(T)
Tel: 614 293-8415 *Fax:* 614 293-4044
E-mail: hackworth-1@medctr.osu.edu
Med Dir: Gahbauer Reinhard, MD
Class Cap: 7 *Begins:* Jul
Length: 12 mos *Award:* Cert
Tuition per yr: $1,000

Owens Community College

Radiation Therapy Prgm
PO Box 10,000
Toledo, OH 43699-1947
Prgm Dir: Roy A Miller, BS RT(T)
Tel: 419 661-7415 *Fax:* 419 661-7665
E-mail: bmiller@owens.cc.oh.us
Class Cap: 9 *Begins:* Jun
Length: 24 mos *Award:* AAS
Tuition per yr: $2,060 res, $3,860 non-res
Evening or weekend classes available

Oklahoma

Univ of Oklahoma Health Sciences Center

Radiation Therapy Prgm
PO Box 26901 Rm 128D
Oklahoma City, OK 73190
Prgm Dir: Lynda N Reynolds, BS RT(R)(T) FAS
Tel: 405 271-2288 *Fax:* 405 271-1424
E-mail: lynda-reynolds@uokhsc.edu
Med Dir: Carl R Bogardus, MD
Class Cap: 11 *Begins:* Aug
Length: 48 mos *Award:* BS
Tuition per yr: $2,610 res, $7,177 non-res
Evening or weekend classes available

Oregon

Oregon Health Sciences University

Radiation Therapy Prgm
3181 SW Sam Jackson Pk Rd
L37
Portland, OR 97201-3098
Prgm Dir: Anne M Maddeford, BS RT(T)
Tel: 503 494-6708 *Fax:* 503 494-2730
E-mail: maddefoa@ohsu.edu
Med Dir: Keaneth Stevens, MD
Begins: Sep
Length: 24 mos *Award:* Dipl, BS
Tuition per yr: $6,792 res, $12,264 non-res
Evening or weekend classes available

Pennsylvania

Mercy Regional Health System

Radiation Therapy Prgm
2500 Seventh Ave
Altoona, PA 16602-2099
Prgm Dir: Sr Rose Mary Modzelewski, BS RT(R)
Tel: 814 949-4280
Class Cap: 5 *Begins:* Sep
Length: 12 mos *Award:* Cert
Tuition per yr: $2,150

Gwynedd-Mercy College

Radiation Therapy Prgm
Sumneytown Pike
Gwynedd Valley, PA 19437
Prgm Dir: Patricia J Giordano, MS RT(R)(T)
Tel: 215 646-7300 *Fax:* 215 641-5559
Med Dir: C Jules Rominler, MD
Class Cap: 43 *Begins:* Jul Sep
Length: 24 mos, 13 mos *Award:* Cert, AS
Tuition per yr: $18,370 res, $12,670 non-res

Comm Coll of Allegheny Cnty-Alleg Campus

Radiation Therapy Prgm
808 Ridge Ave
Pittsburgh, PA 15212-6097
Prgm Dir: Charleen Gombert, BS RT(T)
Tel: 412 237-2752 *Fax:* 412 237-4521
E-mail: cgombert@ccac.edu
Med Dir: Melvin Deutsch, MD
Class Cap: 30 *Begins:* Aug
Length: 12 mos, 24 mos *Award:* Cert, AS
Tuition per yr: $2,040 res, $4,080 non-res
Evening or weekend classes available

Rhode Island

Rhode Island Hospital

Radiation Therapy Prgm
593 Eddy St
Providence, RI 02903
Prgm Dir: Gayle A Sawyer, MEd RT(R)(T)
Tel: 401 444-8311 *Fax:* 901 444-5335
Med Dir: Mohamedyakub A Puthawla, MD
Class Cap: 5 *Begins:* Sep
Length: 12 mos *Award:* Cert
Tuition per yr: $1,500 res, $2,000 non-res

South Carolina

Medical University of South Carolina

Radiation Therapy Prgm
171 Ashley Ave Rm 304
Wachoyia Bank Bldg Rm 403
Charleston, SC 29425
Prgm Dir: Mary Jo Repasky, MHSA RT(T)
Tel: 803 792-3789 *Fax:* 873 792-0506
E-mail: repaskym@musc.edu
Med Dir: Leta Sue Lamb, MD
Class Cap: 12 *Begins:* Aug
Length: 24 mos *Award:* BS
Tuition per yr: $4,401 res, $12,822 non-res

Tennessee

Chattanooga State Technical Comm College

Radiation Therapy Prgm
407 Chestnut St Level B
Chattanooga, TN 37402
Prgm Dir: Lisa Legg, BS RT(R)(T)
Tel: 423 634-7713 *Fax:* 423 634-7706
E-mail: LEGG@CSTCC.CC.TN.US
Med Dir: Deanna Davidson, MD
Class Cap: 52 *Begins:* Aug
Length: 12 mos *Award:* Cert
Tuition per yr: $1,208 res, $4,620 non-res

Baptist Memorial Health Care Systems

Radiation Therapy Prgm
1003 Monroe Ave 3rd Fl
Memphis, TN 38104
Prgm Dir: Beverly K Coker, RT(R)(T)
Tel: 901 227-5152 *Fax:* 901 227-4431
Med Dir: Valerian Chyle, MD
Class Cap: 12 *Begins:* Aug
Length: 13 mos *Award:* Cert
Tuition per yr: $2,500

Methodist Hospitals of Memphis

Radiation Therapy Prgm
1265 Union Ave
Memphis, TN 38104
Prgm Dir: Joan D Simone, BS RT(R)(T)
Tel: 901 726-7367 *Fax:* 901 726-7370
Class Cap: 8 *Begins:* Jul
Length: 12 mos *Award:* Cert
Tuition per yr: $1,450

Vanderbilt University Medical Center

Radiation Therapy Prgm
Center for Radiation Oncology
The Vanderbilt Clinic B 902
Nashville, TN 37232-5671
Prgm Dir: Barbara L Flexner, BS RT(R)(T)
Tel: 615 322-2555 *Fax:* 615 343-0161
Med Dir: Donald R Eisert, MD
Class Cap: 18 *Begins:* Sep
Length: 12 mos *Award:* Cert
Tuition per yr: $3,500

Texas

Amarillo College

Radiation Therapy Prgm
PO Box 447
Amarillo, TX 79178
Prgm Dir: Tony Tackitt, BMEd RT(T)
Tel: 806 354-6063 *Fax:* 806 354-6096
E-mail: tmtackitt@actx.edu
Med Dir: Joe Arko, MD
Class Cap: 10 *Begins:* Aug
Length: 24 mos *Award:* AAS
Tuition per yr: $702 res, $999 non-res

Galveston College-University of Texas

Radiation Therapy Prgm
4015 Ave Q
Galveston, TX 77550-2782
Prgm Dir: Halena Shermer-Hellums, BS
  RT(R)(T)
Tel: 409 772-3042 *Fax:* 409 772-3014
Med Dir: Martin Colman, MD
Class Cap: 8 *Begins:* Sep
Length: 23 mos *Award:* AAS
Tuition per yr: $580 res, $1,600 non-res
Evening or weekend classes available

Univ of Texas M D Anderson Cancer Ctr

Radiation Therapy Prgm
1515 Holcombe Blvd
PO Box 701
Houston, TX 77030
Prgm Dir: Charles M Washington, BS RT(T)
Tel: 713 792-3455 *Fax:* 713 792-0956
E-mail: cwashington@radonc.mdacc.tmc.edu
Med Dir: Eric A Storm, MD
Class Cap: 30 *Begins:* Aug
Length: 24 mos *Award:* Cert
Tuition per yr: $1,800

Methodist Hospital

Radiation Therapy Prgm
3615 19th St PO Box 1201
Lubbock, TX 79408
Prgm Dir: Francess V Lozano, AAS RT(R)(T)
Tel: 806 793-4206 *Fax:* 806 793-4153
Med Dir: John P Lytle
Class Cap: 6 *Begins:* Sep
Length: 12 mos *Award:* Cert

Cancer Therapy & Research Center

Radiation Therapy Prgm
4450 Medical Dr
San Antonio, TX 78229
Prgm Dir: Karen M Cox, RT(R)(T)
Tel: 210 616-5650 *Fax:* 210 692-9822
Class Cap: 12 *Begins:* Aug
Length: 12 mos, 24 mos *Award:* Cert
Tuition per yr: $1,000 res, $1,000 non-res

Vermont

University of Vermont

Radiation Therapy Prgm
302 Rowell Bldg
Burlington, VT 05405-0068
Prgm Dir: Charles H Marschke, BA RT(T)
Tel: 802 656-3455 *Fax:* 802 656-2191
E-mail: cmarschke@cosmos.uvm.edu
Class Cap: 7 *Begins:* Sep
Length: 24 mos *Award:* AS
Tuition per yr: $6,210 res, $15,516 non-res
Evening or weekend classes available

Virginia

Univ of Virginia Health Sciences Center

Radiation Therapy Prgm
Jefferson Park Ave Box 383
Charlottesville, VA 22908
Prgm Dir: Frances R Taylor, BA RT(R)(T)
Tel: 804 924-5191 *Fax:* 804 982-3262
Class Cap: 6 *Begins:* Sep
Length: 12 mos *Award:* Cert
Tuition per yr: $800

Sentara Norfolk General Hospital

Radiation Therapy Prgm
600 Gresham Dr
Norfolk, VA 23507
Prgm Dir: Barbara Murray, BS RT(R)(T)
Tel: 804 628-2907
Class Cap: 8 *Begins:* Aug
Length: 12 mos *Award:* Cert
Tuition per yr: $2,430

Med Coll of VA/Virginia Commonwealth U

Radiation Therapy Prgm
MCV Station Box 495
Box 980495
Richmond, VA 23298-0495
Prgm Dir: Larry G Swafford, BS RT(R)(T)
Tel: 804 828-9104 *Fax:* 804 828-9104
E-mail: lswafford@gems.vcu.edu
Class Cap: 8 *Begins:* Aug
Length: 21 mos *Award:* BS
Tuition per yr: $5,679 res, $16,904 non-res

Carilion Health System/Carilion Roanoke Mem Hosp

Radiation Therapy Prgm
Cancer Center of SWVA
PO Box 13367
Roanoke, VA 24033
Prgm Dir: Alison Cronk, BS RTT
Tel: 540 981-8206 *Fax:* 540 981-7528
Med Dir: Helen Maddux, MD
Class Cap: 8 *Begins:* Aug
Length: 12 mos *Award:* Cert
Tuition per yr: $1,200

Programs

Washington

Bellevue Community College
Radiation Therapy Prgm
3000 Landerholm Circle SE
B-243
Bellevue, WA 98007-6484
Prgm Dir: Julius B Armstrong, MBA RT(T)
Tel: 206 644-5079
Med Dir: Eric Taylor, MD
Class Cap: 28 *Begins:* Sep
Length: 24 mos *Award:* AA
Tuition per yr: $2,600 res, $2,600 non-res
Evening or weekend classes available

West Virginia

West Virginia University Hospitals, Inc
Radiation Therapy Prgm
PO Box 8150 Medical Ctr Dr
Morgantown, WV 26506-8150
Prgm Dir: Christina M Paugh, BA RT(T)
Tel: 304 293-4106 *Fax:* 304 293-4717
Med Dir: Leroy J Korb, MD
Class Cap: 5 *Begins:* Jul
Length: 12 mos *Award:* Cert
Tuition per yr: $1,600

Wisconsin

University of Wisconsin Hosp & Clinics
Radiation Therapy Prgm
600 Highland Ave (K4/B100)
Madison, WI 53792
Prgm Dir: Kristine Saeger, BS RT(R)(T)
Tel: 608 263-8517 *Fax:* 608 263-9167
E-mail: burksaeg@macc.wisc.edu
Med Dir: Daniel Petereit, MD
Class Cap: 8 *Begins:* Sep
Length: 12 mos *Award:* Cert
Tuition per yr: $1,000 res, $1,000 non-res

St Joseph's Hospital
Radiation Therapy Prgm
5000 W Chambers St
Milwaukee, WI 53210
Prgm Dir: Cindy Mueller, BS RT(T)
Tel: 414 447-2289 *Fax:* 414 874-4507
Class Cap: 5 *Begins:* Sep
Length: 12 mos *Award:* Cert
Tuition per yr: $300

St Luke's Medical Center
Radiation Therapy Prgm
2900 W Oklahoma Ave
PO Box 2901
Milwaukee, WI 53201-2901
Prgm Dir: Pamela Kresl-Bauman, RT(T)
Tel: 414 649-6420 *Fax:* 414 649-5309
Med Dir: William Pao
Class Cap: 8 *Begins:* Sep
Length: 12 mos *Award:* Cert

Radiographer

Alabama

Carraway Methodist Medical Center
Radiography Prgm
1600 N 26th St
Birmingham, AL 35234
Prgm Dir: Gina B Slaten, RT(R)
Tel: 205 226-6138 *Fax:* 205 226-5365
Med Dir: Randall Finley, MD
Length: 24 mos *Award:* Cert
Tuition per yr: $325

Jefferson State Community College
Radiography Prgm
2601 Carson Rd
Birmingham, AL 35215-3098
Prgm Dir: John T Leesburg, MA RT(R)
Tel: 205 856-6026 *Fax:* 205 856-7725
Med Dir: Bonnie M Embry, MD
Class Cap: 19 *Begins:* Jan June
Length: 24 mos *Award:* AAS
Tuition per yr: $1,800 res, $3,300 non-res
Evening or weekend classes available

University of Alabama at Birmingham
Radiography Prgm
SHRP 354
1714 Ninth Ave S
Birmingham, AL 35294-1270
Prgm Dir: Steven B Dowd, EdD RT(R)
Tel: 205 934-7382 *Fax:* 205 975-7302
Med Dir: Robert Stanley, MD
Class Cap: 25 *Begins:* Sep
Length: 30 mos *Award:* Cert, BS
Evening or weekend classes available

George C Wallace State Comm College
Radiography Prgm
Rte 6 Box 62
Dothan, AL 36303
Prgm Dir: G Bates Gilmore, BS RT(R)
Tel: 334 983-3521, Ext 299 *Fax:* 334 983-3600
Class Cap: 25
Length: 24 mos *Award:* AAS
Tuition per yr: res, $4,209 non-res
Evening or weekend classes available

Gadsden State Community College
Radiography Prgm
PO Box 227
Gadsden, AL 35902-0227
Prgm Dir: Deborah Gay Golden Utz, MED RT(R)
Tel: 205 549-8468 *Fax:* 205 549-8465
Med Dir: Homer Spencer, MD
Class Cap: 32 *Begins:* Sep
Length: 24 mos *Award:* AAS
Tuition per yr: $1,827 res, $3,402 non-res
Evening or weekend classes available

Wallace State College
Radiography Prgm
PO Box 2000
Hanceville, AL 35077-2000
Prgm Dir: Patricia A Robertson, BS RT(R)(M)
Tel: 205 352-8309 *Fax:* 205 352-8228
Med Dir: Fred Moss, MD
Class Cap: 79
Length: 24 mos *Award:* AAS
Tuition per yr: $1,694 res, $3,388 non-res
Evening or weekend classes available

Huntsville Hospital
Radiography Prgm
101 Sivley Rd
Huntsville, AL 35801
Prgm Dir: Ronald A Murphree, BS RT(R)
Tel: 205 533-8928 *Fax:* 205 517-8004
Med Dir: Robert T Smith, MD
Class Cap: 15 *Begins:* July
Length: 24 mos *Award:* Cert
Tuition per yr: $1,000

University of South Alabama
Radiography Prgm
1504 Springhill Ave
Ste 2515
Mobile, AL 36604
Prgm Dir: Charles W Newell, EdD RT(R)
Tel: 334 434-3456
Class Cap: 83
Length: 27 mos *Award:* Cert

Baptist Medical Center
Radiography Prgm
2105 E South Blvd
PO Box 11010
Montgomery, AL 36111-0010
Prgm Dir: Paul H Littlefield, MS RT(R)
Tel: 334 286-3028 *Fax:* 334 286-2861
Med Dir: David C Montiel, MD
Class Cap: 12 *Begins:* Sep
Length: 24 mos *Award:* Cert
Tuition per yr: $1,300 res, $1,300 non-res

Southern Union State Community College
Radiography Prgm
1701 Lafayette Pkwy
Opelika, AL 36801
Prgm Dir: Judy Carol Southern, EdD RT(R)
Tel: 334 745-6437 *Fax:* 334 741-9795
Class Cap: 30 *Begins:* June
Length: 24 mos *Award:* AAS
Tuition per yr: $1,858 res, $3,408 non-res
Evening or weekend classes available

DCH Regional Medical Center
Radiography Prgm
809 University Blvd E
Tuscaloosa, AL 35401
Prgm Dir: Patricia M Strange, BS RT(R)
Tel: 205 759-6266 *Fax:* 205 759-6012
Med Dir: William A Bright, MD
Class Cap: 12 *Begins:* Sep
Length: 24 mos *Award:* Cert
Tuition per yr: $1,000

Arizona

Pima Medical Institute - Mesa
Radiography Prgm
957 S Dobson Rd
Mesa, AZ 85202
Prgm Dir: Steven L Forshier, MAEd RT(R)
Tel: 602 345-7777
Class Cap: 25
Length: 24 mos *Award:* AS
Tuition per yr: $5,073

Gateway Community College
Radiography Prgm
108 N 40th St
Phoenix, AZ 85034
Prgm Dir: Alex S Backus, MS RT(R)
Tel: 602 392-5033 *Fax:* 602 392-5004
Class Cap: 29
Length: 24 mos *Award:* AAS
Evening or weekend classes available

Pima Community College
Radiography Prgm
2202 W Anklam Rd
HRP 230
Tucson, AZ 85709
Prgm Dir: Dan Giaquinto, MEd RT(R)(T)
Tel: 520 884-6916 *Fax:* 520 884-6632
E-mail: dgiaquinto@pimacc.pima.edu
Class Cap: 27 *Begins:* Fall
Length: 28 mos *Award:* AAS
Tuition per yr: $960 res, $5,220 non-res
Evening or weekend classes available

Pima Medical Institute - Tucson
Radiography Prgm
3350 E Grant Rd
Tucson, AZ 85716
Prgm Dir: Lillian Rossadillo, BS RT(R)
Tel: 520 326-1600
Class Cap: 20
Length: 24 mos *Award:* AS
Tuition per yr: $7,775 res, $7,775 non-res

Arkansas

South Arkansas Community College
Radiography Prgm
300 S West Ave
PO Box 7010 W Campus
El Dorado, AR 71731-7010
Prgm Dir: Deborah M Edney, BS RT(R)
Tel: 501 862-8131 *Fax:* 501 864-7122
Med Dir: Tie Ong, MD
Class Cap: 10 *Begins:* Aug
Length: 24 mos *Award:* AAS
Tuition per yr: $1,332 res, $1,656 non-res
Evening or weekend classes available

Univ of Arkansas for Medical Sciences
Radiography Prgm
AHEC-Northwest
2907 E Joyce St
Fayetteville, AR 72703
Prgm Dir: Stanley R Olejniczak, BHS RT(R)
Tel: 501 587-2668 *Fax:* 501 587-2611
Med Dir: Murray Harris, MD
Class Cap: 28 *Begins:* Aug
Length: 24 mos, 42 mos *Award:* AS, BS
Tuition per yr: $2,538 res, $6,344 non-res

Sparks Regional Medical Center
Radiography Prgm
1311 South I St
PO Box 17006
Ft Smith, AR 72917-7006
Prgm Dir: Robert C Thompson, BS RT(R)
Tel: 501 441-5171 *Fax:* 501 441-4933
Class Cap: 19 *Begins:* July
Length: 24 mos *Award:* Cert
Tuition per yr: $1,450

St Edward Mercy Medical Center
Radiography Prgm
7301 Rogers Ave
PO Box 17000
Ft Smith, AR 72917-7000
Prgm Dir: Paula G Brown, BS RT(R) RDMS
Tel: 501 484-6208 *Fax:* 501 452-0478
Class Cap: 10 *Begins:* July
Length: 24 mos *Award:* Cert
Tuition per yr: $600 res, $600 non-res

North Arkansas Comm and Tech Coll
Radiography Prgm
420 Pioneer Ridge
Harrison, AR 72601
Prgm Dir: Sondra L Richards, MS RT(R)(M)
Tel: 501 743-3000 *Fax:* 501 743-3577
E-mail: srichard@nactc1.nactc.cc.ar.us
Med Dir: Robert Marris, MD
Class Cap: 13 *Begins:* July
Length: 24 mos *Award:* AAS
Tuition per yr: $1,030 res, $2,567 non-res

Garland County Community College
Radiography Prgm
101 College Dr
Hot Springs Natl Pk, AR 71913-7194
Prgm Dir: Timothy J Skaife, MA RT(R)
Tel: 501 767-9371 *Fax:* 501 767-6896
E-mail: tskaife@jill.gccc.cc.ar.us
Class Cap: 20 *Begins:* Aug
Length: 24 mos *Award:* AAS
Tuition per yr: $888 res, $1,104 non-res

Baptist Medical System
Radiography Prgm
11900 Colonel Glenn Rd
Ste 1000
Little Rock, AR 72210-2820
Prgm Dir: Oleta H Copeland, BS RT(R)
Tel: 501 223-7942 Fax: 501 223-7406
Class Cap: 15
Length: 24 mos *Award:* Cert
Tuition per yr: $4,250

St Vincent Infirmary Medical Center
Radiography Prgm
Two St Vincent Circle
Little Rock, AR 72205-5499
Prgm Dir: Frank Porter, RT(R)
Tel: 501 660-2971 *Fax:* 501 671-4226
Med Dir: George Norton, MD
Class Cap: 13 *Begins:* Aug
Length: 24 mos *Award:* Cert
Tuition per yr: $2,400

Univ of Arkansas for Medical Sciences
Radiography Prgm
4301 W Markham Slot 563
Little Rock, AR 72205
Prgm Dir: Joseph R Bittengle, MEd RT(R)
Tel: 501 686-6510 *Fax:* 501 686-6513
E-mail: jrbittngl@chp.uams.edu
Med Dir: Ernest Ferris, MD
Class Cap: 25 *Begins:* Aug
Length: 24 mos, 42 mos *Award:* AS, BS
Tuition per yr: $2,538 res, $6,344 non-res

Jefferson Regional Medical Center
Radiography Prgm
1515 W 42nd Ave
Pine Bluff, AR 71603
Prgm Dir: Jennifer S Thomas, BS RT(R)
Tel: 501 541-7630 *Fax:* 501 541-7618
Class Cap: 10
Length: 24 mos *Award:* Cert
Tuition per yr: $2,000

Arkansas State University
Radiography Prgm
PO Box 69
State University, AR 72467-0069
Prgm Dir: Raymond F Winters, MS RT(R)
Tel: 501 972-3073 *Fax:* 501 972-2040
E-mail: rwinters@crow.astate.edu
Class Cap: 30 *Begins:* Jun
Length: 24 mos, 48 mos *Award:* AAS , BS
Tuition per yr: $2,440 res, $6,300 non-res
Evening or weekend classes available

Univ of Arkansas for Medical Sciences
Radiography Prgm
AHEC-Southwest
600 Walnut St
Texarkana, AR 75502
Prgm Dir: William M Pedigo, MPA RT(R)
Tel: 501 774-5607 *Fax:* 501 773-1002
Med Dir: Allen Jean, MD
Class Cap: 10 *Begins:* Aug
Length: 24 mos, 42 mos *Award:* AS
Tuition per yr: $2,538 res, $6,344 non-res

California

Cabrillo College
Radiography Prgm
6500 Soquel Dr
Aptos, CA 95003
Prgm Dir: Ann S O'Connor, BS RT(R)
Tel: 408 479-6461 *Fax:* 408 479-5748
Med Dir: Fred Chin, MA
Class Cap: 23 *Begins:* Aug
Length: 22 mos *Award:* AS
Evening or weekend classes available

Bakersfield College
Radiography Prgm
1801 Panorama Dr
Bakersfield, CA 93305
Prgm Dir: Nancy J Perkins, MA RT(R)(M)
Tel: 805 395-4284 *Fax:* 805 395-4295
Med Dir: Michael Wells, MD
Class Cap: 20 *Begins:* June
Length: 24 mos *Award:* AS
Tuition per yr: $400 res, $4,000 non-res
Evening or weekend classes available

Programs

Mills - Peninsula Hospitals

Radiography Prgm
1783 El Camino Real
Burlingame, CA 94010
Prgm Dir: Lynn Carlton, BA RT(R) (M)
Tel: 415 696-5519   *Fax:* 415 696-5280
Class Cap: 10
Length: 24 mos   *Award:* Cert

Enloe Hospital

Radiography Prgm
W Fifth Ave and The Esplanade
Chico, CA 95926
Prgm Dir: Charles R Cowan Jr, AA RT(R)
Tel: 916 891-7456   *Fax:* 916 899-2022
Med Dir: George Rawley, MD
Class Cap: 6
Length: 24 mos   *Award:* Cert
Tuition per yr: $1,000

Orange Coast College

Radiography Prgm
2701 Fairview Rd
PO Box 5005
Costa Mesa, CA 92628-5005
Prgm Dir: Linda L Visintainer, BVE RT(R)(M)
Tel: 714 432-5757   *Fax:* 714 432-5534
Med Dir: Robert M Turner, MD
Class Cap: 34   *Begins:* Aug
Length: 24 mos   *Award:* Cert, AA
Tuition per yr: $403 res, $3,937 non-res
Evening or weekend classes available

Cypress College

Radiography Prgm
9200 Valley View St
Cypress, CA 90630-5897
Prgm Dir: Robert J Parelli, MA RT(R)
Tel: 714 826-2220
Med Dir: Stephen Scholkoff, MD
Class Cap: 45
Length: 30 mos   *Award:* Cert, AA
Tuition per yr: $377 res, $3,277 non-res
Evening or weekend classes available

Fresno City College

Radiography Prgm
1101 E University Ave
Fresno, CA 93741
Prgm Dir: Paul N Gonzales, MS RT(R)
Tel: 209 442-4600   *Fax:* 209 244-2626
Class Cap: 18
Length: 29 mos   *Award:* AS
Evening or weekend classes available

Daniel Freeman Memorial Hospital

Radiography Prgm
333 N Prairie Ave
Inglewood, CA 90301
Prgm Dir: Debra S McMahan, BS RT(R)
Tel: 310 674-7050   *Fax:* 310 671-8968
Class Cap: 10   *Begins:* Oct
Length: 24 mos   *Award:* Cert
Tuition per yr: $500

Loma Linda University

Radiography Prgm
School of Allied Health Profs
Loma Linda, CA 92350
Prgm Dir: Mark J Clements, MA RT(R)
Tel: 909 824-4931   *Fax:* 909 824-4291
E-mail: mclements@sabp.iiu.edu
Class Cap: 40   *Begins:* Sep
Length: 27 mos   *Award:* AS, BS
Tuition per yr: $8,208 res, $8,208 non-res

Long Beach City College

Radiography Prgm
4901 E Carson St
Long Beach, CA 90808
Prgm Dir: Vickie D Goodson, PhD RT(R)
Tel: 310 938-4176   *Fax:* 310 938-4191
Med Dir: robert Conroy, MD
Class Cap: 66   *Begins:* Jan
Length: 30 mos   *Award:* Cert, AS
Tuition per yr: $566 res, $5,525 non-res
Evening or weekend classes available

Foothill College

Radiography Prgm
12345 El Monte Rd
Los Altos Hills, CA 94022-4599
Prgm Dir: Eloise J Orrell, BS RT(R)
Tel: 415 949-7469
Med Dir: Volney F VanDalsem III, MD
Class Cap: 35   *Begins:* Aug
Length: 24 mos   *Award:* AS
Tuition per yr: $502 res, $3,984 non-res

Charles R Drew Univ of Med & Science

Radiography Prgm
1621 E 120th St
Los Angeles, CA 90059-3025
Prgm Dir: Morris Hunter, BVE RT(R)
Tel: 213 563-5835
Class Cap: 17
Length: 24 mos   *Award:* AS

Children's Hospital of Los Angeles

Radiography Prgm
4650 Sunset Blvd
Los Angeles, CA 90027
Prgm Dir: Lawrence A Eppich, RT(R)
Tel: 213 669-2285   *Fax:* 213 669-2239
Class Cap: 10   *Begins:* Sep
Length: 24 mos   *Award:* Cert
Tuition per yr: $3,000

Los Angeles City College

Radiography Prgm
855 N Vermont Ave
Los Angeles, CA 90029
Prgm Dir: Edward C Vasquez, BA RT(R)
Tel: 213 953-4325   *Fax:* 213 953-4294
Med Dir: Sherwin M Olken, MD
Class Cap: 34
Length: 27 mos   *Award:* AA
Tuition per yr: $195 res, $2,070 non-res
Evening or weekend classes available

Los Angeles County - USC Medical Center

Radiography Prgm
1200 N State St
PO Box 2082
Los Angeles, CA 90033
Prgm Dir: Lawrence J Szpila, MA RT(R)
Tel: 213 226-7266   *Fax:* 213 226-8064
Med Dir: James Halls, MD
Class Cap: 15   *Begins:* Sep
Length: 24 mos   *Award:* Cert

Veterans Affairs Med Ctr W Los Angeles

Radiography Prgm
11301 Wilshire Blvd
Los Angeles, CA 90073
Prgm Dir: Patricia A Reed, RT CRT (R)(M)
Tel: 310 268-3470   *Fax:* 310 268-4973
Class Cap: 10   *Begins:* Sep
Length: 25 mos   *Award:* Cert

Yuba Community College

Radiography Prgm
2088 N Beale Rd
Marysville, CA 95901
Prgm Dir: Angela Willson, MPA RT(R)(M)
Tel: 916 741-6960   *Fax:* 916 741-3541
E-mail: willson@mako.com
Med Dir: Susan A Lott
Class Cap: 30   *Begins:* Aug
Length: 36 mos   *Award:* AA
Tuition per yr: $550 res, $4,125 non-res
Evening or weekend classes available

Merced College

Radiography Prgm
3600 M St
Merced, CA 95348-2898
Prgm Dir: K Judy Ciuba, MA RT(R)
Tel: 209 384-6132   *Fax:* 209 384-6167
E-mail: kjc@elite.net
Class Cap: 16   *Begins:* Aug
Length: 29 mos   *Award:* Cert, AS
Evening or weekend classes available

Moorpark College

Radiography Prgm
7075 Campus Rd
Moorpark, CA 93021
Prgm Dir: Jo Ann Moore, BVE RTR
Tel: 805 378-1535   *Fax:* 805 378-1548
Med Dir: Ruth Polan, MD
Class Cap: 25
Length: 24 mos   *Award:* Dipl, AS
Tuition per yr: $585 res, $5,130 non-res
Evening or weekend classes available

California State University - Northridge

Radiography Prgm
18111 Nordhoff St
Northridge, CA 91330
Prgm Dir: Anita M Slechta, MS RT(R)(M)
Tel: 818 885-2475   *Fax:* 818 677-2045
E-mail: anita.slechta@csun.edu
Med Dir: Vincent Fennell, MD
Class Cap: 13   *Begins:* Aug
Length: 51 mos   *Award:* BS
Tuition per yr: $1,970 res, $5,904 non-res
Evening or weekend classes available

Merritt College

Radiography Prgm
12500 Campus Dr
Oakland, CA 94619
Prgm Dir: Kistler Osborne, EdD RT(R)
Tel: 510 436-2508   *Fax:* 510 482-9652
Class Cap: 83
Length: 24 mos   *Award:* AS
Tuition per yr: $195
Evening or weekend classes available

St John's Regional Medical Center

Radiography Prgm
1600 N Rose Ave
Oxnard, CA 93030
Prgm Dir: Michael E Gram, BA RT(R)
Tel: 805 988-2872
Class Cap: 5
Length: 24 mos   *Award:* Cert

Huntington Memorial Hospital

Radiography Prgm
100 W California Blvd
Pasadena, CA 91105
Prgm Dir: Michael O Loomis, BS RT(R)
Tel: 818 397-5070   *Fax:* 818 397-3409
Class Cap: 6   *Begins:* Jan
Length: 24 mos   *Award:* Cert

Pasadena City College

Radiography Prgm
1570 E Colorado Blvd
Pasadena, CA 91106-2003
Prgm Dir: Leavon L Spires, RT(R)
Tel: 818 585-7271   *Fax:* 818 585-7912
Class Cap: 24
Length: 24 mos   *Award:* Cert, AS

Chaffey Community College

Radiography Prgm
5885 Haven Ave
Rancho Cucamonga, CA 91737
Prgm Dir: TerriAnn Linn-Watson Norcutt, MEd
   RT(RM) RDMS
Tel: 909 941-2359   *Fax:* 909 941-2783
Med Dir: Robert Stevenson, MD
Class Cap: 64
Length: 24 mos   *Award:* Cert, AS
Tuition per yr: $468 res, $4,644 non-res
Evening or weekend classes available

Canada College

Radiography Prgm
4200 Farm Hill Blvd
Redwood City, CA 94061
Prgm Dir: Pamela D. Jones, AS RT (R)(M)(ST)
Tel: 415 306-3283
Class Cap: 50   *Begins:* Aug
Length: 25 mos   *Award:* AS

Kaiser Permanente Medical Center

Radiography Prgm
901 Nevin Ave
Richmond, CA 94801-3195
Prgm Dir: Gregg Kurita, MA RT(R)
Tel: 510 307-2325   *Fax:* 510 307-2327
E-mail: gregg.kuirita@ncal.kaiperm.org
Med Dir: Lee A Shratter, MD
Class Cap: 25   *Begins:* Oct
Length: 24 mos   *Award:* Cert
Tuition per yr: $4,000

San Bernardino County Medical Center

Radiography Prgm
780 E Gilbert St
San Bernardino, CA 92315-0935
Prgm Dir: Joy A Guy, BA RT(R)
Tel: 909 387-7817   *Fax:* 909 387-0589
Med Dir: Byron Fujimoto, MD
Class Cap: 10   *Begins:* July
Length: 24 mos   *Award:* Cert, AS
Tuition per yr: $1,500

San Diego Mesa College

Radiography Prgm
7250 Mesa College Dr
San Diego, CA 92111
Prgm Dir: Sharon E Huebner, BS RT(R)
Tel: 619 627-2666   *Fax:* 619 279-5668
Class Cap: 35
Length: 24 mos   *Award:* Cert
Tuition per yr: $390 res, $1,500 non-res
Evening or weekend classes available

City College of San Francisco

Radiography Prgm
50 Phelan Ave
San Francisco, CA 94112
Prgm Dir: Richard R Carlton, MS RT(R)(CV)
Tel: 415 239-3431   *Fax:* 415 239-3930
E-mail: carltonr@slip.net
Class Cap: 30   *Begins:* Aug Jan
Length: 32.5 mo , 35.5 mos   *Award:* AS
Tuition per yr: $1,600 res, $4,200 non-res
Evening or weekend classes available

Santa Barbara City College

Radiography Prgm
721 Cliff Dr
Santa Barbara, CA 93109-2394
Prgm Dir: George S Lewis, MEd RT(R)
Tel: 805 965-0581   *Fax:* 805 963-7222
Med Dir: Brian Schnier, MD
Class Cap: 36
Length: 24 mos   *Award:* AS

Santa Rosa Junior College

Radiography Prgm
1501 Mendocino Ave
Santa Rosa, CA 95401-4395
Prgm Dir: Xuan Michael Ho, PhD RT(R)
Tel: 707 527-4346   *Fax:* 707 527-4426
E-mail: xhocployd.santarosa.edu
Med Dir: Gary Shaw, MD
Class Cap: 16   *Begins:* Aug
Length: 25 mos   *Award:* Cert, AS
Evening or weekend classes available

San Joaquin General Hospital

Radiography Prgm
PO Box 1020
Stockton, CA 95201
Prgm Dir: Michael L Walker, BA RT(R)
Tel: 209 468-6233   *Fax:* 209 468-6038
Med Dir: Dennis Jacobsen, MD
Class Cap: 16   *Begins:* July
Length: 24 mos   *Award:* Cert
Tuition per yr: $520 res, $520 non-res

Olive View/UCLA Medical Center

Radiography Prgm
14445 Olive View Dr
Sylmar, CA 91342
Prgm Dir: Maria Warner
Tel: 818 364-1555
Class Cap: 18
Length: 24 mos   *Award:* Cert

El Camino College

Radiography Prgm
16007 S Crenshaw Blvd
Torrance, CA 90506
Prgm Dir: Donald J Visintainer, BVE RT(R)
Tel: 310 660-3249
Class Cap: 20   *Begins:* Aug
Length: 25 mos   *Award:* Cert, AS
Evening or weekend classes available

LA County Harbor UCLA Medical Center

Radiography Prgm
1000 W Carson St Box 27
Torrance, CA 90509-2910
Prgm Dir: Karen Trivedi, BS RT(R)
Tel: 310 222-2825   *Fax:* 310 618-9500
Class Cap: 10   *Begins:* Jul
Length: 24 mos   *Award:* Cert

Mt San Antonio College

Radiography Prgm
1100 N Grand Ave
Walnut, CA 91789-1399
Prgm Dir: Gordon L McMullen, MS RT(R)
Tel: 909 594-5611   *Fax:* 909 468-3938
Med Dir: A Franklin Turner, MD
Class Cap: 40   *Begins:* Jun
Length: 26 mos   *Award:* AS
Tuition per yr: $416 res, $3,648 non-res
Evening or weekend classes available

Colorado

Memorial Hospital

Radiography Prgm
2790 N Academy Blvd Ste 201
Colorado Springs, CO 80917
Prgm Dir: Elaine R Ivan, BS RT(R)(M)
Tel: 719 475-6819   *Fax:* 719 475-5198
Med Dir: Warren Goldsteins
Class Cap: 9   *Begins:* June
Length: 24 mos   *Award:* Cert
Tuition per yr: $1,250

Community Coll of Denver - Auraria Campus

Radiography Prgm
PO Box 173363
Campus Box 950
Denver, CO 80217-3363
Prgm Dir: Linda Forkner, RT(R)
Tel: 303 556-3846   *Fax:* 303 556-4583
Class Cap: 49
Length: 24 mos   *Award:* AAS
Tuition per yr: $2,125 res, $8,786 non-res
Evening or weekend classes available

Pima Medical Institute - Denver
Radiography Prgm
1701 W 72nd Ave
Denver, CO 80221
Prgm Dir: Renee M Crider-Martinez, BS RT(R)
Tel: 303 426-1800 *Fax:* 303 450-4048
Med Dir: Kenneth D Morehead, MD
Class Cap: 24 *Begins:* Every 8 months.
Length: 24 mos *Award:* AS
Tuition per yr: $7,512 res, $7,512 non-res

Provenant - St Anthony Hospitals
Radiography Prgm
1601 Lowell Blvd
Denver, CO 80204-1597
Prgm Dir: William E Kail, PhD RT(R)
Tel: 303 899-5267 *Fax:* 303 595-6097
Med Dir: David Raetz, MD
Class Cap: 15 *Begins:* Sep
Length: 24 mos *Award:* Cert
Tuition per yr: $3,000 res, $3,000 non-res

Mesa State College
Radiography Prgm
1175 Texas Ave
PO Box 2647
Grand Junction, CO 81502
Prgm Dir: Bette A Schans, MS RT(R)
Tel: 970 248-1651 *Fax:* 970 248-1133
E-mail: bschans@mesa5.mesa.colo.edu
Class Cap: 14 *Begins:* Jan
Length: 24 mos *Award:* AAS
Tuition per yr: $1,932 res, $5,902 non-res
Evening or weekend classes available

Aims Community College
Radiography Prgm
5401 W 20th St
PO Box 69
Greeley, CO 80632
Prgm Dir: Diana L Duncan, BS RT(R)
Tel: 970 330-8008 *Fax:* 970 339-6611
Class Cap: 20 *Begins:* Sep
Length: 24 mos *Award:* AAS
Evening or weekend classes available

Red Rocks Community College
Radiography Prgm
13300 W Sixth Ave
Lakewood, CO 80401-5398
Prgm Dir: Wayne Stellick, MA RTR
Tel: 303 914-6320
Class Cap: 15
Length: 24 mos *Award:* AS

Pueblo Community College
Radiography Prgm
900 W Orman Ave
Pueblo, CO 81004
Prgm Dir: Larry E Bontrager, BS RT(R)
Tel: 719 549-3285 *Fax:* 719 549-3136
E-mail: bountrager@pcc.ccoes.edu
Class Cap: 17 *Begins:* Jan
Length: 27 mos *Award:* AAS
Tuition per yr: $2,206 res, $8,987 non-res
Evening or weekend classes available

Connecticut

Danbury Hospital
Radiography Prgm
24 Hospital Ave
Danbury, CT 06810
Prgm Dir: Kristen Johnston, AS RT(R)(CV)(M)
Tel: 203 797-7182 *Fax:* 203 797-7721
Class Cap: 10
Length: 24 mos *Award:* Cert
Tuition per yr: $2,400

Quinnipiac College
Radiography Prgm
Mt Carmel Ave
Hamden, CT 06518-0008
Prgm Dir: Gerald J Conlogue, MHS RT(R)
Tel: 203 281-8683 *Fax:* 203 281-8706
Med Dir: Jack Westcott, MD
Class Cap: 50 *Begins:* Aug
Length: 38 mos *Award:* Cert, BS
Tuition per yr: $12,800 res, $12,800 non-res
Evening or weekend classes available

CCTC/St Francis Hosp & Med Ctr
Radiography Prgm
61 Woodland St
Hartford, CT 06105
Prgm Dir: Paul Creech, MPH RT(R)
Tel: 860 520-7940 *Fax:* 860 520-7906
E-mail: creech@apollo.commnet.edu
Class Cap: 15
Length: 21 mos *Award:* AS
Tuition per yr: $1,700 res, $4,800 non-res
Evening or weekend classes available

Hartford Hospital
Radiography Prgm
560 Hudson St
Hartford, CT 06106
Prgm Dir: Pamela M Cooke, BS RT(R)
Tel: 860 545-3955 *Fax:* 860 545-7066
Med Dir: Stuart K Markowitz
Class Cap: 21 *Begins:* Oct
Length: 24 mos *Award:* Cert
Tuition per yr: $2,000 res, $2,000 non-res

Manchester Memorial Hospital
Radiography Prgm
71 Haynes St
Manchester, CT 06040-4188
Prgm Dir: Frances E Lutzen, AS RT(R)(M)
Tel: 203 645-3624 *Fax:* 203 645-3624
Med Dir: Edward Rosenblatt, MD
Class Cap: 8 *Begins:* Oct
Length: 24 mos *Award:* Cert
Tuition per yr: $2,000 res, $2,000 non-res

Veterans Memorial Medical Center
Radiography Prgm
One King Pl
PO Box 1009
Meriden, CT 06450-1009
Prgm Dir: Linda E Gejda, AS RT(R)
Tel: 203 238-8270
Med Dir: Harry Hajedemos, MD
Class Cap: 10 *Begins:* Oct
Length: 24 mos *Award:* Cert
Tuition per yr: $1,000 res, $1,000 non-res

Middlesex Community - Technical College
Radiography Prgm
100 Training Hill Rd
Middletown, CT 06457
Prgm Dir: Elaine Lisitano, BA RT(R)(M)
Tel: 860 344-6505
Class Cap: 18 *Begins:* June
Length: 27 mos *Award:* AS
Tuition per yr: $1,722 res, $2,421 non-res
Evening or weekend classes available

Gateway Community - Technical College
Radiography Prgm
88 Bassett Rd
North Haven, CT 06473
Prgm Dir: Julie A Mangini, MEd RT(R)
Tel: 203 234-3329 *Fax:* 203 234-3353
Med Dir: Anne M Curtis, MD
Class Cap: 35 *Begins:* Sep
Length: 22 mos *Award:* AS
Tuition per yr: $1,560 res, $4,680 non-res
Evening or weekend classes available

Stamford Hospital
Radiography Prgm
Shelburne Rd W Broad St
Box 9317
Stamford, CT 06904-9317
Prgm Dir: Dorothy A Saia, BS RT(R)
Tel: 203 325-7877
Class Cap: 8 *Begins:* July
Length: 24 mos *Award:* Cert
Tuition per yr: $1,000

Naugatuck Valley Comm - Tech College
Radiography Prgm
750 Chase Pkwy
Waterbury, CT 06708
Prgm Dir: James P Pronovost, MS RT(R)
Tel: 203 575-8266 *Fax:* 203 596-8779
Class Cap: 17 *Begins:* Sep
Length: 22 mos *Award:* AS
Tuition per yr: $2,119 res, $5,963 non-res
Evening or weekend classes available

University of Hartford
Radiography Prgm
200 Bloomfield Ave
Dana Hall Rm 267
West Hartford, CT 06117
Prgm Dir: Susan Morison, BS RT(R)
Tel: 860 768-5289 *Fax:* 860 768-5244
E-mail: bitnet.morison@hartford
Med Dir: Howard Shapiro, MD
Class Cap: 21 *Begins:* Sep
Length: 52 mos, 30 mos *Award:* Cert, BS
Tuition per yr: $14,860 res, $14,860 non-res
Evening or weekend classes available

Windham Community Memorial Hospital
Radiography Prgm
112 Mansfield Ave
Willimantic, CT 06226
Prgm Dir: Mark K Patros, BS RT(R)
Tel: 860 456-6713 *Fax:* 860 456-6858
E-mail: mpatros@mail.snet.net
Med Dir: Robert Daly, MD
Class Cap: 16 *Begins:* Oct
Length: 24 mos *Award:* Cert
Tuition per yr: $8,000 res, $8,000 non-res

Delaware

Delaware Tech & Comm Coll - Owens Campus
Radiography Prgm
PO Box 610
Georgetown, DE 19947
Prgm Dir: David C Ludema, MA RT(R)
Tel: 302 856-5400 *Fax:* 302 856-5773
E-mail: dludema@outland.dtcc.edu
Med Dir: Mortin Cosgiave, MD
Class Cap: 26 *Begins:* Aug
Length: 24 mos *Award:* AAS
Tuition per yr: $1,200 res, $3,000 non-res
Evening or weekend classes available

Delaware Tech & Comm Coll - Wilmington
Radiography Prgm
333 Shipley St
Wilmington, DE 19801
Prgm Dir: Theresa A Foy, BS RT(R)
Tel: 302 428-6945 *Fax:* 302 428-2691
E-mail: +foychopi.dtcc.edu
Med Dir: Allen Evantsh
Class Cap: 16 *Begins:* May
Length: 24 mos *Award:* AAS
Tuition per yr: $1,180 res, $4,725 non-res
Evening or weekend classes available

St Francis Hospital
Radiography Prgm
7th and Clayton Sts
Wilmington, DE 19805-0500
Prgm Dir: Linda J Smith, AS RT(R)
Tel: 302 421-4301 *Fax:* 302 421-4819
Med Dir: Bentley A Hollander, MD
Class Cap: 6 *Begins:* Jun
Length: 24 mos *Award:* Dipl,Cert
Tuition per yr: $1,500

District of Columbia

Bureau of Medicine and Surgery (MED-05)
Radiography Prgm
Accreditation Program Manager
2300 E St NW
Washington, DC 20372-5300
Prgm Dir: Melva M Boatright (MED 537)
Tel: 202 762-3830
Med Dir: John R Wilcox, Capt USN MD
Class Cap: 60 *Begins:* Apr Jul Sep Dec
Length: 12 mos *Award:* Cert

University of the District of Columbia
Radiography Prgm
4200 Connecticut Ave NW
Washington, DC 20008
Prgm Dir: Paul Herring, MA RT(R)
Tel: 202 274-5928
Class Cap: 35
Length: 24 mos *Award:* AAS

Washington Hospital Center
Radiography Prgm
110 Irving St NW
Washington, DC 20010
Prgm Dir: Margaret C Roberts, BS RT(R)
Tel: 202 877-6343
Med Dir: David C Grant Jr, MD
Class Cap: 15 *Begins:* Sep
Length: 22 mos, 24 mos *Award:* Cert
Tuition per yr: $600

Florida

West Boca Medical Center
Radiography Prgm
21644 State Rd 7
Boca Raton, FL 33428
Prgm Dir: Raymond Mata, BS RT(R)
Tel: 407 488-8173 *Fax:* 561 488-8347
Med Dir: Richard Beerman, MD
Class Cap: 21 *Begins:* Oct
Length: 24 mos *Award:* Cert
Tuition per yr: $4,200 res, $4,200 non-res

Bethesda Memorial Hospital
Radiography Prgm
2815 S Seacrest Blvd
Boynton Beach, FL 33435
Prgm Dir: Charles E Lockett Jr, BS RT(R)
Tel: 407 737-7733 *Fax:* 561 737-6758
Med Dir: David Graves, MD
Class Cap: 8 *Begins:* July
Length: 24 mos *Award:* Cert
Tuition per yr: $170

Manatee Community College
Radiography Prgm
5840 26th St W
PO Box 1849
Bradenton, FL 32406-1849
Prgm Dir: Gary P Randle, MS RT(R)
Tel: 813 755-1511 *Fax:* 813 727-8304
Med Dir: Paul J Macchi, MD
Class Cap: 30 *Begins:* June
Length: 24 mos *Award:* AS

Brevard Community College
Radiography Prgm
1519 Clearlake Rd
Cocoa, FL 32922
Prgm Dir: Susan A Sheehan, MS RT(R)(M)
Tel: 407 632-1111 *Fax:* 407 634-3731
Class Cap: 30
Length: 24 mos *Award:* AS
Tuition per yr: $1,702 res, $6,210 non-res

Broward Community College
Radiography Prgm
3501 SW Davie Rd
Davie, FL 33314
Prgm Dir: John H Britt, MEd RT(R)
Tel: 954 475-6917 *Fax:* 954 473-9037
Med Dir: David H Epstein, MD
Class Cap: 39 *Begins:* Aug
Length: 22 mos *Award:* AS
Tuition per yr: $1,415 res, $5,189 non-res
Evening or weekend classes available

Halifax Medical Center
Radiography Prgm
303 N Clyde Morris Blvd
PO Box 2830
Daytona Beach, FL 32120-2830
Prgm Dir: Darcie J Nethery, PhD RT(R)
Tel: 904 254-4075
Med Dir: Charles Burkett
Class Cap: 10 *Begins:* Jan
Length: 30 mos *Award:* Cert

Keiser College of Technology
Radiography Prgm
1500 NW 49th St
Ft Lauderdale, FL 33309
Prgm Dir: Janice Leifer, MS RT(R)
Tel: 954 776-4456 *Fax:* 954 771-4894
Class Cap: 28
Length: 22 mos *Award:* AS
Tuition per yr: $10,500 res, $10,500 non-res

Edison Community College
Radiography Prgm
PO Box 60210
Ft Myers, FL 33906-6210
Prgm Dir: Paul R Monagan, MEd RT(R)
Tel: 941 489-9315 *Fax:* 941 489-9037
Med Dir: Rodger Shaver, MD
Class Cap: 36 *Begins:* Aug
Length: 24 mos *Award:* AS
Tuition per yr: $1,716 res, $6,384 non-res
Evening or weekend classes available

Indian River Community College
Radiography Prgm
3209 Virginia Ave
Ft Pierce, FL 34981-5599
Prgm Dir: Gary W Shaver, MA RT(R)
Tel: 407 462-4368 *Fax:* 407 462-4796
E-mail: gshaver@ircc.cc.fl.us
Class Cap: 28 *Begins:* May
Length: 24 mos *Award:* AAS
Tuition per yr: $1,890 res, $6,130 non-res

Santa Fe Community College
Radiography Prgm
3000 NW 83rd St
Gainesville, FL 32602-6200
Prgm Dir: Edwin J Dice, MS RT(R)(N)
Tel: 352 395-5702 *Fax:* 352 395-5711
E-mail: ed.dice@santafe.cc.fl.us
Med Dir: Edward V Steel, MD
Class Cap: 28 *Begins:* Aug
Length: 22 mos *Award:* AS
Tuition per yr: $1,348 res, $1,348 non-res
Evening or weekend classes available

Baptist Medical Center
Radiography Prgm
800 Prudential Dr
Jacksonville, FL 32207
Prgm Dir: Ginger S Griffin, RT(R)
Tel: 904 202-2004 *Fax:* 904 202-1031
Class Cap: 12 *Begins:* July
Length: 24 mos *Award:* Cert
Tuition per yr: $1,000

St Vincent's Medical Center
Radiography Prgm
1800 Barrs St
PO Box 2982
Jacksonville, FL 32204
Prgm Dir: Karen F Nevins, BS RT(R)
Tel: 904 387-7310 *Fax:* 904 308-7462
Class Cap: 9
Length: 24 mos *Award:* Cert
Tuition per yr: $2,000 res, $2,000 non-res

University Medical Center

Radiography Prgm
655 W Eighth St
Jacksonville, FL 32209
Prgm Dir: Christene W Haddock, BS RT(R)
Tel: 904 549-3274   *Fax:* 904 549-3186
Med Dir: H Martin Northup, MD
Class Cap: 16   *Begins:* Jul
Length: 24 mos   *Award:* Cert
Tuition per yr: $500

Lakeland Regional Medical Center

Radiography Prgm
1324 Lakeland Hills Blvd
PO Box 95448
Lakeland, FL 33804-0448
Prgm Dir: Barbara V Spano, AS RT(R)
Tel: 941 687-1100, Ext 3768   *Fax:* 941 687-1471
Med Dir: Howard A Gorell, MD
Class Cap: 19   *Begins:* July
Length: 24 mos   *Award:* Cert
Tuition per yr: $500

Miami-Dade Community College

Radiography Prgm
Medical Center Campus
950 NW 20th St
Miami, FL 33127
Prgm Dir: Gregory J Ferenchak, MS RT(R)
Tel: 305 237-4034   *Fax:* 305 237-4116
Med Dir: Marjorie Sanders, MD
Class Cap: 40   *Begins:* June
Length: 24 mos, 24 mos   *Award:* AS
Tuition per yr: $1,114 res, $3,915 non-res
Evening or weekend classes available

Univ of Miami/Jackson Memorial Hosp

Radiography Prgm
1611 NW 12th Ave
Miami, FL 33136
Prgm Dir: Howard Schechter, BS RT(R)
Tel: 305 585-6811   *Fax:* 305 585-7866
Med Dir: Albert Weinfeld, MD
Class Cap: 20   *Begins:* June
Length: 24 mos   *Award:* Cert
Tuition per yr: $1,200 res, $1,500 non-res

Mt Sinai Medical Center of Greater Miami

Radiography Prgm
4300 Alton Rd
Miami Beach, FL 33140
Prgm Dir: Douglas D Fuller, MS RT(R)(N)
Tel: 305 674-2670   *Fax:* 305 674-2694
Med Dir: Manuel Viamonte Jr, MD
Class Cap: 8   *Begins:* July
Length: 24 mos   *Award:* Cert
Tuition per yr: $1,200

Marion County School of Radiologic Tech

Radiography Prgm
1014 SW 7th Rd
Ocala, FL 34474
Prgm Dir: Timothy Richardson, RT(R)
Tel: 352 620-7582   *Fax:* 352 629-1117
E-mail: richart5@mail.firm.edu
Med Dir: Mark A Yap, MD
Class Cap: 18   *Begins:* Aug
Length: 24 mos   *Award:* Cert
Tuition per yr: $1,500

Florida Hospital Medical Center

Radiography Prgm
800 Lake Estelle Dr
Orlando, FL 32803
Prgm Dir: Genese M Gibson, MA RT(R)
Tel: 407 895-7747   *Fax:* 407 895-7680
Class Cap: 20
Length: 24 mos   *Award:* AS
Tuition per yr: $4,356 res, $4,356 non-res
Evening or weekend classes available

University of Central Florida

Radiography Prgm
4000 Central Florida Blvd
PO Box 25000
Orlando, FL 32816-0200
Prgm Dir: Thomas J Edwards III, EdD RT(R)
Tel: 407 823-2174   *Fax:* 407 823-6509
E-mail: tedwards@pagasus.cc.ucf.edu
Med Dir: George A Stanley, MD
Class Cap: 16
Length: 51 mos   *Award:* BS
Tuition per yr: $2,730 res, $10,539 non-res

Valencia Community College

Radiography Prgm
925 S Orange Ave
Orlando, FL 32806
Prgm Dir: Julie Anne Guy, BS RT(R)
Tel: 407 841-5111, Ext 5606   *Fax:* 407 423-3204
Med Dir: David R Harding, MD
Class Cap: 5   *Begins:* Aug
Length: 24 mos   *Award:* AS
Tuition per yr: $1,444 res, $4,986 non-res

Palm Beach Community College

Radiography Prgm
3160 PGA Blvd
Palm Beach Gardens, FL 33418-2893
Prgm Dir: Vicki E Shaver, MS RT(R)
Tel: 561 625-2511
Med Dir: Nila Wilbur
Class Cap: 30   *Begins:* Jan
Length: 24 mos   *Award:* AS
Tuition per yr: $1,683
Evening or weekend classes available

Gulf Coast Community College

Radiography Prgm
5230 W US Hwy 98
Panama City, FL 32401-1041
Prgm Dir: Martin A Reed, PhD RT(R)
Tel: 904 872-3827   *Fax:* 904 747-3246
Med Dir: Pual Clifford, MD
Class Cap: 12   *Begins:* May
Length: 23 mos   *Award:* AS
Tuition per yr: $1,460 res, $5,478 non-res
Evening or weekend classes available

Pensacola Junior College

Radiography Prgm
Warrington Campus
5555 W Hwy 98
Pensacola, FL 32507-1097
Prgm Dir: Marilyn K Coseo, MEd RT(R)
Tel: 904 484-2304
Class Cap: 38
Length: 22 mos   *Award:* AS

Hillsborough Community College

Radiography Prgm
PO Box 30030
Tampa, FL 33630-3030
Prgm Dir: Jayme S Rothberg, BA RT(R)
Tel: 813 253-7415   *Fax:* 813 253-7415
Class Cap: 32   *Begins:* Aug
Length: 24 mos   *Award:* AS
Tuition per yr: $1,199 res, $4,467 non-res
Evening or weekend classes available

Polk Community College

Radiography Prgm
999 Ave H NE
Winter Haven, FL 33881-4299
Prgm Dir: Miriam Spisak, MA RT(R)
Tel: 941 297-1020   *Fax:* 941 297-1036
Med Dir: Gerald Luedaman
Class Cap: 16
Length: 25 mos   *Award:* AS
Evening or weekend classes available

Georgia

Albany Technical Institute

Radiography Prgm
1021 Lowe Rd
Albany, GA 31708
Prgm Dir: Shirley M Armstrong, MEd RT(R)
Tel: 912 430-3553   *Fax:* 912 430-5115
Med Dir: Sam Strickland, MD
Class Cap: 26   *Begins:* July
Length: 24 mos   *Award:* Dipl
Tuition per yr: $1,708 res, $2,716 non-res
Evening or weekend classes available

Athens Area Technical Institute

Radiography Prgm
US Hwy 29 N
Athens, GA 30601-1500
Prgm Dir: Gerald R Cummings, BS RT(R)
Tel: 706 355-5052   *Fax:* 706 369-5753
E-mail: cummings@admin1.athens.tec.ga.us
Med Dir: Paul L Davis, MD
Class Cap: 27   *Begins:* Sep
Length: 24 mos   *Award:* AAS
Tuition per yr: $1,132 res, $2,264 non-res
Evening or weekend classes available

Emory University

Radiography Prgm
1364 Clifton Rd NE
Atlanta, GA 30322
Prgm Dir: Dawn C Moore, MMSc RT(R)
Tel: 404 712-5005   *Fax:* 404 712-7256
Med Dir: Richard Colvin
Class Cap: 36   *Begins:* Aug
Length: 24 mos   *Award:* AMSc
Tuition per yr: $5,700 res, $5,700 non-res

Georgia Baptist Medical Center

Radiography Prgm
303 Parkway NE Box 51
Atlanta, GA 30312-1206
Prgm Dir: Dawn Ley, RT(R)
Tel: 404 265-4299   *Fax:* 404 265-4983
Med Dir: Barry Jeffries, MD
Class Cap: 10
Length: 24 mos   *Award:* Cert
Tuition per yr: $2,000

Grady Health System

Radiography Prgm
80 Butler St SE
PO Box 26095
Atlanta, GA 30335-3801
Prgm Dir: Judith K Williams, BMSc RT(R)
Tel: 404 616-3610 *Fax:* 404 616-3512
Med Dir: Turner I Ball, MD
Class Cap: 31 *Begins:* July
Length: 24 mos *Award:* Cert
Tuition per yr: $1,900

Medical College of Georgia

Radiography Prgm
Sch of Allied Health Sciences
AE 1003
Augusta, GA 30912-0600
Prgm Dir: Nancy L Lavin, MEd RT(R)
Tel: 706 721-3691 *Fax:* 706 721-8293
E-mail: nlavin@mail.mcg.edu
Class Cap: 15
Length: 21 mos *Award:* AS
Tuition per yr: $2,820 res, $10,022 non-res

University Hospital

Radiography Prgm
1350 Walton Way
Augusta, GA 30910-3599
Prgm Dir: Patty Frazier, BSRT
Tel: 706 774-8646 *Fax:* 706 774-5079
Med Dir: Jimpsy Johnson, MD
Class Cap: 12 *Begins:* July
Length: 24 mos *Award:* Cert
Tuition per yr: $1,800 res, $1,800 non-res

Coastal Georgia Community College

Radiography Prgm
3700 Altama Ave
Brunswick, GA 31520-3644
Prgm Dir: Dianne T Castor, BS RT(R)
Tel: 912 264-7381 *Fax:* 912 262-3283
E-mail: dcastor@bc9000.bc.teac.peachnet.edu
Med Dir: M.E. Skelton, MD
Class Cap: 15 *Begins:* Sept
Length: 24 mos *Award:* AS
Tuition per yr: $405 res, $1,373 non-res
Evening or weekend classes available

Medical Center Inc

Radiography Prgm
1951 8th Ave
PO Box 951
Columbus, GA 31994-2299
Prgm Dir: Ruby C Montgomery, MSAdm RT(R) F
Tel: 706 571-1155 *Fax:* 706 660-2887
Class Cap: 15
Length: 24 mos *Award:* Cert
Tuition per yr: $1,400

Hamilton Medical Center

Radiography Prgm
Herschel U Martin Sch of Rad
PO Box 1168
Dalton, GA 30722-1168
Prgm Dir: Susan D West, MEd RT(R)
Tel: 706 272-6427 *Fax:* 706 272-6111
Class Cap: 7
Length: 24 mos *Award:* Cert
Tuition per yr: $1,000

DeKalb Medical Center

Radiography Prgm
2701 N Decatur Rd
Decatur, GA 30033
Prgm Dir: Pat A Martin, MEd RT(R)
Tel: 404 501-5306
Class Cap: 19
Length: 24 mos *Award:* Cert
Tuition per yr: $1,200 res, $1,200 non-res

Griffin Technical Institute

Radiography Prgm
501 Varsity Rd
Griffin, GA 30223-2042
Prgm Dir: Lynn McGahee, BS RT(R)
Tel: 770 229-3225 *Fax:* 770 229-3227
Med Dir: Ronald Gay
Class Cap: 20 *Begins:* Oct
Length: 24 mos *Award:* AAT
Tuition per yr: $1,200

West Georgia Technical Institute

Radiography Prgm
303 Fort Dr
LaGrange, GA 30240
Prgm Dir: Sandra W Hood, BSEd RT(R)(M)
Tel: 706 882-2518
Med Dir: Marc Hinrichs
Class Cap: 13 *Begins:* July
Length: 24 mos *Award:* Dipl
Tuition per yr: $1,132 res, $1,132 non-res
Evening or weekend classes available

Gwinnett Technical Institute

Radiography Prgm
5150 Sugarloaf Parkway
PO Box 1505
Lawrenceville, GA 30246
Prgm Dir: James A Sass, MEd RT(R)(M)
Tel: 770 962-7580 *Fax:* 770 962-7985
Class Cap: 50 *Begins:* July
Length: 23 mos *Award:* AAT
Tuition per yr: $1,200 res, $2,200 non-res
Evening or weekend classes available

Medical Center of Central Georgia

Radiography Prgm
777 Hemlock St
PO Box 6000
Macon, GA 31208
Prgm Dir: Barbara B Wright, AS RT(R)(M)
Tel: 912 633-1258 *Fax:* 912 633-5219
Med Dir: Dan Strawn, MD
Class Cap: 14 *Begins:* Oct
Length: 24 mos *Award:* Cert
Tuition per yr: $1,650

Promina Kennestone Hospital

Radiography Prgm
677 Church St
Marietta, GA 30060
Prgm Dir: Barbara L Tamplin, RT(R)
Tel: 770 793-5571 *Fax:* 770 793-7796
Med Dir: James M Tallman, MD
Class Cap: 10 *Begins:* July
Length: 24 mos *Award:* Cert
Tuition per yr: $300

Moultrie Area Technical Institute

Radiography Prgm
PO Box 520
Moultrie, GA 31776-0520
Prgm Dir: Alan Clark Miller, MEd RT(R)
Tel: 912 891-7000 *Fax:* 912 891-9010
Med Dir: Leonard Perrybacoute, MD
Class Cap: 15 *Begins:* July
Length: 24 mos *Award:* Cert
Evening or weekend classes available

Armstrong Atlantic State University

Radiography Prgm
11935 Abercorn St
Savannah, GA 31419
Prgm Dir: Sharyn D Gibson, MHS RT(R)
Tel: 912 927-5360 *Fax:* 912 921-5889
E-mail: aad.scl@mailgate.armstrong.edu
Class Cap: 18
Length: 24 mos *Award:* AS, BS
Tuition per yr: $2,290 res, $5,572 non-res
Evening or weekend classes available

Ogeechee Technical Institute

Radiography Prgm
1 Joe Kennedy Blvd
Statesboro, GA 30458
Prgm Dir: Lynda Tinker, RT(R)(M) BS
Tel: 912 681-5500 *Fax:* 912 871-1162
E-mail: ihnker@adminl.ogeechee.tec.ga.us
Med Dir: Karen Lovett, MD
Class Cap: 12 *Begins:* Oct
Length: 24 mos *Award:* Dipl,Cert
Tuition per yr: $1,120

Thomas Technical Institute

Radiography Prgm
15689 US Hwy North
Thomasville, GA 31792
Prgm Dir: Werner W Waldron, MEd RT(R)
Tel: 912 225-4078 *Fax:* 912 225-5289
Class Cap: 28
Length: 21 mos *Award:* AAT
Tuition per yr: $1,128 res, $2,256 non-res
Evening or weekend classes available

Valdosta Technical Institute

Radiography Prgm
PO Box 928 Val-Tech Rd
Valdosta, GA 31603
Prgm Dir: Linda L Booth, RT(R)
Tel: 912 333-2100 *Fax:* 912 333-2129
Med Dir: DeWey L Barton, MD
Begins: Sep
Length: 24 mos *Award:* Cert
Tuition per yr: $1,008 res, $1,008 non-res
Evening or weekend classes available

Okefenokee Technical Institute

Radiography Prgm
1701 Carswell Ave
Waycross, GA 31501
Prgm Dir: Orie M Pinckard, RT(R)
Tel: 912 287-6584 *Fax:* 912 287-4865
Class Cap: 12
Length: 24 mos *Award:* Cert
Evening or weekend classes available

Hawaii

Kapiolani Community College
Radiography Prgm
4303 Diamond Head Rd
Honolulu, HI 96816
Prgm Dir: Roland W Clements, MS RT(R)
Tel: 808 734-9251 *Fax:* 808 734-9126
Med Dir: Robert D Mauro, MD
Class Cap: 30 *Begins:* Aug
Length: 24 mos *Award:* AS
Tuition per yr: $1,024 res, $6,816 non-res

Idaho

Boise State University
Radiography Prgm
College of Health Science
1910 University Dr
Boise, ID 83725
Prgm Dir: Darlene K Travis, BS RT(R)(T)(CV)
Tel: 208 385-3290 *Fax:* 208 385-4459
Med Dir: John Truska
Class Cap: 22 *Begins:* Aug
Length: 36 mos, 48 mos *Award:* AS, BS
Tuition per yr: $1,964 res, $5,164 non-res
Evening or weekend classes available

Illinois

Northwest Community Hospital
Radiography Prgm
800 W Central Rd
Arlington Heights, IL 60005
Prgm Dir: Sandra L Saletta, BA RT(R)(M)
Tel: 847 618-5790 *Fax:* 847 618-5409
Class Cap: 12 *Begins:* July
Length: 24 mos *Award:* Cert
Tuition per yr: $800

Belleville Area College
Radiography Prgm
2500 Carlyle Ave
Belleville, IL 62221-5899
Prgm Dir: Dorothy A Bowers, MA RT(R)
Tel: 618 235-2700 *Fax:* 618 235-1578
Med Dir: Ribarton Bridges, MD
Class Cap: 40
Length: 24 mos *Award:* AAS
Tuition per yr: $1,785 res, $3,822 non-res

Southern Illinois Univ at Carbondale
Radiography Prgm
Coll of Applied Sciences and Arts
Health Care Professions
Carbondale, IL 62901
Prgm Dir: Steven C Jensen, PhD RT(R)
Tel: 618 453-8882 *Fax:* 618 453-7286
E-mail: sjensen@siu.edu
Class Cap: 50
Length: 24 mos *Award:* AAS
Tuition per yr: $2,500 res, $2,500 non-res
Evening or weekend classes available

Kaskaskia College
Radiography Prgm
27210 College Rd
Centralia, IL 62801
Prgm Dir: Penny L Brinkman, BS RT(R)
Tel: 618 532-1981 *Fax:* 618 532-1990
E-mail: plbrinkman@kc.cc.il.us
Med Dir: Richard Rudman
Class Cap: 59 *Begins:* Aug
Length: 18 mos, 21 mos *Award:* AAS
Tuition per yr: $3,143 res, $6,639 non-res
Evening or weekend classes available

Parkland College
Radiography Prgm
2400 W Bradley Ave
Champaign, IL 61821-1899
Prgm Dir: Thomas B Wagner, MS RT(R)
Tel: 217 351-2436
Class Cap: 17
Length: 23 mos *Award:* AAS
Tuition per yr: $1,575 res, $5,113 non-res
Evening or weekend classes available

Cook County Hospital
Radiography Prgm
1825 W Harrison St
Chicago, IL 60612-9985
Prgm Dir: George N Talge, RT(R)
Tel: 312 633-8522 *Fax:* 312 633-5557
Med Dir: Bradley G Langer, MD
Class Cap: 25 *Begins:* Oct
Length: 24 mos *Award:* Cert
Tuition per yr: $500

Malcolm X College
Radiography Prgm
1900 W Van Buren St
Chicago, IL 60612
Prgm Dir: Geraldine Williams, MEd RT(R)
Tel: 312 850-7373 *Fax:* 312 850-7453
Class Cap: 78
Length: 24 mos *Award:* AAS
Evening or weekend classes available

Ravenswood Hospital Medical Center
Radiography Prgm
4550 N Winchester Ave
Chicago, IL 60640-5205
Prgm Dir: Philis George, BS RT(R)
Tel: 312 878-4300 *Fax:* 312 907-7479
Med Dir: Michael Garcia, MD
Class Cap: 11 *Begins:* Sep
Length: 24 mos *Award:* Cert
Tuition per yr: $700

Trinity Hospital
Radiography Prgm
2320 E 93rd St
Chicago, IL 60617
Prgm Dir: Joann Kern, BS RT(R)
Tel: 312 978-2000 *Fax:* 312 978-7211
Med Dir: Ari Mintz, MD
Class Cap: 11
Length: 24 mos *Award:* Cert
Tuition per yr: $1,000

Wilbur Wright College
Radiography Prgm
4300 N Narragansett Ave
Chicago, IL 60634
Prgm Dir: Dennis M King, MHS RT(R)
Tel: 312 481-8880 *Fax:* 312 481-8892
E-mail: dking@ccc.edu
Class Cap: 380 *Begins:* Aug
Length: 26 mos *Award:* AAS
Tuition per yr: $170 res, $5,330 non-res
Evening or weekend classes available

United Samaritans Medical Center
Radiography Prgm
812 N Logan Ave
Danville, IL 61832-3788
Prgm Dir: Robert D Verkler, BSEd RT(R)
Tel: 217 443-5245 *Fax:* 217 443-1965
Class Cap: 15
Length: 24 mos *Award:* Dipl
Tuition per yr: $2,300 res, $2,300 non-res

Sauk Valley Community College
Radiography Prgm
173 IL Rte 2
Dixon, IL 61021-9112
Prgm Dir: Stan Shippert, MEd RT(R)(MR)
Tel: 815 288-5511 *Fax:* 815 288-5651
Class Cap: 42
Length: 22 mos *Award:* AAS
Tuition per yr: $1,548 res, $4,235 non-res

St Francis Hospital
Radiography Prgm
355 Ridge Ave
Evanston, IL 60202
Prgm Dir: Mary Ellen Newton, RTR M
Tel: 847 866-5810
Med Dir: Dan Murphy, MD
Class Cap: 12 *Begins:* Aug
Length: 24 mos *Award:* Cert
Tuition per yr: $600

Carl Sandburg College
Radiography Prgm
2232 S Lake Storey Rd
Galesburg, IL 61401
Prgm Dir: Elaine Long, BA RT(R)
Tel: 309 344-2518 *Fax:* 309 344-3526
Med Dir: Subbia Jagannatuau, MD
Class Cap: 20 *Begins:* June
Length: 24 mos *Award:* AAS
Tuition per yr: $1,800 res, $4,290 non-res
Evening or weekend classes available

College of DuPage
Radiography Prgm
22nd St and Lambert Rd
Glen Ellyn, IL 60137-6599
Prgm Dir: Gina M Rigoni, MS RT(R)
Tel: 630 858-2800 *Fax:* 630 858-5409
E-mail: rigoni@conet.cod.edu
Med Dir: Terry K Kushner, MD
Class Cap: 49 *Begins:* Sep
Length: 24 mos *Award:* AAS
Tuition per yr: $1,392 res, $5,664 non-res
Evening or weekend classes available

College of Lake County

Radiography Prgm
19351 W Washington St
Grayslake, IL 60030-1198
Prgm Dir: Thomas M Vogl, MS RT(R)
Tel: 847 223-6601   *Fax:* 847 223-1357
E-mail: tomvogl@clc.cc.il.us
Class Cap: 43   *Begins:* Aug
Length: 24 mos   *Award:* AAS
Tuition per yr: $1,632 res, $6,596 non-res
Evening or weekend classes available

McDonough District Hospital

Radiography Prgm
525 E Grant St
Macomb, IL 61455
Prgm Dir: Richard L Hart, RT(R)
Tel: 309 833-4101   *Fax:* 309 836-1551
Med Dir: Robert E Stallworth, MD
Class Cap: 4   *Begins:* Sep
Length: 24 mos   *Award:* Cert

Kishwaukee College

Radiography Prgm
21193 Malta Rd
Malta, IL 60150-9699
Prgm Dir: Carol Guschl, BS RT(R)
Tel: 815 825-2086   *Fax:* 815 825-2072
Class Cap: 20
Length: 24 mos   *Award:* AAS
Tuition per yr: $1,752 res, $6,379 non-res
Evening or weekend classes available

Trinity Medical Center

Radiography Prgm
501 Tenth Ave
Moline, IL 61265
Prgm Dir: Cheryl A Thompson, BSHA RT(R)
Tel: 309 757-3385   *Fax:* 309 757-2194
Med Dir: Kenneth Andre
Class Cap: 12   *Begins:* June
Length: 24 mos   *Award:* Cert
Tuition per yr: $3,795

Bloomington-Normal School of Radiography

Radiography Prgm
900 Franklin Ave
Normal, IL 61761
Prgm Dir: Beth S Kuhfuss, MS RT(R)
Tel: 309 452-2834
Med Dir: Richard Puckett, MD
Class Cap: 13   *Begins:* July
Length: 24 mos   *Award:* Cert
Tuition per yr: $1,100 res, $1,100 non-res

Olney Central College

Radiography Prgm
RR #3
Olney, IL 62450
Prgm Dir: M Diane Newham, MS RT(R)
Tel: 618 395-7340   *Fax:* 618 392-3228
Class Cap: 24
Length: 24 mos   *Award:* AAS
Tuition per yr: $772
Evening or weekend classes available

Moraine Valley Community College

Radiography Prgm
10900 S 88th Ave
Palos Hills, IL 60465
Prgm Dir: John R Hein, MHS RT(R)
Tel: 708 974-5316   *Fax:* 708 974-1184
E-mail: hein@moraine.cc.il.us
Class Cap: 32
Length: 26 mos   *Award:* AAS
Tuition per yr: $1,354 res, $4,928 non-res

Illinois Central College

Radiography Prgm
Health and Public Svcs Bldg
201 SW Adams St
Peoria, IL 61635-0001
Prgm Dir: Diane L Schulz, MEd RT(R)
Tel: 309 999-4659   *Fax:* 309 673-9626
E-mail: dwchulz@iccnet.icc.cc.il.us
Med Dir: Stephen E Lehnert, MD
Class Cap: 25   *Begins:* Aug
Length: 23 mos   *Award:* AAS
Tuition per yr: $1,554 res, $4,810 non-res
Evening or weekend classes available

St Francis Medical Center

Radiography Prgm
530 NE Glen Oak Ave
Peoria, IL 61637
Prgm Dir: Suzanne M Yezek, RT(R)
Tel: 309 655-2782   *Fax:* 309 655-7404
Med Dir: Clinton J Wentz, MD
Class Cap: 9   *Begins:* June
Length: 24 mos   *Award:* Cert
Tuition per yr: $1,000 res, $1,000 non-res

Blessing Hospital

Radiography Prgm
Box 7005
Broadway at 14th Street
Quincy, IL 62301
Prgm Dir: Pauline M Upper, BS RT(R)
Tel: 217 223-1200, Ext 4292   *Fax:* 217 223-3906
Med Dir: Monty Karoll, MD
Class Cap: 13   *Begins:* July
Length: 24 mos   *Award:* Cert
Tuition per yr: $750

Triton College

Radiography Prgm
2000 Fifth Ave
River Grove, IL 60171
Prgm Dir: Catherine T Lekostaj, MEd RT(R)
Tel: 708 456-0300   *Fax:* 708 583-3121
Med Dir: Donald Waxler
Class Cap: 45   *Begins:* aug
Length: 24 mos   *Award:* AAS
Tuition per yr: $1,462 res, $4,500 non-res

Rockford Memorial Hospital

Radiography Prgm
2400 N Rockton Ave
Rockford, IL 61103
Prgm Dir: Patricia Griesman, RT(R)
Tel: 815 971-5480   *Fax:* 815 968-3407
Med Dir: Bradley Munson, MD
Class Cap: 8   *Begins:* June
Length: 24 mos   *Award:* Cert
Tuition per yr: $1,600 res, $2,000 non-res

Swedish American Hospital

Radiography Prgm
1400 Charles St
Rockford, IL 61104-2298
Prgm Dir: Natalie A Wagner, MS RT(R)
Tel: 815 968-4400, Ext 4966   *Fax:* 815 966-3979
Med Dir: Mark Traill, MD
Class Cap: 12   *Begins:* July
Length: 24 mos   *Award:* Cert
Tuition per yr: $850 res, $850 non-res

South Suburban College of Cook County

Radiography Prgm
15800 S State St
South Holland, IL 60473
Prgm Dir: Jody L Ellis, MPA RT(R)
Tel: 708 596-2000   *Fax:* 708 210-5792
Length: 28 mos   *Award:* AAS
Tuition per yr: $1,519 res, $4,630 non-res

Bristol Community College

Radiography Prgm
Shepherd Rd
Springfield, IL 62794-9256
Prgm Dir: William J Callaway, BA RT(R)
Tel: 217 786-2408   *Fax:* 217 786-2824
E-mail: bcallawa@cabin.llcc.cc.il.us
Med Dir: Jill Sullivan, MD
Class Cap: 48   *Begins:* June
Length: 24 mos   *Award:* AAS
Tuition per yr: $1,443
Evening or weekend classes available

Lincoln Land Community College

Radiography Prgm
Shepherd Rd
Springfield, IL 62794-9256
Prgm Dir: William J Callaway, BA RT(R)
Tel: 217 786-2408   *Fax:* 217 786-2824
E-mail: bcallawa@cabin.llcc.cc.il.us
Med Dir: Jill Sullivan, MD
Class Cap: 48   *Begins:* Jun
Length: 24 mos   *Award:* AAS
Tuition per yr: $1,443
Evening or weekend classes available

Indiana

Columbus Regional Hospital

Radiography Prgm
2400 E 17th St
Columbus, IN 47201
Prgm Dir: Karen A Frazier, BS RT(R)
Tel: 812 376-5354   *Fax:* 812 378-5988
Med Dir: Frederick B Andrews, MD
Class Cap: 6   *Begins:* July
Length: 24 mos   *Award:* Cert
Tuition per yr: $1,250

University of Southern Indiana

Radiography Prgm
8600 University Blvd
Evansville, IN 47712
Prgm Dir: Curt L Serbus, MEd RT(R)
Tel: 812 464-1894   *Fax:* 812 465-7092
E-mail: cserbus.ucs@smtp.usi.edu
Med Dir: Robert R Penkava, MD
Class Cap: 16   *Begins:* July
Length: 28 mos   *Award:* AS
Tuition per yr: $2,880 res, $7,029 non-res
Evening or weekend classes available

Programs

Welborn Cancer Center

Radiography Prgm
401 SE Sixth St
Evansville, IN 47713-1299
Prgm Dir: Rachel E Bailey, RT(R)
Tel: 812 426-8321 *Fax:* 812 426-8935
Med Dir: Thomas Schulloor, MD
Class Cap: 7 *Begins:* Jul
Length: 24 mos *Award:* Cert
Tuition per yr: $500

Ft Wayne School of Radiography

Radiography Prgm
700 Broadway
Ft Wayne, IN 46802
Prgm Dir: Karen S Brehn, RT(R)BS
Tel: 219 425-3990
Med Dir: Daine Daly, MD
Class Cap: 23 *Begins:* June
Length: 24 mos *Award:* Cert, AS
Tuition per yr: $1,800
Evening or weekend classes available

Lutheran College of Health Professions

Radiography Prgm
3024 Fairfield Ave
Ft Wayne, IN 46807-1698
Prgm Dir: Donna J Lyke, MS RT(R)
Tel: 219 458-2024 *Fax:* 219 458-3077
Class Cap: 19
Length: 22 mos *Award:* AS
Tuition per yr: $6,200

Indiana University Northwest

Radiography Prgm
3400 Broadway
Gary, IN 46408-1197
Prgm Dir: Arlene M Adler, MEd RT(R) FAERS
Tel: 219 980-6540 *Fax:* 219 980-6649
E-mail: aadler@iunhaw1.iun.indiana.edu
Med Dir: John Gustaitis, MD
Class Cap: 40 *Begins:* Sep
Length: 24 mos *Award:* AS
Tuition per yr: $3,150 res, $8,150 non-res
Evening or weekend classes available

Hancock Memorial Hospital

Radiography Prgm
801 N State St
Greenfield, IN 46140
Prgm Dir: Vaughn Sutton, BS RT(R)
Tel: 317 462-0468 *Fax:* 317 462-0549
Med Dir: Richard A Silver, MD
Class Cap: 12 *Begins:* July
Length: 24 mos *Award:* Cert
Tuition per yr: $2,500

Community Hospitals of Indianapolis

Radiography Prgm
1500 N Ritter Ave
Indianapolis, IN 46219
Prgm Dir: Meryem Cole, BS RT(R)
Tel: 317 355-5867 *Fax:* 317 351-7864
Med Dir: Gordon McLaughlin
Class Cap: 12 *Begins:* June
Length: 24 mos *Award:* Cert
Tuition per yr: $1,000 res, $1,000 non-res

Indiana University School of Medicine

Radiography Prgm
541 Clinical Dr 120
Indianapolis, IN 46202-5111
Prgm Dir: Emily M Hernandez, MS RT(R)
Tel: 317 274-5252 *Fax:* 317 274-4074
E-mail: ehernand@xray.indyrad.iupui.edu
Med Dir: Mervyn Cohgn, MD
Class Cap: 36 *Begins:* June
Length: 22 mos *Award:* AS
Tuition per yr: $4,188 res, $12,843 non-res
Evening or weekend classes available

Ivy Tech State Coll - Indianapolis

Radiography Prgm
Central Indiana Region
One W 26th St/PO Box 1763
Indianapolis, IN 46206-1763
Prgm Dir: Randall Dings
Tel: 317 921-4414
Class Cap: 26
Length: 24 mos *Award:* AAS

St Joseph Hospital & Health Center

Radiography Prgm
1907 W Sycamore St
Kokomo, IN 46904-9010
Prgm Dir: John O Hughley, MS RT(R)
Tel: 317 456-5144 *Fax:* 317 456-5812
Med Dir: Bill Babchor, MD
Class Cap: 6 *Begins:* June
Length: 24 mos *Award:* Cert

King's Daughter's Hospital

Radiography Prgm
One King's Daughter's Dr
PO Box 447
Madison, IN 47250
Prgm Dir: Carol A Park, BS RT(R)
Tel: 812 265-5211 *Fax:* 812 265-0474
Med Dir: Melvin J Skiles, MD
Class Cap: 6
Length: 24 mos *Award:* Cert
Tuition per yr: $2,000 res, $2,000 non-res

Ball Memorial Hospital

Radiography Prgm
2401 University Ave
Muncie, IN 47303-3499
Prgm Dir: Susan J Hinds, RT(R)
Tel: 317 747-4372 *Fax:* 317 747-4415
Class Cap: 12 *Begins:* June July
Length: 24 mos *Award:* AAS
Tuition per yr: $2,000
Evening or weekend classes available

Ball State University

Radiography Prgm
Phys and Hlth Sciences Dept
Muncie, IN 47306
Prgm Dir: James J Wirrell, MEd RT(R)
Tel: 317 929-8088
E-mail: 3179292102
Class Cap: 20
Length: 24 mos *Award:* AS
Tuition per yr: $3,315 res, $3,315 non-res
Evening or weekend classes available

Reid Hospital & Health Care Services

Radiography Prgm
1401 Chester Blvd
Richmond, IN 47374
Prgm Dir: Roger A Preston, BS RT(R)
Tel: 317 983-3167 *Fax:* 317 983-3176
Med Dir: William Cory Gary, MD
Class Cap: 11 *Begins:* Oct
Length: 24 mos *Award:* Cert
Tuition per yr: $1,000 res, $1,000 non-res

Indiana University - South Bend

Radiography Prgm
1700 Mishawaka Ave
PO Box 7111
South Bend, IN 46634
Prgm Dir: Steven D Walters, MS RT(R)
Tel: 219 284-6532
Class Cap: 16
Length: 24 mos *Award:* AS

Ivy Tech State Coll - Terre Haute

Radiography Prgm
7999 US Hwy 41 S
Terre Haute, IN 47802-4898
Prgm Dir: John A Garner, BS RT(R)
Tel: 812 299-1121 *Fax:* 812 299-5723
Class Cap: 15 *Begins:* Aug
Length: 24 mos *Award:* AAS
Tuition per yr: $2,631 res, $4,624 non-res
Evening or weekend classes available

Porter Memorial Hospital

Radiography Prgm
814 LaPorte Ave
Valparaiso, IN 46383
Prgm Dir: Bridget Burge, BS RT(R)
Tel: 219 465-4883 *Fax:* 219 465-4854
Class Cap: 9 *Begins:* July
Length: 24 mos *Award:* Cert
Tuition per yr: $650

Good Samaritan Hospital

Radiography Prgm
520 S Seventh St
Vincennes, IN 47591
Prgm Dir: Ronald R Weitze, MBA RT(R)
Tel: 812 885-8011 *Fax:* 812 885-8043
Med Dir: John Mathis, DO
Class Cap: 6
Length: 24 mos *Award:* Cert
Tuition per yr: $600

Iowa

Scott Community College

Radiography Prgm
500 Belmont Rd
Bettendorf, IA 52722-5649
Prgm Dir: Donna M Collentine, BS RT(R)
Tel: 319 359-7531 *Fax:* 319 344-0384
E-mail: dcollentine@eiccd.cc.ia.us
Med Dir: Robert Hartung, MD
Class Cap: 20 *Begins:* Aug
Length: 24 mos *Award:* AAS
Tuition per yr: $4,300 res, $6,200 non-res

Mercy/St Luke's Hospitals
Radiography Prgm
1026 A Ave NE
Cedar Rapids, IA 52402
Prgm Dir: Donald J Leonard, BS RT(R)
Tel: 319 369-7097
Class Cap: 19
Length: 24 mos   *Award:* Cert
Tuition per yr: $1,000

Jennie Edmundson Memorial Hospital
Radiography Prgm
933 E Pierce St
Council Bluffs, IA 51503
Prgm Dir: Kristin E Schnitker, RT(R)
Tel: 712 328-6746
Med Dir: Charles H Morris, MD
Class Cap: 6   *Begins:* Aug
Length: 24 mos   *Award:* Cert
Tuition per yr: $2,200 res, $2,200 non-res

Iowa Methodist Medical Center
Radiography Prgm
1200 Pleasant St
Des Moines, IA 50309
Prgm Dir: Margaret J Page, MS RT(R)
Tel: 515 241-6171   *Fax:* 515 241-8015
Class Cap: 13   *Begins:* July
Length: 24 mos   *Award:* Cert
Tuition per yr: $1,000 res, $1,000 non-res

Mercy Hospital Medical Center
Radiography Prgm
928 Sixth Ave
Des Moines, IA 50309
Prgm Dir: Suzanne E Crandall, MS RT(R)
Tel: 515 247-3180
Class Cap: 10
Length: 22 mos   *Award:* Dipl, AS
Tuition per yr: $6,045
Evening or weekend classes available

Iowa Central Community College
Radiography Prgm
330 Ave M
Ft Dodge, IA 50501
Prgm Dir: Jeffrey B Killion, BS RT(R)
Tel: 515 576-7201   *Fax:* 515 576-7206
E-mail: killion@duke.iccc.cc.ia.us
Med Dir: Raymond D Schamel, MD
Class Cap: 28   *Begins:* Sep
Length: 22 mos   *Award:* AAS
Tuition per yr: $3,615 res, $4,221 non-res
Evening or weekend classes available

University of Iowa Hospitals and Clinics
Radiography Prgm
200 Hawkins Dr C-723
Iowa City, IA 52242 1077
Prgm Dir: Marilyn D Holland, BS RT(R)
Tel: 319 356-4332   *Fax:* 319 353-6769
E-mail: marilyn-holland@uiowa.edu
Med Dir: Yutaka Sato, MD
Class Cap: 25   *Begins:* July
Length: 24 mos   *Award:* Cert
Tuition per yr: $1,000

North Iowa Mercy Health Center
Radiography Prgm
84 Beaumont Dr
Mason City, IA 50401
Prgm Dir: Joan Van Osten, MBA RT(R)(M)
Tel: 515 424-7200   *Fax:* 515 424-7943
Med Dir: M W Schularick, MD
Class Cap: 8   *Begins:* June
Length: 24 mos   *Award:* Cert
Tuition per yr: $1,000 res, $1,000 non-res

Indian Hills Community College
Radiography Prgm
525 Grandview
Ottumwa, IA 52501
Prgm Dir: Dana D Schmitz, BS Ed RT(R)
Tel: 515 683-5165   *Fax:* 515 683-5184
Med Dir: Elvin McCarl, MD
Class Cap: 31   *Begins:* Aug
Length: 24 mos   *Award:* AAS
Tuition per yr: $2,332 res, $3,498 non-res

Northeast Iowa Community College
Radiography Prgm
10250 Sundown Rd
Peosta, IA 52068
Prgm Dir: Beverly J Vana, BS RT(R)
Tel: 319 556-5110   *Fax:* 319 556-5058
Med Dir: Donald P Mueller, MD
Class Cap: 22   *Begins:* Aug
Length: 24 mos   *Award:* AAS
Tuition per yr: $3,038 res, $4,686 non-res

Marian Health Center
Radiography Prgm
801 5th St
Sioux City, IA 51101
Prgm Dir: Maryellen Brazzell, BS RT(R)
Tel: 712 279-2251   *Fax:* 712 279-2440
Length: 24 mos   *Award:* Cert
Tuition per yr: $2,500

Allen College
Radiography Prgm
1825 Logan Ave
Waterloo, IA 50703
Prgm Dir: Peggy S Fortsch
Tel: 319 235-3693
Class Cap: 10
Length: 24 mos   *Award:* Cert

Covenant Medical Center
Radiography Prgm
3421 W 9th St
Waterloo, IA 50702
Prgm Dir: Trent L Gerdes, BS RT(R)
Tel: 319 291-3464   *Fax:* 319 291-3433
Med Dir: J V Connell, MD
Class Cap: 9   *Begins:* June
Length: 24 mos   *Award:* Cert
Tuition per yr: $2,000 res, $1,000 non-res

Kansas

Ft Hays State University
Radiography Prgm
600 Park St
Hays, KS 67601-4099
Prgm Dir: Michael E Madden, PhD RT(R)
Tel: 913 628-5678   *Fax:* 913 628-4076
E-mail: bima@fluvm.fhsu.edu
Class Cap: 62
Length: 24 mos   *Award:* AS
Tuition per yr: $3,407 res, $4,190 non-res

Hutchinson Community College
Radiography Prgm
815 N Walnut
Hutchinson, KS 67501
Prgm Dir: Renee Kautzer, MS RT(R)
Tel: 316 665-4954
Med Dir: Theil Bloom
Class Cap: 28   *Begins:* Aug
Length: 24 mos   *Award:* AAS
Tuition per yr: $2,250 res, $2,250 non-res

Bethany Medical Center
Radiography Prgm
51 N 12th St
Kansas City, KS 66102
Prgm Dir: Mary J Renz, BA RT(R)
Tel: 913 281-8874
Med Dir: Ronald Reeb, MD
Class Cap: 6   *Begins:* July
Length: 24 mos   *Award:* Cert
Tuition per yr: $1,500 res, $1,500 non-res

Labette Community College
Radiography Prgm
200 S 14th St
Parsons, KS 67357
Prgm Dir: Paul W Bober, EdD RT(R)
Tel: 316 421-6700   *Fax:* 316 421-0180
Med Dir: William K Smith, Radiologist
Class Cap: 35   *Begins:* Aug
Length: 23 mos   *Award:* AAS
Tuition per yr: $1,295 res, $1,295 non-res
Evening or weekend classes available

Washburn University of Topeka
Radiography Prgm
1700 College Ave
Topeka, KS 66621
Prgm Dir: Jera J Roberts, EdS RT(R)
Tel: 913 231-1010   *Fax:* 913 231-1027
Med Dir: Clay Harvey, MD
Class Cap: 19   *Begins:* Aug
Length: 24 mos   *Award:* AS
Tuition per yr: $3,813 res, $7,831 non-res
Evening or weekend classes available

Kansas Newman College
Radiography Prgm
3100 McCormick Ave
Wichita, KS 67213
Prgm Dir: Ronald Shipley
Tel: 316 942-4291
Class Cap: 40
Length: 24 mos   *Award:* Cert

Programs

Kentucky

King's Daughter's Medical Center
Radiography Prgm
2201 Lexington Ave
Ashland, KY 41105-0151
Prgm Dir: Thomas L Dobbins, RT(R)
Tel: 606 327-4637 *Fax:* 606 327-4707
Class Cap: 8 *Begins:* Sep
Length: 24 mos *Award:* Cert
Tuition per yr: $1,500

Bowling Green State Voc Tech School
Radiography Prgm
1845 Loop Dr
Bowling Green, KY 42101
Prgm Dir: Diane Brett, MA RT(R)(M)
Tel: 502 843-5461 *Fax:* 502 746-7466
Med Dir: Rodney D Veitschegger, MD
Class Cap: 23
Length: 22 mos *Award:* Cert
Tuition per yr: $600 res, $1,200 non-res
Evening or weekend classes available

Ky Tech Elizabethtown State Voc Tech School
Radiography Prgm
505 University Dr
Elizabethtown, KY 42701
Prgm Dir: Penelope Logsdon
Tel: 502 766-5133
Class Cap: 10
Length: 22 mos *Award:* Cert

Hazard Community College
Radiography Prgm
One Community College Dr
Hazard, KY 41701
Prgm Dir: Homer Terry, BS RT(R)
Tel: 606 436-5721 *Fax:* 606 439-1600
Med Dir: Ashook Pated, MD
Class Cap: 19 *Begins:* Aug
Length: 24 mos *Award:* AAS
Tuition per yr: $1,000 res, $3,010 non-res
Evening or weekend classes available

Northern Kentucky University
Radiography Prgm
Albright Health Ctr Rm 227
Highland Heights, KY 41099-2104
Prgm Dir: Diane H Gronefeld
Tel: 606 572-5606 *Fax:* 606 572-6182
Med Dir: James L Schmitt, MD
Class Cap: 28
Length: 23 mos *Award:* AAS
Tuition per yr: $1,960 res, $5,320 non-res
Evening or weekend classes available

Kentucky Tech Central Campus
Radiography Prgm
104 Vo-Tech Rd
Lexington, KY 40511
Prgm Dir: Lynda Norris-Donathan, MS Ed RT(R)
Tel: 606 246-2400 *Fax:* 606 246-2504
Med Dir: Galen Castle, MD
Class Cap: 27 *Begins:* Aug
Length: 24 mos *Award:* Cert
Tuition per yr: $600 res, $1,200 non-res
Evening or weekend classes available

Lexington Community College
Radiography Prgm
Oswald Bldg Cooper Dr
Lexington, KY 40506-0235
Prgm Dir: M Judy McLaughlin, MS RT RNM
  FAERS
Tel: 606 257-6140 *Fax:* 606 257-4339
Med Dir: Margerite Purcell, MD
Class Cap: 50 *Begins:* Aug
Length: 24 mos *Award:* AAS
Tuition per yr: $2,252 res, $6,032 non-res

St Joseph Hospital
Radiography Prgm
One St Joseph Dr
Lexington, KY 40504
Prgm Dir: Karen S Lanphierd, BHS RT(R)
Tel: 606 254-1177 *Fax:* 606 260-8115
Med Dir: Darryl Dochterman
Class Cap: 10 *Begins:* Sep
Length: 24 mos *Award:* Cert
Tuition per yr: $500

University of Louisville
Radiography Prgm
School of Allied Health Sciences
Health Sciences Ctr
Louisville, KY 40292
Prgm Dir: Frances E Campeau, MA RT(R)(M)
  FAERS
Tel: 502 852-5629 *Fax:* 502 852-4597
E-mail: fecamp01@ulkyvm.louisville.edu
Med Dir: Nettie G King, MD
Class Cap: 35 *Begins:* Aug
Length: 24 mos *Award:* AHS

Madisonville Health Technology Center
Radiography Prgm
750 N Laffoon St
Madisonville, KY 42431
Prgm Dir: Meryl A Clements, BS RT(R)
Tel: 502 825-6552
Class Cap: 41
Length: 22 mos *Award:* AAS

Morehead State University
Radiography Prgm
UPO 784 Reed Hall 408
Morehead, KY 40351
Prgm Dir: Jacklynn K Darling, MS RT(R)
Tel: 606 783-5175 Fax: 606 783-5039
E-mail: jdarling@morehead-st.edu
Med Dir: Mircea Lipovan, MD
Class Cap: 50 *Begins:* Aug
Length: 24 mos *Award:* AAS
Tuition per yr: $2,090

Owensboro Community College
Radiography Prgm
4800 New Hartford Rd
Owensboro, KY 42303
Prgm Dir: Debbie J Poelhuis, MS RT(R)
Tel: 502 686-4498 *Fax:* 502 686-4662
Med Dir: Wayne Myers, MD
Class Cap: 15 *Begins:* Aug
Length: 24 mos *Award:* AAS
Tuition per yr: $1,596 res, $4,500 non-res
Evening or weekend classes available

West Kentucky Tech
Radiography Prgm
5200 Blandville Rd
PO Box 7408
Paducah, KY 42002-7408
Prgm Dir: Teresa Mayo, MS RT(R)
Tel: 502 554-6232 *Fax:* 502 445-6227
Med Dir: C Dale Brown, MD
Class Cap: 25 *Begins:* Aug
Length: 24 mos *Award:* Cert
Tuition per yr: $1,200 non-res
Evening or weekend classes available

Cumberland Valley Health Technology Ctr
Radiography Prgm
PO Box 187
Pineville, KY 40977
Prgm Dir: Charles McCary, BS RT(R)
Tel: 606 337-3106 *Fax:* 606 337-5662
Class Cap: 26 *Begins:* Aug
Length: 24 mos *Award:* Cert
Tuition per yr: $600 res, $1,200 non-res

Louisiana

Baton Rouge General Medical Center
Radiography Prgm
3600 Florida Blvd
PO Box 2511
Baton Rouge, LA 70806
Prgm Dir: Catherine W Lennier, RT(R)
Tel: 504 387-7157 *Fax:* 504 381-6168
Med Dir: J Sidney Lawton, MD
Class Cap: 12
Length: 24 mos *Award:* Cert
Tuition per yr: $1,500

Our Lady of the Lake Coll
Radiography Prgm
5345 Brittany Dr
Baton Rouge, LA 70808
Prgm Dir: Debbie Gallerson, MEd RT(R)
Tel: 504 768-1737 *Fax:* 504 768-1726
Med Dir: Robert C McReynolds Jr, MD
Class Cap: 16 *Begins:* Aug
Length: 22 mos *Award:* AD
Tuition per yr: $7,260
Evening or weekend classes available

Louisiana State University at Eunice
Radiography Prgm
PO Box 1129
Eunice, LA 70535
Prgm Dir: Rob McLaughlin, MA RT
Tel: - *Fax:* 318 546-6620
Med Dir: John Higgins, MD
Class Cap: 23 *Begins:* June
Length: 24 mos *Award:* AS
Tuition per yr: $1,584 res, $3,084 non-res
Evening or weekend classes available

North Oaks Health System
Radiography Prgm
PO Box 2668 Hwy 51 S
Hammond, LA 70404
Prgm Dir: Judith D Bennett, BS RT
Tel: 504 543-6504
Med Dir: Sephen M Williams, MD
Class Cap: 12
Length: 24 mos *Award:* Cert
Tuition per yr: $8,000

Lafayette General Medical Center
Radiography Prgm
1214 Coolidge Ave
PO Box 52009 OCS
Lafayette, LA 70505
Prgm Dir: Charlotte S Powell, BS LRT
Tel: 318 289-7457 *Fax:* 318 289-8136
Med Dir: Vidyadhar Akkaraju, MD
Class Cap: 8 *Begins:* July
Length: 24 mos *Award:* Cert
Tuition per yr: $3,000

University Medical Center
Radiography Prgm
2390 W Congress
PO Box 4016-C
Lafayette, LA 70502
Prgm Dir: Carl J Fontenot, RT(R)
Tel: 318 261-6208 *Fax:* 318 261-6660
Med Dir: Leonard Bok, MD
Class Cap: 6 *Begins:* Jul
Length: 24 mos *Award:* Cert
Tuition per yr: $1,800

McNeese State University
Radiography Prgm
PO Box 92000
Lake Charles, LA 70609-2000
Prgm Dir: Gregory L Bradley, MEd RT(R)
Tel: 318 475-5657 *Fax:* 318 475-5677
Med Dir: J R Romero, MD
Class Cap: 26 *Begins:* Aug
Length: 45 mos *Award:* BS
Tuition per yr: $2,012 res, $3,530 non-res
Evening or weekend classes available

Northeast Louisiana University
Radiography Prgm
700 University Ave
Monroe, LA 71209-0450
Prgm Dir: Jerry E McNeil, MA RT(R)
Tel: 318 342-1630 *Fax:* 318 342-1635
Med Dir: Lionel Barraza, MD
Class Cap: 47 *Begins:* Aug
Length: 48 mos *Award:* BS
Tuition per yr: $965 res, $2,136 non-res
Evening or weekend classes available

Northwestern State University
Radiography Prgm
Dept of Life Sciences
Natchitoches, LA 71497
Prgm Dir: Arnold Young, RT(R)
Tel: 318 681-4347
Class Cap: 20
Length: 21 mos *Award:* BS

Alton Ochsner Medical Foundation
Radiography Prgm
1516 Jefferson Hwy
New Orleans, LA 70121
Prgm Dir: Kenneth W Jones, MEd RT(R)
Tel: 504 842-3705
Med Dir: Christopher Merritt, MD
Begins: July
Length: 24 mos *Award:* Cert
Tuition per yr: $1,560 res, $1,560 non-res

Delgado Community College
Radiography Prgm
615 City Park Ave
New Orleans, LA 70119-4399
Prgm Dir: Ray A Gisclair, MS RT(R)
Tel: 504 483-4015 *Fax:* 504 483-4609
Med Dir: Mario Calonje, MD FACR
Class Cap: 115 *Begins:* Aug
Length: 25 mos *Award:* AS
Tuition per yr: $1,689 res, $4,299 non-res
Evening or weekend classes available

Southern Univ at Shreveport - Bossier City
Radiography Prgm
610 Texas St
Shreveport, LA 71101
Prgm Dir: Sharon Fisher Green, MART(R)
Tel: 318 674-3358 *Fax:* 318 676-5308
Med Dir: Richard Handley, MD
Length: 27 mos *Award:* AAS
Tuition per yr: res, $555 non-res

Maine

Eastern Maine Technical College
Radiography Prgm
354 Hogan Rd
Bangor, ME 04401
Prgm Dir: Sue Roeder, MEd RT(R)(N)
Tel: 207 941-4659 *Fax:* 207 941-4608
Med Dir: David Wakner, MD
Class Cap: 17 *Begins:* Aug
Length: 24 mos *Award:* AAS
Tuition per yr: res, $2,610 non-res
Evening or weekend classes available

Central Maine Medical Center
Radiography Prgm
300 Main St
Lewiston, ME 04240-0305
Prgm Dir: Judith M Ripley, RT(R)
Tel: 207 795-2428 *Fax:* 207 795-5539
Class Cap: 9 *Begins:* Aug
Length: 24 mos *Award:* Cert
Tuition per yr: $1,260

Mercy Hospital
Radiography Prgm
144 State St
Portland, ME 04101
Prgm Dir: Catherine A Munroe, RT(R)
Tel: 207 879-3501 *Fax:* 207 879-3167
Med Dir: Payson S Adams Jr, MD
Class Cap: 9 *Begins:* July
Length: 24 mos *Award:* Cert, AS
Tuition per yr: $2,000 res, $2,000 non-res

Southern Maine Technical College
Radiography Prgm
Fort Rd
South Portland, ME 04106
Prgm Dir: Sally A Doe, BS RT(R)
Tel: 207 767-9596
Class Cap: 0
Length: 23 mos *Award:* AAS
Evening or weekend classes available

Mid Maine Medical Center Thayer Unit
Radiography Prgm
149 North St
Waterville, ME 04901
Prgm Dir: Charlotte N Roberge, RT(R)
Tel: 207 872-1227 *Fax:* 207 872-1127
Class Cap: 9
Length: 24 mos *Award:* Dipl
Tuition per yr: $3,886

Maryland

Anne Arundel Community College
Radiography Prgm
101 College Pkwy
Arnold, MD 21012-1895
Prgm Dir: Thomas A Luby Jr, MBA RT(R)
Tel: 410 315-7311 *Fax:* 410 315-7099
E-mail: ztal@aacci.aacc.md.us
Med Dir: Mark Radovich, MD
Class Cap: 25
Length: 24 mos *Award:* AAS
Tuition per yr: $5,400
Evening or weekend classes available

Essex Community College
Radiography Prgm
7201 Rossville Blvd
Baltimore, MD 21237-9987
Prgm Dir: Linda Caplis, MS RT(R)
Tel: 410 682-7414 *Fax:* 410 682-7987
E-mail: linda@helix.org
Med Dir: Edward B Mishner, MD
Class Cap: 16 *Begins:* July
Length: 24 mos *Award:* AAS
Tuition per yr: $2,040 res, $3,604 non-res
Evening or weekend classes available

Greater Baltimore Medical Center
Radiography Prgm
6701 N Charles St
Baltimore, MD 21204
Prgm Dir: Pat J Wolfe, BA RT(R)
Tel: 410 828-2463 *Fax:* 410 828-2866
Med Dir: Alexander Manitz
Class Cap: 15 *Begins:* July
Length: 24 mos *Award:* Cert
Tuition per yr: $1,500 res, $1,500 non-res

Johns Hopkins Hospital
Radiography Prgm
600 N Wolfe St
Baltimore, MD 21287
Prgm Dir: Dixon C Barthel, MA RT(R)
Tel: 410 955-5968 *Fax:* 410 955-0589
E-mail: dbarthel@rod.jhu.edu
Class Cap: 30
Length: 24 mos *Award:* Cert
Tuition per yr: $3,000 res, $3,000 non-res

Maryland General Hospital
Radiography Prgm
827 Linden Ave
Baltimore, MD 21202
Prgm Dir: Earl S Ramp, RT(R)
Tel: 410 225-8080 *Fax:* 410 669-8710
Med Dir: Ronald Stanfiels, MD
Class Cap: 11
Length: 24 mos *Award:* Cert
Tuition per yr: $1,200

Mercy Medical Center
Radiography Prgm
301 St Paul Pl
Baltimore, MD 21202-2165
Prgm Dir: Brenda Ann Schuette, BA RT(R)
Tel: 410 332-9266 *Fax:* 410 783-5609
Med Dir: Frank Twardzik, MD
Class Cap: 10
Length: 24 mos *Award:* Cert
Tuition per yr: $1,500 res, $1,500 non-res

Allegany College of Maryland
Radiography Prgm
12401 Willowbrook Rd SE
Cumberland, MD 21502-2596
Prgm Dir: Ester L Verhovsek, MEd RT(R)
Tel: 301 724-7700 *Fax:* 301 724-6892
E-mail: [ester@ac.cc.md.us]@int
Med Dir: Jong Kim
Class Cap: 15 *Begins:* Sep
Length: 22 mos *Award:* AAS
Tuition per yr: $1,241 res, $1,581 non-res
Evening or weekend classes available

Hagerstown Junior College
Radiography Prgm
11400 Robinwood Dr
Hagerstown, MD 21742-6590
Prgm Dir: Brenda J Hassinger, MS RT(R)(M)
Tel: 301 790-2800 *Fax:* 301 739-0737
E-mail: hassinger.b@hjc.cc.md.us
Med Dir: Allan M Wexler
Class Cap: 20 *Begins:* June
Length: 24 mos *Award:* AAS
Tuition per yr: $2,240 res, $3,150 non-res
Evening or weekend classes available

Prince George's Community College
Radiography Prgm
301 Largo Rd
Largo, MD 20772-2199
Prgm Dir: Barbara K Walton, BS RT(R)(M)
Tel: 301 322-0745
Class Cap: 57
Length: 24 mos *Award:* AA

Wor-Wic Community College
Radiography Prgm
32000 Campus Dr
Salisbury, MD 21801
Prgm Dir: Andrew P Woodward, MA RT(R)
Tel: 410 548-5115 *Fax:* 410 543-7087
Med Dir: Peter Libby, MD
Class Cap: 16 *Begins:* July
Length: 24 mos *Award:* AAS
Tuition per yr: $2,173 res, $5,371 non-res
Evening or weekend classes available

Holy Cross Hospital
Radiography Prgm
1500 Forest Glen Rd
Silver Spring, MD 20910
Prgm Dir: Sambra J Flanagan, BS RT(R)
Tel: 301 754-7367 *Fax:* 301 754-7371
Med Dir: Harendra Rupani, MD
Class Cap: 12
Length: 24 mos *Award:* Cert
Tuition per yr: $1,500

Montgomery College
Radiography Prgm
Takoma Ave and Fenton St
Takoma Park, MD 20912
Prgm Dir: Angela M Pickwick, MS RT(R)(M)
Tel: 301 650-1341 *Fax:* 301 650-1335
Med Dir: Sydney Pion
Class Cap: 30 *Begins:* Sep
Length: 24 mos *Award:* AA
Tuition per yr: $2,750 res, $5,260 non-res
Evening or weekend classes available

Washington Adventist Hospital
Radiography Prgm
7600 Carroll Ave
Takoma Park, MD 20912
Prgm Dir: James E Mayhew, BS RT(R)
Tel: 301 891-3450 *Fax:* 301 891-3520
Class Cap: 11 *Begins:* Oct
Length: 24 mos *Award:* Cert
Tuition per yr: $1,000

Chesapeake College
Radiography Prgm
PO Box 8
Wye Mills, MD 21679
Prgm Dir: Linda Burchett Blythe, AA RT(R)
Tel: 410 827-5814 *Fax:* 410 827-9466
Med Dir: H Gilmore Greg, MD
Class Cap: 9 *Begins:* June
Length: 25 mos *Award:* AAS
Tuition per yr: $2,376 res, $4,250 non-res
Evening or weekend classes available

Massachusetts

Middlesex Community College - Bedford
Radiography Prgm
Springs Rd
Bedford, MA 01730
Prgm Dir: Dale Trudo, MEd RT(R)
Tel: 617 275-8910 *Fax:* 617 275-4911
E-mail: trudod@admin.mcc.mass.edu
Class Cap: 50
Length: 22 mos *Award:* AS
Tuition per yr: $3,008 res, $3,328 non-res

Bunker Hill Community College
Radiography Prgm
250 New Rutherford Ave
Boston, MA 02129-2991
Prgm Dir: Judith D Burnett, MEd RT(R)
Tel: 617 228-2027 *Fax:* 617 228-2120
Med Dir: Miriam Vincent, MD
Class Cap: 30
Length: 24 mos *Award:* AS
Tuition per yr: $1,016

Northeastern University
Radiography Prgm
266 Ryder Hall
Boston, MA 02115
Prgm Dir: Valerie A Lamb, BS RT(R)
Tel: 617 373-2818
Class Cap: 87
Length: 27 mos *Award:* AS

Massasoit Community College
Radiography Prgm
One Massasoit Blvd
Brockton, MA 02402
Prgm Dir: Nancy J Sutcliffe, Equiv RT(R)
Tel: 508 588-9100 *Fax:* 508 427-1250
Med Dir: Phillip Arena, MD
Class Cap: 40 *Begins:* Sep
Length: 21 mos *Award:* AS
Tuition per yr: $2,822 res, $6,392 non-res
Evening or weekend classes available

North Shore Community College
Radiography Prgm
1 Ferncroft Rd PO Box 3340
Danvers, MA 01923-0840
Prgm Dir: Christine E Wiley, BS RT(R)(N)
Tel: 508 762-4163 *Fax:* 508 762-4022
Med Dir: Philip Thomason, MD
Class Cap: 18 *Begins:* Sep
Length: 21 mos *Award:* AS
Tuition per yr: $2,844 res, $8,316 non-res
Evening or weekend classes available

Northern Essex Community College
Radiography Prgm
100 Elliot Way
Haverhill, MA 01830-2399
Prgm Dir: Carol D Wallace, BA RT(R)
Tel: 508 374-3826 *Fax:* 508 374-3723
Med Dir: Arthur Lathrop Zerbey III, MD
Class Cap: 24 *Begins:* Aug
Length: 22 mos *Award:* AS

Holyoke Community College
Radiography Prgm
303 Homestead Ave
Holyoke, MA 01040
Prgm Dir: Kathryn C Root, MEd RT(R)
Tel: 413 538-7000
E-mail: kroot@hcc.mass.edu
Class Cap: 20
Length: 23 mos *Award:* AS
Tuition per yr: $2,890 res, $5,200 non-res

Springfield Technical Community College
Radiography Prgm
One Armory Sq PO Box 9000
Springfield, MA 01101-9000
Prgm Dir: Richard J Pushkin, AS RT(R)
Tel: 413 781-7822 *Fax:* 413 781-5805
E-mail: pushkin@stccadm.stcc.mass.edu
Med Dir: Eckart Sachsse, MD
Class Cap: 22 *Begins:* Sep
Length: 23 mos *Award:* AS
Tuition per yr: $1,520 res, $7,164 non-res

Massachusetts Bay Community College
Radiography Prgm
50 Oakland St
Wellesley Hills, MA 02181-5399
Prgm Dir: James V Lampka, MS RT(R)
Tel: 617 239-2238
Class Cap: 45
Length: 20 mos *Award:* AS

Quinsigamond Community College
Radiography Prgm
670 W Boylston St
Worcester, MA 01606-2092
Prgm Dir: Sandra D Ostresh, MEd RT(R)
Tel: 508 854-4289   *Fax:* 508 852-6943
E-mail: sandieo@qcc.hass.edu
Class Cap: 49   *Begins:* July
Length: 22 mos   *Award:* AS
Evening or weekend classes available

Michigan

Washtenaw Community College
Radiography Prgm
4800 E Huron River Dr
Ann Arbor, MI 48106-0978
Prgm Dir: Gerald A Baker, MEd RT(R)
Tel: 313 973-3333
Class Cap: 28
Length: 24 mos   *Award:* AAS
Tuition per yr: $2,340 res, $3,375 non-res
Evening or weekend classes available

Kellogg Community College
Radiography Prgm
450 North Ave
Battle Creek, MI 49017-3397
Prgm Dir: Carl W Brockman, BS RT(R)
Tel: 616 965-3931, Ext 1315   *Fax:* 616 965-4133
E-mail: kathy@rad.hgh.edu
Med Dir: William P Sanders, MD
Class Cap: 23
Length: 24 mos   *Award:* AAS
Tuition per yr: $1,911 res, $2,902 non-res
Evening or weekend classes available

Lake Michigan College
Radiography Prgm
2755 E Napier Ave
Benton Harbor, MI 49022-1899
Prgm Dir: Edna Jones-Holmes, MPA RT(R)
Tel: 616 927-8100
Class Cap: 25
Length: 24 mos   *Award:* AS

Ferris State University
Radiography Prgm
901 S State St
Big Rapids, MI 49307-9989
Prgm Dir: Robert T Holihan, BS RT(R)
Tel: 616 592-2326   *Fax:* 616 592-3788
Class Cap: 72
Length: 24 mos   *Award:* AAS
Tuition per yr: $1,824 res, $2,740 non-res
Evening or weekend classes available

Oakwood Hospital and Medical Center
Radiography Prgm
18101 Oakwood Blvd
PO Box 2500
Dearborn, MI 48124
Prgm Dir: Susan C Jabara, BS RT(R)
Tel: 313 593-7660   *Fax:* 313 439-2039
Med Dir: David S Yates, MD
Class Cap: 15
Length: 24 mos   *Award:* Cert
Tuition per yr: $2,500

Grace Hospital
Radiography Prgm
6071 W Outer Dr
Detroit, MI 48235
Prgm Dir: Mary L Seib, RT(R)
Tel: 313 966-6816   *Fax:* 313 966-6855
Med Dir: Burt T Weying III, MD FACR
Class Cap: 9   *Begins:* July
Length: 24 mos   *Award:* Cert
Tuition per yr: $600

Henry Ford Hospital
Radiography Prgm
2799 W Grand Blvd
Detroit, MI 48202
Prgm Dir: Kathleen Kath, RT(R)
Tel: 313 876-1348   *Fax:* 313 876-9119
Med Dir: William P. Sanders, MD
Class Cap: 27   *Begins:* Sept
Length: 24 mos   *Award:* Cert
Tuition per yr: $500 res, $500 non-res

Marygrove College
Radiography Prgm
8425 W McNichols Rd
Detroit, MI 48221-2599
Prgm Dir: John W High, BS RT(R)
Tel: 313 862-8000   *Fax:* 313 864-6670
Med Dir: Michael L Schwartz, MD
Class Cap: 15
Length: 24 mos   *Award:* Cert, AS
Tuition per yr: $11,369
Evening or weekend classes available

St John Hospital and Medical Center
Radiography Prgm
22101 Moross Rd
Detroit, MI 48236-2172
Prgm Dir: Sean P Skinner, BAS RT(R)
Tel: 313 343-3549   *Fax:* 313 343-7305
Length: 24 mos   *Award:* Cert
Tuition per yr: $1,000

Genesys Regional Medical Center
Radiography Prgm
302 Kensington Ave
Flint, MI 48503-2000
Prgm Dir: Lewis R Geyer, RT(R)
Tel: 313 762-8780
Med Dir: Anthony Pawillo, MD
Class Cap: 12   *Begins:* July
Length: 24 mos   *Award:* Cert
Tuition per yr: $300 res, $300 non-res

Hurley Medical Center
Radiography Prgm
One Hurley Plaza
Flint, MI 48503-5993
Prgm Dir: Dawn Sturk, BS RT(R) RCVT
Tel: 810 257-9835   *Fax:* 810 257-9009
Class Cap: 10
Length: 24 mos   *Award:* Cert
Tuition per yr: $2,200

Grand Rapids Community College
Radiography Prgm
143 Bostwick NE
Grand Rapids, MI 49503
Prgm Dir: John F Godisak, MA RT(R)
Tel: 616 771-4233   *Fax:* 616 771-4234
E-mail: jgodisak@raider.grcc.cc.mi.us
Class Cap: 28
Length: 24 mos   *Award:* AAS
Tuition per yr: $2,025 res, $3,000 non-res
Evening or weekend classes available

Mid Michigan Community College
Radiography Prgm
1375 S Clare Ave
Harrison, MI 48625-9447
Prgm Dir: John Skinner, MEd RT(R)
Tel: 517 386-6646   *Fax:* 517 386-2411
Class Cap: 28   *Begins:* Aug
Length: 24 mos   *Award:* AAS
Tuition per yr: $1,395 res, $2,108 non-res
Evening or weekend classes available

Jackson Community College
Radiography Prgm
2111 Emmons Rd
Jackson, MI 49201
Prgm Dir: Edwin W Martin Jr, BS RT(R)
Tel: 517 796-8533   *Fax:* 517 796-8633
E-mail: emartin@jackson.cc
Class Cap: 20   *Begins:* May
Length: 24 mos   *Award:* AAS
Tuition per yr: $1,164 res, $1,502 non-res
Evening or weekend classes available

Lansing Community College
Radiography Prgm
Dept 3400 PO Box 40010
Lansing, MI 48901-7210
Prgm Dir: Lucy Smythe, MA RT(R)
Tel: 517 483-1428
Class Cap: 24   *Begins:* Aug Jan
Length: 24 mos   *Award:* AAS
Tuition per yr: $1,700 res, $2,700 non-res
Evening or weekend classes available

Marquette General Hospital
Radiography Prgm
420 W Magnetic St
Marquette, MI 49855
Prgm Dir: John R Howko, MEd RT(R)
Tel: 906 225-4916   *Fax:* 906 225-4678
Class Cap: 6   *Begins:* Aug
Length: 24 mos   *Award:* Cert
Tuition per yr: $1,200 res, $1,200 non-res

Baker College of Owosso
Radiography Prgm
1020 S Washington St
Owosso, MI 48867-4400
Prgm Dir: Brian W Pickford, BS RT(R)
Tel: 517 723-5251   *Fax:* 517 723-3355
E-mail: pickfo_b@owosso.baker.edu
Med Dir: Konstantin R Loewig, MD
Class Cap: 45   *Begins:* Sep
Length: 24 mos   *Award:* AAS
Tuition per yr: $8,710
Evening or weekend classes available

Programs

Port Huron Hospital

Radiography Prgm
1001 Kearney St
PO Box 5011
Port Huron, MI 48061-5011
Prgm Dir: Monica S Rowling, BAS RT(R)
Tel: 810 989-3163 *Fax:* 810 985-2672
Class Cap: 7 *Begins:* Sep
Length: 24 mos *Award:* Cert
Tuition per yr: $1,700

William Beaumont Hospital

Radiography Prgm
3601 W 13 Mile Rd
Royal Oak, MI 48073
Prgm Dir: Terese A Trost-Price, BAS RT(R)
Tel: 810 551-6048 *Fax:* 810 551-5490
Med Dir: Henrietta Juras, MD
Class Cap: 16 *Begins:* Jul
Length: 24 mos *Award:* Cert
Tuition per yr: $350

Oakland Community College

Radiography Prgm
22322 Rutland Dr
Southfield, MI 48075
Prgm Dir: Carolyn Nacy, BS RT(R)
Tel: 810 552-2610 *Fax:* 810 552-2661
Med Dir: Hugh H Kerr, MD
Class Cap: 30 *Begins:* May
Length: 26 mos *Award:* AAS
Tuition per yr: $1,610 res, $2,730 non-res
Evening or weekend classes available

Providence Hospital and Medical Centers

Radiography Prgm
16001 W Nine Mile Rd
PO Box 2043
Southfield, MI 48037
Prgm Dir: Mary Holzman
Tel: 810 424-3293
Med Dir: Cynthia Wheeler, MD
Class Cap: 10 *Begins:* Sept
Length: 24 mos *Award:* Cert
Tuition per yr: $550

Delta College

Radiography Prgm
University Center, MI 48710
Prgm Dir: Kathleen M Gavalas, MEd RT(R)
Tel: 517 686-9533 *Fax:* 517 686-3736
Class Cap: 18 *Begins:* Aug
Length: 24 mos *Award:* AAS
Tuition per yr: $1,666 res, $2,170 non-res
Evening or weekend classes available

Oakwood-United Hospitals Inc

Radiography Prgm
33155 Annapolis Rd
Wayne, MI 48184
Prgm Dir: Dawn M Baker, BAS RT(R)(M)
Tel: 313 467-4115 *Fax:* 313 467-4191
Class Cap: 5
Length: 24 mos *Award:* Cert
Tuition per yr: $1,000

Minnesota

Minnesota Riverland Tech College-Austin

Radiography Prgm
Medical Imaging
1600 8th Ave NW
Austin, MN 55912
Prgm Dir: Rebecca Lee Waters, BS RT(R)
Tel: 507 433-0645 *Fax:* 507 433-0665
Class Cap: 25 *Begins:* Sep
Length: 24 mos *Award:* AAS
Tuition per yr: $3,000

Medical Institute of Minnesota

Radiography Prgm
5503 Green Valley Dr
Bloomington, MN 55437
Prgm Dir: Michael C Stori, BS RT(R)
Tel: 612 844-0064 *Fax:* 612 755-0671
Class Cap: 40 *Begins:* Oct Jan Apr
Length: 21 mos *Award:* AAS
Tuition per yr: $7,275
Evening or weekend classes available

Lake Superior College

Radiography Prgm
2101 Trinity Rd
Duluth, MN 55811-2741
Prgm Dir: Nancy A Fredrickson, Equiv RT(R)
Tel: 218 725-7714 *Fax:* 218 723-4921
E-mail: n.fredrickson@lsc.cc.mn.us
Med Dir: William Schwartan, MD
Class Cap: 25 *Begins:* Sep
Length: 24 mos *Award:* AS
Tuition per yr: $2,392 res, $4,784 non-res
Evening or weekend classes available

Northwest Technical Coll - E Grand Forks

Radiography Prgm
Hwy 220 N PO Box 111
East Grand Forks, MN 56721
Prgm Dir: Darrell Hinger, RT(R)
Tel: 218 773-3441 *Fax:* 218 773-4502
E-mail: hinger@adm.egf.tec.mn.us
Med Dir: Bradley C Aqfedt, MD
Class Cap: 16
Length: 24 mos *Award:* AAS
Tuition per yr: $3,286

College of St Catherine

Radiography Prgm
601 25th Ave S
Minneapolis, MN 55454
Prgm Dir: Alan Bode, MA RT(R)
Tel: 612 690-7887
Class Cap: 48
Length: 24 mos *Award:* AAS

Minneapolis Veterans Affairs Medical Ctr

Radiography Prgm
One Veterans Dr
Minneapolis, MN 55417
Prgm Dir: Gwen Wawers, MEd RT(R)
Tel: 612 725-2000, Ext 2546 *Fax:* 612 727-5635
Med Dir: Reinke
Class Cap: 12
Length: 24 mos *Award:* Cert
Evening or weekend classes available

Univ of Minnesota Hosp and Clinic

Radiography Prgm
Harvard at East River Rd
Box 292
Minneapolis, MN 55455
Prgm Dir: Patricia A Skundberg, BAS RT(R)
Tel: 612 626-0602 *Fax:* 612 624-8495
E-mail: skund001@maroon.tc.umn.edu
Med Dir: William M Thompson, MD
Length: 27 mos *Award:* AAS
Tuition per yr: $1,080 res, $2,067 non-res
Evening or weekend classes available

North Memorial Medical Center

Radiography Prgm
3300 N Oakdale
Robbinsdale, MN 55422
Prgm Dir: Richard M Amundson, AA RT(R)
Tel: 612 520-5337 *Fax:* 612 520-5297
Class Cap: 10 *Begins:* March Oct
Length: 24 mos *Award:* Cert

Mayo Clinic/Mayo Foundation

Radiography Prgm
Sch of Hlth Related Sciences
Siebens 1119
Rochester, MN 55905
Prgm Dir: Eugene D Frank, MA RT(R)
Tel: 507 284-3169 *Fax:* 507 284-3640
E-mail: efrank@mayo.edu
Class Cap: 30 *Begins:* Sep
Length: 24 mos *Award:* Cert, AS
Tuition per yr: $1,800
Evening or weekend classes available

St Cloud Hospital

Radiography Prgm
1406 Sixth Ave N
St Cloud, MN 56303
Prgm Dir: John Falconer, BA RT(R)
Tel: 320 255-5719 *Fax:* 320 255-5730
Class Cap: 8
Length: 24 mos *Award:* Cert
Tuition per yr: $3,000

Health System Minnesota/Methodist Hospital

Radiography Prgm
6500 Excelsior Blvd
St Louis Park, MN 55426
Prgm Dir: Linda C Olson, RT(R)
Tel: 612 993-5410 *Fax:* 612 993-5404
Med Dir: Frank Mork, MD
Class Cap: 6
Length: 24 mos *Award:* Cert
Tuition per yr: $300

Century Community and Technical College

Radiography Prgm
3300 Century Ave N
White Bear Lake, MN 55110
Prgm Dir: Diane J Fleury, MA RT(R)
Tel: 612 779-3334 *Fax:* 612 779-3417
E-mail: d.fleuryjcctc.cc.mn.us
Class Cap: 40
Length: 24 mos *Award:* AAS
Evening or weekend classes available

Rice Memorial Hospital
Radiography Prgm
301 Becker Ave SW
Willmar, MN 56201-3395
Prgm Dir: Luther Linn, RT(R)
Tel: 320 231-4530
Class Cap: 6
Length: 24 mos   *Award:* Cert
Tuition per yr: $950

Mississippi

Northeast Mississippi Community College
Radiography Prgm
Cunningham Blvd
Booneville, MS 38829
Prgm Dir: Carl Simms
Tel: 601 728-7751
Class Cap: 12
Length: 24 mos   *Award:* AAS

Jones County Junior College
Radiography Prgm
900 Court St
Ellisville, MS 39437
Prgm Dir: Timothy S Cochran, BS RT(R)
Tel: 601 477-4159   *Fax:* 601 477-4152
Med Dir: Clyde R Allen, MD
Class Cap: 10
Length: 24 mos   *Award:* AAS
Tuition per yr: $392 res, $792 non-res
Evening or weekend classes available

Itawamba Community College
Radiography Prgm
602 W Hill St
Fulton, MS 38843-0999
Prgm Dir: William H May, AS RT(R)
Tel: 601 862-3101   *Fax:* 601 862-7697
Med Dir: Doug Clark, MD
Class Cap: 18   *Begins:* Aug
Length: 24 mos   *Award:* AAS
Tuition per yr: $1,120 res, $1,130 non-res
Evening or weekend classes available

Mississippi Gulf Coast Community College
Radiography Prgm
PO Box 100
Gautier, MS 39553
Prgm Dir: Mary E Trichell, BS RT(R)
Tel: 601 497-9602   *Fax:* 601 497-7670
Med Dir: Paul H Moore
Class Cap: 21   *Begins:* July
Length: 24 mos   *Award:* AAS
Tuition per yr: $1,320 res, $3,189 non-res
Evening or weekend classes available

Hattiesburg Radiology Group
Radiography Prgm
5000 W 4th St
Hattiesburg, MS 39402
Prgm Dir: C David Armstrong, MEd RT(R)
Tel: 601 288-4241   *Fax:* 601 288-1657
Class Cap: 14   *Begins:* Aug
Length: 24 mos   *Award:* Cert
Tuition per yr: $3,150 res, $3,150 non-res

Mississippi Baptist Medical Center
Radiography Prgm
1225 N State St
Jackson, MS 39202-0231
Prgm Dir: Stephen C Compton, RT(R)
Tel: 601 968-4199   *Fax:* 601 968-1748
Med Dir: Gary Cirilli, MD
Class Cap: 14   *Begins:* July
Length: 24 mos   *Award:* Cert
Tuition per yr: $900

University of Mississippi Medical Center
Radiography Prgm
2500 N State St
Jackson, MS 39216-4505
Prgm Dir: Ann W Fox, BS RT(R)(M)
Tel: 601 984-2605   *Fax:* 601 984-2542
Med Dir: Ramesh Patel, MD
Class Cap: 20   *Begins:* Jul
Length: 24 mos   *Award:* Cert
Tuition per yr: $110

Meridian Community College
Radiography Prgm
910 Hwy 19 N
Meridian, MS 39307
Prgm Dir: Darlene G Withers, AA RT(R)
Tel: 601 483-8241   *Fax:* 601 482-3936
Med Dir: Mary Ann Cowart, MD
Class Cap: 19   *Begins:* Aug
Length: 24 mos   *Award:* AA
Tuition per yr: $1,310 res, $1,310 non-res
Evening or weekend classes available

Mississippi Delta Community College
Radiography Prgm
PO Box 668
Moorehead, MS 38761
Prgm Dir: Alice K Pyles, BS RT(R)
Tel: 601 246-5631   *Fax:* 601 246-6517
Class Cap: 19   *Begins:* June
Length: 25 mos   *Award:* AAS
Tuition per yr: $890 res, $980 non-res
Evening or weekend classes available

Copiah - Lincoln Community College
Radiography Prgm
PO Box 649
Wesson, MS 39191
Prgm Dir: Laura C Williams, AA RT(R)
Tel: 601 643-8392   *Fax:* 601 643-8214
Class Cap: 20
Length: 24 mos   *Award:* AAS
Tuition per yr: $1,500 res, $1,500 non-res

Missouri

University of Missouri - Columbia
Radiography Prgm
518 Lewis Hall
Columbia, MO 65211
Prgm Dir: Mary C Sebacher, MEd RT(R)
Tel: 573 882-8405   *Fax:* 573 884-8000
E-mail: sebachem@ext.missouri.edu
Med Dir: Clive Levine, MD
Class Cap: 12
Length: 42 mos   *Award:* BHS
Tuition per yr: res, $3,836 non-res

Mineral Area Regional Medical Center
Radiography Prgm
1212 Weber Rd
Farmington, MO 63640-3398
Prgm Dir: Henry Y Cashion, BS RT(R)
Tel: 573 756-4581   *Fax:* 573 756-6007
Med Dir: Raymond A Murphy, MD
Class Cap: 12   *Begins:* Aug
Length: 24 mos   *Award:* Cert
Tuition per yr: $2,210 res, $2,210 non-res

Penrose-St Francis Health System
Radiography Prgm
1212 Weber Rd
Farmington, MO 63640-3398
Prgm Dir: Henry Y Cashion, BS RT(R)
Tel: 573 756-4581   *Fax:* 573 756-6007
Med Dir: Raymond A Murphy
Class Cap: 12   *Begins:* Aug
Length: 24 mos   *Award:* Cert
Tuition per yr: $2,210 res, $2,210 non-res

Independence Regional Health Center
Radiography Prgm
1509 W Truman Rd
Independence, MO 64050
Prgm Dir: Joan Hedrick, RT(R)
Tel: 816 836-8100
Med Dir: Jon Gustafson, MD
Begins: Sep
Length: 24 mos   *Award:* Cert
Tuition per yr: $200

Nichols Career Center
Radiography Prgm
609 Union
Jefferson City, MO 65101
Prgm Dir: Stephanie L Patrick, BS RT(R)(M)
Tel: 573 659-3238   *Fax:* 573 659-3154
E-mail: stefpatrik@aol.com
Med Dir: Sid Belshe, MD
Class Cap: 14   *Begins:* Aug
Length: 24 mos   *Award:* Cert
Tuition per yr: $3,900 res, $3,900 non-res

Missouri Southern State College
Radiography Prgm
3950 E Newman Rd
Joplin, MO 64801-1595
Prgm Dir: Wiley A Beals, AS RT(R)
Tel: 417 625-9322
Class Cap: 6
Length: 24 mos   *Award:* AS
Tuition per yr: $2,660 res, $5,320 non-res

Avila College
Radiography Prgm
11901 Wornall Rd
Kansas City, MO 64145-9990
Prgm Dir: Carole A Urbanski, MS RT(R)
Tel: 816 942-8400   *Fax:* 816 942-3362
E-mail: urbanskica@mail.avila.edu
Class Cap: 15
Length: 40 mos   *Award:* BS
Tuition per yr: $10,100 res, $10,100 non-res
Evening or weekend classes available

Penn Valley Community College
Radiography Prgm
3201 SW Trafficway
Kansas City, MO 64111
Prgm Dir: Judith E Taylor, MEd RT(R)
Tel: 816 759-4243
Med Dir: Gerald Finke, DO
Class Cap: 39   *Begins:* July
Length: 24 mos   *Award:* AAS
Tuition per yr: $5,365 res, $7,615 non-res
Evening or weekend classes available

Research Medical Center
Radiography Prgm
2316 E Meyer Blvd
Kansas City, MO 64132-1199
Prgm Dir: Cheryl S Johnson, BS RT(R)
Tel: 816 276-3390   *Fax:* 816 276-4439
Med Dir: Jay Rozen
Class Cap: 15   *Begins:* July
Length: 24 mos   *Award:* Cert
Tuition per yr: $2,000 res, $2,000 non-res

North Kansas City Hospital
Radiography Prgm
2800 Clay Edwards Dr
North Kansas City, MO 64116-3281
Prgm Dir: Peggy Stephens, MEd RT(R)
Tel: 816 691-1861
Class Cap: 9
Length: 24 mos   *Award:* Cert

Rolla Technical Institute
Radiography Prgm
1304 E Tenth St
Rolla, MO 65401-3699
Prgm Dir: Waneta M Odgen, MEd RT(R)(M)
Tel: 573 364-3726   *Fax:* 573 365-0767
Med Dir: Wendell Henderson
Class Cap: 24   *Begins:* July
Length: 24 mos   *Award:* Cert
Tuition per yr: $3,200

Cox Medical Centers
Radiography Prgm
1423 N Jefferson Ave
Springfield, MO 65802
Prgm Dir: Laura M Murney, MEd RT(R)
Tel: 417 836-8987   *Fax:* 417 269-5556
Med Dir: Lanny Brent
Class Cap: 22   *Begins:* Oct
Length: 24 mos   *Award:* Cert
Tuition per yr: $1,200 res, $1,200 non-res
Evening or weekend classes available

St John's Regional Health Center
Radiography Prgm
1235 E Cherokee St
Springfield, MO 65804-2263
Prgm Dir: Joan Hedrick, BA RT(R)
Tel: 417 885-2982   *Fax:* 417 888-7864
Med Dir: Thomas Sweeney, MD
Class Cap: 18
Length: 24 mos   *Award:* Cert
Tuition per yr: $1,300

Barnes-Jewish Hospital
Radiography Prgm
One Barnes Hospital Plaza
St Louis, MO 63110
Prgm Dir: Johnnie B Moore, BS RT(R)
Tel: 314 362-2977   *Fax:* 314 747-1573
Class Cap: 25
Length: 24 mos   *Award:* Cert
Tuition per yr: $1,250

St John's Mercy Medical Center
Radiography Prgm
615 S New Ballas Rd
St Louis, MO 63141-8221
Prgm Dir: Rachelle M Brenton, RT(R)
Tel: 314 569-6031   *Fax:* 314 569-6343
Med Dir: Donald B Spalding, MD
Class Cap: 12
Length: 24 mos   *Award:* Cert
Tuition per yr: $2,400

St Louis Comm College at Forest Park
Radiography Prgm
5600 Oakland Ave
St Louis, MO 63110
Prgm Dir: Darrell E McKay, PhD RT(R)
Tel: 314 644-9325   *Fax:* 314 644-9752
E-mail: dmckay@dalink.com
Med Dir: Joseph M Ziegler, MD
Class Cap: 35
Length: 24 mos   *Award:* AAS
Tuition per yr: $2,968 res, $3,760 non-res
Evening or weekend classes available

Montana

St Vincent Hospital & Health Center
Radiography Prgm
1233 N 30th St
PO Box 35200
Billings, MT 59107-5200
Prgm Dir: Guy A Copeman, RT(R)(T)
Tel: 406 657-7119   *Fax:* 406 657-8752
Med Dir: John Hanson, MD
Class Cap: 9   *Begins:* July
Length: 24 mos   *Award:* Cert
Tuition per yr: $450 res, $450 non-res

Benefits Health Care-West Campus
Radiography Prgm
500 15th Ave S
Great Falls, MT 59405
Prgm Dir: Thomas M Liston, RT(R)
Tel: 406 771-5146   *Fax:* 406 771-5162
Med Dir: John C. Hackethorn, MD
Class Cap: 6   *Begins:* July   *Award:* Cert
Tuition per yr: $500

St Patrick Hospital
Radiography Prgm
500 W Braodway
PO Box 4587
Missoula, MT 59801
Prgm Dir: Pamela J Liechti, BS RT(R)
Tel: 406 329-5829   *Fax:* 406 329-5690
Med Dir: Michael Stewart
Class Cap: 5   *Begins:* July
Length: 24 mos   *Award:* Cert
Tuition per yr: $800 res, $800 non-res

Nebraska

Mary Lanning Memorial Hospital
Radiography Prgm
715 N St Joseph Ave
Hastings, NE 68901
Prgm Dir: Jean M Korth, RT(R)
Tel: 402 461-5177   *Fax:* 402 461-5040
Med Dir: Jerry Adler
Class Cap: 10   *Begins:* July
Length: 24 mos   *Award:* Dipl
Tuition per yr: $1,500 res, $1,500 non-res

Southeast Community College
Radiography Prgm
8800 O St
Lincoln, NE 68520
Prgm Dir: Beverly Meidlinger, MEd RT(R)
Tel: 402 437-2775   *Fax:* 402 437-2404
Med Dir: Van Marcus
Class Cap: 24
Length: 24 mos   *Award:* AAS
Tuition per yr: $1,594 res, $1,906 non-res
Evening or weekend classes available

Alegent Health/Immanuel Medical Center
Radiography Prgm
6901 N 72nd St
Omaha, NE 68122
Prgm Dir: Luann Baylor, RT(R)
Tel: 402 572-2043   *Fax:* 402 572-2422
Class Cap: 12   *Begins:* Sep
Length: 24 mos   *Award:* Cert
Tuition per yr: $3,200 res, $2,400 non-res

Clarkson College
Radiography Prgm
101 S 42nd St
Omaha, NE 68131-2739
Prgm Dir: James L Zwieg, BS RT(R)
Tel: 402 552-6140   *Fax:* 402 552-6058
E-mail: zwieg@clrkcol.crhsnet.edu
Med Dir: N Nelson
Class Cap: 20   *Begins:* Aug
Length: 24 mos   *Award:* AS
Tuition per yr: $10,218 res, $10,218 non-res

St Joseph Hospital
Radiography Prgm
601 N 30th St
Omaha, NE 68103-0630
Prgm Dir: Janet L Moore, BSRT(R,M)
Tel: 402 449-4530   *Fax:* 402 449-4270
Med Dir: Peter Doris, MD
Class Cap: 10   *Begins:* Aug
Length: 24 mos   *Award:* Cert
Tuition per yr: $3,000 res, $3,000 non-res

University of Nebraska Medical Center
Radiography Prgm
600 S 42nd St
Omaha, NE 68198-1045
Prgm Dir: James B Temme, MPA RT(R)
Tel: 402 559-6954   *Fax:* 402 559-1011
E-mail: jtemme@unmc.edu
Class Cap: 10   *Begins:* Aug
Length: 36 mos   *Award:* Dipl, BS
Tuition per yr: $2,534 res, $6,909 non-res

Regional West Medical Center
Radiography Prgm
4021 Ave B
Scottsbluff, NE 69361
Prgm Dir: Daniel R Gilbert, RT(R)
Tel: 308 632-1140 *Fax:* 308 630-1120
Med Dir: John Strobel
Class Cap: 5 *Begins:* Aug
Length: 24 mos *Award:* Cert

Nevada

University of Nevada Las Vegas
Radiography Prgm
4505 Maryland Pkwy
Las Vegas, NV 89154-3017
Prgm Dir: Patrick Apsel
Tel: 702 895-0985
Class Cap: 40 *Begins:* Aug
Length: 24 mos *Award:* Cert
Tuition per yr: $2,272

Truckee Meadows Community College
Radiography Prgm
7000 Dandini Blvd
Reno, NV 89512-3999
Prgm Dir: Deborah K Baker, BS RT(R)
Tel: 702 673-7121 *Fax:* 702 673-7034
Med Dir: Lynn Learey
Class Cap: 14 *Begins:* Aug
Length: 24 mos *Award:* AAS
Tuition per yr: $1,205 res, $4,405 non-res

New Hampshire

New Hampshire Technical Institute
Radiography Prgm
11 Institute Dr
Concord, NH 03301-7412
Prgm Dir: Kevin P Barry, BS RT(R)
Tel: 603 225-1234 *Fax:* 603 225-1895
Med Dir: Gerard Smith, PhD
Class Cap: 26 *Begins:* July
Length: 24 mos *Award:* AS
Tuition per yr: $3,816 res, $5,616 non-res
Evening or weekend classes available

New Jersey

Atlantic City Medical Center
Radiography Prgm
1925 Pacific Ave
Atlantic City, NJ 08401
Prgm Dir: Theodore C Vanderlaan, BS RT(R)
Tel: 609 441-8010 *Fax:* 609 441-2166
E mail:
    tvanderlaan@acmco1.ccmail.compuserve.com
Class Cap: 17
Length: 24 mos *Award:* Cert
Tuition per yr: $2,000

Hudson Area School of Radiologic Tech
Radiography Prgm
29 E 29th St
Bayonne, NJ 07002
Prgm Dir: Kenneth Lee, BS RT(R)(M)
Tel: 201 858-5348 *Fax:* 201 858-7363
Med Dir: Eileen Coullnovon
Class Cap: 14
Length: 24 mos *Award:* Cert
Tuition per yr: $4,000

S Jersey Hosp System/Bridgeton Hosp Div
Radiography Prgm
333 Irving Ave
Bridgeton, NJ 08302
Prgm Dir: Edith K Rodriguez, RT(R)
Tel: 609 451-6600 *Fax:* 609 451-0335
Med Dir: Paul Chase, DO
Class Cap: 9 *Begins:* Sep
Length: 24 mos *Award:* Cert
Tuition per yr: $1,500

Cooper Hospital/University Medical Ctr
Radiography Prgm
One Cooper Plaza
Camden, NJ 08103
Prgm Dir: Francis V Williams, BS RT(R)
Tel: 609 342-2397 *Fax:* 609 868-0381
Class Cap: 25 *Begins:* Sep
Length: 24 mos *Award:* Cert
Tuition per yr: $2,000

West Jersey Hospital System
Radiography Prgm
1000 Atlantic Ave
Camden, NJ 08104
Prgm Dir: Barbara Hoffrichter, MEd RT(R)
Tel: 609 342-4629 *Fax:* 609 342-4336
Class Cap: 16
Length: 24 mos *Award:* Cert
Tuition per yr: $1,000

Burdette Tomlin Memorial Hospital
Radiography Prgm
Rte 9 and Stone Harbor Blvd
Cape May CourtHouse, NJ 08210
Prgm Dir: Kathleen E McGarry, PhD RT(R)
Tel: 609 463-2000
Med Dir: Marvin Podolnick, MD
Class Cap: 8 *Begins:* Jul
Length: 24 mos *Award:* Cert
Tuition per yr: $1,500 res, $1,500 non-res

Middlesex County College
Radiography Prgm
155 Mill Rd
PO Box 3050
Edison, NJ 08818-3050
Prgm Dir: Albert M Snopek, BS RT(R)
Tel: 908 548-6000 *Fax:* 908 907-7784
Med Dir: F D Wald, MD FACR
Class Cap: 53 *Begins:* Aug
Length: 24 mos *Award:* AAS
Tuition per yr: $1,337 res, $2,602 non-res

Elizabeth General Medical Center
Radiography Prgm
925 E Jersey St
Elizabeth, NJ 07201
Prgm Dir: Alice F Harris, BS RT(R)(M)
Tel: 908 629-8046 *Fax:* 908 629-8219
Class Cap: 20
Length: 24 mos *Award:* Cert
Tuition per yr: $3,892

Englewood Hospital and Medical Center
Radiography Prgm
350 Engle St
Englewood, NJ 07631
Prgm Dir: Pamela Woodward, MS RT(R)(M)(MR)
Tel: 201 894-3481 *Fax:* 201 894-1924
Med Dir: Mark Shepiro
Class Cap: 10
Length: 24 mos *Award:* Cert

Hackensack Medical Center
Radiography Prgm
30 Prospect Ave
Hillcrest Bldg
Hackensack, NJ 07601
Prgm Dir: Beverly M Patrizze, AAS RT(R)
Tel: 201 996-3680
Class Cap: 15
Length: 24 mos *Award:* Cert
Tuition per yr: $3,000

Morristown Memorial Hospital
Radiography Prgm
100 Madison Ave CN 1956
Morristown, NJ 07962-1956
Prgm Dir: Deborah J Dougless, BA RT(R)
Tel: 201 971-4082 *Fax:* 201 540-8407
Class Cap: 10 *Begins:* Sep
Length: 24 mos *Award:* Cert
Tuition per yr: $3,000

Memorial Hospital of Burlington County
Radiography Prgm
175 Madison Ave
Mt Holly, NJ 08060
Prgm Dir: Sharon L Grovatt, AAS RT(R)
Tel: 609 267-0700
Class Cap: 15
Length: 24 mos *Award:* Cert
Tuition per yr: $2,752 res, $5,342 non-res

Essex County College
Radiography Prgm
303 University Ave
Newark, NJ 07102
Prgm Dir: Kathleen Guyton, MA RT(R)
Tel: 201 877-3497 *Fax:* 201 623-6449
Class Cap: 24
Length: 27 mos *Award:* AAS
Tuition per yr: $1,800 res, $3,600 non-res
Evening or weekend classes available

Bergen Community College
Radiography Prgm
400 Paramus Rd
Paramus, NJ 07652
Prgm Dir: William L Leonard, MA RT(R)
Tel: 201 447-7178 *Fax:* 201 612-8225
Class Cap: 56
Length: 24 mos *Award:* AAS
Tuition per yr: $2,908 res, $5,816 non-res

Passaic County Community College
Radiography Prgm
College Blvd
Paterson, NJ 07509
Prgm Dir: Eileen M Maloney, MEd RT(R)
Tel: 201 684-5280 *Fax:* 201 684-5843
Med Dir: Frank R Schell, MD
Class Cap: 36 *Begins:* Sep
Length: 24 mos *Award:* AAS
Tuition per yr: $738 res, $738 non-res
Evening or weekend classes available

Muhlenberg Regional Medical Center

Radiography Prgm
Park Ave and Randolph Rd
Plainfield, NJ 07061
Prgm Dir: Susan J Fisler, RT(R)
Tel: 908 668-2844 *Fax:* 908 668-3164
Med Dir: Gordon Melville, MD
Class Cap: 31
Length: 27 mos *Award:* Dipl, AS
Tuition per yr: $8,500

Riverview Medical Center

Radiography Prgm
1 Riverview Plaza
Red Bank, NJ 07701
Prgm Dir: Jeffrey P Keane, BS RT(R)
Tel: 908 530-2284 *Fax:* 908 224-7214
Med Dir: John Parrella, MD
Class Cap: 12 *Begins:* July
Length: 24 mos *Award:* Cert
Tuition per yr: $2,500

The Valley Hospital

Radiography Prgm
223 N Van Dien Ave
Ridgewood, NJ 07450
Prgm Dir: Denise Hampson, BS RT(R)
Tel: 201 447-8221 *Fax:* 201 447-8429
Med Dir: Louis E Rambler, MD
Class Cap: 13 *Begins:* Sep
Length: 24 mos *Award:* Cert, AAS

Shore Memorial Hospital

Radiography Prgm
644 Shore Rd
Somers Point, NJ 08244
Prgm Dir: Richard Eric Olson, BS RT(R)
Tel: 609 653-3924 *Fax:* 609 926-1987
E-mail: ericolson@smh1.cmail.compuserve.com
Med Dir: Richard Menghetti, MD
Class Cap: 13 *Begins:* July
Length: 24 mos *Award:* Cert
Tuition per yr: $2,000

Marriott Health Care/Helene Fuld Med Ctr

Radiography Prgm
750 Brunswick Ave
Trenton, NJ 08638
Prgm Dir: Gail J Hoffman, BS RT(R)
Tel: 609 394-6068 *Fax:* 609 989-1512
Med Dir: Michael Stebbins, MD
Class Cap: 10 *Begins:* Jun
Length: 24 mos *Award:* Cert
Tuition per yr: $2,000

Mercer County Community College

Radiography Prgm
1200 Old Trenton Rd
PO Box B
Trenton, NJ 08690
Prgm Dir: Sandra L Kerr, MA RT(R)
Tel: 609 586-4800 *Fax:* 609 586-2318
Med Dir: Gregory Kaufman, MD
Class Cap: 31 *Begins:* Aug
Length: 24 mos *Award:* AAS
Tuition per yr: $2,275 res, $3,415 non-res

St Francis Medical Center

Radiography Prgm
601 Hamilton Ave
Trenton, NJ 08629-1986
Prgm Dir: Theresa M Levitsky, AAS RT(R)
Tel: 609 599-5234 *Fax:* 609 599-6254
Med Dir: Joel Namm, MD
Class Cap: 12 *Begins:* Jul
Length: 24 mos *Award:* Dipl,Cert
Tuition per yr: $1,250

Cumberland County College

Radiography Prgm
College Dr PO Box 517
Vineland, NJ 08360
Prgm Dir: Jane Leggieri, MS RT(R)
Tel: 609 691-8600 *Fax:* 609 691-9489
Med Dir: Ernesto Go, MD
Class Cap: 33 *Begins:* Sep
Length: 24 mos *Award:* AAS
Tuition per yr: $2,287 res, $4,573 non-res
Evening or weekend classes available

Pascack Valley Hospital

Radiography Prgm
Old Hook Rd
Westwood, NJ 07675-3181
Prgm Dir: Diane C DeVos, RT(R)
Tel: 201 358-3219 *Fax:* 201 358-3216
Med Dir: Anna B Kelly, MD MACR
Class Cap: 14 *Begins:* Sep
Length: 24 mos *Award:* Cert
Tuition per yr: res, $1,500 non-res

New Mexico

PIMA Medical Institute - Albuquerque

Radiography Prgm
2201 San Pedro NE
Bldg 3 Ste 100
Albuquerque, NM 87110
Prgm Dir: Sherry M Floerchinger, BS RT(R)(N)
Tel: 505 881-1234 *Fax:* 505 884-8371
Class Cap: 31 *Begins:* Aug
Length: 23 mos *Award:* AS
Tuition per yr: $4,750 res, $4,750 non-res

Univ of New Mexico School of Medicine

Radiography Prgm
Hlth Sciences and Svc Bldg
Rm 217
Albuquerque, NM 87131-5656
Prgm Dir: Robert A Fosbinder, BA RT(R)
Tel: 505 277-5254 *Fax:* 505 277-7011
Med Dir: Fred A Mettler Jr, MD
Class Cap: 15
Length: 24 mos *Award:* AS
Tuition per yr: $998 res, $3,771 non-res
Evening or weekend classes available

Clovis Community College

Radiography Prgm
417 Schepps Blvd
Clovis, NM 88101
Prgm Dir: Jeannie Kilgore, MEd RT(R)
Tel: 505 769-4996 *Fax:* 505 769-4190
Med Dir: Martin Goodwin
Class Cap: 16
Length: 24 mos *Award:* AAS
Tuition per yr: $486 res, $508 non-res
Evening or weekend classes available

Northern New Mexico Community College

Radiography Prgm
1002 N Onate St
Espanola, NM 87532
Prgm Dir: Donna Foster, AAS RT(R)
Tel: 505 747-2218 *Fax:* 505 747-2180
E-mail: foster@nnm.cc.nm.edu
Med Dir: Robin Gaupp, MD
Class Cap: 14 *Begins:* June Aug
Length: 24 mos *Award:* AAS
Tuition per yr: $615 res, $1,798 non-res
Evening or weekend classes available

Dona Ana Branch Community College

Radiography Prgm
3400 S Espina St
Las Cruces, NM 88003-8001
Prgm Dir: Joyce M Ortego, MS RT(R)
Tel: 505 527-7581 *Fax:* 505 527-7515
E-mail: jortego@nmsu.edu
Med Dir: Eduardo Martinez
Class Cap: 18 *Begins:* Fall Sem
Length: 22 mos *Award:* AS
Tuition per yr: $961 res, $1,116 non-res
Evening or weekend classes available

New York

Albany Memorial Hospital

Radiography Prgm
600 Northern Blvd
Albany, NY 12204
Prgm Dir: Colleen A Carnegie, RT(R)
Tel: 518 471-3238 *Fax:* 518 471-3064
Class Cap: 10 *Begins:* July
Length: 24 mos *Award:* Cert
Tuition per yr: $600 res, $600 non-res

Broome Community College

Radiography Prgm
Upper Front St
PO Box 1017
Binghamton, NY 13902
Prgm Dir: Nancy E Button, MS RT(R)
Tel: 607 778-5070 *Fax:* 607 778-5345
E-mail: button_n@sunybroome.edu
Class Cap: 30
Length: 24 mos *Award:* AAS

CUNY Bronx Community College

Radiography Prgm
University Ave and W 181st St
Bronx, NY 10453
Prgm Dir: Virginia M Mishkin, MS RT(R)(M)
Tel: 718 289-5396 *Fax:* 718 289-6373
Class Cap: 33 *Begins:* Sep
Length: 24 mos *Award:* Dipl, AAS
Tuition per yr: $2,400 res, $3,076 non-res

Hostos Community College of CUNY

Radiography Prgm
475 Grand Concourse
Bronx, NY 10451
Prgm Dir: Allen Solomon, MSEd RT(R)
Tel: 718 518-4123
Class Cap: 73
Length: 24 mos *Award:* AAS

CUNY New York City Technical College

Radiography Prgm
300 Jay St
Brooklyn, NY 11201-2983
Prgm Dir: Sonja L Jackson, EdD RT(R)
Tel: 718 260-5362
Class Cap: 64
Length: 24 mos *Award:* AAS

Long Island College Hospital

Radiography Prgm
340 Henry St
Brooklyn, NY 11201
Prgm Dir: Evans Lespinasse, BS RT(R)
Tel: 718 780-1681
Med Dir: R T Bergeron, MD
Class Cap: 12 *Begins:* Sep
Length: 24 mos *Award:* Cert
Tuition per yr: $3,938

New York Methodist Hospital

Radiography Prgm
506 Sixth St
Brooklyn, NY 11215
Prgm Dir: William J Brennan Jr, BA RT(R)
Tel: 718 780-3887 *Fax:* 718 780-3414
Med Dir: Joseph Giovannello
Class Cap: 14 *Begins:* Sep
Length: 24 mos *Award:* Cert
Tuition per yr: $4,000

SUNY Health Science Center - Brooklyn

Radiography Prgm
450 Clarkson Ave
Box 1226
Brooklyn, NY 11203
Prgm Dir: Kenneth P Martinucci, BS RT(R)
Tel: 718 270-2929 *Fax:* 718 270-7751
E-mail: kmartinucci@netmail.nscbklyn.edu
Med Dir: Joshua A Becker, MD
Class Cap: 40
Length: 24 mos *Award:* Cert
Tuition per yr: $2,150

Long Island Univ - C W Post Campus

Radiography Prgm
720 Northern Blvd
Brookville, NY 11548-1300
Prgm Dir: James F Joyce, BS RT(R)
Tel: 516 299-3075 *Fax:* 516 299-3081
E-mail: radtech@titan.liu.net.edu
Med Dir: Gerald Irwin, MD CM FACH
Class Cap: 56 *Begins:* Sep
Length: 48 mos *Award:* BS
Tuition per yr: $13,120
Evening or weekend classes available

Millard Fillmore Health Systems

Radiography Prgm
3 Gates Circle
Buffalo, NY 14209
Prgm Dir: Cynthia A Sciera, BS RT(R)
Tel: 716 887-5129
Length: 24 mos *Award:* Cert
Tuition per yr: $4,400

Trocaire College

Radiography Prgm
110 Red Jacket Pkwy
Buffalo, NY 14220-2094
Prgm Dir: Nancy L Augustyn, MSEd RT(R)
Tel: 716 826-1200 *Fax:* 716 826-0059
Med Dir: Noel M Chaintella, MD
Class Cap: 40 *Begins:* Aug
Length: 24 mos *Award:* AAS
Tuition per yr: $5,850
Evening or weekend classes available

Arnot Ogden Medical Center

Radiography Prgm
600 Roe Ave
Elmira, NY 14905-1676
Prgm Dir: Ellen R Richards, BS RT(R)
Tel: 607 737-4289 *Fax:* 607 737-4116
Med Dir: Renato H Rojas, MD
Class Cap: 7 *Begins:* Aug
Length: 24 mos *Award:* Cert
Tuition per yr: $2,550 res, $2,550 non-res

Peninsula Hospital Center

Radiography Prgm
51-15 Beach Channel Dr
Far Rockaway, NY 11691-1074
Prgm Dir: Ellen R Klinsky, BA LRT
Tel: 718 945-7100, Ext 891 *Fax:* 718 954-6828
Med Dir: Stanley Sprecher, MD
Class Cap: 12
Length: 24 mos *Award:* Cert
Tuition per yr: $5,000

Nassau Community College

Radiography Prgm
One Education Dr
Garden City, NY 11530
Prgm Dir: Jeffrey T Miller, BS RT(R)
Tel: 516 572-7559
Med Dir: Howard Gelber, MD
Class Cap: 30
Length: 24 mos *Award:* AAS
Tuition per yr: $1,950 res, $3,900 non-res
Evening or weekend classes available

Glens Falls Hospital

Radiography Prgm
100 Park St
Glens Falls, NY 12801
Prgm Dir: Mitch Bieber
Tel: 518 792-3151 *Fax:* 518 761-5288
Med Dir: John Tata, MD
Class Cap: 10 *Begins:* Aug
Length: 24 mos *Award:* Cert
Tuition per yr: $1,500 res, $1,500 non-res

St James Mercy Hospital

Radiography Prgm
411 Canisteo St
Hornell, NY 14843
Prgm Dir: Lynne M Freeland, BS RT(R)
Tel: 607 324-8265 *Fax:* 607 324-8070
Med Dir: Iddo Netamyshu, MD
Class Cap: 5 *Begins:* July
Length: 24 mos *Award:* Dipl,Cert
Tuition per yr: $3,000

Cayuga Medical Center at Ithaca

Radiography Prgm
101 Dates Dr
Ithaca, NY 14850
Prgm Dir: Thomas Kleckner, RT(R)
Tel: 607 274-4376
Class Cap: 6 *Begins:* Sep
Length: 24 mos *Award:* Cert
Tuition per yr: $1,000 res, $1,000 non-res

Woman's Christian Association Hospital

Radiography Prgm
207 Foote Ave
Jamestown, NY 14701-0840
Prgm Dir: Cheryl A Macey, BS RT(R)
Tel: 716 664-8238
Med Dir: James G Dahlie, MD
Class Cap: 6 *Begins:* Aug
Length: 22 mos, 24 mos *Award:* Cert
Tuition per yr: $750

Orange County Community College

Radiography Prgm
115 South St
Middletown, NY 10940
Prgm Dir: Robert M Misiak, BS RT(R)
Tel: 914 341-4275 *Fax:* 914 343-1228
Med Dir: K Schwartz, MD
Class Cap: 47 *Begins:* Sep
Length: 24 mos *Award:* AAS
Tuition per yr: $4,536 res, $9,072 non-res
Evening or weekend classes available

Winthrop University Hospital

Radiography Prgm
259 First St
Mineola, NY 11501
Prgm Dir: Virginia M Edele, MBA RT(R)
Tel: 516 663-2536 *Fax:* 516 663-3884
Class Cap: 10
Length: 24 mos *Award:* Cert
Tuition per yr: $3,500

Bellevue Hospital Center

Radiography Prgm
First Ave and 27th St
New York, NY 10016
Prgm Dir: James L Bain, BS RT(R)
Tel: 212 561-4895
Class Cap: 30
Length: 24 mos *Award:* Cert
Tuition per yr: $5,400

Harlem Hospital Center

Radiography Prgm
506 Lenox Ave
Kountz Pavilion Rm 415
New York, NY 10037
Prgm Dir: George A Ramsay, BS RT(R)
Tel: 212 939-3475
Class Cap: 18
Length: 24 mos *Award:* Cert
Tuition per yr: $3,000

Northport VA Medical Center #632C

Radiography Prgm
79 Middleville Rd (632/153)
Northport, NY 11768
Prgm Dir: Joseph E Whitton, BS RT(R)
Tel: 516 261-4400 *Fax:* 516 266-6012
Med Dir: Paul Boneheim, MD
Class Cap: 20
Length: 24 mos *Award:* Dipl,Cert
Tuition per yr: $500 res, $500 non-res

Programs

Hochstim Sch Radiography/S Nassau Hosp

Radiography Prgm
2445 Oceanside Rd
Oceanside, NY 11572
Prgm Dir: Robert Dacker, MAd RT(R)
Tel: 516 763-2030   *Fax:* 516 763-3949
Med Dir: Stewart R. Bakst, MD
Class Cap: 10
Length: 24 mos   *Award:* Cert
Tuition per yr: $4,000 res, $4,000 non-res

Champlain Valley Phys Hospital Med Ctr

Radiography Prgm
100 Beekman St
Plattsburgh, NY 12901
Prgm Dir: Fayrene M Ashline, BS RT(R)
Tel: 518 562-7510   *Fax:* 518 562-7505
Med Dir: David Hammack, MD
Class Cap: 12   *Begins:* July
Length: 24 mos   *Award:* Cert, AS
Tuition per yr: $4,000 res, $4,000 non-res

United Hospital Medical Center

Radiography Prgm
406 Boston Post Rd
Port Chester, NY 10573
Prgm Dir: Rose P LaBate, BS RT(R)(M)
Tel: 914 934-3000   *Fax:* 914 934-3199
Class Cap: 10
Length: 24 mos   *Award:* Cert
Tuition per yr: $6,000

Central Suffolk Hospital

Radiography Prgm
1300 Roanoke Ave
Riverhead, NY 11901
Prgm Dir: William L DeCamp, BS RT(R)
Tel: 516 548-6173   *Fax:* 516 548-6751
Class Cap: 17
Length: 24 mos   *Award:* Cert
Tuition per yr: $1,400

Monroe Community College

Radiography Prgm
1000 E Henrietta Rd
Rochester, NY 14623-5780
Prgm Dir: Betty J Grabowski, BS RT(R)
Tel: 716 292-2378
Med Dir: James Haggerty, MD
Class Cap: 32   *Begins:* Sep
Length: 24 mos   *Award:* AAS
Tuition per yr: $2,410 res, $4,820 non-res

Mercy Medical Center

Radiography Prgm
1000 N Village Ave
Rockville Centre, NY 11570-1098
Prgm Dir: Regina M Friedman, MS RT(R)
Tel: 516 255-2602   *Fax:* 516 764-3662
Med Dir: Joseph J Macy, MD FACR
Class Cap: 11   *Begins:* Sep
Length: 24 mos   *Award:* Cert
Tuition per yr: $3,000

Niagara County Community College

Radiography Prgm
3111 Saunders Settlement Rd
Sanborn, NY 14132
Prgm Dir: Carolyn Cianciosa, MS RT(R)
Tel: 716 731-3271   *Fax:* 716 731-4053
Med Dir: Brian Block
Class Cap: 24
Length: 24 mos   *Award:* AAS
Tuition per yr: $2,250 res, $2,250 non-res
Evening or weekend classes available

North Country Community College

Radiography Prgm
20 Winona Ave
PO Box 89
Saranac Lake, NY 12983-0089
Prgm Dir: Andrea M Trigg Stevens, MS RT(R)
Tel: 518 891-2915   *Fax:* 518 891-2915
Med Dir: Richard Moccia
Length: 24 mos   *Award:* AAS
Tuition per yr: $3,800 res, $3,600 non-res

SUNY Health Science Center at Syracuse

Radiography Prgm
750 E Adams St
Syracuse, NY 13210
Prgm Dir: Patricia J Duffy, MPS RT(R)
Tel: 315 464-4464   *Fax:* 315 464-6914
E-mail: duffyp@vax.cs.hscsyr.edu
Med Dir: Stephen Kieffer, MD
Class Cap: 49   *Begins:* Aug
Length: 23 mos   *Award:* AAS
Tuition per yr: $4,574 res, $11,225 non-res

Hudson Valley Community College

Radiography Prgm
80 Vandenburgh Ave
Troy, NY 12180
Prgm Dir: Jeanne S Kelleher, BS RT(R)
Tel: 518 270-7123   *Fax:* 518 270-7452
Class Cap: 40   *Begins:* Aug
Length: 24 mos   *Award:* AAS
Tuition per yr: $2,150 res, $5,000 non-res
Evening or weekend classes available

St Elizabeth Hospital

Radiography Prgm
2209 Genesee St
Utica, NY 13501
Prgm Dir: Mary Louise Ecret, RT(R) LRT
Tel: 315 798-8258   *Fax:* 315 798-8382
Class Cap: 13
Length: 24 mos   *Award:* Cert
Tuition per yr: $2,000

St Luke's Memorial Hospital Center

Radiography Prgm
Champlin Ave
PO Box 479
Utica, NY 13503-0479
Prgm Dir: Rosemary Morin, MS RT(R)
Tel: 315 798-6136   *Fax:* 315 798-6295
Class Cap: 20
Length: 24 mos   *Award:* Cert
Tuition per yr: $2,600

Westchester Community College

Radiography Prgm
75 Grasslands Rd
Valhalla, NY 10595-1698
Prgm Dir: Melvin D Thornhill, MPA RT(R)
Tel: 914 785-6882
Class Cap: 99
Length: 24 mos   *Award:* AAS

Catholic Medical Center

Radiography Prgm
89-15 Woodhaven Blvd
Woodhaven, NY 11421
Prgm Dir: Barbara Wilson- Chakmakjian, MS RT(R)
Tel: 718 805-7099   *Fax:* 718 805-7189
Med Dir: Joseph N Savino, MD
Begins: Sep
Length: 24 mos   *Award:* Cert
Tuition per yr: $5,000

North Carolina

Asheville Buncombe Technical Comm Coll

Radiography Prgm
340 Victoria Rd
Asheville, NC 28801
Prgm Dir: Debra J Reese, MPH RT(R)
Tel: 704 254-1921   *Fax:* 704 667-3660
E-mail: debreese@prodigy.com
Med Dir: Thomas Kennedy, MD
Class Cap: 20   *Begins:* Sep
Length: 21 mos   *Award:* AAS
Tuition per yr: $742
Evening or weekend classes available

Univ of North Carolina at Chapel Hill

Radiography Prgm
CB 7130 E Wing
Medical School
Chapel Hill, NC 27599-7130
Prgm Dir: Joy J Renner, MA RT(R)
Tel: 919 966-5146   *Fax:* 919 966-3678
E-mail: jrenner@css.unc.edu
Class Cap: 12   *Begins:* July
Length: 48 mos   *Award:* BS
Tuition per yr: $1,450 res, $1,450 non-res

Presbyterian Hospital

Radiography Prgm
200 Hawthorne Ln
PO Box 33549
Charlotte, NC 28233-3549
Prgm Dir: Shelley J Sumpter, BA RT(R)
Tel: 704 384-4056   *Fax:* 704 358-9691
Med Dir: Bennett R Hollenberg, MD
Class Cap: 10   *Begins:* July
Length: 24 mos   *Award:* Cert
Tuition per yr: $850

Fayetteville Technical Community College

Radiography Prgm
PO Box 35236
Fayetteville, NC 28303-0236
Prgm Dir: Mary Jane Gentry, EdD RT(R)
Tel: 910 678-8303   *Fax:* 910 484-6600
Med Dir: Gerald Ellison, MD
Class Cap: 18
Length: 21 mos   *Award:* AAS
Tuition per yr: $742 res, $6,020 non-res

Gaston Memorial Hospital
Radiography Prgm
2525 Court Dr
PO Box 1747
Gastonia, NC 28053-1747
Prgm Dir: Ernest C Griffith Jr, PhD RT(R)
Tel: 704 834-2949   *Fax:* 704 834-2282
Med Dir: Carlos Vargas, MD
Class Cap: 10
Length: 24 mos   *Award:* Cert
Tuition per yr: $400

Moses H Cone Memorial Hospital
Radiography Prgm
1200 N Elm St
Greensboro, NC 27401-1020
Prgm Dir: Elizabeth S Shields, BS RT(R)
Tel: 910 574-7528   *Fax:* 910 574-7381
E-mail: shieldb1@mosescone.com
Med Dir: Arthur F Kriner, MD
Class Cap: 15   *Begins:* July
Length: 24 mos   *Award:* Cert
Tuition per yr: $250

Pitt Community College
Radiography Prgm
PO Drawer 7007
Hwy 11 S
Greenville, NC 27835-7007
Prgm Dir: Louise R Cox, BA RT(R)
Tel: 919 355-4254   *Fax:* 919 321-4451
Med Dir: Julian R Vainright Jr, MD
Class Cap: 31   *Begins:* Sep
Length: 24 mos   *Award:* AAS
Tuition per yr: $742 res, $6,020 non-res
Evening or weekend classes available

Vance Granville Community College
Radiography Prgm
PO Box 917
Henderson, NC 27536
Prgm Dir: Angela R Ballentine, MEd RT(R)
Tel: 919 492-2061   *Fax:* 919 430-0460
Class Cap: 32
Length: 24 mos   *Award:* AAS
Tuition per yr: $778 res, $6,020 non-res

Caldwell Comm College & Tech Institute
Radiography Prgm
2855 Hickory Blvd
Hudson, NC 28638
Prgm Dir: Rosanne Y Annas, RT(R)
Tel: 704 726-2356   *Fax:* 704 726-2216
Med Dir: Richard Curtis, MD
Class Cap: 15   *Begins:* June
Length: 24 mos   *Award:* AAS
Tuition per yr: $742 res, $6,020 non-res
Evening or weekend classes available

Lenoir Memorial Hospital
Radiography Prgm
100 Airport Rd
Box 1678
Kinston, NC 28501-0678
Prgm Dir: Johnny H Graham, RT(R)
Tel: 919 522-7088   *Fax:* 919 522-7167
Med Dir: Lewis B Gilpin, MD
Class Cap: 5   *Begins:* Sep
Length: 24 mos   *Award:* Cert
Tuition per yr: $150

Carteret Community College
Radiography Prgm
3505 Arendell St
Morehead City, NC 28557-2989
Prgm Dir: Larry H Miller, RT(R)
Tel: 919 247-3097   *Fax:* 919 247-2514
E-mail: miller/@ncccs.cc.nc.us
Med Dir: William Rickey, MD
Class Cap: 16   *Begins:* Sep
Length: 24 mos   *Award:* AAS
Tuition per yr: $763 res, $6,041 non-res

Wilkes Regional Medical Center
Radiography Prgm
West D St/PO Box 609
North Wilkesboro, NC 28659
Prgm Dir: Betty S Winslow, MA RT(R)
Tel: 910 651-8431   *Fax:* 910 651-8437
Med Dir: Lawrence Bennett, MD
Class Cap: 9
Length: 24 mos   *Award:* Cert
Tuition per yr: $2,500 res, $2,500 non-res

Sandhills Community College
Radiography Prgm
2200 Airport Rd
Pinehurst, NC 28374
Prgm Dir: Michael D Emery, BS RT(R)
Tel: 910 695-3841   *Fax:* 910 692-2756
Med Dir: Daniel Clark, MD
Class Cap: 18   *Begins:* Sep
Length: 24 mos   *Award:* AAS
Tuition per yr: $768 res, $6,048 non-res

Wake Technical Community College
Radiography Prgm
9101 F9101 Fayetteville Rd
Raleigh, NC 27603
Prgm Dir: Anita R Phillips, RTR BS
Tel: 919 231-4500   *Fax:* 919 779-3360
E-mail: alpblp@aol.com
Med Dir: Donald G Detweiler, MD
Class Cap: 24   *Begins:* Sep
Length: 21 mos   *Award:* AAS
Tuition per yr: $742 res, $6,020 non-res
Evening or weekend classes available

Edgecombe Community College
Radiography Prgm
225 Tarboro St
Rocky Mount, NC 27801
Prgm Dir: Fonda H Worthington, BS RT(R)
Tel: 919 446-0436   *Fax:* 919 985-2212
Med Dir: Frederick Williams
Class Cap: 30
Length: 24 mos   *Award:* AAS
Tuition per yr: $742 res, $6,020 non-res
Evening or weekend classes available

Rowan-Cabarrus Community College
Radiography Prgm
PO Box 1595
Salisbury, NC 28145-1595
Prgm Dir: Terry N Chapman, MS RT(R)
Tel: 704 637-0760   *Fax:* 704 642-0750
Class Cap: 21   *Begins:* Aug
Length: 24 mos   *Award:* AAS
Tuition per yr: $185 res, $1,505 non-res

Cleveland Community College
Radiography Prgm
137 S Post Rd
Shelby, NC 28150
Prgm Dir: JoAnn Schilling, EdS RT(R)
Tel: 704 484-4091   *Fax:* 704 484-4036
Med Dir: Thomas Blackburn, MD
Class Cap: 9   *Begins:* Sep
Length: 24 mos   *Award:* AAS
Tuition per yr: $186 res, $9,505 non-res

Johnston Community College
Radiography Prgm
PO Box 2350
Smithfield, NC 27577-2350
Prgm Dir: Shelia W Smith, MEd RT(R)
Tel: 919 934-3051   *Fax:* 919 934-2823
Med Dir: Bradley Brenton
Class Cap: 26   *Begins:* Sep
Length: 24 mos   *Award:* AAS
Tuition per yr: $770 res, $6,048 non-res

Southwestern Community College
Radiography Prgm
275 Webster Rd
Sylva, NC 28779
Prgm Dir: Gene C Couch Jr, EdS RT(R)
Tel: 704 586-4091   *Fax:* 704 586-3129
Class Cap: 21
Length: 24 mos   *Award:* AAS
Tuition per yr: $766 res, $6,044 non-res
Evening or weekend classes available

Forsyth Technical Community College
Radiography Prgm
2100 Silas Creek Pkwy
Winston-Salem, NC 27103
Prgm Dir: Carolyn M Holland, BA RT(R)(T)
Tel: 910 723-0371   *Fax:* 910 748-9395
Class Cap: 41   *Begins:* Sep
Length: 24 mos   *Award:* AAS
Tuition per yr: $742 res, $6,020 non-res
Evening or weekend classes available

North Dakota

Medcenter One Health Systems
Radiography Prgm
300 N 7th St
Bismarck, ND 58506-5525
Prgm Dir: Mary Jo Bergman, MEd MS RT(R) RN
Tel: 701 222-5470   *Fax:* 701 222-5479
Med Dir: W H Cain
Class Cap: 9   *Begins:* Aug
Length: 24 mos   *Award:* Cert

St Alexius Medical Center
Radiography Prgm
900 E Broadway
Bismarck, ND 58502-5510
Prgm Dir: Dan Johannes, BS RT(R)
Tel: 701 224-7533   *Fax:* 701 224-7284
Med Dir: Lee Podoll, MD
Class Cap: 8   *Begins:* July
Length: 24 mos   *Award:* Cert
Tuition per yr: $8,500

MeritCare

Radiography Prgm
720 4th St N
Fargo, ND 58122
Prgm Dir: Dan T Jensen, BS RT(R)
Tel: 701 234-5165
Class Cap: 8
Length: 24 mos   *Award:* Cert
Tuition per yr: $4,000

Minot School for Allied Health

Radiography Prgm
401 S Main Ste C
Minot, ND 58701
Prgm Dir: Debbie K Hornbacher, BS RT(R)
Tel: 701 857-5620   *Fax:* 701 857-5245
Class Cap: 4
Length: 24 mos   *Award:* Cert
Tuition per yr: $1,300 res, $1,300 non-res

Ohio

Children's Hospital Medical Ctr of Akron

Radiography Prgm
One Perkins Square
Akron, OH 44308
Prgm Dir: David L Whipple, MEd RT(R)
Tel: 330 379-8849
Med Dir: Richard A Krams, MD
Class Cap: 7   *Begins:* July
Length: 24 mos   *Award:* Cert
Tuition per yr: $3,000

Summa Health System

Radiography Prgm
525 E Market St
Akron, OH 44309-2090
Prgm Dir: Bonnie J Rutledge, AAS RT(R)
Tel: 330 375-3696   *Fax:* 330 375-4759
Class Cap: 15   *Begins:* July
Length: 24 mos   *Award:* Dipl
Tuition per yr: $3,194

Aultman Hospital

Radiography Prgm
2600 Sixth St SW
Canton, OH 44710
Prgm Dir: John Zuppe, RT(R)
Tel: 330 438-7415   *Fax:* 330 438-7415
Med Dir: William Wallace
Class Cap: 14
Length: 24 mos   *Award:* Cert
Tuition per yr: $1,700

Timken Mercy Medical Center

Radiography Prgm
1320 Timken Mercy Dr NW
Canton, OH 44708
Prgm Dir: Gary F Greathouse, BS RT(R)
Tel: 330 489-1273   *Fax:* 330 489-1341
Med Dir: Laura Cawthon, MD
Class Cap: 8
Length: 24 mos   *Award:* Cert
Tuition per yr: $3,500

Univ of Cincinnati

Radiography Prgm
234 Goodman St ML 579
Cincinnati, OH 45267-0579
Prgm Dir: Tracy L Herrmann, MEd RT(R)
Tel: 513 558-7231   *Fax:* 513 558-0300
E-mail: tracy.herrmann@uc.edu
Med Dir: Gary Merhar, MD
Class Cap: 24   *Begins:* Sep
Length: 24 mos   *Award:* AAS
Tuition per yr: $4,628 res, $1,166 non-res
Evening or weekend classes available

Xavier University

Radiography Prgm
3800 Victory Pkwy
Cincinnati, OH 45207-4331
Prgm Dir: Donna J Endicott, BS RT(R)
Tel: 513 745-3358   *Fax:* 513 745-1954
E-mail: endicott@admin.xu.edu
Med Dir: Charles McCarthy, MD
Class Cap: 21   *Begins:* Aug
Length: 23 mos   *Award:* AS
Tuition per yr: $4,580 res, $4,580 non-res

Ohio State University

Radiography Prgm
1583 Perry St
Columbus, OH 43210-1234
Prgm Dir: William F Finney, MA RT(R)
Tel: 614 292-0571   *Fax:* 614 292-0210
E-mail: finney.1@osu.edu
Class Cap: 20   *Begins:* Sep
Length: 48 mos   *Award:* BS
Tuition per yr: $4,364 res, $13,084 non-res

Sinclair Community College

Radiography Prgm
444 W Third St
Dayton, OH 45402-1460
Prgm Dir: Denise E Moore, BS RT(R)
Tel: 513 226-2842   *Fax:* 513 449-5175
E-mail: dmoore@sinclaire.edu
Class Cap: 70   *Begins:* June Sep
Length: 24 mos   *Award:* AAS
Tuition per yr: $1,643 res, $2,491 non-res
Evening or weekend classes available

Lorain County Community College

Radiography Prgm
1005 N Abbe Rd
ST 210
Elyria, OH 44035
Prgm Dir: Jeffrey J Walmsley, BA RT(R)
Tel: 216 365-5222   *Fax:* 216 366-4116
Med Dir: Peter Fanton, DO
Class Cap: 43   *Begins:* Sep
Length: 24 mos   *Award:* AAS
Tuition per yr: res, $3,500 non-res
Evening or weekend classes available

Meridia Health System

Radiography Prgm
18901 Lakeshore Blvd
Euclid, OH 44119
Prgm Dir: Fred E Truesdail, AAS RT(R)
Tel: 216 692-8708   *Fax:* 216 692-7453
Med Dir: Jeffrey S Umger, MD
Class Cap: 7   *Begins:* July
Length: 24 mos   *Award:* Cert
Tuition per yr: $2,000

Kettering College of Medical Arts

Radiography Prgm
3737 Southern Blvd
Kettering, OH 45429
Prgm Dir: Larry Beneke, MSEd RT(R)
Tel: 513 296-7201   *Fax:* 513 296-4238
Class Cap: 22   *Begins:* Aug
Length: 20 mos, 24 mos   *Award:* Dipl, AS
Tuition per yr: $8,400

Lakeland Community College

Radiography Prgm
7700 Clocktower Dr
Kirtland, OH 44094-5198
Prgm Dir: Jack A Thomas, BS RT(R)
Tel: 216 953-7074   *Fax:* 216 975-4733
Med Dir: Victor J Demayrco, MD
Class Cap: 31
Length: 24 mos   *Award:* AAS
Tuition per yr: $2,377 res, $2,916 non-res
Evening or weekend classes available

Lima Technical College

Radiography Prgm
4240 Campus Dr
Lima, OH 45804-3597
Prgm Dir: Dennis F Spragg, MSEd RT(R)
Tel: 419 995-8257   *Fax:* 419 995-8818
E-mail: spraggdeltc.tec.oh.us
Class Cap: 30
Length: 24 mos   *Award:* AAS
Tuition per yr: $3,688 res, $7,346 non-res
Evening or weekend classes available

North Central Technical College

Radiography Prgm
2441 Kenwood Circle
PO Box 698
Mansfield, OH 44901-0698
Prgm Dir: Addie M Tackett, BS RT(R)
Tel: 419 755-4886   *Fax:* 419 755-5630
Med Dir: Joel E Kaye, MD
Class Cap: 13
Length: 24 mos   *Award:* AAS
Tuition per yr: $3,108 res, $5,830 non-res

Marietta Memorial Hospital

Radiography Prgm
401 Matthew St
Marietta, OH 45750
Prgm Dir: Paul E Richards Jr, BA RT(R)
Tel: 614 374-1640   *Fax:* 614 374-1480
Med Dir: Paul Prachun, MD FRCP(C)FACR
Class Cap: 7   *Begins:* Sep
Length: 24 mos   *Award:* Cert
Tuition per yr: $600 res, $600 non-res

Marion General Hospital

Radiography Prgm
McKinley Park Dr
Marion, OH 43302
Prgm Dir: Sharon W Wu, BA RT(R)
Tel: 614 383-8417   *Fax:* 614 929-8623
Class Cap: 6   *Begins:* Sep
Length: 24 mos   *Award:* Dipl,Cert, AAS
Tuition per yr: $2,100
Evening or weekend classes available

Southwest General Health Center

Radiography Prgm
18697 E Bagley Rd
Middleburg Hts, OH 44130
Prgm Dir: Judy A Buzas, MEd RT(R)
Tel: 216 816-8779 *Fax:* 216 816-8806
Med Dir: Walter George, MD
Class Cap: 6 *Begins:* July
Length: 24 mos *Award:* Cert
Tuition per yr: $2,000

Central Ohio Technical College

Radiography Prgm
1179 University Dr
Newark, OH 43055-1767
Prgm Dir: Linnea A Hopewell, MEd RT(R)(M)
Tel: 614 366-9387 *Fax:* 614 366-5047
Med Dir: Fearle Meyer, MD
Class Cap: 25 *Begins:* Sep
Length: 23 mos *Award:* AAS
Tuition per yr: $2,798 res, $6,038 non-res

Cuyahoga Community College

Radiography Prgm
Western Campus
11000 Pleasant Valley Rd
Parma, OH 44130-5199
Prgm Dir: Marilyn A Rep, BA RT(R)
Tel: 216 987-5363 *Fax:* 216 987-5066
Med Dir: Craig Irish, MD
Class Cap: 108
Length: 24 mos *Award:* AAS
Tuition per yr: $2,008 res, $2,668 non-res
Evening or weekend classes available

Shawnee State University

Radiography Prgm
940 Second St
Portsmouth, OH 45662-4344
Prgm Dir: William W Sykes, MBA RT(R)(M)(CT)
Tel: 614 355-2253 *Fax:* 614 355-2354
E-mail: bsykes@shawnee.edu
Class Cap: 22
Length: 24 mos *Award:* AAS
Tuition per yr: $4,276 res, $7,176 non-res
Evening or weekend classes available

Kent State University

Radiography Prgm
2491 SR 45 S
Salem, OH 44460-9412
Prgm Dir: Janice J Gibson, BS RT(R)
Tel: 330 332-0361 *Fax:* 330 332-9256
E-mail: gibson@salem.kent.edu
Med Dir: James Silverman, MD
Class Cap: 39 *Begins:* June
Length: 23 mos *Award:* AAS
Tuition per yr: $4,498 res, $10,930 non-res

Providence Hospital, Inc

Radiography Prgm
1912 Hayes Ave
Sandusky, OH 44870
Prgm Dir: Cynthia S Felske, RT(R)
Tel: 419 621-7124 *Fax:* 419 621-7209
Med Dir: James D Frank, MD
Class Cap: 8 *Begins:* Sep
Length: 24 mos *Award:* Cert
Tuition per yr: $1,600

Comm Hosp of Springfield & Clark County

Radiography Prgm
2615 E High St
Springfield, OH 45501
Prgm Dir: Bonnie G Young, Equiv RT(R)
Tel: 513 328-9354 *Fax:* 513 328-9220
Med Dir: Rick Kulkulka
Class Cap: 4 *Begins:* July
Length: 24 mos *Award:* Cert
Tuition per yr: $500

Jefferson Community College

Radiography Prgm
4000 Sunset Blvd
Steubenville, OH 43952-3598
Prgm Dir: Linda M Cipriani, MSEd RT(R)
Tel: 614 264-5591, Ext 233 *Fax:* 614 264-1338
Med Dir: Hunter Vallghan, MD
Class Cap: 16 *Begins:* Aug
Length: 24 mos *Award:* AAS
Tuition per yr: $2,223 res, $2,418 non-res
Evening or weekend classes available

Owens Community College

Radiography Prgm
PO Box 10,000
Toledo, OH 43699-1947
Prgm Dir: Linda R Myers, MEd RT(R)
Tel: 419 661-7261 *Fax:* 419 661-7665
E-mail: lmyers@owens.cc.oh.us
Class Cap: 20 *Begins:* Jan June
Length: 23 mos *Award:* AAS
Tuition per yr: $2,060 res, $3,860 non-res
Evening or weekend classes available

St Vincent Medical Center

Radiography Prgm
2213 Cherry St
Toledo, OH 43608-2691
Prgm Dir: Gaspar Hernandez, BS RT(R)
Tel: 419 321-2851 *Fax:* 419 321-3863
Med Dir: Richard Siders, MD
Class Cap: 12
Length: 24 mos *Award:* Cert
Tuition per yr: $850

St Elizabeth Health Center

Radiography Prgm
1044 Belmont Ave
Youngstown, OH 44501-1790
Prgm Dir: Francis E Potts, BART RT(R)(M)
Tel: 330 480-3265 *Fax:* 330 480-2912
Med Dir: Daniel Lauman, MD
Class Cap: 6 *Begins:* July
Length: 24 mos *Award:* Cert
Tuition per yr: $1,000 res, $1,000 non-res

Western Reserve Care System

Radiography Prgm
500 Gypsy Ln
Youngstown, OH 44501
Prgm Dir: Ruth Creighton, BA RT(R)
Tel: 330 740-3394 *Fax:* 330 740-5658
Class Cap: 10
Length: 24 mos *Award:* Cert
Tuition per yr: $1,000 res, $1,000 non-res

Muskingum Area Technical College

Radiography Prgm
1555 Newark Rd
Zanesville, OH 43701
Prgm Dir: Julia A Gill, MEd RT(R)
Tel: 614 454-2501 *Fax:* 614 454-0035
Class Cap: 21 *Begins:* June
Length: 24 mos *Award:* AAS
Tuition per yr: $2,490 res, $4,000 non-res
Evening or weekend classes available

Oklahoma

O T Autry Area Voc Tech Center

Radiography Prgm
1201 W Willow
Enid, OK 73703
Prgm Dir: Donna L Pruneau, RT(R)
Tel: 405 242-2750 *Fax:* 405 233-8262
Class Cap: 9 *Begins:* Aug
Length: 24 mos *Award:* Cert
Tuition per yr: $1,340 res, $5,745 non-res

Great Plains Area Voc Tech School

Radiography Prgm
4500 W Lee Blvd
Lawton, OK 73505
Prgm Dir: Carrie L Baxter, BS RT(R)(M)
Tel: 405 250-5577 *Fax:* 405 250-5583
Med Dir: Richard Roberts, MD CCMH
Class Cap: 19 *Begins:* Aug
Length: 24 mos *Award:* Cert
Tuition per yr: $1,300 res, $2,300 non-res
Evening or weekend classes available

Rose State College

Radiography Prgm
6420 SE 15th St
Midwest City, OK 73110-2799
Prgm Dir: Henry L Townsend, MEd RT(R)
Tel: 405 733-7568 *Fax:* 405 736-0338
Med Dir: Susan Edwards, MD
Class Cap: 25
Length: 24 mos *Award:* AAS

Bacone College

Radiography Prgm
2299 Old Bacone Rd
Muskogee, OK 74403-1597
Prgm Dir: Marian Maloney
Tel: 918 683-4581 *Fax:* 918 687-5913
Med Dir: Rodney Cave, MD
Class Cap: 26
Length: 24 mos *Award:* AAS
Tuition per yr: $3,670 res, $3,670 non-res

Metro Area Vocational - Technical School

Radiography Prgm
1720 Springlake Dr
Oklahoma City, OK 73111
Prgm Dir: Barbara J Harper, BS RT(R)
Tel: 405 424-8324, Ext 634 *Fax:* 405 424-9403
Class Cap: 10 *Begins:* Aug
, 22 mos *Award:* Cert
Tuition per yr: $1,450

Univ of Oklahoma Health Sciences Center
Radiography Prgm
801 NE 13th St
PO Box 26901
Oklahoma City, OK 73190
Prgm Dir: Barbara M Curcio, MEd RT(R)
Tel: 405 271-6477 *Fax:* 405 271-1424
E-mail: barbara-curcio@uokhsc.edu
Med Dir: Timothy Tytle, MD
Class Cap: 28 *Begins:* Aug
Length: 48 mos *Award:* BS
Tuition per yr: $2,635 res, $7,177 non-res
Evening or weekend classes available

Southwestern Oklahoma State University
Radiography Prgm
409 E Mississippi
Sayre, OK 73662-1236
Prgm Dir: Peggy A Robbins, MEd RT(R)(M)
Tel: 405 928-5533 *Fax:* 405 928-5533
E-mail: robbinp@host1.swou.edu
Med Dir: James E Milton, MD
Class Cap: 18 *Begins:* Aug
Length: 24 mos *Award:* AAS
Evening or weekend classes available

Meridian Technology Center
Radiography Prgm
1312 S Sangre St
Stillwater, OK 74074
Prgm Dir: Mary J Reagan, RT(R)
Tel: 405 377-3333 *Fax:* 405 377-9604
Class Cap: 10
Length: 24 mos *Award:* Cert
Tuition per yr: $1,800

Tulsa Community College
Radiography Prgm
909 S Boston Ave
Tulsa, OK 74119-2094
Prgm Dir: Ronald L Boodt, MS RT(R)
Tel: 918 595-7004 *Fax:* 918 595-2798
Med Dir: John Kawth, MD
Class Cap: 102
Length: 24 mos *Award:* AAS
Tuition per yr: $1,288 res, $3,150 non-res
Evening or weekend classes available

Tulsa Technology Center
Radiography Prgm
3420 S Memorial Dr
Tulsa, OK 74145-1390
Prgm Dir: Kathleen M Davis, MS RT(R)
Tel: 918 579-3288 *Fax:* 918 628-1406
Class Cap: 10
Length: 24 mos *Award:* Cert
Tuition per yr: $500 res, $500 non-res

Oregon

Oregon Institute of Technology
Radiography Prgm
3201 Campus Dr
Klamath Falls, OR 97601-8801
Prgm Dir: Alberto Bello Jr, MA RT(R)
Tel: 541 885-1824 *Fax:* 541 885-1849
E-mail: belloa@mail.osshe.edu
Med Dir: William Tamplen, MD
Begins: Sep *Award:* , BS
Tuition per yr: $3,129 res, $10,065 non-res

Portland Community College
Radiography Prgm
12000 SW 49th Ave
PO Box 19000
Portland, OR 97280-0990
Prgm Dir: Betty L Palmer, AAS RT(R)
Tel: 503 977-4917 *Fax:* 503 977-4869
Med Dir: Michael Vervarka, MD ABR
Class Cap: 30 *Begins:* Sep
Length: 24 mos *Award:* AAS
Tuition per yr: $2,231 res, $7,256 non-res
Evening or weekend classes available

Pennsylvania

Univ of Pittsburgh Med Ctr - Beaver Valley
Radiography Prgm
2500 Hospital Dr
Aliquippa, PA 15001
Prgm Dir: Debra A Majetic, AS RT(R)
Tel: 412 857-1246 *Fax:* 412 857-1254
Med Dir: Morteza Eyaderani, MD
Class Cap: 12
Length: 24 mos *Award:* Cert
Tuition per yr: $2,000

Lehigh Valley Hospital
Radiography Prgm
17th and Chew Sts
PO Box 1110
Allentown, PA 18105-1110
Prgm Dir: Charles W Natterman, BS RT(R)
Tel: 610 402-2300
Class Cap: 6
Length: 24 mos *Award:* Cert
Tuition per yr: $100

Mercy Regional Health System
Radiography Prgm
2500 7th Ave
Altoona, PA 16602-2099
Prgm Dir: Jane Merklin, BS RT(R)
Tel: 814 949-4478 *Fax:* 814 949-5882
Med Dir: Steven Diehl, MD
Class Cap: 10 *Begins:* Jul
Length: 24 mos *Award:* Cert
Tuition per yr: $4,295 res, $4,295 non-res
Evening or weekend classes available

The Medical Center Beaver PA, Inc
Radiography Prgm
1000 Dutch Ridge Rd
Beaver, PA 15009
Prgm Dir: JoAnn M Kosto, BS RT(R)
Tel: 412 773-4998 *Fax:* 412 728-7429
Med Dir: Joel I Cossrow, MD
Class Cap: 9 *Begins:* June or July
Length: 24 mos *Award:* Cert
Tuition per yr: $800

Northampton Community College
Radiography Prgm
3835 Green Pond Rd
Bethlehem, PA 18017
Prgm Dir: Zoland Z Zile III, MS RT(R)
Tel: 610 861-5387 *Fax:* 610 861-4581
E-mail: zzz@pmail.nrhm.cc.pa.us
Med Dir: Jeffrey Blinder
Class Cap: 28 *Begins:* Aug
Length: 24 mos *Award:* AAS
Tuition per yr: $1,960 res, $4,088 non-res

Bradford Regional Medical Center
Radiography Prgm
116 Interstate Pkwy
Bradford, PA 16701
Prgm Dir: Joann M Piatko, BA RT(R)
Tel: 814 362-8292 *Fax:* 814 368-7750
Med Dir: Ross A Horsley, MD
Class Cap: 6
Length: 24 mos *Award:* Dipl
Tuition per yr: $1,000 res, $1,000 non-res

Holy Spirit Hospital
Radiography Prgm
503 N 21st St
Camp Hill, PA 17011-2288
Prgm Dir: Genevieve B Conrad, BS RT(R)
Tel: 717 763-2123
Med Dir: Barbara Kunkle, MD
Class Cap: 8 *Begins:* Jan
Length: 24 mos *Award:* Cert, AA
Tuition per yr: $2,000

Chambersburg Hospital
Radiography Prgm
112 N Seventh St
PO Box 6005
Chambersburg, PA 17201-0187
Prgm Dir: Deborah K Zenefski, BS RT(R)(N)
Tel: 717 267-3000
Class Cap: 10
Length: 24 mos *Award:* Cert
Tuition per yr: $2,400

Clearfield Hospital
Radiography Prgm
809 Turnpike Ave
PO Box 992
Clearfield, PA 16830
Prgm Dir: Sandra L Alsop, RT(R)
Tel: 814 768-2230 *Fax:* 814 768-2279
Class Cap: 6 *Begins:* Sep
Length: 24 mos *Award:* Cert
Tuition per yr: $1,075 res, $1,075 non-res

Brandywine Hospital
Radiography Prgm
201 Reeceville Rd
Coatesville, PA 19320-1536
Prgm Dir: George D Heiser, RT(R)
Tel: 610 383-8122 *Fax:* 610 383-8092
Med Dir: James J Holstein, MD
Class Cap: 8
Length: 24 mos *Award:* Cert
Tuition per yr: $1,800

College Misericordia
Radiography Prgm
301 Lake St
Dallas, PA 18612
Prgm Dir: Elaine Halesey, MS RT(R)
Tel: 717 674-6480 *Fax:* 717 675-2441
E-mail: eholesey@misericordia.edu
Med Dir: Ron Koneche
Class Cap: 42 *Begins:* Aug
Length: 42 mos *Award:* BS
Tuition per yr: $15,560 res, $12,260 non-res
Evening or weekend classes available

Geisinger Medical Center
Radiography Prgm
100 N Academy Ave
Danville, PA 17822-2007
Prgm Dir: Freeman H Betz, BS RT(R)
Tel: 717 271-6301
Med Dir: Franklin J Rothermel, MD
Class Cap: 18 *Begins:* Aug
Length: 24 mos *Award:* Cert
Tuition per yr: $1,350 res, $1,350 non-res

Allegheny University Hospitals Elkins Park
Radiography Prgm
60 E Township Line Rd
Elkins Park, PA 19117
Prgm Dir: Celestine Coleman, BS RT(R)
Tel: 215 663-6083
Class Cap: 24
Length: 24 mos *Award:* Cert
Tuition per yr: $2,000

Gannon University
Radiography Prgm
University Square
Erie, PA 16541
Prgm Dir: Cynthia L Liotta, MS RT(R)
Tel: 814 871-5644 *Fax:* 814 871-5662
E-mail: gclli@mail1.gamnon.edu
Med Dir: Stephen Witchel, MD
Class Cap: 24 *Begins:* Aug
Length: 24 mos *Award:* AS
Tuition per yr: $11,520 res, $11,520 non-res

Northwest Medical Center-Franklin Campus
Radiography Prgm
One Spruce St
Franklin, PA 16323
Prgm Dir: Walter G Jones Sr, RT(R)
Tel: 814 437-7000 *Fax:* 814 437-3036
Med Dir: John V O'Connor, MD
Class Cap: 7
Length: 24 mos *Award:* Cert
Tuition per yr: $750 res, $750 non-res

Health Hospitals/Polyclinic Hospital
Radiography Prgm
2601 N Third St
Harrisburg, PA 17110
Prgm Dir: Kevin L Otb, BS RT(R)
Tel: 717 782-2416 *Fax:* 717 782-4256
Med Dir: Richard J Pawelski, MD
Class Cap: 10 *Begins:* July
Length: 24 mos *Award:* Cert
Tuition per yr: $1,000

Hazleton-St Joseph Medical Center
Radiography Prgm
687 N Church St
Hazleton, PA 18201-3198
Prgm Dir: Jandra J Sackrison, MHA RT(R)(M)
Tel: 717 459-4444 *Fax:* 717 489-4477
Med Dir: Joseph Kalowsky
Class Cap: 5 *Begins:* July
Length: 24 mos *Award:* Cert
Tuition per yr: $500

Penn State University - Hershey
Radiography Prgm
500 University Dr
PO Box 850
Hershey, PA 17033
Prgm Dir: Joanne S Bakel, BS RT(R)(N)
Tel: 717 531-8321 *Fax:* 717 531-4445
Med Dir: David Hartman, MD
Class Cap: 16 *Begins:* Jul
Length: 24 mos *Award:* AS
Tuition per yr: $5,434 res, $11,774 non-res

Monsour Medical Center
Radiography Prgm
70 Lincoln Way E
Jeannette, PA 15644
Prgm Dir: Gloria J Mongelluzzo, MEd RT(R)(M)
Tel: 412 527-0427 *Fax:* 412 527-3711
Med Dir: K S Shetly, MD
Class Cap: 6
Length: 24 mos *Award:* Cert
Tuition per yr: $600

Conemaugh Valley Memorial Hospital
Radiography Prgm
1086 Franklin St
Johnstown, PA 15905-4398
Prgm Dir: Elaine M Fuge, MEd RT(R)
Tel: 814 533-9582 *Fax:* 814 534-3110
Class Cap: 14 *Begins:* Sep
Length: 24 mos *Award:* Cert
Tuition per yr: $750 res, $750 non-res

Lee Hospital
Radiography Prgm
320 Main St
Johnstown, PA 15901-1694
Prgm Dir: John B Reitz, BS RT(R)
Tel: 814 533-0571 *Fax:* 814 533-0088
Med Dir: William Palmer, MD
Class Cap: 16 *Begins:* July
Length: 24 mos *Award:* Cert
Tuition per yr: $1,000

Armstrong County Memorial Hospital
Radiography Prgm
One Nolte Dr
Kittanning, PA 16201
Prgm Dir: Paula Keister, RT(R)
Tel: 412 543-8206 *Fax:* 412 543-3052
Class Cap: 8 *Begins:* July
Length: 24 mos *Award:* Cert
Tuition per yr: $2,500

Lancaster Institute for Health Education
Radiography Prgm
Lancaster General Hospital
143 E Lemon St
Lancaster, PA 17602
Prgm Dir: Robin L Harlclerode, BS RT(R)
Tel: 717 290-4912 *Fax:* 717 290-5970
Class Cap: 20
Length: 24 mos *Award:* Cert
Tuition per yr: $4,000 res, $4,000 non-res

Robert Morris Coll/Ohio Valley Gen Hosp
Radiography Prgm
Chris Valley Gen Hospital
Narrows Run Rd
McRees Rocks, PA 15134
Prgm Dir: Barbara J O'Connor, MS RT(R)
Tel: 412 777-6210 *Fax:* 412 777-6866
Class Cap: 9
Length: 24 mos *Award:* Cert, AS
Tuition per yr: $6,000
Evening or weekend classes available

Comm Coll of Allegheny Cnty-Boyce Campus
Radiography Prgm
595 Beatty Rd
Monroeville, PA 15146-1395
Prgm Dir: August B Kellermann III, MS RT(R)
Tel: 412 733-4334 *Fax:* 412 325-6799
E-mail: akellerm@ccac.edu
Med Dir: Peter Bonadio
Class Cap: 50
Length: 24 mos *Award:* AS
Tuition per yr: $980 res, $1,960 non-res
Evening or weekend classes available

Allegheny Valley Hospital
Radiography Prgm
1301 Carlisle St
Natrona Heights, PA 15065
Prgm Dir: Judith Ann Ostrowski, BA RT(R)
Tel: 412 226-7318 *Fax:* 412 226-7385
Med Dir: James E Bauer
Class Cap: 10 *Begins:* July
Length: 24 mos *Award:* Cert
Tuition per yr: $1,250

St Francis Hospital of New Castle
Radiography Prgm
1000 S Mercer St
New Castle, PA 16101
Prgm Dir: Trudi Anne Nottingham, RT(R)
Tel: 412 656-6134 *Fax:* 412 656-6167
Med Dir: Wan Jo Kim, MD
Class Cap: 10 *Begins:* Aug
Length: 24 mos *Award:* Cert
Tuition per yr: $2,000

Penn State Univ - New Kensington Campus
Radiography Prgm
3550 7th St Rd
New Kensington, PA 15068
Prgm Dir: Ronald Becker, MS RT(R)
Tel: 412 623-2091
Class Cap: 45
Length: 28 mos *Award:* AS

Albert Einstein Medical Center
Radiography Prgm
5501 Old York Rd
Philadelphia, PA 19141
Prgm Dir: Mary Susan Kane, BS RT(R)
Tel: 215 456-6234 *Fax:* 215 456-8996
Med Dir: Jay MacMoran
Class Cap: 20 *Begins:* Sep
Length: 24 mos *Award:* Cert
Tuition per yr: $1,500

Programs

Allegheny University of the Health Sciences
Radiography Prgm
Broad and Vine Sts
Mail Stop 206
Philadelphia, PA 19102-1192
Prgm Dir: Dorothy M Gray, BS RT(R)
Tel: 215 762-8744
Class Cap: 25
Length: 24 mos   *Award:* Cert, AAS
Tuition per yr: $1,650

Community College of Philadelphia
Radiography Prgm
1700 Spring Garden St
Philadelphia, PA 19130
Prgm Dir: Wanda E Wesolowski, MAEd RT(R)
Tel: 215 751-8424   *Fax:* 215 751-8937
Med Dir: Amy K Lansman, MD
Class Cap: 31   *Begins:* July
Length: 24 mos   *Award:* AAS
Tuition per yr: $2,376 res, $4,653 non-res

Germantown Hospital & Medical Center
Radiography Prgm
One Penn Blvd
Philadelphia, PA 19144
Prgm Dir: Bonnie L Benson, RT(R)
Tel: 215 951-8829   *Fax:* 215 951-8258
Med Dir: Amy K Lansman, MD
Class Cap: 5   *Begins:* Sep
Length: 24 mos   *Award:* Cert
Tuition per yr: $2,500

Holy Family College
Radiography Prgm
Grant and Frankford Aves
Philadelphia, PA 19114
Prgm Dir: Joanne Niewood, MEd RTR CT
Tel: 215 637-7202   *Fax:* 215 637-7377
Med Dir: Michael Kates, MD
Class Cap: 33   *Begins:* Jul
Length: 22 mos   *Award:* AS
Tuition per yr: $9,800 res, $9,800 non-res
Evening or weekend classes available

Temple University Hospital
Radiography Prgm
3401 N Broad St
Philadelphia, PA 19140
Prgm Dir: Patricia F Clark, BS RT(R)
Tel: 215 221-3734
Med Dir: Francis J Shea, MD
Class Cap: 12
Length: 24 mos   *Award:* Cert
Tuition per yr: $4,000

Thomas Jefferson University
Radiography Prgm
130 S Ninth St Rm 1004
Philadelphia, PA 19107-5233
Prgm Dir: Albert D Herbert Jr, MS RT(R)
Tel: 215 503-6678   *Fax:* 215 503-1031
E-mail: herber1@jeflin.tju.edu
Med Dir: Robert Steiner, MD
Class Cap: 63   *Begins:* Sept
Length: 16 mos   *Award:* BS
Tuition per yr: $13,800

Robert Morris College/Allegheny Gen Hosp
Radiography Prgm
320 E North Avenue
Pittsburgh, PA 15212
Prgm Dir: Connie D Stanish, BA RT(R)
Tel: 412 359-3774   *Fax:* 412 321-8033
Med Dir: Rodf Schapiro
Class Cap: 12   *Begins:* July
Length: 24 mos   *Award:* Cert, AS
Tuition per yr: $6,368
Evening or weekend classes available

University of Pittsburgh Medical Center
Radiography Prgm
200 Lothrop St
Pittsburgh, PA 15213-2582
Prgm Dir: Denise Csonika Lake, RT(R)(M)
Tel: 412 647-3528
Med Dir: Dave C Strolls, MD
Class Cap: 33   *Begins:* July
Length: 24 mos   *Award:* Cert
Tuition per yr: $3,000

Western Sch of Hlth & Business Careers
Radiography Prgm
327 Fifth Ave
Landmark Bldg
Pittsburgh, PA 15222
Prgm Dir: Charles W Phaneuf, MEd RT(R)
Tel: 412 281-2600   *Fax:* 412 281-0819
Med Dir: Edward Urbanik, MD
Class Cap: 60   *Begins:* Sep
Length: 24 mos   *Award:* AS
Tuition per yr: $9,000 res, $9,000 non-res

Community General Hospital
Radiography Prgm
145 N Sixth St
PO Box 1728
Reading, PA 19603-1728
Prgm Dir: Elizabeth W Price, AAS RT(R)
Tel: 610 376-2100   *Fax:* 610 373-8093
Med Dir: Jonathan Stolz, MD
Class Cap: 9   *Begins:* July
Length: 24 mos   *Award:* Cert
Tuition per yr: $800 res, $800 non-res

Reading Hospital and Medical Center
Radiography Prgm
PO Box 16052
Reading, PA 19612-6052
Prgm Dir: Jeanne L Sandel, RT(R)
Tel: 610 378-6993   *Fax:* 610 378-6400
Class Cap: 15   *Award:* Cert
Tuition per yr: $2,600

St Joseph Hospital
Radiography Prgm
12th and Walnut Sts
PO Box 316
Reading, PA 19603
Prgm Dir: Cynthia L Kolakowski, RT(R)
Tel: 610 378-2230   *Fax:* 610 378-2803
Class Cap: 10   *Begins:* July
Length: 24 mos   *Award:* Cert
Tuition per yr: $2,000

Mansfield University
Radiography Prgm
Guthrie Square
Sayre, PA 18840
Prgm Dir: Terry L Lutz, BS RT(R)(CV)
Tel: 717 882-4007   *Fax:* 717 882-4413
E-mail: tlutz@inet.guthrie.org
Med Dir: Ralph Zehr, MD
Class Cap: 15   *Begins:* Aug
Length: 24 mos   *Award:* AAS
Tuition per yr: $4,206 res, $9,404 non-res

Penn State University - Schuylkill
Radiography Prgm
200 University Dr
Schuylkill Haven, PA 17972-0308
Prgm Dir: Christine M Mehlbaum, BS RT(R)
Tel: 717 385-6108   *Fax:* 717 385-3672
Med Dir: William Connolly, DO
Class Cap: 16
Length: 28 mos   *Award:* AS
Tuition per yr: $6,528 res, $10,224 non-res

Community Medical Center
Radiography Prgm
1800 Mulberry St
Scranton, PA 18510
Prgm Dir: Barbara A Brush, RT(R)
Tel: 717 969-8151   *Fax:* 717 969-8387
Med Dir: Robert Schuman, MD
Class Cap: 4   *Begins:* July
Length: 24 mos   *Award:* Cert

Sewickley Valley Hospital
Radiography Prgm
720 Blackburn Rd
Sewickley, PA 15143-1498
Prgm Dir: Kathleen L Kapsin, BS RT(R)
Tel: 412 749-7245   *Fax:* 412 749-7747
Class Cap: 4
Length: 24 mos   *Award:* Dipl
Tuition per yr: $2,500

Sharon Regional Health System
Radiography Prgm
740 E State St
Sharon, PA 16146-3395
Prgm Dir: Shirley J Cherry, BS RT(R)
Tel: 412 983-3911   *Fax:* 412 983-5614
Class Cap: 7   *Begins:* Sep
Length: 24 mos   *Award:* Cert

Somerset Hospital
Radiography Prgm
225 S Center Ave
Somerset, PA 15501-2088
Prgm Dir: Evelyn R Bunja, BA RT(R)
Tel: 814 443-5028   *Fax:* 814 443-5042
Length: 24 mos   *Award:* Cert
Tuition per yr: $3,500

Crozer-Chester Med Ctr/Delaware Co CC
Radiography Prgm
One Medical Center Blvd
Upland, PA 19013
Prgm Dir: Lisa M Jacovelli, BS RT(R)
Tel: 610 447-2578
Class Cap: 24
Length: 24 mos   *Award:* Cert
Tuition per yr: $2,400 res, $2,400 non-res

Washington Hospital
Radiography Prgm
155 Wilson Ave
Washington, PA 15301
Prgm Dir: Karen C Williams, BA RT(R)
Tel: 412 223-3326
Class Cap: 12
Length: 24 mos   *Award:* Cert
Tuition per yr: $6,000

Wyoming Valley Health Care System Inc
Radiography Prgm
N River and Auburn Sts
Wilkes-Barre, PA 18764
Prgm Dir: Kathleen A Smith, BA RT(R)
Tel: 717 552-1760   *Fax:* 717 552-1707
Med Dir: Satish Patel, MD
Class Cap: 9   *Begins:* Sep
Length: 24 mos   *Award:* Cert
Tuition per yr: $1,600

Pennsylvania College of Technology
Radiography Prgm
One College Ave
Williamsport, PA 17701-5799
Prgm Dir: Robert J Slothus, MS RT(R)
Tel: 717 326-3761   *Fax:* 717 321-5538
E-mail: rslothos@pct.edu
Med Dir: Harshad Patel, MD
Class Cap: 43
Length: 24 mos   *Award:* AAS
Tuition per yr: $7,517
Evening or weekend classes available

Abington Memorial Hospital
Radiography Prgm
2500 Maryland Rd
Willow Grove, PA 19090-1284
Prgm Dir: Mark B Ness, BS RT(R)
Tel: 215 881-5526   *Fax:* 215 881-5579
E-mail: maxness@aol.com
Med Dir: Richard Weiss, MD
Class Cap: 22
Length: 24 mos   *Award:* Cert
Tuition per yr: $1,500

Lankenau Hospital
Radiography Prgm
100 Lancaster Ave
W of City Line
Wynnewood, PA 19096
Prgm Dir: Joan A Zacharko, BS RT(R)
Tel: 610 645-2840   *Fax:* 610 645-3325
Length: 24 mos   *Award:* Cert
Tuition per yr: $5,000

York Hospital
Radiography Prgm
1001 S George St
York, PA 17405
Prgm Dir: Kathleen E Valetsky, EdM RT(R)
Tel: 717 771-2466
Med Dir: C Ronald Duncan, MD
Class Cap: 20   *Begins:* Sep
Length: 22 mos   *Award:* Cert
Tuition per yr: $3,000 res, $3,000 non-res

Puerto Rico

Universidad Central del Caribe
Radiography Prgm
Call Box 60 327
Bayamon, PR 00960-6032
Prgm Dir: Jose Rafael Moscoso, MPH LT
Tel: 787 798-3006   *Fax:* 787 785-3425
E-mail: rinforma@caribe.net
Med Dir: Lorraine Vazquez, MD
Class Cap: 36
Length: 24 mos   *Award:* AS
Tuition per yr: $3,225

University of Puerto Rico
Radiography Prgm
GPO Box 5067
PO Box 3655067
San Juan, PR 00936
Prgm Dir: Haydee Encarnacion, MPHE LRT
Tel: 787 753-8541   *Fax:* 787 763-7256
Med Dir: Heriberto Pagan Saez, MD
Class Cap: 25   *Begins:* Aug
Length: 24 mos   *Award:* AS
Tuition per yr: $1,200 res, $2,000 non-res

Rhode Island

Community College of Rhode Island
Radiography Prgm
Flanagan Campus
1762 Louisquisset Pike
Lincoln, RI 02865-4585
Prgm Dir: Sharon E Perkins, MEd RT(R)(M)
Tel: 401 333-7025   *Fax:* 401 333-7260
E-mail: sperkins@ccri.cc.ri.us
Med Dir: Alan M Schwartz, MD
Class Cap: 83   *Begins:* June
Length: 24 mos   *Award:* AAS
Tuition per yr: $2,133 res, $6,537 non-res
Evening or weekend classes available

Rhode Island Hospital
Radiography Prgm
593 Eddy St
Providence, RI 02903
Prgm Dir: Ann Matthews, MEd RTR
Tel: 401 277-5177   *Fax:* 401 444-6308
Class Cap: 15   *Begins:* July
Length: 24 mos   *Award:* Cert
Tuition per yr: $2,000 res, $2,000 non-res

South Carolina

Anderson Area Medical Center
Radiography Prgm
800 N Fant St
Anderson, SC 29621
Prgm Dir: Gaye Nichols, RT(R)
Tel: 864 260-3705   *Fax:* 864 261-1415
Med Dir: Thomas U Tuten, MD
Class Cap: 19   *Begins:* July
Length: 24 mos   *Award:* Cert
Tuition per yr: $650

Trident Technical College
Radiography Prgm
7000 Rivers Ave
PO Box 118067
Charleston, SC 29423-8067
Prgm Dir: Linus Brown, MHSA RT(R)
Tel: 803 572-6077   *Fax:* 803 569-6585
E-mail: zpbrownl@trident.tec.sc.us
Med Dir: Charles Griffin, MD
Class Cap: 30   *Begins:* May
Length: 24 mos   *Award:* AHS
Tuition per yr: $1,536 res, $1,776 non-res
Evening or weekend classes available

Baptist Medical Center at Columbia
Radiography Prgm
Taylor at Marion St
Columbia, SC 29220
Prgm Dir: Judy B Weathersbee, BS RT(R)
Tel: 803 771-5323
Class Cap: 11
Length: 24 mos   *Award:* Cert
Tuition per yr: $700

Midlands Technical College
Radiography Prgm
PO Box 2408
Columbia, SC 29202
Prgm Dir: C William Mulkey, EdD RT(R)
Tel: 803 434-6343   *Fax:* 803 434-4500
Class Cap: 18   *Begins:* May
Length: 24 mos   *Award:* AS
Tuition per yr: $1,620 res, $2,016 non-res
Evening or weekend classes available

Horry-Georgetown Technical College
Radiography Prgm
Hwy 501 E
PO Box 260004
Conway, SC 29528-6004
Prgm Dir: Arthur R Galbraith, BA RT(R)
Tel: 803 347-3186   *Fax:* 803 347-4207
Med Dir: James C Hewitt, MD
Class Cap: 18   *Begins:* Aug
Length: 24 mos   *Award:* AS
Tuition per yr: $551 res, $603 non-res

Florence-Darlington Technical College
Radiography Prgm
PO Box 100548
Florence, SC 29501-0548
Prgm Dir: E Yancy Wells, BS RT(R)
Tel: 803 667-2804   *Fax:* 803 678-5251
Class Cap: 32   *Begins:* Aug
Length: 24 mos   *Award:* AHS
Tuition per yr: $550 res, $625 non-res
Evening or weekend classes available

Greenville Technical College
Radiography Prgm
PO Box 5616
Greenville, SC 20606-5616
Prgm Dir: Theresa Harris, BHS RT(R)
Tel: 864 250-8290
Class Cap: 28
Length: 24 mos   *Award:* AHS

Programs

Piedmont Technical College
Radiography Prgm
Emerald Rd Drawer 1467
Greenwood, SC 29648
Prgm Dir: Joyce A Hunter, MHS RT(R)
Tel: 864 941-8523 *Fax:* 864 941-8555
E-mail: hunter@al@frodo
Med Dir: W A Kitchens Jr
Class Cap: 15 *Begins:* Aug
Length: 24 mos *Award:* AS
Tuition per yr: $1,744 res, $2,174 non-res
Evening or weekend classes available

Orangeburg Calhoun Technical College
Radiography Prgm
3250 St Matthews Rd
Orangeburg, SC 29115
Prgm Dir: Fran Andrews, BHS RT(R)
Tel: 803 536-0311 *Fax:* 803 535-1388
E-mail: fandrews@org.tech.sc.us.@smtp
Class Cap: 11 *Begins:* Aug
Length: 24 mos *Award:* AAS
Tuition per yr: $1,235 res, $1,544 non-res
Evening or weekend classes available

York Technical College
Radiography Prgm
452 S Anderson Rd
Rock Hill, SC 29730
Prgm Dir: Debra L Caldwell, MA RT(R)
Tel: 803 981-7036 *Fax:* 803 327-8059
E-mail: dcaldwell@york.tec.sc.us
Class Cap: 16 *Begins:* Jun
Length: 24 mos *Award:* AS
Tuition per yr: $1,224 res, $1,512 non-res
Evening or weekend classes available

Spartanburg Technical College
Radiography Prgm
PO Drawer 4386
Spartanburg, SC 29305-4386
Prgm Dir: Dorothy A Kiser, MHS RT(R)
Tel: 864 591-3720 *Fax:* 864 591-3708
E-mail: kiser@spt.tec.sc.us
Med Dir: Robert Mitchell, MD
Class Cap: 21 *Begins:* July
Length: 24 mos *Award:* AAS
Tuition per yr: $1,500 res, $1,875 non-res

South Dakota

St Luke's-Midland Regional Medical Ctr
Radiography Prgm
305 S State St
PO Box 4450
Aberdeen, SD 57402-4450
Prgm Dir: Nancy J Vander Hoek, BS RT(R)
Tel: 605 622-5582 *Fax:* 605 622-5217
Med Dir: Caroline Lundell, MD
Class Cap: 8 *Begins:* July
Length: 24 mos *Award:* Cert
Tuition per yr: $500

Queen of Peace Hospital
Radiography Prgm
525 N Foster
Mitchell, SD 57301-2999
Prgm Dir: Gwen Wawers, MEd RT(R)
Tel: 605 995-2407
Class Cap: 8
Length: 24 mos *Award:* Cert
Tuition per yr: $3,500

Rapid City Regional Hospital
Radiography Prgm
353 Fairmont Blvd
PO Box 6000
Rapid City, SD 57709-6000
Prgm Dir: Deborah L Martin, BS RT(R)
Tel: 605 341-8433 *Fax:* 605 341-8983
Med Dir: Thomas Krafka, MD
Class Cap: 10 *Begins:* June
Length: 24 mos *Award:* Cert
Tuition per yr: $1,250

McKennan Hospital
Radiography Prgm
800 E 21st St
PO Box 5045
Sioux Falls, SD 57117-5045
Prgm Dir: Susan R Calmus, MA RT(R)
Tel: 605 322-1720 *Fax:* 605 322-1657
Med Dir: Lynn Henrickson
Class Cap: 8
Length: 24 mos *Award:* Cert
Tuition per yr: $500

Sioux Valley Hospital
Radiography Prgm
1100 S Euclid Ave
PO Box 5039
Sioux Falls, SD 57117-5039
Prgm Dir: Kenneth G Lee, BS RT(R)
Tel: 605 333-6466 *Fax:* 605 333-1554
Med Dir: Daryl R Wierda, MD
Class Cap: 14
Length: 24 mos *Award:* Cert
Tuition per yr: $500 res, $500 non-res

Sacred Heart Hospital
Radiography Prgm
501 Summit St
Yankton, SD 57078-9967
Prgm Dir: Robin R Berke, BS RT(R)
Tel: 605 665-9371 *Fax:* 605 665-0402
Med Dir: Frank Messner, MD
Class Cap: 8 *Begins:* Sep
Length: 24 mos *Award:* Cert
Tuition per yr: $600

Tennessee

Chattanooga State Technical Comm College
Radiography Prgm
4501 Amnicola Hwy
Chattanooga, TN 37406-1097
Prgm Dir: Glenda Kay Thurman, MEd RT(R)
Tel: 423 697-4450 *Fax:* 423 634-3071
E-mail: kthusman@cstllo.cc.tn.us
Med Dir: Deloris Rissling, MD
Class Cap: 77
Length: 24 mos *Award:* AAS
Tuition per yr: $1,288 res, $4,812 non-res
Evening or weekend classes available

Columbia State Community College
Radiography Prgm
PO Box 1315
Hwy 412 W
Columbia, TN 38402-1315
Prgm Dir: Brenda M Coleman, BS RT(R)
Tel: 615 540-2745 *Fax:* 615 540-2798
E-mail: coleman@coscc.cc.tn.us
Med Dir: Gary Podgorski, MD
Class Cap: 33 *Begins:* Aug
Length: 24 mos *Award:* AAS
Tuition per yr: $1,350 res, $5,170 non-res
Evening or weekend classes available

East Tennessee State University
Radiography Prgm
1000 West E St
ETSU Nave Center
Elizabethton, TN 37643
Prgm Dir: Donna R Shehane, MA RT(R) EdD
Tel: 423 547-4912 *Fax:* 423 547-4921
Class Cap: 57 *Begins:* June
Length: 23 mos *Award:* AAS
Tuition per yr: $2,892 res, $9,396 non-res
Evening or weekend classes available

Volunteer State Community College
Radiography Prgm
1480 Nashville Pike
Gallatin, TN 37066-3188
Prgm Dir: Monica M White, MS RT(R)
Tel: 615 452-8600, Ext 3651 *Fax:* 615 230-3224
E-mail: mwhite@vscc.cc.tn.us
Class Cap: 25 *Begins:* Jul
Length: 24 mos *Award:* AAS
Tuition per yr: $1,491 res, $5,880 non-res
Evening or weekend classes available

Roane State Community College
Radiography Prgm
Patton Ln
Harriman, TN 37748
Prgm Dir: Gail H Porter, BA RT(R)
Tel: 423 481-3496 *Fax:* 423 483-0447
Med Dir: William Prater, MD
Class Cap: 49
Length: 24 mos *Award:* AS
Tuition per yr: $1,491 res, $1,491 non-res

Jackson State Community College
Radiography Prgm
2046 N Parkway St
Jackson, TN 38301-3797
Prgm Dir: Neta B McKnight, BA RT(R)
Tel: 901 424-3520 *Fax:* 901 425-2647
E-mail: NMcKnight@JSCC.CC.TN.US
Med Dir: Thomas R Thompson, MD
Class Cap: 30 *Begins:* Sept
Length: 25 mos *Award:* AAS
Tuition per yr: $1,491 res, $5,880 non-res

Univ of Tennessee Med Ctr at Knoxville
Radiography Prgm
1924 Alcoa Hwy
Knoxville, TN 37920-6999
Prgm Dir: Patti C Armstrong, AS RT(R)
Tel: 615 544-9005
Class Cap: 15
Length: 24 mos *Award:* Cert
Tuition per yr: $200

Baptist Memorial Health Care Systems
Radiography Prgm
899 Madison Ave
Memphis, TN 38146
Prgm Dir: Wanda Lillie, BS RT(R)
Tel: 901 227-5006 *Fax:* 901 227-4310
Med Dir: James E Machin, MD
Class Cap: 20 *Begins:* Sept
Length: 24 mos *Award:* Cert
Tuition per yr: $2,000 res, $2,000 non-res

Methodist Hospitals of Memphis
Radiography Prgm
1265 Union Ave
Memphis, TN 38104
Prgm Dir: Peggy D Franklin, BS
Tel: 901 726-7358 *Fax:* 901 726-7490
E-mail: franklip@mhsgate_meth_mem.org
Med Dir: John M. Dobson, MD
Class Cap: 16
Length: 24 mos *Award:* Cert
Tuition per yr: $2,000

Shelby State Community College
Radiography Prgm
PO Box 40568
Memphis, TN 38174-0568
Prgm Dir: Glenn Swinny, MA RT(R)
Tel: 901 544-5417 *Fax:* 901 544-5391
Class Cap: 30 *Begins:* July
Length: 24 mos *Award:* AAS
Tuition per yr: $512 res, $2,048 non-res
Evening or weekend classes available

St Joseph Hospital
Radiography Prgm
220 Overton Ave
Memphis, TN 38105
Prgm Dir: Rhonda Harris Willcox, BS RT(R)
Tel: 901 577-3081 *Fax:* 901 577-3083
Med Dir: Fred Hamilton, MD
Class Cap: 9 *Begins:* July
Length: 24 mos *Award:* Cert
Tuition per yr: $1,000
Evening or weekend classes available

Metropolitan Nashville General Hospital
Radiography Prgm
72 Hermitage Ave
Nashville, TN 37210
Prgm Dir: James Murray Dozier, BS RT(R)
Tel: 615 862-4181
Class Cap: 8
Length: 24 mos *Award:* Cert

Texas

Hendrick Medical Center
Radiography Prgm
1242 N 19th
Abilene, TX 79601-2316
Prgm Dir: Richard K Bower, MEd RT(R)
Tel: 915 670-2427 *Fax:* 915 670-2575
Med Dir: Johnny Bliznak, MD
Class Cap: 10
Length: 24 mos *Award:* Cert
Tuition per yr: $2,500

Amarillo College
Radiography Prgm
PO Box 447
Amarillo, TX 79178
Prgm Dir: Howard Bacon, BS RT(R)
Tel: 806 354-6071
Class Cap: 37
Length: 24 mos *Award:* AAS

Austin Community College
Radiography Prgm
1020 Grove Blvd
Austin, TX 78741
Prgm Dir: Rudy L Garza, MS RT(R)
Tel: 512 223-6146
Class Cap: 42
Length: 24 mos *Award:* AAS
Tuition per yr: $1,454 res, $2,222 non-res
Evening or weekend classes available

Baptist Hospital of Southeast Texas
Radiography Prgm
PO Drawer 1591
Beaumont, TX 77704
Prgm Dir: Carolyn M Nicholas, RT(R)
Tel: 409 654-6024 *Fax:* 409 654-6195
Class Cap: 14
Length: 24 mos *Award:* Cert
Tuition per yr: $3,800

Lamar Univ Institute of Tech - Beaumont
Radiography Prgm
PO Box 10061
Beaumont, TX 77710
Prgm Dir: W David Short, MEd RT(R)
Tel: 409 880-8845 *Fax:* 409 880-8955
Class Cap: 34
Length: 24 mos *Award:* AAS
Tuition per yr: $963 res, $963 non-res

Scenic Mountain Medical Center
Radiography Prgm
1601 W 11th Pl
Big Spring, TX 79720-9990
Prgm Dir: Vivian R Gordon, BS RT(R)
Tel: 915 263-1211 *Fax:* 915 263-7502
Med Dir: Stanton S Kremsky, MD
Class Cap: 5 *Begins:* July
Length: 24 mos *Award:* Cert
Tuition per yr: $400

Univ Tx at Brownsville/TX Southmost Coll
Radiography Prgm
80 Ft Brown
Brownsville, TX 78520-4993
Prgm Dir: Manuel Gavito, BS RT(R)
Tel: 210 544-8248 *Fax:* 210 844-8910
Med Dir: William McKinney, MD
Class Cap: 28
Length: 24 mos *Award:* AAS
Tuition per yr: $1,931 res, $2,488 non-res

Blinn College
Radiography Prgm
301 Post Office St
Bryan, TX 77801-2142
Prgm Dir: Maria E Flores, MEd RT(R)
Tel: 409 821-0203 *Fax:* 409 821-0219
Med Dir: Ernest Elmendorf, MD
Class Cap: 18 *Begins:* Sep
Length: 24 mos *Award:* AAS
Tuition per yr: $950 res, $1,200 non-res

Del Mar College
Radiography Prgm
101 Baldwin
Corpus Christi, TX 78404
Prgm Dir: Patricia R Paris, MS RT(R)
Tel: 512 886-1102 *Fax:* 512 886-1598
Class Cap: 25
Length: 24 mos *Award:* AAS
Tuition per yr: $1,000 res, $1,500 non-res
Evening or weekend classes available

Baylor University Medical Center
Radiography Prgm
3500 Gaston Ave
Dallas, TX 75246
Prgm Dir: Eunice Irene Camp, BS RT(R)
Tel: 214 820-3780
Med Dir: Roger Rian
Class Cap: 15 *Begins:* July
Length: 24 mos *Award:* Cert

El Centro College
Radiography Prgm
Main and Lamar Sts
Dallas, TX 75202-3604
Prgm Dir: Jolayne Jackson, BA RT(R)
Tel: 214 860-2278 *Fax:* 214 860-2268
E-mail: jxj5540@dcccd.edu
Class Cap: 35 *Begins:* Aug
Length: 24 mos *Award:* AAS
Evening or weekend classes available

El Paso Community College
Radiography Prgm
PO Box 20500
El Paso, TX 79998
Prgm Dir: Christl E Thompson, MA RT(R)
Tel: 915 594-2000 *Fax:* 915 534-4114
Med Dir: Barbara Gainer, MD
Class Cap: 16 *Begins:* May
Length: 27 mos *Award:* AAS
Tuition per yr: $1,380 res, $3,855 non-res

Army Medical Dept Center and School
Radiography Prgm
HSHA-ML (Radiology Branch)
3151 Scott Rd
Ft Sam Houston, TX 78234-6137
Prgm Dir: Janet E Cook, MSG BS RT(R)
Tel: 210 221-8597 *Fax:* 210 221-6501
Class Cap: 440
Length: 12 mos *Award:* Cert

JPS Health Network
Radiography Prgm
2400 Circle Dr Suite 100
Ft Worth, TX 76104
Prgm Dir: Donna J Mitchell, BS RT(R)
Tel: 817 927-3724 *Fax:* 817 536-3812
Med Dir: Richard Rome
Class Cap: 37 *Begins:* July
Length: 24 mos *Award:* Cert
Tuition per yr: $3,600 res, $3,600 non-res

Galveston College-University of Texas

Radiography Prgm
4015 Ave Q
Galveston, TX 77550-2782
Prgm Dir: Belinda Escamilla, MA RT(R)
Tel: 409 772-9467 *Fax:* 409 772-3014
E-mail: bescamil%sahs@mhost.utmb.edu
Med Dir: Eric VanSonnernberg, MD
Class Cap: 37 *Begins:* Sept
Length: 24 mos *Award:* AAS
Tuition per yr: $580 res, $1,600 non-res
Evening or weekend classes available

Harris County Hosp Dist/Ben Taub Hosp

Radiography Prgm
1504 Taub Loop
Houston, TX 77030
Prgm Dir: Hazel E Bourne, MS RT(R)
Tel: 713 793-2276 *Fax:* 713 793-2416
Class Cap: 30
Length: 24 mos *Award:* Cert
Tuition per yr: $500 res, $550 non-res

Houston Community College Central

Radiography Prgm
5514 Clara
Houston, TX 77041
Prgm Dir: Teresa Zullo Rice, BS RT(R)
Tel: 713 718-5531 *Fax:* 713 466-8491
Med Dir: Stanford Goldman, MD
Class Cap: 83 *Begins:* Aug Jan
Length: 24 mos *Award:* AAS
Tuition per yr: $1,110 res, $1,900 non-res

Memorial Hospital System

Radiography Prgm
7600 Beechnut
Houston, TX 77074
Prgm Dir: Rita J Robinson, BS RT(R)
Tel: 713 776-4079 *Fax:* 713 776-5472
Class Cap: 18
Length: 24 mos *Award:* Cert
Tuition per yr: $2,200 res, $2,200 non-res

Tarrant Junior College

Radiography Prgm
828 Harwood Rd
Hurst, TX 76054
Prgm Dir: Judy Espino, MA RT(R)
Tel: 817 788-6569 *Fax:* 817 788-6601
Med Dir: Paxton Daniel, MD
Class Cap: 24 *Begins:* Summer
Length: 24 mos *Award:* AAS
Tuition per yr: $840 res, $1,260 non-res
Evening or weekend classes available

Kilgore College

Radiography Prgm
1100 Broadway
Kilgore, TX 75662
Prgm Dir: Louise Wiley, BS RT(R)
Tel: 903 983-8636 *Fax:* 903 983-8600
Med Dir: E E Zvolanek, MD
Class Cap: 20 *Begins:* July
Length: 24 mos *Award:* AAS
Tuition per yr: $600 res, $1,200 non-res

Laredo Community College

Radiography Prgm
W End Washington St
Laredo, TX 78040-4935
Prgm Dir: Carlos Valle Jr, MEd RT(R)
Tel: 210 721-5386
Class Cap: 9
Length: 24 mos *Award:* AAS

Methodist Hospital

Radiography Prgm
3615 19th St
PO Box 1201
Lubbock, TX 79408-1201
Prgm Dir: Lori Joran, BS RT(NR)
Tel: 806 793-4056
Med Dir: Brian Bruening
Class Cap: 20 *Begins:* June
Length: 24 mos *Award:* Cert

South Plains College

Radiography Prgm
1302 Main St
Lubbock, TX 79401
Prgm Dir: Denny Barnes, BS RT(R)
Tel: 806 747-0576 *Fax:* 806 765-2775
Med Dir: J Max Word, MD
Class Cap: 17 *Begins:* Aug
Length: 24 mos *Award:* AAS
Tuition per yr: $688 res, $1,376 non-res
Evening or weekend classes available

Angelina College

Radiography Prgm
PO Box 1768
Lufkin, TX 75902-1768
Prgm Dir: Freeman J Heck III, MEd RT(R)
Tel: 409 633-5267 *Fax:* 409 639-4299
E-mail: hexter@tcac.com
Med Dir: B G Kistler, MD
Class Cap: 26 *Begins:* May
Length: 23 mos *Award:* AAS
Tuition per yr: $684 res, $864 non-res
Evening or weekend classes available

Midland College

Radiography Prgm
3600 N Garfield
Midland, TX 79705-6399
Prgm Dir: Quinn B Carroll, MEd RT(R)
Tel: 915 685-4600 *Fax:* 915 585-4762
E-mail: eskimo@mc.midland.tx.us
Med Dir: Roberto R Spencer, MD
Class Cap: 11 *Begins:* Aug
Length: 24 mos *Award:* AAS
Tuition per yr: $895 res, $959 non-res
Evening or weekend classes available

Odessa College

Radiography Prgm
201 W University Blvd
Odessa, TX 79764
Prgm Dir: Carolyn Sue Leach, BS RT(R)
Tel: 915 335-6449 *Fax:* 915 335-6846
Med Dir: James Sheehan, MD
Class Cap: 13 *Begins:* July
Length: 24 mos *Award:* AAS
Tuition per yr: $1,158 res, $1,356 non-res

San Jacinto College Central Campus

Radiography Prgm
8060 Spencer Hwy
PO Box 2007
Pasadena, TX 77501-2007
Prgm Dir: Christopher J Gould, MS RT(R)
Tel: 713 476-1871 *Fax:* 713 478-2364
E-mail: cgould@central.sjcd.cc.tx.
Class Cap: 98 *Begins:* Aug Jan
Length: 24 mos *Award:* AAS
Tuition per yr: $532 res, $988 non-res
Evening or weekend classes available

Baptist Memorial

Radiography Prgm
111 Dallas St
San Antonio, TX 78205-1230
Prgm Dir: Anna Y Flores, RT(R)
Tel: 210 302-2386
Med Dir: Gregory Godwin, MD
Class Cap: 40 *Begins:* Jun
Length: 24 mos *Award:* Cert
Tuition per yr: $1,000

St Philip's College

Radiography Prgm
1801 Martin Luther King Dr
San Antonio, TX 78203-2098
Prgm Dir: Gaynell S Gainer, MS RT(R)
Tel: 210 531-3422 *Fax:* 210 531-3459
E-mail: ggainer@accd.edu
Med Dir: Edwell Clarke, MD
Class Cap: 57 *Begins:* May
Length: 24 mos *Award:* AAS
Tuition per yr: $816 res, $1,554 non-res

882 Training Group

Radiography Prgm
381 TRS/CSX
917 Missile Rd
Sheppard AFB, TX 76311-2246
Prgm Dir: Frank A Dunai, Msgt BS RT(R)
Tel: 817 676-3808 *Fax:* 817 676-2210
E-mail: dunaif@win.spd.qetc.qf.mil
Class Cap: 288 *Begins:* All
Length: 24 mos *Award:* Cert, AAS

Wadley Regional Medical Center

Radiography Prgm
1000 Pine St
PO Box 1878
Texarkana, TX 75501
Prgm Dir: Linda Hodge, RT(R)(M)(CV)
Tel: 903 798-7229 *Fax:* 903 798-7980
Med Dir: Robert Mack, MD
Class Cap: 9
Length: 24 mos *Award:* Cert
Tuition per yr: $1,000

Tyler Junior College

Radiography Prgm
PO Box 9020
Tyler, TX 75711
Prgm Dir: Nancy A Wardlow, MS RT(R)
Tel: 903 510-2346 *Fax:* 903 510-2592
Med Dir: E Maxey Abernathy, MD
Class Cap: 26 *Begins:* Aug
Length: 24 mos *Award:* AAS
Tuition per yr: $1,096 res, $1,711 non-res
Evening or weekend classes available

Citizens Medical Center

Radiography Prgm
2701 Hospital Dr
Victoria, TX 77901
Prgm Dir: Jonnye C Griffin, BS RT(R)
Tel: 512 572-5062   *Fax:* 512 572-5091
Med Dir: Frank Wilson, DO
Class Cap: 5
Length: 24 mos   *Award:* Cert
Tuition per yr: $1,000
Evening or weekend classes available

McLennan Community College

Radiography Prgm
1400 College Dr
Waco, TX 76708
Prgm Dir: Brenda Dobelbower, BS RT(R)
Tel: 817 299-8342   *Fax:* 817 299-8435
E-mail: bjd@mcc.cc.tx.us
Med Dir: Charles Huffman, MD
Class Cap: 46   *Begins:* Aug
Length: 24 mos   *Award:* AAS
Tuition per yr: $660 res, $825 non-res

Wharton County Junior College

Radiography Prgm
911 Boling Hwy
Wharton, TX 77488
Prgm Dir: James N Johnston, BS RT(R)(CV)
Tel: 409 532-6379   *Fax:* 409 532-6489
Med Dir: O Preston Copeland, MD
Class Cap: 16   *Begins:* Aug
Length: 24 mos   *Award:* AAS
Tuition per yr: $455 res, $455 non-res
Evening or weekend classes available

Midwestern State University

Radiography Prgm
3410 Taft Blvd
Wichita Falls, TX 76308-2099
Prgm Dir: Valerie Showalter, MS RT(R)
Tel: 817 689-4608   *Fax:* 817 689-4513
E-mail: fshwltrv@nexus.mwsu.edu
Med Dir: Walter Carmoney, MD
Class Cap: 40   *Begins:* Jan Aug
Length: 24 mos   *Award:* AAS
Tuition per yr: $2,000 res, $7,000 non-res
Evening or weekend classes available

Utah

Utah Valley Regional Medical Center

Radiography Prgm
1034 N 500 W
Provo, UT 84603
Prgm Dir: Dottie Winterton, BA RT(R)
Tel: 801 373-7850   *Fax:* 801 371-7585
Med Dir: Brent Chandler
Class Cap: 12   *Begins:* Sep
Length: 24 mos   *Award:* Cert
Tuition per yr: $900

Salt Lake Community College

Radiography Prgm
South City Campus
1575 S State St
Salt Lake City, UT 84121
Prgm Dir: Marlene M Tucker, MEd RT(R)
Tel: 801 957-3255   *Fax:* 801 957-3300
E-mail: tuckerma@slcc.edu
Med Dir: David Bragg
Class Cap: 58
Length: 21 mos   *Award:* AAS
Tuition per yr: $1,446 res, $4,506 non-res
Evening or weekend classes available

Vermont

Champlain College

Radiography Prgm
163 S Willard St
PO Box 670
Burlington, VT 05402-0670
Prgm Dir: Michelle G Miller, MEd RT(R)(M)
Tel: 802 860-2700   *Fax:* 802 860-2750
E-mail: miller@champlain.edu
Class Cap: 23   *Begins:* Aug
Length: 21 mos, 45 mos   *Award:* AS, BS
Tuition per yr: $9,225
Evening or weekend classes available

Rutland Regional Medical Center

Radiography Prgm
160 Allen St
Rutland, VT 05701-4595
Prgm Dir: Robert DeAngelis, BS RT(R)
Tel: 802 747-1712   *Fax:* 802 747-6200
Class Cap: 9
Length: 24 mos   *Award:* Cert
Tuition per yr: $900 res, $900 non-res

Virginia

Northern Virginia Community College

Radiography Prgm
8333 Little River Trnpk
Annandale, VA 22003
Prgm Dir: Marilyn B Sinderbrand, BS RT(R)
Tel: 703 323-3037   *Fax:* 703 323-4576
Class Cap: 30   *Begins:* Aug
Length: 21 mos   *Award:* AAS
Tuition per yr: $48 res, $157 non-res
Evening or weekend classes available

Univ of Virginia Health Sciences Center

Radiography Prgm
Jefferson Park Ave
Radiology Box 170
Charlottesville, VA 22908
Prgm Dir: Mitchell R Bieber, BA RT(R)
Tel: 804 924-9344   *Fax:* 804 982-4019
Med Dir: Hubert Shafer Jr., MD
Class Cap: 20   *Begins:* July
Length: 24 mos   *Award:* Cert
Tuition per yr: $1,800

Mary Washington Hospital

Radiography Prgm
1001 Sam Perry Blvd
Fredericksburg, VA 22401
Prgm Dir: Jan G Clark, MEd RT(R)(CV)
Tel: 540 899-1892   *Fax:* 540 899-1586
Class Cap: 10   *Begins:* Aug
Length: 22.5 mos   *Award:* Cert
Tuition per yr: $1,200 res, $1,200 non-res

Rockingham Memorial Hospital

Radiography Prgm
235 Cantrell Ave
Harrisonburg, VA 22801-3293
Prgm Dir: Jon A Lough, RTR
Tel: 540 433-4532   *Fax:* 540 433-4423
Med Dir: Charles H Henderson
Class Cap: 12   *Begins:* June
Length: 24 mos   *Award:* Cert, AAS
Tuition per yr: $3,000
Evening or weekend classes available

Central Virginia Community College

Radiography Prgm
3506 Wards Rd
Lynchburg, VA 24502-2498
Prgm Dir: Gene Blair, MEd RT(R)
Tel: 804 386-4695   *Fax:* 804 386-4681
Class Cap: 17   *Begins:* Aug
Length: 24 mos   *Award:* AAS
Tuition per yr: $1,679 res, $5,616 non-res

Riverside School of Health Occupations

Radiography Prgm
12420 Warwick Blvd/Ste 6-G
Newport News, VA 23606
Prgm Dir: Pamela C Gebhart-Cline, BA RT(R)
Tel: 804 594-2722
Class Cap: 13
Length: 24 mos   *Award:* Cert
Tuition per yr: $3,200

DePaul Medical Center

Radiography Prgm
150 Kingsley Ln
Norfolk, VA 23505
Prgm Dir: Conwell E Boccia, BS RT(RN)
Tel: 757 889-5227   *Fax:* 757 889-4230
Med Dir: Felix A Hughes III, MD
Length: 24 mos   *Award:* Cert
Tuition per yr: $3,200 res, $3,200 non-res

Southside Regional Medical Center

Radiography Prgm
801 S Adams St
Petersburg, VA 23803
Prgm Dir: Pamela J G Shelton, BBA RT(R)
Tel: 804 862-5883   *Fax:* 804 862-5937
Med Dir: John Grizzard, MD
Class Cap: 12   *Begins:* Aug
Length: 24 mos   *Award:* Cert
Tuition per yr: $1,500

Southwest Virginia Community College

Radiography Prgm
PO Box SVCC
Richlands, VA 24641-1510
Prgm Dir: Ron E Proffitt, MEd RT(R)
Tel: 703 964-7306   *Fax:* 703 964-9307
Class Cap: 24
Length: 24 mos   *Award:* AAS
Tuition per yr: $2,084 res, $6,785 non-res
Evening or weekend classes available

Programs

Med Coll of VA/Virginia Commonwealth U
Radiography Prgm
Box 980495
1200 E Broad St Rm 632
Richmond, VA 23298-0495
Prgm Dir: Joanne S Greathouse, EdS RT(R) FA
Tel: 804 828-9104   *Fax:* 804 828-5778
E-mail: jgreathouse@gems.vcu.edu
Med Dir: Uma Prasad, MD
Class Cap: 24   *Begins:* Aug
Length: 33 mos   *Award:* BS
Tuition per yr: $4,707 res, $13,952 non-res
Evening or weekend classes available

St Mary's Hospital
Radiography Prgm
5801 Bremo Rd
Richmond, VA 23226
Prgm Dir: Joyce O Hawkins, BS RT(R)
Tel: 804 281-8478   *Fax:* 804 285-2772
Med Dir: Karsten Konerding, MD
Class Cap: 9   *Begins:* Sep
Length: 24 mos   *Award:* Cert
Tuition per yr: $1,800

Carilion Health System/Carilion Roanoke Mem Hosp
Radiography Prgm
PO Box 13367
Carilion Roanoke Memorial Hospital
Roanoke, VA 24033-3367
Prgm Dir: Norma F Arthur, MSEd RT(R)
Tel: 540 981-7731
Med Dir: Roger P Wiley
Class Cap: 15   *Begins:* Aug
Length: 24 mos   *Award:* Cert
Tuition per yr: $1,700 res, $1,700 non-res

Virginia Western Community College
Radiography Prgm
3095 Colonial Ave SW
PO Box 14007
Roanoke, VA 24038
Prgm Dir: Shirl Duke Lamanca, MS Ed RT(R)
Tel: 540 857-7306   *Fax:* 540 857-7544
Class Cap: 24   *Begins:* Aug
Length: 24 mos   *Award:* AAS
Tuition per yr: res, $2,050 non-res
Evening or weekend classes available

Tidewater Community College
Radiography Prgm
1700 College Crescent
Virginia Beach, VA 23456
Prgm Dir: Kim M Burford, MS RT(R)
Tel: 804 427-7253   *Fax:* 804 427-1338
Med Dir: David Bridges, MD
Class Cap: 65   *Begins:* May
Length: 24 mos   *Award:* AAS
Tuition per yr: $2,028

Winchester Medical Center
Radiography Prgm
1840 Amherst St
PO Box 3340
Winchester, VA 22603
Prgm Dir: John D Orndorff, BS RT(R)
Tel: 540 722-8750
E-mail: nmcms@global.com.net
Class Cap: 15
Length: 24 mos   *Award:* Cert
Tuition per yr: $3,000

Washington

Bellevue Community College
Radiography Prgm
3000 Landerholm Circle SE
Bellevue, WA 98007-6484
Prgm Dir: Ronald S Radvilas, MS RT(R)
Tel: 206 641-2507
Med Dir: John Harley, MD
Class Cap: 30   *Begins:* July
Length: 24 mos   *Award:* AA
Tuition per yr: $1,831 res, $7,038 non-res
Evening or weekend classes available

Pima Medical Institute - Seattle
Radiography Prgm
1627 Eastlake Ave E
Seattle, WA 98102
Prgm Dir: Janis Stiewing, MS RT(R)
Tel: 206 322-6100   *Fax:* 206 324-1985
Class Cap: 42   *Begins:* March June Oct
Length: 24 mos   *Award:* AS
Tuition per yr: $9,327 res, $9,327 non-res

Holy Family Hospital
Radiography Prgm
N 5633 Lidgerwood Ave
Spokane, WA 99207
Prgm Dir: Earlene S Riggins, RT(R)
Tel: 509 482-2384   *Fax:* 509 482-2176
Class Cap: 8
Length: 24 mos   *Award:* Cert
Tuition per yr: $2,000

Tacoma Community College
Radiography Prgm
6501 S 19th St
Tacoma, WA 98466
Prgm Dir: Royal W Domingo, BA RT(R)
Tel: 206 566-5168   *Fax:* 206 566-5273
E-mail: r.domingo@tcc.tacoma.ctc.edu
Class Cap: 45
Length: 27 mos   *Award:* AAS
Tuition per yr: $1,869 res, $7,349 non-res
Evening or weekend classes available

Wenatchee Valley College
Radiography Prgm
1300 Fifth St
Wenatchee, WA 98801-1799
Prgm Dir: Shirely R King, MS RT(R)
Tel: 509 662-1651   *Fax:* 509 664-2538
Med Dir: David Weber, MD
Class Cap: 28   *Begins:* Sep
Length: 22 mos   *Award:* AAS
Tuition per yr: $467 res, $1,837 non-res
Evening or weekend classes available

Yakima Valley Community College
Radiography Prgm
16th Ave and Nob Hill Blvd
PO Box 1647
Yakima, WA 98907
Prgm Dir: Marcy Barnes, BA RT(R)
Tel: 509 571-4928   *Fax:* 509 571-4604
Med Dir: David Stepanek
Class Cap: 30
Length: 24 mos   *Award:* AS
Tuition per yr: $477 res, $1,847 non-res
Evening or weekend classes available

West Virginia

Bluefield State College
Radiography Prgm
219 Rock St
Bluefield, WV 24701
Prgm Dir: Melissa Oxley Haye, BS RT(R)
Tel: 304 327-4145   *Fax:* 304 327-4219
E-mail: mhaye@bscvax:wvnet.edu
Med Dir: Maurice Bassall
Class Cap: 34   *Begins:* May or June
Length: 24 mos   *Award:* AS
Tuition per yr: $2,450 res, $5,886 non-res
Evening or weekend classes available

University of Charleston
Radiography Prgm
2300 MacCorkle Ave SE
Charleston, WV 25304
Prgm Dir: David J Goddin, MA RT(R)
Tel: 304 357-4854   *Fax:* 304 357-4965
Med Dir: J L Leef Jr, MD
Class Cap: 20   *Begins:* June
Length: 23 mos   *Award:* AS
Tuition per yr: $14,670 res, $14,670 non-res
Evening or weekend classes available

United Hospital Center
Radiography Prgm
3 Hospital Plaza
PO Box 1680
Clarksburg, WV 26301
Prgm Dir: Rosemary V Trupo, BA RT(R)
Tel: 304 624-2895   *Fax:* 304 624-2856
Med Dir: Gerald J Murphy, MD
Class Cap: 10   *Begins:* June
Length: 24 mos   *Award:* Cert
Tuition per yr: $2,000

St Mary's Hospital
Radiography Prgm
2900 First Ave
Huntington, WV 25702
Prgm Dir: Mark E Adkins, MSEd RT(R)
Tel: 304 526-1259   *Fax:* 304 526-1487
Class Cap: 23   *Begins:* July
Length: 24 mos   *Award:* Cert
Tuition per yr: $750 res, $750 non-res

West Virginia University Hospitals, Inc
Radiography Prgm
Box 8062
Morgantown, WV 26505-8062
Prgm Dir: Janice S Shock, BA RT(R)(T)(M)
Tel: 304 598-4251   *Fax:* 304 598-4702
Class Cap: 15
Length: 24 mos   *Award:* Cert
Tuition per yr: $1,600

Southern West Virginia Community College
Radiography Prgm
PO Box 2900
Mt Gay, WV 25637
Prgm Dir: Mary M Holder, MS RT(R)
Tel: 304 792-7098   *Fax:* 304 792-7028
E-mail: maryh@wvnet.
Class Cap: 15
Length: 24 mos   *Award:* AS
Tuition per yr: $1,202 res, $1,202 non-res
Evening or weekend classes available

Camden-Clark Memorial Hospital

Radiography Prgm
800 Garfield Ave
PO Box 718
Parkersburg, WV 26102
Prgm Dir: Teresa Jean Woollard, BS RT(R)
Tel: 304 424-2974   *Fax:* 304 424-2722
Class Cap: 10   *Begins:* July
Length: 24 mos   *Award:* Cert
Tuition per yr: $500

Ohio Valley Medical Center

Radiography Prgm
2000 Eoff St
Wheeling, WV 26003
Prgm Dir: Lisa K Firestone, BS RT(R)
Tel: 304 234-8781   *Fax:* 304 234-8410
Med Dir: Mark Kenamond
Class Cap: 10   *Begins:* July
Length: 24 mos   *Award:* Cert
Tuition per yr: $1,000
Evening or weekend classes available

Wheeling Hospital

Radiography Prgm
Medical Park
Wheeling, WV 26003
Prgm Dir: Misty D Kahl, AS RT(R)
Tel: 304 243-3173   *Fax:* 304 243-3130
Med Dir: Terry L Stake
Class Cap: 20   *Begins:* July
Length: 24 mos   *Award:* Cert
Tuition per yr: $1,000

Wisconsin

Beloit Memorial Hospital

Radiography Prgm
1969 W Hart Rd
Beloit, WI 53511
Prgm Dir: Joseph W Ipsen, BS RT(R)
Tel: 608 364-5645
Length: 24 mos   *Award:* Cert
Tuition per yr: $500

Lakeshore Technical College

Radiography Prgm
1290 North Ave
Cleveland, WI 53015-1414
Prgm Dir: James R Odau, BS RT(R)
Tel: 414 458-4183
Class Cap: 15   *Begins:* Jan
Length: 22 mos   *Award:* AS
Tuition per yr: $2,375 res, $18,253 non-res
Evening or weekend classes available

Chippewa Valley Technical College

Radiography Prgm
620 W Clairemont Ave
Eau Claire, WI 54701-6162
Prgm Dir: Stephen R Schreiner, Equiv RT(R)
Tel: 715 833-6428   *Fax:* 715 833-6470
E-mail: sschreiner@mail.chippewa.tec.wi.us
Class Cap: 16   *Begins:* Aug
Length: 22 mos   *Award:* AAS
Tuition per yr: $2,028 res, $2,028 non-res
Evening or weekend classes available

Bellin Memorial Hospital

Radiography Prgm
744 S Webster
PO Box 23400
Green Bay, WI 54305-3400
Prgm Dir: Linda L Joppe, BS RT(R)
Tel: 414 433-3497   *Fax:* 414 433-5811
Class Cap: 8
Length: 24 mos   *Award:* Dipl
Tuition per yr: $1,000

Western Wisconsin Technical College

Radiography Prgm
304 N 6th St
PO Box 908
LaCrosse, WI 54601-7194
Prgm Dir: Gary Heintz, BS RT(R)
Tel: 608 785-9255   *Fax:* 608 785-7194
Med Dir: Brian Manske, MD
Class Cap: 28   *Begins:* Aug
Length: 24 mos   *Award:* AAS
Tuition per yr: $2,100 res, $13,789 non-res
Evening or weekend classes available

Madison Area Technical College

Radiography Prgm
3550 Anderson St
Madison, WI 53704-2599
Prgm Dir: Jami Skaar, BS RT(R)
Tel: 608 258-2478   *Fax:* 608 258-2480
Class Cap: 18   *Begins:* Aug
Length: 24 mos   *Award:* AAS

University of Wisconsin Hosp & Clinics

Radiography Prgm
600 Highland Ave
E3/311 Radiology
Madison, WI 53792-3252
Prgm Dir: Gregory L Spicer, MA RT(R)
Tel: 608 263-9030   *Fax:* 608 268-0876
E-mail: glspicer@facstaff.wisc.edu
Med Dir: Ian Sproat, MD
Class Cap: 24
Length: 24 mos   *Award:* Cert
Tuition per yr: $1,200 res, $1,200 non-res

St Joseph's Hospital

Radiography Prgm
611 St Joseph Ave
Marshfield, WI 54449
Prgm Dir: Eugene Wawrzyniak, BS RT(R)
Tel: 715 387-7184   *Fax:* 715 387-9846
E-mail: wawrzyng@mfld.clin.edu
Class Cap: 17
Length: 24 mos   *Award:* Cert
Tuition per yr: $1,500

Columbia Hospital

Radiography Prgm
2025 E Newport Ave
Milwaukee, WI 53211
Prgm Dir: Paula S Maramonte, MEd RT(R)
Tel: 414 961-3817   *Fax:* 414 961-4359
Class Cap: 8   *Begins:* Sep
Length: 24 mos   *Award:* Cert
Tuition per yr: $550 res, $550 non-res

Froedtert Memorial Lutheran Hospital

Radiography Prgm
9200 W Wisconsin Ave
Milwaukee, WI 53226
Prgm Dir: Susan Lura Sanson, BS RT(R)
Tel: 414 257-6115   *Fax:* 414 259-9290
Med Dir: Katherine Shaffer, MD
Class Cap: 30   *Begins:* Jul
Length: 24 mos   *Award:* Cert
Tuition per yr: $1,000 res, $1,000 non-res

Milwaukee Area Technical College

Radiography Prgm
700 W State St
Milwaukee, WI 53233-1443
Prgm Dir: Jane Powell, BA RT(R)
Tel: 414 297-7156
Med Dir: Douglas Olen, MD
Class Cap: 30
Length: 24 mos   *Award:* AAS
Tuition per yr: $1,992 res, $1,992 non-res
Evening or weekend classes available

St Luke's Medical Center

Radiography Prgm
2900 W Oklahoma Ave
PO Box 2901
Milwaukee, WI 53201-2901
Prgm Dir: Jean M Schultz, BS RT(R)
Tel: 414 649-6762
Length: 24 mos   *Award:* Cert
Tuition per yr: $600 res, $600 non-res

St Mary's Hospital

Radiography Prgm
2323 N Lake Dr
Milwaukee, WI 53211
Prgm Dir: Linda K Martens, RT(R)
Tel: 414 291-1030
Class Cap: 10
Length: 24 mos   *Award:* Cert
Tuition per yr: $800

St Michael Hospital

Radiography Prgm
2400 W Villard Ave
Milwaukee, WI 53209
Prgm Dir: Donna M Lawien, RT(R)
Tel: 414 527-5149   *Fax:* 414 527-5149
Class Cap: 10   *Begins:* Oct
Length: 24 mos   *Award:* Cert
Tuition per yr: $375

Theda Clark Regional Medical Center

Radiography Prgm
130 Second St
PO Box 2021
Neenah, WI 54957-2021
Prgm Dir: Carliss M Lau, RT(R)
Tel: 414 729-3146   *Fax:* 414 729-2219
Med Dir: Donald Furnez
Class Cap: 10   *Begins:* Sep
Length: 24 mos   *Award:* Cert
Tuition per yr: $1,500 res, $1,500 non-res

Mercy Medical Center

Radiography Prgm
631 Hazel St
PO Box 1100
Oshkosh, WI 54902
Prgm Dir: James R Werner, BS RT(R)
Tel: 414 236-2253   *Fax:* 414 236-1373
Class Cap: 12
Length: 24 mos   *Award:* Cert
Tuition per yr: $4,000

All Saints Healthcare System Inc

Radiography Prgm
1320 Wisconsin Ave
Racine, WI 53403
Prgm Dir: Cheri A Dyke, RT(R)BS
Tel: 414 636-2846   *Fax:* 414 636-8834
Med Dir: Thomas Schuster, MD
Class Cap: 23   *Begins:* July
Length: 24 mos   *Award:* Cert
Tuition per yr: $1,200
Evening or weekend classes available

Northcentral Technical College

Radiography Prgm
1000 Campus Dr
Wausau, WI 54401-1899
Prgm Dir: Steven J Hommerding, MEd RT(R)
Tel: 715 675-3331   *Fax:* 715 675-9776
Med Dir: James Collison
Class Cap: 18   *Begins:* Aug
Length: 24 mos   *Award:* AAS
Tuition per yr: $1,600 res, $1,600 non-res

Wyoming

Casper College

Radiography Prgm
125 College Dr
Casper, WY 82601
Prgm Dir: Deborah K Bauert, MS RT(R)
Tel: 307 268-2544   *Fax:* 307 268-2087
E-mail: dbauert@acad.cc.whecn.edu
Med Dir: Steven Horn, MD
Class Cap: 11
Length: 24 mos   *Award:* AS
Tuition per yr: $1,416 res, $1,416 non-res

Laramie County Community College

Radiography Prgm
1400 E College Dr
Cheyenne, WY 82007
Prgm Dir: Starla L Mason, MS RT(R)
Tel: 307 778-1391   *Fax:* 307 778-1399
Med Dir: James G Hubbard, MD
Class Cap: 14   *Begins:* Aug
Length: 24 mos   *Award:* AAS
Tuition per yr: $1,236 res, $1,854 non-res
Evening or weekend classes available

West Park Hospital

Radiography Prgm
707 Sheridan Ave
Cody, WY 82414
Prgm Dir: Kenneth K Helfrick, BA RT(R)
Tel: 307 578-2278   *Fax:* 307 578-2389
Med Dir: Thomas Pettinger, MD
Class Cap: 3   *Begins:* Jul
Length: 24 mos   *Award:* Cert
Tuition per yr: $2,000 res, $2,000 non-res

Rehabilitation Counselor

History

History of the Profession

Initially, rehabilitation professionals were recruited from a variety of human service disciplines, including public health nursing, social work, and school counseling. Although educational programs began to appear in the 1940s, it was not until the availability of federal funding for rehabilitation counseling programs in 1954 that the profession began to grow and establish its own identity.

Historically, rehabilitation counselors primarily served working-age adults with disabilities. Today, the need for rehabilitation counseling services extends to children and the elderly. Rehabilitation counselors also may provide general and specialized counseling to people with disabilities in public human service programs and private practice settings.

Accreditation History

In 1969, a group of rehabilitation professionals met to discuss the need for accreditation of rehabilitation counselor education (RCE) programs. After 2 years of planning, the Council on Rehabilitation Education (CORE) was formed in 1971 and incorporated in 1972. Five professional rehabilitation organizations were represented by CORE:

- American Rehabilitation Association (ARA), formerly the International Association of Rehabilitation Facilities
- American Rehabilitation Counseling Association (ARCA)
- Council of State Administrators of Vocational Rehabilitation (CSAVR)
- National Council on Rehabilitation Education (NCRE), formerly the Council on Rehabilitation Educators
- National Rehabilitation Counseling Association (NRCA).

Today, these five organizations—except ARA, which has been replaced by the National Council of State Agencies of the Blind (NCSAB)—comprise CORE and as such represent the professional and organizational constituencies concerned with the training, evaluation, and employment of rehabilitation counselors. CORE accredits approximately 80 university- and college-based rehabilitation counselor educational programs at the master's degree level. Accreditation serves to promote the effective delivery of rehabiltation services to people with disabilities by stimulating and fostering continual review and improvement of master's degree rehabilitation counselor educational programs.

Occupational Description

Working directly with an individual with a disability, the rehabilitation counselor determines and coordinates services to assist people with disabilities in moving from psychological and economic dependence to independence.

Job Description

Rehabilitation counselors assist people with physical, mental, emotional, or social disabilities to become or remain self-sufficient, productive citizens. Disabilities may result from birth defects, illness and disease, work-related injuries, automobile accidents, the stresses of war, work, and daily life, and the aging process. Rehabilitation counselors help individuals with disabilities deal with societal and personal problems, plan careers, and find and keep satisfying jobs. They also may work with individuals, professional organizations, and advocacy groups to address the environmental and social barriers that create obstacles for people with disabilities. The rehabilitation counselor builds bridges between the often isolated world of people with disabilities and their families, communities, and work environments.

Other responsibilities for the rehabilitation counselor include

- evaluating an individual's potential for independent living and employment and arranging for medical and psychological care and vocational assessment, training, and job placement;
- evaluating medical and psychological reports and conferring with physicians and psychologists about the types of work individuals can perform; and
- working with employers to identify and/or modify job responsibilities to accommodate individuals with disabilities.

The rehabilitation counselor draws on knowledge from several fields, including psychology, medicine, psychiatry, sociology, social work, education, and law. Their specialized knowledge of disabilities and environmental factors that interact with disabilities, as well as specific knowledge and skills, differentiate rehabilitation counselors from other types of counselors.

Employment Characteristics

Most rehabilitation counselors work in state or federal rehabilitation agencies. Because all state rehabilitation agencies follow the same general procedures, a rehabilitation counselor has geographical mobility and can find employment throughout the United States and its territories. Other potential employers include comprehensive rehabilitation centers, universities and academic settings, insurance companies, substance abuse rehabilitation centers, correctional facilities, halfway houses, and independent living centers. Reflecting this wide range of job opportunities, rehabilitation counselors are often employed in positions with different job titles, such as counselor, job placement specialist, substance abuse counselor, probation and parole officer, mental health counselor, marriage and family counselor, and independent living specialist.

According to the NCRE, the average starting salary for rehabilitation counselors in the public sector is more than $23,000 and can range between $16,000 and $32,000; the salary ranges in the private sector are considerably higher. The average overall salary is estimated at more than $30,000.

Employment Outlook

Rehabilitation counselors serve a large portion of the United States population. An estimated 43 million Americans have physical, mental, or psychological disabilities that restrict their activities and prevent them from obtaining or maintaining jobs.

Consequently, the employment outlook for the profession is excellent: Based on national employment outlook studies and regional and state surveys, hundreds of rehabilitation counselor positions are expected to be available throughout the 1990s and into the next century for qualified master's level professionals. Recent studies show that RCE programs are not graduating sufficient numbers of qualified students to meet current and anticipated marketplace needs.

Recently the roles and responsibilities of rehabilitation counselors have expanded, further increasing the attractiveness of a career in the profession. Rehabilitation counselors, for example, have begun to determine, coordinate, and arrange for rehabilitation and transition services for children within school systems. In addition, rehabilitation counselors are providing geriatric rehabilitation services to older persons with health problems, and workers injured on the job are increasingly receiving rehabilitation services through private rehabilition counseling companies and employers' disability management and employment assistance programs.

Many former teachers, attorneys, nurses, physical therapists, occupational therapists, clergy, and businesspeople have found second careers as rehabilitation counselors.

Certification, Licensure, and Registration

Certification and licensure of rehabilitation counselors help protect the public and provide a means of identifying those individuals who possess the minimum training and meet supervised work experience standards established by professional groups and governmental agencies.

Certification. The Commission on Rehabilitation Counselor Certification (CRCC), an independent credentialing body incorporated in 1974, certifies rehabilitation counselors throughout the United States and in several other countries who meet educational and work experience requirements, pass an examination, and maintain certification by completing 100 hours of acceptable continuing education credit every 5 years.

Licensure. A counseling license is a credential authorized by a state legislature that regulates the title and/or practice of professional counselors. Rehabilitation counselors are eligible for licensure as professional counselors in nearly all states that regulate counselors; licensure requirements include passing an examination, acquiring needed supervised counseling experience, and, in some states, completing specified coursework.

Registration. A number of state workers' compensation laws or regulations specify education, training, and/or credentials requirements for people providing rehabilitation counseling services to workers with disabilities. In these states, rehabilitation counselors pay a fee and provide proof of education and/or certification to register with the state workers' compensation agency. Most of these states also require the certified rehabilitation counselor (CRC) credential, although the permitted scope of services may vary from one state to the next.

Educational Programs

Length. Rehabilitation counselor education programs typically provide between 18 and 24 months of academic and field-based clinical training. Clinical training consists of a practicum and a minimum of 600 hours of supervised internship experience. Clinical field experiences are available in a variety of community, state, federal, and private rehabiltation-related programs.

Prerequisites. Although no formal requirements exist, most rehabilitation counseling graduate students have undergraduate degrees in rehabilitation services, psychology, sociology, or other human services-related fields.

Curriculum. Rehabilitation counselors are trained in counseling theory, skills, and techniques; individual, group, and environmental assessment; psychosocial and medical aspects of disability, including human growth and development; principles of psychiatric rehabilitation; case management and rehabilitation planning; issues and ethics in rehabilitation service delivery; technological adaptation; vocational evaluation and work adjustment; career counseling; and job development and placement. In addition, students often take required or elective courses in such areas as group counseling, marriage and family counseling, substance abuse rehabilitation, juvenile and adult offender rehabilitation, mental retardation, communication disorders, sign language, stress management, psychological testing, and rehabilitation administration.

Standards. Each new rehabilitation counseling education program is assessed in accordance with the *Standards for Rehabilitation Counselor Education Programs*, and accredited programs are periodically reviewed to ensure that they remain in substantial compliance. The *Standards* are not intended to limit program creativity or limit variability; programs may adopt innovative procedures or experiences that meet the standards in a different manner. The *Standards* are available from CORE.

Programs

Inquiries

Accreditation

Inquiries regarding accreditation should be directed to

Jeanne Patterson, Executive Director
Council on Rehabilitation Education (CORE)
1835 Rohlwing Rd/Ste E
Rolling Meadows, IL 60008
847 394-1785
847 394-2108 Fax
E-mail: patters@polaris.net

Careers

Inquiries regarding careers should be directed to

National Rehabilitation Counseling Association (NRCA)
8807 Sudley Rd/#102
Manassas, VA 22110-4719
703 361-2077
American Rehabilitation Counseling Association (ARCA)
5999 Stevenson Ave
Alexandria, VA 22304
703 620-4404

National Association of Rehabilitation Professionals in the Private
Sector (NARPPS)
PO Box 697
Brookline, MA 02146
617 566-4432

National Council on Rehabilitation Education (NCRE)
c/o Dr Garth Eldredge
Department of Special Education and Rehabilitation
Utah State University
Logan, UT 84322-2870
801 797-3241

Certification

Inquiries regarding certification should be directed to

Commission on Rehabilitation Counselor Certification (CRCC)
1835 Rohlwing Rd/Ste E
Rolling Meadows, IL 60008
847 394-2104

Rehabilitation Counselor

Alabama

Auburn University

Rehabilitation Counseling Prgm
Counseling and Counseling Psych
Haley Center Rm 2014
Auburn, AL 36849-5222
Prgm Dir: E Keith Byrd
Tel: 205 844-2882

University of Alabama at Birmingham

Rehabilitation Counseling Prgm
School of Education Rm 107
901 S 13th St
Birmingham, AL 35294-1250
Prgm Dir: William A Crunk Jr, PhD
Tel: 205 934-3701   *Fax:* 205 975-8040

University of Alabama

Rehabilitation Counseling Prgm
318 Graves Hall
PO Box 870231
Tuscaloosa, AL 35487-0231
Prgm Dir: David W Head, PhD
Tel: 205 348-7575   *Fax:* 205 348-6873

Arizona

University of Arizona

Rehabilitation Counseling Prgm
Dept of Spec Educ and Rehab
College of Education
Tucson, AZ 85721
Prgm Dir: Amos Sales
Tel: 520 621-0941   *Fax:* 520 621-3821
Class Cap: 40
Length: 24 mos   *Award:* Dipl, BA, MA
Tuition per yr: $970 res, $2,440 non-res
Evening or weekend classes available

Arkansas

University of Arkansas Main Campus

Rehabilitation Counseling Prgm
Rehabilitation Education
346 North West Ave
Fayetteville, AR 72701
Prgm Dir: Jason Andrew
Tel: 501 575-6412   *Fax:* 501 575-3253
E-mail: JANDREW@COMP.UARK.EDUC
Class Cap: 15   *Begins:* Aug Jan June July
Length: 18 mos   *Award:* Dipl, MS
Tuition per yr: $3,384 res, $7,752 non-res
Evening or weekend classes available

Arkansas State University

Rehabilitation Counseling Prgm
Dep of Psychology and Counseling
PO Box 1560
State University, AR 72467
Prgm Dir: Mark Stebnicki, RhD CRC LPC CCM
Tel: 501 972-3064   *Fax:* 501 972-3828
Class Cap: 60   *Begins:* Aug Jan May
Length: 24 mos   *Award:* MRC
Tuition per yr: $1,170 res, $1,170 non-res
Evening or weekend classes available

California

California State University - Fresno

Rehabilitation Counseling Prgm
5005 N Maple/MS 3
Fresno, CA 93740
Prgm Dir: Charles Arokiasamy, RhD
Tel: 209 278-0325   *Fax:* 209 278-0404
E-mail: charlesa@csufresno.edu
Begins: Jan Aug
Length: 24 mos   *Award:* MS
Tuition per yr: $1,806 res, $9,000 non-res
Evening or weekend classes available

California State University - Los Angeles

Rehabilitation Counseling Prgm
5151 State University Dr
King Hall C1065
Los Angeles, CA 90032
Prgm Dir: Martin Brodwin, PhD CRC
Tel: 213 343-4440   *Fax:* 213 343-4318
Class Cap: 25   *Begins:* Jan Apr Jun Sep
Length: 24 mos   *Award:* MS
Tuition per yr: $1,600, res, $4,500 non-res
Evening or weekend classes available

California State University - Sacramento

Rehabilitation Counseling Prgm
School of Education Rm 437
6000 J St
Sacramento, CA 95819-6079
Prgm Dir: Richard A Koch, EdD
Tel: 916 278-6622   *Fax:* 916 278-5904

California State Univ - San Bernardino

Rehabilitation Counseling Prgm
School of Education
5500 University Pkwy
San Bernardino, CA 92407
Prgm Dir: Margaret Cooney, PhD CRC
Tel: 909 880-5662   *Fax:* 909 880-5992
Class Cap: 26   *Begins:* Sep Mar
Length: 24 mos   *Award:* MS
Tuition per yr: $1,900, res, $6,396 non-res
Evening or weekend classes available

San Diego State University

Rehabilitation Counseling Prgm
Interwork Institute
5850 Hardy Ave/Ste 112
San Diego, CA 92182-5313
Prgm Dir: Fred R McFarlane, PhD
Tel: 619 594-6406   *Fax:* 619 594-4208
E-mail: fmcfarla@mail.sdsu.edu
Class Cap: 30   *Begins:* Aug
Length: 36 mos   *Award:* MS
Tuition per yr: $1,902, res, $4,920 non-res
Evening or weekend classes available

San Francisco State University

Rehabilitation Counseling Prgm
Dept of Counseling
1600 Holloway Ave
San Francisco, CA 94132
Prgm Dir: Alice Nemon
Tel: 415 338-7869   *Fax:* 415 338-0594
E-mail: anemon@sfsu.edu
Class Cap: 25   *Begins:* Sep
Length: 18 mos   *Award:* MS
Tuition per yr: $1,982, res, $1,982 non-res
Evening or weekend classes available

Colorado

University of Northern Colorado

Rehabilitation Counseling Prgm
Dept of Human Services
Greeley, CO 80639
Prgm Dir: Richard R Wolfe, PhD CRC
Tel: 970 351-1541   *Fax:* 970 351-1255
Length: 24 mos   *Begins:* Sep
E-mail: rrwolfe@bentley.univnorthco.edu

District of Columbia

Gallaudet University

Rehabilitation Counseling Prgm
Dept of Counseling
800 Florida Ave NE
Washington, DC 20002
Prgm Dir: Marita Danek, PhD CRC
Tel: 202 651-5515   *Fax:* 202 651-5657
E-mail: mmdanek@gallua

George Washington University

Rehabilitation Counseling Prgm
Dept of Human Services
Washington, DC 20052
Prgm Dir: Jorge Garcia, RhD CRC LPC
Tel: 202 994-7126   *Fax:* 202 994-3436
E-mail: garcia@gwis2.circ.gwu.edu
Class Cap: 20   *Begins:* Sep
Length: 48 mos   *Award:* MS
Evening or weekend classes available

Florida

University of Florida

Rehabilitation Counseling Prgm
Dept of Rehabilitation Counseling
PO Box 100175
Gainesville, FL 32610-0175
Prgm Dir: Horace W Sawyer, EdD CRC
Tel: 352 392-6946   *Fax:* 352 392-6529
E-mail: hsawyer.hrp@mail.health.ufl.edu

Florida State University

Rehabilitation Counseling Prgm
215 Stone Bldg
Tallahassee, FL 32306
Prgm Dir: E Jane Burkhead, PhD CRC
Tel: 904 644-3854   *Fax:* 904 644-4335
Class Cap: 7   *Begins:* Aug
Length: 18 mos   *Award:* MS
Tuition per yr: $3,549, res, $11,671 non-res
Evening or weekend classes available

University of South Florida

Rehabilitation Counseling Prgm
Dept of Rehabilitation Counseling
SOC 107/4202 E Fowler Ave
Tampa, FL 33620-8100
Prgm Dir: John D Rasch, PhD CRC
Tel: 813 974-2855   *Fax:* 813 974-2668
E-mail: rasch@luna.cas.usf.edu

Georgia

University of Georgia

Rehabilitation Counseling Prgm
413 Aderhold Hall
Athens, GA 30602-7142
Prgm Dir: Jerold D Bozarth, PhD
Tel: 706 542-2597   *Fax:* 706 542-4130
E-mail: jbozarth@moe.coe.uga.edu
Class Cap: 12   *Begins:* Sep
Length: 21 mos   *Award:* MEd, MA
Tuition per yr: $0
Evening or weekend classes available

Georgia State University

Rehabilitation Counseling Prgm
Counseling and Psych Services Dept
9th Fl COE
Atlanta, GA 30303
Prgm Dir: Roger Weed, PhD CRC CIRS
Tel: 404 651-2550   *Fax:* 404 651-1160
E-mail: rweed@gsu.edu
Class Cap: 20   *Begins:* Jun Sep
Length: 24 mos   *Award:* MS
Tuition per yr: $0
Evening or weekend classes available

Fort Valley State College

Rehabilitation Counseling Prgm
1005 State College Dr
PO Box 4899
Ft Valley, GA 31030-3298
Prgm Dir: Perry L Hall, EdD CRC LPC
Tel: 912 825-6237   *Fax:* 912 825-6192
Class Cap: 20
Award: MS
Tuition per yr: $0 res, $2,024 non-res
Evening or weekend classes available

Hawaii

University of Hawaii at Manoa

Rehabilitation Counseling Prgm
Dept of Counselor Education
1776 University Ave/WA2-221
Honolulu, HI 96822
Prgm Dir: E Aiko Oda
Tel: 808 956-7904   *Fax:* 808 956-3814
E-mail: oda@hawaii.edu
Class Cap: 20   *Begins:* Jan Aug
Length: 24 mos   *Award:* MEd
Tuition per yr: $2,194, res, $6,842 non-res
Evening or weekend classes available

Programs

Idaho

University of Idaho

Rehabilitation Counseling Prgm
Div of Adult, Counselor and Tech Educ
College of Education Rm 211-B
Moscow, ID 83844-3081
Prgm Dir: Jerry Fischer, RhD CRC LPC
Tel: 208 885-5947   *Fax:* 208 885-6869
E-mail: jfischer@uidaho.edu
Class Cap: 7
Length: 24 mos   *Award:* MEd , MS
Tuition per yr: $4,950 res, $9,450 non-res
Evening or weekend classes available

Illinois

Southern Illinois Univ at Carbondale

Rehabilitation Counseling Prgm
Rehabilitation Institute
Carbondale, IL 62901-4609
Prgm Dir: Donna Falvo, PhD CRC
Tel: 618 453-8262   *Fax:* 618 453-8271
E-mail: dfalvo@siu.edu
Class Cap: 50   *Begins:* Aug Jan
Length: 24 mos   *Award:* MS
Tuition per yr: $2,040 res, $6,120 non-res
Evening or weekend classes available

Univ of Illinois at Urbana - Champaign

Rehabilitation Counseling Prgm
1206 S 4th, 121 Hoff
Champaign, IL 61820
Prgm Dir: Reginald J Alston, PhD
Tel: 217 333-6877   *Fax:* 217 333-2766
E-mail: alston@uiuc.edu

Illinois Institute of Technology

Rehabilitation Counseling Prgm
Inst of Psych/Rm 252 Life Science Bldg
3101 S Dearborn St
Chicago, IL 60616
Prgm Dir: Chow S Lam, PhD
Tel: 312 567-3515   *Fax:* 312 567-3493
E-mail: psychlam@iitvax.bitnet

Northern Illinois University

Rehabilitation Counseling Prgm
Dept of Communicative Disorders
DeKalb, IL 60115
Prgm Dir: Greg Long, PhD
Tel: 815 753-6508   *Fax:* 815 753-9123
E-mail: glong@niu.edu
Class Cap: 15   *Begins:* Aug Jan May
Length: 22 mos   *Award:* BS, MA
Tuition per yr: $1,698, res, $3,900 non-res
Evening or weekend classes available

Iowa

Drake University

Rehabilitation Counseling Prgm
Spec Educ, Counseling and Rehab
3206 University
Des Moines, IA 50311
Prgm Dir: Robert Stensrud
Tel: 515 271-3061   *Fax:* 515 271-4140
E-mail: bs6991r@acad.drake.edu
Class Cap: 18   *Begins:* Aug Jan
Length: 24 mos, 33 mos   *Award:* MS
Tuition per yr: $6,120 res, $6,120 non-res
Evening or weekend classes available

University of Iowa

Rehabilitation Counseling Prgm
N356 Lindquist Center N
Iowa City, IA 52242-1529
Prgm Dir: Vilia M Tarvydas, PhD CRC
Tel: 319 335-5284   *Fax:* 319 335-5386
E-mail: vilia-tarvydas@uiowa.edu
Class Cap: 24   *Begins:* Jun Aug
Length: 23 mos   *Award:* MA, PhD
Tuition per yr: $4,572, res, $14,730 non-res

Kansas

Emporia State University

Rehabilitation Counseling Prgm
Campus Box 4036
1200 Commerical
Emporia, KS 66801
Prgm Dir: Marvin D Kuehn, EdD
Tel: 316 341-5220   *Fax:* 316 341-5785
E-mail: kuehnmar@esuvm.bitnet
Begins: Aug Jan May
Length: 24 mos   *Award:* MS
Tuition per yr: $2,130, res, $5,626 non-res
Evening or weekend classes available

Kentucky

University of Kentucky

Rehabilitation Counseling Prgm
124 Taylor Education Bldg
Lexington, KY 40506
Prgm Dir: Ralph M Crystal
Tel: 606 257-3834   *Fax:* 606 257-3835
E-mail: REC002@pop.uky.edu
Class Cap: 15   *Begins:* Aug Jan May June
Length: 16 mos   *Award:* M.E.C.
Tuition per yr: $1,458 res, $4,038 non-res
Evening or weekend classes available

Louisiana

Southern Univ and A & M College

Rehabilitation Counseling Prgm
Baton Rouge, LA 70813
Prgm Dir: Madan M Kundu, PhD CRC NCC LRC
Tel: 504 771-2990   *Fax:* 504 771-2993
E-mail: kundusubr@aol.com
Class Cap: 25   *Begins:* Aug
Length: 24 mos   *Award:* MS
Tuition per yr: $1,023, res, $1,751 non-res
Evening or weekend classes available

Louisiana State Univ Med Ctr - New Orleans

Rehabilitation Counseling Prgm
School of Allied Health Professions
1900 Gravier St/Ste 8A1
New Orleans, LA 70112-2262
Prgm Dir: Douglas C Strohmer, PhD CRC
Tel: 504 568-4315   *Fax:* 504 568-4324
E-mail: dstroh@lsumc.edu
Class Cap: 18   *Begins:* Aug
Length: 20 mos   *Award:* MHS
Tuition per yr: $1,111, res, $1,250 non-res
Evening or weekend classes available

Maine

University of Southern Maine

Rehabilitation Counseling Prgm
400 Bailey Hall
Gorham, ME 04038
Prgm Dir: Stephen T Murphy, PhD CRC
Tel: 207 780-5319   *Fax:* 207 780-5043
E-mail: smurphy@usm.maine.edu
Class Cap: 15   *Begins:* Sep Jan May
Length: 18 mos   *Award:* MS
Evening or weekend classes available

Maryland

Coppin State College

Rehabilitation Counseling Prgm
2500 W North Ave
Baltimore, MD 21216
Prgm Dir: Leroy Fitzgerald
Tel: 410 383-5797   *Fax:* 410 383-9606

University of Maryland

Rehabilitation Counseling Prgm
Counseling and Personnel Services Dept
Coll of Education/Benjamin Bldg Rm 3214
College Park, MD 20742
Prgm Dir: Paul W Power
Tel: 301 405-2863   *Fax:* 301 405-9995
Class Cap: 15   *Begins:* Sep Jan   *Award:*
Tuition per yr: $2,777 res, $3,977 non-res
Evening or weekend classes available

Massachusetts

Boston University

Rehabilitation Counseling Prgm
Dept of Rehabilitation Counseling
635 Commonwealth Ave
Boston, MA 02215
Prgm Dir: Arthur E Dell Orto, PhD CRC
Tel: 617 353-2725   *Fax:* 617 353-7814
E-mail: abo@bu.edu
Class Cap: 30   *Begins:* Sep
Length: 24 mos, 48 mos   *Award:* Cert, BS MS ,
  ScD
Tuition per yr: $20,570 res, $20,570 non-res
Evening or weekend classes available

Northeastern University
Rehabilitation Counseling Prgm
Counseling Psych, Rehab and Spec Educ
203 Lake Hall
Boston, MA 02115
Prgm Dir: James F Scorzelli, PhD
Tel: 617 373-5919 *Fax:* 617 373-8892
E-mail: jscorzel@lynx.neu.edu
Class Cap: 15 *Begins:* Sep
Length: 48 mos *Award:* MS
Tuition per yr: $12,000 res, $12,000 non-res
Evening or weekend classes available

University of Massachusetts at Boston
Rehabilitation Counseling Prgm
Counseling and School Psychology
Graduate College of Education
Boston, MA 02125-3393
Prgm Dir: Rick Houser
Tel: 617 287-7668 *Fax:* 617 287-7664
E-mail: houser@umbsky
Class Cap: 12 *Begins:* Sept Jan
Length: 48 mos *Award:*
Tuition per yr: $1,044 res, $3,213 non-res
Evening or weekend classes available

Springfield College
Rehabilitation Counseling Prgm
Rehabilitation Services Dept
210 Alden St
Springfield, MA 01109-3797
Prgm Dir: Thomas J Ruscio
Tel: 413 748-3318 *Fax:* 413 748-3787
Class Cap: 35 *Begins:* Sept Jan May
Length: 16 mos, 24 mos *Award:* MEd , MS
Tuition per yr: $9,984 res, $12,480 non-res
Evening or weekend classes available

Assumption College
Rehabilitation Counseling Prgm
Inst for Social and Rehab Services
500 Salisbury St
Worcester, MA 01615-0005
Prgm Dir: George S Elias, EdD CRC
Tel: 508 755-0677 *Fax:* 508 756-1780

Michigan

Wayne State University
Rehabilitation Counseling Prgm
Theoretical and Behavioral Foundation
337 College of Education
Detroit, MI 48202
Prgm Dir: Barbara Wayne
Tel: 313 577-1619 *Fax:* 313 577-3606

Michigan State University
Rehabilitation Counseling Prgm
Counseling, Educ Psych and Spec Educ
332 Erickson Hall
East Lansing, MI 48824-1034
Prgm Dir: Nancy M Crewe, PhD
Tel: 517 355-1838 *Fax:* 517 353-6393
E-mail: ncrewe@msu.edu
Class Cap: 24
Length: 60 mos
Tuition per yr: $5,451 res, $10,449 non-res
Evening or weekend classes available

Minnesota

Mankato State University
Rehabilitation Counseling Prgm
College of Allied Health and Nursing
MSU Box 50/PO Box 8400
Mankato, MN 56002-8400
Prgm Dir: Gerald Schneck, PhD CRC NCC
Tel: 507 389-1318 *Fax:* 507 389-5888
E-mail: gschneck@vax1.mankato.msus.edu
Class Cap: 25 *Begins:* Aug
Length: 21 mos *Award:* MS
Tuition per yr: $3,000 res, $6,000 non-res

St Cloud State University
Rehabilitation Counseling Prgm
Dept of Applied Psychology
St Cloud, MN 56301
Prgm Dir: John C Hotz, RhD CRC
Tel: 320 255-2240 *Fax:* 320 255-4237
E-mail: jhotz@tigger.stcloud.msus.edu
Class Cap: 15 *Begins:* Sep
Length: 18 mos *Award:* MS
Tuition per yr: $4,088 res, $6,474 non-res
Evening or weekend classes available

Mississippi

Jackson State University
Rehabilitation Counseling Prgm
PO Box 17501
Jackson, MS 39217-7501
Prgm Dir: Frank L Giles, CRC
Tel: 601 968-2370 *Fax:* 601 968-2213
E-mail: fgiles@ccaix.jsums.edu

Mississippi State University
Rehabilitation Counseling Prgm
Counselor Educ and Educ Psych
Mail Stop 9727
Mississippi State, MS 39762
Prgm Dir: Glen R Hendren
Tel: 601 325-7918 *Fax:* 601 325-3263
E-mail: glen@ra.msstate.edu
Class Cap: 30 *Begins:* Jun Sep
Length: 24 mos *Award:* MS
Tuition per yr: $998 res, $2,408 non-res
Evening or weekend classes available

Missouri

University of Missouri - Columbia
Rehabilitation Counseling Prgm
Dept of Educ and Counseling Psych
16 Hill Hall
Columbia, MO 65211
Prgm Dir: John F Kosciulek, PhD CRC CVE
Tel: 314 882-3558 *Fax:* 314 882-5071

Montana

Montana State University-Billings
Rehabilitation Counseling Prgm
Dept of Counseling and Human Services
1500 N 30th St
Billings, MT 59101-0298
Prgm Dir: Alan Davis
Tel: 406 657-2094 *Fax:* 406 657-2807
Class Cap: 25 *Begins:* May Aug Jun
Length: 24 mos *Award:* MSRC
Tuition per yr: $977 res, $2,318 non-res

New York

SUNY at Albany
Rehabilitation Counseling Prgm
School of Education Rm 220
1400 Washington Ave
Albany, NY 12222
Prgm Dir: Sheldon A Grand, PhD CRC
Tel: 518 442-5050 *Fax:* 518 442-4953
Class Cap: 20 *Begins:* June
Length: 18 mos *Award:* MS
Tuition per yr: $5,100 res, $8,416 non-res
Evening or weekend classes available

SUNY at Buffalo
Rehabilitation Counseling Prgm
Dept of Counseling and Educ Psych
409 Baldy Hall
Buffalo, NY 14260-1000
Prgm Dir: Dwight R Kauppi, PhD CRC
Tel: 716 645-2476 *Fax:* 716 645-3837
E-mail: kauppi@acsu.buffalo.edu
Class Cap: 10 *Begins:* Aug
Length: 48 mos *Award:* MS
Tuition per yr: $2,870 res, $4,528 non-res

Hofstra University
Rehabilitation Counseling Prgm
Rehabilitation Counselor Education
124 Hofstra University/111 Mason
Hempstead, NY 11550-1090
Prgm Dir: Joseph S Lechowicz, PhD
Tel: 516 463-5782 *Fax:* 516 463-6503
E-mail: edajsl@vaxc.hofstra.edu
Class Cap: 20 *Begins:* Sep Jan
Length: 21 mos *Award:* MS
Evening or weekend classes available

CUNY Hunter College
Rehabilitation Counseling Prgm
Dept of Educ Found and Counseling Prgms
695 Park Ave
New York, NY 10021
Prgm Dir: John H O'Neill, PhD
Tel: 212 772-4755 *Fax:* 212 772-4941
Class Cap: 50 *Begins:* Sep Jan
Length: 24 mos *Award:* MSEd
Tuition per yr: $4,875

New York University
Rehabilitation Counseling Prgm
35 W Fourth St/Rm 1200
New York, NY 10012
Prgm Dir: Nancy Esibill, PhD CRC
Tel: 212 998-5290 *Fax:* 212 995-4192
Class Cap: 30 *Begins:* Sep Jan
Length: 24 mos *Award:* MA, PhD
Tuition per yr: $14,500 res, $14,500 non-res
Evening or weekend classes available

Syracuse University Main Campus
Rehabilitation Counseling Prgm
259 Huntington Hall
Syracuse, NY 13244
Prgm Dir: Paul R Salomone, PhD
Tel: 315 443-9643   *Fax:* 315 443-5732
E-mail: sued.edu
Class Cap: 25   *Begins:* Aug Jan
Length: 24 mos   *Award:* MS
Tuition per yr: $12,360
Evening or weekend classes available

North Carolina

Univ of North Carolina at Chapel Hill
Rehabilitation Counseling Prgm
118 Medical School Wing E
CB 7205
Chapel Hill, NC 27599-7205
Prgm Dir: Robert T Sakata, PhD
Tel: 919 966-3351   *Fax:* 919 966-3678
E-mail: rsakata@css.unc.edu

East Carolina University
Rehabilitation Counseling Prgm
Dept of Rehabilitation Studies
School of Allied Health Sciences
Greenville, NC 27858-4353
Prgm Dir: Paul P Alston, PhD CRC
Tel: 919 328-4455   *Fax:* 919 328-4470
Class Cap: 25
Length: 24 mos   *Award:* MS
Tuition per yr: $950
Evening or weekend classes available

Ohio

Ohio University Main Campus
Rehabilitation Counseling Prgm
201 McCracken Hall
Athens, OH 45701
Prgm Dir: Jerry A Olsheski, PhD CRC LPC
Tel: 614 593-0032   *Fax:* 614 593-0799
E-mail: olsheski@oak.cats.ohiou.edu
Class Cap: 15   *Begins:* Sep
Length: 20 mos   *Award:* MEd
Tuition per yr: $4,890 res, $9,384 non-res
Evening or weekend classes available

Bowling Green State University
Rehabilitation Counseling Prgm
Dept of Special Education
Bowling Green, OH 43403-0255
Prgm Dir: Jay R Stewart, PhD
Tel: 419 372-7301   *Fax:* 419 372-8265

Ohio State University
Rehabilitation Counseling Prgm
356 Arps Hall
1945 N High St
Columbus, OH 43210-1172
Prgm Dir: Michael Klein, PhD CRC
Tel: 614 292-8174   *Fax:* 614 292-4255
E-mail: klein.3@osu.edu
Begins: Sep
Length: 24 mos   *Award:* MA, PhD
Tuition per yr: $1,569 res, $4,074 non-res
Evening or weekend classes available

Wright State University
Rehabilitation Counseling Prgm
M052 Creative Arts Center
Dayton, OH 45435-0001
Prgm Dir: Jan La Forge, PhD CRC LPC
Tel: 513 873-2150   *Fax:* 513 873-3301
E-mail: jlaforge@nova.wright.edu

Kent State University
Rehabilitation Counseling Prgm
310 White Hall
Kent, OH 44242
Prgm Dir: Rita Myers, PhD
Tel: 330 672-2294   *Fax:* 330 672-2512
Class Cap: 30   *Begins:* Sep Jan Jun
Length: 16 mos   *Award:* MA, PhD
Tuition per yr: $2,284 res, $4,428 non-res
Evening or weekend classes available

Oklahoma

East Central University
Rehabilitation Counseling Prgm
Box C-1
Ada, OK 74820
Prgm Dir: Randal Elston, CRC CVE
Tel: 405 332-8000, Ext 463   *Fax:* 405 436-3329
E-mail: relston@mailclerk.ecok.edu
Class Cap: 15   *Begins:* Aug
Length: 20 mos   *Award:* MS
Tuition per yr: $1,690 res, $5,464 non-res
Evening or weekend classes available

Oregon

Western Oregon State College
Rehabilitation Counseling Prgm
Education Bldg 220
Monmouth, OR 97361
Prgm Dir: Joseph Sendelbaugh, EdD
Tel: 503 838-8444   *Fax:* 503 838-8228
E-mail: rrcd@fsa.wosc.osshe.edu
Class Cap: 15   *Begins:* Sep
Length: 22 mos   *Award:* M.S.
Tuition per yr: $5,509 res, $9,319 non-res

Portland State University
Rehabilitation Counseling Prgm
PO Box 751
Portland, OR 97207-0751
Prgm Dir: Hanoch Livneh
Tel: 503 725-4719   *Fax:* 503 725-5599
E-mail: hanoch@psu.pdx.edu
Class Cap: 12   *Begins:* Sep
Length: 32 mos   *Award:* MS/MA
Tuition per yr: $3,600 res, $3,600 non-res
Evening or weekend classes available

Pennsylvania

Edinboro University of Pennsylvania
Rehabilitation Counseling Prgm
131 Butterfield Hall
Edinboro, PA 16444
Prgm Dir: Brenda Fling, PhD CRC NCC
Tel: 814 732-2410   *Fax:* 814 732-2268
Class Cap: 40   *Begins:* Aug Jan Jun
Length: 24 mos   *Award:* MRC
Tuition per yr: $5,443 res, $9,019 non-res
Evening or weekend classes available

University of Pittsburgh
Rehabilitation Counseling Prgm
5C01 Forges Quadrangle
Pittsburgh, PA 15260
Prgm Dir: Richard Desmond, PhD
Tel: 412 648-7090   *Fax:* 412 648-5911

University of Scranton
Rehabilitation Counseling Prgm
Dept of Counseling and Human Services
Scranton, PA 18510-4523
Prgm Dir: David W Hall, PhD
Tel: 717 941-4127   *Fax:* 717 941-4201
E-mail: hall@uofs.edu

Penn State University - Main Campus
Rehabilitation Counseling Prgm
313 Cedar Bldg
University Park, PA 16802
Prgm Dir: David A Rosenthal, PhD CRC
Tel: 814 863-2411   *Fax:* 814 863-7750
E-mail: dar13@psu.edu
Class Cap: 15   *Begins:* Jun
Length: 15 mos   *Award:* MEd, MS
Tuition per yr: $3,039 res, $6,258 non-res
Evening or weekend classes available

Puerto Rico

University of Puerto Rico
Rehabilitation Counseling Prgm
College of Social Science
PO Box 23345
San Juan, PR 00931-3345
Prgm Dir: Jose E Mas Castro, PhD CRC NCC
Tel: 787 764-0000, Ext 4206   *Fax:* 787 763-4199
Class Cap: 30   *Begins:* Aug
Length: 24 mos   *Award:* MRC
Tuition per yr: $2,350
Evening or weekend classes available

South Carolina

University of South Carolina
Rehabilitation Counseling Prgm
School of Medicine
3555 Harden St Ext/Ste B20
Columbia, SC 29208
Prgm Dir: Robert A Chubon, PhD
Tel: 803 434-4296   *Fax:* 803 434-4231
E-mail: rchubon@npsy.ceb.sc.edu
Class Cap: 20   *Begins:* Aug
Length: 16 mos, 72 mos   *Award:* MRC
Tuition per yr: $6,636 res, $13,460 non-res
Evening or weekend classes available

South Carolina State University

Rehabilitation Counseling Prgm
Dept of Human Services
300 College St
Orangeburg, SC 29117-0001
Prgm Dir: C Brannon Underwood, PhD CRC
Tel: 803 536-8908   *Fax:* 803 533-3636
E-mail: UNDERWOOD@SCSU.SCSU.EDU
Begins: Aug Jan May
Length: 18 mos   *Award:* MA
Tuition per yr: $2,730 res, $2,730 non-res
Evening or weekend classes available

Tennessee

University of Tennessee - Knoxville

Rehabilitation Counseling Prgm
133 Claxton Addition
Knoxville, TN 37996-3400
Prgm Dir: James H Miller, EdD CRC
Tel: 423 974-8090   *Fax:* 423 974-8674
E-mail: millerjh@utk.edu
Class Cap: 10   *Begins:* Aug
Length: 16 mos   *Award:* MS, PhD
Tuition per yr: $0 res, $6,000 non-res
Evening or weekend classes available

University of Memphis

Rehabilitation Counseling Prgm
Dept Counseling, Educ Psych and Research
102 Ball Educ Bldg
Memphis, TN 38152
Prgm Dir: William M Jenkins, EdD
Tel: 901 678-2841   *Fax:* 901 678-4778
Class Cap: 15   *Begins:* Aug Jan May
Length: 24 mos   *Award:* MS
Tuition per yr: $1,337 res, $3,505 non-res
Evening or weekend classes available

Texas

University of Texas at Austin

Rehabilitation Counseling Prgm
Special Education/EDB 306/D5300
Austin, TX 78712
Prgm Dir: Randall M Parker
Tel: 512 471-4161   *Fax:* 512 471-4061
E-mail: rparker@mail.utexas.edu
Class Cap: 20
Length: 16 mos   *Award:*
Tuition per yr: $1,350 res, $4,000 non-res
Evening or weekend classes available

Univ of Tx Southwestern Med Ctr - Dallas

Rehabilitation Counseling Prgm
5323 Harry Hines Blvd
Dallas, TX 75235-9088
Prgm Dir: Donald A Pool, PhD
Tel: 214 648-1740   *Fax:* 214 648-1771
E-mail: dpool@mednet.swmed.edu
Class Cap: 8   *Begins:* Aug
Length: 24 mos   *Award:* MS
Tuition per yr: $960 res, $7,380 non-res

University of North Texas

Rehabilitation Counseling Prgm
Center for Rehabilitation Studies
PO Box 13438
Denton, TX 76203-3438
Prgm Dir: Eugenia Bodenhamer-Davis, PhD
Tel: 817 565-2488   *Fax:* 817 565-3960
E-mail: SUE@UNTVAX

Stephen F Austin State University

Rehabilitation Counseling Prgm
Dept of Counseling and Spec Educ Prgms
PO Box 13019/SFA Station
Nacogdoches, TX 75962-3019
Prgm Dir: Robert O Choate, EdD
Tel: 409 468-1145   *Fax:* 409 468-1342
E-mail: rchoate@sfasu.edu
Class Cap: 10   *Begins:* Aug Jan
Length: 2 mo , 6 mos   *Award:* MA
Tuition per yr: $1,257 res, $2,597 non-res
Evening or weekend classes available

Utah

Utah State University

Rehabilitation Counseling Prgm
Dept of Special Educ and Rehab
Logan, UT 84322-2865
Prgm Dir: Garth M Eldredge, PhD
Tel: 801 797-3241   *Fax:* 801 797-3572
E-mail: GARTHE@FSI.ED.USU.EDU
Class Cap: 30   *Begins:* Sep Jan Mar
Length: 18 mos   *Award:* MS
Tuition per yr: $0 res, $2,000 non-res
Evening or weekend classes available

Virginia

Med Coll of VA/Virginia Commonwealth U

Rehabilitation Counseling Prgm
Dept of Rehab Counseling
408 N 12th St/MCV Box 980330
Richmond, VA 23298
Prgm Dir: E Davis Martin
Tel: 804 828-1132   *Fax:* 804 828-1321
E-mail: edmartin@gems.ucu.edu
Class Cap: 50
Length: 24 mos   *Award:* MS
Tuition per yr: $4,592 res, $4,592 non-res
Evening or weekend classes available

West Virginia

West Virginia University

Rehabilitation Counseling Prgm
502 Allen Hall
PO Box 6122
Morgantown, WV 26506-6122
Prgm Dir: Robert P Marinelli, EdD CRC
Tel: 304 293-3807   *Fax:* 304 293-7388
E-mail: rmarinel@wvu.edu
Class Cap: 16   *Begins:* Aug   *Award:* MS
Tuition per yr: $1,206 res, $3,683 non-res
Evening or weekend classes available

Wisconsin

University of Wisconsin - Madison

Rehabilitation Counseling Prgm
Rehab Psych and Special Educ
432 N Murray St
Madison, WI 53706
Prgm Dir: Norman L Berven
Tel: 608 263-7917   *Fax:* 608 262-8108
E-mail: BERVEN@MACC.WISC.EDU

University of Wisconsin - Stout

Rehabilitation Counseling Prgm
Dept of Rehabilitation
403 Education and Human Services Bldg
Menomonie, WI 54751
Prgm Dir: Robert Peters, PhD CRC
Tel: 715 232-1983
E-mail: petersb@uwstout.edu
Class Cap: 50
Length: 24 mos   *Award:* MA

University of Wisconsin - Milwaukee

Rehabilitation Counseling Prgm
Dept of Educational Psych
PO Box 413/Enderis Hall 773
Milwaukee, WI 53201
Prgm Dir: Brian T McMahon, PhD CRC
Tel: 414 229-5681   *Fax:* 414 229-4939
E-mail: BRIANTMC@CSD.UWM.EDU
Med Dir: William Harvey, PhD
Class Cap: 25   *Begins:* Sep
Length: 24 mos, 60 mos   *Award:* MS
Tuition per yr: $4,000 res, $12,000 non-res
Evening or weekend classes available

Programs

Respiratory Care

History

In 1957, a resolution to develop schools of inhalation therapy was introduced to the American Medical Association (AMA) House of Delegates by the Medical Society of New York. Following approval, the resolution was referred to the Council on Medical Education (CME) and subsequently resulted in the proposed report titled *Standards (Essentials) for an Approved School of Inhalation Therapy Technicians*. The proposed *Standards* were tested during the next few years, after which they were recommended for adoption by the CME and formally approved by the AMA House of Delegates in December 1962. The *Standards* were revised in 1967 and included the requirements of an 18-month program.

In 1970, the Board of Schools was reorganized and incorporated as the Joint Review Committee for Inhalation Therapy Education. In 1972, the American Thoracic Society became another sponsor of the Joint Review Committee. In 1972, the *Standards* underwent a third revision, and additional *Standards* were developed for a shorter educational program for training individuals to function as technicians. The *Standards* were approved by the sponsors of the Board of Schools for Inhalation Therapy, the American Society of Anesthesiologists, the American College of Chest Physicians, the American Association of Inhalation Therapy, and the AMA CME and were adopted by the AMA House of Delegates in June 1972. In 1977, the review committee's name was changed to the Joint Review Committee for Respiratory Therapy Education (JRCRTE).

In 1986, *Standards* for both the respiratory therapy technician and the respiratory therapist were consolidated and the revision was adopted by the sponsors of the JRCRTE and by the AMA.

Respiratory Therapist

Occupational Description

The respiratory therapist applies scientific knowledge and theory to practical clinical problems of respiratory care. The respiratory therapist is qualified to assume primary responsibility for all respiratory care modalities, including the supervision of respiratory therapy technician functions. The respiratory therapist may be required to exercise considerable independent clinical judgment, under the supervision of a physician, in the respiratory care of patients.

Job Description

In fulfillment of the therapist role, the respiratory therapist may
1. Review, collect, and recommend obtaining additional data. The therapist evaluates all data to determine the appropriateness of the prescribed respiratory care and participates in the development of the respiratory care plan.
2. Select, assemble, and check all equipment used in providing respiratory care.
3. Initiate and conduct therapeutic procedures and modify prescribed therapeutic procedures to achieve one or more specific objectives.
4. Maintain patient records and communicate relevant information to other members of the health care team.
5. Assist the physician in performing special procedures in a clinical laboratory, procedure room, or operating room.

Employment Characteristics

Respiratory therapy personnel are employed in hospitals, nursing care facilities, clinics, physicians' offices, companies providing emergency oxygen services, and municipal organizations.

According to 1996 data from the American Association for Respiratory Care, a respiratory therapist, on average, earns $32,926.

Educational Programs

Length. Programs are usually 2 years, leading to an associate degree or, in a few instances, to a baccalaureate degree. Programs of 1 year or less usually require 1 year of prior education in respiratory care.

Prerequisite. High school diploma or equivalent.

Curriculum. The knowledge and skills for performing these functions are achieved through formal programs of didactic, laboratory, and clinical preparation. Biological and physical sciences basic to understanding the functioning of the human breathing system are included—anatomy, physiology, medical terminology, chemistry, mathematics, microbiology, physics, therapeutic procedures, clinical medicine, and clinical expressions. The program of study also includes social sciences basic to understanding how to relate to patients—psychology, communication skills, and medical ethics. Clinical training in routine and special procedures applicable to pediatric, adult, and geriatric patients also is provided.

Standards. *Standards* are minimum educational standards adopted by the several collaborating organizations. Each new program is assessed in accordance with the *Standards*, and accredited programs are periodically reviewed to determine whether they remain in substantial compliance. The *Standards and Guidelines* are available on written request from the Division of Allied Health Education and Accreditation.

Respiratory Therapy Technician

Occupational Description

The respiratory therapy technician administers general respiratory care. Technicians may assume clinical responsibility for specified respiratory care modalities involving the application of well-defined therapeutic techniques under the supervision of a respiratory therapist and a physician.

Job Description

In fulfillment of the technician role, the respiratory therapy technician may
1. Review clinical data, history, and respiratory therapy orders.
2. Collect clinical data by interview and examination of the patient. This includes collecting portions of the data by inspection, palpation, percussion, and auscultation of the patient.
3. Recommend and/or perform and review additional bedside procedures, x-rays, and laboratory tests.
4. Evaluate data to determine the appropriateness of the prescribed respiratory care.
5. Assemble and maintain equipment used in respiratory care.
6. Assure cleanliness and sterility by the selection and/or performance of appropriate disinfecting techniques and monitor their effectiveness.
7. Initiate, conduct, and modify prescribed therapeutic procedures.

Employment Characteristics

Respiratory therapy personnel are employed in hospitals, nursing care facilities, clinics, doctors' offices, companies providing emergency oxygen services, and municipal organizations.

According to 1996 data from the American Association for Respiratory Care, a respiratory therapy technician, on average, earns $26,707.

Educational Programs

Length. Programs are usually 12 to 18 months, leading to a certificate of completion and occasionally an associate degree.
Prerequisites. High school diploma or equivalent.
Curriculum. The knowledge and skills of the technician are acquired through formal programs of didactic, laboratory, and clinical preparation. Courses include biological and physical sciences basic to understanding the functioning of the human breathing system, such as anatomy, physiology, medical terminology, chemistry, mathematics, microbiology, physics, therapeutic procedures, clinical medicine, and clinical expressions. Clinical training in routine and special procedures applicable to pediatric, adult, and geriatric patients also is provided.
Standards. *Standards* are minimum educational standards adopted by the several collaborating organizations. Each new program is assessed in accordance with the *Standards*, and accredited programs are periodically reviewed to determine whether they remain in substantial compliance. The *Standards and Guidelines* are available on written request from the Joint Review Committee for Respiratory Therapy Education.

Inquiries

Accreditation

Requests for information on program accreditation, including *Standards*, preparing the self-study report, and arranging a site visit, should be submitted to

Joint Review Committee for Respiratory Therapy Education
1701 W Euless Blvd/Ste 300
Euless, TX 76040
817 283-2835

Careers

Inquiries regarding careers should be addressed to

American Association for Respiratory Care
11030 Ables Ln
Dallas, TX 75229
214 243-2272

Certification/Registration

Inquiries regarding certification may be addressed to

National Board for Respiratory Care
8310 Nieman Rd
Lenexa, KS 66214

Respiratory Therapist

Alabama

University of Alabama at Birmingham
Respiratory Therapist Prgm
School of Hlth Related Profs
1714 9th Ave S SHRP-317
Birmingham, AL 35294-1270
Prgm Dir: Wesley M Granger, PhD RRT
Tel: 205 934-3783   *Fax:* 205 975-7302
E-mail: grangerw@admin.shrp.uab.edu
Med Dir: James H Strickland Jr, MD
Class Cap: 25   *Begins:* Mar
Length: 27 mos   *Award:* BS
Tuition per yr: $3,680 res, $7,360 non-res
Evening or weekend classes available

George C Wallace State Comm College
Respiratory Therapist Prgm
Dothan, AL 36303
Prgm Dir: Timothy H Turney, BS RRT
Tel: 334 983-3521   *Fax:* 334 983-3600
Med Dir: Allen Latimer, MD
Class Cap: 25   *Begins:* Sep
Length: 24 mos   *Award:* AAS
Tuition per yr: $1,880 res, $3,290 non-res

Wallace State College
Respiratory Therapist Prgm
PO Box 2000
Hanceville, AL 35077-2000
Prgm Dir: Paul D Taylor, BS RRT
Tel: 205 352-8310   *Fax:* 205 352-8228
Med Dir: Russell Beaty, MD
Class Cap: 50   *Begins:* Sep
Length: 24 mos   *Award:* Dipl, AAS
Tuition per yr: $1,409 res, $2,818 non-res
Evening or weekend classes available

University of South Alabama
Respiratory Therapist Prgm
1504 Springhill Ave
Mobile, AL 36604
Prgm Dir: William V Wojciechowski, MS RRT
Tel: 334 434-3405   *Fax:* 334 434-3941
E-mail: wwojciec@jaguar1.usouth.al.edu
Med Dir: Ronald Allison, MD
Class Cap: 18   *Begins:* Sep
Length: 18 mos   *Award:* Dipl, BS
Tuition per yr: $2,808 res, $4,608 non-res

Arizona

Apollo College
Respiratory Therapist Prgm
630 W Southern Ave
Mesa, AZ 85210
Prgm Dir: Valerie S Spear, RRT
Tel: 602 831-6585   *Fax:* 503 670-3351
Med Dir: Walter McEarchern, MD
Class Cap: 15   *Begins:* Jan July
Length: 16 mos   *Award:* Dipl
Tuition per yr: $14,723 res, $14,723 non-res

Programs

Pima Medical Institute - Mesa
Respiratory Therapist Prgm
957 S Dobson Rd
Mesa, AZ 85202
Prgm Dir: Cynthia Smathers, MEd RRT
Tel: 602 345-7777   *Fax:* 602 649-5249
Med Dir: David Drachler, MD
Class Cap: 44   *Begins:* Feb May Jun Jul
Length: 11 mos   *Award:* AS
Tuition per yr: $4,447

Apollo College
Respiratory Therapist Prgm
8503 N 27th Ave
Phoenix, AZ 85021
Prgm Dir: Mark L Anderson, RRT
Tel: 602 864-1571   *Fax:* 602 864-8207
Med Dir: Walter W McEarchern, MD
Class Cap: 25   *Begins:* Varies
Length: 16 mos   *Award:* Dipl, AS
Tuition per yr: $14,648

Gateway Community College
Respiratory Therapist Prgm
108 N 40th St
Phoenix, AZ 85034
Prgm Dir: Marie A Fenske, EdD RRT
Tel: 602 392-5062   *Fax:* 602 392-5329
Med Dir: Robert G Hooper, MD
Class Cap: 35   *Begins:* Aug Jan
Length: 8 mo , 12 mos   *Award:* Cert, AAS
Tuition per yr: $1,054 res, $4,867 non-res

Pima Community College
Respiratory Therapist Prgm
2202 W Anklam Rd
Tucson, AZ 85709
Prgm Dir: Richard A Patze Jr, RRT
Tel: 520 884-6916   *Fax:* 520 884-6225
E-mail: rpatze@pimacc.pima.edu
Med Dir: Linda S Snyder, MD
Class Cap: 28   *Begins:* Aug
Length: 21 mos   *Award:* AAS
Tuition per yr: $724 res, $5,080 non-res

Pima Medical Institute - Tucson
Respiratory Therapist Prgm
3350 E Grant
Tucson, AZ 85716
Prgm Dir: Leanna Konechne, BS RRT
Tel: 520 326-1600   *Fax:* 520 795-3463
Med Dir: Anthony D Chavis, MD
Class Cap: 80   *Begins:* Mar Jul Sep Nov
Length: 15 mos, 12 mos   *Award:* AA
Tuition per yr: $11,185

Arkansas

Univ of Arkansas for Medical Sciences
Respiratory Therapist Prgm
VA Med Ctr VAMS/UAMC
4301 W Markham/Slot 704
Little Rock, AR 72205
Prgm Dir: Erna Boone, MEd RRT
Tel: 501 661-1202   *Fax:* 501 370-6691
E-mail: elboone@uams.edu
Med Dir: James Rasch, MD
Class Cap: 48   *Begins:* Aug
Length: 16 mos   *Award:* AS
Tuition per yr: $2,800 res, $6,998 non-res
Evening or weekend classes available

Univ of Arkansas for Medical Sciences
Respiratory Therapist Prgm
AHEC-SW
PO Box 2871
Texarkana, AR 75504
Prgm Dir: Patrick Evans, RRT MEd
Tel: 501 773-4181   *Fax:* 501 772-5417
Med Dir: Stanley R Collins, MD
Class Cap: 12   *Begins:* Aug
Length: 16 mos   *Award:* AS
Tuition per yr: $2,800 res, $6,998 non-res
Evening or weekend classes available

California

Orange Coast College
Respiratory Therapist Prgm
2701 Fairview Rd
PO Box 8005
Costa Mesa, CA 92628
Prgm Dir: Daniel S Adelmann, MEd RRT
Tel: 714 432-5541   *Fax:* 714 432-5534
Med Dir: Archie F Wilson, MD PhD
Class Cap: 30   *Begins:* Aug
Length: 24 mos   *Award:* Cert, AA
Tuition per yr: $358 res, $3,500 non-res
Evening or weekend classes available

Grossmont College
Respiratory Therapist Prgm
8800 Grossmont College Dr
El Cajon, CA 92020
Prgm Dir: Lorenda Seibold-Phalan, MA RRT RCP
Tel: 619 465-1700   *Fax:* 619 461-3396
Med Dir: David Burns, MD
Class Cap: 40   *Begins:* Aug
Length: 22 mos   *Award:* Cert, AS
Tuition per yr: $400 res, $3,400 non-res

Ohlone College
Respiratory Therapist Prgm
43600 Mission Blvd
PO Box 3909
Fremont, CA 94539
Prgm Dir: Carol Mc Namee-Cole, MA RRT
Tel: 510 659-6029   *Fax:* 510 659-6070
Med Dir: Francis C Johnson, MD
Class Cap: 24   *Begins:* Aug
Length: 22 mos   *Award:* Cert, AS
Tuition per yr: $384

Fresno City College
Respiratory Therapist Prgm
1101 E University Ave
Fresno, CA 93741
Prgm Dir: Morris W Ramay, RRT
Tel: 209 442-4600
Med Dir: Enok Lohne, MD
Class Cap: 50   *Begins:* Aug
Length: 18 mos   *Award:* AS
Tuition per yr: $332 res, $3,456 non-res

Loma Linda University
Respiratory Therapist Prgm
Nichols Hall 1926
Loma Linda, CA 92350
Prgm Dir: Robert L Wilkins, MA RRT
Tel: 909 824-4932   Fax: 909 824-4701
Med Dir: N Leonard Specht, MD
Class Cap: 25   *Begins:* Sep
Length: 11 mos   *Award:* Dipl, AS
Tuition per yr: $9,936

Foothill College
Respiratory Therapist Prgm
12345 El Monte Rd
Los Altos Hills, CA 94022
Prgm Dir: Shirley Treanor, EdD RRT
Tel: 415 949-7292   *Fax:* 415 949-7375
E-mail: treanor@admin.fhda.edu
Med Dir: Lawrence E Shapiro, MD
Class Cap: 25   *Begins:* Sep Jan
Length: 6 mo , 20 mos   *Award:* Dipl,Cert, AS
Tuition per yr: $441 res, $2,000 non-res

Modesto Junior College
Respiratory Therapist Prgm
435 College Ave
Modesto, CA 95350
Prgm Dir: Terry P Lyle, MA RRT
Tel: 209 575-6388
E-mail: hyle@ix.netcom
Med Dir: Robert Tanaka, MD
Class Cap: 24   *Begins:* Jan
Length: 18 mos   *Award:* Cert, AS
Tuition per yr: $120 res, $5,096 non-res
Evening or weekend classes available

East Los Angeles College
Respiratory Therapist Prgm
1301 Avenida Cesar Chavez
Monterey, CA 91754
Prgm Dir: Michael R Carr, RCP RRT BA
Tel: 213 265-8612   *Fax:* 213 265-8829
Med Dir: Robert S Eisenberg, MD
Begins: Sep
Length: 24 mos   *Award:* Cert, AS
Tuition per yr: $403 res, $3,937 non-res
Evening or weekend classes available

Napa Valley College
Respiratory Therapist Prgm
2277 Napa Vallejo Hwy
Napa, CA 94558
Prgm Dir: Robert S Chudnofsky, BS RRT
Tel: 707 253-3147   *Fax:* 707 259-8068
E-mail: chudrt.cnuc.cc.ca.edu
Med Dir: Nazir Habib, MD
Class Cap: 30   *Begins:* Aug
Length: 19 mos   *Award:* Cert, AS
Tuition per yr: $143 res, $1,352 non-res
Evening or weekend classes available

California College for Health Sciences
Respiratory Therapist Prgm
222 W 24th St
National City, CA 92050
Prgm Dir: Dale K Bean, RRT
Tel: 619 477-4800   *Fax:* 619 477-4360
E-mail: dalebean@cchs.edu
Med Dir: Jerry E Fein, MD
Begins: Apr Sep
Length: 18 mos   *Award:* Cert, AS
Tuition per yr: $13,875 res, $1,955 non-res

Butte College
Respiratory Therapist Prgm
3536 Butte Campus Dr
Oroville, CA 95965
Prgm Dir: Daniel J Solomon, MA RRT
Tel: 916 895-2423   *Fax:* 916 895-2472
Med Dir: Gerrard Valcarenghi, MD
Class Cap: 26   *Begins:* Aug
Length: 21 mos   *Award:* Cert, AS
Tuition per yr: $833 res, $833 non-res
Evening or weekend classes available

College of the Desert

Respiratory Therapist Prgm
43-500 Monterey Ave
Palm Desert, CA 92260
Prgm Dir: Thomas A Ciastko, RRT RCP
Tel: 619 773-2578
Med Dir: Ronald Sneider, MD
Class Cap: 30 *Begins:* Jun
Length: 24 mos *Award:* Cert, AS
Tuition per yr: $300 res, $2,200 non-res

Calif Paramedical & Tech Coll-Riverside

Respiratory Therapist Prgm
4550 La Sierra Ave
Riverside, CA 92505
Prgm Dir: Jeffrey Welsh, PhD
Tel: 909 687-9006 *Fax:* 909 687-9739
E-mail: jwelsh@pe.net
Med Dir: Luis Taylor, MD
Class Cap: 90 *Begins:* Varies
Length: 15 mos *Award:* Cert
Tuition per yr: $14,995

American River College

Respiratory Therapist Prgm
4700 College Oak Dr
Sacramento, CA 95841
Prgm Dir: James L Warman, PhD RRT
Tel: 916 484-8876 *Fax:* 916 484-8674
Med Dir: Theodore Bacharach, MD
Class Cap: 24 *Begins:* Aug
Length: 21 mos *Award:* AS
Tuition per yr: $240 res, $2,376 non-res

Skyline College

Respiratory Therapist Prgm
3300 College Dr
San Bruno, CA 94066
Prgm Dir: Michael Williamson, RRT
Tel: 415 738-4382
Med Dir: Allan Hotti, MD
Class Cap: 25 *Begins:* Aug
Length: 21 mos *Award:* Cert, AS
Tuition per yr: $334 res, $2,938 non-res

Santa Monica College

Respiratory Therapist Prgm
Health Science Dept
1900 Pico Blvd
Santa Monica, CA 90405-1628
Prgm Dir: Melvin A Welch Jr, RRT
Tel: 310 450-5150, Ext 9823 *Fax:* 310 451-0377
E-mail: melwelch@prodigy.
Med Dir: Paul Eric Bellamy, MD
Class Cap: 22 *Begins:* Jun
Length: 24 mos *Award:* Cert, AA
Tuition per yr: $455 res, $4,515 non-res
Evening or weekend classes available

El Camino College

Respiratory Therapist Prgm
16007 Crenshaw Blvd
Torrance, CA 90506
Prgm Dir: Louis M Sinopoli, EdD RRT
Tel: 310 715-3248 *Fax:* 310 660-3378
Med Dir: Darryl Sue, MD
Class Cap: 15 *Begins:* Jan Feb
Length: 28 mos *Award:* Cert, AS
Tuition per yr: $100 res, $1,000 non-res
Evening or weekend classes available

Los Angeles Valley College

Respiratory Therapist Prgm
5800 Fulton Ave
Van Nuys, CA 91401-4096
Prgm Dir: Virginia M Ettinger, MPH RRT RCP
Tel: 818 781-1200 *Fax:* 818 785-4672
Med Dir: Alan Rothfeld, MD
Class Cap: 30 *Begins:* Varies
Length: 20 mos *Award:* Cert, AA
Tuition per yr: $416 res, $4,125 non-res
Evening or weekend classes available

Victor Valley College

Respiratory Therapist Prgm
PO Drawer 00
Victorville, CA 92392-9699
Prgm Dir: James S Previte, MA RRT
Tel: 619 245-4271
Med Dir: Mohinder P Ahluwalia, MD
Class Cap: 30 *Begins:* Jun
Length: 24 mos *Award:* Cert, AS
Tuition per yr: $300 res, $2,910 non-res

San Joaquin Valley College

Respiratory Therapist Prgm
8400 W Mineral King
Visalia, CA 93291
Prgm Dir: Barry M Westling, MEd RRT RPFT
Tel: 209 651-2500 *Fax:* 209 651-0574
Med Dir: William R Winn, MD
Class Cap: 20 *Begins:* Jan Aug
Length: 7 mo , 14 mos *Award:* Cert, AS
Tuition per yr: $6,060
Evening or weekend classes available

Mt San Antonio College

Respiratory Therapist Prgm
1100 N Grand Ave
Walnut, CA 91789
Prgm Dir: Terrance M Krider, BS RRT RCP
Tel: 909 594-5611 *Fax:* 909 468-3938
Med Dir: Earl S Young, MD
Class Cap: 30 *Begins:* Aug
Length: 24 mos *Award:* Cert, AS
Tuition per yr: $150 res, $3,600 non-res
Evening or weekend classes available

Crafton Hills College

Respiratory Therapist Prgm
11711 Sand Canyon Rd
Yucaipa, CA 92399
Prgm Dir: Kenneth R Bryson, BVE RRT
Tel: 909 794-2161 *Fax:* 909 794-0423
Med Dir: Richard Sheldon, MD
Class Cap: 40 *Begins:* Aug
Length: 27 mos *Award:* Cert, AS
Tuition per yr: $770 res, $6,754 non-res
Evening or weekend classes available

Colorado

Pima Medical Institute - Denver

Respiratory Therapist Prgm
1701 W 72nd Ave
Denver, CO 80221
Prgm Dir: C Allen Wentworth, RRT
Tel: 303 426-1800 *Fax:* 303 430-4048
Med Dir: Joseph Heit, MD
Class Cap: 75 *Begins:* Jan thru Dec
Length: 24 mos *Award:* AS
Tuition per yr: $11,335 res, $11,335 non-res

Pueblo Community College

Respiratory Therapist Prgm
900 W Orman Ave
Pueblo, CO 81004
Prgm Dir: Thomas W Trujillo, BS RRT
Tel: 719 549-3265 *Fax:* 719 549-3136
E-mail: trujillo_t@pcc.colorado.edu
Med Dir: Dumont Clark, MD
Class Cap: 20 *Begins:* Jun
Length: 24 mos *Award:* AAS
Tuition per yr: $2,450 res, $9,025 non-res

Front Range Comm College - Westminster

Respiratory Therapist Prgm
3645 W 112th Ave
Westminster, CO 80030
Prgm Dir: Lisa R Elstun, RRT
Tel: 303 404-5217 *Fax:* 303 404-2178
E-mail: FR_USA@mash.colorado.edu
Med Dir: Philip Ziporin, MD
Class Cap: 24 *Begins:* Sep
Length: 24 mos *Award:* Dipl,Cert, AAS
Tuition per yr: $2,354 res, $10,725 non-res
Evening or weekend classes available

Connecticut

Sacred Heart Univ/St Vincent Med Ctr

Respiratory Therapist Prgm
5151 Park Ave
Fairfield, CT 06432
Prgm Dir: Cecelia K Szakolczay, MA RRT CPFT
Tel: 203 576-5329
E-mail: shuresp@connix.com
Med Dir: Robert Brown, MD
Class Cap: 15 *Begins:* Sep
Length: 24 mos *Award:* Cert, AS
Tuition per yr: $12,212

Quinnipiac College

Respiratory Therapist Prgm
Mt Carmel Ave
Hamden, CT 06518
Prgm Dir: Ronald G Beckett, RRT PhD
Tel: 203 281-8682 *Fax:* 203 281-8706
Med Dir: Michael J McNamee, MD
Class Cap: 24 *Begins:* Sep
Length: 38 mos *Award:* Dipl,Cert, BS
Tuition per yr: $13,440 res, $13,440 non-res
Evening or weekend classes available

Manchester Community - Technical College

Respiratory Therapist Prgm
60 Bidwell St
Manchester, CT 06045-1046
Prgm Dir: Karen Milikowski, MS RRT
Tel: 860 647-6193 *Fax:* 860 647-6238
Med Dir: Richard L ZuWallack, MD
Class Cap: 18 *Begins:* Sep
Length: 21 mos *Award:* AS
Tuition per yr: $2,032 res, $5,152 non-res
Evening or weekend classes available

Programs

Norwalk Hospital
Respiratory Therapist Prgm
24 Maple St
Norwalk, CT 06856
Prgm Dir: Edward A Reardon, RRT
Tel: 203 852-2479
Med Dir: Stephen M Winter, MD
Class Cap: 15 *Begins:* Sep
Length: 24 mos *Award:* Cert, AS
Tuition per yr: $1,722 res, $4,842 non-res

University of Hartford
Respiratory Therapist Prgm
200 Bloomfield Ave
West Hartford, CT 06117-1559
Prgm Dir: Peter W Kennedy, MA RRT
Tel: 860 768-4823 *Fax:* 860 768-5244
E-mail: pkenedy@uhavax.harford.edu
Med Dir: Robert E Mueller, MD
Class Cap: 15 *Begins:* Sep
Length: 48 mos *Award:* Cert, BS
Tuition per yr: $15,600
Evening or weekend classes available

Delaware

Delaware Tech & Comm Coll - Owens Campus
Respiratory Therapist Prgm
PO Box 610
Georgetown, DE 19947
Prgm Dir: James G Little, MEd RRT
Tel: 302 856-5400 *Fax:* 302 856-5773
E-mail: jlittle2outland.ctcc.edu
Med Dir: Pedro Cardona, MD
Class Cap: 18 *Begins:* Jun
Length: 23 mos *Award:* AAS
Tuition per yr: $1,890 res, $4,725 non-res

Delaware Tech & Comm Coll - Wilmington
Respiratory Therapist Prgm
333 Shipley St
Wilmington, DE 19801
Prgm Dir: Robert M Lang, RRT
Tel: 302 428-2678 *Fax:* 302 428-2691
E-mail: blang@hopi.dtcc.edu
Med Dir: Albert Rizzo, MD
Class Cap: 15 *Begins:* Jun
Length: 24 mos *Award:* AAS
Tuition per yr: $1,890 res, $4,725 non-res
Evening or weekend classes available

District of Columbia

University of the District of Columbia
Respiratory Therapist Prgm
4200 Connecticut Ave NW
Washington, DC 20008
Prgm Dir: Susan D Lockwood, MA RN RRT
Tel: 202 274-5925 *Fax:* 202 274-5952
Med Dir: Bernard Grand, MD
Class Cap: 30 *Begins:* Aug Jan
Length: 19 mos *Award:* Dipl, AAS
Tuition per yr: $2,198 res, $6,446 non-res
Evening or weekend classes available

Florida

Manatee Community College
Respiratory Therapist Prgm
5840 26th St W
PO Box 1849
Bradenton, FL 34206
Prgm Dir: J Lynn Haines, MPH RRT
Tel: 941 755-1511
Med Dir: Terrence P Kane, MD
Class Cap: 20 *Begins:* Aug
Length: 21 mos *Award:* AS
Tuition per yr: $2,660 res, $9,652 non-res
Evening or weekend classes available

Brevard Community College
Respiratory Therapist Prgm
1519 Clearlake Rd
Cocoa, FL 32922
Prgm Dir: Carol Szewczyk, MS RRT
Tel: 407 632-1111 *Fax:* 407 634-3731
E-mail: szewczyk.c@a1.brevard.cc.fl.us
Med Dir: John F Jessup, MD FCCP
Class Cap: 16 *Begins:* Aug
Length: 24 mos *Award:* AS
Tuition per yr: $1,700 res, $5,130 non-res
Evening or weekend classes available

Daytona Beach Community College
Respiratory Therapist Prgm
PO Box 2811
Daytona Beach, FL 32120
Prgm Dir: Charles Carroll, EdD RRT
Tel: 904 255-8131 *Fax:* 404 254-4491
Med Dir: Michael A Diamond, MD
Class Cap: 28 *Begins:* Aug
Length: 21 mos *Award:* AS
Tuition per yr: $3,363 res, $12,638 non-res

Indian River Community College
Respiratory Therapist Prgm
3209 Virginia Ave
Fort Pierce, FL 34981-5599
Prgm Dir: Georgette Rosenfeld, BS RRT
Tel: 407 462-4358
Med Dir: Donald Hoffman, MD
Class Cap: 16 *Begins:* Aug
Length: 22 mos *Award:* AS
Tuition per yr: $1,452 res, $5,808 non-res
Evening or weekend classes available

Broward Community College
Respiratory Therapist Prgm
3501 SW Davie Rd
Ft Lauderdale, FL 33314
Prgm Dir: John Prince, RRT
Tel: 954 969-2082 *Fax:* 954 973-2348
Med Dir: Milton Braunstein, MD
Begins: Aug
Length: 24 mos *Award:* Dipl,Cert, AS
Tuition per yr: $1,700 res, $5,325 non-res

Edison Community College
Respiratory Therapist Prgm
College Pkwy
Ft Myers, FL 33906-6210
Prgm Dir: William A O'Neill, MA RRT
Tel: 941 489-9252 *Fax:* 941 489-9037
Med Dir: George Mestas, MD
Class Cap: 30 *Begins:* Aug
Length: 20 mos *Award:* AS
Tuition per yr: $1,455 res, $5,410 non-res

Santa Fe Community College
Respiratory Therapist Prgm
Gainesville, FL 32606-6200
Prgm Dir: David N Yonutas, MS RRT
Tel: 352 395-5703 *Fax:* 352 395-5711
E-mail: dave.yonutas@santafe.cc.fl.us
Med Dir: T James Gallagher, MD
Class Cap: 25 *Begins:* Jan
Length: 24 mos *Award:* Dipl,Cert, AS
Tuition per yr: $2,907 res, $10,819 non-res
Evening or weekend classes available

Flagler Career Institute - Jacksonville
Respiratory Therapist Prgm
3225 University Blvd S
Jacksonville, FL 32216
Prgm Dir: Penny Campbell, RRT
Tel: 904 721-1622 *Fax:* 904 723-3117
Med Dir: Charles D Burger, MD
Class Cap: 75 *Begins:* Jul Nov Mar
Length: 9 mo , 18 mos *Award:* AAS
Tuition per yr: $6,440

Florida Community College - Jacksonville
Respiratory Therapist Prgm
North Campus
4501 Capper Rd
Jacksonville, FL 32218
Prgm Dir: Beverly L T Edwards, BHS RRT
Tel: 904 766-6513 *Fax:* 904 766-6654
Med Dir: Isabella K Sharpe, MD
Class Cap: 30 *Begins:* Aug
Length: 18 mos *Award:* AS
Tuition per yr: $1,528 res, $5,768 non-res
Evening or weekend classes available

ATI Health Education Centers
Respiratory Therapist Prgm
1395 NW 167th St Ste 200
Miami, FL 33169
Prgm Dir: Jules Clavan, BS RRT
Tel: 305 628-1000
Med Dir: Edgar Bolton Jr, DO FCCP
Class Cap: 50 *Begins:* Aug Dec Apr
Length: 21 mos *Award:* AS
Tuition per yr: $7,995

Miami-Dade Community College
Respiratory Therapist Prgm
Medical Center Campus
950 NW 20th St
Miami, FL 33127
Prgm Dir: Carol J Miller, EdD RT
Tel: 305 237-4031 *Fax:* 305 237-4278
E-mail: milleo@mdcc.edu
Med Dir: Bruce Krieger, MD
Class Cap: 40 *Begins:* Aug
Length: 24 mos *Award:* AS
Tuition per yr: $2,063 res, $7,250 non-res
Evening or weekend classes available

University of Central Florida
Respiratory Therapist Prgm
Dept of Health Professions and P.T.
Orlando, FL 32816
Prgm Dir: L Timothy Worrell, MPH RRT
Tel: 407 823-2214 *Fax:* 407 823-6138
E-mail: worrell@pegasus.cc.ucf.edu
Med Dir: Lawrence M Gilliard, MD
Class Cap: 16 *Begins:* Aug
Length: 20 mos *Award:* Dipl, BS
Tuition per yr: $2,182 res, $4,129 non-res
Evening or weekend classes available

Valencia Community College

Respiratory Therapist Prgm
PO Box 3028
Orlando, FL 32802-9961
Prgm Dir: Lynn W Capraun, MS RRT
Tel: 407 299-5000, Ext 1550 *Fax:* 407 293-8839
Med Dir: Robert C Snyder, MD
Class Cap: 24 *Begins:* Aug
Length: 20 mos *Award:* Dipl, AS
Tuition per yr: $1,690 res, $6,160 non-res
Evening or weekend classes available

Palm Beach Community College

Respiratory Therapist Prgm
3160 PGA Blvd
Palm Beach Gardens, FL 33410
Prgm Dir: Edward W Willey, MS RRT
Tel: 561 625-2587 *Fax:* 561 625-2305
Med Dir: Rogelio Choy, MD
Class Cap: 25 *Begins:* Aug
Length: 21 mos *Award:* AS
Tuition per yr: $1,360 res, $5,062 non-res
Evening or weekend classes available

Pensacola Junior College

Respiratory Therapist Prgm
5555 W Hwy 98
Pensacola, FL 32507
Prgm Dir: Sheila R Peterson, RRT BS
Tel: 904 484-2214
Med Dir: John Bray, MD
Class Cap: 25 *Begins:* May
Length: 24 mos *Award:* AS
Tuition per yr: $4,500 res, $12,150 non-res
Evening or weekend classes available

Seminole Community College

Respiratory Therapist Prgm
100 Weldon Blvd
Sanford, FL 32773
Prgm Dir: Steve Shideler, MS RRT
Tel: 407 328-2293 *Fax:* 407 328-2139
E-mail: s.shidelea@ipu.seminole.cc.fl.us
Med Dir: Alan R Varraux, MD
Class Cap: 25 *Begins:* Aug
Length: 20 mos *Award:* AS
Tuition per yr: $2,000 res, $2,800 non-res
Evening or weekend classes available

St Petersburg Junior College

Respiratory Therapist Prgm
PO Box 13489
St Petersburg, FL 33733
Prgm Dir: Stephen P Mikles, EdS RRT
Tel: 813 341-3627 *Fax:* 813 341-3744
E-mail: mikless@email.spjc.cc.fl.us
Med Dir: Anthony N Ottaviani, DO
Class Cap: 24 *Begins:* Aug
Length: 24 mos *Award:* Cert, AS
Tuition per yr: $1,555 res, $5,600 non-res

Florida A & M University

Respiratory Therapist Prgm
Ware-Rhaney Bldg
Tallahassee, FL 32307
Prgm Dir: Patrick L Johnson, MA RRT
Tel: 904 561-2186 *Fax:* 904 561-2457
E-mail: pjohnson@mailer.fsu.edu
Med Dir: Kenneth Wasson, MD
Class Cap: 20 *Begins:* Aug
Length: 24 mos *Award:* BS
Tuition per yr: $1,892 res, $7,286 non-res
Evening or weekend classes available

Tallahassee Community College

Respiratory Therapist Prgm
444 Appleyard Dr
Tallahassee, FL 32301
Prgm Dir: Dewey Streetman, RRT
Tel: 904 922-8103
Med Dir: Kenneth Wasson, MD
Class Cap: 30 *Begins:* Aug
Length: 22 mos *Award:* AS
Tuition per yr: $1,200 res, $4,600 non-res

Georgia

Darton College

Respiratory Therapist Prgm
2400 Gillionville Rd
Albany, GA 31707
Prgm Dir: Brian J Parker, MPH RRT
Tel: 912 430-6900 *Fax:* 912 430-6794
Med Dir: Mark M Shoemaker, MD
Class Cap: 20 *Begins:* Jun
Length: 24 mos *Award:* AS
Tuition per yr: $1,360 res, $3,204 non-res

Athens Area Technical Institute

Respiratory Therapist Prgm
Hwy 29 N
Athens, GA 30610-0399
Prgm Dir: Bruce A Ott, EdD RRT
Tel: 706 355-5084 *Fax:* 706 369-5753
E-mail: ott@admin1.athens.tcc.ga.us
Med Dir: Dale Green, MD
Class Cap: 25 *Begins:* Sep
Length: 24 mos *Award:* AAT
Tuition per yr: $1,068

Georgia State University

Respiratory Therapist Prgm
University Plaza
Atlanta, GA 30303
Prgm Dir: Joseph L Rau Jr, PhD RRT
Tel: 404 651-3037 *Fax:* 404 651-1531
Med Dir: Robert Aranson, MD
Class Cap: 30 *Begins:* Sep
Length: 22 mos *Award:* Cert, BS
Tuition per yr: $3,021 res, $11,917 non-res
Evening or weekend classes available

Augusta Technical Institute

Respiratory Therapist Prgm
3116 Deans Bridge Rd
Augusta, GA 30906
Prgm Dir: Rita Waller, BS BSN RN RTT
Tel: 706 771-4194 *Fax:* 706 771-4181
Med Dir: A Darrell McDaniel, BS RTT CRTT
Class Cap: 20 *Begins:* Jul
Length: 24 mos *Award:* AS
Tuition per yr: $932 res, $1,748 non-res

Medical College of Georgia

Respiratory Therapist Prgm
Augusta, GA 30912
Prgm Dir: Shelley C Mishoe, PhD RRT
Tel: 706 721-3554 *Fax:* 706 721-0495
E-mail: smishoe@mail.mcg.edu
Med Dir: Bashir Ahmad Chaudhary, MD
Class Cap: 22 *Begins:* Sep
Length: 22 mos *Award:* BS
Tuition per yr: $2,703 res, $6,393 non-res

Columbus State University

Respiratory Therapist Prgm
2400 Gillionville Rd
Albany, GA 31707
Prgm Dir: Brian J Parker, MPH RRT
Tel: 912 430-6900 *Fax:* 912 430-6794
Med Dir: Mark M Shoemaker, MD
Class Cap: 20 *Begins:* Jun
Length: 24 mos *Award:* AS
Tuition per yr: $1,360 res, $3,204 non-res

Darton College

Respiratory Therapist Prgm
4225 University Ave
Columbus, GA 31907-5645
Prgm Dir: David W Chang, EdD RRT
Tel: 706 568-2130 *Fax:* 706 568-2313
E-mail: chang_david@colstate.edu
Med Dir: Kenny C. Nall, MD
Begins: Jun
Length: 21 mos *Award:* Cert, AS
Tuition per yr: $2,460 res, $7,632 non-res

Armstrong Atlantic State University

Respiratory Therapist Prgm
11935 Abercorn St
Savannah, GA 31406
Prgm Dir: Ross L Bowers III, MHS RRT
Tel: 912 927-5204 *Fax:* 912 921-5585
Med Dir: Robert J DiBenedetto, MD
Class Cap: 20 *Begins:* Sep
Length: 21 mos *Award:* Dipl, AS
Tuition per yr: $2,292 res, $6,572 non-res
Evening or weekend classes available

Hawaii

Kapiolani Community College

Respiratory Therapist Prgm
4303 Diamond Head Rd
Honolulu, HI 96816
Prgm Dir: Stephen F Wehrman, RRT
Tel: 808 734-9243 *Fax:* 808 734-9126
E-mail: swehrman@leahi.kcchawcui.edu
Med Dir: Christine Fukui, MD
Class Cap: 16 *Begins:* Aug
Length: 22 mos *Award:* AS
Tuition per yr: $790 res, $7,485 non-res

Idaho

Boise State University

Respiratory Therapist Prgm
College of Health Science
Boise, ID 83725
Prgm Dir: Lonny J Ashworth, MEd RRT
Tel: 208 385-3383 *Fax:* 208 385-4093
E-mail: lashwor@bsu.idbsu.edu
Med Dir: David Merrick, MD
Class Cap: 16 *Begins:* Aug
Length: 27 mos, 36 mos *Award:* AS, BS
Tuition per yr: $1,964 res, $7,310 non-res
Evening or weekend classes available

Illinois

Southern Illinois Univ at Carbondale
Respiratory Therapist Prgm
Health Care Professions
Carbondale, IL 62901-6604
Prgm Dir: Stanley M Pearson II, MSEd RRT
Tel: 618 453-7221 *Fax:* 618 453-7286
Med Dir: Parvis Sanjabi, MD
Class Cap: 35 *Begins:* Aug
Length: 16 mos, 28 mos *Award:* Cert, AAS
Tuition per yr: $4,006 res, $9,556 non-res

Parkland College
Respiratory Therapist Prgm
2400 W Bradley Ave
Champaign, IL 61821
Prgm Dir: Terry Des Jardins, MEd RRT
Tel: 217 351-2224 *Fax:* 217 351-2581
E-mail: tdesjardins@parkland.cc.il.us
Med Dir: Maury Topolosky, MD
Class Cap: 25 *Begins:* Aug
Length: 20 mos *Award:* Cert, AAS
Tuition per yr: $1,476 res, $4,021 non-res

Malcolm X College
Respiratory Therapist Prgm
1900 W Van Buren St
Chicago, IL 60612
Prgm Dir: Dorian Hampton, MS RRT
Tel: 312 850-7486 *Fax:* 312 850-7453
Med Dir: Naresh K Upahyay, MD
Class Cap: 35 *Begins:* Sep
Length: 21 mos *Award:* Cert, AAS
Tuition per yr: $2,905 res, $8,462 non-res

National-Louis University
Respiratory Therapist Prgm
2840 Sheridan Rd
Evanston, IL 60201
Prgm Dir: Stephen L Thompson, MS RRT
Tel: 847 256-5150 *Fax:* 847 256-1057
Med Dir: John H Buehler, MD
Class Cap: 12 *Begins:* Sep
Length: 15 mos, 24 mos *Award:* Cert, BA
Tuition per yr: $11,250
Evening or weekend classes available

College of DuPage
Respiratory Therapist Prgm
Advanced Practitioner
22nd St and Lambert Rd
Glen Ellyn, IL 60137-6599
Prgm Dir: Kenneth M Bretl, MA RRT
Tel: 630 942-2518 *Fax:* 630 858-9399
E-mail: bretlk@cdnet.cod.edu
Med Dir: Robert T Zeck, MD
Class Cap: 20 *Begins:* Sept
Length: 12 mos *Award:* AAS
Tuition per yr: $1,363 res, $4,277 non-res
Evening or weekend classes available

Black Hawk College
Respiratory Therapist Prgm
Quad Cities Campus
6600 34th Ave
Moline, IL 61265
Prgm Dir: Nancy M Smith, BA RRT
Tel: 309 796-1311 *Fax:* 309 792-3418
E-mail: smithn@bhc1bhc.edu
Med Dir: Edward L Ebert, DO
Class Cap: 12 *Begins:* Aug
Length: 9 mos *Award:* Dipl,Cert, AAS
Tuition per yr: $1,349 res, $5,488 non-res
Evening or weekend classes available

Moraine Valley Community College
Respiratory Therapist Prgm
10900 S 88th Ave
Palos Hills, IL 60465
Prgm Dir: Raymond F Lehner, RRT
Tel: 708 974-5380
Med Dir: Richard Earle, MD
Class Cap: 32 *Begins:* Aug
Length: 21 mos *Award:* AAS
Tuition per yr: $1,533 res, $5,876 non-res

Illinois Central College
Respiratory Therapist Prgm
201 SW Adams
Peoria, IL 61635-0001
Prgm Dir: Margaret A Swanson, MS RRT
Tel: 309 999-4663 *Fax:* 309 673-9626
Med Dir: Stanley Bugaieski, MD
Class Cap: 15 *Begins:* Aug
Length: 21 mos *Award:* AAS
Tuition per yr: $1,554 res, $4,810 non-res
Evening or weekend classes available

Triton College
Respiratory Therapist Prgm
2000 N Fifth Ave
River Grove, IL 60171
Prgm Dir: Kristine Anderson, MEd RRT CPFT
Tel: 708 456-0300
Med Dir: Patrick J Fahey, MD
Class Cap: 30 *Begins:* Sep
Length: 22 mos *Award:* AAS
Tuition per yr: $891 res, $2,850 non-res

Rock Valley College
Respiratory Therapist Prgm
3301 N Mulford Rd
Rockford, IL 61114-5699
Prgm Dir: James R Sills, MEd CPFT RRT
Tel: 815 654-4413 *Fax:* 815 654-5359
E-mail: fahe3js@rvcux1.rvc.cc.il.us
Med Dir: John Foster, MD
Class Cap: 15 *Begins:* Aug
Length: 22 mos *Award:* AAS
Tuition per yr: $1,435 res, $4,674 non-res
Evening or weekend classes available

Lincoln Land Community College
Respiratory Therapist Prgm
Shepherd Rd
Springfield, IL 62794-9256
Prgm Dir: Randel A Prather, BA RRT
Tel: 217 786-2814
Med Dir: Lanie E Eagleton, MD
Class Cap: 20 *Begins:* Jun
Length: 22 mos *Award:* Cert, AAS
Tuition per yr: $1,482
Evening or weekend classes available

Indiana

University of Southern Indiana
Respiratory Therapist Prgm
8600 University Blvd
Evansville, IN 47712
Prgm Dir: Robert Hooper, RRT
Tel: 812 464-1702 *Fax:* 812 465-7092
Med Dir: James S Dunnick, MD FACC
Class Cap: 14 *Begins:* Aug
Length: 24 mos *Award:* Dipl, AAS
Tuition per yr: $2,840 res, $6,825 non-res
Evening or weekend classes available

Ivy Tech State Coll NE - Ft Wayne
Respiratory Therapist Prgm
3800 N Anthony Blvd
Ft Wayne, IN 46805
Prgm Dir: Candace Schladenhauffen, RRT RPFT
Tel: 219 482-9171 *Fax:* 219 480-4149
Med Dir: Thomas Hayhurst, MD
Class Cap: 28 *Begins:* Aug
Length: 21 mos *Award:* AAS
Tuition per yr: $4,353 res, $7,921 non-res
Evening or weekend classes available

Indiana University Northwest
Respiratory Therapist Prgm
3400 Broadway NW Campus
Gary, IN 46408
Prgm Dir: Cheryl Oprisko, JD RRT
Tel: 219 980-6955 *Fax:* 219 980-6649
E-mail: copnsko@iunhaw1.iun.indiana.edu
Med Dir: Raja G Devanathan, MD
Class Cap: 18 *Begins:* Aug
Length: 26 mos *Award:* AS
Tuition per yr: $2,214 res, $8,414 non-res

Ball State University
Respiratory Therapist Prgm
1701 N Senate Blvd
Indianapolis, IN 46202
Prgm Dir: Linda I Van Scoder, EdD RRT
Tel: 317 929-8475 *Fax:* 317 929-2102
Med Dir: Michael Niemeier, MD
Class Cap: 12 *Begins:* Aug
Length: 24 mos *Award:* AS
Tuition per yr: $3,264 res, $3,264 non-res
Evening or weekend classes available

Indiana University School of Medicine
Respiratory Therapist Prgm
1140 W Michigan St
CF 224
Indianapolis, IN 46223
Prgm Dir: Deborah L Cullen, EdD RRT
Tel: 317 274-7381 *Fax:* 317 278-7383
Med Dir: Alvin M LoSasso, MD
Class Cap: 20 *Begins:* Aug
Length: 24 mos, 48 mos *Award:* Cert, BS
Tuition per yr: $3,421 res, $10,500 non-res
Evening or weekend classes available

Ivy Tech State Coll - Indianapolis

Respiratory Therapist Prgm
Central Indiana Region
One W 26th St/PO Box 1763
Indianapolis, IN 46206-1763
Prgm Dir: Kathleen F Lee, MS RRT
Tel: 317 921-4402   *Fax:* 317 921-4753
Med Dir: James D Pike, DO FCCP
Class Cap: 10   *Begins:* Sep Jan
Length: 21 mos, 31 mos   *Award:* AAS
Tuition per yr: $2,894 res, $5,268 non-res
Evening or weekend classes available

Vincennes University

Respiratory Therapist Prgm
1002 N First Street
Vincennes, IN 47591
Prgm Dir: Everett Wood Jr, MS RRT
Tel: 812 888-4421   *Fax:* 812 888-4550
E-mail: twood@vunet.vinu.edu
Med Dir: Richard H Stein, MD
Class Cap: 24   *Begins:* Aug
Length: 23 mos   *Award:* Dipl, AS
Tuition per yr: $2,870 res, $6,956 non-res

Iowa

Des Moines Area Community College

Respiratory Therapist Prgm
2006 Ankeny Blvd
Ankeny, IA 50021
Prgm Dir: Kerry E George, RRT
Tel: 515 964-6298   *Fax:* 515 964-6440
Med Dir: John Glazier, MD
Class Cap: 24   *Begins:* Aug
Length: 23 mos   *Award:* AAS
Tuition per yr: $2,350 res, $4,700 non-res
Evening or weekend classes available

Kirkwood Community College

Respiratory Therapist Prgm
6301 Kirkwood Blvd SW
PO Box 2068
Cedar Rapids, IA 52406-9973
Prgm Dir: H Kenneth Bronkhorst, MBA RRT
Tel: 319 398-4987   *Fax:* 319 398-1293
E-mail: kbronho@kirkwood.cc.ia.us
Med Dir: Jeffrey S Wilson, MD
Class Cap: 25   *Begins:* May
Length: 24 mos   *Award:* AAS
Tuition per yr: $2,393 res, $4,786 non-res

Northeast Iowa Community College

Respiratory Therapist Prgm
10250 Sundown Rd
Peosta, IA 52068
Prgm Dir: Sue E Meade, RRT
Tel: 800 728-7367   *Fax:* 319 556-5058
E-mail: meades@nicc.cc.ia.us
Med Dir: Mark Janes, MD
Class Cap: 25   *Begins:* Aug
Length: 21 mos   *Award:* Dipl, AAS
Tuition per yr: $5,084 res, $7,118 non-res
Evening or weekend classes available

Kansas

Bethany Med Ctr/Kansas City Kansas Comm Coll

Respiratory Therapist Prgm
51 N 12th St
Kansas City, KS 66102
Prgm Dir: C Michael Parrett, MBA RPFT RRT
Tel: 913 281-8768   *Fax:* 913 281-7875
Med Dir: Ajit Parekh, MD
Begins: Sep
Length: 24 mos   *Award:* Cert, AS
Tuition per yr: $3,850 res, $5,200 non-res

University of Kansas Medical Center

Respiratory Therapist Prgm
3901 Rainbow Blvd
5003 Hinch Hall
Kansas City, KS 66160-7606
Prgm Dir: Barbara A Ludwig, MA RRT
Tel: 913 588-4634   *Fax:* 913 588-4631
E-mail: bludwig@kumc.edu
Med Dir: Hugh S Mathewson, MD
Class Cap: 30   *Begins:* Aug
Length: 22 mos   *Award:* Dipl,Cert, BS
Tuition per yr: $2,394 res, $10,070 non-res

Seward County Community College

Respiratory Therapist Prgm
PO Box 1137
Liberal, KS 67905-1137
Prgm Dir: Ken Killion, RRT
Tel: 316 626-3080   *Fax:* 316 626-3026
Med Dir: Frank W Hansen, MD
Class Cap: 16   *Begins:* Aug
Length: 24 mos   *Award:* Dipl, AAS
Tuition per yr: $1,134 res, $2,100 non-res
Evening or weekend classes available

Johnson County Community College

Respiratory Therapist Prgm
Respiratory Care
12345 College Blvd
Overland Park, KS 66210
Prgm Dir: Clarissa M Craig, MA RRT
Tel: 913 469-8500   *Fax:* 913 469-2518
E-mail: ccraig@jcccnet.johncd.cc.ks.us
Med Dir: Larry D Botts, MD
Class Cap: 20   *Begins:* Jun
Length: 24 mos   *Award:* Cert, AS
Tuition per yr: $1,702 res, $4,514 non-res
Evening or weekend classes available

Labette Community College

Respiratory Therapist Prgm
200 S 14th St
Parsons, KS 67357
Prgm Dir: Connie S Crooks, BS RRT
Tel: 316 421-6700   *Fax:* 316 421-0180
E-mail: connie@computer-services.com
Med Dir: Daniel Pauls, MD
Class Cap: 30   *Begins:* Aug
Length: 24 mos   *Award:* AAS
Tuition per yr: $1,287 res, $1,287 non-res
Evening or weekend classes available

Washburn University of Topeka

Respiratory Therapist Prgm
1700 College Ave SW
Topeka, KS 66621
Prgm Dir: Patricia M Munzer, MS RRT
Tel: 913 231-1010   *Fax:* 913 231-1027
E-mail: zzmunz@sace.wuacc.edu
Med Dir: Ted W Daughety, MD
Class Cap: 18   *Begins:* Aug
Length: 22 mos   *Award:* Cert, AS
Tuition per yr: $3,456 res, $8,018 non-res
Evening or weekend classes available

Wichita State University

Respiratory Therapist Prgm
Campus Box 43
Wichita, KS 67208
Prgm Dir: Alphonso Baldwin, PhD RRT RPFT
Tel: 316 689-3619   *Fax:* 316 978-3025
Med Dir: Douglas R Livingston, DO AFACA
Class Cap: 20   *Begins:* Aug
Length: 28 mos   *Award:* Dipl,Cert, AS
Tuition per yr: $2,162 res, $7,442 non-res
Evening or weekend classes available

Kentucky

Southeast Community College

Respiratory Therapist Prgm
300 College Rd
Cumberland, KY 40823-1099
Prgm Dir: Michael Good, RRT
Tel: 606 589-2145   *Fax:* 606 337-5662
Med Dir: Abdi Vazey, MD FCCP
Class Cap: 12
Length: 24 mos   *Award:* AAS

Northern Kentucky University

Respiratory Therapist Prgm
Nunn Dr
Highland, KY 41099-8002
Prgm Dir: Robert Langenderfer
Tel: 606 572-5557   *Fax:* 606 572-6182
E-mail: Langenderfer@nku.edu
Med Dir: Roy Moser III, MD
Class Cap: 18   *Begins:* Aug
Length: 21 mos   *Award:* AAS
Tuition per yr: $2,500 res, $6,770 non-res
Evening or weekend classes available

Lexington Community College

Respiratory Therapist Prgm
Cooper Dr
Oswald Bldg
Lexington, KY 40506-0235
Prgm Dir: James K Matchuny, BS RRT
Tel: 606 257-6154   *Fax:* 606 257-4339
E-mail: jkmatc1.uky.edu
Med Dir: James McCormick
Class Cap: 48   *Begins:* Jun
Length: 24 mos   *Award:* AAS
Tuition per yr: $2,382 res, $6,432 non-res
Evening or weekend classes available

Programs

Jefferson Community College
Respiratory Therapist Prgm
109 E Broadway
Louisville, KY 40202
Prgm Dir: Carolyn O'Daniel, EdD RRT
Tel: 502 584-0181, Ext 2491   *Fax:* 502 584-0181
Med Dir: Judah Skolnick, MD
Class Cap: 25   *Begins:* Jun
Length: 24 mos   *Award:* AAS
Tuition per yr: $1,252 res, $3,756 non-res

University of Louisville
Respiratory Therapist Prgm
KBLDG 4th Floor
Louisville, KY 40292
Prgm Dir: Jerome Walker, EdD RRT
Tel: 502 852-8280   *Fax:* 502 852-4597
E-mail: jfwalkoi@ulkyvm.louisville.edu
Med Dir: Lynell Collins, MD
Class Cap: 25   *Begins:* May Aug
Length: 24 mos   *Award:* Dipl, AHS , BHS
Tuition per yr: $3,705 res, $10,875 non-res
Evening or weekend classes available

Madisonville Community College
Respiratory Therapist Prgm
Consortium for Resp Care Educ
College Dr
Madisonville, KY 42431
Prgm Dir: David F Pennaman, MS RRT
Tel: 502 824-7552
Med Dir: Frank H Taylor, MD
Class Cap: 15   *Begins:* Aug Jan
Length: 22 mos   *Award:* AAS
Tuition per yr: $980 res, $2,940 non-res
Evening or weekend classes available

Louisiana

Bossier Parish Community College
Respiratory Therapist Prgm
2719 Airline Dr
Bossier City, LA 71111
Prgm Dir: Beth Hamilton, MHS RRT
Tel: 318 675-6814   *Fax:* 318 675-6937
E-mail: ehamil@mail-sh.isumc.edu
Med Dir: Keith Payne, MD
Class Cap: 15   *Begins:* Jun
Length: 28 mos   *Award:* Dipl, AD
Tuition per yr: $1,400

Delgado Community College
Respiratory Therapist Prgm
615 City Park Ave
New Orleans, LA 70119
Prgm Dir: Diane M Olsen, MHS RRT
Tel: 504 483-4007   *Fax:* 504 483-4609
E-mail: dolsen@pop3.dcc.edu
Med Dir: Mack Thomas, MD
Class Cap: 25   *Begins:* Aug
Length: 24 mos   *Award:* AS
Tuition per yr: $1,455 res, $3,255 non-res
Evening or weekend classes available

Alton Ochsner Medical Foundation
Respiratory Therapist Prgm
1516 Jefferson Hwy
New Orleans, LA 70121
Prgm Dir: Mary LaBiche, MEd RRT
Tel: 504 842-3267   *Fax:* 504 842-9129
Med Dir: John M Onofrio, MD
Class Cap: 6   *Begins:* Sep
Length: 14 mos   *Award:* Cert
Tuition per yr: $1,820 res, $1,820 non-res

Louisiana State Univ Med Ctr - New Orleans
Respiratory Therapist Prgm
1900 Gravier St
New Orleans, LA 70112
Prgm Dir: James M Cairo, PhD RRT
Tel: 504 568-4229   *Fax:* 504 568-4248
E-mail: jcairo@lsumc.edu
Med Dir: Mack Thomas, MD
Class Cap: 53   *Begins:* Jun
Length: 24 mos   *Award:* Dipl, BS
Tuition per yr: $2,050 res, $5,050 non-res

Southern Univ at Shreveport - Bossier City
Respiratory Therapist Prgm
3050 Martin Luther King Jr Dr
Shreveport, LA 71107
Prgm Dir: JoAnn Warren, BA RRT
Tel: 318 674-3452
Med Dir: Shawn A Milligan, MD
Begins: Aug
Length: 24 mos   *Award:* AS
Tuition per yr: $1,110 res, $2,240 non-res
Evening or weekend classes available

Nicholls State University
Respiratory Therapist Prgm
Dept of Allied Health Sciences
PO Box 2090
Thibodaux, LA 70310
Prgm Dir: Errol J Champagne, BS RRT
Tel: 504 448-4495   *Fax:* 504 448-4923
Med Dir: John C King, MD
Class Cap: 10   *Begins:* Aug
Length: 12 mos   *Award:* Cert
Tuition per yr: $1,349 res, $3,077 non-res

Maine

Kennebec Valley Technical College
Respiratory Therapist Prgm
92 Western Ave
Fairfield, ME 04937-1367
Prgm Dir: Barbara A Larsson, MEd RRT
Tel: 207 453-5161   *Fax:* 207 453-5194
E-mail: kblar.sso@kvtc.mtcs.tec.me.us
Med Dir: Dennis McCann, MD
Class Cap: 19   *Begins:* Aug
Length: 13 mos   *Award:* AAS
Tuition per yr: $2,623 res, $6,063 non-res
Evening or weekend classes available

Southern Maine Technical College
Respiratory Therapist Prgm
2 Fort Rd
South Portland, ME 04106
Prgm Dir: Walter C Chop, MS RRT
Tel: 207 767-9592   *Fax:* 207 767-9690
E-mail: wchop@smtc.mtcs.tec.me.us
Med Dir: Paul Cox, MD
Class Cap: 15   *Begins:* Aug
Length: 21 mos   *Award:* AAS
Tuition per yr: $2,200 res, $4,400 non-res

Maryland

Allegany College of Maryland
Respiratory Therapist Prgm
12401 Willowbrook Rd SE
Cumberland, MD 21502-2596
Prgm Dir: William R Rocks, MEd RRT
Tel: 301 724-7700   *Fax:* 301 724-1727
E-mail: billr@ac.cc.md.us
Med Dir: Robert J Orlino, MD
Class Cap: 24   *Begins:* Aug Sep
Length: 17 mos   *Award:* AAS
Tuition per yr: $2,590 res, $3,255 non-res
Evening or weekend classes available

Frederick Community College
Respiratory Therapist Prgm
7932 Opossumtown Pike
Frederick, MD 21702
Prgm Dir: Mark L Paugh, PhD
Tel: 301 846-2528   *Fax:* 301 846-2498
Med Dir: Allen Gilson, MD
Class Cap: 24   *Begins:* Aug
Length: 21 mos   *Award:* AAS
Tuition per yr: $2,100 res, $4,200 non-res
Evening or weekend classes available

Prince George's Community College
Respiratory Therapist Prgm
301 Largo Rd
Largo, MD 20772
Prgm Dir: Marie D York, RRT BS
Tel: 301 322-0747   *Fax:* 301 386-7504
E-mail: myl@pqstumail.pq.cc.us
Med Dir: Joseph J Colella, MD
Class Cap: 24   *Begins:* Sep
Length: 22 mos   *Award:* AAS
Tuition per yr: $3,031 res, $6,766 non-res
Evening or weekend classes available

Salisbury State University
Respiratory Therapist Prgm
College and Camden Aves
Salisbury, MD 21801
Prgm Dir: Theodore R Wiberg, PhD RRT
Tel: 410 543-6418   *Fax:* 410 548-3313
E-mail: trwiberg@ssu.edu
Med Dir: Rodney Layton, MD
Class Cap: 20   *Begins:* Sep Feb
Length: 24 mos   *Award:* Cert, BS
Tuition per yr: $2,566 res, $5,876 non-res

Columbia Union College

Respiratory Therapist Prgm
7600 Flower Ave
Takoma Park, MD 20912
Prgm Dir: Alvin R Tucker, BS RRT
Tel: 301 891-4188   *Fax:* 301 891-4191
Med Dir: Joseph Mizgerd, MD
Class Cap: 25   *Begins:* Sep
Length: 20 mos   *Award:* AAS
Tuition per yr: $10,950

Massachusetts

Northeastern University

Respiratory Therapist Prgm
100 Dockser Hall
360 Huntington Ave
Boston, MA 02115
Prgm Dir: Thomas A Barnes, EdD RRT
Tel: 617 373-3667   *Fax:* 617 373-2968
Med Dir: Alan Lisbon, MD
Class Cap: 16   *Begins:* Jan Apr Jun Sep
Length: 57 mos   *Award:* Cert, BS
Tuition per yr: $15,015

Massasoit Community College

Respiratory Therapist Prgm
One Massasoit Blvd
Brockton, MA 02402
Prgm Dir: Martha DeSilva, BS RRT
Tel: 508 588-9100, Ext 1787   *Fax:* 508 427-1250
Med Dir: Ronald Coutu, MD
Class Cap: 28   *Begins:* Sep
Length: 18 mos   *Award:* Cert, AS
Tuition per yr: $2,822 res, $6,392 non-res
Evening or weekend classes available

Newbury College

Respiratory Therapist Prgm
129 Fisher Ave
Brookline, MA 02146
Prgm Dir: Geraldine Twomey, MEd RRT
Tel: 617 730-7058   *Fax:* 617 730-7182
Med Dir: Jonathan D Strongin, MD PhD
Class Cap: 35   *Begins:* Sep Jan
Length: 20 mos   *Award:* AAS
Tuition per yr: $11,110

North Shore Community College

Respiratory Therapist Prgm
One Ferncroft Rd
PO Box 3340
Danvers, MA 01923-0840
Prgm Dir: William W Goding, MEd RRT
Tel: 508 762-4160   *Fax:* 508 762-4022
E-mail: wgoding@meen.mass.edu
Med Dir: Neil S Shore, MD
Class Cap: 20   *Begins:* Sep
Length: 21 mos   *Award:* Cert, AS
Tuition per yr: $2,822 res, $7,718 non-res
Evening or weekend classes available

Northern Essex Community College

Respiratory Therapist Prgm
100 Elliot Way
Haverhill, MA 01830
Prgm Dir: Christopher Rowse, MS RRT
Tel: 508 374-3828
Med Dir: Daniel Coleman, MD
Class Cap: 15   *Begins:* Sep
Length: 13 mos, 18 mos   *Award:* AS
Tuition per yr: $2,805 res, $3,399 non-res

Berkshire Community College

Respiratory Therapist Prgm
West St
Pittsfield, MA 01201
Prgm Dir: Thomas P Carey Jr, RRT MPH
Tel: 413 499-4660   *Fax:* 413 448-2700
E-mail: tpcarry@cbcc.bcwan.net
Med Dir: Jack Ringler, MD
Class Cap: 20   *Begins:* Sep Jan Jun
Length: 21 mos   *Award:* Dipl,Cert, AS
Tuition per yr: $3,310 res, $7,810 non-res
Evening or weekend classes available

Springfield Technical Community College

Respiratory Therapist Prgm
One Armory Square
Springfield, MA 01105
Prgm Dir: Lee J Robinson, MEd RRT
Tel: 413 781-7822   *Fax:* 413 781-5805
Med Dir: Bruce M Meth, MD
Class Cap: 0   *Begins:* Sep
Length: 10 mos   *Award:* Dipl,Cert, AS
Tuition per yr: $1,939 res, $7,119 non-res
Evening or weekend classes available

Quinsigamond Community College

Respiratory Therapist Prgm
670 W Boylston St
Worcester, MA 01606
Prgm Dir: Lynda A Nesbitt, RRT
Tel: 508 853-2300   *Fax:* 508 852-6943
Med Dir: Richard Rosiello, MD
Class Cap: 20   *Begins:* Aug
Length: 20 mos   *Award:* AS
Tuition per yr: $1,008
Evening or weekend classes available

Michigan

Washtenaw Community College

Respiratory Therapist Prgm
4800 E Huron River Dr
Ann Arbor, MI 48106
Prgm Dir: Mimi Y Norwood, MA RRT
Tel: 313 973-3331   *Fax:* 313 677-5078
Med Dir: William Patton, MD
Class Cap: 24   *Begins:* Jan Aug
Length: 21 mos   *Award:* Cert, AD
Tuition per yr: $3,672 res, $5,256 non-res

Ferris State University

Respiratory Therapist Prgm
200 Ferris Dr
VFS 405-A
Big Rapids, MI 49307-2740
Prgm Dir: Julian F Easter, MS RRT
Tel: 616 592-2312   *Fax:* 616 592-3788
E-mail: jeaster@music.ferris.edu
Med Dir: Chaitanya Acharya, MD
Class Cap: 25   *Begins:* Aug
Length: 21 mos   *Award:* Cert, AAS
Tuition per yr: $3,565 res, $7,186 non-res

Oakland Community College

Respiratory Therapist Prgm
2480 Opdyke Rd
Bloomfield Hills, MI 48304-2266
Prgm Dir: David W Sanford, PhD RRT
Tel: 810 552-2655   *Fax:* 810 552-2661
Med Dir: Stanley Sherman, MD
Class Cap: 40   *Begins:* Jul
Length: 14 mos, 24 mos   *Award:* Dipl, AAS
Tuition per yr: $1,935 res, $3,311 non-res
Evening or weekend classes available

Macomb Community College

Respiratory Therapist Prgm
44575 Garfield Rd
Clinton Township, MI 48038-1139
Prgm Dir: Lawrence J Fields, MS RRT
Tel: 810 286-2075   *Fax:* 810 286-2098
Med Dir: Raymond D Sphire, MD
Class Cap: 40   *Begins:* Aug
Length: 21 mos   *Award:* AAS
Tuition per yr: $1,988 res, $3,013 non-res
Evening or weekend classes available

Henry Ford Community College

Respiratory Therapist Prgm
22586 Ann Arbor Trail
Dearborn Heights, MI 48127
Prgm Dir: Debra A Szymanski, MA RRT
Tel: 313 730-5973   *Fax:* 313 359-4601
Med Dir: Bradford K Grassmick, MD
Class Cap: 28   *Begins:* Aug
Length: 21 mos   *Award:* AS
Tuition per yr: $1,771 res, $2,701 non-res
Evening or weekend classes available

Marygrove College

Respiratory Therapist Prgm
8425 W McNichols Rd
Detroit, MI 48221-2599
Prgm Dir: Kathy Miller, RRT
Tel: 313 862-8000   *Fax:* 313 864-6670
Med Dir: Richard S Fine, MD
Class Cap: 15   *Begins:* Jan
Length: 24 mos   *Award:* Cert, AS
Tuition per yr: $9,636
Evening or weekend classes available

Charles Stewart Mott Community College

Respiratory Therapist Prgm
1401 E Court St
Flint, MI 48503
Prgm Dir: David L Panzlau, MA RRT
Tel: 810 232-6563   *Fax:* 810 762-5619
Med Dir: Ahmed Hannan, MD
Class Cap: 24   *Begins:* Sep
Length: 19 mos   *Award:* AAS
Tuition per yr: $2,687 res, $3,875 non-res
Evening or weekend classes available

Kalamazoo Valley Community College

Respiratory Therapist Prgm
6767 W O Ave
Kalamazoo, MI 49009
Prgm Dir: James William Taylor, MA RRT
Tel: 616 372-5356   *Fax:* 616 372-5958
Med Dir: John W Dircks, MD
Class Cap: 24   *Begins:* Aug Sep
Length: 20 mos   *Award:* AAS
Tuition per yr: $1,440 res, $3,920 non-res

Programs

Lansing Community College
Respiratory Therapist Prgm
PO Box 40010
Lansing, MI 48901
Prgm Dir: Jerry A Rocho, BS RRT
Tel: 517 483-1450   *Fax:* 517 483-1410
E-mail: jr1450@lois.cc.mi.us
Med Dir: Alan Atkinson, DO
Class Cap: 18   *Begins:* Aug
Length: 23 mos   *Award:* Dipl, AAS
Tuition per yr: $1,871 res, $3,132 non-res
Evening or weekend classes available

Monroe County Community College
Respiratory Therapist Prgm
1555 S Raisinville Rd
Monroe, MI 48161
Prgm Dir: Bonnie Boggs-Clothier, RRT
Tel: 313 242-7300   *Fax:* 313 242-9711
Med Dir: Milo Engoren, MD
Class Cap: 20   *Begins:* Aug
Length: 21 mos   *Award:* Dipl, AAS
Tuition per yr: $1,978 res, $3,082 non-res
Evening or weekend classes available

Muskegon Community College
Respiratory Therapist Prgm
221 S Quarterline Rd
Muskegon, MI 49442
Prgm Dir: Daniel B Knue, MM RRT
Tel: 616 777-0370   *Fax:* 616 777-0255
E-mail: dkune@aol.com
Med Dir: Mark Ivey, MD
Class Cap: 20   *Begins:* Jan
Length: 12 mos   *Award:* AAS
Tuition per yr: $2,150 res, $3,100 non-res
Evening or weekend classes available

Delta College
Respiratory Therapist Prgm
University Center, MI 48710
Prgm Dir: Earl B Gregory, MS RRT
Tel: 517 686-9489   *Fax:* 517 686-8736
E-mail: ebgregor@alpha.delta.edu
Med Dir: Vincent de las Alas, MD
Class Cap: 15   *Begins:* Aug
Length: 24 mos   *Award:* AAS
Tuition per yr: $1,643 res, $2,100 non-res
Evening or weekend classes available

Minnesota

Lake Superior College
Respiratory Therapist Prgm
West Campus
2101 Trinity Rd
Duluth, MN 55811
Prgm Dir: Mark Schmidt, BS RT
Tel: 218 722-2801   *Fax:* 218 722-2899
Med Dir: Paul Windberg, MD
Class Cap: 28   *Begins:* Sep
Length: 21 mos   *Award:* AAS
Tuition per yr: $3,000 res, $3,000 non-res

Northwest Technical Coll - E Grand Forks
Respiratory Therapist Prgm
Hwy 220 N
PO Box 111
East Grand Forks, MN 56721
Prgm Dir: Tony Sorum, RRT
Tel: 218 773-3441   *Fax:* 218 773-4502
E-mail: solum@adm.egt.mn.us
Med Dir: Wayne Bretweiser, MD
Begins: Aug
Length: 12 mos   *Award:* AAS
Tuition per yr: $2,768 res, $5,983 non-res

College of St Catherine
Respiratory Therapist Prgm
College of St Catherine, MPLS
601 25th Ave S
Minneapolis, MN 55454
Prgm Dir: John E Boatright, RRT
Tel: 612 690-7819   *Fax:* 612 690-7849
E-mail: jeboatnght@alex.stkate.edu
Med Dir: Keith Harmon, MD
Class Cap: 28   *Begins:* Sep
Length: 24 mos   *Award:* AAS
Tuition per yr: $13,000

Rochester Community and Technical College
Respiratory Therapist Prgm
Mayo Foundation
851 30th Ave SE
Rochester, MN 55905
Prgm Dir: Jeffrey J Ward, MEd RRT
Tel: 507 284-0174   *Fax:* 507 284-0656
Med Dir: David J Plevak, MD
Class Cap: 15   *Begins:* Sep
Length: 21 mos   *Award:* Dipl, AS
Tuition per yr: $2,325 res, $4,650 non-res
Evening or weekend classes available

St Paul Technical College
Respiratory Therapist Prgm
235 Marshall Ave
St Paul, MN 55102
Prgm Dir: Duane R Peterson, RRT
Tel: 612 221-1413   *Fax:* 612 221-1416
Med Dir: Kathy R Gromer, MD
Class Cap: 30   *Begins:* Sep
Length: 24 mos   *Award:* AD
Tuition per yr: $2,953 res, $5,907 non-res
Evening or weekend classes available

Mississippi

Itawamba Community College
Respiratory Therapist Prgm
602 W Hill St
Fulton, MS 38843
Prgm Dir: J Harold Plunkett, RRT
Tel: 601 862-3101   *Fax:* 601 862-7697
Med Dir: Benjamin Moore, MD
Class Cap: 16   *Begins:* Aug
Length: 12 mos, 21 mos   *Award:* Dipl, AAS
Tuition per yr: $1,000 res, $1,800 non-res
Evening or weekend classes available

Mississippi Gulf Coast Community College
Respiratory Therapist Prgm
PO Box 100
Gautier, MS 39553
Prgm Dir: Judie A Scott, AS RRT
Tel: 601 497-7711, Ext 290   *Fax:* 601 497-7670
Med Dir: David H Witty, MD
Class Cap: 20   *Begins:* Aug
Length: 24 mos   *Award:* AS
Tuition per yr: $1,400 res, $1,023 non-res

Pearl River Community College
Respiratory Therapist Prgm
Forrest County Voc-Tech Ctr
5448 US Hwy 49 S
Hattiesburg, MS 39401
Prgm Dir: S Lee King, BS MS RRT
Tel: 601 544-7722   *Fax:* 601 545-2976
Med Dir: Steven W Stogner, MD
Class Cap: 25   *Begins:* Aug
Length: 24 mos   *Award:* Cert
Tuition per yr: $1,275 res, $2,725 non-res
Evening or weekend classes available

Hinds Community College District
Respiratory Therapist Prgm
1750 Chadwick Dr
Jackson, MS 39204
Prgm Dir: Diane H Sylvester, RRT
Tel: 601 372-6501   *Fax:* 601 371-3703
E-mail: hccnahc@teclink.net
Med Dir: Graham B Shaw, MD
Class Cap: 30   *Begins:* Aug
Length: 21 mos   *Award:* Dipl, AAS
Tuition per yr: $1,325 res, $2,461 non-res

Copiah - Lincoln Community College
Respiratory Therapist Prgm
Natchez Campus Voc/Tech
30 Campus Dr
Natchez, MS 39120-5398
Prgm Dir: Richard G Waltman, RRT
Tel: 601 445-8299   *Fax:* 601 446-1298
Med Dir: Barry F Tillman, MD
Class Cap: 15   *Begins:* Aug
Length: 16 mos, 21 mos   *Award:* Cert, AS
Tuition per yr: $2,300 res, $4,900 non-res
Evening or weekend classes available

Northwest Mississippi Community College
Respiratory Therapist Prgm
5197 WE Ross Parkway
Southaven, MS 38671
Prgm Dir: Regina K Clark, BS RRT
Tel: 601 342-1570   *Fax:* 601 342-5686
Med Dir: Neal Aguillard, MD
Class Cap: 30   *Begins:* Aug
Length: 22 mos   *Award:* Cert, AAS
Tuition per yr: $1,000 res, $2,050 non-res

Missouri

University of Missouri - Columbia
Respiratory Therapist Prgm
504 Lewis Hall
Columbia, MO 65211
Prgm Dir: Michael W Prewitt, PhD RRT
Tel: 573 882-8034 *Fax:* 573 884-8000
E-mail: prewittm@ext.missouri.edu
Med Dir: R Phillip Dellinger, MD
Class Cap: 16 *Begins:* Aug
Length: 24 mos *Award:* Cert, BHS
Tuition per yr: $3,232 res, $8,980 non-res
Evening or weekend classes available

Ozarks Technical Community College
Respiratory Therapist Prgm
1417 N Jefferson
Springfield, MO 65802
Prgm Dir: Steven I Bishop, RRT PhD
Tel: 417 895-7127 *Fax:* 417 895-7161
Med Dir: John Wolfe, MD
Class Cap: 20 *Begins:* Jun
Length: 21 mos *Award:* AAS
Tuition per yr: $1,677 res, $2,457 non-res
Evening or weekend classes available

St Louis Comm College at Forest Park
Respiratory Therapist Prgm
5600 Oakland Ave
St Louis, MO 63110
Prgm Dir: James R Brennan, MEd RRT
Tel: 314 644-9326 *Fax:* 314 644-9752
Med Dir: Oscar Schwartz, MD
Class Cap: 10 *Begins:* Aug
Length: 22 mos *Award:* AAS
Tuition per yr: $1,700 res, $2,400 non-res
Evening or weekend classes available

Montana

Montana State Univ Coll of Technology
Respiratory Therapist Prgm
2100 16th Ave S
Great Falls, MT 59405
Prgm Dir: Leonard Bates, RRT
Tel: 406 771-4360 *Fax:* 406 771-4313
E-mail: agf6012@maia.oscs.montana.edu
Med Dir: Richard Blevins, MD
Class Cap: 18 *Begins:* Sep
Length: 20 mos *Award:* AAS
Tuition per yr: $2,256 res, $5,302 non-res
Evening or weekend classes available

Nebraska

Southeast Community College
Respiratory Therapist Prgm
8800 O St
Lincoln, NE 68520-1299
Prgm Dir: Dhiren K Chatterji, MS RRT
Med Dir: John Rudersdorf, MD
Class Cap: 18 *Begins:* Jul
Length: 18 mos *Award:* AAS
Tuition per yr: $1,764 res, $2,088 non-res

Alegent Health/Immanuel Medical Center
Respiratory Therapist Prgm
6901 N 72nd St
Omaha, NE 68122
Prgm Dir: Steven L Carper, BA RRT
Tel: 402 572-2312
Med Dir: John D Roehrs, MD
Begins: Sep
Length: 12 mos *Award:* Dipl,Cert, AS, BS
Tuition per yr: $10,990

Metropolitan Community College
Respiratory Therapist Prgm
PO Box 3777
Omaha, NE 68103
Prgm Dir: Jerald A Moss, RRT MPA
Tel: 402 449-8510 *Fax:* 402 449-8532
E-mail: jmoss@metro.mccneb.edu
Med Dir: Lon W Keim, MD
Class Cap: 21 *Begins:* Sep
Length: 24 mos *Award:* AAS
Tuition per yr: $3,519 res, $4,463 non-res
Evening or weekend classes available

NE Methodist Coll Nursing & Allied Hlth
Respiratory Therapist Prgm
8501 W Dodge Rd
Omaha, NE 68114
Prgm Dir: Christine Romeo, BA RRT
Tel: 402 354-4913 *Fax:* 402 354-8875
Med Dir: George Thommi, MD
Class Cap: 14 *Begins:* Aug Jan Jun
Length: 24 mos *Award:* AS
Tuition per yr: $9,348
Evening or weekend classes available

New Hampshire

New Hampshire Community Technical College
Respiratory Therapist Prgm
Hanover St Extension
Claremont, NH 03743
Prgm Dir: Susan M Perry, RRT
Tel: 603 542-7744 *Fax:* 603 543-1844
E-mail: s_perry@tec.nh.us
Med Dir: H Worth Parker, MD
Class Cap: 15 *Begins:* Aug
Length: 20 mos *Award:* AS
Tuition per yr: $2,756 res, $4,134 non-res
Evening or weekend classes available

New Jersey

Univ of Med & Dent of New Jersey
Respiratory Therapist Prgm
UMDNJ Sch of Hlth Related Prgm
PO Box 200
Blackwood, NJ 08012
Prgm Dir: G Woodard Gross, MA RRT
Tel: 609 227-7200 *Fax:* 609 374-4891
E-mail: gross@onyx.umonj.edu
Med Dir: Donald Auerbach, MD
Begins: Sep
Length: 24 mos *Award:* AAS
Tuition per yr: $1,632 res, $1,664 non-res

Northwest NJ Consortium Resp Care Educ
Respiratory Therapist Prgm
c/o NW Covenant Med Ctr
25 Pocono Rd
Denville, NJ 07834
Prgm Dir: Sharon K Shenton, MA RRT
Tel: 201 625-6723 *Fax:* 201 983-2394
Med Dir: Jack Goldshlack, DO
Class Cap: 20 *Begins:* Sep
Length: 24 mos *Award:* Cert, AAS , AS
Tuition per yr: $2,800 res, $5,200 non-res
Evening or weekend classes available

Brookdale Community College
Respiratory Therapist Prgm
765 Newman Springs Rd
Lincroft, NJ 07738
Prgm Dir: Patricia A Fusaro, RRT MSEd
Tel: 908 224-2606 *Fax:* 908 224-2772
Med Dir: J DeTullio, MD
Class Cap: 25 *Begins:* Sep
Length: 18 mos *Award:* AAS
Tuition per yr: $2,736 res, $5,856 non-res
Evening or weekend classes available

Univ of Med & Dent of New Jersey
Respiratory Therapist Prgm
Sch of Hlth Related Professions
65 Bergen St
Newark, NJ 07107-3006
Prgm Dir: Craig L Scanlan, EdD RRT
Tel: 201 982-5503 *Fax:* 201 982-5258
E-mail: scanlan@umdnj.edu
Med Dir: Marc H Lavietes, MD
Class Cap: 24 *Begins:* Sep
Length: 12 mos *Award:* AS
Tuition per yr: $2,310 res, $4,620 non-res

Bergen Community College
Respiratory Therapist Prgm
400 Paramus Rd
Paramus, NJ 07652
Prgm Dir: Robert A Muller, MA RRT
Tel: 201 447-7178
Med Dir: L Denson, MD
Class Cap: 20 *Begins:* Sep
Length: 19 mos *Award:* Dipl, AAS
Tuition per yr: $3,001 res, $6,002 non-res
Evening or weekend classes available

Passaic County Community College
Respiratory Therapist Prgm
One College Blvd
Paterson, NJ 07505-1179
Prgm Dir: Sandra McCleaster, MA RRT
Tel: 201 684-5280 *Fax:* 201 684-5843
Med Dir: Reza Farhangfar, MD
Class Cap: 24 *Begins:* Sep
Length: 22 mos *Award:* AAS

Union County College
Respiratory Therapist Prgm
E Second St
Plainfield, NJ 07060
Prgm Dir: Harlan Andrews, MEd CPFT RRT
Tel: 908 889-8629 *Fax:* 908 754-2798
Med Dir: Peter Goodluck, MD
Class Cap: 20 *Begins:* Sep
Length: 22 mos *Award:* AAS
Tuition per yr: $1,584 res, $3,168 non-res
Evening or weekend classes available

Programs

New Mexico

Dona Ana Branch Community College

Respiratory Therapist Prgm
Box 30001 Dept 3DA
3400 S Espina
Las Cruces, NM 88003-0001
Prgm Dir: Rene Adams, MA RRT
Tel: 505 527-7634 *Fax:* 505 527-7515
E-mail: radams@nmsu.edu
Med Dir: Harry Bass, MD
Class Cap: 20 *Begins:* Aug
Length: 24 mos *Award:* AAS
Tuition per yr: $800 res, $2,000 non-res

New York

Long Island University - Brooklyn Campus

Respiratory Therapist Prgm
University Plaza
Brooklyn, NY 11201
Prgm Dir: Thomas J Johnson, RRT
Tel: 718 488-1492 *Fax:* 718 488-1432
E-mail: tjohnson@titan.liunet.edu
Med Dir: Albert Heurich, MD
Class Cap: 32 *Begins:* Sep
Length: 24 mos *Award:* BS
Tuition per yr: $7,680
Evening or weekend classes available

Erie Community College - City Campus

Respiratory Therapist Prgm
Main and Youngs Rd
Buffalo, NY 14221
Prgm Dir: Marlon B Siegel, RRT MEd
Tel: 716 851-1531 *Fax:* 716 851-1429
E-mail: siegel@nstaff.sunnyerie.edu
Med Dir: Eric Ten Brock, MD
Class Cap: 36 *Begins:* Sep
Length: 24 mos *Award:* AAS
Tuition per yr: $2,600 res, $5,200 non-res
Evening or weekend classes available

Nassau Community College

Respiratory Therapist Prgm
Stewart Ave
Garden City, NY 11530
Prgm Dir: Warren Hostetter, RRT
Tel: 516 572-7550
Med Dir: Stephen Picca, MD
Class Cap: 24 *Begins:* Sep
Length: 24 mos *Award:* Cert, AAS
Tuition per yr: $2,200 res, $4,400 non-res
Evening or weekend classes available

CUNY Borough of Manhattan Community Coll

Respiratory Therapist Prgm
199 Chambers St
New York, NY 10007
Prgm Dir: Everett W Flannery, MPS RRT
Tel: 212 346-8731 *Fax:* 212 346-8730
Med Dir: Paul Goldiner, MD
Class Cap: 200 *Begins:* Aug
Length: 24 mos *Award:* Dipl,Cert, AAS
Tuition per yr: $2,500 res, $3,076 non-res

New York University

Respiratory Therapist Prgm
Basic Science Bldg
342 E 26th St First Fl
New York, NY 10010
Prgm Dir: Carole Smith, RRT
Tel: 212 263-6644
Med Dir: Vincent Donnabella, MD
Class Cap: 45 *Begins:* Sep
Length: 21 mos *Award:* Cert, AAS
Tuition per yr: $17,000 res, $17,000 non-res

Molloy College

Respiratory Therapist Prgm
1000 Hempstead Ave
Rockville Centre, NY 11570
Prgm Dir: Teresa Barrett, MA RRT
Tel: 516 678-5000 *Fax:* 516 256-2252
Med Dir: Joseph Genovese, DO
Class Cap: 26 *Begins:* Sep
Length: 24 mos *Award:* AAS
Tuition per yr: $11,520

SUNY Health Science Ctr at Stony Brook

Respiratory Therapist Prgm
School of Hlth Tech and Mgmt
Stony Brook, NY 11794
Prgm Dir: Kenneth L Axton Jr, RRT
Tel: 516 444-3180 *Fax:* 516 444-7621
Med Dir: Gerald Smaldone, MD PhD
Class Cap: 25 *Begins:* July
Length: 23 mos *Award:* Dipl,Cert, BS
Tuition per yr: $3,948 res, $9,684 non-res

Rockland Community College

Respiratory Therapist Prgm
145 College Rd
Suffern, NY 10901
Prgm Dir: Janice R Close, RRT
Tel: 914 574-4539 *Fax:* 908 224-2772
Med Dir: John D Pellicone, MD
Class Cap: 25 *Begins:* Sep
Length: 24 mos *Award:* Cert, AAS
Tuition per yr: $2,135 res, $5,856 non-res
Evening or weekend classes available

Onondaga Community College

Respiratory Therapist Prgm
Rte 173
Syracuse, NY 13215
Prgm Dir: Daniel V Cleveland, RRT
Tel: 315 469-2458 *Fax:* 315 469-2593
Med Dir: Russell Acevedo, MD
Begins: Jan Sep
Length: 24 mos *Award:* Dipl, AAS
Tuition per yr: $2,686 res, $5,372 non-res

SUNY Health Science Center at Syracuse

Respiratory Therapist Prgm
750 E Adams St
Syracuse, NY 13210
Prgm Dir: Carl P Wiezalis, MS RRT
Tel: 315 464-5580 *Fax:* 315 464-6876
E-mail: wiezalic@vax.cs.hscsyr.edu
Med Dir: Edward D Sivak, MD
Class Cap: 35 *Begins:* Aug
Length: 22 mos, 34 mos *Award:* Dipl, AAS , BS
Tuition per yr: $4,096 res, $10,722 non-res

Hudson Valley Community College

Respiratory Therapist Prgm
80 Vandenburgh Ave
Troy, NY 12180
Prgm Dir: Patricia G Hyland, BS RRT
Tel: 518 270-7454 *Fax:* 518 270-7594
E-mail: hylanpat@hvcc.edu
Med Dir: Anthony Malanga, MD
Class Cap: 40 *Begins:* Aug
Length: 20 mos *Award:* AAS
Tuition per yr: $2,150 res, $4,500 non-res
Evening or weekend classes available

Westchester Community College

Respiratory Therapist Prgm
75 Grasslands Rd
Valhalla, NY 10595
Prgm Dir: Jose Quinones, MS RRT
Tel: 914 785-6883 *Fax:* 914 785-6889
Med Dir: George Maguire, MD
Class Cap: 36 *Begins:* Sep
Length: 24 mos *Award:* AAS
Tuition per yr: $2,150 res, $5,375 non-res
Evening or weekend classes available

North Carolina

Stanly Community College

Respiratory Therapist Prgm
141 College Dr
Albemarle, NC 28001
Prgm Dir: Tammy P Crump, MS RRT
Tel: 704 982-0121 *Fax:* 704 982-0819
Med Dir: William J Messick, MD
Class Cap: 15 *Begins:* Sep
Length: 9 mos *Award:* AAS
Tuition per yr: $578 res, $4,536 non-res
Evening or weekend classes available

Central Piedmont Community College

Respiratory Therapist Prgm
PO Box 35009
Charlotte, NC 28235
Prgm Dir: Thomas R Morris, RRT
Tel: 704 330-6274 *Fax:* 704 330-5930
E-mail: tom.morris@cpcc.cc.nc.us
Med Dir: Richard C Corbin, MD
Class Cap: 24 *Begins:* Sep
Length: 21 mos *Award:* AAS
Tuition per yr: $742 res, $6,020 non-res

Durham Technical Community College

Respiratory Therapist Prgm
1637 Lawson St
Drawer 11307
Durham, NC 27703
Prgm Dir: Richard D Miller, PhD RRT
Tel: 919 598-9243 *Fax:* 919 686-3601
Med Dir: James R Yankaskas, MD
Class Cap: 25 *Begins:* Sep
Length: 12 mos *Award:* Dipl, AAS
Tuition per yr: $742 res, $6,020 non-res
Evening or weekend classes available

Fayetteville Technical Community College

Respiratory Therapist Prgm
2201 Hull Rd
Fayetteville, NC 28303
Prgm Dir: Ruth A Baldwin, MA RRT
Tel: 910 678-8316   *Fax:* 910 484-8254
Med Dir: Hamid Khodaparast, MD
Class Cap: 24   *Begins:* Sep
Length: 21 mos   *Award:* AAS
Tuition per yr: $742 res, $6,020 non-res

Pitt Community College

Respiratory Therapist Prgm
PO Drawer 7007
Greenville, NC 27834
Prgm Dir: R Bruce Steinbach, RRT
Tel: 919 321-4378
E-mail: lung@ohim.pitt.cc.ne.us
Med Dir: Robert Shaw, MD
Class Cap: 18   *Begins:* Sep
Length: 21 mos   *Award:* AAS
Tuition per yr: $742 res, $6,020 non-res
Evening or weekend classes available

Catawba Valley Community College

Respiratory Therapist Prgm
2550 Hwy 70 SE
Hickory, NC 28602
Prgm Dir: Catherine A Bitsche, BS RRT
Tel: 704 327-7000
Med Dir: John Dew, MD
Class Cap: 20   *Begins:* Sep
Length: 12 mos, 24 mos   *Award:* Dipl, AAS
Tuition per yr: $771 res, $6,049 non-res
Evening or weekend classes available

Robeson Community College

Respiratory Therapist Prgm
PO Box 1420
Lumberton, NC 28359
Prgm Dir: William L Croft, BS RRT
Tel: 910 875-8665   *Fax:* 910 671-4143
Med Dir: Charles R Beasley, MD
Class Cap: 20   *Begins:* Aug
Length: 20 mos   *Award:* AAS
Tuition per yr: $742 res, $6,020 non-res

Carteret Community College

Respiratory Therapist Prgm
3505 Arendell St
Morehead City, NC 28557
Prgm Dir: Barbara S Thomas, RRT
Tel: 919 247-3097   *Fax:* 919 247-2514
E-mail: thomasb@ncccs.cc.nc.us
Med Dir: Terrence Goodman, MD
Class Cap: 20   *Begins:* Sep
Length: 24 mos   *Award:* AAS
Tuition per yr: $742 res, $6,020 non-res
Evening or weekend classes available

Sandhills Community College

Respiratory Therapist Prgm
2200 Airport Rd
Pinehurst, NC 28374
Prgm Dir: William A Byrtus, MEd RRT
Tel: 910 695-3835   *Fax:* 910 692-2756
Med Dir: Farrell Collins, MD
Begins: Sep
Length: 24 mos   *Award:* AAS
Tuition per yr: $742 res, $6,020 non-res

Edgecombe Community College

Respiratory Therapist Prgm
225 Tarboro St
Rocky Mount, NC 27801
Prgm Dir: Ralph D Webb, RRT
Tel: 919 446-0436   *Fax:* 919 985-2212
Med Dir: Lindsey E de Guehery, MD
Class Cap: 14   *Begins:* Sep
Length: 24 mos   *Award:* AAS
Tuition per yr: $766 res, $6,044 non-res
Evening or weekend classes available

Southwestern Community College

Respiratory Therapist Prgm
447 College Dr
Sylva, NC 28779-9578
Prgm Dir: Deborah Beck, BS RRT
Tel: 704 586-4091   *Fax:* 704 586-3129
E-mail: debbieb@southwest.cc.nc.us
Med Dir: Harry G Lipham, MD
Class Cap: 18   *Begins:* Sep
Length: 21 mos   *Award:* AS
Tuition per yr: $742 res, $6,020 non-res
Evening or weekend classes available

Forsyth Technical Community College

Respiratory Therapist Prgm
2100 Silas Creek Pkwy
Winston-Salem, NC 27103
Prgm Dir: Perry W Sheppard, BS RPFT RRT
Tel: 910 723-0371   *Fax:* 910 761-2399
Med Dir: Loren Bauman, MD
Class Cap: 18   *Begins:* Sep
Length: 24 mos   *Award:* AAS
Tuition per yr: $742 res, $6,020 non-res

North Dakota

St Alexius Medical Center

Respiratory Therapist Prgm
North Dakota Sch of Resp Care
900 E Broadway/PO Box 1658
Bismarck, ND 58502
Prgm Dir: Wilmer D Beachey, MEd RRT
Tel: 701 224-7526   *Fax:* 701 224-7076
Med Dir: James A Hughes, MD
Class Cap: 10   *Begins:* Aug
Length: 20 mos   *Award:* Cert, BS
Tuition per yr: $8,550

NDSU/Merit Care Hospital RC Prgm

Respiratory Therapist Prgm
720 Fourth St N
Fargo, ND 58722
Prgm Dir: Gary Brown, BA RRCP
Tel: 701 234-6147   *Fax:* 701 234-6942
Med Dir: Patrick Stoy, MD
Begins: June
Length: 12 mos   *Award:* Cert, BSRT
Tuition per yr: $2,110 res, $2,428 non-res

Ohio

University of Akron

Respiratory Therapist Prgm
302 E Buchtel Ave
Akron, OH 44325
Prgm Dir: LaVerne Yousey, MS RRT
Tel: 330 972-7906   *Fax:* 330 972-7906
E-mail: lavarne@uakron.edu
Med Dir: Bradley R Martin, MD
Class Cap: 25   *Begins:* Sep
Length: 24 mos   *Award:* AAS
Tuition per yr: $3,486 res, $8,686 non-res
Evening or weekend classes available

Stark State College of Technology

Respiratory Therapist Prgm
6200 Frank Ave NW
Canton, OH 44720-7299
Prgm Dir: Peter R Castillo, RRT
Tel: 330 494-6170   *Fax:* 330 966-6586
Med Dir: Robert Miller, MD
Class Cap: 20   *Begins:* Aug
Length: 21 mos   *Award:* Dipl, AAS
Tuition per yr: $2,560 res, $3,520 non-res

Cincinnati State Tech and Comm College

Respiratory Therapist Prgm
3520 Central Pkwy
Cincinnati, OH 45223
Prgm Dir: Debra Lierl, MEd RRT
Tel: 513 569-1690   *Fax:* 513 569-1559
Med Dir: Peter Enyeart, MD
Class Cap: 20   *Begins:* Sep
Length: 22 mos   *Award:* AAS
Tuition per yr: $4,012 res, $8,024 non-res
Evening or weekend classes available

Columbus State Community College

Respiratory Therapist Prgm
550 E Spring St
Columbus, OH 43210
Prgm Dir: Leonard J Chmielewski, MA RRT
Tel: 614 227-5151
Med Dir: Thomas Boes, MD
Class Cap: 35   *Begins:* Sep
Length: 21 mos   *Award:* Dipl, AAS
Tuition per yr: $2,736 res, $6,000 non-res
Evening or weekend classes available

Ohio State University

Respiratory Therapist Prgm
1583 Perry St
Columbus, OH 43210
Prgm Dir: F Herbert Douce, MS RRT RPFT
Tel: 614 292-8445   *Fax:* 614 292-0210
E-mail: douce.2@osu.edu
Med Dir: James E Gadek, MD
Class Cap: 16   *Begins:* Sep
Length: 45 mos   *Award:* BS
Tuition per yr: $3,468 res, $10,335 non-res
Evening or weekend classes available

Programs

Sinclair Community College

Respiratory Therapist Prgm
444 W Third St
Dayton, OH 45402
Prgm Dir: Cynthia A Beckett, MS RRT
Tel: 513 226-2849
Med Dir: James P Graham, MD
Class Cap: 45 *Begins:* Sep
Length: 21 mos *Award:* AAS
Tuition per yr: $1,550 res, $2,100 non-res
Evening or weekend classes available

Bowling Green State University

Respiratory Therapist Prgm
901 Rye Beach Rd
Huron, OH 44839-9791
Prgm Dir: Rod C Roark, MS RRT
Tel: 419 433-5560 *Fax:* 419 433-9696
Med Dir: Anthony J Linz, DO
Class Cap: 20 *Begins:* Jun
Length: 24 mos *Award:* AAS
Tuition per yr: $4,096 res, $6,096 non-res
Evening or weekend classes available

Kettering College of Medical Arts

Respiratory Therapist Prgm
3737 Southern Blvd
Kettering, OH 45429
Prgm Dir: Thomas V Hill, MS RRT
Tel: 513 296-7201 *Fax:* 513 296-4238
E-mail: tom_hill@ketthealth.com
Med Dir: George Burton, MD
Class Cap: 24 *Begins:* Aug
Length: 22 mos *Award:* Dipl, AS
Tuition per yr: $7,200

Lakeland Community College

Respiratory Therapist Prgm
Kirtland, OH 44094-5198
Prgm Dir: Catherine J Kenny, BSEd RRT
Tel: 216 953-7343 *Fax:* 216 975-4733
Med Dir: Adi A Gerblich, MD
Class Cap: 20 *Begins:* Sep
Length: 21 mos *Award:* Cert, AAS
Tuition per yr: $2,944 res, $3,549 non-res
Evening or weekend classes available

Lima Technical College

Respiratory Therapist Prgm
4240 Campus Dr
Lima, OH 45804
Prgm Dir: Richard N Woodfield Jr, MS RRT
Tel: 419 995-8366 *Fax:* 419 995-8818
E-mail: woodfier@ltc.tec.oh.us
Med Dir: Rick D Watson, MD
Class Cap: 24 *Begins:* Sep
Length: 21 mos *Award:* AAS
Tuition per yr: $3,735 res, $7,470 non-res
Evening or weekend classes available

North Central Technical College

Respiratory Therapist Prgm
2441 Kenwood Circle
PO Box 698
Mansfield, OH 44901
Prgm Dir: Robert A Slabodnick, BS RRT
Tel: 419 755-4800 *Fax:* 419 755-5630
Med Dir: Henry Heinzmann, MD
Class Cap: 20 *Begins:* Sep
Length: 21 mos *Award:* AAS
Tuition per yr: $3,367 res, $6,325 non-res
Evening or weekend classes available

Cuyahoga Community College

Respiratory Therapist Prgm
11000 Pleasant Valley Rd
Parma, OH 44130
Prgm Dir: David A Lucas, MS RRT
Tel: 216 987-5267 *Fax:* 216 987-5066
E-mail: dave.lucas@tri-c.cc.oh.us
Med Dir: Joseph A Sopko, MD
Class Cap: 25 *Begins:* Sep
Length: 22 mos *Award:* AAS
Tuition per yr: $2,126 res, $2,824 non-res

Shawnee State University

Respiratory Therapist Prgm
940 Second St
Portsmouth, OH 45662
Prgm Dir: Donald L Thomas, BS RRT
Tel: 614 355-2235 *Fax:* 614 355-2354
E-mail: othomas@shawnee.edu
Med Dir: Elle M Saab, MD
Class Cap: 24 *Begins:* Sep
Length: 21 mos *Award:* Dipl, AAS
Tuition per yr: $4,676 res, $7,176 non-res
Evening or weekend classes available

Jefferson Community College

Respiratory Therapist Prgm
4000 Sunset Blvd
Steubenville, OH 43952
Prgm Dir: Cynthia K Carducci, MEd BSRT RRT
Tel: 614 264-5591 *Fax:* 614 264-1338
Med Dir: Narendra Patel, MD
Class Cap: 12 *Begins:* Aug
Length: 22 mos *Award:* AAS
Tuition per yr: $1,995 res, $2,170 non-res
Evening or weekend classes available

University of Toledo

Respiratory Therapist Prgm
Community and Technical Coll
2801 W Bancroft St
Toledo, OH 43606
Prgm Dir: Margaret F Traband, RRT
Tel: 419 530-3373 *Fax:* 419 530-3096
Med Dir: Robert A May, MD
Begins: Sep
Length: 48 mos *Award:* BS
Tuition per yr: $4,302 res, $10,321 non-res
Evening or weekend classes available

Youngstown State University

Respiratory Therapist Prgm
One University Plaza
Youngstown, OH 44555
Prgm Dir: Louis N Harris, EdD RRT
Tel: 330 742-1764 *Fax:* 330 742-1764
E-mail: fr080601@ysub.ysu.edu
Med Dir: Tejinder S Bal, MD
Class Cap: 23 *Begins:* Sep
Length: 44 mos *Award:* BS
Tuition per yr: $3,865 res, $6,553 non-res
Evening or weekend classes available

Oklahoma

Rose State College

Respiratory Therapist Prgm
6420 SE 15th St
Midwest City, OK 73110
Prgm Dir: Nancy J Deck Lorance, BS RRT
Tel: 405 733-7571 *Fax:* 405 736-0338
Med Dir: Jack Reyes, MD
Class Cap: 24 *Begins:* Aug
Length: 24 mos *Award:* Dipl, AAS
Tuition per yr: $924 res, $2,904 non-res
Evening or weekend classes available

Tulsa Community College

Respiratory Therapist Prgm
909 S Boston Ave
Tulsa, OK 74119
Prgm Dir: Lindel W Porter, RRT
Tel: 918 587-6561
Med Dir: Fred Garfinkel, MD
Class Cap: 24 *Begins:* Aug
Length: 24 mos *Award:* Dipl, AS
Tuition per yr: $1,332 res, $3,598 non-res
Evening or weekend classes available

Oregon

Lane Community College

Respiratory Therapist Prgm
4000 E 30th Ave
Eugene, OR 97405
Prgm Dir: Matthew Schubert, RRT
Tel: 541 757-4501 *Fax:* 541 744-4151
E-mail: schubertm@lanecc.edu
Med Dir: Indulal Rughani, MD
Class Cap: 18 *Begins:* Sep
Length: 21 mos *Award:* Dipl, AAS
Tuition per yr: $1,734 res, $5,916 non-res
Evening or weekend classes available

Rogue Community College

Respiratory Therapist Prgm
3345 Redwood Hwy
Grants Pass, OR 97526
Prgm Dir: Pedro G Cabrera, RRT
Tel: 541 471-3500
Med Dir: John Ordal, MD
Class Cap: 18 *Begins:* Sep
Length: 12 mos, 21 mos *Award:* Cert, AS
Tuition per yr: $1,610 res, $2,438 non-res
Evening or weekend classes available

Mt Hood Community College

Respiratory Therapist Prgm
26000 SE Stark St
Gresham, OR 97030
Prgm Dir: Jan E Bohlmann, RRT
Tel: 503 669-6904 *Fax:* 503 492-6047
Med Dir: Alan Barker, MD
Class Cap: 20 *Begins:* Sep
Length: 18 mos *Award:* AAS
Tuition per yr: $1,620 res, $5,950 non-res

Apollo College

Respiratory Therapist Prgm
Portland Campus
2600 SE 98th
Portland, OR 97286-1302
Prgm Dir: Daniel L Harding, BS RRT
Tel: 503 761-6100 *Fax:* 503 761-3351
Med Dir: John C Fowler, MD
Class Cap: 15 *Begins:* Jan Jul
Length: 16 mos *Award:* Dipl
Tuition per yr: $14,723 res, $14,723 non-res

Pennsylvania

West Chester University

Respiratory Therapist Prgm
Bryn Mawr Hosp
Bryn Mawr, PA 19010
Prgm Dir: Douglas Albright, MEd RRT
Tel: 610 526-3347 *Fax:* 610 526-8545
Med Dir: Blair LeRoy, MD
Class Cap: 25 *Begins:* Sep
Length: 24 mos *Award:* Dipl,Cert, AS
Tuition per yr: $4,028 res, $10,250 non-res

Gannon University

Respiratory Therapist Prgm
University Square
Erie, PA 16541
Prgm Dir: Charles Cornfield, MS RRT
Tel: 814 877-5637 *Fax:* 814 871-5662
E-mail: gcsc1@mail2.gamnon.edu
Med Dir: John T Schaaf, MD
Class Cap: 20 *Begins:* Sep
Length: 24 mos, 48 mos *Award:* AS, BS
Tuition per yr: $14,805
Evening or weekend classes available

Gwynedd-Mercy College

Respiratory Therapist Prgm
Sumneytown Pike
Gwynedd Valley, PA 19437
Prgm Dir: William F Galvin, MSEd RRT CPFT
Tel: 215 646-7300 *Fax:* 215 641-5559
Med Dir: William Figueroa, MD
Class Cap: 20 *Begins:* Aug
Length: 21 mos *Award:* Dipl, AS
Tuition per yr: $1,670
Evening or weekend classes available

Harrisburg Area Community College

Respiratory Therapist Prgm
One HACC Dr
Harrisburg, PA 17110
Prgm Dir: Bradley A Leidich, MSEd RRT
Tel: 717 780-2315 *Fax:* 717 780-2351
E-mail: baleidic@hacc01b.hacc.edu
Med Dir: William M Anderson III, MD
Class Cap: 25 *Begins:* Aug
Length: 28 mos, 36 mos *Award:* AS
Tuition per yr: $2,214 res, $4,427 non-res
Evening or weekend classes available

University of Pittsburgh - Johnstown

Respiratory Therapist Prgm
224 Krebs Hall
Johnstown, PA 15904
Prgm Dir: Bruce J Colbert, MS RRT
Tel: 814 269-2958 *Fax:* 814 269-7255
Med Dir: Jean M Weaver, MD
Class Cap: 40 *Begins:* Sep
Length: 20 mos *Award:* Cert, AS
Tuition per yr: $8,760 res, $18,830 non-res

Mansfield University

Respiratory Therapist Prgm
Dept of Hlth Sciences
Home Economics Ctr
Mansfield, PA 16933
Prgm Dir: Larry B Vosburgh, BS RRT
Tel: 717 882-4513 *Fax:* 717 882-4413
Med Dir: Michael Chisdak, MD
Class Cap: 14 *Begins:* Aug
Length: 21 mos *Award:* AAS
Tuition per yr: $3,626 res, $9,224 non-res
Evening or weekend classes available

Millersville University of Pennsylvania

Respiratory Therapist Prgm
Millersville, PA 17551
Prgm Dir: John M Hughes, MEd RRT
Tel: 717 291-8208 *Fax:* 717 390-3804
Med Dir: Robert A Matlin, MD
Class Cap: 15 *Begins:* Aug
Length: 16 mos *Award:* Cert, BS
Tuition per yr: $3,216 res, $7,848 non-res

Community College of Philadelphia

Respiratory Therapist Prgm
1700 Spring Garden St
Philadelphia, PA 19130
Prgm Dir: Frank M Alsis, EdD RRT
Tel: 215 751-8423 *Fax:* 215 751-8937
Med Dir: Paul S Karlin, DO
Begins: Sep
Length: 24 mos *Award:* Cert, AAS
Tuition per yr: $2,500 res, $5,000 non-res

Comm Coll of Allegheny Cnty-Alleg Campus

Respiratory Therapist Prgm
808 Ridge Ave
Pittsburgh, PA 15212
Prgm Dir: Thomas A Roop, RRT
Tel: 412 237-2607 *Fax:* 412 237-4521
E-mail: troop@ccac.edu
Med Dir: David Laman, MD
Class Cap: 25 *Begins:* Aug
Length: 21 mos *Award:* AS
Tuition per yr: $2,040 res, $4,080 non-res
Evening or weekend classes available

Indiana University of Pennsylvania

Respiratory Therapist Prgm
4800 Friendship Ave
Pittsburgh, PA 15224
Prgm Dir: William J Malley, MS RRT
Tel: 412 578-7000 *Fax:* 412 578-4651
Med Dir: Paul C Fiehler, MD
Class Cap: 30 *Begins:* Aug
Length: 36 mos *Award:* Dipl, BS
Tuition per yr: $3,368 res, $8,566 non-res

Western Sch of Hlth & Business Careers

Respiratory Therapist Prgm
327 Fifth Ave
Pittsburgh, PA 15222
Prgm Dir: Kimberly A Crilley, AS RRT
Tel: 412 281-7083, Ext 118 *Fax:* 412 281-0819
Med Dir: Vaughn Strimlan, MD
Class Cap: 40 *Begins:* Sep Apr
Length: 21 mos *Award:* AST
Tuition per yr: $8,285 res, $8,285 non-res

Reading Area Community College

Respiratory Therapist Prgm
Ten S Second St
PO Box 1706
Reading, PA 19603
Prgm Dir: Marie Jacoby, MSA RRT
Tel: 610 372-4721 *Fax:* 610 607-6254
Med Dir: Joseph Mariglio, MD
Class Cap: 12 *Begins:* Sep
Length: 12 mos *Award:* Cert
Tuition per yr: $1,972 res, $3,944 non-res

Lehigh Carbon Community College

Respiratory Therapist Prgm
4525 Education Park Dr
Schnecksville, PA 18078-2598
Prgm Dir: Denise B McCardle, MSEd RRT
Tel: 215 799-1504 *Fax:* 610 799-1537
Med Dir: Joseph M Zasik, DO
Class Cap: 25 *Begins:* Aug
Length: 15 mos *Award:* Cert
Tuition per yr: $1,575 res, $3,150 non-res
Evening or weekend classes available

Crozer-Chester Med Ctr/Delaware Co CC

Respiratory Therapist Prgm
15th and Upland Ave
Upland, PA 19013
Prgm Dir: Kathleen C Day, BS RRT
Tel: 610 447-2435
E-mail: kday@dccnaet.dccc.edu
Med Dir: Jerome Rudnitzky, MD
Class Cap: 18 *Begins:* Sep
Length: 21 mos *Award:* Cert, AAS
Tuition per yr: $1,750 res, $5,250 non-res
Evening or weekend classes available

York College of Pennsylvania

Respiratory Therapist Prgm
York, PA 17403
Prgm Dir: Mark Simmons, MSEd RRT
Tel: 717 851-2464 *Fax:* 717 851-2487
Med Dir: Richard L Keesports, MD
Class Cap: 12 *Begins:* Sep
Length: 26 mos, 48 mos *Award:* AS, BS
Tuition per yr: $6,100 res, $6,100 non-res

Puerto Rico

Universidad Adventista de las Antillas

Respiratory Therapist Prgm
PO Box 118
Mayaguez, PR 00681-0118
Prgm Dir: Vilma Torres, RRT
Tel: 787 834-9595 *Fax:* 787 834-9597
Med Dir: Antonio Padua, MD
Class Cap: 60 *Begins:* Aug
Length: 23 mos, 31 mos *Award:* Dipl, AS
Tuition per yr: $2,375

Universidad Metropolitana

Respiratory Therapist Prgm
PO Box 21150
Rio Piedras, PR 00928
Prgm Dir: Leyda Torres de Marin, MA RRT
Tel: 787 766-1717   *Fax:* 787 759-7663
Med Dir: Juan Jimenez-Vega, MD
Class Cap: 40   *Begins:* Aug
Length: 48 mos   *Award:* BS
Tuition per yr: $3,700

University of Puerto Rico

Respiratory Therapist Prgm
PO Box 365067
San Juan, PR 00936-5067
Prgm Dir: Wanda M Rodriguez Garcia, RRT
Tel: 787 758-2525
Med Dir: Roberto Martinez, MD
Class Cap: 70   *Begins:* Aug
Length: 18 mos   *Award:* Cert
Tuition per yr: $4,000
Evening or weekend classes available

Rhode Island

Community College of Rhode Island

Respiratory Therapist Prgm
1762 Louisquisset Pike
Lincoln, RI 02865-4585
Prgm Dir: Joanne Jacobs, MA RRT
Tel: 401 333-7024   *Fax:* 401 333-7260
E-mail: jjacobs@ccri.cc.ri.us
Med Dir: Thomas J Raimondo, DO
Class Cap: 25   *Begins:* Jun
Length: 24 mos   *Award:* AAS
Tuition per yr: $2,700 res, $7,256 non-res
Evening or weekend classes available

South Carolina

Trident Technical College

Respiratory Therapist Prgm
PO Box 10367
Charleston, SC 29411
Prgm Dir: Ann R Moore, MS RRT CPFT
Tel: 803 572-6101   *Fax:* 803 569-6585
E-mail: zpmoore1@trident.tec.sc.us
Med Dir: Howard R Bromley, MD
Class Cap: 24   *Begins:* Aug
Length: 20 mos   *Award:* AAS
Tuition per yr: $1,527 res, $1,707 non-res
Evening or weekend classes available

Midlands Technical College

Respiratory Therapist Prgm
PO Box 2408
Columbia, SC 29202
Prgm Dir: Linda H Ackerman, RRT
Tel: 803 822-3433   *Fax:* 803 822-3079
E-mail: mtc2.mid.tec.sc.us
Med Dir: J Daniel Love, MD
Begins: Sep
Length: 24 mos   *Award:* AS
Tuition per yr: $1,620 res, $2,016 non-res
Evening or weekend classes available

Florence-Darlington Technical College

Respiratory Therapist Prgm
PO Box 100548
Florence, SC 29501-0548
Prgm Dir: John A Evans, RRT
Tel: 803 661-8148
Med Dir: William M Hazelwood, MD
Begins: Aug
Length: 24 mos   *Award:* AS
Tuition per yr: $1,650 res, $1,815 non-res
Evening or weekend classes available

Greenville Technical College

Respiratory Therapist Prgm
PO Box 5616
Station B
Greenville, SC 29606
Prgm Dir: Thomas D Baxter, MHRD RRT
Tel: 864 250-8373
Med Dir: L Hayes, MD
Begins: Aug
Length: 4 mo , 24 mos   *Award:* Cert, AD
Tuition per yr: $1,500 res, $2,400 non-res

Piedmont Technical College

Respiratory Therapist Prgm
PO Box 1467
Greenwood, SC 29647
Prgm Dir: Sherri Pickelsimmer, RRT
Tel: 864 941-8528   *Fax:* 864 941-8555
Med Dir: O M Cobb, MD
Class Cap: 23   *Begins:* Aug Jan
Length: 16 mos, 24 mos   *Award:* Dipl, AS
Tuition per yr: $1,500 res, $3,157 non-res
Evening or weekend classes available

Spartanburg Technical College

Respiratory Therapist Prgm
PO Drawer 4386
Spartanburg, SC 29305-4386
Prgm Dir: Dot Kiser, RT(R)
Tel: 864 591-3720   *Fax:* 864 591-3708
E-mail: kiser@spt.tec.sc.us
Med Dir: Charles Fogarty, MD
Class Cap: 20   *Begins:* Jan
Length: 24 mos   *Award:* AAS , AS
Tuition per yr: $1,500 res, $1,875 non-res

South Dakota

Dakota State University

Respiratory Therapist Prgm
Madison, SD 57042-1799
Prgm Dir: Bruce A Feistner, MSS RRT
Tel: 605 322-8613   *Fax:* 605 322-6666
E-mail: feistneb@atlas.sfple.sdbor.edu
Med Dir: John Crump, MD
Class Cap: 20   *Begins:* Sep
Length: 21 mos, 39 mos   *Award:* AS, BS
Tuition per yr: $1,650 res, $4,840 non-res

Tennessee

Chattanooga State Technical Comm College

Respiratory Therapist Prgm
4501 Amnicola Hwy
Chattanooga, TN 37406
Prgm Dir: McIver Rountree Jr, BS RRT
Tel: 423 697-4450
E-mail: mrountree@cstcc.cc.tn.us
Med Dir: Suresh Enjeti, MD
Class Cap: 15   *Begins:* Aug
Length: 24 mos   *Award:* AAS
Tuition per yr: $1,584 res, $5,628 non-res
Evening or weekend classes available

Columbia State Community College

Respiratory Therapist Prgm
Hwy 99 W
PO Box 1315
Columbia, TN 38401
Prgm Dir: Bill R Gandy, RRT
Tel: 615 540-2663   *Fax:* 615 540-2795
E-mail: gandy@cosoooc.tn.us
Med Dir: J Brevard Hayes, MD
Class Cap: 48   *Begins:* Aug
Length: 21 mos   *Award:* AAS
Tuition per yr: $1,536 res, $6,144 non-res
Evening or weekend classes available

East Tennessee State University

Respiratory Therapist Prgm
1000 West E St
ETSU Nave Center
Elizabethton, TN 37643
Prgm Dir: Delmar Mack, MS RRT
Tel: 423 547-4916   *Fax:* 423 547-4921
Med Dir: Jeff Farrow, MD FCCP
Class Cap: 10   *Begins:* Aug
Length: 21 mos   *Award:* AAS
Tuition per yr: $2,892 res, $9,396 non-res
Evening or weekend classes available

Roane State Community College

Respiratory Therapist Prgm
Patton Ln
Harriman, TN 37748
Prgm Dir: Gwen Valentine, RRT
Tel: 423 354-3000   *Fax:* 423 282-4549
Med Dir: Richard A Obenour, MD
Class Cap: 20   *Begins:* Aug
Length: 21 mos   *Award:* AAS
Tuition per yr: $1,392 res, $4,017 non-res

Jackson State Community College

Respiratory Therapist Prgm
2046 N Parkway St
Jackson, TN 38301-3797
Prgm Dir: Cathy K Garner, BS RRT
Tel: 901 425-2612   *Fax:* 901 425-2647
E-mail: GGarner@JSCC.CC.TN.US
Med Dir: Thomas Ellis, MD
Class Cap: 16   *Begins:* Sep
Length: 24 mos   *Award:* AAS
Tuition per yr: $1,491 res, $5,880 non-res

Tennessee State University
Respiratory Therapist Prgm
3500 John A Merritt Blvd
Nashville, TN 37209
Prgm Dir: Thomas John, PhD RRT
Tel: 615 963-7431 *Fax:* 615 963-7422
Med Dir: Michael Niedermeyer, MD
Class Cap: 30 *Begins:* Aug
Length: 37 mos *Award:* BS
Tuition per yr: $195 res, $6,280 non-res

Texas

Alvin Community College
Respiratory Therapist Prgm
3110 Mustang Rd
Alvin, TX 77511
Prgm Dir: Diane Flatland, MS RRT CPFT
Tel: 713 388-4695 *Fax:* 713 388-4936
Med Dir: Wayne K Hite, DO
Class Cap: 20 *Begins:* Jun
Length: 24 mos *Award:* Dipl, AAS
Tuition per yr: $588 res, $998 non-res
Evening or weekend classes available

Amarillo College
Respiratory Therapist Prgm
PO Box 447
Amarillo, TX 79178
Prgm Dir: William A Young, MS RRT
Tel: 806 354-6058 *Fax:* 806 354-6076
E-mail: wayoung@actx.edu
Med Dir: Bruce Baker, MD
Class Cap: 20 *Begins:* Sep
Length: 22 mos *Award:* Dipl, AAS
Tuition per yr: $700 res, $2,400 non-res

Lamar Univ Institute of Tech - Beaumont
Respiratory Therapist Prgm
PO Box 10061
Beaumont, TX 77710
Prgm Dir: Paul A Bronson, MEd RRT
Tel: 409 880-8852 *Fax:* 409 880-8955
Med Dir: Paul Shaw, MD
Class Cap: 35 *Begins:* Aug
Length: 24 mos *Award:* AAS
Tuition per yr: $1,392 res, $6,476 non-res

Univ Tx at Brownsville/TX Southmost Coll
Respiratory Therapist Prgm
83 Ft Brown
Brownsville, TX 78520
Prgm Dir: John L McCabe, PhD RRT
Tel: 210 544-8262 *Fax:* 210 544-8916
Med Dir: Lorenzo Pelly
Begins: Sep
Length: 21 mos *Award:* Dipl,Cert, AAS
Tuition per yr: $2,327 res, $3,403 non-res
Evening or weekend classes available

Del Mar College
Respiratory Therapist Prgm
Corpus Christi, TX 78404
Prgm Dir: Jeffrey T Watson, BA RRT
Tel: 512 886-1103
Med Dir: William Burgin, Jr, MD
Class Cap: 12 *Begins:* Jun
Length: 12 mos *Award:* Dipl, AAS
Tuition per yr: $647 res, $968 non-res
Evening or weekend classes available

El Centro College
Respiratory Therapist Prgm
Main and Lamar Sts
Dallas, TX 75202
Prgm Dir: Gary L Peschka, MEd RRT RCP
Tel: 214 746-2279
Med Dir: Peter Heidbrink, MD
Class Cap: 30 *Begins:* Sep
Length: 21 mos *Award:* Dipl, AAS
Tuition per yr: $560 res, $1,360 non-res

El Paso Community College
Respiratory Therapist Prgm
PO Box 20500
El Paso, TX 79998
Prgm Dir: Harry Kirshenbaum, MEd RRT
Tel: 915 534-4072 *Fax:* 915 534-4114
Med Dir: Gonzalo Diaz, MD
Begins: May
Length: 24 mos *Award:* Dipl, AAS
Tuition per yr: $1,128 res, $3,503 non-res
Evening or weekend classes available

Houston Community College Central
Respiratory Therapist Prgm
3100 Shenandoah
Houston, TX 77021
Prgm Dir: Ralph E Bartel, MEd RRT
Tel: 713 746-5356
Med Dir: Fernando Stein, MD
Class Cap: 30 *Begins:* Aug
Length: 24 mos *Award:* Dipl,Cert, AAS
Tuition per yr: $1,260 res, $3,825 non-res
Evening or weekend classes available

Texas Southern University
Respiratory Therapist Prgm
3201 Wheeler St
Houston, TX 77004
Prgm Dir: Jean M Hampton, MS RRT
Tel: 713 313-7265 *Fax:* 713 313-1094
Med Dir: Lectoy Johnson, MD
Class Cap: 40 *Begins:* Jan Jun Sep
Length: 48 mos *Award:* Cert, BS
Tuition per yr: $1,820 res, $9,310 non-res

Tarrant Junior College
Respiratory Therapist Prgm
828 Harwood Rd
Hurst, TX 76054
Prgm Dir: John D Hiser, MEd RRT
Tel: 817 788-6574 *Fax:* 817 788-6426
Med Dir: Woody V Kageler, MD
Class Cap: 24 *Begins:* Aug
Length: 21 mos *Award:* AAS
Tuition per yr: $932 res, $1,272 non-res
Evening or weekend classes available

Kingwood College - NHMCCD
Respiratory Therapist Prgm
20,000 Kingwood Dr
Kingwood, TX 77339
Prgm Dir: Kenny P McCowen, RRT
Tel: 713 359-1608 *Fax:* 713 359-0490
E-mail: kmccowen@kc.nhmccd.cc.tx.us
Med Dir: Edward Flores, MD
Class Cap: 25 *Begins:* Aug
Length: 12 mos *Award:* AAS
Tuition per yr: $668 res, $1,508 non-res

South Plains College
Respiratory Therapist Prgm
1302 Main St
Lubbock, TX 79401
Prgm Dir: Shonni L Collier, RRT
Tel: 806 747-0576 *Fax:* 806 765-2775
Med Dir: Wayne McNeil, MD
Class Cap: 30 *Begins:* Aug
Length: 24 mos *Award:* Dipl, AAS
Tuition per yr: $1,300 res, $1,600 non-res
Evening or weekend classes available

Collin County Community Coll District
Respiratory Therapist Prgm
2200 W University Dr
McKinney, TX 75070
Prgm Dir: Allen W Barbaro, MS RRT
Tel: 214 548-6678 *Fax:* 214 548-6722
E-mail: 255rivers@express.cccd.edu
Med Dir: Timothy Chappell, MD
Class Cap: 22 *Begins:* Aug
Length: 22 mos *Award:* AAS
Tuition per yr: $1,239 res, $1,568 non-res
Evening or weekend classes available

Midland College
Respiratory Therapist Prgm
3600 N Garfield
Midland, TX 79705
Prgm Dir: Robert Weidmann, BS RRT
Tel: 915 685-4595 *Fax:* 915 685-4762
E-mail: rweidmann@midland.cc.tx.us
Med Dir: Dan J Hendrickson, MD
Class Cap: 21 *Begins:* Sep
Length: 21 mos *Award:* Cert, AAS
Tuition per yr: $1,141 res, $1,886 non-res
Evening or weekend classes available

Odessa College
Respiratory Therapist Prgm
201 W University
Odessa, TX 79764
Prgm Dir: Shelia Butler, RRT CPFT
Tel: 915 335-6456 *Fax:* 915 335-6846
Med Dir: John D Bray, MD
Class Cap: 24 *Begins:* Jul
Length: 14 mos, 22 mos *Award:* Dipl,Cert, AAS
Tuition per yr: $1,112 res, $1,370 non-res
Evening or weekend classes available

San Jacinto College Central Campus
Respiratory Therapist Prgm
8060 Spencer Hwy
PO Box 2007
Pasadena, TX 77505-2007
Prgm Dir: Patrick Helton, MS RRT RPFT
Tel: 713 476-1864 *Fax:* 713 478-2754
Med Dir: Joseph Rodarte Jr, DO PhD
Begins: Sep
Length: 24 mos *Award:* AAS
Tuition per yr: $598 res, $978 non-res

Southwest Texas State University
Respiratory Therapist Prgm
San Marcos, TX 78666
Prgm Dir: Cade J Harkins III, MSHP RRT
Tel: 512 245-8243 *Fax:* 512 245-7978
E-mail: cade-harkins@swt.edu
Med Dir: George J Handley, MD
Class Cap: 48 *Begins:* Aug
Length: 48 mos *Award:* BSRC
Tuition per yr: $3,019 res, $11,151 non-res
Evening or weekend classes available

Programs

Temple College
Respiratory Therapist Prgm
2600 S First St
Temple, TX 76504
Prgm Dir: William M Cornelius III, RRT
Tel: 817 773-9961   *Fax:* 817 771-4528
Med Dir: William G Petersen, MD
Begins: Sep
Length: 24 mos   *Award:* AAS
Tuition per yr: $1,140 res, $1,634 non-res
Evening or weekend classes available

Tyler Junior College
Respiratory Therapist Prgm
PO Box 9020
Tyler, TX 75711
Prgm Dir: Paul Weskamp, RRT
Tel: 903 510-2472   *Fax:* 903 510-2592
E-mail: pwes@tjc.tyler.cc.tx.us
Med Dir: James Stocks, MD
Class Cap: 45   *Begins:* Aug
Length: 12 mos, 23 mos   *Award:* AS
Tuition per yr: $966 res, $1,506 non-res
Evening or weekend classes available

Victoria College
Respiratory Therapist Prgm
2200 E Red River
Victoria, TX 77901
Prgm Dir: Chris E Kallus, MEd RRT RCP
Tel: 512 572-6491   *Fax:* 512 572-3850
E-mail: ckallus@vc.cc.tx.us
Med Dir: Bruce E Wheeler, MD
Class Cap: 18   *Begins:* Aug
Length: 16 mos   *Award:* Cert
Tuition per yr: $919 res, $3,800 non-res

Midwestern State University
Respiratory Therapist Prgm
Wichita General Hospital
1600 Eighth St
Wichita Falls, TX 76301
Prgm Dir: Terrance J Gilmore, BS RRT
Tel: 817 723-8970   *Fax:* 817 689-4513
E-mail: fgilnolt@nzxy.law
Med Dir: Edgar Lockett, MD
Class Cap: 20   *Begins:* Sep Jan Jun
Length: 45 mos
Evening or weekend classes available

Utah

Weber State University
Respiratory Therapist Prgm
3750 Harrison Blvd
Ogden, UT 84408-3904
Prgm Dir: Georgine L Bills, MBA RRT
Tel: 801 626-7071   *Fax:* 801 626-7683
E-mail: gbills@weber.edu
Med Dir: Gary K Goucher, MD
Class Cap: 20   *Begins:* Sep
Length: 22 mos   *Award:* Cert, AS, BS
Tuition per yr: $1,863 res, $5,550 non-res

Vermont

Champlain College
Respiratory Therapist Prgm
163 S Willard St
Burlington, VT 05402
Prgm Dir: Faye Bacon, RRT
Tel: 802 658-0800
E-mail: baconf@champlain.edu
Med Dir: Robert Deane, MD
Class Cap: 15   *Begins:* Aug
Length: 18 mos   *Award:* AS
Tuition per yr: $8,400
Evening or weekend classes available

Virginia

Northern Virginia Community College
Respiratory Therapist Prgm
8333 Little River Trnpk
Annandale, VA 22003
Prgm Dir: Mark L Diana, MBA RRT
Tel: 703 323-3280   *Fax:* 703 323-4576
E-mail: nudiannenn.cc.va.us
Med Dir: Frank Fusco, MD
Class Cap: 24   *Begins:* Aug
Length: 21 mos, 12 mos   *Award:* Dipl,Cert, AAS
Tuition per yr: $2,160 res, $7,081 non-res
Evening or weekend classes available

Southwest Virginia Community College
Respiratory Therapist Prgm
Box SVCC
Richlands, VA 24641-1510
Prgm Dir: Joseph S DiPietro, MS RRT
Tel: 540 964-2555   *Fax:* 540 964-9307
Med Dir: Randy Forehand, MD
Class Cap: 24   *Begins:* Sep
Length: 22 mos   *Award:* Dipl,Cert
Tuition per yr: $3,168 res, $10,224 non-res

J Sargeant Reynolds Community College
Respiratory Therapist Prgm
PO Box 85622
Richmond, VA 23285-5622
Prgm Dir: Donald K O'Donohue, RRT
Tel: 804 786-1375
Med Dir: Clifton L Parker, MD
Class Cap: 36   *Begins:* Aug
Length: 7 mos   *Award:* Cert
Tuition per yr: $1,165 res, $3,790 non-res
Evening or weekend classes available

College of Health Sciences
Respiratory Therapist Prgm
PO Box 13186
920 S Jefferson St
Roanoke, VA 24031
Prgm Dir: Paul M Lemons, MEd RRT
Tel: 540 985-8268
Med Dir: Kirk Hippensteel, MD
Class Cap: 25   *Begins:* Sep
Length: 21 mos   *Award:* Dipl, AS
Tuition per yr: $3,120
Evening or weekend classes available

Tidewater Community College
Respiratory Therapist Prgm
1700 College Crescent
Virginia Beach, VA 23456
Prgm Dir: Barry S Anderson, MBA RRT
Tel: 804 427-7263   *Fax:* 804 427-1338
E-mail: tcandeb%vccscent.edu
Med Dir: James F Fussell, MD
Class Cap: 16   *Begins:* May
Length: 24 mos   *Award:* AAS
Tuition per yr: $2,205 res, $6,872 non-res

Shenandoah University
Respiratory Therapist Prgm
1775 N Sector Ct
Winchester, VA 22601-5195
Prgm Dir: Karen K Schultz, MBA RRT
Tel: 540 665-5516   *Fax:* 540 665-5519
E-mail: kschultz@su.edu
Med Dir: Vicken V Kalbian, MD
Class Cap: 20   *Begins:* Aug
Length: 24 mos   *Award:* Cert, AS, BS
Tuition per yr: $15,700

Washington

Highline Community College
Respiratory Therapist Prgm
2400 S 240th St
Des Moines, WA 98198-9800
Prgm Dir: Robert W Hirnle, MS RRT
Tel: 206 878-3710   *Fax:* 206 870-3780
E-mail: bhirnle@hcc.ctc.edu
Med Dir: Jon S Huseby, MD
Class Cap: 25   *Begins:* Jun
Length: 21 mos   *Award:* Cert, AAS
Tuition per yr: $1,296 res, $5,094 non-res
Evening or weekend classes available

Seattle Central Community College
Respiratory Therapist Prgm
1701 Broadway
Seattle, WA 98122
Prgm Dir: Thomasa R McCown, BS RRT
Tel: 206 587-4056   *Fax:* 206 344-4390
E-mail: tmccow@seaccc.sccd.ctc.edu
Med Dir: Kenneth Steinberg, MD
Class Cap: 25   *Begins:* Sep
Length: 20 mos   *Award:* AAS
Tuition per yr: $1,774 res, $7,038 non-res
Evening or weekend classes available

Spokane Community College
Respiratory Therapist Prgm
N 1810 Greene St
Spokane, WA 99207
Prgm Dir: Gary C White, MEd RRT
Tel: 509 533-7307   *Fax:* 509 533-8621
Med Dir: James C Bonvallet, MD
Class Cap: 22   *Begins:* Sep
Length: 22 mos   *Award:* Dipl, AAS
Tuition per yr: $1,800 res, $7,064 non-res

Tacoma Community College

Respiratory Therapist Prgm
5900 S 12th St
Tacoma, WA 98465
Prgm Dir: Bill M Leffler, BA RRT
Tel: 206 566-5163
Med Dir: James R Taylor, MD
Begins: Jun
Length: 15 mos, 9 mos *Award:* AAS
Tuition per yr: $1,800 res, $7,060 non-res

West Virginia

College of West Virginia

Respiratory Therapist Prgm
609 S Kanawha St
Beckley, WV 25802-2830
Prgm Dir: Leisa K Bowden, MS RRT
Tel: 304 253-7351 *Fax:* 304 253-0789
Med Dir: Norma Mullins, MD
Class Cap: 24 *Begins:* Jun
Length: 24 mos *Award:* Cert, AS
Tuition per yr: $4,200
Evening or weekend classes available

University of Charleston

Respiratory Therapist Prgm
2300 MacCorkle Ave SE
Charleston, WV 25304
Prgm Dir: Anna W Parkman, MBA RRT
Tel: 304 357-4837 *Fax:* 304 357-4965
E-mail: awp@aol.com
Med Dir: Dominic Gaziano, MD
Class Cap: 20 *Begins:* Aug
Length: 20 mos, 48 mos *Award:* Dipl, AS
Tuition per yr: $11,700 res, $15,125 non-res
Evening or weekend classes available

West Virginia Northern Community College

Respiratory Therapist Prgm
College Square
Wheeling, WV 26003
Prgm Dir: Ralph C Lucki, MA RRT
Tel: 304 233-5900
E-mail: rlucki@nccvax.wvnet.edu
Med Dir: Michael Blatt, MD
Class Cap: 24 *Begins:* Aug
Length: 21 mos *Award:* AAS
Tuition per yr: $4,830 non-res
Evening or weekend classes available

Wheeling Jesuit University

Respiratory Therapist Prgm
316 Washington Ave
Wheeling, WV 26003
Prgm Dir: Allen H Marangoni, MMS RRT
Tel: 304 243-2372 *Fax:* 304 243-4441
E-mail: amaran.wjc.edu
Med Dir: Mike Blatt, MD
Class Cap: 12 *Begins:* Sep
Length: 37 mos *Award:* BS
Tuition per yr: $11,000

Wisconsin

Northeast Wisconsin Technical College

Respiratory Therapist Prgm
2740 W Mason St
PO Box 19042
Green Bay, WI 54307
Prgm Dir: Diana Luder, PhD RRT
Tel: 414 498-5533 *Fax:* 414 498-5673
Med Dir: John Andrews, MD
Begins: Aug
Length: 20 mos *Award:* AAS
Tuition per yr: $1,852 res, $12,854 non-res

Western Wisconsin Technical College

Respiratory Therapist Prgm
304 N Sixth St
PO Box 908
La Crosse, WI 54602-0908
Prgm Dir: Robert A Milisch, MEd RRT
Tel: 608 785-9244 *Fax:* 608 785-9794
E-mail: milisch@al.ucstern.tec.wiius
Med Dir: Edward Winga, MD
Class Cap: 22 *Begins:* Aug
Length: 21 mos *Award:* AS
Tuition per yr: $1,744 res, $24,177 non-res

Madison Area Technical College

Respiratory Therapist Prgm
3550 Anderson St
Madison, WI 53704
Prgm Dir: Glenn N Hojem, RRT
Tel: 608 246-6686 *Fax:* 608 246-6013
Med Dir: Louis Chosy, MD
Class Cap: 26 *Begins:* Aug
Length: 23 mos *Award:* AAS
Tuition per yr: $2,048 res, $14,048 non-res
Evening or weekend classes available

Mid-State Technical College

Respiratory Therapist Prgm
2600 W 5th St
Marshfield, WI 54449
Prgm Dir: Scott S Osborne, MEd RRT
Tel: 715 387-2538 *Fax:* 715 389-2664
E-mail: midstate@wctc.net
Med Dir: John A Campbell, PhD MD
Begins: Aug
Length: 22 mos *Award:* Dipl, AS
Tuition per yr: $1,800 res, $12,495 non-res
Evening or weekend classes available

Milwaukee Area Technical College

Respiratory Therapist Prgm
700 W State St
Milwaukee, WI 53233
Prgm Dir: Mark J Hoffman, MS RRT
Tel: 414 297-7130 *Fax:* 414 297-6851
E-mail: hoffmanm@milwaukee.tec.wi.us
Med Dir: Glenn F Ragalie, MD
Class Cap: 36 *Begins:* Sep
Length: 20 mos *Award:* Dipl, AAS
Tuition per yr: $1,792 res, $12,033 non-res
Evening or weekend classes available

Wyoming

Western Wyoming Community College

Respiratory Therapist Prgm
2500 College Dr
PO Box 428
Rock Springs, WY 82902-0428
Prgm Dir: Bruce W Robinson, RRT
Tel: 307 382-1799 *Fax:* 307 382-7665
Med Dir: John Guicheateau, MD
Class Cap: 10 *Begins:* Aug
Length: 10 mos *Award:* Cert
Tuition per yr: $1,022 res, $2,670 non-res
Evening or weekend classes available

Programs

Respiratory Therapy Technician

Arizona

Pima Medical Institute - Mesa
Respiratory Therapy Tech Prgm
957 S Dobson Rd
Mesa, AZ 85202
Prgm Dir: Cynthia Smathers, MEd RRT
Tel: 602 345-7777 *Fax:* 602 649-5249
Med Dir: David Drachler, MD
Class Cap: 44 *Begins:* Feb May Jun Jul
Length: 11 mos
Tuition per yr: $4,447

Gateway Community College
Respiratory Therapy Tech Prgm
108 N 40th St
Phoenix, AZ 85034
Prgm Dir: Marie A Fenske, EdD RRT
Tel: 602 392-5062
Med Dir: Robert G Hooper, MD FACP FCCP
Class Cap: 40 *Begins:* Jan
Length: 12 mos *Award:* Cert
Tuition per yr: $1,326 res, $6,123 non-res

Long Medical Institute
Respiratory Therapy Tech Prgm
4126 N Black Canyon Hwy
Phoenix, AZ 85017
Prgm Dir: Ronda D Anderson, RRT
Tel: 602 279-9333
Med Dir: Alan Schwartz, MD
Class Cap: 150 *Begins:* Quarterly
Length: 10 mos *Award:* Dipl
Tuition per yr: $8,190
Evening or weekend classes available

Pima Medical Institute - Tucson
Respiratory Therapy Tech Prgm
3350 E Grant
Tucson, AZ 85716
Prgm Dir: Leanna R Konechne, BS RRT
Tel: 520 326-1600 *Fax:* 520 795-3463
Med Dir: Anthony Chavis, MD
Class Cap: 80 *Begins:* Mar Jul Sep Nov
Length: 15 mos *Award:* Cert
Tuition per yr: $11,185

Arkansas

Northwest Arkansas Community College
Respiratory Therapy Tech Prgm
One College Dr
Bentonville, AR 72712
Prgm Dir: Alan Clark, BA RRT
Tel: 501 619-4250 *Fax:* 501 619-4254
Med Dir: David M Halinski, MD
Class Cap: 16 *Begins:* Jun
Length: 15 mos *Award:* AAS
Tuition per yr: $1,250 res, $2,450 non-res
Evening or weekend classes available

Arkansas Valley Tech Institute
Respiratory Therapy Tech Prgm
1311 S I St
Ft Smith, AR 72901
Prgm Dir: F Ross Payne, RRT RPFT
Tel: 501 441-5256 *Fax:* 501 441-4823
Med Dir: David Nichols, MD
Class Cap: 18 *Begins:* Jan
Length: 14 mos *Award:* Cert
Tuition per yr: $840
Evening or weekend classes available

Univ of Arkansas Comm Coll at Hope
Respiratory Therapy Tech Prgm
Hwy 29 S
PO Box 140
Hope, AR 71801
Prgm Dir: Ken LeJuene, BSE RRT
Tel: 501 777-5722
Med Dir: Michael R Downs, MD
Class Cap: 25 *Begins:* Aug
Length: 15 mos, 24 mos *Award:* Cert, AAS
Tuition per yr: $1,748 res, $2,760 non-res

Univ of Arkansas for Medical Sciences
Respiratory Therapy Tech Prgm
4301 W Markham
Slot 704
Little Rock, AR 72205
Prgm Dir: Erna Boone, MEd RRT
Tel: 501 661-1202 *Fax:* 501 370-6691
E-mail: elboone@uams.edu
Med Dir: Clyde Campbell, MD
Class Cap: 12 *Begins:* Jan
Length: 12 mos *Award:* Cert
Tuition per yr: $2,975 res, $7,438 non-res

Pulaski Technical College
Respiratory Therapy Tech Prgm
3000 W Scenic Dr
North Little Rock, AR 72118
Prgm Dir: Jim C Davis, BS RRT
Tel: 501 771-1000 *Fax:* 501 771-2844
Med Dir: Anthony R Giglia, MD
Class Cap: 24 *Begins:* Aug
Length: 10 mos *Award:* Cert
Tuition per yr: $1,230

Black River Technical College
Respiratory Therapy Tech Prgm
PO Box 468
Pocahontas, AR 72455
Prgm Dir: Cindy Smith, RRT
Tel: 501 892-4565 *Fax:* 501 892-3546
Med Dir: William S Hubbard, MD
Class Cap: 24 *Begins:* Aug
Length: 9 mos *Award:* Cert, AAS
Tuition per yr: $912 res, $1,128 non-res
Evening or weekend classes available

California

San Joaquin Valley College
Respiratory Therapy Tech Prgm
201 New Stine Rd
Bakersfield, CA 93309
Prgm Dir: Barbara Slater
Tel: 805 834-0126
Med Dir: Hans Einstein, MD
Class Cap: 30 *Begins:* Varies
Length: 21 mos *Award:* AS
Tuition per yr: $19,800

Hacienda LaPuente Unified School Dist
Respiratory Therapy Tech Prgm
15540 E Fairgrove Ave
La Puente, CA 91744
Prgm Dir: Sidney Coffin, MS RRT
Tel: 818 968-4638 *Fax:* 818 855-3833
Med Dir: Kamalakar Rambhatla, MD
Class Cap: 110 *Begins:* Sep Jan Jun
Length: 18 mos *Award:* Cert
Tuition per yr: $450

California Paramedical & Tech College
Respiratory Therapy Tech Prgm
3745 Long Beach Blvd
Long Beach, CA 90807
Prgm Dir: Robert R Eriksen, RRT RCP
Tel: 310 426-9359 *Fax:* 310 427-2920
Med Dir: William Klein, MD
Class Cap: 100 *Begins:* Jan Apr Jul Oct
Length: 12 mos *Award:* Cert
Tuition per yr: $9,495

California College for Health Sciences
Respiratory Therapy Tech Prgm
222 W 24th St
National City, CA 92050
Prgm Dir: Dale K Bean, RRT
Tel: 619 477-4800 *Fax:* 619 477-4360
E-mail: dalebean@cchs.edu
Med Dir: Jerry Fein, MD
Class Cap: 60 *Begins:* Apr Sep
Length: 11 mos, 18 mos *Award:* Cert, AS
Tuition per yr: $13,875 res, $1,955 non-res

ConCorde Career Institute
Respiratory Therapy Tech Prgm
4150 Lankershim Blvd
North Hollywood, CA 91602
Prgm Dir: Marlyn H Haberwood, RRT
Tel: 818 766-8151 *Fax:* 818 766-1587
Med Dir: Earl S Young, MD FACP FCCP
Class Cap: 120 *Begins:* Varies
Length: 10 mos *Award:* Cert, 10286
Tuition per yr: $10,286

ConCorde Career Institute
Respiratory Therapy Tech Prgm
1290 N First
San Jose, CA 95112
Prgm Dir: Mark Strausbaugh, BSEd RRT
Tel: 408 441-6411 *Fax:* 408 441-7818
Med Dir: Greg MacDonnell, MD
Class Cap: 25 *Begins:* Sep Dec Mar Jul
Length: 10 mos *Award:* Dipl
Tuition per yr: $10,995

Simi Valley Adult School
Respiratory Therapy Tech Prgm
3192 Los Angeles Ave
Simi Valley, CA 93065
Prgm Dir: Christine R Kingston, BS RRT
Tel: 805 579-6262 *Fax:* 805 522-8902
Med Dir: Michael Littner, MD
Class Cap: 30 *Begins:* Aug
Length: 12 mos *Award:* Cert
Tuition per yr: $60
Evening or weekend classes available

San Joaquin Valley College

Respiratory Therapy Tech Prgm
8400 W Mineral King
Visalia, CA 93291
Prgm Dir: Barry M Westling, MEd RRT RPFT
Tel: 209 651-2500 *Fax:* 209 651-0574
Med Dir: William R Winn, MD
Class Cap: 30 *Begins:* Jan Aug
Length: 7 mos *Award:* Cert
Tuition per yr: $5,333

Crafton Hills College

Respiratory Therapy Tech Prgm
11711 Sand Canyon Rd
Yucaipa, CA 92399
Prgm Dir: Kenneth R Bryson, BVE RRT
Tel: 909 794-2161 *Fax:* 909 794-0423
Med Dir: Richard Sheldon, MD
Begins: Aug
Length: 12 mos *Award:* Cert
Tuition per yr: $770 res, $6,754 non-res

Colorado

T H Pickens Technical Center

Respiratory Therapy Tech Prgm
500 Airport Blvd
Aurora, CO 80011
Prgm Dir: Gary S Schroeder, MA RRT
Tel: 303 344-4910 *Fax:* 303 340-1898
Med Dir: James Ellis, MD
Class Cap: 40 *Begins:* Aug Jan
Length: 14 mos, 12 mos *Award:* Cert, AAS
Tuition per yr: $2,627 res, $5,254 non-res

Pima Medical Institute - Denver

Respiratory Therapy Tech Prgm
1701 W 72nd Ave
Denver, CO 80221
Prgm Dir: C Allen Wentworth, RRT
Tel: 303 426-1800 *Fax:* 303 430-4048
Med Dir: Joseph Heit, MD
Class Cap: 75 *Begins:* Jun Oct Apr
Length: 12 mos *Award:* Cert
Tuition per yr: $11,335 res, $11,335 non-res

Connecticut

Naugatuck Valley Comm - Tech College

Respiratory Therapy Tech Prgm
750 Chase Pkwy
Waterbury, CT 06708
Prgm Dir: Sharon Baer, MBA RRT CPFT
Tel: 203 596-8662
Med Dir: Janet Hilbert, MD
Class Cap: 20 *Begins:* Sep
Length: 12 mos *Award:* Cert
Tuition per yr: $1,873 res, $4,842 non-res
Evening or weekend classes available

Florida

Daytona Beach Community College

Respiratory Therapy Tech Prgm
PO Box 2811
Daytona Beach, FL 32120
Prgm Dir: Charles Carroll, EdD RRT
Tel: 904 255-8131
Med Dir: Michael A Diamond, MD
Begins: Aug
Length: 12 mos *Award:* Cert
Tuition per yr: $1,977 res, $7,426 non-res

Broward Community College

Respiratory Therapy Tech Prgm
3501 SW Davie Rd
Ft Lauderdale, FL 33314
Prgm Dir: John Prince, RRT
Tel: 954 969-2082 *Fax:* 954 973-2348
Med Dir: Milton Braunstein, MD
Begins: Aug
Length: 12 mos *Award:* Cert
Tuition per yr: $1,700 res, $5,325 non-res

Flagler Career Institute - Jacksonville

Respiratory Therapy Tech Prgm
3225 University Blvd S
Jacksonville, FL 32216
Prgm Dir: Penny Campbell, RRT
Tel: 904 721-1622 *Fax:* 904 723-3117
Med Dir: Charles D Burger, MD
Class Cap: 50 *Begins:* Varies
Length: 16 mos *Award:* Cert
Tuition per yr: $6,768
Evening or weekend classes available

ATI Health Education Centers

Respiratory Therapy Tech Prgm
1395 NW 167th St/2nd Fl
Miami, FL 33169
Prgm Dir: Jules Clavan, BS RRT
Tel: 305 628-1000
Med Dir: Edgar Bolton Jr, DO FCCP
Class Cap: 250 *Begins:* Aug Dec Apr
Length: 14 mos *Award:* Dipl,Cert, AS
Tuition per yr: $14,795

Miami-Dade Community College

Respiratory Therapy Tech Prgm
Medical Ctr Campus
950 NW 20th St
Miami, FL 33127
Prgm Dir: Carol J Miller, RRT EdD
Tel: 305 237-4031 *Fax:* 305 237-4278
E-mail: millerc@mdcc.edu
Med Dir: Bruce Krieger, MD
Class Cap: 40 *Begins:* Aug
Length: 12 mos *Award:* Cert
Tuition per yr: $2,063 res, $7,250 non-res
Evening or weekend classes available

Palm Beach Community College

Respiratory Therapy Tech Prgm
3160 PGA Blvd
Palm Beach Gardens, FL 33410
Prgm Dir: Edward W Willey, MS RRT
Tel: 561 625-2587 *Fax:* 561 625-2305
Med Dir: Rogelio Choy, MD
Class Cap: 25 *Begins:* Aug
Length: 10 mos *Award:* Cert
Tuition per yr: $1,503 res, $5,595 non-res
Evening or weekend classes available

Gulf Coast Community College

Respiratory Therapy Tech Prgm
5230 W US Hwy 98
Panama City, FL 32401
Prgm Dir: Robert E Moore, BS RRT
Tel: 904 872-3837 *Fax:* 904 747-3246
Med Dir: S A Daffin III, MD
Class Cap: 16 *Begins:* Aug
Length: 10 mos, 20 mos *Award:* Cert, AS
Tuition per yr: $1,365 res, $4,936 non-res
Evening or weekend classes available

Seminole Community College

Respiratory Therapy Tech Prgm
100 Weldon Blvd
Sanford, FL 32773
Prgm Dir: Steve Shideler, MSHS RRT
Tel: 407 328-2293
E-mail: s.shideler@ipo.sminole.cc.fl.us
Med Dir: Alan Varraux, MD
Class Cap: 25 *Begins:* Aug
Length: 16 mos *Award:* Cert
Tuition per yr: $2,000 res, $2,800 non-res
Evening or weekend classes available

Pinellas Tech Educ Ctr - St Petersburg

Respiratory Therapy Tech Prgm
901 34th St S
St Petersburg, FL 33711
Prgm Dir: Marsha E Karkheck, RRT
Tel: 813 893-2500
Med Dir: Lynn Feaster III, MD
Class Cap: 46 *Begins:* Varies
Length: 13 mos *Award:* Dipl
Tuition per yr: $705 res, $3,175 non-res

David G Erwin Technical Center

Respiratory Therapy Tech Prgm
2010 E Hillsborough Ave
Tampa, FL 33610-8299
Prgm Dir: Arlen K Black, RRT
Tel: 813 231-1800 *Fax:* 813 231-1820
Med Dir: Mark A Smith, MD
Class Cap: 35 *Begins:* Varies
Length: 14 mos *Award:* Dipl
Tuition per yr: $650 res, $4,884 non-res
Evening or weekend classes available

Georgia

Georgia State University

Respiratory Therapy Tech Prgm
University Plaza
Atlanta, GA 30303
Prgm Dir: Joseph L Rau Jr, PhD RRT
Tel: 404 651-3037 *Fax:* 404 651-1531
Med Dir: Robert Aranson, MD
Class Cap: 25 *Begins:* Sep
Length: 15 mos *Award:* Cert
Tuition per yr: $3,021 res, $11,917 non-res
Evening or weekend classes available

Programs

Gwinnett Technical Institute
Respiratory Therapy Tech Prgm
5150 Sugarloaf Parkway
PO Box 1505
Lawrenceville, GA 30246-1505
Prgm Dir: Robert P De Lorme, EdS RRT
Tel: 770 962-7580 *Fax:* 770 962-7985
Med Dir: Gregory L Mauldin, MD
Class Cap: 20 *Begins:* Sept
Length: 24 mos *Award:* Cert, AAT
Tuition per yr: $1,200 res, $2,208 non-res
Evening or weekend classes available

Coosa Valley Technical Institute
Respiratory Therapy Tech Prgm
785 Cedar Ave
Rome, GA 30161-6757
Prgm Dir: Leann I Papp, RRT RN BA
Tel: 706 235-6756
Med Dir: Tony Warren, MD
Class Cap: 18 *Begins:* Oct
Length: 15 mos *Award:* Dipl
Tuition per yr: $600 res, $1,200 non-res

Thomas Technical Institute
Respiratory Therapy Tech Prgm
PO Box 1578
Thomasville, GA 31799
Prgm Dir: Tammy A Miller, MEd RRT
Tel: 912 225-4078 *Fax:* 912 225-5289
Med Dir: Craig Wolff, MD
Begins: Jul
Length: 24 mos *Award:* Dipl, AAT
Tuition per yr: $1,260 res, $2,520 non-res

Okefenokee Technical Institute
Respiratory Therapy Tech Prgm
1701 Carswell Ave
Waycross, GA 31501
Prgm Dir: Faye Mathis, RRT RCP
Tel: 912 287-6584 *Fax:* 912 284-2508
E-mail: faye@admin1.waycross-tec.ga.us
Med Dir: Manel Nayak, MD
Class Cap: 19 *Begins:* Varies
Length: 15 mos *Award:* Dipl
Tuition per yr: $1,000

Idaho

Boise State University
Respiratory Therapy Tech Prgm
College of Technology
1910 University Dr
Boise, ID 83725
Prgm Dir: Vera A Mc Crink, MEd RRT
Tel: 208 467-5707 *Fax:* 208 466-2933
Med Dir: Charles E Reed, MD
Class Cap: 15 *Begins:* Jul
Length: 13 mos *Award:* Cert
Tuition per yr: $2,434 res, $10,609 non-res

Illinois

Belleville Area College
Respiratory Therapy Tech Prgm
St Elizabeth's Hospital
211 S Third St
Belleville, IL 62222
Prgm Dir: Margaret J McMillin, BS RRT
Tel: 618 234-8911, Ext 989 *Fax:* 618 234-9025
Med Dir: Douglas W Dothager, MD
Class Cap: 28 *Begins:* Aug
Length: 12 mos *Award:* Cert
Tuition per yr: $1,360 res, $2,890 non-res
Evening or weekend classes available

Kaskaskia College
Respiratory Therapy Tech Prgm
27210 College Rd
Centralia, IL 62801
Prgm Dir: Sharon Urban, RRT
Tel: 618 532-1981 *Fax:* 618 532-1990
Med Dir: Aziz Rahman, MD
Class Cap: 20 *Begins:* Jun
Length: 12 mos *Award:* Cert
Tuition per yr: $1,584 res, $3,696 non-res
Evening or weekend classes available

St Augustine College
Respiratory Therapy Tech Prgm
1333 W Argyle
Chicago, IL 60640
Prgm Dir: Watson Stewart, RRT
Tel: 312 878-8756
Med Dir: Raoul L Wolf, MD
Class Cap: 40 *Begins:* Jan Sep
Length: 20 mos *Award:* Dipl, AAS
Tuition per yr: $4,800
Evening or weekend classes available

Trinity Hospital
Respiratory Therapy Tech Prgm
Trinity Hospital
2320 E 93rd St
Chicago, IL 60617
Prgm Dir: Goldie May Belk, RRT CPPT
Tel: 773 978-2000 *Fax:* 773 933-6436
Med Dir: Prentiss Taylor, MD
Class Cap: 25 *Begins:* Aug
Length: 14 mos *Award:* Cert
Tuition per yr: $1,701 res, $1,701 non-res
Evening or weekend classes available

College of DuPage
Respiratory Therapy Tech Prgm
22nd St and Lambert Rd
Glen Ellyn, IL 60137-6599
Prgm Dir: Kenneth M Bretl, MA RRT
Tel: 630 942-2518 *Fax:* 630 858-9399
E-mail: bretlk@cdnet.cod.edu
Med Dir: Robert T Zeck, MD
Class Cap: 30 *Begins:* Jun
Length: 12 mos *Award:* Cert
Tuition per yr: $1,421 res, $4,459 non-res
Evening or weekend classes available

Black Hawk College
Respiratory Therapy Tech Prgm
Quad Cities Campus
6600 34th Ave
Moline, IL 61265
Prgm Dir: Nancy M Smith, BA RRT
Tel: 309 796-1311 *Fax:* 309 792-3418
E-mail: sm.thn@bhc1bhc.edu
Med Dir: Edward L Ebert, DO
Class Cap: 25 *Begins:* Aug
Length: 18 mos *Award:* Cert
Tuition per yr: $1,344 res, $5,488 non-res
Evening or weekend classes available

Illinois Central College
Respiratory Therapy Tech Prgm
201 SW Adams
Peoria, IL 61635-0001
Prgm Dir: Margaret A Swanson, MS RRT
Tel: 309 999-4663 *Fax:* 309 673-9626
Med Dir: Stanley Bugaieski, MD
Class Cap: 5 *Begins:* Aug
Length: 12 mos *Award:* Cert
Tuition per yr: $1,596 res, $4,940 non-res
Evening or weekend classes available

Rock Valley College
Respiratory Therapy Tech Prgm
3301 N Mulford Rd
Rockford, IL 61114-5699
Prgm Dir: James R Sills, MEd CPFT RRT
Tel: 815 654-4413 *Fax:* 815 654-5359
E-mail: fahe3js@rvcux1.rvc.cc.il.us
Med Dir: John Foster, MD
Class Cap: 19 *Begins:* Jun
Length: 14 mos, 19 mos *Award:* Cert
Tuition per yr: $1,435 res, $4,674 non-res
Evening or weekend classes available

St John's Hospital
Respiratory Therapy Tech Prgm
800 E Carpenter
Springfield, IL 62769
Prgm Dir: T A Venters-Poe, BA RRT CPFT
Tel: 217 757-6788 *Fax:* 217 535-3996
Med Dir: Pradeep S Kulkarni, MD
Class Cap: 8 *Begins:* Jun
Length: 12 mos *Award:* Dipl
Tuition per yr: $3,715

Waubonsee Community College
Respiratory Therapy Tech Prgm
Rte 47 at Harter Rd
Sugar Grove, IL 60554
Prgm Dir: Carleton A Solarski, BS RRT
Tel: 630 466-7900 *Fax:* 630 466-9414
E-mail: carletons@wccb.cucc.cc.il.us
Med Dir: Thomas Liske, MD
Class Cap: 15 *Begins:* Aug
Length: 10 mos *Award:* Cert
Tuition per yr: $1,542 res, $7,317 non-res

Indiana

Ivy Tech State Coll NE - Ft Wayne
Respiratory Therapy Tech Prgm
3800 N Anthony Blvd
Ft Wayne, IN 46805
Prgm Dir: Candace Schladenhauffen, RRT RPFT
Tel: 219 482-9171 *Fax:* 219 480-4149
Med Dir: Thomas Hayhurst, MD
Class Cap: 28 *Begins:* Aug
Length: 15 mos *Award:* Cert
Tuition per yr: $2,580 res, $4,694 non-res
Evening or weekend classes available

Ivy Tech State Coll - Lafayette
Respiratory Therapy Tech Prgm
3208 Ross Rd
PO Box 6299
Lafayette, IN 47903
Prgm Dir: Peggy S James, MBA RRT
Tel: 317 772-9207
Med Dir: David Emery, MD
Class Cap: 20 *Begins:* Aug
Length: 16 mos, 21 mos *Award:* Dipl,Cert, AS
Tuition per yr: $2,580 res, $4,694 non-res
Evening or weekend classes available

Ivy Tech State Coll - Valparaiso
Respiratory Therapy Tech Prgm
2401 Valley Dr
Valparaiso, IN 46383
Prgm Dir: Susan Layhew, BS RRT
Tel: 219 464-8514 *Fax:* 219 464-9751
Med Dir: Charles Rebesco, MD
Class Cap: 25 *Begins:* Aug
Length: 12 mos *Award:* Cert
Tuition per yr: $3,195 res, $6,390 non-res
Evening or weekend classes available

Iowa

Northeast Iowa Community College
Respiratory Therapy Tech Prgm
10250 Sundown Rd
Peosta, IA 52068
Prgm Dir: Sue E Meade, RRT
Tel: 319 556-5110 *Fax:* 319 556-5058
E-mail: medes@nicc.cc.ia.us
Med Dir: Mark Janes, MD
Class Cap: 25 *Begins:* Aug
Length: 12 mos *Award:* Dipl
Tuition per yr: $2,976 res, $4,166 non-res
Evening or weekend classes available

Hawkeye Community College
Respiratory Therapy Tech Prgm
1501 E Orange Rd
PO Box 8015
Waterloo, IA 50704
Prgm Dir: Lawrence A Dahl, EdD RRT
Tel: 319 296-2320 *Fax:* 319 296-2874
Med Dir: Russell Adams, MD
Class Cap: 24 *Begins:* Aug
Length: 12 mos *Award:* Dipl
Tuition per yr: $3,262 res, $6,525 non-res
Evening or weekend classes available

Kansas

Bethany Med Ctr/Kansas City Kansas CC
Respiratory Therapy Tech Prgm
51 N 12th St
Kansas City, KS 66102
Prgm Dir: C Michael Parrett, RRT
Tel: 913 281-8768 *Fax:* 913 281-7875
Med Dir: Ajit Parekh, MD
Class Cap: 10 *Begins:* Sep
Length: 12 mos *Award:* Cert
Tuition per yr: $3,850 res, $5,200 non-res

Seward County Community College
Respiratory Therapy Tech Prgm
PO Box 1137
Liberal, KS 67901-1137
Prgm Dir: Ken Killion, RRT
Tel: 316 626-3080 *Fax:* 316 626-3026
Med Dir: Frank Hansen, MD
Class Cap: 16 *Begins:* Aug
Length: 12 mos *Award:* Cert
Tuition per yr: $1,134 res, $2,100 non-res
Evening or weekend classes available

Washburn University of Topeka
Respiratory Therapy Tech Prgm
1700 College Ave SW
Topeka, KS 66621
Prgm Dir: Patricia M Munzer, MS RRT
Tel: 913 231-1010 *Fax:* 913 231-1027
E-mail: zzmunz@sace.wuacc.edu
Med Dir: Ted W Daughety, MD
Class Cap: 18 *Begins:* Aug
Length: 15 mos *Award:* Cert
Tuition per yr: $2,976 res, $6,541 non-res
Evening or weekend classes available

Kentucky

Bowling Green State Voc Tech School
Respiratory Therapy Tech Prgm
1845 Loop Dr
Bowling Green, KY 42101
Prgm Dir: Brian Harlan, RRT
Tel: 502 746-7461 *Fax:* 502 746-7466
Med Dir: Randall Hansbrough, MD
Class Cap: 24 *Begins:* Apr
Length: 15 mos *Award:* Dipl
Tuition per yr: $750 res, $1,500 non-res
Evening or weekend classes available

Kentucky Tech Central Campus
Respiratory Therapy Tech Prgm
104 Vo-Tech Rd
Region 15
Lexington, KY 40510
Prgm Dir: Rebecca Simms, CRTT RRT
Tel: 606 246-2417
Med Dir: Andrew Daniel, MD
Class Cap: 20 *Begins:* Apr
Length: 15 mos *Award:* Dipl
Tuition per yr: $750 res, $1,250 non-res
Evening or weekend classes available

Kentucky Tech/Jefferson State Campus
Respiratory Therapy Tech Prgm
800 W Chestnut
Louisville, KY 40203
Prgm Dir: Anthony W Schmitt, BS RRT
Tel: 502 595-4275 *Fax:* 502 595-2387
Med Dir: Kenneth C Anderson, MD
Class Cap: 20 *Begins:* Varies
Length: 18 mos *Award:* Dipl
Tuition per yr: $500 res, $1,000 non-res
Evening or weekend classes available

Madisonville Health Technology Center
Respiratory Therapy Tech Prgm
Consortium for Resp Care Educ
750 N Laffoon St
Madisonville, KY 42431
Prgm Dir: David F Pennaman, MS RRT
Tel: 502 824-7552 *Fax:* 502 824-7069
Med Dir: Frank H Taylor, MD
Class Cap: 20 *Begins:* Aug Jan
Length: 18 mos *Award:* Dipl
Tuition per yr: $600 res, $1,200 non-res
Evening or weekend classes available

Rowan State Voc Tech School
Respiratory Therapy Tech Prgm
100 Voc-Tech Dr
KY 32 - 5 Miles N
Morehead, KY 40351
Prgm Dir: Kayla D Dolan, BS RRT
Tel: 606 783-1538 *Fax:* 606 784-9876
Med Dir: Jeffrey W Dickerson, MD
Class Cap: 25 *Begins:* Aug
Length: 15 mos *Award:* Dipl,Cert
Tuition per yr: $500 res, $1,000 non-res
Evening or weekend classes available

KY Tech-Rockcastle County Area Tech Ctr
Respiratory Therapy Tech Prgm
PO Box 275
Mt Vernon, KY 40456
Prgm Dir: Jess Hoskins, RRT
Tel: 606 256-4346 *Fax:* 606 256-4337
Med Dir: Abdi Vaezy, MD
Class Cap: 30 *Begins:* Varies
Length: 15 mos *Award:* Dipl
Tuition per yr: $500 res, $600 non-res

West Kentucky Tech
Respiratory Therapy Tech Prgm
Blandville Rd
PO Box 7408
Paducah, KY 42001
Prgm Dir: Ruth Thompson, MS RRT
Tel: 502 554-6244 *Fax:* 502 554-4227
Med Dir: Bradley T Rankin, MD
Class Cap: 20 *Begins:* Aug Jan
Length: 15 mos, 21 mos *Award:* Dipl
Tuition per yr: $500 res, $1,000 non-res
Evening or weekend classes available

KY Tech - Mayo Regional Tech Ctr
Respiratory Therapy Tech Prgm
513 Third St
Paintsville, KY 41240
Prgm Dir: Melissa B Steele, CRTT RRT CPFT
Tel: 606 789-5321 *Fax:* 606 789-9753
Med Dir: Raghy Sunduram, MD
Class Cap: 30 *Begins:* Aug
Length: 15 mos *Award:* Dipl
Tuition per yr: $605 res, $1,205 non-res

Cumberland Valley Health Technology Ctr
Respiratory Therapy Tech Prgm
US 25E S
PO Box 187
Pineville, KY 40977
Prgm Dir: Michael S Good, RRT
Tel: 606 337-3106 *Fax:* 606 337-5662
Med Dir: Abdi Vaezy, MD
Class Cap: 20 *Begins:* Aug
Length: 12 mos, 15 mos *Award:* Cert
Tuition per yr: $600 res, $1,200 non-res
Evening or weekend classes available

Louisiana

Bossier Parish Community College
Respiratory Therapy Tech Prgm
2719 Airline Dr
Bossier City, LA 71111
Prgm Dir: Beth Hamilton, BS RRT
Tel: 318 675-6814 *Fax:* 318 675-6937
E-mail: ehamil@mail-sh.isumc.edu
Med Dir: Keith Payne, MD
Class Cap: 15 *Begins:* Jan
Length: 16 mos *Award:* Cert
Tuition per yr: $1,400

Louisiana State University at Eunice
Respiratory Therapy Tech Prgm
PO Box 1129
Eunice, LA 70535
Prgm Dir: Edward Calloway, MHS RRT
Tel: 318 457-7311 *Fax:* 318 546-6620
E-mail: ecallowa@lsue.edu
Med Dir: Gary Guidry, MD
Begins: Aug,Jan,Jun
Length: 24 mos *Award:* AAS
Tuition per yr: $1,320 res, $2,820 non-res

LA Tech College-West Jefferson Campus
Respiratory Therapy Tech Prgm
475 Manhattan Blvd
Harvey, LA 70058
Prgm Dir: Toy B Smoot, RRT
Tel: 504 361-6388
Med Dir: Thomas Grimstad, MD
Class Cap: 15 *Begins:* Varies
Length: 18 mos *Award:* Dipl
Tuition per yr: $420

Alton Ochsner Medical Foundation
Respiratory Therapy Tech Prgm
1516 Jefferson Hwy
New Orleans, LA 70121
Prgm Dir: Mary LaBiche, MEd RRT
Tel: 504 842-3267 *Fax:* 504 842-9129
Med Dir: John M Onofrio, MD
Class Cap: 6 *Begins:* Sep
Length: 10 mos *Award:* Cert
Tuition per yr: $1,235 res, $1,235 non-res

Delgado Community College
Respiratory Therapy Tech Prgm
615 City Park Ave
New Orleans, LA 70119
Prgm Dir: Diane M Olsen, MHS RRT
Tel: 504 483-4007
Med Dir: Mack Thomas, MD
Class Cap: 30 *Begins:* Aug
Length: 12 mos, 12 mos *Award:* Cert
Tuition per yr: $1,455 res, $3,255 non-res

Nicholls State University
Respiratory Therapy Tech Prgm
PO Box 2090
Thibodaux, LA 70310
Prgm Dir: Errol J Champagne, RRT
Tel: 504 448-4495 *Fax:* 504 448-4923
Med Dir: John C. King, MD
Class Cap: 20 *Begins:* Aug
Length: 24 mos *Award:* Cert, AS
Tuition per yr: $2,761 res, $6,325 non-res

Massachusetts

Newbury College
Respiratory Therapy Tech Prgm
129 Fisher Ave
Brookline, MA 02146
Prgm Dir: Geraldine Twomey, MEd RRT
Tel: 617 730-7058 *Fax:* 617 730-7182
Med Dir: Jonathan D Strongin, MD PhD
Class Cap: 35 *Begins:* Sep Jan
Length: 16 mos *Award:* Cert
Tuition per yr: $11,110

Northern Essex Community College
Respiratory Therapy Tech Prgm
100 Elliot Way
Haverhill, MA 01830
Prgm Dir: Christopher Rowse, MS RRT
Tel: 508 374-3828
Med Dir: Daniel Coleman, MD
Class Cap: 20 *Begins:* Sep
Length: 13 mos *Award:* Cert
Tuition per yr: $2,805 res, $3,399 non-res

Michigan

St John Hospital and Medical Center
Respiratory Therapy Tech Prgm
22101 Moross Rd
Detroit, MI 48236
Prgm Dir: Madeleine K Dwaihy, BS RRT
Tel: 313 343-3769 *Fax:* 313 343-6052
Med Dir: Mario S Benvenuto, MD
Class Cap: 12 *Begins:* Jul
Length: 12 mos *Award:* Cert
Tuition per yr: $400

Monroe County Community College
Respiratory Therapy Tech Prgm
1555 S Rasinville Rd
Monroe, MI 48161
Prgm Dir: Bonnie Boggs-Clothier, RRT
Tel: 313 242-7300 *Fax:* 313 242-9711
Med Dir: Milo Engoren, MD
Class Cap: 20 *Begins:* Aug
Length: 12 mos, 16 mos *Award:* Cert
Tuition per yr: $2,064 res, $3,216 non-res
Evening or weekend classes available

Muskegon Community College
Respiratory Therapy Tech Prgm
221 S Quarterline Rd
Muskegon, MI 49442
Prgm Dir: Daniel B Knue, MM RRT
Tel: 616 777-0370 *Fax:* 616 777-0255
E-mail: dknue@aol.com
Med Dir: Mark Ivey, MD
Class Cap: 30 *Begins:* Sep
Length: 16 mos *Award:* Cert
Tuition per yr: $2,150 res, $3,100 non-res
Evening or weekend classes available

Minnesota

Northwest Technical Coll - E Grand Forks
Respiratory Therapy Tech Prgm
Hwy 220 N
East Grand Forks, MN 56721
Prgm Dir: Tony Sorum, RRT
Tel: 218 773-3441 *Fax:* 218 773-4502
E-mail: sorum@adm.egf.mn.us
Med Dir: Wayne Bretweiser, MD
Class Cap: 25 *Begins:* Aug
Length: 13 mos *Award:* Dipl
Tuition per yr: $2,768 res, $5,983 non-res
Evening or weekend classes available

Mississippi

Northeast Mississippi Community College
Respiratory Therapy Tech Prgm
Cunningham Blvd
Booneville, MS 38829
Prgm Dir: Beverly D Prince, RRT
Tel: 601 720-7307 *Fax:* 601 728-1165
Med Dir: Angel R Rodriquez, MD
Class Cap: 17 *Begins:* Aug
Length: 12 mos, 10 mos *Award:* Cert, AAS
Tuition per yr: $950 res, $2,050 non-res
Evening or weekend classes available

Itawamba Community College
Respiratory Therapy Tech Prgm
602 W Hill St
Fulton, MS 38843
Prgm Dir: J Harold Plunkett, RRT
Tel: 601 862-3101 *Fax:* 601 862-7697
Med Dir: Benjamin Moore, MD
Class Cap: 16 *Begins:* Aug
Length: 12 mos *Award:* Cert
Tuition per yr: $1,000 res, $1,800 non-res

Pearl River Jr College - Forest Cty Branch
Respiratory Therapy Tech Prgm
5448 Hwy 49
Hattiesburg, MS 39401
Prgm Dir: S Lee King, MS RRT
Tel: 601 544-7722 *Fax:* 601 545-2976
Med Dir: Steven Warren Stogner, MD
Class Cap: 30 *Begins:* Aug
Length: 21 mos, 24 mos *Award:* Cert, AAS
Tuition per yr: $1,275 res, $2,775 non-res
Evening or weekend classes available

Hinds Community College District
Respiratory Therapy Tech Prgm
1750 Chadwick Dr
Jackson, MS 39204
Prgm Dir: Diane H Sylvester, RRT
Tel: 601 372-6507 *Fax:* 601 371-3703
E-mail: hccnahc@teclink.net
Med Dir: William C Pinkston, MD
Class Cap: 30 *Begins:* Aug
Length: 12 mos *Award:* Cert
Tuition per yr: $1,325 res, $2,461 non-res

Meridian Community College
Respiratory Therapy Tech Prgm
910 Hwy 19 N
Meridian, MS 39307
Prgm Dir: Steve W Arinder, BS MPH, RRT
Tel: 601 483-8241
Med Dir: Luis Borrell, MD
Class Cap: 21 *Begins:* Aug
Length: 12 mos *Award:* Cert
Tuition per yr: $1,440 res, $3,000 non-res

Copiah - Lincoln Community College
Respiratory Therapy Tech Prgm
Natchez Campus Voc/Tech
30 Campus Dr
Natchez, MS 39120-5398
Prgm Dir: Richard G Waltman, RRT
Tel: 601 445-8299 *Fax:* 601 446-1298
Med Dir: Barry F Tillman, MD
Class Cap: 15 *Begins:* Aug
Length: 16 mos *Award:* Cert
Tuition per yr: $2,900 res, $4,900 non-res

Missouri

Cape Girardeau Area Voc Tech School
Respiratory Therapy Tech Prgm
301 N Clark Ave
Cape Girardeau, MO 63701
Prgm Dir: Kenneth L Pfau, BS RRT
Tel: 573 334-0826 *Fax:* 573 334-5930
Med Dir: Richard E Moore, MD
Class Cap: 22 *Begins:* Aug
Length: 12 mos *Award:* Cert
Tuition per yr: $3,465

Hannibal Area Voc Tech School
Respiratory Therapy Tech Prgm
4550 McMasters Ave
Hannibal, MO 63401
Prgm Dir: David D Bach, RRT CRTT
Tel: 573 221-4430 *Fax:* 573 221-7971
E-mail: dbach@hannibal.k12.edu
Med Dir: Richard Ha, MD
Class Cap: 20 *Begins:* Sep
Length: 16 mos *Award:* Dipl
Tuition per yr: $5,100 res, $5,300 non-res

ConCorde Career Institute
Respiratory Therapy Tech Prgm
3239 Broadway
Kansas City, MO 64111
Prgm Dir: Lana Falls, BS RRT RCP
Tel: 816 531-5223 *Fax:* 816 756-3231
Med Dir: Lida Osbern, MD
Class Cap: 50 *Begins:* Jun Dec
Length: 10 mos *Award:* Dipl
Tuition per yr: $6,761 res, $6,761 non-res

Rolla Technical Institute
Respiratory Therapy Tech Prgm
1304 E 10th St
Rolla, MO 65401-3699
Prgm Dir: Jerry Joiner, BS RRT
Tel: 573 364-3726 *Fax:* 573 364-0767
E-mail: jjoiner@rollanet.org
Med Dir: Edward Bruns, DO
Class Cap: 20 *Begins:* Aug
Length: 12 mos *Award:* Cert
Tuition per yr: $4,000

State Fair Community College
Respiratory Therapy Tech Prgm
3201 W 16th
Sedalia, MO 65301
Prgm Dir: Susan E Whitcomb, RRT
Tel: 816 826-7100
Class Cap: 18 *Begins:* May
Length: 12 mos *Award:* Cert
Tuition per yr: $1,947 res, $3,127 non-res

Ozarks Technical Community College
Respiratory Therapy Tech Prgm
1417 N Jefferson
Springfield, MO 65802
Prgm Dir: Steven I Bishop, PhD RRT
Tel: 417 895-7127 *Fax:* 417 895-7161
Med Dir: John Wolfe, MD
Class Cap: 20 *Begins:* Jun
Length: 12 mos *Award:* Dipl
Tuition per yr: $1,677 res, $2,457 non-res
Evening or weekend classes available

Montana

Montana State Univ Coll of Technology
Respiratory Therapy Tech Prgm
2100 16th Ave S
Great Falls, MT 59405
Prgm Dir: Leonard Bates, RRT
Tel: 406 771-4360 *Fax:* 406 771-4317
E-mail: zgf6012@maia.oscs.montana.edu
Med Dir: Richard Blevins, MD
Class Cap: 18 *Begins:* Sep
Length: 12 mos *Award:* Cert
Tuition per yr: $2,256 res, $5,302 non-res
Evening or weekend classes available

University of Montana-Missoula
Respiratory Therapy Tech Prgm
College of Technology
University of Montana-Missoula
Missoula, MT 59801
Prgm Dir: Robert W Wafstet, MS RRT
Tel: 406 243-7821 *Fax:* 406 243-7899
Med Dir: William B Bekemeyer, MD
Class Cap: 25 *Begins:* Sep
Length: 13 mos *Award:* Cert
Tuition per yr: $3,081 res, $6,519 non-res

Nebraska

Metropolitan Community College
Respiratory Therapy Tech Prgm
PO Box 3777
Omaha, NE 68103
Prgm Dir: Jerald A Moss, MPA RRT
Tel: 402 449-8510 *Fax:* 402 449-8532
E-mail: jmoss@metro.mccneb.edu
Med Dir: Lon W Keim, MD
Class Cap: 21 *Begins:* Sep
Length: 18 mos *Award:* Cert
Tuition per yr: $2,652 res, $3,315 non-res
Evening or weekend classes available

New Jersey

Univ of Med & Dent of New Jersey
Respiratory Therapy Tech Prgm
Sch of Hlth Professions
65 Bergen St
Newark, NJ 07107-3006
Prgm Dir: Craig L Scanlan, EdD RRT
Tel: 201 982-5503 *Fax:* 201 982-5258
E-mail: scanlan@umdnj.edu
Med Dir: Marc H Lavietes, MD
Class Cap: 32 *Begins:* Sep
Length: 12 mos *Award:* Cert
Tuition per yr: $2,590 res, $5,180 non-res

Passaic County Community College
Respiratory Therapy Tech Prgm
One College Blvd
Paterson, NJ 07505
Prgm Dir: Sandra McCleaster, RRT
Tel: 201 684-5280 *Fax:* 201 684-5832
Med Dir: Reza Farhangfar, MD
Class Cap: 24 *Begins:* Sep
Length: 15 mos *Award:* Dipl
Tuition per yr: $2,500 res, $2,500 non-res

Gloucester County College
Respiratory Therapy Tech Prgm
1400 Tanyard Rd
Sewell, NJ 08080
Prgm Dir: Anna P Leder, RRT
Tel: 609 468-5000 *Fax:* 607 464-8463
Med Dir: Donald Auerbach, MD
Class Cap: 30 *Begins:* Sep
Length: 10 mos *Award:* Cert
Tuition per yr: $1,800 res, $5,000 non-res
Evening or weekend classes available

New York

Molloy College
Respiratory Therapy Tech Prgm
1000 Hempstead Ave
Rockville Centre, NY 11570
Prgm Dir: Teresa Barrett, MA RRT
Tel: 516 678-5000 *Fax:* 516 256-2252
Med Dir: Joseph Genovese, DO
Class Cap: 26 *Begins:* Sep
Length: 10 mos *Award:* Cert
Tuition per yr: $11,520

Onondaga Community College
Respiratory Therapy Tech Prgm
Rte 173
Syracuse, NY 13215
Prgm Dir: Daniel V Cleveland, RRT
Tel: 315 469-2458 *Fax:* 315 469-2593
Med Dir: Russell Acevedo, MD
Begins: Jan
Length: 12 mos *Award:* Cert
Tuition per yr: $2,686 res, $5,372 non-res
Evening or weekend classes available

Mohawk Valley Community College
Respiratory Therapy Tech Prgm
1101 Sherman Dr
Payne Hall 368
Utica, NY 13501
Prgm Dir: Lorie L Phillips, MS RRT
Tel: 315 792-5664 *Fax:* 315 792-5666
Med Dir: James Kohan, MD
Class Cap: 36 *Begins:* Aug
Length: 12 mos *Award:* Dipl,Cert
Evening or weekend classes available

North Carolina

Stanly Community College
Respiratory Therapy Tech Prgm
141 College Dr
Albermarle, NC 28001
Prgm Dir: Tammy P Crump, MS RRT
Tel: 704 982-0121 *Fax:* 704 982-0819
Med Dir: William J Messick, MD
Class Cap: 24 *Begins:* Sep
Length: 12 mos *Award:* Dipl
Tuition per yr: $770 res, $6,048 non-res
Evening or weekend classes available

Durham Technical Community College
Respiratory Therapy Tech Prgm
PO Box 11307
Durham, NC 27703
Prgm Dir: Richard D Miller, PhD RRT
Tel: 919 598-9243 *Fax:* 919 686-3601
Med Dir: James R Yankaskas, MD
Class Cap: 25 *Begins:* Sep
Length: 12 mos *Award:* Dipl
Tuition per yr: $742 res, $6,020 non-res
Evening or weekend classes available

Catawba Valley Community College
Respiratory Therapy Tech Prgm
2550 Hwy 70 SE
Hickory, NC 28602-9699
Prgm Dir: Catherine A Bitsche, BS RRT
Tel: 704 327-7000, Ext 7391 *Fax:* 704 327-7276
Med Dir: John Dew, MD
Class Cap: 20 *Begins:* Sep
Length: 12 mos *Award:* Dipl
Tuition per yr: $771 res, $6,049 non-res
Evening or weekend classes available

Carteret Community College
Respiratory Therapy Tech Prgm
3505 Arendell St
Morehead City, NC 28557
Prgm Dir: Barbara S Thomas, RRT
Tel: 919 247-6000 *Fax:* 919 247-2514
E-mail: thomasb@ncccs.ce.nc.us
Med Dir: Terrence Goodman, MD
Class Cap: 20 *Begins:* Sep
Length: 12 mos *Award:* Dipl,Cert
Tuition per yr: $742 res, $6,020 non-res
Evening or weekend classes available

Edgecombe Community College
Respiratory Therapy Tech Prgm
225 Tarboro St
Rocky Mount, NC 27801
Prgm Dir: Ralph D Webb, RRT
Tel: 919 446-0436 *Fax:* 919 985-2212
Med Dir: Lindsey E de Guehery, MD
Class Cap: 14 *Begins:* Sep
Length: 12 mos *Award:* Dipl
Tuition per yr: $766 res, $6,044 non-res
Evening or weekend classes available

Southwestern Community College
Respiratory Therapy Tech Prgm
275 Webster Rd
Sylva, NC 28779-9578
Prgm Dir: Deborah Beck, RRT
Tel: 704 586-4091 *Fax:* 704 586-3129
E-mail: debbieb@southwest.cc.nc.us
Med Dir: Harry G Lipham, MD
Class Cap: 18 *Begins:* Sep
Length: 12 mos *Award:* Dipl
Tuition per yr: $742 res, $6,020 non-res

Ohio

Collins Career Center
Respiratory Therapy Tech Prgm
Collins Career Ctr
11627 State Rte 243
Chesapeake, OH 45619
Prgm Dir: Kathy J Bentley, CRTT RCP
Tel: 614 867-6641 *Fax:* 614 867-6641
Med Dir: Randall L McCollister, MD RRT
Class Cap: 35 *Begins:* Aug
Length: 11 mos *Award:* Dipl,Cert
Tuition per yr: $3,300
Evening or weekend classes available

Columbus State Community College
Respiratory Therapy Tech Prgm
550 E Spring St
Columbus, OH 43215
Prgm Dir: Leonard J Chmielewski, MA RRT
Tel: 614 227-5151
Med Dir: Thomas Boes, MD
Class Cap: 25 *Begins:* Mar
Length: 12 mos *Award:* Cert
Tuition per yr: $2,736 res, $6,000 non-res
Evening or weekend classes available

Lima Technical College
Respiratory Therapy Tech Prgm
4240 Campus Dr
Lima, OH 45804
Prgm Dir: Richard N Woodfield Jr, MS RRT
Tel: 419 995-8366 *Fax:* 419 995-8818
Med Dir: Rick D Watson, MD
Class Cap: 25 *Begins:* Sep
Length: 12 mos *Award:* Cert
Tuition per yr: $2,941 res, $5,883 non-res

University of Toledo
Respiratory Therapy Tech Prgm
2801 W Bancroft St
Toledo, OH 43606
Prgm Dir: Margaret F Traband, MEd RRT
Tel: 419 530-3373 *Fax:* 419 530-3096
Med Dir: Robert A May, MD
Class Cap: 25 *Begins:* Sep
Length: 18 mos *Award:* Dipl, AS
Tuition per yr: $4,302 res, $10,321 non-res
Evening or weekend classes available.

Oklahoma

Great Plains Area Voc Tech School
Respiratory Therapy Tech Prgm
4500 W Lee Blvd
Lawton, OK 73505
Prgm Dir: Jack A Powers, RRT
Tel: 405 355-6371 *Fax:* 405 250-5583
E-mail: jpowers@ionet.net
Med Dir: Patrick KC Chun, MD
Class Cap: 12 *Begins:* Feb
Length: 12 mos *Award:* Cert
Tuition per yr: $1,250 res, $2,250 non-res

Francis Tuttle Vocational Technical Ctr
Respiratory Therapy Tech Prgm
12777 N Rockwell Ave
Oklahoma City, OK 73142
Prgm Dir: Lezli Heyland, BS RRT
Tel: 405 720-4269 *Fax:* 405 720-4789
Med Dir: Stephen Adler, MD
Class Cap: 44 *Begins:* Sep
Length: 12 mos, 24 mos *Award:* Cert
Tuition per yr: $1,150

Tulsa Community College
Respiratory Therapy Tech Prgm
909 S Boston Ave
Tulsa, OK 74119
Prgm Dir: Lindel W Porter, RRT
Tel: 918 587-6561 *Fax:* 918 595-7298
Med Dir: Fred Garfinkel, MD
Class Cap: 24 *Begins:* Aug
Length: 12 mos *Award:* Cert
Tuition per yr: $1,332 res, $3,598 non-res

Oregon

Rogue Community College

Respiratory Therapy Tech Prgm
3345 Redwood Hwy
Grants Pass, OR 97526
Prgm Dir: Pedro G Cabrera, RRT
Tel: 541 479-5541 *Fax:* 541 471-3566
Med Dir: John Ordal, MD
Class Cap: 18 *Begins:* Sep
Length: 12 mos *Award:* Dipl,Cert
Tuition per yr: $1,785 res, $2,704 non-res
Evening or weekend classes available

Pennsylvania

Thiel College

Respiratory Therapy Tech Prgm
75 College Ave
Greenville, PA 16125
Prgm Dir: Elaine K Allen, RRT
Tel: 412 589-2186
Med Dir: John S Belany, DO
Class Cap: 16 *Begins:* Aug
Length: 12 mos *Award:* Cert, BA
Tuition per yr: $9,950

Gwynedd-Mercy College

Respiratory Therapy Tech Prgm
Sumneytown Pike
Gwynedd Valley, PA 19437
Prgm Dir: William F Galvin, MSEd RRT CPFT
Tel: 610 646-7300 *Fax:* 610 641-5559
Med Dir: William Figueroa, MD
Class Cap: 20 *Begins:* Aug
Length: 13 mos *Award:* Cert
Tuition per yr: $12,670
Evening or weekend classes available

Harrisburg Area Community College

Respiratory Therapy Tech Prgm
One HACC Dr
Harrisburg, PA 17110
Prgm Dir: Bradley A Leidich, MSEd RRT
Tel: 717 780-2315
Med Dir: William M Anderson III, MD
Class Cap: 25 *Begins:* Jun
Length: 18 mos *Award:* Cert, AA
Tuition per yr: $2,498 res, $4,996 non-res

Greater Johnstown Area Voc - Tech School

Respiratory Therapy Tech Prgm
445 Schoolhouse Rd
Johnstown, PA 15904-2998
Prgm Dir: Mary Jane Johnson, RRT
Tel: 814 269-3874 *Fax:* 814 269-4586
Med Dir: George D Hanzel, MD
Class Cap: 20 *Begins:* Sep
Length: 12 mos *Award:* Dipl
Tuition per yr: $5,300
Evening or weekend classes available

Luzerne County Community College

Respiratory Therapy Tech Prgm
Prospect St and Middle Rd
Nanticoke, PA 18634
Prgm Dir: Christopher Tino, BS RRT
Tel: 717 829-7467 *Fax:* 717 821-1525
Med Dir: James Yarnal, DO PhD
Class Cap: 30 *Begins:* Jun
Length: 18 mos *Award:* Cert
Tuition per yr: $2,491 res, $4,982 non-res

Point Park College/St Francis Med Ctr

Respiratory Therapy Tech Prgm
School of Respiratory Care
400 45th St
Pittsburgh, PA 15201-1198
Prgm Dir: Albert M Gameos, BS RRT
Tel: 412 622-4475
Med Dir: Sukhdev S Grover, MD
Class Cap: 19 *Begins:* Aug
Length: 13 mos *Award:* Dipl
Tuition per yr: $6,000

Reading Area Community College

Respiratory Therapy Tech Prgm
Ten S Second St
PO Box 1706
Reading, PA 19603
Prgm Dir: Marie Jacoby, MSA RRT
Tel: 610 372-4721 *Fax:* 610 607-6254
Med Dir: Joseph Mariglio, MD
Class Cap: 60 *Begins:* Jun
Length: 24 mos *Award:* AAS
Tuition per yr: $1,972 res, $3,944 non-res

Lehigh Carbon Community College

Respiratory Therapy Tech Prgm
4525 Education Park Dr
Schnecksville, PA 18078-2598
Prgm Dir: Denise B McCardle, MSEd RRT
Tel: 215 799-1504 *Fax:* 610 799-1527
Med Dir: Joseph M Zasik, DO
Class Cap: 25 *Begins:* Aug
Length: 21 mos *Award:* AAS
Tuition per yr: $2,016 res, $4,032 non-res

York College of Pennsylvania

Respiratory Therapy Tech Prgm
York, PA 17403
Prgm Dir: Mark Simmons, MSEd RRT
Tel: 717 851-2464 *Fax:* 717 851-2487
Med Dir: Richard L Keesports, MD
Class Cap: 10 *Begins:* Jun
Length: 14 mos *Award:* Cert
Tuition per yr: $6,100 res, $6,100 non-res

Puerto Rico

Ponce Paramedical College

Respiratory Therapy Tech Prgm
Villa Flores Urbanization
L-15 Acacia St
Ponce, PR 00731
Prgm Dir: Efrain Gonzalez, BS RRT CPFT
Tel: 787 848-1589 *Fax:* 787 259-0169
Med Dir: Pedro J Rodriguez, MD FAAP
Class Cap: 120 *Begins:* Jul Sep Jan Apr
Length: 15 mos, 22 mos *Award:* Dipl
Tuition per yr: $6,480

South Carolina

Midlands Technical College

Respiratory Therapy Tech Prgm
PO Box 2408
Columbia, SC 29200
Prgm Dir: Linda H Ackerman, RRT
Tel: 803 822-3433 *Fax:* 803 822-3079
E-mail: mtc2.mid.tec.sc.us
Med Dir: J Daniel Love, MD
Class Cap: 30 *Begins:* Sep
Length: 15 mos *Award:* Dipl
Tuition per yr: $1,620 res, $2,016 non-res
Evening or weekend classes available

Florence-Darlington Technical College

Respiratory Therapy Tech Prgm
PO Box 100548
Florence, SC 29501-0548
Prgm Dir: John A Evans, RRT
Tel: 803 661-8148
Med Dir: William M Hazelwood, MD
Class Cap: 20 *Begins:* Aug
Length: 16 mos *Award:* Dipl
Tuition per yr: $1,650 res, $1,875 non-res
Evening or weekend classes available

Greenville Technical College

Respiratory Therapy Tech Prgm
PO Box 5616
Station B
Greenville, SC 29606
Prgm Dir: Thomas D Baxter, MHRD RRT
Tel: 864 250-8373
Med Dir: L Hayes, MD
Begins: Aug
Length: 6 mo , 15 mos *Award:* Dipl,Cert
Tuition per yr: $1,500 res, $2,400 non-res

Piedmont Technical College

Respiratory Therapy Tech Prgm
Emerald Rd
PO Drawer 1467
Greenwood, SC 29646
Prgm Dir: Sherri Pickelsimmer, RRT
Tel: 864 223-8357 *Fax:* 864 941-8555
Med Dir: O M Cobb Jr, MD
Class Cap: 23 *Begins:* Aug
Length: 16 mos, 16 mos *Award:* Dipl, AS
Tuition per yr: $1,584 res, $2,542 non-res
Evening or weekend classes available

Orangeburg Calhoun Technical College

Respiratory Therapy Tech Prgm
3250 St Matthews Rd
Orangeburg, SC 29118
Prgm Dir: Audrey T Stinchcomb, BHS RRT
Tel: 803 536-0311 *Fax:* 803 535-1344
E-mail: stinch@org.tec.sc.us
Med Dir: Thomas E Northrup, MD
Class Cap: 25 *Begins:* Aug
Length: 16 mos *Award:* Dipl
Tuition per yr: $1,260 res, $1,500 non-res
Evening or weekend classes available

Programs

Spartanburg Technical College

Respiratory Therapy Tech Prgm
PO Drawer 4386
Spartanburg, SC 29305-4386
Prgm Dir: Dot Kiser, RT(R)
Tel: 864 591-3720   *Fax:* 864 591-3708
E-mail: kiser@spt.tec.sc.us
Med Dir: Charles Fogarty, MD
Class Cap: 20   *Begins:* Aug
Length: 16 mos   *Award:* Dipl
Tuition per yr: $1,500 res, $1,875 non-res

Tennessee

East Tennessee State University

Respiratory Therapy Tech Prgm
1000 West E St
ETSU Nave Center
Elizabethton, TN 37643
Prgm Dir: Delmar L Mack, RRT
Tel: 423 547-4916   *Fax:* 423 547-4921
Med Dir: Jeff R Farrow, MD
Class Cap: 21   *Begins:* Aug
Length: 12 mos   *Award:* Cert
Tuition per yr: $2,892 res, $9,396 non-res
Evening or weekend classes available

Volunteer State Community College

Respiratory Therapy Tech Prgm
Nashville Pike
Gallatin, TN 37066
Prgm Dir: Emmy L Wishum, BS RRT
Tel: 615 452-8600   *Fax:* 615 230-3224
E-mail: ewishum@vscc.cc.tn.us
Med Dir: James H Haynes, MD
Class Cap: 20   *Begins:* Aug
Length: 12 mos, 8 mos   *Award:* Cert
Tuition per yr: $1,491 res, $4,389 non-res

Tennessee Technology Center - Memphis

Respiratory Therapy Tech Prgm
550 Alabama Ave
Memphis, TN 38105
Prgm Dir: William Parker, BS RRT
Tel: 901 543-6100
Med Dir: Kenneth V Leeper, MD
Class Cap: 30   *Begins:* Jul
Length: 12 mos   *Award:* Dipl,Cert
Tuition per yr: $400

Walters State Community College

Respiratory Therapy Tech Prgm
500 S Davy Crockett Pkwy
Morristown, TN 37813-6899
Prgm Dir: Robert G McGee, RRT
Tel: 423 787-1501   *Fax:* 423 787-1504
E-mail: robert.mcgee@wscc.cc.tn.us
Med Dir: Thomas F Beckner, MD
Class Cap: 24   *Begins:* Aug
Length: 12 mos   *Award:* Cert
Tuition per yr: $1,596

Texas

Alvin Community College

Respiratory Therapy Tech Prgm
3110 Mustang Rd
Alvin, TX 77511
Prgm Dir: Diane Flatland, MS RRT
Tel: 713 388-4695   *Fax:* 713 388-4936
Med Dir: Wayne K Hite, DO
Class Cap: 20   *Begins:* Jun
Length: 18 mos   *Award:* Cert
Tuition per yr: $854 res, $1,444 non-res
Evening or weekend classes available

Lamar Univ Institute of Tech - Beaumont

Respiratory Therapy Tech Prgm
PO Box 10061
Beaumont, TX 77710
Prgm Dir: Paul A Bronson, MEd RRT
Tel: 409 880-8852   *Fax:* 409 880-8955
Med Dir: Paul B Shaw, MD
Class Cap: 35   *Begins:* Aug
Length: 16 mos   *Award:* Cert
Tuition per yr: $1,392 res, $6,476 non-res

Univ Tx at Brownsville/TX Southmost Coll

Respiratory Therapy Tech Prgm
80 Ft Brown
Brownsville, TX 78520
Prgm Dir: John L McCabe, PhD RRT
Tel: 210 544-8262   *Fax:* 210 544-8910
Med Dir: Lorenzo Pelly, MD
Begins: Sep
Length: 12 mos   *Award:* Cert
Tuition per yr: $1,721 res, $2,461 non-res

Del Mar College

Respiratory Therapy Tech Prgm
Baldwin and Ayers
Corpus Christi, TX 78404
Prgm Dir: Jeffrey T Watson, RRT
Tel: 512 886-1103
Med Dir: William Burgin, Jr, MD
Class Cap: 24   *Begins:* Jun
Length: 12 mos   *Award:* Cert
Tuition per yr: $647 res, $968 non-res
Evening or weekend classes available

Houston Community College Central

Respiratory Therapy Tech Prgm
3100 Shenandoah
Houston, TX 77021
Prgm Dir: Mildred L C Bartel, MEd RRT RCP
Tel: 713 718-7380   *Fax:* 713 718-7401
Med Dir: Fernando Stein, MD
Class Cap: 30   *Begins:* Aug Jan
Length: 12 mos   *Award:* Cert
Tuition per yr: $1,300 res, $2,115 non-res
Evening or weekend classes available

Kingwood College - NHMCCD

Respiratory Therapy Tech Prgm
20,000 Kingwood Dr
Kingwood, TX 77339
Prgm Dir: Kenny P McCowen, RRT
Tel: 713 359-1608   *Fax:* 713 359-0490
E-mail: kmccowen@kc.nhmcc.cc.tx.us
Med Dir: Edward Flores, MD
Class Cap: 25   *Begins:* Jun
Length: 12 mos   *Award:* Cert
Tuition per yr: $606 res, $1,366 non-res

South Plains College

Respiratory Therapy Tech Prgm
1302 Main St
Lubbock, TX 79401
Prgm Dir: Shonni L Collier, RRT
Tel: 806 747-0576   *Fax:* 806 765-2775
Med Dir: Wayne McNeil, MD
Class Cap: 30   *Begins:* Aug
Length: 16 mos   *Award:* Cert
Tuition per yr: $1,300 res, $1,600 non-res
Evening or weekend classes available

Angelina College

Respiratory Therapy Tech Prgm
PO Box 1768
Lufkin, TX 75902-1768
Prgm Dir: William M Parks, MEd RRT
Tel: 409 639-1301   *Fax:* 409 639-4299
Med Dir: Mannoor Thomas, MD
Class Cap: 42   *Begins:* Aug
Length: 12 mos, 9 mos   *Award:* Dipl,Cert, AAS
Tuition per yr: $546 res, $1,096 non-res
Evening or weekend classes available

Midland College

Respiratory Therapy Tech Prgm
3600 N Garfield
Midland, TX 79705
Prgm Dir: Robert Weidmann, BS RRT
Tel: 915 685-4595   *Fax:* 915 685-4762
E-mail: rweidmann@midland.cc.tx
Med Dir: Dan J Hendrickson, MD
Class Cap: 21   *Begins:* Sep
Length: 12 mos   *Award:* Cert
Tuition per yr: $1,141 res, $1,221 non-res
Evening or weekend classes available

Odessa College

Respiratory Therapy Tech Prgm
201 W University
Odessa, TX 79764
Prgm Dir: Shelia Butler, RRT CPFT
Tel: 915 335-6456   *Fax:* 915 335-6846
Med Dir: John D Bray, MD
Class Cap: 24   *Begins:* Jul
Length: 14 mos   *Award:* Cert
Tuition per yr: $1,112 res, $1,307 non-res
Evening or weekend classes available

San Jacinto College Central Campus

Respiratory Therapy Tech Prgm
8060 Spencer Hwy
PO Box 2007
Pasadena, TX 77505-2007
Prgm Dir: Patrick Helton
Tel: 713 476-1864
Med Dir: Anna Marie Harkins, PhD DO
Class Cap: 36   *Begins:* Sep
Length: 12 mos   *Award:* Cert
Tuition per yr: $580 res, $940 non-res

Howard College

Respiratory Therapy Tech Prgm
3197 Executive Dr
San Angelo, TX 76904
Prgm Dir: Alfred S Allen Jr, BS RRT
Tel: 915 947-9516, Ext 25   *Fax:* 915 947-9524
Med Dir: Daniel Parsons, MD
Class Cap: 24   *Begins:* Aug Jan
Length: 15 mos, 24 mos   *Award:* Dipl,Cert
Tuition per yr: res, $1,900 non-res
Evening or weekend classes available

Army Medical Dept Center and School
Respiratory Therapy Tech Prgm
Medical Science Div
PE Branch Bldg 609/610
San Antonio, TX 78234-6100
Prgm Dir: J P O'Hora, RRT
Tel: 210 221-2080   *Fax:* 210 916-7304
Med Dir: Gregg T Anders, DO
Class Cap: 210   *Begins:* Feb May Sep
Length: 8 mos   *Award:* Dipl

St Philip's College
Respiratory Therapy Tech Prgm
1801 Martin Luther King Dr
San Antonio, TX 78203-2098
Prgm Dir: Bruce Fisher, MS RRT RCP
Tel: 210 531-3457   *Fax:* 210 531-3459
E-mail: bfisher@accd.edu
Med Dir: Carlos Orozco, MD
Class Cap: 30   *Begins:* Sep
Length: 12 mos, 12 mos   *Award:* Dipl,Cert, AAS
Tuition per yr: $1,200 res, $3,900 non-res

Southwest Texas State University
Respiratory Therapy Tech Prgm
San Marcos, TX 78666
Prgm Dir: Cade J Harkins III, RRT MSHP
Tel: 512 245-8243   *Fax:* 512 245-7978
E-mail: cade-harkins@swt.edu
Med Dir: George Handley, MD
Class Cap: 48   *Begins:* Aug
Length: 30 mos   *Award:* Cert
Tuition per yr: $3,019 res, $3,019 non-res
Evening or weekend classes available

Tyler Junior College
Respiratory Therapy Tech Prgm
PO Box 9020
Tyler, TX 75711
Prgm Dir: Paul Weskamp, RRT
Tel: 903 531-2472   *Fax:* 903 510-2592
E-mail: pwes@tjc.tyler.cc.tx.us
Med Dir: James Stocks, MD
Class Cap: 45   *Begins:* Aug
Length: 12 mos   *Award:* Cert
Tuition per yr: $966 res, $1,506 non-res
Evening or weekend classes available

Victoria College
Respiratory Therapy Tech Prgm
2220 E Red River
Victoria, TX 77901
Prgm Dir: Chris E Kallus, MED RRT RCP
Tel: 512 572-6491   *Fax:* 512 572-3850
E-mail: ckallus@vc.cc.tx.us
Med Dir: Bruce E Wheeler, MD
Class Cap: 18   *Begins:* Aug
Length: 20 mos   *Award:* AAS
Tuition per yr: $919 res, $3,800 non-res

McLennan Community College
Respiratory Therapy Tech Prgm
1400 College Dr
Waco, TX 76708
Prgm Dir: Douglas Gibson, BA RRT
Tel: 817 299-8369
Med Dir: Robert R Springer, MD
Class Cap: 24   *Begins:* Jun
Length: 15 mos   *Award:* Cert
Tuition per yr: $880 res, $1,100 non-res
Evening or weekend classes available

Utah

Weber State University
Respiratory Therapy Tech Prgm
3750 Harrison Blvd
Ogden, UT 84408-3904
Prgm Dir: Georgine L Bills, MBA RRT
Tel: 801 626-7071   *Fax:* 801 626-7683
E-mail: gbills@weber.edu
Med Dir: Gary K Goucher, MD
Class Cap: 24   *Begins:* Sep
Length: 18 mos, 21 mos   *Award:* Cert, AAS
Tuition per yr: $1,863 res, $5,550 non-res

Virginia

Northern Virginia Community College
Respiratory Therapy Tech Prgm
8333 Little River Trnpk
Annandale, VA 22003
Prgm Dir: Mark L Diana, MBA RRT
Tel: 703 323-3280   *Fax:* 703 323-4576
E-mail: nudianmenv.cc.va.us
Med Dir: Frank Fusco, MD
Class Cap: 24   *Begins:* Aug
Length: 12 mos   *Award:* Cert
Tuition per yr: $2,160 res, $7,081 non-res
Evening or weekend classes available

Mountain Empire Community College
Respiratory Therapy Tech Prgm
Drawer 700
Big Stone Gap, VA 24219
Prgm Dir: Michael W Cook, MA
Tel: 540 523-2400   *Fax:* 540 523-8220
E-mail: mecookm@me.cc.va.us
Med Dir: Lawrence Fleenor, MD
Class Cap: 25   *Begins:* Jun
Length: 14 mos   *Award:* Dipl
Tuition per yr: $2,781 res, $9,014 non-res
Evening or weekend classes available

Central Virginia Community College
Respiratory Therapy Tech Prgm
3506 Wards Rd
Lynchburg, VA 24502
Prgm Dir: Martha N Crawley, RRT
Tel: 804 386-4599   *Fax:* 804 386-4681
E-mail: cvcrqwm@vccscent.binet
Med Dir: Michael G Milam, MD
Class Cap: 20   *Begins:* Aug
Length: 11 mos   *Award:* Cert
Tuition per yr: $2,238 res, $7,488 non-res
Evening or weekend classes available

Southwest Virginia Community College
Respiratory Therapy Tech Prgm
PO Box SVCC
Richlands, VA 24641
Prgm Dir: Joseph S DiPietro, MS RRT
Tel: 540 964-2555   *Fax:* 540 964-9307
Med Dir: John R Forehand, MD
Begins: Aug
Length: 15 mos, 7 mos   *Award:* Dipl,Cert
Tuition per yr: $2,552 res, $8,410 non-res

J Sargeant Reynolds Community College
Respiratory Therapy Tech Prgm
PO Box 85622
Richmond, VA 23285-5622
Prgm Dir: Donald K O'Donahue, RRT
Tel: 804 786-1375
Med Dir: Clifton L Parker, MD
Class Cap: 36   *Begins:* Aug
Length: 16 mos   *Award:* AAS
Tuition per yr: $3,447 res, $11,211 non-res
Evening or weekend classes available

Tidewater Community College
Respiratory Therapy Tech Prgm
1700 College Crescent
Virginia Beach, VA 23456
Prgm Dir: Barry S Anderson, MBA RRT
Tel: 804 427-7263   *Fax:* 804 427-1338
E-mail: tcandeb%vccscent.bitnet@vtbit.cc.vt.edu
Med Dir: Ignacio Ripoll, MD
Class Cap: 25   *Begins:* May
Length: 12 mos   *Award:* Cert
Tuition per yr: $2,069 res, $6,532 non-res

Washington

Tacoma Community College
Respiratory Therapy Tech Prgm
5900 S 12th St Bldg 19
Tacoma, WA 98465
Prgm Dir: Bill M Leffler, BA RRT
Tel: 206 566-5163   *Fax:* 206 566-5273
E-mail: bleffler@tcc.tacoma.ctc.edu
Med Dir: James R Taylor, MD
Class Cap: 20   *Begins:* Jun
Length: 15 mos   *Award:* Cert
Tuition per yr: $1,800 res, $7,060 non-res

West Virginia

Carver Career & Tech Education Center
Respiratory Therapy Tech Prgm
4799 Midland Dr
Charleston, WV 25306
Prgm Dir: Kym Chaffin, RRT
Tel: 304 348-1965   *Fax:* 304 348-1965
E-mail: kchaffin@access.klz.wv.us
Med Dir: Mahendra Patel, MD
Class Cap: 25   *Begins:* Aug
Length: 11 mos   *Award:* Cert
Tuition per yr: $1,530 res, $1,530 non-res
Evening or weekend classes available

Wyoming

Western Wyoming Community College
Respiratory Therapy Tech Prgm
2500 College Dr
PO Box 428
Rock Springs, WY 82901-0428
Prgm Dir: Bruce W Robinson, RRT
Tel: 307 382-1799   *Fax:* 307 382-7665
Med Dir: John Guicheteau, MD
Class Cap: 15   *Begins:* Aug
Length: 24 mos, 24 mos   *Award:* Cert, AAS
Tuition per yr: $1,022 res, $2,670 non-res
Evening or weekend classes available

Programs

Surgical Technologist

History

The profession of surgical technology was developed during World War II when there was a critical need for assistance in performing surgical procedures and a shortage of qualified personnel to meet that need. Individuals were educated specifically to assist in surgical procedures and to function in the operative theater.

The Association of Surgical Technologists (AST) was organized in July 1969, with an advisory board of representatives from the American College of Surgeons (ACS), the Association of Operating Room Nurses (AORN), the American Hospital Association (AHA), and the American Medical Association (AMA).

In December 1972, the AMA's Council on Medical Education (CME) adopted the recommended educational standards for this field, and the Accreditation Review Committee on Education in Surgical Technology (ARC-ST) was formed. The ARC-ST is jointly sponsored by the AST, ACS, and AHA, in collaboration with the AMA.

The accreditation policies and processes of the ARC-ST comply with the standards for nationally recognized agencies established by the US Department of Education and the Commission on Recognition of Postsecondary Accreditation.

Occupational Description

Surgical technologists are health professionals who are an integral part of the team of medical practitioners providing surgical care to patients in a variety of settings.

Job Description

Surgical technologists prepare the operating room by selecting and opening sterile supplies. Preoperative duties also include assembling, adjusting, and checking nonsterile equipment to ensure that it is in proper working order. Common duties include operating sterilizers, lights, suction machines, electrosurgical units, and diagnostic equipment.

When patients arrive in the surgical suite, surgical technologists assist in preparing them for surgery by providing physical and emotional support, checking charts, and observing vital signs. They have been educated to properly position the patient on the operating table, assist in connecting and applying surgical equipment and/or monitoring devices, and prepare the incision site. Surgical technologists have primary responsibility for maintaining the sterile field, being constantly vigilant that all members of the team adhere to aseptic technique.

They most often function as the sterile member of the surgical team who passes instruments, sutures, and sponges during surgery. After "scrubbing," they don gown and gloves and prepare the sterile setup for the appropriate procedure. After other members of the sterile team have scrubbed, they assist them with gowning and gloving and with the application of sterile drapes that isolate the operative site.

In order that surgery may proceed smoothly, surgical technologists anticipate the needs of surgeons, passing instruments and providing sterile items in an efficient manner. They share with the circulator the responsibility for accounting for sponges, needles, and instruments before, during, and after surgery.

Surgical technologists may hold retractors or instruments, sponge or suction the operative site, or cut suture materials as directed by the surgeon. They connect drains and tubing and receive and prepare specimens for subsequent pathologic analysis. They are responsible for preparing and applying sterile dressings following the procedure and may assist in the application of nonsterile dressings, including plaster or synthetic casting materials. After surgery, they prepare the operating room for the next patient.

Surgical technologists are most often members of the sterile team but may function in the nonsterile role of circulator. The circulator is not gowned and gloved during the surgical procedure but is available to respond to the needs of the individual providing anesthesia, keep a written account of the surgical procedure, and participate jointly with the scrubbed person in counting sponges, needles, and instruments before, during, and after surgery. In operating rooms where local anesthetics are administered, they meet the needs of the conscious patient.

Certified surgical technologists with additional specialized education or training also may act in the role of the surgical first assistant. The surgical first assistant provides aid in exposure, hemostasis, and other technical functions under the surgeon's direction that will help the surgeon carry out a safe operation with optimal results for the patient.

Surgical technologists also may provide staffing in postoperative recovery rooms where patients' responses are carefully monitored in the critical phases following general anesthesia.

Employment Characteristics

A majority of surgical technologists work in hospitals, principally in the surgical suite and also in emergency rooms and other settings that call for knowledge of, and ability in, maintaining asepsis, such as materials management and central service. A number work in a wide variety of settings and arrangements, including outpatient surgicenters, private employment by physicians, or as self-employed technologists.

Those who work in hospital and other institutional settings are usually expected to work rotating shifts or to accommodate on-call assignments to ensure adequate staffing for emergency surgical procedures during evening, night, weekend, and holiday hours. Otherwise, surgical technologists follow a standard hospital workday.

Salaries vary depending on the experience and education of the individual, the economy of a given region, the responsibilities of the position, and the working hours.

According to the AST, salaries for certified surgical technologists average $22,786 per year.

Job Outlook

According to a recent study conducted by the US Bureau of Labor Statistics, the forecast for employment opportunities for surgical technologists is one of rapid growth. Demand for technologists varies among communities and geographic regions. Prospective students are advised to assess the market for graduates within the region in which they would like to work before matriculating in an educational program. Such information is likely to be available through local employment offices, local accredited programs, and hospital councils or hospitals.

Educational Programs

Length. Programs vary from 9 to 24 months.

Prerequisites. High school diploma or equivalent.

Curriculum. Accreditation standards require didactic instruction and supervised clinical practice. Subject areas include medical terminology, professional ethics, and legal aspects of surgical patient care; anatomy and physiology, microbiology, anesthesia, and pharmacology; sterilization methods and aseptic technique; instruments, supplies, and equipment used in surgery; surgical patient care and safety precautions; and operative procedures. Supervised clinical practice in the operating room must include commonly performed procedures in general surgery, obstetrics and gynecology, ophthalmology, otorhinolaryngology, plastic surgery, urology, orthopedics, neurosurgery, thoracic surgery, and cardiovascular and peripheral vascular surgery.

Standards. *Standards* are minimum education standards adopted by the four collaborating organizations. Each new program is assessed in accordance with the *Standards*. Accredited programs are reviewed at least every sixth year to determine whether they remain in substantial compliance. The *Standards and Guidelines* are available on written request from the ARC-ST.

Inquiries

Accreditation

Requests for information on program accreditation, including *Standards*, preparing the self-study report, and arranging a site visit, should be submitted to

Accreditation Review Committee on Education
   in Surgical Technology (ARC-ST)
7108-C S Alton Way/Ste 150
Englewood, CO 80112
303 694-9262

Careers

Inquiries regarding careers and curriculum should be addressed to

Association of Surgical Technologists
7108-C S Alton Way/Ste 100
Englewood, CO 80112-2106
800 637-7433
303 741-3655 Fax

Certification/Registration

Inquiries regarding certification as a certified surgical technologist (CST) or a CST certified first assistant (CST/CFA) may be addressed to

Liaison Council on Certification for the Surgical Technologist
7790 E Arapahoe Rd/Ste 240
Englewood, CO 80112-1274
800 707-0057

Surgical Technologist

Arkansas

Westark Community College

Surgical Technologist Prgm
PO Box 3649
Ft Smith, AR 72913
Prgm Dir: Carrie Mullens, ST LPN
Tel: 501 788-7855   *Fax:* 501 788-7869
Class Cap: 18   *Begins:* Aug
Length: 9 mo , 18 mos   *Award:* Cert, AAS
Tuition per yr: $1,100 res, $1,860 non-res
Evening or weekend classes available

Univ of Arkansas for Medical Sciences

Surgical Technologist Prgm
2200 Fort Roots Dr
Slot 14B/NLR
North Little Rock, AR 72114-1706
Prgm Dir: Cindy Crumb, MEd RN BSN CNOR
Tel: 501 661-1202   *Fax:* 501 370-6691
E-mail: cdbagwell@chrp.uam.edu
Med Dir: Raymond C Read, MD
Class Cap: 20   *Begins:* Aug
Length: 10 mos, 20 mos   *Award:* Cert, AS
Tuition per yr: $2,275 res, $5,688 non-res

California

Hospital Consortium Education Network

Surgical Technologist Prgm
1600 Trousdale Dr
Burlingame, CA 94010
Prgm Dir: Alice Erskine, RN CST CNOR
Tel: 415 696-7872   *Fax:* 415 696-7864
Class Cap: 20   *Begins:* Sep
Length: 10 mos, 24 mos   *Award:* Cert, AS
Tuition per yr: $3,800

Southwestern College

Surgical Technologist Prgm
900 Otay Lakes Rd
Chula Vista, CA 91910
Prgm Dir: Terry Davis, BS MHA
Tel: 619 421-6700   *Fax:* 619 482-6439
Med Dir: Jon Grief, DO
Class Cap: 35   *Begins:* Aug
Length: 12 mos, 24 mos   *Award:* Dipl,Cert, AS
Tuition per yr: $340

Loma Linda University

Surgical Technologist Prgm
Nichol Hall Rm 1926
Loma Linda, CA 92350
Prgm Dir: Elizabeth Dickenson, RN MPH
Tel: 909 824-4932   *Fax:* 909 824-4701
Class Cap: 25   *Begins:* Sep
Length: 24 mos   *Award:* AS
Tuition per yr: $11,000 res, $11,000 non-res

Programs

California Paramedical & Tech College
Surgical Technologist Prgm
3745 Long Beach Blvd
Long Beach, CA 90807
Prgm Dir: Keith R Orloff, AA CST
Tel: 310 595-6630 *Fax:* 310 427-2920
Class Cap: 25 *Begins:* Jan May Sep
Length: 12 mos *Award:* Dipl
Tuition per yr: $11,995

ConCorde Career Institute
Surgical Technologist Prgm
4150 Lankershim Blvd
North Hollywood, CA 91602
Prgm Dir: Arthur C Martinez Jr, CST CSMM
Tel: 818 766-8151, Ext 122 *Fax:* 818 766-0833
E-mail: amartinez@aol.com
Class Cap: 110 *Begins:* Feb July Aug Dec
Length: 11 mos *Award:* Dipl
Tuition per yr: $10,995 res, $10,995 non-res

Naval School of Hlth Sciences - San Diego
Surgical Technologist Prgm
San Diego, CA 92134-5291
Prgm Dir: Deborah S McCain
Tel: 619 532-7821
Med Dir: CDR Charles Landon, MD
Class Cap: 30 *Begins:* Oct Jan Apr Jul
Length: 6 mos *Award:* Cert

Simi Valley Adult School & Career Institute
Surgical Technologist Prgm
3192 Los Angeles Ave
Simi Valley, CA 93065
Prgm Dir: Ronald O Kruzel, CST
Tel: 805 579-6200 *Fax:* 805 522-8902
Class Cap: 22 *Begins:* Sep
Length: 12 mos *Award:* Dipl
Tuition per yr: $1,600
Evening or weekend classes available

Colorado

Community Coll of Denver - Auraria Campus
Surgical Technologist Prgm
1111 W Colfax Ave
Denver, CO 80204
Prgm Dir: Mary L Centa, RN BA CNOR
Tel: 303 556-2464 *Fax:* 303 556-4583
E-mail: cd_mary@mash.colorado.edu
Class Cap: 20 *Begins:* Jun
Length: 12 mos *Award:* Cert
Tuition per yr: $2,063 res, $7,680 non-res
Evening or weekend classes available

ConCorde Career Institute
Surgical Technologist Prgm
770 Grant St
Denver, CO 80203
Prgm Dir: Christine Moran, CST AD
Tel: 303 861-1151 *Fax:* 303 839-5478
Class Cap: 36 *Begins:* Jan Jul
Length: 14 mos *Award:* Dipl
Tuition per yr: $10,998

Pueblo Community College
Surgical Technologist Prgm
900 W Orman Ave
Pueblo, CO 81004
Prgm Dir: Bonnie J Powell, BSN RN
Tel: 719 549-3279 *Fax:* 719 549-3136
E-mail: powell_b@pcc.colorado.edu
Class Cap: 15 *Begins:* Aug
Length: 11 mos *Award:* Cert
Tuition per yr: $2,635 res, $11,008 non-res
Evening or weekend classes available

Connecticut

Danbury Hospital
Surgical Technologist Prgm
24 Hospital Ave
Danbury, CT 06810
Prgm Dir: Mary E Janell, MS RN
Tel: 203 797-7724 *Fax:* 203 731-8602
Med Dir: John DeFrance, MD
Class Cap: 11 *Begins:* Sep
Length: 12 mos *Award:* Dipl
Tuition per yr: $2,400 res, $2,400 non-res

Manchester Community - Technical College
Surgical Technologist Prgm
MS 19/PO Box 1046
Manchester, CT 06040
Prgm Dir: Judith T Parmelee, PhD RN
Tel: 860 647-6186 *Fax:* 860 647-6214
E-mail: ma_parmelee@commnet.edu
Med Dir: David Crombie, MD
Class Cap: 20 *Begins:* Sep
Length: 21 mos *Award:* AS
Tuition per yr: $1,722 res, $4,842 non-res
Evening or weekend classes available

Florida

Daytona Beach Community College
Surgical Technologist Prgm
PO Box 2811
Daytona Beach, FL 32120
Prgm Dir: Marilyn A Hunter, RN CNOR
Tel: 904 255-8131 *Fax:* 904 254-4491
Class Cap: 15 *Begins:* Aug
Length: 10 mos *Award:* Cert
Tuition per yr: $1,058 res, $3,621 non-res

Traviss Technical Center
Surgical Technologist Prgm
3225 Winter Lake Rd
Lakeland, FL 33803
Prgm Dir: Susan Bogel, RN BSN
Tel: 941 499-2700 *Fax:* 941 499-2706
Class Cap: 12 *Begins:* Aug
Length: 1 mos *Award:* Cert
Tuition per yr: $765 res, $1,345 non-res
Evening or weekend classes available

Lindsey Hopkins Tech Education Center
Surgical Technologist Prgm
750 NW 20th St
Miami, FL 33127
Prgm Dir: Ibia Bustelo, RN
Tel: 305 324-6070 *Fax:* 305 326-1408
Class Cap: 16 *Begins:* Aug
Length: 12 mos *Award:* Cert
Tuition per yr: $600 res, $4,131 non-res

Central Florida Community College
Surgical Technologist Prgm
PO Box 1388
3001 SW College Rd
Ocala, FL 34474
Prgm Dir: Brenda Frazier, MEd RN CNOR
Tel: 352 237-2111, Ext 271 *Fax:* 352 854-2322
Class Cap: 16 *Begins:* Aug
Length: 10.5 mos *Award:* Cert
Tuition per yr: $1,188 res, $3,299 non-res
Evening or weekend classes available

Orlando Technical Education Centers
Surgical Technologist Prgm
301 W Amelia St
Orlando, FL 32801
Prgm Dir: Betty Arnett, RMA CST
Tel: 407 246-7060, Ext 4887 *Fax:* 407 317-3372
E-mail: wyvetts@aol.com
Begins: Jul Aug
Length: 12 mos *Award:* Dipl
Evening or weekend classes available

David G Erwin Technical Center
Surgical Technologist Prgm
2010 E Hillsborough Ave
Tampa, FL 33610-8299
Prgm Dir: Deborah Pearson, CST CRCST
Tel: 813 231-1800 *Fax:* 813 231-1820
Class Cap: 48 *Begins:* Oct Jun
Length: 12 mos *Award:* Dipl
Tuition per yr: $585 res, $4,329 non-res
Evening or weekend classes available

Georgia

Albany Technical Institute
Surgical Technologist Prgm
1021 Lowe Rd
Albany, GA 31708
Prgm Dir: Dana Higginbotham, CST
Tel: 912 430-3552 *Fax:* 912 430-5115
Class Cap: 30 *Begins:* Oct
Length: 12 mos *Award:* Dipl
Tuition per yr: $1,410 res, $2,820 non-res

Athens Area Technical Institute
Surgical Technologist Prgm
US Hwy 29N
Athens, GA 30610
Prgm Dir: Beth Jackson
Tel: 706 355-5069 *Fax:* 706 369-5753
Med Dir: Steve Shirley, MD
Class Cap: 15 *Begins:* Sep
Length: 15 mos *Award:* Dipl
Tuition per yr: $1,132 res, $2,264 non-res
Evening or weekend classes available

Augusta Technical Institute
Surgical Technologist Prgm
3116 Deans Bridge Rd
900 Bldg
Augusta, GA 30906
Prgm Dir: Helene Thomas, BSN CNOR
Tel: 706 771-4191 *Fax:* 706 771-4181
E-mail: hthomas@adminl.augusta.tec.ga.us
Med Dir: Thomas Howdie Shell, MD
Class Cap: 15 *Begins:* Jul
Length: 15 mos *Award:* Dipl
Tuition per yr: $1,130

De Kalb Technical Institute
Surgical Technologist Prgm
495 N Indian Creek Dr
Clarkston, GA 30021
Prgm Dir: Carolyn R Stone, RN, CNOR
Tel: 404 297-9522   *Fax:* 404 294-4234
Class Cap: 20   *Begins:* Jul
Length: 15 mos   *Award:* Dipl
Tuition per yr: $1,260 res, $2,520 non-res
Evening or weekend classes available

Savannah Technical Institute
Surgical Technologist Prgm
5717 White Bluff Rd
Savannah, GA 31499
Prgm Dir: Emily H Boegli, MA RN
Tel: 912 351-4564   *Fax:* 912 352-4362
Class Cap: 30   *Begins:* Jul
Length: 15 mos   *Award:* Dipl, AAT
Tuition per yr: $1,104 res, $2,112 non-res
Evening or weekend classes available

Thomas Technical Institute
Surgical Technologist Prgm
15689 US Hwy 19 N
Thomasville, GA 31792
Prgm Dir: Sherrie Holliman, ADN RN CNOR
  RNFA
Tel: 912 225-4078   *Fax:* 912 225-5289
E-mail: cooksey@aol.com
Class Cap: 12   *Begins:* Sep
Length: 15 mos   *Award:* Dipl
Tuition per yr: $1,104 res, $2,208 non-res
Evening or weekend classes available

Okefenokee Technical Institute
Surgical Technologist Prgm
1701 Carswell Ave
Waycross, GA 31501
Prgm Dir: Sally M Smith, RN
Tel: 912 287-6584   *Fax:* 912 287-4865
E-mail: sally@admin1.tech.ga.us
Med Dir: Michael O'Connell, MD
Class Cap: 16   *Begins:* Jul
Length: 15 mos   *Award:* Dipl
Tuition per yr: $1,377
Evening or weekend classes available

Idaho

Boise State University
Surgical Technologist Prgm
College of Technology
Boise State University
Boise, ID 83725
Prgm Dir: Sandra Schorzman, RN BSN
Tel: 208 385-1519   *Fax:* 208 385-3155
E-mail: sschorz@bsuidbsu.edu
Class Cap: 16   *Begins:* Aug
Length: 9 mos   *Award:* Cert
Tuition per yr: $2,504 res, $7,450 non-res

Illinois

Parkland College
Surgical Technologist Prgm
2400 W Bradley Ave
Champaign, IL 61821
Prgm Dir: Jody Randolph, BSN RN
Tel: 217 351-2375
E-mail: jrandolph@parkbnd.cc.ilus
Class Cap: 18   *Begins:* Aug
Length: 11 mos   *Award:* Cert
Tuition per yr: $1,755 res, $5,698 non-res
Evening or weekend classes available

Malcolm X College
Surgical Technologist Prgm
1900 W Van Buren
Chicago, IL 60612
Prgm Dir: Lacy Brown, CST
Tel: 312 850-7381   *Fax:* 312 850-7056
Med Dir: Keith O Roper, MD
Class Cap: 12   *Begins:* Sep
Length: 12 mos   *Award:* Cert
Tuition per yr: $3,600

Elgin Community College
Surgical Technologist Prgm
1700 Spartan Dr
Elgin, IL 60123
Prgm Dir: Maureen Lange, RNC MS CNOR
Tel: 847 697-1000
Class Cap: 24   *Begins:* Jan
Length: 12 mos   *Award:* Cert
Tuition per yr: $1,560 res, $6,357 non-res
Evening or weekend classes available

Trinity Medical Center
Surgical Technologist Prgm
Trinity School East Campus
501 Tenth Ave
Moline, IL 61265
Prgm Dir: Mary Smith, BSN RN
Tel: 309 757-3450   *Fax:* 309 757-2194
Class Cap: 10   *Begins:* July
Length: 10 mos   *Award:* Cert
Tuition per yr: $2,960
Evening or weekend classes available

Illinois Central College
Surgical Technologist Prgm
Career Education Div
Peoria, IL 61635-0001
Prgm Dir: Ruth Ann Briggs, MSN RN
Tel: 309 999-4673   *Fax:* 309 673-9626
Class Cap: 13   *Begins:* Aug
Length: 12 mos   *Award:* Cert
Tuition per yr: $1,715

Triton College
Surgical Technologist Prgm
2000 N Fifth Ave
River Grove, IL 60171
Prgm Dir: Judith A Bohn
Tel: 708 456-0300   *Fax:* 708 583-3121
Class Cap: 40   *Begins:* Sep
Length: 11 mos   *Award:* Cert
Tuition per yr: $1,634 res, $4,816 non-res
Evening or weekend classes available

College of DuPage
Surgical Technologist Prgm
550 Washington St
West Chicago, IL 60185
Prgm Dir: Dorothy Caracciolo, CST CFA
Tel: 630 293-4115   *Fax:* 630 293-4129
Med Dir: Eddie Joe Reddick, MD
Class Cap: 30   *Begins:* Jan
Length: 12 mos   *Award:* Dipl
Tuition per yr: $3,300

Indiana

Bloomington Hospital
Surgical Technologist Prgm
PO Box 1149
Bloomington, IN 47402
Prgm Dir: Marilyn Bourke, CST RN BSN
Tel: 812 335-5571
Class Cap: 12   *Begins:* Feb
Length: 11 mos   *Award:* Cert
Tuition per yr: $3,850

Ivy Tech State Coll SW - Evansville
Surgical Technologist Prgm
3501 First Ave
Evansville, IN 47710
Prgm Dir: Roma A Leach
Tel: 812 429-1490   *Fax:* 812 429-1483
Class Cap: 34   *Begins:* Aug
Length: 24 mos   *Award:* AAS
Tuition per yr: $1,811 res, $3,309 non-res
Evening or weekend classes available

Lutheran College of Health Professions
Surgical Technologist Prgm
3024 Fairfield Ave
Fort Wayne, IN 46807-1697
Prgm Dir: Elizabeth Slagle, MS RN
Tel: 219 458-2392
Class Cap: 22   *Begins:* Aug
Length: 18 mos   *Award:* AS
Tuition per yr: $5,920 res, $5,920 non-res
Evening or weekend classes available

Ivy Tech State Coll - Indianapolis
Surgical Technologist Prgm
Central Indiana Region
One W 26th St/PO Box 1763
Indianapolis, IN 46206-1763
Prgm Dir: Wanda L Haver
Tel: 317 921-4404
Med Dir: Richard Eisenhut, MD
Class Cap: 21   *Begins:* Aug
Length: 24 mos   *Award:* AAS
Tuition per yr: $2,766 res, $5,032 non-res

Ivy Tech State Coll - Lafayette
Surgical Technologist Prgm
3101 S Creasy Ln
PO Box 6299
Lafayette, IN 47903
Prgm Dir: Dorothy S Hall, BSN AAS
Tel: 317 772-9208   *Fax:* 317 772-9107
Class Cap: 40   *Begins:* Aug
Length: 24 mos   *Award:* AAS
Tuition per yr: $1,817 res, $3,309 non-res
Evening or weekend classes available

Programs

Ivy Tech State Coll - Valparaiso

Surgical Technologist Prgm
2401 Valley Dr
Valparaiso, IN 46383
Prgm Dir: Lora Plank, RN CNOR CST
Tel: 219 464-8514 *Fax:* 219 464-9751
Med Dir: Nicholas Retson, PhD
Class Cap: 25 *Begins:* Aug
Length: 24 mos *Award:* Cert, AAS
Tuition per yr: $1,817 res, $3,309 non-res

Vincennes University

Surgical Technologist Prgm
1002 N First St
WAB-1
Vincennes, IN 47591
Prgm Dir: Chris Keegan, CST MS
Tel: 812 888-5893 *Fax:* 812 888-4550
E-mail: ckeegan@vunet.vinu.edu
Class Cap: 20 *Begins:* Aug
Length: 11 mos, 24 mos *Award:* Cert, AS
Tuition per yr: $3,108 res, $7,520 non-res
Evening or weekend classes available

Iowa

Marshalltown Community College

Surgical Technologist Prgm
3700 S Ctr St
Marshalltown, IA 50158
Prgm Dir: Kathryne Balmer, CST
Tel: 515 752-7106 *Fax:* 515 754-1445
Class Cap: 25 *Begins:* Aug
Length: 11 mos, 24 mos *Award:* Dipl, AAS
Tuition per yr: $2,271 res, $5,742 non-res
Evening or weekend classes available

Western Iowa Tech Community College

Surgical Technologist Prgm
4647 Stone Ave
Po Box 265
Sioux City, IA 51102-0265
Prgm Dir: Beverly A Baker, DA CST
Tel: 712 274-6400 *Fax:* 712 274-6412
Class Cap: 20 *Begins:* Aug Jan
Length: 9 mos *Award:* Dipl
Tuition per yr: $1,643 res, $3,410 non-res
Evening or weekend classes available

Kansas

Wichita Area Technical College

Surgical Technologist Prgm
324 N Emporia
Wichita, KS 67202
Prgm Dir: Aven Cumbie, RN
Tel: 316 833-4370 *Fax:* 316 833-4332
Class Cap: 20 *Begins:* Aug
Length: 10 mos, 24 mos *Award:* Dipl, AAS
Tuition per yr: $1,082 res, $7,200 non-res

Kentucky

Kentucky Tech - Ashland Campus

Surgical Technologist Prgm
4818 Roberts Dr
Ashland, KY 41102-9046
Prgm Dir: Kay Swartzwelder, RN BSN CNOR
Tel: 606 928-6427
Class Cap: 15 *Begins:* April
Length: 11 mos *Award:* Dipl
Tuition per yr: $600 res, $1,200 non-res

Bowling Green State Voc Tech School

Surgical Technologist Prgm
1845 Loop Dr
Bowling Green, KY 42101
Prgm Dir: Linda Kinser, RN
Tel: 502 843-5461 Fax: 502 746-7466
Med Dir: William Daniel, MD
Class Cap: 15 *Begins:* Aug
Length: 11 mos *Award:* Dipl
Tuition per yr: $600 res, $1,200 non-res

Kentucky Tech Central Campus

Surgical Technologist Prgm
104 Vo-Tech Rd
Lexington, KY 40501
Prgm Dir: Robert A Goodwin, CST/CFA BA
Tel: 606 246-2400 *Fax:* 606 246-2504
Class Cap: 30 *Begins:* Aug
Length: 11 mos, 15 mos *Award:* Dipl
Tuition per yr: $600 res, $1,200 non-res
Evening or weekend classes available

Madisonville Health Technology Center

Surgical Technologist Prgm
750 Laffoon St
Madisonville, KY 42431
Prgm Dir: Teresa Vincent, RN
Tel: 502 824-7552 *Fax:* 502 824-7069
Med Dir: Jack L Hamman, MD
Class Cap: 12 *Begins:* Aug
Length: 11 mos *Award:* Dipl
Tuition per yr: $600 res, $1,200 non-res

Kentucky Tech - Owensboro Campus

Surgical Technologist Prgm
1501 Frederica St
Owensboro, KY 42301
Prgm Dir: Linda Kemp, RN
Tel: 502 686-3255 *Fax:* 502 687-7223
Class Cap: 12 *Begins:* Aug
Length: 11 mos *Award:* Dipl
Tuition per yr: $500 res, $1,000 non-res

West Kentucky Tech

Surgical Technologist Prgm
Blandville Rd
PO Box 7408
Paducah, KY 42001
Prgm Dir: Ruth Taylor, RN
Tel: 502 554-6291
Med Dir: William G Wheeler II, MD
Class Cap: 12 *Begins:* Aug
Length: 11 mos *Award:* Dipl
Tuition per yr: $600 res, $1,200 non-res

Cumberland Valley Health Technology Ctr

Surgical Technologist Prgm
US 25E S
PO Box 187
Pineville, KY 40977
Prgm Dir: Roberta Dean, BS
Tel: 606 337-3106 *Fax:* 606 337-5662
Med Dir: Talmadge V Hays
Class Cap: 12 *Begins:* Aug
Length: 11 mos *Award:* Cert
Tuition per yr: $600 res, $1,200 non-res
Evening or weekend classes available

Louisiana

Our Lady of the Lake Coll

Surgical Technologist Prgm
5345 Brittany
Baton Rouge, LA 70808
Prgm Dir: Lydia Arriaga, RH BSN CNOR
Tel: 504 768-1750 *Fax:* 504 768-1726
E-mail: larriaga@ololcollege.cc.la.us
Class Cap: 12 *Begins:* Jan
Length: 12 mos, 24 mos *Award:* Cert, AS
Tuition per yr: $2,005
Evening or weekend classes available

Alton Ochsner Medical Foundation

Surgical Technologist Prgm
1516 Jefferson Hwy
New Orleans, LA 70123-3335
Prgm Dir: Susan H Austin, CST
Tel: 504 842-3267
Med Dir: Martha B Roach, MD
Class Cap: 6 *Begins:* Jul
Length: 12 mos *Award:* Cert

Delgado Community College

Surgical Technologist Prgm
615 City Park Ave
New Orleans, LA 70119-4399
Prgm Dir: Carolyn Polk Bowman, BSN RN MA
Tel: 504 568-6559 *Fax:* 504 568-5494
Med Dir: M Naraghi, MD
Class Cap: 50 *Begins:* Jan Aug
Length: 14 mos *Award:* Cert
Tuition per yr: $1,518 res, $3,168 non-res

Maine

Southern Maine Tech Coll/Maine Med Ctr

Surgical Technologist Prgm
School of Surgical Technology
SMTC Fort Road
Portland, ME 04106
Prgm Dir: Diane A Dussault, RN
Tel: 207 767-9589 *Fax:* 207 767-9690
Class Cap: 18 *Begins:* Mar Sep
Length: 12 mos *Award:* Dipl
Tuition per yr: $2,500

Maryland

Naval School of Health Sciences - MD
Surgical Technologist Prgm
Bethesda, MD 20889-5611
Prgm Dir: Kathryn Cadwell, CDR NC USN
Tel: 301 295-1399 *Fax:* 301 295-0621
E-mail: kcadwell@nsh20.mnavy.mi
Class Cap: 32 *Begins:* Jul Oct Feb Jun
Length: 6 mos *Award:* Cert

Massachusetts

Quincy College
Surgical Technologist Prgm
Sch of Allied Hlth
50 Saville Ave
Quincy, MA 02169
Prgm Dir: Meryl Lemeshow, RN
Tel: 617 984-1718 *Fax:* 617 984-1792
Class Cap: 50 *Begins:* Sep
Length: 9 mos *Award:* Cert
Tuition per yr: $3,600

Springfield Technical Community College
Surgical Technologist Prgm
One Armory Square
Springfield, MA 01105
Prgm Dir: Kathleen T Flynn, MS RN
Tel: 413 781-7822
Class Cap: 25 *Begins:* Sep
Length: 16 mos *Award:* AS
Tuition per yr: $1,320 res, $16,204 non-res
Evening or weekend classes available

Worcester Technical Institute
Surgical Technologist Prgm
251 Belmont St
Worcester, MA 01605
Tel: 508 799-1945 *Fax:* 508 799-1932
Class Cap: 14 *Begins:* Aug
Length: 9 mos *Award:* Dipl
Tuition per yr: $1,600 res, $3,000 non-res

Michigan

Highland Park Community College
Surgical Technologist Prgm
Glendale at Third
Highland Park, MI 48203
Prgm Dir: Beatrice M Franklin, MEd CST
Tel: 313 252-0475
Class Cap: 30 *Begins:* Aug Jan
Length: 12 mos, 18 mos *Award:* Cert, AAS
Tuition per yr: $2,265

Baker College of Muskegon
Surgical Technologist Prgm
123 Apple Ave
Muskegon, MI 49442
Prgm Dir: Ruth Deters, RN CHOR CST
Tel: 616 726-4904 *Fax:* 616 728-4417
E-mail: deters_4@muskegon.baker.edu
Class Cap: 15 *Begins:* Sep Jan Mar June
Length: 18 mos *Award:* AAS
Tuition per yr: $6,240
Evening or weekend classes available

Delta College
Surgical Technologist Prgm
University Center, MI 48710
Prgm Dir: Margrethe May, MS CST
Tel: 517 686-9505 *Fax:* 517 686-8736
Class Cap: 15 *Begins:* Aug
Length: 16 mos, 16 mos *Award:* Cert, AAS
Tuition per yr: $1,774 res, $2,310 non-res
Evening or weekend classes available

Minnesota

Anoka-Hennepin Technical College
Surgical Technologist Prgm
1355 W Hwy 10
Anoka, MN 55303
Prgm Dir: Rita M Schutz, RN
Tel: 612 576-4974 *Fax:* 612 576-4715
E-mail: @amk.tec.mn.us
Class Cap: 45 *Begins:* Sep
Length: 12 mos *Award:* Dipl
Tuition per yr: $2,963 res, $5,926 non-res

Northwest Technical Coll - E Grand Forks
Surgical Technologist Prgm
Hwy 220 N
East Grand Forks, MN 56721
Prgm Dir: Beverly Wirth, RN
Tel: 218 773-3441 *Fax:* 218 773-4502
E-mail: wirth@adm.egf.tec.mn.us
Class Cap: 36 *Begins:* Sep
Length: 11 mos, 20 mos *Award:* Dipl, AAS
Tuition per yr: $2,108 res, $4,216 non-res

Rochester Community and Technical College
Surgical Technologist Prgm
University Center Rochester
851 30th Avenue SE
Rochester, MN 55904
Prgm Dir: Katherine Jacobson
Tel: 507 285-7143
Class Cap: 25 *Begins:* Sep
Length: 18 mos *Award:* AAS
Tuition per yr: $2,579 res, $4,826 non-res
Evening or weekend classes available

St Cloud Technical College
Surgical Technologist Prgm
1540 Northway Dr
St Cloud, MN 56301
Prgm Dir: Terry Olson, RN, MED
Tel: 320 654-5921 *Fax:* 320 654-5981
Class Cap: 24 *Begins:* Jun
Length: 12 mos *Award:* Dipl, AAS
Tuition per yr: $2,864 res, $5,522 non-res
Evening or weekend classes available

Mississippi

Hinds Community College District
Surgical Technologist Prgm
1750 Chadwick Dr
Jackson, MS 39204
Prgm Dir: Martha Thomas, BSEd RN
Tel: 601 372-6507 *Fax:* 601 371-3529
Class Cap: 26 *Begins:* Aug
Length: 12 mos *Award:* Cert
Tuition per yr: $1,425 res, $1,425 non-res

Missouri

St Louis Comm College at Forest Park
Surgical Technologist Prgm
5600 Oakland Ave
St Louis, MO 63110
Prgm Dir: Diane Gerardot, CST/CFA BA
Tel: 314 644-9340 *Fax:* 314 644-9752
Med Dir: Stan Thawley, MD
Begins: Aug
Length: 11 mos *Award:* Cert
Tuition per yr: $1,240 res, $2,080 non-res
Evening or weekend classes available

Montana

University of Montana-Missoula
Surgical Technologist Prgm
College of Technology
909 South Ave W
Missoula, MT 59801
Prgm Dir: Bobette K Pattee, BSN RN
Tel: 406 243-7860 *Fax:* 406 243-7899
Class Cap: 17 *Begins:* Aug
Length: 14 mos *Award:* Cert
Tuition per yr: $3,081 res, $6,519 non-res

Nebraska

Southeast Community College
Surgical Technologist Prgm
8800 O St
Lincoln, NE 68520
Prgm Dir: Ruth E Walsh, BS RN
Tel: 402 437-2785
Class Cap: 36 *Begins:* Mar Sep
Length: 12 mos, 18 mos *Award:* Dipl, AAS
Tuition per yr: $1,764 res, $2,088 non-res
Evening or weekend classes available

Metropolitan Community College
Surgical Technologist Prgm
PO Box 3777
Omaha, NE 68103
Prgm Dir: Catherine Kallhoff, RN
Tel: 402 449-8367 *Fax:* 402 448-8333
E-mail: ckallhof@metro.mccneb.edu
Class Cap: 22 *Begins:* Sep
Length: 15 mos *Award:* Cert
Tuition per yr: $1,691 res, $2,152 non-res
Evening or weekend classes available

New Jersey

Univ of Med & Dent of New Jersey
Surgical Technologist Prgm
Sch of Hlth Related Professions
65 Bergen St
Newark, NJ 07107-3006
Prgm Dir: Jane M Verpent, RN BA
Tel: 201 982-5311 *Fax:* 908 889-2487
Class Cap: 15 *Begins:* Sep
Length: 9 mos *Award:* Cert
Tuition per yr: $1,450 res, $2,175 non-res

Programs

Bergen Community College

Surgical Technologist Prgm
400 Paramus Rd
Paramus, NJ 07652
Prgm Dir: Joan Ann Verderame, MA RN
Tel: 201 447-7178
Class Cap: 25 *Begins:* Sep
Length: 10 mos *Award:* Cert
Tuition per yr: $2,669 res, $5,338 non-res
Evening or weekend classes available

Univ of Med & Dent of New Jersey

Surgical Technologist Prgm
160 Fries Mill Rd
Turnersville, NJ 08012
Prgm Dir: Jane M Verpent, RN BA
Tel: 908 889-2403 *Fax:* 908 889-2487
Class Cap: 15 *Begins:* Sep
Length: 9 mos *Award:* Cert
Tuition per yr: $1,450 res, $2,175 non-res

New York

Trocaire College

Surgical Technologist Prgm
110 Red Jacket Pkwy
Buffalo, NY 14220
Prgm Dir: Ann J Williams, MSN RN
Tel: 716 826-1200 *Fax:* 716 826-0059
Class Cap: 30 *Begins:* Sep
Length: 9 mo , 18 mos *Award:* Cert, AAS
Tuition per yr: $5,850

Nassau Community College

Surgical Technologist Prgm
One Education Dr
Garden City, NY 11530
Prgm Dir: Alice Jones, MS RN CNOR
Tel: 516 572-7912
Class Cap: 64 *Begins:* Sep
Length: 24 mos *Award:* AAS
Tuition per yr: $1,950 res, $3,900 non-res
Evening or weekend classes available

New York University Medical Center

Surgical Technologist Prgm
Ctr for Allied Hlth Educ
550 First Ave
New York, NY 10016
Prgm Dir: Zaida Jacoby
Tel: 212 263-5007 *Fax:* 212 263-6107
Class Cap: 25 *Begins:* Sep
Length: 12 mos *Award:* Dipl

Onondaga Community College

Surgical Technologist Prgm
4941 Onondaga Rd
Syracuse, NY 13215
Prgm Dir: Julia A Halpin, MSEd RN CNOR
Tel: 315 469-7741 *Fax:* 315 469-2593
Med Dir: Ronald A Naumann, MD
Class Cap: 24 *Begins:* Jan Aug
Length: 11 mos, 12 mos *Award:* Cert
Tuition per yr: $3,014 res, $6,028 non-res
Evening or weekend classes available

North Carolina

Carolinas College of Health Sciences

Surgical Technologist Prgm
PO Box 32861
1200 Blythe Rd
Charlotte, NC 28232-2861
Prgm Dir: Mary W Proctor, RN
Tel: 704 355-6146 *Fax:* 704 355-5967
Med Dir: Michael H Thomason, MD
Class Cap: 15 *Begins:* May
Length: 12 mos *Award:* Dipl
Tuition per yr: $3,570

Presbyterian Hospital

Surgical Technologist Prgm
PO Box 33549
Charlotte, NC 28233-3549
Prgm Dir: Marylee Sumrell, RN CNOR
Tel: 704 384-4822 *Fax:* 704 384-5839
Med Dir: E Craig Evans, MD
Class Cap: 8 *Begins:* Sep
Length: 12 mos *Award:* Cert
Tuition per yr: $2,200

Fayetteville Technical Community College

Surgical Technologist Prgm
PO Box 35236
Fayetteville, NC 28303
Prgm Dir: Rachel A Addison, BS RN
Tel: 910 678-8358
Begins: Sep
Length: 12 mos *Award:* Dipl
Tuition per yr: $729 res, $5,912 non-res

Catawba Valley Community College

Surgical Technologist Prgm
2550 Hwy 70 SE
Hickory, NC 28602
Prgm Dir: Brenda Knight-Kanipe, RN
Tel: 704 327-7000 *Fax:* 704 327-7301
Class Cap: 20 *Begins:* Sep
Length: 12 mos *Award:* Dipl
Tuition per yr: $742 res, $6,020 non-res
Evening or weekend classes available

Coastal Carolina Community College

Surgical Technologist Prgm
444 Western Blvd
Jacksonville, NC 28546-6877
Prgm Dir: Diana E Reagen, BSN RN CNOR
Tel: 910 938-6274
Class Cap: 16 *Begins:* June
Length: 12 mos *Award:* Dipl
Tuition per yr: $742 res, $6,020 non-res

Lenoir Community College

Surgical Technologist Prgm
PO Box 188
Kinston, NC 28501
Prgm Dir: Shirley H Taylor, RN
Tel: 919 527-6223 *Fax:* 919 527-1199
Class Cap: 20 *Begins:* Sep
Length: 9 mos *Award:* Dipl,Cert
Tuition per yr: $779 res, $4,545 non-res
Evening or weekend classes available

Sandhills Community College

Surgical Technologist Prgm
2200 Airport Rd
Pinehurst, NC 28374
Prgm Dir: Barbara McCullough, MEd RN CNOR
Tel: 910 695-3838 *Fax:* 910 692-2756
Class Cap: 18 *Begins:* Sep
Length: 12 mos *Award:* Dipl
Tuition per yr: $742 res, $6,020 non-res

Ohio

University of Akron

Surgical Technologist Prgm
Polsky Bldg Rm 124 H
Akron, OH 44325-3703
Prgm Dir: Melanie A Ditchey, CST CSA
Tel: 330 972-6514 *Fax:* 330 972-6952
E-mail: ditchey@vakron.edu
Class Cap: 22 *Begins:* Sep
Length: 12 mos, 24 mos *Award:* Dipl,Cert, AAS
Tuition per yr: $3,486 res, $8,686 non-res
Evening or weekend classes available

Cincinnati State Tech and Comm College

Surgical Technologist Prgm
3520 Central Pkwy
Cincinnati, OH 45223
Prgm Dir: Judith A Spraley, MEd RN
Tel: 513 569-1677 *Fax:* 513 569-1659
Class Cap: 30 *Begins:* Sep
Length: 20 mos *Award:* AAS
Tuition per yr: $3,360 res, $6,720 non-res
Evening or weekend classes available

Owens State Community College

Surgical Technologist Prgm
PO Box 10,000
Oregon Rd
Toledo, OH 43699
Prgm Dir: Elizabeth M Ream, MSN RN
Tel: 419 661-7338 *Fax:* 419 661-7665
E-mail: eream@owens.cc.oh.us
Class Cap: 20 *Begins:* Aug
Length: 20 mos *Award:* AAS
Tuition per yr: $2,370 res, $2,370 non-res
Evening or weekend classes available

Youngstown Pub Sch/Choffin Career Center

Surgical Technologist Prgm
200 E Wood St
Youngstown, OH 44501
Prgm Dir: Olivia Jones, RN CNOR
Tel: 330 744-8763
Med Dir: Janet Carpenter, RN MEd
Class Cap: 25 *Begins:* Sep
Length: 10 mos *Award:* Cert
Tuition per yr: $4,200

Oklahoma

Autry Technology Center

Surgical Technologist Prgm
1201 W Willow
Enid, OK 73703
Prgm Dir: Virginia Rodriguez, RN CST CNOR
Tel: 405 242-2750 *Fax:* 405 233-8262
Med Dir: Barry Pollard, MD
Class Cap: 10 *Begins:* Aug
Length: 11 mos *Award:* Cert
Tuition per yr: $1,185

Great Plains Area Voc Tech School
Surgical Technologist Prgm
4500 W Lee Blvd
Lawton, OK 73505
Prgm Dir: Ann Tahah, LPN
Tel: 405 355-6371 *Fax:* 405 250-5583
Class Cap: 12 *Begins:* Aug
Length: 9 mo , 1 mos *Award:* Cert
Tuition per yr: $1,000
Evening or weekend classes available

Northeastern Oklahoma A & M College
Surgical Technologist Prgm
PO Box 3907
Miami, OK 74354-6497
Prgm Dir: Judy K Hancock, BSN MS CNOR CST
Tel: 918 542-8441 *Fax:* 918 542-2680
Med Dir: Mark S Cotner, MD
Class Cap: 16 *Begins:* Jun
Length: 12 mos *Award:* Cert
Tuition per yr: $1,350

Metro Area Vocational - Technical School
Surgical Technologist Prgm
Health Careers Center
1720 Springlake Dr
Oklahoma City, OK 73111
Prgm Dir: Vicki Bushey, CST
Tel: 405 424-8324, Ext 620 *Fax:* 405 424-9403
Class Cap: 15 *Begins:* Aug
Length: 10 mos *Award:* Cert
Tuition per yr: $1,250 res, $1,250 non-res

Tulsa Technology Center
Surgical Technologist Prgm
3420 S Memorial Dr
Tulsa, OK 74145
Prgm Dir: Carol Dollar, RN
Tel: 918 627-7200 *Fax:* 918 628-1406
Class Cap: 20 *Begins:* Aug
Length: 9 mos *Award:* Cert
Tuition per yr: $330

Oregon

Mt Hood Community College
Surgical Technologist Prgm
26000 SE Stark St
Gresham, OR 97030
Prgm Dir: Jacqueline Morfitt, RN CNOR
Tel: 503 667-7179 *Fax:* 503 492-6047
Class Cap: 25 *Begins:* Sep
Length: 18 mos *Award:* AAS
Tuition per yr: $1,485 res, $4,995 non-res
Evening or weekend classes available

Pennsylvania

Mt Aloysius College
Surgical Technologist Prgm
7373 Admiral Peary Hwy
Cresson, PA 16630-1999
Prgm Dir: Clifford W Smith, RN
Tel: 814 886-6340 *Fax:* 814 886-2978
E-mail: smithcli@mtaloy.edu
Class Cap: 30 *Begins:* Jul
Length: 11 mos *Award:* Dipl
Tuition per yr: $8,360

Conemaugh Valley Memorial Hospital
Surgical Technologist Prgm
1086 Franklin St
Johnstown, PA 15905
Prgm Dir: Patricia Pavlikowski, MA CNOR
Tel: 814 534-9770 *Fax:* 814 534-3244
Med Dir: Kenneth W Rowe, MD
Class Cap: 20 *Begins:* Sep
Length: 12 mos *Award:* Cert
Tuition per yr: $2,400 res, $2,400 non-res

Lancaster Institute for Health Education
Surgical Technologist Prgm
555 N Duke St
Lancaster, PA 17604
Prgm Dir: Luanne McDonald, RN AS CNOR
Tel: 717 290-5511
Class Cap: 12 *Begins:* July
Length: 12 mos *Award:* Cert
Tuition per yr: $4,000

Delaware County Community College
Surgical Technologist Prgm
901 S Media Line Rd
Media, PA 19063-1094
Prgm Dir: Jane Rothrock, DNSc RN CNOR
Tel: 610 359-5286 *Fax:* 610 359-7350
Class Cap: 16 *Begins:* Sep
Length: 12 mos, 24 mos *Award:* Cert, AAS
Tuition per yr: $2,313 res, $4,581 non-res
Evening or weekend classes available

Comm Coll of Allegheny Cnty-Boyce Campus
Surgical Technologist Prgm
595 Beatty Rd
Monroeville, PA 15146
Prgm Dir: Mary Lou Fragale, BSN RN
Tel: 412 325-6779 *Fax:* 412 325-6799
E-mail: mfragale@ccac.edu
Class Cap: 40 *Begins:* Aug
Length: 16 mos *Award:* AAS
Tuition per yr: $2,040 res, $4,080 non-res
Evening or weekend classes available

Rhode Island

New England Institute of Technology
Surgical Technologist Prgm
2500 Post Rd
Warwick, RI 02886-2266
Prgm Dir: Jo-Ann Fielding, RN BSN
Tel: 401 739-5000 *Fax:* 401 738-5122
Class Cap: 48 *Begins:* Apr Oct
Length: 18 mos *Award:* AS
Tuition per yr: $9,200 res, $9,200 non-res

South Carolina

Tri-County Technical College
Surgical Technologist Prgm
c/o Anderson Area Medical Ctr
800 N Fant St
Anderson, SC 29621
Prgm Dir: Margaret Thomas, BS RN CNOR
Tel: 864 261-1169 *Fax:* 864 646-8256
Med Dir: Audra McPeak, MSN
Class Cap: 22 *Begins:* Aug
Length: 12 mos *Award:* Dipl
Tuition per yr: $1,350 res, $1,638 non-res
Evening or weekend classes available

Midlands Technical College
Surgical Technologist Prgm
PO Box 2408
Columbia, SC 29202
Prgm Dir: Linda Oliver, RN CNOR
Tel: 803 822-3438 *Fax:* 803 822-3079
E-mail: oliverl@mtc2.mio.tec.s.c.us
Class Cap: 21 *Begins:* Aug
Length: 12 mos *Award:* Dipl
Tuition per yr: $1,575 res, $2,776 non-res
Evening or weekend classes available

Florence-Darlington Technical College
Surgical Technologist Prgm
PO Box 100548
Florence, SC 29501-0548
Prgm Dir: Nelda S Coleman, RN CNOR
Tel: 803 662-8151 *Fax:* 803 661-8041
Class Cap: 25 *Begins:* Aug
Length: 12 mos *Award:* Dipl
Tuition per yr: $1,650 res, $1,875 non-res
Evening or weekend classes available

Greenville Technical College
Surgical Technologist Prgm
PO Box 5616
Greenville, SC 29606-8616
Prgm Dir: Patricia Caldwell, BSN RN
Tel: 864 250-8294 *Fax:* 864 250-8549
E-mail: caldwephc@gultec.edu
Class Cap: 30 *Begins:* Aug
Length: 12 mos *Award:* Dipl
Tuition per yr: $1,500 res, $1,620 non-res
Evening or weekend classes available

Spartanburg Technical College
Surgical Technologist Prgm
PO Drawer 4386
Spartanburg, SC 29305
Prgm Dir: Emily W Rogers, BS RN CNOR
Tel: 864 591-3870 *Fax:* 864 591-3708
E-mail: rogerse@spt.tec.sc.us
Class Cap: 22 *Begins:* Aug
Length: 12 mos *Award:* Dipl
Tuition per yr: $1,500 res, $1,875 non-res
Evening or weekend classes available

South Dakota

Presentation College
Surgical Technologist Prgm
1500 N Main
Aberdeen, SD 57401
Prgm Dir: Katherine C Snyder, CST
Tel: 605 229-8415 *Fax:* 605 229-8430
E-mail: ksnyder@mail.pbvm.edu
Class Cap: 14 *Begins:* Aug
Length: 18 mos *Award:* AS
Tuition per yr: $6,820

Programs

Tennessee

East Tennessee State University

Surgical Technologist Prgm
1000 West E St
ETSU Nave Center
Elizabethton, TN 37643
Prgm Dir: Alan G Ballard, PA-C
Tel: 423 547-4908   *Fax:* 423 547-4921
Med Dir: Phillip J Hinton, MD
Class Cap: 14   *Begins:* Aug
Length: 12 mos   *Award:* Cert
Tuition per yr: $2,892 res, $9,396 non-res
Evening or weekend classes available

Tennessee Technology Center - Memphis

Surgical Technologist Prgm
550 Alabama Ave
Memphis, TN 38105-3799
Prgm Dir: Paul A Holmes, CST
Tel: 901 543-6177   *Fax:* 901 543-6197
Class Cap: 30   *Begins:* Jul
Length: 12 mos   *Award:* Cert
Tuition per yr: $448

Texas

Amarillo College

Surgical Technologist Prgm
PO Box 447
Amarillo, TX 79178
Prgm Dir: Deborah Inman, MSN RN CNOR
Tel: 806 356-3663   *Fax:* 806 354-6076
E-mail: djinman@actx.edu
Class Cap: 30   *Begins:* Aug
Length: 12 mos   *Award:* Cert
Tuition per yr: $1,100

Austin Community College

Surgical Technologist Prgm
7748 Hwy 290 W
Austin, TX 78736
Prgm Dir: Kathleen Baumbach, CST RN CNOR
Tel: 512 223-8084   *Fax:* 512 288-8016
Med Dir: Tim Faulkenberry, MD
Class Cap: 21   *Begins:* Sep
Length: 24 mos   *Award:* Cert, AAS
Tuition per yr: $1,610 res, $3,080 non-res
Evening or weekend classes available

Del Mar College

Surgical Technologist Prgm
Baldwin and Ayers
Corpus Christi, TX 78404
Prgm Dir: Elena Mendieta, MS RN
Tel: 512 886-1105   *Fax:* 512 886-1598
Class Cap: 20   *Begins:* Aug
Length: 12 mos   *Award:* Cert, AAS
Tuition per yr: $676

El Centro College

Surgical Technologist Prgm
Main and Lamar Sts
Dallas, TX 75202
Prgm Dir: Cindy Calcaterra, MBA RN CNOR
Tel: 214 860-2281   *Fax:* 214 860-2268
E-mail: clc5545@dcccd.edu
Class Cap: 30   *Begins:* Aug
Length: 11 mos   *Award:* Cert
Tuition per yr: $908 res, $1,611 non-res
Evening or weekend classes available

El Paso Community College

Surgical Technologist Prgm
PO Box 20500
El Paso, TX 79998
Prgm Dir: Cynthia Rivera, RN
Tel: 915 534-4086   *Fax:* 915 534-4114
Class Cap: 12   *Begins:* Jun
Length: 24 mos   *Award:* AAS
Tuition per yr: $1,290 res, $4,303 non-res
Evening or weekend classes available

Houston Community College Central

Surgical Technologist Prgm
3100 Shenandoah
Houston, TX 77021
Prgm Dir: Vera Edwards, RN MSN
Tel: 713 718-7362   *Fax:* 713 746-5370
Class Cap: 36   *Begins:* Aug
Length: 12 mos   *Award:* Cert
Tuition per yr: $955 res, $2,650 non-res

Tarrant Junior College

Surgical Technologist Prgm
828 Harwood Rd
Hurst, TX 76054
Prgm Dir: Robin Thacker, RN CNOR CST
Tel: 817 515-6568   *Fax:* 817 515-6601
Class Cap: 24   *Begins:* Sep
Length: 11 mos   *Award:* Cert
Tuition per yr: $931 res, $1,271 non-res

Trinity Valley Community College

Surgical Technologist Prgm
Hlth Science Ctr
800 Hwy 243 W
Kaufman, TX 75142
Prgm Dir: Nancy L Couch, RN CNOR
Tel: 214 932-4309   *Fax:* 214 932-5010
Class Cap: 14   *Begins:* Aug
Length: 9 mos   *Award:* Cert
Tuition per yr: $576 res, $2,676 non-res

Kilgore College

Surgical Technologist Prgm
1100 Broadway
Kilgore, TX 75662
Prgm Dir: Lane J Barnett, RN MSN CNOR
Tel: 903 983-8163   *Fax:* 903 983-8600
Class Cap: 14   *Begins:* Jul
Length: 12 mos   *Award:* Cert
Tuition per yr: $1,104 res, $1,932 non-res
Evening or weekend classes available

South Plains College

Surgical Technologist Prgm
1302 Main St
Lubbock, TX 79401
Prgm Dir: Paul Price, CST
Tel: 806 747-0576   *Fax:* 806 765-2775
Class Cap: 40   *Begins:* Sep Jan
Length: 12 mos   *Award:* Cert
Tuition per yr: $964 res, $1,394 non-res

Odessa College

Surgical Technologist Prgm
201 W University
Odessa, TX 79764
Prgm Dir: Leola Rutledge, BSN RN
Tel: 915 335-6470   *Fax:* 915 335-6846
E-mail: irutledge@odessa.edu
Class Cap: 15   *Begins:* Aug
Length: 11 mos, 24 mos   *Award:* Cert, AAS
Tuition per yr: $1,148 res, $1,384 non-res
Evening or weekend classes available

San Jacinto College Central Campus

Surgical Technologist Prgm
8060 Spencer Hwy
PO Box 2007
Pasadena, TX 77505-2007
Prgm Dir: Diane DeYoung, MEd BS RN
Tel: 713 478-2759   *Fax:* 713 478-2754
E-mail: ddeyou@central.sjcd.cc.tx.us
Med Dir: Benny Cleveland, MD
Class Cap: 70   *Begins:* Sep Jan
Length: 10 mos   *Award:* Cert
Tuition per yr: $848

Baptist Health System Institute of Health Education

Surgical Technologist Prgm
111 Dallas St
San Antonio, TX 78205-1230
Prgm Dir: Christallia Starks, RN, CNOR
Tel: 210 302-2955   *Fax:* 210 302-3609
Med Dir: Marcus Dalkowitz, MD
Class Cap: 12   *Begins:* July
Length: 9 mos   *Award:* Cert
Tuition per yr: $2,000 res, $2,000 non-res

St Philip's College

Surgical Technologist Prgm
1801 Martin Luther King Dr
San Antonio, TX 78203-2098
Prgm Dir: Mary Leonard, RN CNOR
Tel: 210 531-3424   *Fax:* 210 531-3459
E-mail: mcoy@accd.edu
Class Cap: 26   *Begins:* Aug
Length: 12 mos   *Award:* Cert
Tuition per yr: $1,542 res, $3,500 non-res

Temple College

Surgical Technologist Prgm
2600 S First St
Temple, TX 76504
Prgm Dir: Carol A Reinking
Tel: 817 773-9961   *Fax:* 817 771-3726
Class Cap: 20   *Begins:* Aug Jan
Length: 12 mos   *Award:* Cert
Tuition per yr: $1,323 res, $1,960 non-res

882 Training Group

Surgical Technologist Prgm
383 TS/NTED
Sheppard Air Force Base
Wichita Falls, TX 76311-2262
Prgm Dir: Danny A Morgan, Maj USAF NC
Tel: 817 676-3849
Class Cap: 320   *Begins:* Bi-monthly
Length: 2 mos   *Award:* Cert

Utah

Salt Lake Community College

Surgical Technologist Prgm
PO Box 31808
Salt Lake City, UT 84130
Prgm Dir: Ray Liddell, BSN LNOR
Tel: 801 957-4161   *Fax:* 801 957-4444
E-mail: liddelra@slcc.edu
Class Cap: 25   *Begins:* Sep
Length: 9 mos   *Award:* Cert
Tuition per yr: $1,446 res, $4,202 non-res

Virginia

Riverside School of Health Occupations
Surgical Technologist Prgm
12420 Warwick Blvd
Bldg #6G
Newport News, VA 23606
Prgm Dir: Carolyn M Branson, CST RN
Tel: 804 594-2721
Class Cap: 12 *Begins:* Jan
Length: 11 mos *Award:* Cert
Tuition per yr: $1,600 res, $1,950 non-res

Sentara Norfolk General Hospital
Surgical Technologist Prgm
600 Gresham Dr
Norfolk, VA 23507
Prgm Dir: Jill Nester, RN CNOR CST
Tel: 757 668-4240 *Fax:* 757 668-2905
Class Cap: 15 *Begins:* Aug
Length: 12 mos *Award:* Cert
Tuition per yr: $2,600

Naval School of Health Sciences
Surgical Technologist Prgm
1001 Holcomb Rd
Portsmouth, VA 23708-5200
Prgm Dir: Doris J Safran, CDR NC USN
Tel: 757 398-7270 *Fax:* 757 398-5033
E-mail: pnhadijs@pnhio.med.nav.mi
Class Cap: 40 *Begins:* Jan Apr Aug
Length: 6 mos *Award:* Cert

Winchester Medical Center
Surgical Technologist Prgm
1840 Amherst St
PO Box 3340
Winchester, VA 22601
Prgm Dir: Mae S Ball, RN
Tel: 540 722-8720 *Fax:* 540 722-8973
Med Dir: Terry Sinclair, MD
Class Cap: 8 *Begins:* Jan
Length: 12 mos *Award:* Cert
Tuition per yr: $2,000
Evening or weekend classes available

Washington

Renton Technical College
Surgical Technologist Prgm
3000 NE Fourth St
Renton, WA 98056
Prgm Dir: Rosemary Thurston
Tel: 206 235-7812 *Fax:* 206 235-7832
Med Dir: Melvin Freeman, MD
Class Cap: 18 *Begins:* Sep Jan
Length: 11 mos *Award:* Cert, AAS
Tuition per yr: $2,180 res, $2,180 non-res
Evening or weekend classes available

Seattle Central Community College
Surgical Technologist Prgm
1701 Broadway
Seattle, WA 98122
Prgm Dir: Carol Denckla, RN CNOR
Tel: 206 587-6950 *Fax:* 206 344-4390
Class Cap: 25 *Begins:* Sep
Length: 9 mos *Award:* Cert
Tuition per yr: $1,379 res, $5,489 non-res
Evening or weekend classes available

Spokane Community College
Surgical Technologist Prgm
N 1810 Green St
Spokane, WA 99207
Prgm Dir: Jeannie Hurd, RN BS CNOR
Tel: 509 533-7303 *Fax:* 509 533-8621
E-mail: jhurd@ctc.edu
Med Dir: Geofrey Nunes, MD
Class Cap: 22 *Begins:* Sep
Length: 18 mos *Award:* AAS
Tuition per yr: $1,350 res, $5,298 non-res
Evening or weekend classes available

West Virginia

Monongalia County Tech Education Center
Surgical Technologist Prgm
1000 Mississippi St
Morgantown, WV 26505
Prgm Dir: Eleanor Jessen
Tel: 304 291-9240 *Fax:* 304 291-9247
Med Dir: Lynda J Overking, RN BSN
Class Cap: 20 *Begins:* Aug
Length: 9 mos *Award:* Cert
Tuition per yr: $5,070

West Virginia Northern Community College
Surgical Technologist Prgm
15th and Jacob Sts
Wheeling, WV 26003
Prgm Dir: Fritzie Grossenbacher, CST
Tel: 304 233-5900
Class Cap: 16 *Begins:* Aug
Length: 12 mos *Award:* Cert
Tuition per yr: $1,770 res, $1,770 non-res

Wisconsin

Northeast Wisconsin Technical College
Surgical Technologist Prgm
2740 W Mason St
PO Box 19042
Green Bay, WI 54307-9042
Prgm Dir: Georgia Peterson, BSN
Tel: 414 498-5430 *Fax:* 414 498-5673
Med Dir: Per R Anderas
Class Cap: 26 *Begins:* Jun
Length: 12 mos *Award:* Dipl
Tuition per yr: $2,424 res, $1,812 non-res

Gateway Technical College
Surgical Technologist Prgm
3520 30th Ave
Kenosha, WI 53142-1690
Prgm Dir: Nellie Frazee, MS RN
Tel: 414 656-6956
Class Cap: 20 *Begins:* Aug
Length: 9 mos *Award:* Dipl
Tuition per yr: $2,655 res, $2,655 non-res
Evening or weekend classes available

Western Wisconsin Technical College
Surgical Technologist Prgm
304 N Sixth St
PO Box 908
La Crosse, WI 54601
Prgm Dir: Ruth Wills, BSN RN
Tel: 608 785-9193 *Fax:* 608 785-9194
E-mail: willsr@al.western.tec.wi.us
Class Cap: 16 *Begins:* Aug
Length: 10 mos *Award:* Dipl
Tuition per yr: $2,829 res, $13,463 non-res

Madison Area Technical College
Surgical Technologist Prgm
Hlth Human & Protective Svcs
3550 Anderson St
Madison, WI 53704
Prgm Dir: Alda S Preston, MSN MA RN
Tel: 608 246-6877 *Fax:* 608 246-6013
E-mail: asp9002@madison.tec.wi.us
Class Cap: 20 *Begins:* Aug
Length: 9 mos *Award:* Dipl
Tuition per yr: $2,159 res, $2,159 non-res
Evening or weekend classes available

Mid-State Technical College
Surgical Technologist Prgm
2600 W Fifth St
Marshfield, WI 54449
Prgm Dir: Raquel L Kluge-Mayer, RN
Tel: 715 387-2538 *Fax:* 715 389-2864
E-mail: midstate@wctc.net
Med Dir: Bruce E Brink, MD
Class Cap: 19 *Begins:* Aug
Length: 9 mos *Award:* Dipl
Tuition per yr: $1,900
Evening or weekend classes available

Milwaukee Area Technical College
Surgical Technologist Prgm
700 W State St
Milwaukee, WI 53233
Prgm Dir: Janet Miller, BSN RN
Tel: 414 297-7153
Med Dir: Marvin Wagner, MD
Class Cap: 13 *Begins:* Aug Jan
Length: 24 mos *Award:* Dipl, AAS
Tuition per yr: $1,440 res, $1,440 non-res
Evening or weekend classes available

Waukesha County Technical College
Surgical Technologist Prgm
800 Main St
Pewaukee, WI 53072
Prgm Dir: Kay Braaten, MS RN
Tel: 414 691-5563 *Fax:* 414 691-5451
E-mail: kbraaten@waukesha.tec.wi.us
Med Dir: David Schmitt, MD
Class Cap: 24 *Begins:* Aug
Length: 9 mos *Award:* Dipl
Tuition per yr: $2,008
Evening or weekend classes available

Northcentral Technical College
Surgical Technologist Prgm
1000 Campus Dr
Wausau, WI 54401
Prgm Dir: Ellen Kafka, MSN RN
Tel: 715 675-3331   *Fax:* 715 675-9776
E-mail: kafka?ntc@mail.northcentral.tec.wi.us
Class Cap: 24   *Begins:* Aug Jan
Length: 9 mos   *Award:* Dipl
Tuition per yr: $1,638 res, $1,638 non-res
Evening or weekend classes available

Therapeutic Recreation Specialist

Occupational Description

Practiced in clinical, residential, and community settings, the therapeutic recreation profession uses treatment, education, and recreation services to help people with illnesses, disabilities, and other conditions develop and use leisure activities to enhance health, independence, and well-being.

Job Description

The day-to-day work experience of therapeutic recreation specialists can vary dramatically, depending on the setting and clients they serve. All therapeutic recreation specialists, however, conduct assessments of physical, mental, emotional, and social functioning to determine the client's needs, interests, and abilities. The therapeutic recreation specialist works with the client, family, and others to design and implement an individualized treatment, education, or program plan.

Professional therapeutic recreation services are divided into three specific service areas, which represent a comprehensive continuum approach based on individual needs:

- *Therapy* is intended to improve functional skills for individuals with disabilities who require treatment or remediation of functional skills as a prerequisite to their involvement in meaningful leisure experiences.
- *Leisure education* provides persons in clinical, residential, and community settings—including individuals with disabilities—opportunities to attain skills, knowledge, and attitudes of leisure involvement.
- *Recreation participation* provides opportunities for voluntary involvement in recreation interests and activities. Specialized recreation participation programs are provided when assistance and/or adapted recreation equipment are needed or when appropriate community recreation opportunities are not available.

During a typical day, a therapeutic recreation specialist will be responsible for one or more group activities. These might include a stress management group, a high or low ropes course activity, a community outing, a family activity, an exercise group, or a leisure education group. The therapeutic recreation specialist also might meet with individual clients to conduct an assessment, develop a leisure discharge plan, or plan evening and weekend activities. Charting client progress and communicating with professionals in other disciplines and family members are also part of a typical day.

A therapeutic recreation specialist working in a community recreation agency also conducts assessments to determine client needs and interests and is responsible for adapting activities as needed and for providing adaptive equipment to enable individuals with disabilities or limitations to participate. In addition, the therapeutic recreation specialist provides in-service training for recreation staff who have individuals with disabilities in their programs to orient them to the needs of these individuals and to promote general sensitivity. The therapeutic recreation specialist will generally seek to integrate clients into existing recreation programs, activities, and classes when possible.

An important responsibility for a therapeutic recreation specialist in both community and clinical settings is to serve as an advocate on behalf of individuals with disabilities. This includes addressing such issues as limited transportation resources, inaccessible facilities, and legislation that affects people with disabilities or limitations. A therapeutic recreation specialist frequently serves on advisory committees and consults with outside agencies to ensure that resources and services are provided for people with disabilities.

One of the most attractive qualities of the therapeutic recreation profession is the opportunity for variety and diversity. The many changes in the health care delivery system have provided—and will continue to offer—an array of challenges and opportunities for continued growth in therapeutic recreation. In addition, the opportunity to positively affect the quality of life of an individual with a disability or limitation is extremely rewarding.

Employment Characteristics

In clinical settings, such as hospitals and rehabilitation centers, therapeutic recreation specialists treat and rehabilitate individuals with specific medical problems, usually in cooperation with physicians, nurses, psychologists, social workers, and physical and occupational therapists. In nursing homes, residential facilities, and community recreation departments, they use leisure activities—mostly group-oriented—to improve general health and well-being, but also may treat medical problems.

Therapeutic recreation specialists assess patients, based on information from medical records, medical staff, family, and patients themselves. They then develop therapeutic activity programs consistent with patient needs and interests. For instance, a patient having trouble socializing may be helped to play games with others, or a client with right-side paralysis may be helped to use the left arm to throw a ball or swing a racket. Therapeutic recreation specialists observe and record patients' participation, reactions, and progress. These records are used by the medical staff and others to monitor progress, to justify changes or end treatment, and for billing.

Community-based therapeutic recreation specialists work in park and recreation departments, special education programs, or programs for older adults or people with disabilities. In these programs, therapeutic recreation specialists help clients develop leisure activities and provide them with opportunities for exercise, mental stimulation, creativity, and fun.

Therapeutic recreation specialists often lift and carry equipment as well as participate in activities. They generally work a 40-hour week, which may include some evenings, weekends, and holidays.

Therapeutic recreation specialists held about 32,000 jobs in 1990. Two-fifths were in hospitals and one-third were in nursing homes. Others were in community mental health centers, adult day care programs, correctional facilities, residential facilities, community programs for people with disabilities, and substance abuse centers. Some were self-employed, generally contracting with nursing homes or community agencies to develop and oversee programs.

According to a 1994 study of members of the National Therapeutic Recreation Society, the average salary of therapeutic recreation specialists was $31,472. In nursing homes, where therapeutic recreation specialists are often classified as activity directors, the average annual salary was $28,720 in 1994. Average annual earnings for therapeutic recreation specialists in the federal government were $30,559 in 1991.

Employment Outlook

Employment of therapeutic recreation specialists is expected to grow faster than the average for all occupations through the year 2005, because of anticipated expansion in long-term care, physical and psychiatric rehabilitation, and services for people with disabilities.

Hospital-based adult day care and outpatient programs and units offering short-term mental health and alcohol or drug abuse services will provide a large number of jobs through the year 2005.

The rapidly growing number of older people is expected to spur job growth for activity directors in nursing homes, retirement communities, adult day care programs, and social service agencies. Continued growth is expected in community residential facilities, as well as day care programs for people with disabilities.

Employment Requirements

A bachelor's degree in therapeutic recreation (or in recreation with an option in therapeutic recreation) is required for hospital and other clinical positions. An associate degree in therapeutic recreation; training in art, drama, or music therapy; or qualifying work experience may be sufficient for activity director positions in nursing homes.

Therapeutic recreation specialists should be comfortable working with people with disabilities and be patient, tactful, and persuasive. Ingenuity and imagination are needed in adapting activities to individual needs, and good physical coordination is necessary when demonstrating or participating in recreational activities.

Licensure, Certification, and Registration

A few states regulate the therapeutic recreation profession through licensure, certification, or registration of titles. Applicants for licensure must pass a state examination. Licensure is required in Utah. For more information, contact

Division of Occupational and Professional Licensure
160 East 300 South
Salt Lake City, UT 84145-0801
801 530-6628

National certification is available through the National Council for Therapeutic Recreation Certification (NCTRC), which awards the title of Certified Therapeutic Recreation Specialist (CTRS).

Through registration, qualified individuals are listed on an official roster maintained by a governmental or nongovernmental agency. Information regarding registration requirements may be obtained from state recreation and park associations.

Educational Programs

Length. A major in therapeutic recreation or recreation with an option in therapeutic recreation entails completion of a degree including a minimum of 18 semester or 24 quarter units in therapeutic recreation and general recreation content course work; completion of supportive courses to include a minimum of 18 semester units or 27 quarter units; and completion of a minimum 360-hour, 10-consecutive-week field placement experience in a clinical, residential, or community-based therapeutic recreation program.

Curriculum. In addition to therapeutic recreation courses in clinical practice and helping skills, program design, management, and professional issues, students study human anatomy, physiology, abnormal psychology, medical and psychiatric terminology, characteristics of illness and disabilities, and the concepts of mainstreaming and normalization. Additional courses cover professional ethics, assessment and referral procedures, and the use of adaptive and medical equipment. In addition, 360 hours of internship under the supervision of a certified therapeutic recreation specialist are required.

Standards. *Standards and Evaluative Criteria for Baccalaureate Programs in Recreation, Park Resources and Leisure Services* established by the NRPA/AALR Council on Accreditation. Each new educational program is assessed in accordance with the *Standards*, and accredited programs are periodically reviewed to determine whether they remain in substantial compliance.

Programs

Career Planning Publications

The *1996-97 SPRE Curriculum Catalog* (published by the Society for Park and Recreation Educators) provides valuable information on curricula and faculty in the parks, recreation, and leisure studies profession. Degree levels offered and accreditation status are indicated for each program. Each listing includes the location and mailing address for each program, enrollment data, a description of the character of the campus and community, and a detailed listing of the faculty and specialties.

The *Job Bulletin* newsletter, published twice each month, details job opportunities in parks, recreation, and therapeutic recreation across the United States and abroad, including internships and seasonal positions. Annual 22-issue subscriptions are available only to NRPA members for a fee of $45. Individual issues are available to members and nonmembers for $5 each (prepaid).

Preparing for a Career in Therapeutic Recreation describes the continuum of services within therapeutic recreation and standards for certification and includes a listing of colleges and universities that offer therapeutic recreation programs, including those accredited by the NRPA/AALR Council on Accreditation. Available for $5.25 (NRPA member) and $7.50 (nonmember).

Inquiries

Accreditation

Inquiries regarding accreditation should be addressed to

Jeanne Houghton, Accreditation Coordinator
Professional Services Division
National Recreation and Park Association (NRPA)
2775 S Quincy St/Ste 300
Arlington, VA 22206
703 578-5570

Careers

Inquiries regarding careers should be addressed to

National Therapeutic Recreation Society (NTRS)
2775 S Quincy St/Ste 300
Arlington, VA 22206-2236
703 820-4940
703 578-5548 (Rikki Epstein, NTRS director)
800 626-NRPA (for membership information and other services)
703 671-6772 Fax
E-mail: Info@NRPA.org
Internet: http://www.nrpa.org

Certification

For information on national certification, contact

National Council for Therapeutic Recreation Certification
PO Box 479
Thiells, NY 10984-0479
914 947-4346
914 947-1634

Therapeutic Recreation Specialist

California

California State University - Chico
Therapeutic Recreation Specialist Prgm
Dept of Recreation and Parks Mgmt
Rm 130 Aymer J Hamilton
Chico, CA 95929-0560
Tel: 916 898-6408 *Fax:* 916 898-6557

California State University - Long Beach
Therapeutic Recreation Specialist Prgm
Dept of Recreation and Leisure Studies
1250 Bellflower Blvd
Long Beach, CA 90840-4903
Prgm Dir: Michael Blazey, PhD
Tel: 310 985-4071 *Fax:* 310 985-8154
E-mail: mblazey@csulb.edu
Begins: Aug Jan
Length: 30 mos *Award:* BA, MS
Tuition per yr: $2,270 res, $7,872 non-res
Evening or weekend classes available

California State University - Northridge
Therapeutic Recreation Specialist Prgm
Dept of Leisure Studies and Recreation
18111 Nordhoff St
Northridge, CA 91330
Prgm Dir: Robert Winslow
Tel: 818 885-3202 *Fax:* 818 677-2695
E-mail: bwinslow@csun.edu
Class Cap: 20 *Begins:* Aug
Length: 24 mos *Award:* BS, MS
Tuition per yr: $1,970 res, $17,468 non-res
Evening or weekend classes available

California State University - Sacramento
Therapeutic Recreation Specialist Prgm
Dept of Recreation and Leisure Studies
600 J St
Sacramento, CA 95819-6110
Prgm Dir: Carol Stensrud, CTRS RTC EdD
Tel: 916 278-5668 *Fax:* 916 278-5053
E-mail: stensrud@csus.edu
Begins: Aug Jan
Length: 30 mos *Award:* BS, MS
Tuition per yr: $2,438 res, $15,252 non-res
Evening or weekend classes available

San Diego State University
Therapeutic Recreation Specialist Prgm
Dept of Recreation
5900 Campanile Dr
San Diego, CA 92182-0368
Prgm Dir: Gene Lamke
Tel: 619 594-5110 *Fax:* 619 594-6974

Colorado

University of Northern Colorado
Therapeutic Recreation Specialist Prgm
Dept of Human Services
Gunter 1250
Greeley, CO 80639
Prgm Dir: N R Van Dinter
Tel: 970 351-2403   *Fax:* 970 351-1255
Class Cap: 50   *Begins:* Jan Aug
Length: 48 mos   *Award:* BS
Tuition per yr: $1,914 res, $8,416 non-res
Evening or weekend classes available

Connecticut

University of Connecticut
Therapeutic Recreation Specialist Prgm
Sport, Leisure and Exercise Science
U-110 2095 Hillside Rd
Storrs, CT 06269-1110
Prgm Dir: Jay S Shivers
Tel: 860 486-3625   *Fax:* 860 486-1123
E-mail: shivers@uconnvm.uconn.edu
Begins: Sep Jan
Length: 30 mos   *Award:* BS, MA
Evening or weekend classes available

District of Columbia

Gallaudet University
Therapeutic Recreation Specialist Prgm
Health, Physical Educ and Recreation
800 Florida Ave NE/Field House
Washington, DC 20002
Prgm Dir: Anne Simonsen, CTRS CLP
Tel: 202 651-5591   *Fax:* 202 651-5861
E-mail: alsimonsen@gallus.gallaudet.edu
Class Cap: 25   *Begins:* Sep Jan
Length: 81 mos   *Award:* Dipl
Tuition per yr: $2,805 res, $2,805 non-res

Florida

University of Florida
Therapeutic Recreation Specialist Prgm
Dept of Recreation, Parks and Tourism
229 Florida Gymnasium
Gainesville, FL 32611-2034
Tel: 352 392-4042   *Fax:* 352 392-7588

Florida State University
Therapeutic Recreation Specialist Prgm
Leisure Services and Studies
215 Stone Bldg
Tallahassee, FL 32306-3001
Prgm Dir: Cheryl Beeler
Tel: 904 644-3061   *Fax:* 904 644-4335

Georgia

Georgia Southern University
Therapeutic Recreation Specialist Prgm
Dept of Recreation and Leisure Studies
Landrum Box 8077/Anderson Hall
Statesboro, GA 30460-8077
Prgm Dir: Henry Eisenhart
Tel: 912 681-5462   *Fax:* 912 681-0386
Class Cap: 65   *Begins:* Sep Jan Mar
Length: 48 mos   *Award:*
Tuition per yr: $0 res, $1,422 non-res
Evening or weekend classes available

Illinois

Southern Illinois Univ at Carbondale
Therapeutic Recreation Specialist Prgm
Dept of Health Educ and Recreation
Pulliam Hall 307/Postal Code 4632
Carbondale, IL 62901
Prgm Dir: Regina B Glover
Tel: 618 453-4331   *Fax:* 618 453-1829
Begins: Aug Dec
Length: 23 mos   *Award:* BS, MS
Tuition per yr: $927 res, $2,781 non-res
Evening or weekend classes available

Eastern Illinois University
Therapeutic Recreation Specialist Prgm
Recreation and Leisure Studies
Rm 10 McAfee Bldg
Charleston, IL 61920
Prgm Dir: William Higelmire
Tel: 217 581-3018   *Fax:* 217 581-7013
E-mail: cfwfh@uxa.ecn.bgu.edu
Class Cap: 45
Length: 48 mos   *Award:* BS
Tuition per yr: $3,028 res, $7,276 non-res

Western Illinois University
Therapeutic Recreation Specialist Prgm
Recreation, Park and Tourism Admin
400 Currens Hall
Macomb, IL 61455
Prgm Dir: Nick DiGrino
Tel: 309 298-1967   *Fax:* 309 298-2967

Illinois State University
Therapeutic Recreation Specialist Prgm
Recreation and Park Admin Prgm
101 McCormick Hall
Normal, IL 61790-5121
Prgm Dir: Norma J Stumbo
Tel: 309 438-5608   *Fax:* 309 438-5561

Indiana

Indiana University - Bloomington
Therapeutic Recreation Specialist Prgm
Dept of Recreation and Park Admin
133 HPER Bldg
Bloomington, IN 47405
Prgm Dir: David Austen, PhD CTRS
Tel: 812 855-4711   *Fax:* 812 855-3998
E-mail: daustin@indiana.edu
Begins: Sep
Length: 30 mos   *Award:* BS, MS
Evening or weekend classes available

Iowa

University of Northern Iowa
Therapeutic Recreation Specialist Prgm
Leisure Services Div
School of HPELS/203 E Gym
Cedar Falls, IA 50614-0161
Prgm Dir: Jane Mertesdorf
Tel: 319 273-6840   *Fax:* 319 273-5833

University of Iowa
Therapeutic Recreation Specialist Prgm
Sport, Health, Leisure and Phys Studies
Field House E 102
Iowa City, IA 52242-1111
Prgm Dir: Bonnie Slatton
Tel: 319 335-9335   *Fax:* 319 335-8669
Begins: Aug
Length: 24 mos   *Award:* BS
Tuition per yr: $2,470 res, $9,068 non-res
Evening or weekend classes available

Kentucky

Eastern Kentucky University
Therapeutic Recreation Specialist Prgm
Dept of Recreation and Park Admin
Begley Bldg Rm 402
Richmond, KY 40475
Prgm Dir: Larry Belknap, ReD CLP
Tel: 606 622-1833   *Fax:* 606 622-1020
E-mail: recbelkn@acs.eku.edu
Begins: Aug Jan
Length: 30 mos   *Award:* BS
Tuition per yr: $5,760 res, $17,280 non-res

Louisiana

Grambling State University
Therapeutic Recreation Specialist Prgm
Recreation Careers Program
Dept of HPER/PO Box 4244
Grambling, LA 71245
Prgm Dir: Wallace Bly
Tel: 318 274-2294   *Fax:* 318 274-6053

Massachusetts

Springfield College
Therapeutic Recreation Specialist Prgm
Dept of Recreation and Leisure Studies
263 Alden St/215 Schoo Hall
Springfield, MA 01109
Prgm Dir: Matthew J Pantera
Tel: 413 748-3693

Michigan

Central Michigan University
Therapeutic Recreation Specialist Prgm
Dept of Recreation and Park Admin
Mount Pleasant, MI 48859
Prgm Dir: Roger Coles
Tel: 517 774-3858   *Fax:* 517 774-2161
Class Cap: 25
Award: BS, BAA
Tuition per yr: $5,946 res, $15,441 non-res

Programs

Minnesota

University of Minnesota - Twin Cities

Therapeutic Recreation Specialist Prgm
Recreation, Park and Leisure Studies
203 Cooke Hall/1900 University SE
Minneapolis, MN 55455
Tel: 612 625-5887

Mississippi

University of Southern Mississippi

Therapeutic Recreation Specialist Prgm
Schl of Human Performance and Recreation
Box 5142 Southern Station
Hattiesburg, MS 39406-5142
Prgm Dir: Sandra Gangstead
Tel: 601 266-5386   *Fax:* 601 266-4445
Begins: Jan Jun Aug
Length: 36 mos   *Award:* BS, MS
Tuition per yr: $1,234 res, $2,644 non-res
Evening or weekend classes available

Missouri

University of Missouri - Columbia

Therapeutic Recreation Specialist Prgm
Dept of Parks, Recreation and Tourism
624 Clark Hall
Columbia, MO 65211
Prgm Dir: C Randal Vessell
Tel: 573 882-7086   *Fax:* 573 882-9526

New York

SUNY College at Cortland

Therapeutic Recreation Specialist Prgm
Recreation and Leisure Studies Dept
PO Box 2000
Cortland, NY 13045
Prgm Dir: Anderson B Young
Tel: 607 753-4941   *Fax:* 607 753-5982
E-mail: young@snycorva.cortland.edu
Class Cap: 45   *Begins:* Aug Jan
Length: 48 mos, 18 mos   *Award:* BS.BSE,MSE
Tuition per yr: $3,400 res, $8,300 non-res
Evening or weekend classes available

North Carolina

Univ of North Carolina at Greensboro

Therapeutic Recreation Specialist Prgm
Dept of Leisure Studies
420-HHP Bldg
Greensboro, NC 27412-5001
Prgm Dir: Kathleen Williams
Tel: 910 334-5327   *Fax:* 910 334-3238
E-mail: k_williams@uncg.edu
Begins: Jan May Aug
Length: 4 mos   *Award:* BS, MS
Tuition per yr: $948 res, $8,904 non-res
Evening or weekend classes available

Univ of North Carolina - Wilmington

Therapeutic Recreation Specialist Prgm
Parks and Recreation Mgmt Curriculum
PO Box 1425/601 S College Rd
Wilmington, NC 28403-3297
Prgm Dir: Charles Lewis, PhD
Tel: 919 395-3250   *Fax:* 919 350-7073
E-mail: lewisc@uncwil.edu
Begins: Aug Jan
Length: 30 mos   *Award:* BA
Tuition per yr: $2,080 res, $10,633 non-res

Ohio

University of Toledo

Therapeutic Recreation Specialist Prgm
Div of Recreation and Leisure Studies
2801 W Bancroft St
Toledo, OH 43606
Prgm Dir: Steven L Ranck
Tel: 419 537-2757   *Fax:* 419 537-4759

Oklahoma

Oklahoma State University Main Campus

Therapeutic Recreation Specialist Prgm
Dept of Leisure Studies
Colvin Center
Stillwater, OK 74078
Prgm Dir: Jerry Jordan
Tel: 405 744-5479   *Fax:* 405 744-6507

Pennsylvania

Lincoln University

Therapeutic Recreation Specialist Prgm
Health, Physical Educ and Athletics
Rivero Hall
Lincoln, PA 19352
Prgm Dir: James L DeBoy, PhD
Tel: 610 932-8300, Ext 385   *Fax:* 610 932-0815
Class Cap: 25   *Begins:* Aug Jan
Length: 32 mos   *Award:* BS
Tuition per yr: $3,300 res, $5,280 non-res

Temple University

Therapeutic Recreation Specialist Prgm
Sport Mgmt and Leisure Studies
Seltzer Hall 3rd Fl/Broad & Columbia
Philadelphia, PA 19122
Prgm Dir: John Shank, EdD
Tel: 215 204-6278   *Fax:* 215 204-1455
E-mail: jshank@thunder.temple.edu
Class Cap: 30   *Begins:* Sep Jan
Length: 24 mos, 48 mos   *Award:* BS, EdM
Tuition per yr: $5,314 res, $10,096 non-res

South Carolina

Clemson University

Therapeutic Recreation Specialist Prgm
Parks, Recreation and Tourism Mgmt
263 Lehotsky Hall/PO Box 341005
Clemson, SC 29634-1005
Prgm Dir: Ann James
Tel: 863 656-3400   *Fax:* 864 656-2226
E-mail: ajms@clemson.edu
Class Cap: 20   *Begins:* Aug Jan May Jul
Award: BS, MS
Tuition per yr: $2,922 res, $8,126 non-res

Texas

University of North Texas

Therapeutic Recreation Specialist Prgm
Kinesiology, Health Promo and Recreation
UNT Box 13857
Denton, TX 76203-3857
Prgm Dir: James R Morrow
Tel: 817 565-2651   *Fax:* 817 565-4904

Utah

Brigham Young University

Therapeutic Recreation Specialist Prgm
Recreation Mgmt and Youth Leadership
273 Richards Bldg
Provo, UT 84602
Prgm Dir: S Harold Smith
Tel: 801 378-4369   *Fax:* 801 378-7461
E-mail: smithh@byu.edu
Class Cap: 60   *Award:* BS
Tuition per yr: $2,530 res, $3,800 non-res

Univ of Utah Health Sciences Center

Therapeutic Recreation Specialist Prgm
Dept of Recreation and Leisure
College of Health/HPR N-226
Salt Lake City, UT 84112
Prgm Dir: Gary Ellis
Tel: 801 581-3220   *Fax:* 801 581-4930
E-mail: gellis@health.utah.edu
Class Cap: 50
Award: BS
Tuition per yr: $2,117 res, $6,461 non-res

Virginia

Longwood College

Therapeutic Recreation Specialist Prgm
Dept of HPER
201 High St
Farmville, VA 23909-1899
Prgm Dir: Patricia Shrank
Tel: 804 395-2545   *Fax:* 804 395-2568
E-mail: pshank@logwood.lwc.edu
Class Cap: 120   *Begins:* Aug Jan
Length: 36 mos   *Award:* BS
Tuition per yr: $2,684 res, $8,156 non-res
Evening or weekend classes available

Radford University

Therapeutic Recreation Specialist Prgm
Dept of Recreation and Leisure Studies
Box 6963
Radford, VA 24142
Prgm Dir: Gerald O'Morrow, PhD
Tel: 540 831-5221   *Fax:* 540 831-6487
E-mail: gomorrow@runet.edu
Begins: Aug Jan
Length: 30 mos   *Award:* BS
Tuition per yr: $3,893 res, $9,610 non-res

Med Coll of VA/Virginia Commonwealth U

Therapeutic Recreation Specialist Prgm
Dept of Recreation, Parks and Tourism
817 W Franklin St/Box 842015
Richmond, VA 23284-2015
Prgm Dir: Michael S Wise, EdD CLP
Tel: 804 828-1948   *Fax:* 804 828-1946
E-mail: mwise@saturn.vcu.edu
Begins: Aug Jan
Length: 30 mos   *Award:* BS
Tuition per yr: $7,995 res, $28,290 non-res
Evening or weekend classes available

Washington

Eastern Washington University

Therapeutic Recreation Specialist Prgm
Physical Educ, Health and Recreation
MS #66
Cheney, WA 99004
Prgm Dir: Howard Uibel
Tel: 509 359-2341   *Fax:* 509 359-4833

Wisconsin

University of Wisconsin - LaCrosse

Therapeutic Recreation Specialist Prgm
Recreation Mgmt and Therapeutic Rec
128 Wittich Hall
LaCrosse, WI 54601
Prgm Dir: Nancy Navar, CTRS
Tel: 608 785-8207   *Fax:* 608 785-8206
E-mail: navar@mail.vwlax.edu
Length: 36 mos, 18 mos   *Award:* BS, MS
Tuition per yr: $1,317 res, $4,049 non-res

Section III

Institutions Sponsoring Accredited Programs

Alabama

Auburn

Auburn University
William V Muse, President
Auburn, AL 36849
205 826-4000
- Audiologist
- Dietitian/Nutritionist
- Rehabilitation Counselor
- Speech Language Pathologist

Bay Minette

James Faulkner State Community College
Gary L Branch, President
1900 Hwy 31S
Bay Minette, AL 36507-2619
334 580-2100
- Dental Assistant

Bessemer

Bessemer State Technical College
W Michael Bailey, President
Hwy 11 S PO Box 308
Bessemer, AL 35021
205 428-6391
- Dental Assistant

Birmingham

Baptist Health System Inc
Dennis A Hall, FACHE, President
PO Box 830605
Birmingham, AL 35283-0605
205 715-5319
- Clin Lab Scientist/Med Tech
- Histologic Technician-Cert

Carraway Methodist Medical Center
Warren E Calloway, Administrator
1600 N 26th St
Birmingham, AL 35234
205 226-6000
- Radiographer

Jefferson State Community College
Judy M Merritt, PhD, President
2601 Carson Rd
Birmingham, AL 35215
205 853-1200
- Clin Lab Tech/Med Lab Tech-AD
- Occupational Therapy Asst
- Radiographer

Samford University
Thomas E Corts, President
800 Lakeshore Dr
Birmingham, AL 35229
205 870-2011
- Dietitian/Nutritionist

Univ of Alabama at Birmingham Hospital
Kevin Lofton, MBA FACHE, Exec Director
619 S 19th St
Birmingham, AL 35223
205 934-4011
- Specialist in BB Tech

Institutions

University of Alabama at Birmingham

J Claude Bennett, MD, President
Administration Bldg/Rm 1070
Birmingham, AL 35294-0110
205 934-4636
- Clin Lab Scientist/Med Tech
- Cytotechnologist
- Dental Assistant
- Dietitian/Nutritionist
- Emergency Med Tech-Paramedic
- Health Information Admin
- Nuclear Medicine Tech
- Occupational Therapist
- Physician Assistant
- Radiation Therapist
- Radiographer
- Rehabilitation Counselor
- Respiratory Therapist

University of Alabama at Birmingham

J Claude Bennett, MD, President
Office of the President
701 South 20th Street, AB1070
Birmingham, AL 35294-0101
205 943-4636
- Emergency Med Tech-Paramedic

Decatur

John Calhoun State Community College

Richard Carpenter, President
PO Box 2216
Decatur, AL 35609-2216
205 306-2500
- Dental Assistant

Dothan

George C Wallace State Comm College

Larry Beaty, EdD, President
Office of the President
Rte 6 Box 62
Dothan, AL 36303
334 983-3521
- Clin Lab Tech/Med Lab Tech-AD
- Emergency Med Tech-Paramedic
- Medical Assistant
- Radiographer
- Respiratory Therapist

Gadsden

Gadsden State Community College

Victor B Ficker, EdD MEd EdS BA, President
PO Box 227
1001 George Wallace Dr
Gadsden, AL 35902-0227
205 549-8463
- Clin Lab Tech/Med Lab Tech-AD
- Emergency Med Tech-Paramedic
- Radiographer

Hanceville

Wallace State College

James C Bailey, EdD, President
Commerce Bldg
PO Box 2000
Hanceville, AL 35077-2000
205 352-8180
- Clin Lab Tech/Med Lab Tech-AD
- Dental Assistant
- Dental Hygienist
- Diagnostic Med Sonographer
- Emergency Med Tech-Paramedic
- Health Information Tech
- Medical Assistant
- Occupational Therapy Asst
- Radiographer
- Respiratory Therapist

Huntsville

Huntsville Hospital

Edward D Boston, MHA, Administrator
101 Sivley Rd
Huntsville, AL 35801
205 533-8123
- Radiographer

Oakwood College

Benjamin F Reaves, President
Huntsville, AL 35896
205 726-7000
- Dietitian/Nutritionist

Jacksonville

Jacksonville State University

Harold J McGee, President
Jacksonville, AL 36265
205 782-5781
- Dietitian/Nutritionist

Mobile

Bishop State Community College

Yvonne Kennedy, PhD, President
351 N Broad St
Mobile, AL 36603-5898
205 690-6416
- Health Information Tech

Mobile Infirmary Medical Center

E Chandler Bramlett, President/CEO
PO Box 2144
Mobile, AL 36652
334 431-4444
- Radiation Therapist

University of South Alabama

Frederick P Whiddon, PhD DLitt, President
Office of the President
307 N University Blvd
Mobile, AL 36688-0002
334 460-6111
- Audiologist
- Clin Lab Scientist/Med Tech
- Emergency Med Tech-Paramedic
- Occupational Therapist
- Radiographer
- Respiratory Therapist
- Speech Language Pathologist

Montevallo

University of Montevallo

Robert M McChesney, President
Station 6001
Montevallo, AL 35115
205 665-6000
- Audiologist
- Dietitian/Nutritionist
- Speech Language Pathologist

Montgomery

Alabama Reference Laboratories, Inc

Robert B Adams, MD, President
543 S Hull St PO Box 4600
Montgomery, AL 36103-4600
334 263-5745
- Clin Lab Scientist/Med Tech

Auburn University at Montgomery

Roy Saigo, PhD, Chancellor
Montgomery, AL 36193
334 244-3601
- Clin Lab Scientist/Med Tech

Baptist Medical Center

Michael D DeBoer, CEO
2105 E South Blvd
Montgomery, AL 36111
334 288-2100
- Clin Lab Scientist/Med Tech
- Radiographer

Draughons Junior College

Victor Biebighauser, BA, President
122 Commerce St
Montgomery, AL 36104
334 263-1013
- Medical Assistant

H Councill Trenholm State Technical College

Leroy Bell, Jr., Interim President
1225 Air Base Blvd PO Box 9000
Montgomery, AL 36108
334 832-9000
- Dental Assistant
- Dental Lab Technician
- Emergency Med Tech-Paramedic
- Medical Assistant

Normal

Alabama A & M University

David B Henson, President
PO Box 1357
Normal, AL 35762
205 851-5000
- Dietitian/Nutritionist
- Speech Language Pathologist

Opelika

Southern Union State Community College

Roy W Johnson, LLT, President
1701 LaFayette Pkwy
Opelika, AL 36803-2268
334 745-6437
- Radiographer

Tuscaloosa

DCH Regional Medical Center
Bryan N Kindred, MBA, President/CEO
809 University Blvd E
Tuscaloosa, AL 35401
205 759-7177
- Clin Lab Scientist/Med Tech
- Radiographer

Shelton St Comm Coll/Alabama Fire Coll
Thomas Umphrey, EdD, President
2015 McFarland Blvd E
Tuscaloosa, AL 35405
205 391-2253
- Emergency Med Tech-Paramedic

University of Alabama
Roger Sayers, PhD, President
Office of the President
PO Box 870100
Tuscaloosa, AL 35487
205 348-5100
- Athletic Trainer
- Audiologist
- Dietitian/Nutritionist
- Music Therapist
- Rehabilitation Counselor
- Speech Language Pathologist

Tuskegee

Tuskegee University
Benjamin F Payton, PhD, President
Kresge Ctr
Tuskegee, AL 36088-1677
334 727-8530
- Clin Lab Scientist/Med Tech
- Dietitian/Nutritionist
- Occupational Therapist

Alaska

Anchorage

University of Alaska Anchorage
Lee Gorsuch, PhD, Chancellor
3211 Providence Dr
Anchorage, AK 99508
907 786-1101
- Dental Assistant
- Dental Hygienist
- Dietitian/Nutritionist
- Medical Assistant

Juneau

University of Alaska Southeast
Marshall L Lind, Chancellor
Office of the Chancellor/UAS
11120 Glacier Hwy
Juneau, AK 99801-8697
907 789-4472
- Health Information Tech

Arizona

Coolidge

Central Arizona College
Kathleen Arns, PhD, President
Woodruff at Overfield Rd
Coolidge, AZ 85228
602 426-4444
- Dietetic Technician

Flagstaff

Northern Arizona University
Clara Lovett, PhD, President
PO Box 4092
Flagstaff, AZ 86011
520 523-3232
- Dental Hygienist
- Dietitian/Nutritionist
- Speech Language Pathologist

Phoenix

Apollo College
Margaret M Carlson, President
2701 W Bethany Home Rd
Phoenix, AZ 85017-1705
602 433-1333
- Occupational Therapy Asst
- Respiratory Therapist

Focus on Nutrition
Ste 26-113
3923 E Thunderbird Rd
Phoenix, AZ 85032
602 788-7096
- Dietitian/Nutritionist

Gateway Community College
Phil Randolph, EdD, President
108 N 40th St
Phoenix, AZ 85034
602 392-5000
- Diagnostic Med Sonographer
- Nuclear Medicine Tech
- Radiographer
- Respiratory Therapist
- Respiratory Therapy Tech

Long Medical Institute
Gary Kerber, MBA, CEO
4126 N Black Canyon Hwy
Phoenix, AZ 85017
602 279-9333
- Respiratory Therapy Tech

Paradise Valley Unified School District
20621 N 32nd St
Phoenix, AZ 85032
602 493-2600
- Dietitian/Nutritionist

Phoenix College
Marie Pepicello, PhD, President
1202 W Thomas Rd
Phoenix, AZ 85013
602 285-7364
- Clin Lab Tech/Med Lab Tech-AD
- Dental Assistant
- Dental Hygienist
- Health Information Tech

The Bryman School
Dennis Pobiak, President
4343 N 16th St
Phoenix, AZ 85016
602 274-4300
- Medical Assistant

Prescott

Yavapai County Health Department
930 Division St
Prescott, AZ 86301
602 771-3122
- Dietitian/Nutritionist

Sun City

Walter O Boswell Memorial Hospital
10401 W Thunderbird Blvd
Sun City, AZ 85372
602 977-7211
- Dietitian/Nutritionist

Tempe

Arizona State University
Lattie F Coor, PhD, President
Box 872203
Tempe, AZ 85287-2203
602 965-5606
- Audiologist
- Clin Lab Scientist/Med Tech
- Dietitian/Nutritionist
- Music Therapist
- Speech Language Pathologist

Maricopa County Dept of Public Health
Office of Nutrition Services
1414 W Broadway Ste 237
Tempe, AZ 85282
602 966-3090
- Dietitian/Nutritionist

Tucson

Carondelet St Mary's Hospital
Morrisons Custom Management Company
1601 W St Mary's Rd
Tucson, AZ 85745
520 622-5833
- Dietitian/Nutritionist

Pima Community College
Robert D Jensen, Chancellor
4905-C E Broadway
Tucson, AZ 85709-1005
520 748-4747
- Dental Assistant
- Dental Hygienist
- Dental Lab Technician
- Radiographer
- Respiratory Therapist

Institutions

Pima Medical Institute - Denver
Richard L Luebke, Sr, President
3350 E Grant Rd #200
Tucson, AZ 85716
800 456-7462
- Radiographer
- Respiratory Therapist
- Respiratory Therapy Tech

Pima Medical Institute - Mesa
Richard L Luebke Sr, President
3350 E Grant Rd #200
Tucson, AZ 85716
520 326-1600
- Radiographer
- Respiratory Therapist
- Respiratory Therapy Tech

Pima Medical Institute - Tucson
Richard L Luebke, Sr, President
3350 E Grant Rd #200
Tucson, AZ 85716
520 326-1600
- Diagnostic Med Sonographer
- Radiographer
- Respiratory Therapist
- Respiratory Therapy Tech

Univ Medical Center/Univ of Arizona
Gregory Pivirotto, CEO
1501 N Campbell Ave
Tucson, AZ 85724
520 694-4660
- Dietitian/Nutritionist

University of Arizona
Manuel T Pacheco, PhD, President
Adminstration Bldg Rm 712
Tucson, AZ 85721
520 621-5511
- Audiologist
- Clin Lab Scientist/Med Tech
- Dietitian/Nutritionist
- Perfusionist
- Rehabilitation Counselor
- Speech Language Pathologist

Arkansas

Arkadelphia

Ouachita Baptist University
Arkadelphia, AR 71998-0001
501 245-5000
- Dietitian/Nutritionist

Beebe

Arkansas State University-Beebe
Eugene McKay, PhD, Chancellor
PO Drawer H
Beebe, AR 72012
501 882-6458
- Clin Lab Tech/Med Lab Tech-AD

Bentonville

Northwest Arkansas Community College
Bob Burns, PhD, President
One College Dr
Bentonville, AR 72712-5091
501 636-9222
- Radiation Therapist
- Respiratory Therapy Tech

Burdette

Cotton Boll Technical Institute
William Nelson, President
Box 36
Burdette, AR 72321
501 763-1486
- Dental Assistant

Conway

University of Central Arkansas
Winfred L Thompson, PhD, President
201 Donaghey Ave
Conway, AR 72035-0001
501 450-3170
- Dietitian/Nutritionist
- Occupational Therapist
- Speech Language Pathologist

El Dorado

South Arkansas Community College
Ben T Whitfield, PhD, President
PO Box 7010 W Campus
El Dorado, AR 71731-7010
501 862-8131
- Clin Lab Tech/Med Lab Tech-AD
- Radiographer

Fayetteville

University of Arkansas Main Campus
Daniel E Ferritor, Chancellor
Fayetteville, AR 72701
501 575-2000
- Dietitian/Nutritionist
- Rehabilitation Counselor
- Speech Language Pathologist

Ft Smith

Arkansas Valley Tech Institute
Carl Jones, MSEd, President
1311 S I St
Ft Smith, AR 72901
501 441-5256
- Respiratory Therapy Tech

Sparks Regional Medical Center
Charles Shuffield, FACHE, President
1311 S I St Box 17006
Ft Smith, AR 72917-7006
501 441-5407
- Radiographer

St Edward Mercy Medical Center
Judith Marie Keith, RSM, Administrator
7301 Rogers Ave PO Box 17000
Ft Smith, AR 72917-7000
501 484-6100
- Radiographer

Westark Community College
Joel R Stubblefield, MBA, President
PO Box 3649
Ft Smith, AR 72913
501 788-7004
- Clin Lab Tech/Med Lab Tech-AD
- Surgical Technologist

Harrison

North Arkansas Comm and Tech Coll
Bill Baker, EdD, President
420 Pioneer Ridge Dr
Harrison, AR 72601
501 743-3000
- Clin Lab Tech/Med Lab Tech-AD
- Radiographer

Helena

Phillips County Community College
Steven Jones, EdD, Chancellor
PO Box 785
Helena, AR 72342
501 338-6474
- Clin Lab Tech/Med Lab Tech-AD

Hope

Univ of Arkansas Comm Coll at Hope
Johnny Rapert, MS, Director
2500 S Main
Hope, AR 71801
501 777-5722
- Respiratory Therapy Tech

Hot Springs

Garland County Community College
Tom Spencer, PhD, President
101 College Dr
Hot Springs, AR 71913-9174
501 767-9371
- Clin Lab Tech/Med Lab Tech-AD
- Health Information Tech
- Radiographer

Little Rock

Baptist Medical System
Russell D Harrington Jr, FACHE, Pres
9601 Interstate 630 Exit 7
Little Rock, AR 72205-7299
501 227-2274
- Clin Lab Scientist/Med Tech
- Histologic Technician-Cert
- Nuclear Medicine Tech
- Radiographer

Central Arkansas Radiation Therapy Inst
Janice Burford, CEO/President
PO Box 55050
Little Rock, AR 72215
501 664-8573
- Radiation Therapist

St Vincent Infirmary Medical Center
Diana T Hueter, CEO
Two St Vincent Circle
Little Rock, AR 72205-5499
501 660-3910
- Nuclear Medicine Tech
- Radiographer

Univ of Ark for Med Sci/St Vincent Infirmary
Harry P Ward, MD, Chancellor
4301 W Markham/Slot 704
Little Rock, AR 72205
501 686-5681
- Nuclear Medicine Tech

Univ of Arkansas for Medical Sciences
Harry P Ward, MD, Chancellor
4301 W Markham Slot 541
Little Rock, AR 72205
501 686-5681
- Clin Lab Scientist/Med Tech
- Cytotechnologist
- Dietitian/Nutritionist
- Nuclear Medicine Tech
- Radiographer
- Respiratory Therapist
- Respiratory Therapy Tech
- Surgical Technologist

University of Arkansas & VA Medical Ctr
Harry P Ward, MD, CEO
U of Arkansas for Medical Sciences
4301 W Markham Slot 541
Little Rock, AR 72205-7199
501 686-5681
- Dental Hygienist

University of Arkansas at Little Rock
Charles E Hathaway, Chancellor
2801 S University Ave
Little Rock, AR 72204
501 569-3000
- Audiologist
- Speech Language Pathologist

North Little Rock

Pulaski Technical College
Ben Wyatt, MEd, President
3000 W Scenic Rd
North Little Rock, AR 72118
501 771-1000
- Dental Assistant
- Respiratory Therapy Tech

Pine Bluff

Jefferson Regional Medical Center
Robert P Atkinson, MHA, CEO
1515 W 42nd Ave
Pine Bluff, AR 71603
501 541-7269
- Radiographer

University of Arkansas at Pine Bluff
Lawrence A Davis, Chancellor
Pine Bluff, AR 71601
501 543-8000
- Dietitian/Nutritionist

Pocahontas

Black River Technical College
Richard Gaines, MS, Director
PO Box 468
Pocahontas, AR 72455
501 892-4565
- Dietetic Technician
- Respiratory Therapy Tech

Russellville

Arkansas Tech University
Robert Charles Brown, PhD, President
Administration 210
Russellville, AR 72801
501 968-0237
- Health Information Admin
- Medical Assistant

Searcy

Harding University Main Campus
David B Burks, President
Searcy, AR 72149
501 279-4000
- Dietitian/Nutritionist

State University

Arkansas State University
L Leslie Wyatt, PhD, President
Administration PO Box 10
State University, AR 72467-0010
501 972-3030
- Clin Lab Scientist/Med Tech
- Clin Lab Tech/Med Lab Tech-AD
- Radiographer
- Rehabilitation Counselor
- Speech Language Pathologist

California

Alameda

College of Alameda
George Herring, President
555 Atlantic Ave
Alameda, CA 94501
415 522-7221
- Dental Assistant

Anaheim

ConCorde Career Institute
Garo Ghaxarian, MD, Executive Director
1717 S Brookhurst
Anaheim, CA 92804
714 635-3450
- Medical Assistant

Angwin

Pacific Union College
D Malcolm Maxwell, President
Angwin, CA 94508
707 965-6311
- Dietitian/Nutritionist

Aptos

Cabrillo College
John D Hurd, President/Supt
6500 Soquel Dr
Aptos, CA 95003
408 479-6306
- Dental Hygienist
- Radiographer

Bakersfield

Bakersfield College
Richard L Wright, PhD, President
1801 Panorama Dr
Bakersfield, CA 93305
805 395-4211
- Radiographer

California State University - Bakersfield
Thomas Arciniega, PhD, President
9001 Stockdale Hwy
Bakersfield, CA 93311
805 833-2241
- Clin Lab Scientist/Med Tech

Belmont

College of Notre Dame
Margaret Huber, President
Ralston Ave
Belmont, CA 94002
415 593-1601
- Art Therapist

Berkeley

University of California Berkeley
Chang-Lin Tien, Chancellor
Berkeley, CA 94720
510 642-6000
- Dietitian/Nutritionist

Burlingame

Hospital Consortium of San Mateo County
Frank E Gibson, President/CEO
1600 Trousdale Dr
Burlingame, CA 94010
415 696-7838
- Surgical Technologist

Mills - Peninsula Hospitals
Robert W Merwin, CEO
1783 El Camino Real
Burlingame, CA 94010
415 696-5678
- Radiographer

Carson

California State Univ-Dominguez Hills
Robert Detweiler, PhD, President
1000 E Victoria St
Carson, CA 90747
310 243-3301
- Clin Lab Scientist/Med Tech
- Nuclear Medicine Tech
- Orthotist/Prosthetist

Chico

California State University - Chico
Manuel A Esteban, President
Chico, CA 95929-0222
916 898-5871
- Dietitian/Nutritionist
- Speech Language Pathologist
- Therapeutic Recreation Specialist

Institutions

Enloe Hospital
Philip R Wolfe, MS, Executive Director
W Fifth Ave and The Esplanade
Chico, CA 95926
916 891-7300
• Radiographer

Chula Vista

Southwestern Community College
Joseph M Conte, MS, Superintendent/President
900 Otay Lakes Rd
Chula Vista, CA 91910
619 482-6301
• Surgical Technologist

Costa Mesa

Orange Coast College
Margaret A Gratton, MS MA, President
2701 Fairview Rd
Costa Mesa, CA 92628-0120
714 432-5712
• Dental Assistant
• Diagnostic Med Sonographer
• Dietetic Technician
• Electroneurodiagnostic Tech
• Medical Assistant
• Radiographer
• Respiratory Therapist

Culver City

West Los Angeles College
Evelyn C Wong, President
4800 Freshman Dr
Culver City, CA 90230
310 287-4200
• Dental Hygienist

Cupertino

De Anza College
Martha Kanter, PhD, President
21250 Stevens Creek Blvd
Cupertino, CA 95014
408 864-8705
• Medical Assistant

Cypress

Cypress College
Christine Johnson, EdD, President
9200 Valley View St
Cypress, CA 90630
714 826-2220
• Dental Assistant
• Dental Hygienist
• Health Information Tech
• Radiographer

Davis

University of California - Davis
Gerald S Lazarus, MD, Dean
School of Medicine
Davis, CA 95616
916 752-0321
• Dietitian/Nutritionist
• Physician Assistant

Duarte

City of Hope National Medical Center
Charles M. Bach, MD, CEO
1500 E Duarte Rd
Duarte, CA 91010
818 359-8111
• Radiation Therapist

El Cajon

Grossmont College
Richard Sanchez, EdD, President
8800 Grossmont College Dr
El Cajon, CA 92020
619 465-1700
• Cardiovascular Technologist
• Dietetic Technician
• Occupational Therapy Asst
• Respiratory Therapist

Emeryville

Kaiser Permanente Medical Center
Donald Oxley, Area Manager
2200 Powell St
Tower II 4th Fl, Ste 450
Emeryville, CA 94608
510 596-6618
• Radiographer

Eureka

College of the Redwoods
Cedric A Sampson, President
Tompkins Hill Rd
Eureka, CA 95501
707 445-6700
• Dental Assistant

Fremont

Ohlone College
Floyd Hogue, PhD, Supt/President
43600 Mission Blvd
PO Box 3909
Fremont, CA 94539
510 659-6200
• Respiratory Therapist

Fresno

California State University - Fresno
John D Welty, President
5048 N Jackson
Fresno, CA 93740-0080
209 278-2423
• Dietitian/Nutritionist
• Rehabilitation Counselor
• Speech Language Pathologist

Comm Hospital of Central California
Fresno and R Sts
Fresno, CA 93715
209 442-3946
• Dietitian/Nutritionist

Fresno City College
Arthur Ellish, EdD, Interim President
1101 E University Ave
Fresno, CA 93741
209 442-4600
• Dental Hygienist
• Health Information Tech
• Radiographer
• Respiratory Therapist

Fresno Community Hospital & Medical Ctr
Bruce Perry, President
PO Box 1232
Fresno, CA 93715
209 442-3911
• Clin Lab Scientist/Med Tech

Valley Children's Hospital
Rex Riley, CEO
3151 N Millbrook Ave
Fresno, CA 93703
209 225-3000
• Clin Lab Scientist/Med Tech

Fullerton

California State University - Fullerton
Milton A Gordon, President
800 N State College Blvd
Fullerton, CA 92634
714 773-3617
• Speech Language Pathologist

Glendale

Uni Health America/Glendale Mem Hosp
1420 S Central Ave
Glendale, CA 91204
818 502-2334
• Dietitian/Nutritionist

Glendora

Citrus College
Louis E Zellers,
1000 W Foothill
Glendora, CA 91740
818 963-0323
• Dental Assistant

Hayward

California State University - Hayward
Norma S Rees, President
25800 Carlos Bee Blvd
Hayward, CA 94542
510 881-3086
• Speech Language Pathologist

Chabot College
Raul J Cardoza, EdD, President
25555 Hesperian Blvd
PO Box 5001
Hayward, CA 94545-5001
510 786-6640
• Dental Assistant
• Dental Hygienist
• Health Information Tech
• Medical Assistant

Inglewood

Daniel Freeman Memorial Hospital
Joseph W Dunn, PhD, CEO
333 N Prairie Ave
Inglewood, CA 90301
310 674-7050
- Emergency Med Tech-Paramedic
- Radiographer

Irwindale

Public Health Foundation
WIC Program
12781 Schabarum Ave
Irwindale, CA 91706-6802
818 856-6376
- Dietitian/Nutritionist

Kentfield

College of Marin
James E Middleton, Superintendent/Pres
College Ave
Kentfield, CA 94904
415 457-8811
- Dental Assistant

La Jolla

Scripps Memorial Hospitals
Martin Buser, MHA, President/CEO
9888 Genesee Ave
La Jolla, CA 92037
619 457-6100
- Clin Lab Scientist/Med Tech

La Puente

Hacienda LaPuente Unified School Dist
John E Rieckewald, PhD, Asst Supt
Adult and Alternative Education
15540 E Fairgrove Ave
La Puente, CA 91744
818 968-4638
- Dental Assistant
- Respiratory Therapy Tech

Loma Linda

Loma Linda University
B Lyn Behrens, MS, President and CEO
Magan Hall Room 111
Loma Linda, CA 92350
909 824-4540
- Clin Lab Scientist/Med Tech
- Cytotechnologist
- Dental Hygienist
- Diagnostic Med Sonographer
- Dietitian/Nutritionist
- Dietetic Technician
- Health Information Admin
- Nuclear Medicine Tech
- Occupational Therapist
- Occupational Therapy Asst
- Radiation Therapist
- Radiographer
- Respiratory Therapist
- Speech Language Pathologist
- Surgical Technologist

Long Beach

California Paramedical & Tech College
Julia Morally, President/Owner
3745 Long Beach Blvd
Long Beach, CA 90807
310 595-6630
- Respiratory Therapy Tech
- Surgical Technologist

California State University - Long Beach
Robert Maxson, EdD, President
1250 Bellflower Blvd SS/AD 300
Long Beach, CA 90840-0115
310 985-4121
- Audiologist
- Dietitian/Nutritionist
- Radiation Therapist
- Speech Language Pathologist
- Therapeutic Recreation Specialist

Long Beach City College
Barbara A Adams, MA, Supt/Pres
4901 E Carson St
Long Beach, CA 90808
310 938-4121
- Dietetic Technician
- Radiographer

St Mary Medical Center
David Tillman, MD, Administrator
1050 Linden Ave
Long Beach, CA 90813
310 491-9010
- Clin Lab Scientist/Med Tech

Veterans Affairs Medical Center
Jerry B Boyd, Director
5901 E Seventh St
Long Beach, CA 90822
310 494-5400
- Clin Lab Scientist/Med Tech

Los Altos Hills

Foothill College
Bernadine Fong, PhD, President
12345 El Monte Rd
Los Altos Hills, CA 94022
415 949-7200
- Dental Assistant
- Dental Hygienist
- Radiation Therapist
- Radiographer
- Respiratory Therapist

Los Angeles

California State University - Los Angeles
James M Rosser, President
5151 State University Dr
Los Angeles, CA 90032
213 343-4690
- Audiologist
- Dietitian/Nutritionist
- Rehabilitation Counselor
- Speech Language Pathologist

Cedars Sinai Medical Center
Thomas Priselac, Exec Vice Pres
8700 Beverly Blvd
Los Angeles, CA 90048
310 855-6211
- Clin Lab Scientist/Med Tech

Charles R Drew Univ of Med & Science
Reed V Tuckson, MD, President
1621 E 120th St
Los Angeles, CA 90059
213 563-4987
- Clin Lab Scientist/Med Tech
- Dietitian/Nutritionist
- Health Information Tech
- Nuclear Medicine Tech
- Physician Assistant
- Radiographer

Children's Hospital of Los Angeles
Walter W Noce Jr, MPH, President & CEO
4650 Sunset Blvd
Los Angeles, CA 90027
213 669-2301
- Dietitian/Nutritionist
- Radiographer

East Los Angeles Occupational Center
2100 Marengo St
Los Angeles, CA 90033
213 223-1283
- Dental Assistant

Los Angeles City College
Jose L Robledo, MA, President
855 N Vermont Ave
Los Angeles, CA 90029
213 953-4201
- Dental Lab Technician
- Dietetic Technician
- Radiographer

Los Angeles County - USC Medical Center
Douglas D Bagley, MS, Interim Exec Dir
1200 N State St Rm 112
Los Angeles, CA 90033
213 226-6501
- Clin Lab Scientist/Med Tech
- Cytotechnologist
- Dietitian/Nutritionist
- Nuclear Medicine Tech
- Radiation Therapist
- Radiographer

Loyola Marymount University
Thomas P O'Malley, SJ, President
Loyola Blvd at W 80th St
Los Angeles, CA 90045
310 338-2700
- Art Therapist

Mt St Mary's College
Sr Karen Kennelly, PhD, President
Chalon Campus
12001 Chalon Rd
Los Angeles, CA 90049-1599
310 471-9500
- Occupational Therapy Asst

UCLA Center for Health Sciences
Sheldon King, MD, Interim Med Ctr Dir
Administration 17-165 CHS
10833 Le Conte Ave
Los Angeles, CA 90024-1730
310 825-5041
- Cytotechnologist

Institutions

University of Southern California
Steven B Sample, PhD, President
University Park Campus
Los Angeles, CA 90089
213 740-2111
- Dental Hygienist
- Occupational Therapist
- Physician Assistant

Veterans Affairs Med Ctr W Los Angeles
Kenneth J Clark, MA JD, Director
11301 Wilshire Blvd
Los Angeles, CA 90073
310 268-3132
- Clin Lab Scientist/Med Tech
- Dietitian/Nutritionist
- Nuclear Medicine Tech
- Radiographer

Malibu

Pepperdine University
David Davenport, President
24255 Pacific Coast Hwy
Malibu, CA 90263
310 456-4000
- Dietitian/Nutritionist

Marysville

Yuba Community College
Stephen Epler, Superintendent
2088 N Beal Rd
Marysville, CA 95901
916 741-6716
- Radiographer

Merced

Merced College
Jan Moser, PhD, President/Supt
3600 M St
Merced, CA 95348-2898
209 384-6101
- Radiographer

Modesto

Modesto Junior College
Maria Sheehan, PhD, President
435 College Ave
Modesto, CA 95350-9977
209 575-6067
- Dental Assistant
- Emergency Med Tech-Paramedic
- Medical Assistant
- Respiratory Therapist

Monterey

Monterey Peninsula College
Edward O Gould, Superindentent/Pres
980 Fremont Ave
Monterey, CA 93940
408 646-4010
- Dental Assistant

Monterey Park

East Los Angeles College
Ernest H Moreno, MA, President
1301 Avenida Cesar Chavez
Monterey Park, CA 91754
213 265-8662
- Health Information Tech
- Respiratory Therapist

Moorpark

Moorpark College
James Walker, PhD, President
7075 Campus Rd
Moorpark, CA 93021
805 378-1400
- Radiographer

Napa

ARAMARK Healthcare Support Services
477 Devlin Rd Ste 108
Napa, CA 94558
707 254-1130
- Dietitian/Nutritionist

Napa State Hospital
2100 Napa Vallejo Hwy
Napa, CA 94558
707 253-5428
- Dietitian/Nutritionist

Napa Valley College
Diane Carey, PhD, President/Supt
2277 Napa Vallejo Hwy
Napa, CA 94558
707 253-3360
- Respiratory Therapist

National City

California College for Health Sciences
Roy Winter, MBA, President/CEO
222 W 24th St
National City, CA 91950
619 477-4800
- Respiratory Therapist
- Respiratory Therapy Tech

North Hollywood

ConCorde Career Institute
Jeanne Thompson, Director
4150 Lankershim Blvd
North Hollywood, CA 91602
818 766-8151
- Respiratory Therapy Tech
- Surgical Technologist

Northridge

California State University - Northridge
Blenda J Wilson, PhD, President
18111 Nordhoff St
Northridge, CA 91330
818 677-2121
- Athletic Trainer
- Audiologist
- Dietitian/Nutritionist
- Music Therapist
- Radiographer
- Speech Language Pathologist
- Therapeutic Recreation Specialist

Norwalk

Cerritos College
Fred Gaskin, Superintendent/Pres
11110 E Alondra Blvd
Norwalk, CA 90650
310 860-2451
- Dental Assistant
- Dental Hygienist

Oakland

Merritt College
Wise Allen, PhD, President
12500 Campus Dr
Oakland, CA 94619
510 436-2414
- Radiographer

Samuel Merritt College
Sharon Diaz, MS RN, President
370 Hawthorne Ave
Oakland, CA 94609-3108
510 420-6011
- Occupational Therapist

Orange

Chapman University
James L Doti, President
333 N Glassell St
Orange, CA 92666
714 997-6815
- Music Therapist

CSi Bryman College
Pamela Burns, BA, Executive Director
1120 W La Veta Ave/Ste 100
Orange, CA 92668
714 953-6500
- Medical Assistant

St Joseph Hospital
Larry Ainsworth, President/CEO
1100 Stewart Dr
Orange, CA 92668
714 771-8111
- Clin Lab Scientist/Med Tech

Univ of California Irvine Med Ctr
Mark Laret, Executive Dir
UCI Medical Ctr
101 City Dr S
Orange, CA 92868-3298
714 456-5678
- Clin Lab Scientist/Med Tech

Oroville

Butte College
Betty Dean, EdD, President
3536 Butte Campus Dr
Oroville, CA 95965
916 895-2484
- Respiratory Therapist

Oxnard

St John's Regional Medical Center
Daniel Herlinger, President
1600 N Rose Ave
Oxnard, CA 93030
805 988-2500
- Radiographer

Palm Desert

College of the Desert

David George, PhD, President
43-500 Monterey Ave
Palm Desert, CA 92260
619 346-8041
- Respiratory Therapist

Pasadena

Huntington Memorial Hospital

Stephen A Ralph, President/CEO
100 W California Blvd
PO Box 7013
Pasadena, CA 91109-7013
818 397-5000
- Clin Lab Scientist/Med Tech
- Radiographer

Pasadena City College

James Kossler, PhD, Supt/President
1570 E Colorado Blvd
Pasadena, CA 91106
818 585-7201
- Dental Assistant
- Dental Hygienist
- Dental Lab Technician
- Medical Assistant
- Radiographer

Patton

Patton State Hospital

3102 E Highland Ave
Patton, CA 92369
909 425-7297
- Dietitian/Nutritionist

Pleasant Hill

Diablo Valley College

Mark Edelstein, President
321 Golf Club Rd
Pleasant Hill, CA 94523
510 685-1230
- Dental Assistant
- Dental Hygienist

Pomona

California State Polytechnic University

Bob H Suzuki, President
3801 W Temple Ave
Pomona, CA 91768
909 869-2000
- Dietitian/Nutritionist

Western Univ of Health Sciences

Philip Pumerantz, PhD, President
College Plaza
Pomona, CA 91766-1889
909 469-5200
- Physician Assistant

Porterville

Porterville Development Center

Porterville, CA 93258
209 782-2753
- Dietitian/Nutritionist

Rancho Cucamonga

Chaffey Community College

Jerry W Young, PhD, Supt/President
5885 Haven Ave
Rancho Cucamonga, CA 91737
909 941-2100
- Dental Assistant
- Dietetic Technician
- Radiographer

Rancho Mirage

Eisenhower Memorial Hospital

Andrew Deems, President/CEO
39000 Bob Hope Dr
Rancho Mirage, CA 92270
619 340-3911
- Clin Lab Scientist/Med Tech

Redlands

University of Redlands

James R Appleton, President
PO Box 3080
1200 E Colton Ave
Redlands, CA 92373-0999
714 335-4061
- Speech Language Pathologist

Redwood City

Canada College

Marie E Rosenwasser, President
4200 Farm Hill Blvd
Redwood City, CA 94061
415 364-1212
- Radiographer

Riverside

Calif Paramedical & Tech Coll-Riverside

Julia Morally, President
4550 LaSierra Ave
Riverside, CA 92505
909 687-9006
- Respiratory Therapist

Rosemead

National Education Ctr - Bryman Campus

Roger Gugelmeyer, Executive Director
3505 N Hart Ave
Rosemead, CA 91770
818 573-5470
- Medical Assistant

Sacramento

American River College

Marie Smith, EdD, President
4700 College Oak Dr
Sacramento, CA 95841
916 484-8211
- Respiratory Therapist

California State University - Sacramento

Donald Gerth, PhD, President
CSUS 6000 J St
Sacramento, CA 95819
916 278-7737
- Athletic Trainer
- Audiologist
- Dietitian/Nutritionist
- Rehabilitation Counselor
- Speech Language Pathologist
- Therapeutic Recreation Specialist

Cosumnes River College

Merrilee Lewis, PhD, President
8401 Ctr Pkwy
Sacramento, CA 95823
916 688-7321
- Health Information Tech
- Medical Assistant

Sacramento City College

Robert M Harris, PhD, President
3835 Freeport Blvd
Sacramento, CA 95822-1386
916 558-2100
- Dental Assistant
- Dental Hygienist
- Occupational Therapy Asst

Sacramento Medical Foundation Blood Ctr

Paul V Holland, MD, CEO
1625 Stockton Blvd
Sacramento, CA 95816
916 456-1500
- Specialist in BB Tech

Univ of California Davis Med Ctr

Frank J Loge, Administrator
2315 Stockton Blvd
Sacramento, CA 95817
916 453-3096
- Clin Lab Scientist/Med Tech

Western Career College

Richard G Nathanson, BS, CEO
8909 Folsom Blvd
Sacramento, CA 95826
916 361-1660
- Medical Assistant

Western Career College of San Leandro

Richard G Nathanson, BS, CEO
8909 Folsom Blvd
Sacramento, CA 95826
916 361-1660
- Medical Assistant

San Bernardino

California State Univ - San Bernardino

Anthony H Evans, President
5500 University Pkwy
San Bernardino, CA 92407
909 880-5000
- Dietitian/Nutritionist
- Rehabilitation Counselor

National Education Ctr - Skadron Campus

David W Corson, BA MBA, President
825 E Hospitality Ln
San Bernardino, CA 92408
909 885-3896
- Medical Assistant

Institutions

San Bernardino County Medical Center
Charles Jervis, MBA, Administrator
780 E Gilbert St
San Bernardino, CA 92415-0935
909 387-8185
- Clin Lab Scientist/Med Tech
- Radiographer

San Bernardino Valley College
Donald L Singer, President
701 S Mount Vernon Ave
San Bernardino, CA 92410
909 888-6511
- Dietetic Technician

San Bruno

Skyline College
Linda Salters, MS, President
3300 College Dr
San Bruno, CA 94066
415 738-4111
- Respiratory Therapist

San Diego

Maric College of Medical Careers
Gerry M Taylor, BS, Director of Operations
8880 Rio San Diego Dr/Ste 370
San Diego, CA 92108-1634
619 908-3600
- Occupational Therapy Asst

Naval School of Dental Technology
W A Rathbun, Commanding Officer
4170 Norman Scott Rd
San Diego, CA 92136-5597
615 556-7987
- Dental Lab Technician

Naval School of Hlth Sciences - San Diego
Cynthia E Perry, Capt NC USN, CO Officer
Naval School of Hlth Sciences-San Diego
34101 Farenholt Ave
San Diego, CA 92134-5291
619 532-7700
- Clin Lab Tech/Med Lab Tech-C
- Physician Assistant
- Surgical Technologist

San Diego Mesa College
Constance M Carroll, MA, President
7250 Mesa College Dr
San Diego, CA 92111
619 627-2721
- Dental Assistant
- Health Information Tech
- Medical Assistant
- Radiographer

San Diego State University
Thomas B Day, President
San Diego, CA 92182
619 594-7746
- Audiologist
- Dietitian/Nutritionist
- Rehabilitation Counselor
- Speech Language Pathologist
- Therapeutic Recreation Specialist

Sharp Memorial Hospital
Peter K Ellsworth, President/CEO
San Diego Hospital Assoc
3131 Berger Ave
San Diego, CA 92123
619 541-4000
- Cytotechnologist

Univ of California San Diego Med Ctr
Sumi Kastelic, Director
200 W Arbor Dr/H-910C
San Diego, CA 92103-8970
619 543-6654
- Nuclear Medicine Tech
- Radiation Therapist

Veterans Affairs Medical Center
3350 La Jolla Village Dr
San Diego, CA 92161
619 552-8585
- Dietitian/Nutritionist

San Francisco

California Pacific Medical Center
G Aubrey Serfling, MBA MPH, CEO
3700 California St
San Francisco, CA 94118
415 387-8700
- Clin Lab Scientist/Med Tech

City College of San Francisco
Del Anderson, Chancellor
50 Phelan Ave
San Francisco, CA 94112
415 239-3000
- Dental Assistant
- Health Information Tech
- Medical Assistant
- Radiation Therapist
- Radiographer

National Education Ctr - Bryman Campus
Albert H Plante, BA MA, Executive Director
731 Market St
San Francisco, CA 94103
415 777-2500
- Medical Assistant

San Francisco State University
Robert A Corrigan, PhD, President
1600 Holloway Ave
San Francisco, CA 94132
415 338-1381
- Audiologist
- Clin Lab Scientist/Med Tech
- Dietitian/Nutritionist
- Rehabilitation Counselor
- Speech Language Pathologist

University of California - San Francisco
William B Kerr, MPH, Dir Med Ctr
505 Parnassus Ave
San Francisco, CA 94143
415 476-1405
- Dental Hygienist
- Dietitian/Nutritionist
- Nuclear Medicine Tech

San Jose

Columbia San Jose Medical Center
Mary Schwird, President
675 E Santa Clara St
San Jose, CA 95112
408 977-4540
- Clin Lab Scientist/Med Tech

ConCorde Career Institute
Cheryl Smith, Director
1290 N First St
San Jose, CA 95112
408 441-6411
- Respiratory Therapy Tech

National Education Ctr - Bryman Campus
Janice L Coble, Executive Director
2015 Naglee Ave
San Jose, CA 95128
408 275-8800
- Medical Assistant

San Jose City College
Chui Tsang, President
2100 Moorpark Ave
San Jose, CA 95128
408 298-2181
- Dental Assistant

San Jose State University
Robert L Caret, PhD, President
Coll of Applied Sciences and Arts
One Washington Square
San Jose, CA 95192-0002
408 924-1177
- Audiologist
- Dietitian/Nutritionist
- Occupational Therapist
- Speech Language Pathologist

San Luis Obispo

California Polytechnic State University
Warren J Baker, President
San Luis Obispo, CA 93407
805 756-1111
- Dietitian/Nutritionist

San Marcos

Palomar Community College
George R Boggs, Superintendent/Pres
1140 W Mission Rd
San Marcos, CA 92069
619 744-1150
- Dental Assistant

San Mateo

College of San Mateo
Peter J Landsberger, President
1700 W Hillsdale Blvd
San Mateo, CA 94402
415 574-6161
- Dental Assistant

San Pablo

Contra Costa College
D Candy Rose, President
2600 Mission Bell Dr
San Pablo, CA 94806
510 235-7800
● Dental Assistant

Santa Barbara

Cancer Foundation of Santa Barbara
Richard Scott, BA CPA, Executive Director
300 W Pueblo St
Santa Barbara, CA 93105
805 682-7300
● Nuclear Medicine Tech
● Radiation Therapist

Santa Barbara City College
Peter R MacDougall, Supt/President
721 Cliff Dr
Santa Barbara, CA 93109
805 965-0581
● Radiographer

Santa Barbara Cottage Hospital
James L Ash, President/CEO
PO Box 689 Pueblo at Bath Sts
Santa Barbara, CA 93102
805 569-7290
● Clin Lab Scientist/Med Tech

Santa Maria

Coastal Valley College
Stella P Martin, CMA BS, Associate Director
731 S Lincoln St
Santa Maria, CA 93454
805 925-1478
● Medical Assistant

Santa Monica

Santa Monica College
Piedad F Robertson, PhD, President
1900 Pico Blvd
Santa Monica, CA 90405
310 450-5150
● Respiratory Therapist

Santa Rosa

Santa Rosa Junior College
Robert F Agrella, EdD, Supt/President
1501 Mendocino Ave
Santa Rosa, CA 95401
707 527-4431
● Dental Assistant
● Radiographer

Saratoga

West Valley Community College District
Leo Chavez, PhD, President
14000 Fruitvale Ave
Saratoga, CA 95070
408 867-2200
● Medical Assistant

Simi Valley

Simi Valley Adult School
Sondra Jones, MA, Director
3192 Los Angeles Ave
Simi Valley, CA 93065
805 579-6200
● Respiratory Therapy Tech
● Surgical Technologist

Stanford

Stanford University School of Medicine
Eugene Bauer, MD, Dean
SU Medical Ctr Rm M121
Stanford, CA 94305-5302
415 723-6436
● Physician Assistant

Stockton

San Joaquin General Hospital
Stephen Ebert, Hospital Director
PO Box 1020
Stockton, CA 95201
209 468-6600
● Radiographer

University of the Pacific
3601 Pacific Ave
Stockton, CA 95211
209 946-2381
● Music Therapist
● Speech Language Pathologist

Sylmar

Olive View/UCLA Medical Center
14445 Olive View Dr
Sylmar, CA 91342
818 364-4224
● Dietitian/Nutritionist
● Radiographer

Taft

Taft College
David Cothrum, President
29 Emmons Park Dr Box 1437
Taft, CA 93268
805 763-4282
● Dental Hygienist

Torrance

El Camino College
Thomas M Fallo, Superintendent/President
16007 Crenshaw Blvd
Torrance, CA 90506
310 532-3670
● Radiographer
● Respiratory Therapist

LA County Harbor UCLA Medical Center
Tecla Mickoseff, MBA, Acting Hosp Admin
1000 W Carson St Box 1
Torrance, CA 90509-2910
310 222-2101
● Clin Lab Scientist/Med Tech
● Radiographer

National Education Ctr - Bryman Campus
Judy Kavanaugh, Director
4212 W Artesia Blvd
Torrance, CA 90504
310 542-6951
● Medical Assistant

Van Nuys

Los Angeles Valley College
Tyree Weider, MS, President
5800 Fulton Ave
Van Nuys, CA 91401-4096
818 781-1200
● Respiratory Therapist

Victorville

Victor Valley College
Nicholas Halisky, CEO
18422 Bear Valley Rd
Victorville, CA 92392-9699
619 245-4271
● Respiratory Therapist

Visalia

Golden State Business College Inc
Gary Yasuda, BSBA, President
3356 S Fairway
Visalia, CA 93277
209 733-4040
● Medical Assistant

San Joaquin Valley College
Michael D Perry, CEO
8400 W Mineral King
Visalia, CA 93291
209 651-2500
● Respiratory Therapist
● Respiratory Therapy Tech

Walnut

Mt San Antonio College
William H Feddersen, EdD, Supt/President
1100 N Grand Ave
Walnut, CA 91789
909 594-5611
● Radiographer
● Respiratory Therapist

Yucaipa

Crafton Hills College
Louis Gomez, PhD, President
11711 Sand Canyon Rd
Yucaipa, CA 92399
909 389-3200
● Emergency Med Tech-Paramedic
● Respiratory Therapist
● Respiratory Therapy Tech

Colorado

Aurora

T H Pickens Technical Center
Dan R Lucero, PhD, Executive Director
Vocational Education
500 Airport Blvd
Aurora, CO 80011
303 344-4910
- Clin Lab Tech/Med Lab Tech-C
- Dental Assistant
- Medical Assistant
- Respiratory Therapy Tech

Boulder

University of Colorado
Campus Box 409
Boulder, CO 80309-0409
303 492-6445
- Audiologist
- Speech Language Pathologist

Colorado Springs

Blair Junior College
Pat Draper-Hardy, Director
828 Wooten Rd
Colorado Springs, CO 80915
719 574-1082
- Medical Assistant

Memorial Hospital
J Robert Peters, MBA, Exec Director
2790 N Academy Blvd Ste 201
Colorado Springs, CO 80917
719 475-5000
- Radiographer

Penrose-St Francis Health System
Donna Bertram, MBA, COO
Penrose Hospital, Member Centura Health
2215 N Cascade Ave/PO Box 7021
Colorado Springs, CO 80933
719 776-5111
- Clin Lab Scientist/Med Tech
- Diagnostic Med Sonographer
- Dietitian/Nutritionist
- Histologic Technician-Cert
- Radiographer

Pike's Peak Community College
Marijane A Paulsen, President
5765 S Academy Blvd
Colorado Springs, CO 80906
719 576-7711
- Dental Assistant

Denver

Community Coll of Denver - Auraria Campus
Byron McClenney, EdD, President
Campus Box 250 PO Box 173363
Denver, CO 80217-3363
303 556-2411
- Nuclear Medicine Tech
- Radiographer
- Surgical Technologist

Community College of Denver
Byron N McClenney, President
PO Box 173363
Denver, CO 80217
303 556-2600
- Dental Hygienist
- Medical Assistant

ConCorde Career Institute
Gene Johnson, VP of Operations
770 Grant St
Denver, CO 80203
303 861-1151
- Surgical Technologist

Denver Institute of Technology
James Z Turner, MBA, Vice President
7350 N Broadway
Denver, CO 80221-3653
303 650-5050
- Medical Assistant
- Occupational Therapy Asst

Emily Griffith Opportunity School
Sharon Johnson,
1250 Welton St
Denver, CO 80204
303 575-4721
- Dental Assistant
- Medical Assistant

HealthONE Ctr for Health Sciences Educ
Jeanette Mladenovic, MD, President
1719 E 19th Ave
Denver, CO 80218
303 869-2278
- Clin Lab Scientist/Med Tech

Parks College
Janis Y Schoonmaker, BS, Director
9065 Grant St
Denver, CO 80229
303 457-2757
- Medical Assistant

Provenant - St Anthony Hospitals
Michael H Erne, CEO
4231 W 16th Ave
Denver, CO 80204
303 629-4350
- Emergency Med Tech-Paramedic
- Radiographer

Regis University
Michael J Sheeran, SJ, President
3333 Regis Blvd
Denver, CO 80221-1099
303 458-4190
- Health Information Admin

Swedish Medical Center
Jeffery Dorsey, President/CEO
Columbia/Denver Region
4343 S Ulster St #1200
Denver, CO 80237
303 779-4993
- Emergency Med Tech-Paramedic

University of Colorado Hlth Science Ctr
Vincent Fulginiti, MD, Chancellor
4200 E Ninth Ave/PO Box A095
Denver, CO 80262
303 315-7682
- Clin Lab Scientist/Med Tech
- Dental Hygienist
- Diagnostic Med Sonographer
- Physician Assistant

Englewood

Tri-County Health Nutrition Services
7000 E Bellview Ave Ste 301
Englewood, CO 80111-1628
303 220-9200
- Dietitian/Nutritionist

Fort Collins

Colorado State University
Albert C Yates, PhD, President
102 Administration Bldg
Fort Collins, CO 80523
970 491-6211
- Dietitian/Nutritionist
- Music Therapist
- Occupational Therapist

Front Range Comm College - Ft Collins
Rom Gonzales, President
Larimer Campus PO Box 270490
Fort Collins, CO 80527
303 226-2500
- Dental Assistant

Fort Morgan

Morgan Community College
John R McKay, PhD, President
17800 Rd 20
Fort Morgan, CO 80701-4399
970 867-3081
- Occupational Therapy Asst

Grand Junction

Mesa State College
Michael Gallagher, PhD, President
PO Box 2647
Grand Junction, CO 81502
970 248-1020
- Radiographer

Greeley

Aims Community College
George R Conger, PhD, President
PO Box 69
Greeley, CO 80632
303 330-8008
- Radiographer

University of Northern Colorado
Howard Skinner, President
Carter Hall 4000
President's Office
Greeley, CO 80639
970 351-1890
- Athletic Trainer
- Audiologist
- Dietitian/Nutritionist
- Rehabilitation Counselor
- Speech Language Pathologist
- Therapeutic Recreation Specialist

Lakewood

Red Rocks Community College
Dorothy A Horrell, President
13300 W Sixth Ave
Lakewood, CO 80401-5398
303 988-6160
- Radiographer

Littleton

Arapahoe Community College
James F Weber, PhD, President
2500 W College Dr PO Box 9002
Littleton, CO 80160-9002
303 797-5701
- Clin Lab Tech/Med Lab Tech-AD
- Health Information Tech
- Occupational Therapy Asst

Pueblo

Parkview Episcopal Medical Center
C W Smith, MBA, President/CEO
400 W 16th St
Pueblo, CO 81003
719 584-4573
- Clin Lab Scientist/Med Tech

Pueblo Community College
Joe D May, EdD, President
900 W Orman Ave
Pueblo, CO 81004-1499
719 549-3213
- Dental Assistant
- Dental Hygienist
- Health Information Tech
- Occupational Therapy Asst
- Radiographer
- Respiratory Therapist
- Surgical Technologist

Rangley

Colorado Northwestern Community College
Robert A Anderson, President
500 Kennedy Dr
Rangley, CO 81648
970 675-2261
- Dental Hygienist

Thornton

Colorado Assn of Paramedical Educ, Inc
Donald Massey, DO, Medical Director
9191 Grant St
Thornton, CO 80229
303 451-7800
- Emergency Med Tech-Paramedic

Westminster

Front Range Comm College - Westminster
Thomas Gonzales, PhD, President
3645 W 112th Ave
Westminster, CO 80030
303 404-5422
- Dental Assistant
- Dietetic Technician
- Medical Assistant
- Respiratory Therapist

Connecticut

Branford

Branford Hall Career Institute
Michael D Bouman, COO
One Summit Pl
Branford, CT 06405
203 488-2525
- Medical Assistant

Bridgeport

Bridgeport Hospital
Robert Trefry, President
267 Grant St
Bridgeport, CT 06610
203 384-3464
- Clin Lab Scientist/Med Tech

Housatonic Community Technical College
Janis M Wertz, EdD, President
510 Barnum Ave
Bridgeport, CT 06608
203 579-6464
- Clin Lab Tech/Med Lab Tech-AD

St Vincent's Medical Center
William J Riordan, MHA, President
2800 Main St
Bridgeport, CT 06606
203 576-5455
- Clin Lab Scientist/Med Tech
- Nuclear Medicine Tech

Univ of Bridgeport/Fones School
Richard L Rubenstein, President
30 Hazel St
Bridgeport, CT 06601
203 576-4000
- Dental Hygienist

Danbury

Danbury Hospital
Frank Kelly, President/CEO
24 Hospital Ave
Danbury, CT 06810
203 797-7210
- Clin Lab Scientist/Med Tech
- Dietitian/Nutritionist
- Radiation Therapist
- Radiographer
- Surgical Technologist

Danielson

Quinebaug Valley Comm - Tech College
Dianne E Williams, BS MS, President
742 Upper Maple St
Danielson, CT 06239
860 774-1160
- Medical Assistant

East Hartford

Data Institute Business School
Mark E Scheinberg, BA, President
745 Burnside Ave
East Hartford, CT 06108
860 528-4111
- Medical Assistant

Enfield

Porter and Chester Institute - Chicopee
Joseph Doering, VP and Executive Director
138 Weymouth Rd
Enfield, CT 06082
203 741-2561
- Medical Assistant

Porter and Chester Institute - Enfield
Joseph Doering, Executive Director
138 Weymouth Rd
Enfield, CT 06082
203 741-2561
- Medical Assistant

Fairfield

Sacred Heart Univ/St Vincent Med Ctr
Anthony Cernera, PhD, President
5151 Park Ave
Fairfield, CT 06432-1000
203 371-7999
- Respiratory Therapist

Farmington

Tunxis Community Technical College
Cathryn L Addy, President
271 Scott Swamp Rd
Farmington, CT 06032-3187
203 677-7701
- Dental Assistant
- Dental Hygienist

University of Connecticut Health Center
Leslie S Cutler, DDS PhD, Exec Director
Farmington Ave
Farmington, CT 06030
860 679-2111
- Cytotechnologist

Hamden

Eli Whitney Regional Voc Tech School
71 Jones Rd
Hamden, CT 06514
203 397-4037
- Dental Assistant

Quinnipiac College

John L Lahey, PhD, President
275 Mt Carmel Ave
Hamden, CT 06518-0008
203 288-5251
- Clin Lab Scientist/Med Tech
- Occupational Therapist
- Perfusionist
- Physician Assistant
- Radiographer
- Respiratory Therapist

Stone Academy

Janet S Arena, President
1315 Dixwell Ave
Hamden, CT 06514
203 288-7474
- Medical Assistant

Hartford

A I Prince Regional Vocational Technical

500 Bookfield St
Hartford, CT 06106
203 246-8594
- Dental Assistant

CCTC/St Francis Hosp & Med Ctr

Ira Rubenzahl, PhD
61 Woodland St
Hartford, CT 06105-2354
203 520-7801
- Emergency Med Tech-Paramedic
- Radiographer

Hartford Hospital

John J Meehan, MHA, President/CEO
80 Seymour St PO Box 5037
Hartford, CT 06102-5037
860 545-2100
- Clin Lab Scientist/Med Tech
- Histologic Technician-Cert
- Radiation Therapist
- Radiographer

Morse School of Business

Michael S Taub, MEd, President
275 Asylum St
Hartford, CT 06103
203 522-2261
- Medical Assistant

Manchester

Manchester Community - Technical College

Jonathan Daube, EdD, President
60 Bidwell St - Mail Station #1
PO Box 1046
Manchester, CT 06045-1046
860 647-6005
- Clin Lab Tech/Med Lab Tech-AD
- Occupational Therapy Asst
- Respiratory Therapist
- Surgical Technologist

Manchester Memorial Hospital

Michael R Gallacher, MS, President
71 Haynes St
Manchester, CT 06040-4188
203 646-1222
- Radiographer

Meriden

Veterans Memorial Medical Center

Theodore H Horwitz, MBA, President
One King Pl PO Box 1009
Meriden, CT 06450-1009
203 238-8202
- Radiographer

Middletown

Middlesex Community - Technical College

Dianne Loilliams, MS, Acting President
100 Training Hill Rd
Middletown, CT 06457
860 343-5701
- Nuclear Medicine Tech
- Ophthalmic Dispenser
- Radiographer

New Haven

Gateway Community - Technical College

Diana VanDerPloeg, PhD, President
60 Sargent Dr
New Haven, CT 06511
203 789-7028
- Dietetic Technician
- Nuclear Medicine Tech
- Radiation Therapist
- Radiographer

Southern Connecticut State University

Michael Adanti, MS, President
501 Crescent St
New Haven, CT 06515
203 397-4234
- Athletic Trainer
- Audiologist
- Speech Language Pathologist

Yale University School of Medicine

Gerard N Burrow, MD, Dean
333 Cedar St
New Haven, CT 06510
203 785-4672
- Physician Assistant

Yale-New Haven Hospital

20 York St GBB
New Haven, CT 06504
203 785-5074
- Dietitian/Nutritionist

Newington

Connecticut Children's Medical Center

Scott Goodspeed, FACHE, President/CEO
181 E Cedar St
Newington, CT 06111
203 667-5580
- Orthotist/Prosthetist

Norwalk

Norwalk Hospital

David W Osborne, MS, CEO
Maple St
Norwalk, CT 06856
203 852-2211
- Respiratory Therapist

Southington

Briarwood College

Richard G Rausch, EdD, President
2279 Mt Vernon Rd
Southington, CT 06489
203 628-4751
- Dental Assistant
- Dietetic Technician
- Health Information Tech

Stamford

Stamford Hospital

Philip D Cusano, MA, President/CEO
Shelburne Rd PO Box 9317
Stamford, CT 06904-9317
203 325-7500
- Radiographer

Storrs

University of Connecticut

Harry J Hartley, President
Storrs, CT 06269
203 486-2000
- Audiologist
- Dietitian/Nutritionist
- Speech Language Pathologist
- Therapeutic Recreation Specialist

Stratford

Porter and Chester Institute - Stratford

Raymond R Clark, Executive Director
670 Lordship Blvd
Stratford, CT 06497
203 375-4463
- Medical Assistant

Waterbury

Naugatuck Valley Comm - Tech College

Richard L Sanders, EdD, President
750 Chase Pkwy
Waterbury, CT 06708
203 575-0328
- Radiographer
- Respiratory Therapy Tech

St Mary's Hospital

Sr Margurite Waite, CSJ MHA FACHE, President
56 Franklin St
Waterbury, CT 06702
203 574-6300
- Clin Lab Scientist/Med Tech

Watertown

Porter and Chester Institute - Watertown

Louis Giannelli, VP and Executive Director
320 Sylvan Lake Rd
Watertown, CT 06779
203 274-9294
- Medical Assistant

West Hartford

Fox Institute of Business
Patrick J Fox, BS, Director
99 South St
West Hartford, CT 06110
860 947-2299
- Medical Assistant

Saint Joseph College
Winifred E Coleman, President
1678 Asylum Ave
West Hartford, CT 06117
203 232-4571
- Dietitian/Nutritionist

University of Hartford
Humphrey Tonkin, PhD, President
200 Bloomfield Ave
West Hartford, CT 06117-1599
860 768-4417
- Clin Lab Scientist/Med Tech
- Occupational Therapist
- Radiographer
- Respiratory Therapist

West Haven

University of New Haven
Lawrence J Denardis, President
300 W Orange Ave
West Haven, CT 06516
203 932-7000
- Dental Hygienist
- Dietitian/Nutritionist

Wethersfield

Porter and Chester Institute
John D Mashia, BS, Executive Director
125 Silas Deane Hwy
Wethersfield, CT 06109
203 529-2519
- Medical Assistant

Willimantic

Windham Community Memorial Hospital
Duane Carlberg, President/CEO
112 Mansfield Ave
Willimantic, CT 06226
860 456-9116
- Radiographer

Windham Regional Vocational Tech School
210 Birch St
Willimantic, CT 06226
203 456-3789
- Dental Assistant

Winsted

Northwestern Connecticut Comm College
R Eileen Baccus, PhD, President
Park Place E
Winsted, CT 06098
203 738-6410
- Medical Assistant

Delaware

Dover

Delaware State University
William B Delauder, President
Dover, DE 19901
302 739-4924
- Dietitian/Nutritionist

Delaware Tech & Comm Coll - Owens Campus
G Timothy Kavel, EdD, VP/Campus Dir
Owens Campus
PO Box 610 Rte 18
Dover, DE 19947
302 856-5400
- Clin Lab Tech/Med Lab Tech-AD
- Occupational Therapy Asst
- Radiographer
- Respiratory Therapist

Delaware Tech & Comm Coll - Wilmington
Orlando J George Jr, EdD, President
President's Office PO Box 897
Dover, DE 19903
302 739-4621
- Dental Hygienist
- Diagnostic Med Sonographer
- Histologic Technician-AD
- Nuclear Medicine Tech
- Radiographer
- Respiratory Therapist

Kent General Central Delaware Hosp
Dennis E Klima, MHA, Pres/CEO
640 S State St
Dover, DE 19901
302 674-7001
- Emergency Med Tech-Paramedic

Newark

University of Delaware
David P Roselle, PhD, President
Office of the President
104A Hullihen Hall
Newark, DE 19716
302 831-2111
- Athletic Trainer
- Clin Lab Scientist/Med Tech
- Dietitian/Nutritionist

Wilmington

Medical Center of Delaware
Allen L Johnson, MHA, President
PO Box 1668
Wilmington, DE 19899
302 428-2571
- Emergency Med Tech-Paramedic

St Francis Hospital
Paul C King, MBA, President
Seventh and Clayton Sts
Wilmington, DE 19805
302 421-4801
- Radiographer

District of Columbia

Washington

Bureau of Medicine and Surgery (MED-05)
2300 E St W
Washington, DC 20372-5300
202 762-3830
- Radiographer

Gallaudet University
I Sr King Jordan, President
800 Florida Ave NE
Washington, DC 20002
202 651-5329
- Audiologist
- Rehabilitation Counselor
- Speech Language Pathologist
- Therapeutic Recreation Specialist

George Washington University
Allan B Weingold, MD, CEO
School of Medicine and Health Sciences
2300 Eye St NW/Ross Hall/Rm #713
Washington, DC 20037
202 994-3727
- Art Therapist
- Audiologist
- Clin Lab Scientist/Med Tech
- Diagnostic Med Sonographer
- Nuclear Medicine Tech
- Physician Assistant
- Radiation Therapist
- Rehabilitation Counselor
- Speech Language Pathologist

Georgetown University Medical Center
Sam Wiesel, MD, Exec VP Hlth Sciences
120 Bldg D/4000 Reservoir Dr NW
Washington, DC 20007
202 687-4601
- Ophthalmic Med Technician

Howard University
H Patrick Swygert, President
Mordecai Wyatt Johnson Bldg
2400 Sixth St NW
Washington, DC 20059
202 806-2500
- Audiologist
- Clin Lab Scientist/Med Tech
- Dental Hygienist
- Dietitian/Nutritionist
- Music Therapist
- Occupational Therapist
- Physician Assistant
- Radiation Therapist
- Speech Language Pathologist

M M Washington Career High School
27 O St NW
Washington, DC 20001
202 673-7478
- Dental Assistant

Marriott Corp/Marriott Hlthcare Mid-Atlantic
One Marriott Dr
Washington, DC 20058
301 380-2454
- Dietitian/Nutritionist

Institutions

University of the District of Columbia

Tilden J Le Melle, PhD, President
4200 Connecticut Ave NW
Washington, DC 20008
202 274-5100
- Dietitian/Nutritionist
- Radiographer
- Respiratory Therapist
- Speech Language Pathologist

Walter Reed Army Medical Center

Michael J Kussman, Col, MC Commander
Washington, DC 20307-5001
202 782-6104
- Clin Lab Scientist/Med Tech
- Dietitian/Nutritionist
- Perfusionist
- Specialist in BB Tech

Washington Hospital Center

Kenneth Samet, MHSA, President & CEO
110 Irving St NW
Washington, DC 20010
202 877-6101
- Clin Lab Scientist/Med Tech
- Radiographer

Florida

Boca Raton

Florida Atlantic University

Anthony Catanese, PhD, President
777 Glades Rd
Boca Raton, FL 33431
561 367-3450
- Clin Lab Scientist/Med Tech
- Speech Language Pathologist

West Boca Medical Center

Richard Gold, CEO
21644 State Rd 7
Boca Raton, FL 33428
407 488-8000
- Radiographer

Boynton Beach

Bethesda Memorial Hospital

Robert Hill, MHA, President
2815 S Seacrest Blvd
Boynton Beach, FL 33435
407 737-7733
- Radiographer

Bradenton

Manatee Area Vocational-Technical Center

Royce Williams, Interim Director
5603 34th St W
Bradenton, FL 34210
941 751-7903
- Dental Assistant
- Emergency Med Tech-Paramedic

Manatee Community College

Stephen J Korcheck, EdD, President
5840 26th St W
PO Box 1849
Bradenton, FL 34206
941 755-1511
- Radiographer
- Respiratory Therapist

Cocoa

Brevard Community College

Maxwell C King, EdD, President
1519 Clearlake Rd
Cocoa, FL 32922
407 632-1111
- Clin Lab Tech/Med Lab Tech-AD
- Dental Assistant
- Dental Hygienist
- Emergency Med Tech-Paramedic
- Radiographer
- Respiratory Therapist

Coral Gables

University of Miami

Edward T Foote II, President
University Station
Coral Gables, FL 33124
305 284-2211
- Music Therapist

Davie

McFatter Vocational Technical Center

D Robert Boegli, Director
6500 Nova Dr
Davie, FL 33317
305 370-8324
- Dental Lab Technician

Daytona Beach

Bethune-Cookman College

Oswald P Bronson Sr, PhD, President
640 Second Ave
Daytona Beach, FL 32114-3099
904 255-1401
- Clin Lab Scientist/Med Tech

Daytona Beach Community College

Philip R Day Jr, EdD, President
PO Box 2811
Daytona Beach, FL 32120-2811
904 255-8131
- Dental Assistant
- Dental Hygienist
- Emergency Med Tech-Paramedic
- Health Information Tech
- Occupational Therapy Asst
- Respiratory Therapist
- Respiratory Therapy Tech
- Surgical Technologist

Halifax Medical Center

Dan Lang, MHA, Chief Operating Officer
303 N Clyde Morris Blvd
PO Box 2830
Daytona Beach, FL 32120-2830
904 254-4065
- Nuclear Medicine Tech
- Radiation Therapist
- Radiographer

Eustis

Lake County Vocational Technical Center

Steve Hand, MEd, Director
2001 Kurt St
Eustis, FL 32726
904 742-6486
- Emergency Med Tech-Paramedic

Ft Lauderdale

Broward Community College

Willis N Holcombe, PhD, President
225 E Las Olas Blvd
Ft Lauderdale, FL 33301
954 761-7401
- Dental Assistant
- Dental Hygienist
- Diagnostic Med Sonographer
- Emergency Med Tech-Paramedic
- Health Information Tech
- Medical Assistant
- Nuclear Medicine Tech
- Radiation Therapist
- Radiographer
- Respiratory Therapist
- Respiratory Therapy Tech

Flagler Career Institute - Jacksonville

Louis Wangberg, PhD, President
2727 E Oakland Pk Blvd
Ste 205D and F
Ft Lauderdale, FL 33306
305 327-9860
- Respiratory Therapist
- Respiratory Therapy Tech

Keiser College of Technology

Arthur Keiser, BA, President
1500 NW 49th St
Ft Lauderdale, FL 33309
954 776-4456
- Clin Lab Tech/Med Lab Tech-AD
- Medical Assistant
- Radiographer

Nova Southeastern University

Ovid C Lewis, JSD, President
3301 College Ave
Ft Lauderdale, FL 33314-7796
954 475-7575
- Occupational Therapist
- Physician Assistant
- Speech Language Pathologist

Ft Myers

Edison Community College

Kenneth P Walker, PhD, President
8099 College Pkwy SW
PO Box 60210
Ft Myers, FL 33906-6210
941 941-9211
- Cardiovascular Technologist
- Dental Hygienist
- Emergency Med Tech-Paramedic
- Radiographer
- Respiratory Therapist

Radiation Therapy Regional Center

Daniel E Dosoretz, MD ABR, CEO
7341 Gladiolus Dr
Ft Myers, FL 33908
941 489-3420
- Radiation Therapist

Ft Pierce

Indian River Community College

Edwin R Massey, PhD, President
3209 Virginia Ave
Ft Pierce, FL 34981-5599
561 462-4700
- Clin Lab Tech/Med Lab Tech-AD
- Dental Assistant
- Dental Hygienist
- Dental Lab Technician
- Emergency Med Tech-Paramedic
- Health Information Tech
- Radiographer
- Respiratory Therapist

Gainesville

Santa Fe Community College

Lawrence W Tyree, EdD, President
3000 NW 83rd St
Gainesville, FL 32606-6200
352 395-5164
- Dental Assistant
- Dental Hygienist
- Emergency Med Tech-Paramedic
- Nuclear Medicine Tech
- Radiographer
- Respiratory Therapist

University of Florida

John V Lombardi, PhD, President
PO Box 113150
Gainesville, FL 32611-3150
352 392-1311
- Audiologist
- Dietitian/Nutritionist
- Occupational Therapist
- Ophthalmic Med Technician
- Physician Assistant
- Rehabilitation Counselor
- Speech Language Pathologist
- Therapeutic Recreation Specialist

Hollywood

Sheridan Vocational Technical Center

Horace F McLeod, Director
5400 Sheridan St
Hollywood, FL 33021
954 985-3220
- Clin Lab Tech/Med Lab Tech-C

Jacksonville

Baptist Medical Center

A Hugh Greene, FACHE, Executive Vice President
800 Prudential Dr
Jacksonville, FL 32207
904 393-2001
- Radiographer

Florida Community College - Jacksonville

Edgar C Napier, EdD, Interim President
501 W State St
Jacksonville, FL 32202
904 632-3000
- Clin Lab Tech/Med Lab Tech-AD
- Dental Hygienist
- Dietetic Technician
- Emergency Med Tech-Paramedic
- Health Information Tech
- Histologic Technician-AD
- Respiratory Therapist

St Luke's Hosp/Mayo Clinic Jacksonville

4201 Belfort Rd
Jacksonville, FL 32216-1431
904 296-3733
- Dietitian/Nutritionist

St Vincent's Medical Center

Everett Devaney, MHA, President/CEO
1800 Barrs St PO Box 2982
Jacksonville, FL 32203
904 387-7300
- Clin Lab Scientist/Med Tech
- Radiation Therapist
- Radiographer

University Medical Center

Mac McGriff, President/CEO
655 W Eighth St
Jacksonville, FL 32209
904 549-3000
- Clin Lab Scientist/Med Tech
- Cytotechnologist
- Radiographer

University of North Florida

Adam W Herbert Jr, President
4567 St Johns Bluff Rd S
Jacksonville, FL 32224
904 646-2666
- Dietitian/Nutritionist

Lake City

Lake City Community College

Muriel Kay Heimer, EdD, President
Rte 19 Box 1030
Lake City, FL 32025
904 752-1822
- Clin Lab Tech/Med Lab Tech-AD
- Emergency Med Tech-Paramedic

Lake Worth

Palm Beach Community College

Edward M Eissey, PhD, President
4200 Congress Ave
Lake Worth, FL 33461-4796
407 439-8080
- Dental Assistant
- Dental Hygienist
- Dietetic Technician
- Emergency Med Tech-Paramedic
- Occupational Therapy Asst
- Radiographer
- Respiratory Therapist
- Respiratory Therapy Tech

Lakeland

Lakeland Regional Medical Center

Jack T Stephens, President/CEO
1324 Lakeland Hills Blvd
PO Box 95448
Lakeland, FL 33804
813 687-1100
- Radiographer

Traviss Technical Center

Charles D Paulk, Director
3225 Winter Lake Rd
Lakeland, FL 33803
941 449-2700
- Surgical Technologist

Melbourne

Orlando College-Melbourne Campus

Sharlee Brittingham, President
2401 N Harbor City Blvd
Melbourne, FL 32935
407 253-2929
- Medical Assistant
- Respiratory Therapy Tech

Miami

Florida International University

Modesto Maidique, PhD, President
Office of Academic Affairs
University Park Campus
Miami, FL 33199
305 348-2111
- Clin Lab Scientist/Med Tech
- Dietitian/Nutritionist
- Health Information Admin
- Occupational Therapist

Lindsey Hopkins Tech Education Center

John J Leyva, Principal
750 NW 20th St
Miami, FL 33127
305 324-6070
- Dental Assistant
- Dental Lab Technician
- Surgical Technologist

Miami-Dade Community College

Eduardo Padron, PhD, College President
Medical Ctr Campus
950 NW 20th St
Miami, FL 33127
305 237-4026
- Clin Lab Tech/Med Lab Tech-AD
- Dental Hygienist
- Diagnostic Med Sonographer
- Dietetic Technician
- Emergency Med Tech-Paramedic
- Health Information Tech
- Ophthalmic Dispenser
- Radiation Therapist
- Radiographer
- Respiratory Therapist
- Respiratory Therapy Tech

R Morgan Vocational Technical Institute

18180 SW 122nd Ave
R Morgan Vocational Technical Institute
Miami, FL 33177
305 253-9920
- Dental Assistant

Univ of Miami/Jackson Memorial Hosp

Ira Clark, MA, President
Public Health Trust
1611 NW 12th Ave
Miami, FL 33136
305 585-6754
- Histologic Technician-Cert
- Nuclear Medicine Tech
- Radiographer

University of Miami School of Medicine

Bernard J Fogel, MD, Vice Pres/Dean
1600 NW 10th Ave R-699
Miami, FL 33136
305 585-6545
- Cytotechnologist

Miami Beach

Mt Sinai Medical Center of Greater Miami

Fred Hirt, MS, President/CEO
4300 Alton Rd
Miami Beach, FL 33140
305 674-2222
- Nuclear Medicine Tech
- Radiographer

Miami Shores

Barry University

Jeanne O'Laughlin, OP PhD, President
11300 NE 2nd Ave
Miami Shores, FL 33161-6695
305 899-3010
- Athletic Trainer
- Occupational Therapist
- Perfusionist

Naples

International College

Terry P McMahan, JD, President
2654 E Tamiami Trail
Naples, FL 33962
813 774-4700
- Health Information Tech

J Walker Vocational Technical Center

President ,
3702 Estey Ave
Naples, FL 34102-4587
941 643-0919
- Dental Assistant

New Port Richey

HRS Pasco County Public Health Unit

10841 Little Rd
New Port Richey, FL 34654-2533
813 869-3900
- Dietitian/Nutritionist

Pasco-Hernando Community College

Robert W Judson Jr, EdD, President
10230 Ridge Rd
New Port Richey, FL 34654-5199
904 567-6701
- Dental Hygienist
- Emergency Med Tech-Paramedic

Ocala

Central Florida Community College

Charles Dassance, PhD, President
3001 SW College Rd/PO Box 1388
Ocala, FL 34474
352 237-2111
- Emergency Med Tech-Paramedic
- Occupational Therapy Asst
- Surgical Technologist

Marion County School of Radiologic Tech

Sam Lauff Jr, MEd, Administrator
1014 SW 7th Rd
Ocala, FL 34474-3172
352 620-7582
- Radiographer

Orlando

Central Florida Blood Bank

Edward O Carr, MT(ASCP) SBB, President/CEO
32 W Gore St
Orlando, FL 32806
407 849-6100
- Specialist in BB Tech

Florida Hospital Coll of Health Sciences

David E Greenlaw, DMin, President
800 Lake Estelle Dr
Orlando, FL 32803
407 895-7747
- Diagnostic Med Sonographer

Florida Hospital Medical Center

Dave Greenlaw, PhD, President
Florida Hospital Col of Health Sciences
800 Lake Stelle Dr
Orlando, FL 32803
- Clin Lab Scientist/Med Tech
- Radiation Therapist
- Radiographer

Orlando Technical Education Centers

Nancy Cordill, Senior Director
301 W Amelia St
Orange Technical Educational Centers
Orlando, FL 32801
407 246-7060
- Dental Assistant
- Surgical Technologist

Southern College

David L Peoples, President
5600 Lake Underhill Rd
Orlando, FL 32807
407 273-1000
- Dental Assistant
- Dental Lab Technician

University of Central Florida

John C Hitt, PhD, President
Office of the President
PO Box 25000
Orlando, FL 32816
407 823-1823
- Clin Lab Scientist/Med Tech
- Health Information Admin
- Radiographer
- Respiratory Therapist
- Speech Language Pathologist

Valencia Community College

Paul C Gianini Jr, EdD, President
PO Box 3028
Orlando, FL 32802-3028
407 299-5000
- Dental Hygienist
- Diagnostic Med Sonographer
- Emergency Med Tech-Paramedic
- Nuclear Medicine Tech
- Radiographer
- Respiratory Therapist

Panama City

Gulf Coast Community College

Robert L McSpadden, EdD, President
5230 W US Hwy 98
Panama City, FL 32401-1041
904 769-1551
- Dental Assistant
- Dental Hygienist
- Emergency Med Tech-Paramedic
- Radiographer
- Respiratory Therapy Tech

Pensacola

Pensacola Junior College

Horace E Hartsell, EdD, President
1000 College Blvd
Pensacola, FL 32501
904 484-1700
- Dental Assistant
- Dental Hygienist
- Dietetic Technician
- Emergency Med Tech-Paramedic
- Health Information Tech
- Medical Assistant
- Radiographer
- Respiratory Therapist

University of West Florida

Morris Marx, PhD, President
11000 University Pkwy
Pensacola, FL 32514-5750
904 474-2202
- Clin Lab Scientist/Med Tech

Port Charlotte

Charlotte Vocational Technical Center

18300 Toledo Blade Blvd
Port Charlotte, FL 33948-3399
813 629-6819
- Dental Assistant

Sanford

Seminole Community College

E Ann McGee, EdD, President
100 Weldon Blvd
Sanford, FL 32773
423 328-4722
- Emergency Med Tech-Paramedic
- Respiratory Therapist
- Respiratory Therapy Tech

Sarasota

Sarasota County Technical Institute
Steve I Harvey, MA, Director
4748 Beneva Rd
Sarasota, FL 34233-1798
813 924-1365
• Emergency Med Tech-Paramedic
• Medical Assistant

Sarasota Memorial Hospital
1700 S Tamiami Trail
Sarasota, FL 34239-3555
813 917-1080
• Dietitian/Nutritionist

St Augustine

St Augustine Technical Center
Ernie Matthews, EdD, Director
2980 Collins Ave
St Augustine, FL 32095-1919
904 824-4401
• Emergency Med Tech-Paramedic

St Petersburg

Bayfront Medical Center
Sue S Brody, MHA, President/CEO
701 Sixth St S
St Petersburg, FL 33701
813 893-6085
• Clin Lab Scientist/Med Tech

Pinellas Tech Educ Ctr - St Petersburg
Warren Laux, EdD, Director
901 34th St S
St Petersburg, FL 33711-2298
813 893-2500
• Dental Assistant
• Medical Assistant

St Petersburg Junior College
Carl M Kuttler Jr, JD, President
PO Box 13489
St Petersburg, FL 33733
813 341-3241
• Clin Lab Tech/Med Lab Tech-AD
• Dental Hygienist
• Emergency Med Tech-Paramedic
• Health Information Tech
• Respiratory Therapist

Transfusion Med Acad Ctr FL Blood Svcs
German F Leparc, MD, President
445 31st St N
St Petersburg, FL 33713
813 977-5433
• Specialist in BB Tech

Tallahassee

Florida A & M University
Fredrick S Humphries, PhD, President
Tallahassee, FL 32307
904 599-3225
• Health Information Admin
• Occupational Therapist
• Respiratory Therapist

Florida State University
Talbot D'Alemberte, President
Tallahassee, FL 32306
904 644-2525
• Dietitian/Nutritionist
• Music Therapist
• Rehabilitation Counselor
• Speech Language Pathologist
• Therapeutic Recreation Specialist

Tallahassee Community College
T K Wetherell, PhD, President
444 Appleyard Dr
Tallahassee, FL 32304
904 488-9200
• Dental Assistant
• Dental Hygienist
• Emergency Med Tech-Paramedic
• Respiratory Therapist

Tallahassee Memorial Regional Med Center
Duncan Moore, MS, President/CEO
Magnolia Dr and Miccosukee Rd
Tallahassee, FL 32308
904 681-5385
• Clin Lab Scientist/Med Tech

Tampa

David G Erwin Technical Center
Michael D Donohue, MEd, Principal
2010 E Hillsborough Ave
Tampa, FL 33610-8299
813 231-1800
• Clin Lab Tech/Med Lab Tech-C
• Dental Assistant
• Electroneurodiagnostic Tech
• Medical Assistant
• Respiratory Therapy Tech
• Surgical Technologist

Hillsborough Community College
Andreas Paloumpis, PhD, President
PO Box 31127
Tampa, FL 33631-3127
813 253-7050
• Diagnostic Med Sonographer
• Emergency Med Tech-Paramedic
• Nuclear Medicine Tech
• Occupational Therapy Asst
• Ophthalmic Dispenser
• Radiation Therapist
• Radiographer

James A Haley Veteran's Hospital
13000 N Bruce B Downs Blvd
Tampa, FL 33612-4745
813 972-2000
• Dietitian/Nutritionist

Tampa General Hospital
Bruce Siegel, MD, President & CEO
PO Box 1289
Tampa, FL 33601
813 251-7383
• Clin Lab Scientist/Med Tech

University of South Florida
Betty Castor, President
BEH 255
Tampa, FL 33620-8150
813 974-2006
• Audiologist
• Rehabilitation Counselor
• Speech Language Pathologist

West Palm Beach

New England Institute of Tech at Palm Beach
Charles Halliday, President
1126 53rd Ct
West Palm Beach, FL 33407
561 842-8324
• Medical Assistant

South College
John T South III, President
1760 N Congress Ave
West Palm Beach, FL 33409
407 651-8100
• Medical Assistant

Winter Haven

Polk Community College
Maryly VanLeer Peck, PhD, President
999 Ave H NE
Winter Haven, FL 33881
941 297-1000
• Emergency Med Tech-Paramedic
• Radiographer

Winter Park

Winter Park Adult Vocational Center
Joseph McCoy, Director
901 Webster Ave
Winter Park, FL 32789
407 647-6366
• Medical Assistant

Georgia

Albany

Albany Technical Institute
Anthony Parker, PhD, President
1021 Lowe Rd
Albany, GA 31708
912 430-3500
• Dental Assistant
• Radiographer
• Surgical Technologist

Darton College
Peter J Sireno, EdD, President
2400 Gillionville Rd
Albany, GA 31707
912 430-6705
• Clin Lab Tech/Med Lab Tech-AD
• Dental Hygienist
• Health Information Tech
• Respiratory Therapist

Institutions

Athens

Athens Area Technical Institute
Kenneth C Easom, EdD, President
Hwy 29 N
Athens, GA 30601
706 355-5000
- Radiographer
- Respiratory Therapist
- Surgical Technologist

University of Georgia
Charles B Knapp, President
Athens, GA 30602
706 542-3030
- Audiologist
- Dietitian/Nutritionist
- Music Therapist
- Rehabilitation Counselor
- Speech Language Pathologist

Atlanta

American RC Southern Region
Roger Svoboda, MBA MS MT(ASCP), Principal
Officer
1925 Monroe Dr NE
Atlanta, GA 30324
404 881-9800
- Specialist in BB Tech

Atlanta Area Technical School
Brenda W Jones, PhD, President
1560 Stewart Ave SW
Atlanta, GA 30310
404 756-3700
- Clin Lab Tech/Med Lab Tech-C
- Dental Lab Technician
- Medical Assistant

Clark Atlanta University
Thomas W Cole Jr, PhD, President
James P Brawley Dr at Fair St SW
Atlanta, GA 30314
404 880-8500
- Health Information Admin

Div of Pub Hlth/Georgia Dept of Hum Res
2 Peachtree St NE
Atlanta, GA 30303-3141
404 657-2884
- Dietitian/Nutritionist

Emory University
Willaim M Chace, PhD, President
1300 E Oxford Dr
Atlanta, GA 30322
404 727-6012
- Anesthesiologist Asst
- Physician Assistant
- Radiographer

Emory University Hospital
John D Henry Sr, FACHE, CEO
1364 Clifton Rd NE/Rm B216
Atlanta, GA 30322
404 712-4881
- Clin Lab Scientist/Med Tech

Emory University System of Health Care
John Henry, Administrator
1364 Clifton Rd NE
Atlanta, GA 30322
404 712-7397
- Clin Lab Scientist/Med Tech

Georgia Baptist Medical Center
Jo Kicker, President/CEO
303 Parkway NE
Atlanta, GA 30312
404 265-4203
- Radiographer

Georgia State University
Carl V Patton, PhD, President
University Plaza
Atlanta, GA 30303-3090
404 651-3111
- Clin Lab Scientist/Med Tech
- Dietitian/Nutritionist
- Rehabilitation Counselor
- Respiratory Therapist
- Respiratory Therapy Tech
- Speech Language Pathologist

Grady Health System
Edward J Renford, MBA, President/CEO
PO Box 26189
Atlanta, GA 30335-3801
404 616-4252
- Clin Lab Scientist/Med Tech
- Cytotechnologist
- Diagnostic Med Sonographer
- Radiation Therapist
- Radiographer

St Joseph Hospital
Brue Chandler, President
5665 Peachtree Dunwoody Rd NE
Atlanta, GA 30342-1764
404 851-7120
- Histologic Technician-Cert

Augusta

Augusta Area Dietetic Internship
University Hospital
1350 Walton Way (10)
Augusta, GA 30901-2629
706 774-8897
- Dietitian/Nutritionist

Augusta Technical Inst/University Hosp
Terry Elam, MEd BA, President
3116 Deans Bridge Rd
Augusta, GA 30906
706 771-4000
- Cardiovascular Technologist

Augusta Technical Institute
Jack B Patrick, EdS MEd BS, President
3116 Deans Bridge Rd
Augusta, GA 30906
706 771-4005
- Clin Lab Tech/Med Lab Tech-AD
- Dental Assistant
- Medical Assistant
- Respiratory Therapist
- Surgical Technologist

Medical College of Georgia
Francis J Tedesco, MD, President
1120 15th St AA-311
Augusta, GA 30912-0700
706 721-2301
- Clin Lab Scientist/Med Tech
- Dental Hygienist
- Diagnostic Med Sonographer
- Health Information Admin
- Health Information Tech
- Medical Illustrator
- Nuclear Medicine Tech
- Occupational Therapist
- Occupational Therapy Asst
- Physician Assistant
- Radiation Therapist
- Radiographer
- Respiratory Therapist

University Hospital
Donald C Bray, MS, President/CEO
1350 Walton Way
Augusta, GA 30901
706 722-9011
- Radiographer

Brunswick

Coastal Georgia Community College
Dorothy L Lord, PhD, President
3700 Altama Ave
Brunswick, GA 31520
912 264-7201
- Clin Lab Tech/Med Lab Tech-AD
- Radiographer

Clarkesville

North Georgia Technical Institute
Judy H Hulsey, EdD, President
Hwy 197 N PO Box 65
Clarkesville, GA 30523
706 754-7701
- Clin Lab Tech/Med Lab Tech-C

Clarkston

De Kalb Technical Institute
Paul M Starnes, PhD, President
495 N Indian Creek Dr
Clarkston, GA 30021
404 297-9522
- Clin Lab Tech/Med Lab Tech-C
- Ophthalmic Dispenser
- Surgical Technologist

Cochran

Middle Georgia College
Joe Ben Welch, EdD, President
1100 Second St SE
Cochran, GA 31014-1599
912 934-3011
- Occupational Therapy Asst

Columbus

Columbus State University
Frank D Brown, PhD, President
4225 University Ave
Columbus, GA 31907-5645
706 568-2211
- Clin Lab Scientist/Med Tech
- Dental Hygienist
- Respiratory Therapist

Columbus Technical Institute
Eugene M Demonet, MBA, President
928 45th St
Columbus, GA 31995
404 649-1837
- Medical Assistant

Medical Center Inc
Robert J Corey, FACHE, President
1951 Eighth Ave PO Box 951
Columbus, GA 31994-2299
706 571-1200
- Radiographer

Dalton

Dalton College
James A Burran, PhD, President
213 N College Dr
Dalton, GA 30720
404 278-4215
- Clin Lab Tech/Med Lab Tech-AD

Hamilton Medical Center
Ned Wilford, CEO
Herschel U Martin School of Radiography
PO Box 1168
Dalton, GA 30720-1168
706 278-2105
- Radiographer

Decatur

DeKalb College
Jacquelyn M Belcher, President
3251 Panthersville Rd
Decatur, GA 30034
404 244-2365
- Dental Hygienist

DeKalb Medical Center
John R Gerlach, MHA, Acting CEO
2701 N Decatur Rd
Decatur, GA 30033
404 501-5206
- Radiographer

Douglasville

Carroll Technical Institute
4600 Timber Ridge Dr
Douglasville, GA 30135
770 947-7300
- Dental Hygienist

Dublin

Heart of Georgia Technical Institute
Ron Henderson, EdD, President
560 Pinehill Rd
Dublin, GA 31021
912 275-6589
- Medical Assistant

Fort Valley

Fort Valley State College
Oscar L Prater, President
1005 State College Dr
Fort Valley, GA 31030
912 825-6315
- Dietitian/Nutritionist
- Rehabilitation Counselor

Griffin

Griffin Technical Institute
Coy L Hodges, EdD, CEO
501 Varsity Rd
Griffin, GA 30223
770 228-7365
- Radiographer

LaGrange

West Georgia Technical Institute
William Sellers, PhD, Interim President
Fort Dr
LaGrange, GA 30240
706 882-3273
- Radiographer

Lawrenceville

Gwinnett Technical Institute
Sharon Rigsby, Interim President
5150 Sugarloaf Parkway
PO Box 1505
Lawrenceville, GA 30246-1505
770 962-7580
- Dental Assistant
- Dental Lab Technician
- Radiographer
- Respiratory Therapy Tech

Macon

Macon College
S Aaron Hyatt, President
100 College Station Dr
Macon, GA 31297
912 471-2700
- Dental Hygienist

Macon Technical Institute
Melton Palmer Jr, PhD, President
3300 Macon Tech Dr
Macon, GA 31206
912 757-3400
- Clin Lab Tech/Med Lab Tech-C

Medical Center of Central Georgia
Don Faulk, FACHA, President
777 Hemlock St/PO Box 6000
Macon, GA 31208
912 744-1451
- Radiographer

Marietta

Life College
Sid E Williams, President
1269 Barclay Circle
Marietta, GA 30060
404 424-0554
- Dietitian/Nutritionist

Promina Kennestone Hospital
Edward J Bonn, BA MS, President/CEO
677 Church St
Marietta, GA 30060
770 793-5170
- Radiographer

Midgeville

Georgia College and State University
Edwin G Speir, President
Midgeville, GA 31061
912 453-5350
- Music Therapist

Morrow

Clayton State College
Richard A Skinner, President
5900 N Lee St
Morrow, GA 30260
770 961-3400
- Dental Hygienist

Moultrie

Moultrie Area Technical Institute
Michael Moye, EdD, President
PO Box 520
Moultrie, GA 31776-0520
912 891-7000
- Radiographer

Oakwood

Lanier Technical Institute
Joe E Hill, EdD, President
PO Box 58
Oakwood, GA 30566-0058
770 531-6304
- Clin Lab Tech/Med Lab Tech-C
- Dental Assistant
- Dental Hygienist

Riverdale

Southern Regional Medical Center
11 Upper Riverdale Rd SW
Riverdale, GA 30274-2600
770 991-8053
- Dietitian/Nutritionist

Rome

Coosa Valley Technical Institute
Ronald Swanson, PhD, President
785 Cedar Ave
Rome, GA 30161-6757
706 295-6702
- Respiratory Therapy Tech

Savannah

Armstrong Atlantic State University
Robert A Burnett, PhD, President
11935 Abercorn St
Savannah, GA 31419-1997
912 927-5258
- Clin Lab Scientist/Med Tech
- Dental Hygienist
- Radiation Therapist
- Radiographer
- Respiratory Therapist

Institutions

Savannah Technical Institute
John D Stewart, EdD, Assistant Superintendent
5717 White Bluff Rd
Savannah, GA 31405-5594
912 351-4404
• Dental Assistant
• Medical Assistant
• Surgical Technologist

South College
John T South III, BS, CEO
709 Mall Blvd
Savannah, GA 31406
912 651-8100
• Medical Assistant

Smyrna

Medix School
Wesley J Henry, President
2108 Cobb Pkwy
Smyrna, GA 30080
770 980-0002
• Dental Assistant
• Medical Assistant

Statesboro

Georgia Southern University
Nicholas L Henry, President
Statesboro, GA 30460
912 681-5611
• Dietitian/Nutritionist
• Therapeutic Recreation Specialist

Ogeechee Technical Institute
Stephen A Deraney,
1 Joe Kennedy Blvd
Statesboro, GA 30458
912 681-5500
• Radiographer

Swainsboro

Swainsboro Technical Institute
Donald Speir, MEd, President
346 Kite Rd
Swainsboro, GA 30401
912 237-6465
• Medical Assistant

Thomasville

Thomas Technical Institute
Charles R DeMott, EdS, President
15689 US Hwy 19 N
PO Box 1578
Thomasville, GA 31792
912 225-5069
• Clin Lab Tech/Med Lab Tech-AD
• Clin Lab Tech/Med Lab Tech-C
• Medical Assistant
• Radiation Therapist
• Radiographer
• Respiratory Therapy Tech
• Surgical Technologist

Valdosta

Valdosta State University
Hugh C Bailey, PhD, President
Office of the President
West Hall
Valdosta, GA 31698
912 333-5952
• Athletic Trainer
• Speech Language Pathologist

Valdosta Technical Institute
James Bridges, President
4089 Valtech Rd
PO Box 928
Valdosta, GA 31603-0928
912 333-2100
• Medical Assistant
• Radiographer

Waycross

Okefenokee Technical Institute
Joseph Ray Miller, SEd, President
1701 Carswell Ave
Waycross, GA 31501
912 287-6584
• Clin Lab Tech/Med Lab Tech-C
• Radiographer
• Respiratory Therapy Tech
• Surgical Technologist

Hawaii

Honolulu

Kapiolani Community College
John Morton, MS, Provost
4303 Diamond Head Rd/Kauila 210
Honolulu, HI 96816
808 734-9565
• Clin Lab Tech/Med Lab Tech-AD
• Medical Assistant
• Occupational Therapy Asst
• Radiographer
• Respiratory Therapist

University of Hawaii at Manoa
Kenneth P Mortimer, PhD, President
2444 Dole St Bachman 202
Honolulu, HI 96822
808 956-5280
• Audiologist
• Clin Lab Scientist/Med Tech
• Dental Hygienist
• Dietitian/Nutritionist
• Rehabilitation Counselor
• Speech Language Pathologist

Idaho

Boise

American Institute of Health Technology
Judy L Groothuis, President and Acad Dean
6600 Emerald
Boise, ID 83704-8738
208 377-8080
• Occupational Therapy Asst

Boise State University
Charles P Ruch, PhD, President
1910 Universiey Dr
Boise, ID 83725
208 385-1491
• Athletic Trainer
• Dental Assistant
• Health Information Tech
• Radiographer
• Respiratory Therapist
• Respiratory Therapy Tech
• Surgical Technologist

St Alphonsus Regl Medical Center
Karl Kurtz, Interim President
1055 N Curtis Rd
Boise, ID 83706
208 378-2000
• Clin Lab Scientist/Med Tech

Moscow

University of Idaho
Thomas O Bell, Interim President
Moscow, ID 83844
208 885-6111
• Dietitian/Nutritionist
• Rehabilitation Counselor

Pocatello

Idaho State University
Richard L Bowen, PhD, President
Campus Box 8310
Pocatello, ID 83209-0009
208 236-3440
• Audiologist
• Clin Lab Scientist/Med Tech
• Dental Hygienist
• Dental Lab Technician
• Dietitian/Nutritionist
• Health Information Tech
• Speech Language Pathologist

Rexburg

Ricks College
Steven D Bennion, President
Rexburg, ID 83460
208 356-2011
• Dietetic Technician

Twin Falls

College of Southern Idaho
Gerald R Meyerhoeffer, MS, President
PO Box 1238
Twin Falls, ID 83303-1238
208 733-9554
• Medical Assistant

Illinois

Arlington Heights

Northwest Community Hospital
Bruce K Crowther, MBA, President
800 W Central Rd
Arlington Heights, IL 60005
847 618-1000
• Radiographer

Belleville

Belleville Area College

Joseph Cipfl, PhD, President
2500 Carlyle Ave
Belleville, IL 62221
618 235-2700
- Clin Lab Tech/Med Lab Tech-AD
- Health Information Tech
- Medical Assistant
- Radiographer
- Respiratory Therapy Tech

St Elizabeth Hospital

Gerald M Harman, MBA FACHE, Exec VP
211 S Third St
Belleville, IL 62222
618 234-2120
- Clin Lab Scientist/Med Tech

Carbondale

Southern Illinois Univ at Carbondale

Donald L Beggs, PhD, Chancellor
Southern Illinois Univ. at Carbondale
Health Care Professions
Carbondale, IL 62901
618 453-2341
- Athletic Trainer
- Dental Hygienist
- Dental Lab Technician
- Dietitian/Nutritionist
- Radiographer
- Rehabilitation Counselor
- Respiratory Therapist
- Speech Language Pathologist
- Therapeutic Recreation Specialist

Carterville

John A Logan College

Ray Hancock, President
Rural Rte 2
Carterville, IL 62918
618 985-3741
- Dental Assistant

Centralia

Kaskaskia College

Alice Mumaw-Jacobs, PhD, President
27210 College Rd
Centralia, IL 62801
618 532-1981
- Dental Assistant
- Radiographer
- Respiratory Therapy Tech

Champaign

Parkland College

Zelema Harris, EdD, President
2400 W Bradley Ave
Champaign, IL 61821-1899
217 351-2231
- Dental Assistant
- Dental Hygienist
- Occupational Therapy Asst
- Radiographer
- Respiratory Therapist
- Surgical Technologist

Charleston

Eastern Illinois University

David L Jorns, PhD, President
Charleston, IL 61920
217 581-2011
- Athletic Trainer
- Dietitian/Nutritionist
- Speech Language Pathologist
- Therapeutic Recreation Specialist

Chicago

Chicago State University

Dolores E Cross, PhD, President
9501 S King Dr
Chicago, IL 60628-1598
773 995-2400
- Health Information Admin
- Occupational Therapist

Cook County Hospital

Ruth M Rothstein, Director
1825 W Harrison St
Chicago, IL 60612
312 633-8533
- Radiographer

Illinois Institute of Technology

Lewis M Collens, President
3300 S Federal St
Chicago, IL 60616
773 567-3000
- Rehabilitation Counselor

Kennedy-King College/University of Illinois

6800 S Wentworth Ave
Chicago, IL 60621
773 602-5229
- Dental Hygienist

Loyola University of Chicago

John J Piderit, President
820 N Michigan Ave
Chicago, IL 60611
312 915-6000
- Dietitian/Nutritionist

Malcolm X College

Zerrie D Campbell, MS MA, President
1900 W Van Buren St
Chicago, IL 60612
312 850-7031
- Clin Lab Tech/Med Lab Tech-AD
- Dietetic Technician
- Physician Assistant
- Radiographer
- Respiratory Therapist
- Surgical Technologist

Michael Reese Hospital

Bruce Elegant, COO
2929 S Ellis Ave
Chicago, IL 60616-3390
773 791-5362
- Cytotechnologist

Northwestern Business College

Lawrence W Schumacher, BA, President
4829 N Lipps Ave
Chicago, IL 60630
773 777-4220
- Medical Assistant

Ravenswood Hospital Medical Center

John E Blair, President
4550 N Winchester Ave
Chicago, IL 60640
773 878-4300
- Radiographer

Robert Morris College

Michael Viollt, President
180 N LaSalle St
Chicago, IL 60401
312 836-4888
- Health Information Tech
- Medical Assistant

Rush University

Leo M Henikoff, MD, President
Rush Presbyterian St Luke's Med Ctr
1653 W Harrison St
Chicago, IL 60612
312 942-5474
- Audiologist
- Clin Lab Scientist/Med Tech
- Dietitian/Nutritionist
- Occupational Therapist
- Perfusionist
- Speech Language Pathologist

Saint Xavier University

Richard A Yanikoski, President
3700 W 103rd St
Chicago, IL 60655
773 298-3561
- Speech Language Pathologist

School of the Art Institute of Chicago

Carol Becker, Dean of Faculty
37 S Wabash
Chicago, IL 60603
312 899-1236
- Art Therapist

St Augustine College

Fr Carlos A Plazas, PhD, President
1333 W Argyle
Chicago, IL 60640
773 878-8756
- Respiratory Therapy Tech

Trinity Hospital

John N Schwartz, MHA, President
2320 E 93rd St
Chicago, IL 60617
773 978-2000
- Radiographer
- Respiratory Therapy Tech

Truman College

Donald Smith, EdD, Interim President
1145 W Wilson
Chicago, IL 60640
773 907-4450
- Health Information Tech

Univ of Chicago Hosp/Roosevelt Univ

Ralph W Mueller, President
University of Chicago Hospital
5841 S Maryland PO Box 442
Chicago, IL 60637
773 702-6240
- Radiation Therapist

Univ of Illinois at Chicago
David C Broski, PhD, Chancellor
University Hall
601 S Morgan St M/C 102
Chicago, IL 60607
312 413-3350
● Art Therapist
● Clin Lab Scientist/Med Tech
● Dietitian/Nutritionist
● Health Information Admin
● Medical Illustrator
● Occupational Therapist
● Specialist in BB Tech

Wilbur Wright College
Raymond F LeFevour, MA, President
4300 N Narragansett Ave
Chicago, IL 60634
773 777-7900
● Diagnostic Med Sonographer
● Occupational Therapy Asst
● Radiographer

Chicago Heights

Prairie State College
E Timothy Lightfield, President
202 S Halsted
Chicago Heights, IL 60411
708 756-3110
● Dental Hygienist

Cicero

Morton College
John A Neuhaus, President
3801 S Central Ave
Cicero, IL 60804
708 656-8000
● Dental Assistant

Danville

United Samaritans Medical Center
Dennis J Doran, MBA, President
812 N Logan Ave
Danville, IL 61832-3788
217 443-5201
● Radiographer

Decatur

Decatur Memorial Hospital
Kenneth Smithmier, President/CEO
Medical Administration
2300 N Edward St
Decatur, IL 62526
217 876-2331
● Clin Lab Scientist/Med Tech

DeKalb

Northern Illinois University
John E La Tourette, PhD, President
DeKalb, IL 60115
815 753-9501
● Audiologist
● Clin Lab Scientist/Med Tech
● Dietitian/Nutritionist
● Rehabilitation Counselor
● Speech Language Pathologist

Des Plaines

Oakton Community College
Margaret B Lee, PhD, President
1600 E Golf Rd
Des Plaines, IL 60016
847 635-1732
● Clin Lab Tech/Med Lab Tech-AD
● Health Information Tech

Dixon

Sauk Valley Community College
Richard L Behrendt, PhD, President
173 IL Rt 2
Dixon, IL 61021-9110
815 288-5511
● Clin Lab Tech/Med Lab Tech-AD
● Radiographer

Downers Grove

Midwestern University
Kathleen Goepplinger, PhD, President
555 31st St
Downers Grove, IL 60515
630 515-6300
● Physician Assistant

East Peoria

Illinois Central College
Thomas K Thomas, EdD, President
One College Dr
East Peoria, IL 61635-0001
309 694-5431
● Clin Lab Tech/Med Lab Tech-AD
● Dental Assistant
● Dental Hygienist
● Occupational Therapy Asst
● Radiographer
● Respiratory Therapist
● Respiratory Therapy Tech
● Surgical Technologist

Edwardsville

Southern Illinois Univ at Edwardsville
Nancy G Belck, PhD, President
Edwardsville, IL 62026
618 692-2000
● Art Therapist
● Speech Language Pathologist

Elgin

Elgin Community College
Roy Flores, MS PhD, CEO
1700 Spartan Dr
Elgin, IL 60123-7193
847 697-1000
● Clin Lab Tech/Med Lab Tech-AD
● Dental Assistant
● Surgical Technologist

St Joseph Hospital
Larry Narum, MA, President
77 N Airlite St
Elgin, IL 60123
847 695-3200
● Radiation Therapist

Evanston

National-Louis University
Orley R Herron, PhD, President
2840 N Sheridan Rd
Evanston, IL 60201
847 256-5150
● Clin Lab Scientist/Med Tech
● Radiation Therapist
● Respiratory Therapist

Northwestern University
Henry S Bienen, President
2299 Sheridan Rd
Evanston, IL 60201
847 491-3741
● Audiologist
● Speech Language Pathologist

St Francis Hospital
James Gizzi, Administrator
355 Ridge Ave
Evanston, IL 60202
847 492-4000
● Radiographer

Galesburg

Carl Sandburg College
Donald C Crist, EdD, President
2232 S Lake Storey Rd
PO Box 1407
Galesburg, IL 61402
309 344-2518
● Radiographer

Glen Ellyn

College of DuPage
Michael T Murphy, EdD, President
22nd St and Lambert Rd
Glen Ellyn, IL 60137-6599
630 942-2800
● Health Information Tech
● Nuclear Medicine Tech
● Occupational Therapy Asst
● Radiographer
● Respiratory Therapist
● Respiratory Therapy Tech

Godfrey

Lewis & Clark Community College
Dale T Chapman, EdD, President
5800 Godfrey Rd
Godfrey, IL 62035
618 466-3411
● Clin Lab Tech/Med Lab Tech-AD
● Dental Assistant
● Dental Hygienist

Grayslake

College of Lake County
Gretchen Naff, PhD, President
19351 W Washington St
Grayslake, IL 60030-1198
847 223-6601
● Clin Lab Tech/Med Lab Tech-AD
● Health Information Tech
● Radiographer

Harvey

Ingalls Memorial Hospital

Onc Ingalls Dr
Harvey, IL 60426
708 333-2300
- Dietitian/Nutritionist

Herrin

Southern Illinois Collegiate Common Mkt

Ronald K House, PhD, Executive Director
3213 S Park Ave
Herrin, IL 62948
618 942-6902
- Clin Lab Tech/Med Lab Tech-C
- Health Information Tech
- Occupational Therapy Asst

Hines

Edward Hines Jr VA Hospital

John Denardo, Director
Fifth Ave and Roosevelt Rd
PO Box 5000
Hines, IL 60141
708 216-2153
- Clin Lab Scientist/Med Tech
- Dietitian/Nutritionist
- Nuclear Medicine Tech
- Radiation Therapist

Kankakee

Kankakee Community College

Larry D Huffman, PhD, President
PO Box 888
Kankakee, IL 60901-0888
815 933-0211
- Clin Lab Tech/Med Lab Tech-AD

Olivet Nazarene University

John C Bowling, President
Kankakee, IL 60901
815 939-5011
- Dietitian/Nutritionist
- Dietetic Technician

Lisle

Illinois Benedictine College

William J Carroll, President
5700 College Rd
Lisle, IL 60532
708 960-1500
- Dietitian/Nutritionist

Macomb

McDonough District Hospital

Stephen R Hopper, MS, President
525 E Grant St
Macomb, IL 61455
309 833-4101
- Radiographer

Western Illinois University

Donald S Spencer, President
1 University Circle
Macomb, IL 61455
309 295-1414
- Audiologist
- Dietitian/Nutritionist
- Music Therapist
- Speech Language Pathologist
- Therapeutic Recreation Specialist

Malta

Kishwaukee College

Norman L Jenkins, PhD, President
21193 Malta Rd
Malta, IL 60150
815 825-2086
- Radiographer

Mattoon

Lake Land College

Robert K Luther, President
5001 Lake Land Blvd
Mattoon, IL 61938-9366
217 234-5253
- Dental Hygienist

Maywood

Foster G McGaw Hosp of Loyola University

Anthony Barbato, MD, Executive Vice President
2160 S First Ave
Maywood, IL 60153
708 216-9000
- Clin Lab Scientist/Med Tech
- Emergency Med Tech-Paramedic
- Perfusionist

Moline

Black Hawk College

Judith A Redwine, PhD, President
6600 34th Ave
Moline, IL 61265
309 796-1311
- Respiratory Therapist
- Respiratory Therapy Tech

Trinity Medical Center

Eric Crowell, MS, President
501 10th Ave
Moline, IL 61265
309 757-3222
- Emergency Med Tech-Paramedic
- Radiographer
- Surgical Technologist

Normal

Bloomington-Normal School of Radiography

Scott Kaminski, Sr Vice President
900 Franklin Ave
Normal, IL 61761
309 452-2834
- Radiographer

Illinois State University

David Strand, PhD, President
Hovey Hall 308G
Normal, IL 61761
309 438-5677
- Audiologist
- Dietitian/Nutritionist
- Health Information Admin
- Music Therapist
- Speech Language Pathologist
- Therapeutic Recreation Specialist

North Chicago

Finch U of Hlth Science/Chicago Med Sch

Herman M Finch, President/CEO
3333 Green Bay Rd
North Chicago, IL 60064
708 578-3000
- Clin Lab Scientist/Med Tech
- Physician Assistant

Oglesby

Illinois Valley Community College

Jean Goodnow, President
815 N Orlando Smith Ave
Oglesby, IL 61348-9691
815 224-2720
- Dental Assistant

Olney

Olney Central College

Hans Andrews, PhD, President
R R #3
Olney, IL 62450
618 395-4351
- Radiographer

Palatine

William Rainey Harper College

Paul Thompson, PhD, President
1200 W Algonquin Rd
Palatine, IL 60067
847 925-6000
- Dental Hygienist
- Dietetic Technician
- Medical Assistant

Palos Hills

Moraine Valley Community College

Vernon Crawley, PhD, President/CEO
10900 S 88th Ave
Palos Hills, IL 60465
708 974-5201
- Clin Lab Tech/Med Lab Tech-AD
- Health Information Tech
- Radiographer
- Respiratory Therapist

Peoria

Bradley University

John R Brazil, President
Peoria, IL 61625
309 676-7611
- Dietitian/Nutritionist

Institutions

Methodist Medical Center of Illinois
James Knoble, President
Executive Offices
221 NE Glen Oak
Peoria, IL 61636
309 672-4826
- Histologic Technician-Cert

Midstate College
R Dale Bunch, President
244 SW Jefferson
Peoria, IL 61602
309 673-6365
- Medical Assistant

St Francis Medical Center
Sr Mary Canisia, OSF, Administrator
530 NE Glen Oak Ave
Peoria, IL 61637
309 655-2020
- Clin Lab Scientist/Med Tech
- Dietitian/Nutritionist
- Histologic Technician-Cert
- Nuclear Medicine Tech
- Radiographer

Quincy

Blessing Hospital
Lawrence L Swearingen, MHA, President
Broadway at 11th St
Quincy, IL 62305
217 223-8400
- Clin Lab Tech/Med Lab Tech-C
- Radiographer

River Forest

Rosary College
Donna M Carroll, President
7900 W Division
River Forest, IL 60305
708 366-2490
- Dietitian/Nutritionist

River Grove

Triton College
George Jorndt, PhD, President
2000 N Fifth Ave
River Grove, IL 60171
708 456-0300
- Clin Lab Tech/Med Lab Tech-AD
- Dental Lab Technician
- Diagnostic Med Sonographer
- Nuclear Medicine Tech
- Ophthalmic Med Technician
- Radiographer
- Respiratory Therapist
- Surgical Technologist

Rockford

Rock Valley College
Karl Jacobs, EdD, President
3301 N Mulford Rd
Rockford, IL 61114-5699
815 654-4260
- Respiratory Therapist
- Respiratory Therapy Tech

Rockford Business College
David G Swank, BS, President and CEO
730 N Church
Rockford, IL 61103
815 965-8616
- Medical Assistant

Rockford Memorial Hospital
Thomas DeFauw, MS, President
2400 N Rockton Ave
Rockford, IL 61103
815 971-5000
- Clin Lab Scientist/Med Tech
- Radiographer

St Anthony Medical Center
David Schertz, Administrator
5666 E State St
Rockford, IL 61108
815 226-2000
- Clin Lab Scientist/Med Tech

Swedish American Hospital
Robert Klint, MD, President/CEO
1400 Charles St
Rockford, IL 61104-2298
815 968-4400
- Clin Lab Scientist/Med Tech
- Radiation Therapist
- Radiographer

South Holland

South Suburban College of Cook County
Robert T Marshall Jr, Interim President
15800 S State St
South Holland, IL 60473-1262
708 596-2000
- Occupational Therapy Asst
- Radiographer

Springfield

Lincoln Land Community College
Norman L Stephens Jr, PhD, President
Shepherd Rd
Springfield, IL 62794-9256
217 786-2274
- Radiographer
- Respiratory Therapist

St John's Hospital
Allison Laabs, FACHE, Exec VP
800 E Carpenter
Springfield, IL 62769
217 544-6464
- Clin Lab Scientist/Med Tech
- Dietitian/Nutritionist
- Electroneurodiagnostic Tech
- Histotechnologist
- Respiratory Therapy Tech

University of Illinois at Springfield
Naomi B Lynn, PhD, Chancellor
Shepherd Rd
Springfield, IL 62794
217 786-6634
- Clin Lab Scientist/Med Tech

Sugar Grove

Waubonsee Community College
John J Swalec, PhD, President
Rt 47 at Harter Rd
Sugar Grove, IL 60554
630 466-7900
- Respiratory Therapy Tech

University Park

Governors State University
Paula Wolff, PhD, President
Rte 54 and Stuenkel Rd
University Park, IL 60466
708 534-5000
- Speech Language Pathologist

Urbana

Univ of Illinois at Urbana - Champaign
James J Stukel, PhD, President
506 S Wright St
364 Henry Admin Bldg
Urbana, IL 61801
217 333-3071
- Athletic Trainer
- Audiologist
- Dietitian/Nutritionist
- Rehabilitation Counselor
- Speech Language Pathologist

West Chicago

Central Medical Education Inc
Steve Lakner, Vice President
550 Washington St
West Chicago, IL 60185
708 682-1600
- Surgical Technologist

Indiana

Anderson

Anderson University
James L Edwards, PhD, President
1100 E 5th St
Anderson, IN 46012
317 641-4011
- Athletic Trainer

Beech Grove

St Francis Hospital and Health Centers
Kevin D Leahy, MBA MHA, President/CEO
1600 Albany St
Beech Grove, IN 46107
317 783-8220
- Clin Lab Scientist/Med Tech

Bloomington

Bloomington Hospital
Nancy Carlstedt, BS MS, President
PO Box 1149
Bloomington, IN 47402
812 336-6821
- Surgical Technologist

Indiana University - Bloomington

Kenneth R R Gros Louis, VP & Chancellor
2931 E 10th St
Bloomington, IN 47405
812 855-4848
- Audiologist
- Dietitian/Nutritionist
- Speech Language Pathologist
- Therapeutic Recreation Specialist

Columbus

Columbus Regional Hospital

Douglas J Leonard, Vice President
2400 E 17th St
Columbus, IN 47201
812 376-5439
- Radiographer

Ivy Tech State Coll - Columbus

Gregory K Flood, MA, Exec Dean
4475 Central Ave
Columbus, IN 47203
812 372-9925
- Medical Assistant

Evansville

Ivy Tech State Coll SW - Evansville

Daniel Schenk, MBA, Executive Dean
3501 First Ave
Evansville, IN 47710
812 426-2865
- Medical Assistant
- Surgical Technologist

Ivy Tech/Evansville Adv Life Support Consort

Douglas French, MS, President and CEO
3700 Washington Ave
Evansville, IN 47750-0001
812 479-4000
- Emergency Med Tech-Paramedic

University of Evansville

James C Vinson, President
1800 Lincoln Ave
Evansville, IN 47722
812 479-2000
- Music Therapist

University of Southern Indiana

H Ray Hoops, PhD, President
8600 University Blvd
Evansville, IN 47712-3534
812 464-1756
- Dental Assistant
- Dental Hygienist
- Occupational Therapist
- Radiographer
- Respiratory Therapist

Welborn Cancer Center

Marjorie Soyugenc, MBA, President
401 SE Sixth St
Evansville, IN 47713
812 426-8264
- Radiation Therapist
- Radiographer

Ft Wayne

Ft Wayne School of Radiography

Frank Byrne, MD, CEO
Parkview Memorial Hosp
700 Broadway
Ft Wayne, IN 46802
219 484-6636
- Radiographer

Indiana Univ/Purdue Univ Ft Wayne

Michael A Wartell, PhD, Chancellor
2101 Coliseum Blvd E
Ft Wayne, IN 46805
219 481-6103
- Dental Assistant
- Dental Hygienist
- Dental Lab Technician
- Health Information Tech
- Music Therapist

International Business Coll - Ft Wayne

3811 Illinois Rd
Ft Wayne, IN 46804-1298
219 432-8702
- Medical Assistant

Ivy Tech State Coll NE - Ft Wayne

Jon L Rupright, MS, Vice Pres/Chancellor
3800 N Anthony Blvd
Ft Wayne, IN 46805
219 482-9171
- Medical Assistant
- Respiratory Therapist
- Respiratory Therapy Tech

Lutheran College of Health Professions

Marilyn Wilson, EdD, Executive Dean
3024 Fairfield Ave
Ft Wayne, IN 46807
219 458-2452
- Radiographer
- Surgical Technologist

Lutheran Hospital of Indiana, Inc

William Andrson, CEO
7950 W Jefferson Blvd
Ft Wayne, IN 46804-1677
219 435-7101
- Clin Lab Scientist/Med Tech

Parkview Memorial Hospital

Frank Byrne, MD, President
2200 Randallia Dr
Ft Wayne, IN 46805
219 484-6636
- Clin Lab Scientist/Med Tech

Gary

Indiana University Northwest

Hilda Richards, EdD, Chancellor
3400 Broadway
Gary, IN 46408
219 980-6700
- Clin Lab Tech/Med Lab Tech-AD
- Dental Assistant
- Dental Hygienist
- Health Information Admin
- Health Information Tech
- Radiation Therapist
- Radiographer
- Respiratory Therapist

Greenfield

Hancock Memorial Hospital

Bobby Keen, President
801 N State St
Greenfield, IN 46140
317 462-0457
- Radiographer

Hammond

Purdue University-Calumet

James Yackel, Chancellor
Hammond, IN 46323
219 989-2993
- Dietitian/Nutritionist
- Dietetic Technician

St Margaret Hospital & Health Centers

Gene Diamond, President/CEO
Mercy Healthcare Ctrs
5454 Hohman Ave
Hammond, IN 46320
219 932-2300
- Clin Lab Scientist/Med Tech

Hobart

St Mary Medical Center

Elizabeth Kaminski, CEO
1500 S Lake Park Ave
Hobart, IN 46342
219 947-6000
- Clin Lab Scientist/Med Tech

Indianapolis

Butler University/Methodist Hosp of Indiana

Geoffrey Bannister, PhD, President
Butler University
4600 Sunset Ave
Indianapolis, IN 46208-3485
317 940-9900
- Physician Assistant

Community Hospitals of Indianapolis

William E Corley, President
1500 N Ritter Ave
Indianapolis, IN 46219
317 355-5529
- Radiographer

Indiana Business College

Ken Konesco, MS, President
802 N Meridian St
Indianapolis, IN 46204
317 783-5100
- Medical Assistant

Indiana University School of Medicine
Robert W Holden, MD, Dean
1120 South Dr
Fesler Hall Rm 302
Indianapolis, IN 46202-5113
317 274-8157
● Clin Lab Scientist/Med Tech
● Cytotechnologist
● Dental Assistant
● Dental Hygienist
● Dietitian/Nutritionist
● Health Information Admin
● Nuclear Medicine Tech
● Occupational Therapist
● Radiation Therapist
● Radiographer
● Respiratory Therapist

International Business Coll - Indianapolis
Eric Stovall, President
7205 Shadeland Station
Indianapolis, IN 46256
317 841-6400
● Medical Assistant

Ivy Tech State Coll - Indianapolis
Gerald I Lamkin, President
One W 26th St/PO Box 1763
Indianapolis, IN 46206-1763
317 921-4750
● Medical Assistant
● Occupational Therapy Asst
● Radiographer
● Respiratory Therapist
● Surgical Technologist

Marian College
Daniel A Felicetti, PhD, President
3200 Cold Spring Rd
Indianapolis, IN 46222
317 929-0237
● Dietitian/Nutritionist

Methodist Hospital of Indiana, Inc
William J Loveday, MBA, President/CEO
1701 N Senate Blvd PO Box 1367
Indianapolis, IN 46206
317 929-5900
● Clin Lab Scientist/Med Tech
● Emergency Med Tech-Paramedic
● Radiation Therapist

Professional Careers Institute
Richard Weiss, BS, President
2611 Waterfront Pkwy East Dr
Indianapolis, IN 46214
317 299-6001
● Dental Assistant
● Medical Assistant

St Vincent Hosp & Health Care Ctr, Inc
Douglas French, President
2001 W 86th St
Indianapolis, IN 46260
317 338-7073
● Clin Lab Scientist/Med Tech

University of Indianapolis
Benjamin C Lantz, PhD, President
1400 E Hanna Ave
Indianapolis, IN 46227-3697
317 788-3211
● Occupational Therapist

Kokomo

Ivy Tech State Coll - Kokomo
Steve Daili, BS MS, Executive Dean
1815 E Morgan St
Kokomo, IN 46901
317 459-0561
● Medical Assistant

St Joseph Hospital & Health Center
Sr M Martin McEntee, President
1907 W Sycamore St
Kokomo, IN 46901
317 452-5611
● Clin Lab Scientist/Med Tech
● Radiographer

Lafayette

Ivy Tech State Coll - Lafayette
Elizabeth Doversberger, PhD, Chancellor
3101 S Creasy Ln
Lafayette, IN 47903
317 772-9138
● Dental Assistant
● Medical Assistant
● Respiratory Therapy Tech
● Surgical Technologist

Madison

Ivy Tech State Coll SE - Madison
Jonathan Thomas, Exec Dean
Ivy Tech SE
590 Ivy Tech Dr
Madison, IN 47250
812 265-2580
● Medical Assistant

King's Daughter's Hospital
Roger J Allman, MHA, President/CEO
One King's Daughter's
PO Box 447
Madison, IN 47250
812 265-5211
● Radiographer

Marion

Indiana Wesleyan University
James Barnes, EdD, President
4201 S Washington St
Marion, IN 46953
317 677-2100
● Clin Lab Tech/Med Lab Tech-AD

Michigan City

Lakeshore Med Laboratory Training Prgm
Thomas H Roberts, MD, Chair
402 Franklin St
Michigan City, IN 46360
219 872-7032
● Clin Lab Tech/Med Lab Tech-C

Muncie

Ball Memorial Hospital
Robert T Brodhead, MHA, President
2401 University Ave
Muncie, IN 47303-3499
317 747-3393
● Clin Lab Scientist/Med Tech
● Dietitian/Nutritionist
● Radiographer

Ball State University
John E Worthen, EdD, President
Administration Bldg 101
Muncie, IN 47306
317 285-5555
● Athletic Trainer
● Audiologist
● Dietitian/Nutritionist
● Dietetic Technician
● Nuclear Medicine Tech
● Radiographer
● Respiratory Therapist
● Speech Language Pathologist

Ivy Tech State Coll EC - Muncie
J Robert Jeffs, Executive Dean
PO Box 3100
Muncie, IN 47307
317 289-2291
● Medical Assistant

Richmond

Ivy Tech State Coll - Richmond
James L Steck, BS MS, Executive Dean
2325 Chester Blvd
Richmond, IN 47374
317 966-2656
● Medical Assistant

Reid Hospital & Health Care Services
Barry S MacDowell, MHA, President
1401 Chester Blvd
Richmond, IN 47374
317 983-3122
● Radiographer

Sellersburg

Ivy Tech State Coll SC - Sellersburg
Jeff Puttman, BS MS, Exec Dean
8204 Hwy 311
Sellersburg, IN 47172
812 246-3301
● Medical Assistant

South Bend

Indiana University - South Bend
Lester Lamon, PhD, Chancellor
1700 Mishawaka Ave Box 7111
South Bend, IN 46634
219 237-4220
● Dental Assistant
● Dental Hygienist
● Radiographer

Ivy Tech State Coll NC - South Bend

Carl Lutz, PhD, Vice President
1534 W Sample St
South Bend, IN 46619
219 289-7001
● Clin Lab Tech/Med Lab Tech-AD
● Medical Assistant

Michiana College

David M Krueper, BBA, President
1030 E Jefferson Blvd
South Bend, IN 46617
219 237-0774
● Medical Assistant

Terre Haute

Indiana State University

John Moore, PhD, President
Condit House
Terre Haute, IN 47809
812 237-4000
● Clin Lab Tech/Med Lab Tech-AD
● Dietitian/Nutritionist
● Speech Language Pathologist

Ivy Tech State Coll - Terre Haute

Sam Borden, PhD, Vice Pres/Chancellor
7999 US Hwy 41 S
Terre Haute, IN 47802-4894
812 299-1121
● Clin Lab Tech/Med Lab Tech-AD
● Medical Assistant
● Radiographer

Valparaiso

Ivy Tech State Coll - Valparaiso

Darnell Cole, PhD, Vice Pres/Chancellor
2401 Valley Dr
Valparaiso, IN 46383
219 464-8514
● Medical Assistant
● Respiratory Therapy Tech
● Surgical Technologist

Porter Memorial Hospital

Wiley Carr, FACHE, President/CEO
814 La Porte Ave
Valparaiso, IN 46383
219 465-4600
● Radiographer

Vincennes

Good Samaritan Hospital

John Hidde, MHA, Exec Director
520 S Seventh St
Vincennes, IN 47591
812 885-3195
● Clin Lab Scientist/Med Tech
● Radiographer

Vincennes University

Phillip M Summers, PhD, President
1002 N First Street
Vincennes, IN 47591
812 888-4201
● Clin Lab Tech/Med Lab Tech-AD
● Health Information Tech
● Respiratory Therapist
● Surgical Technologist

West Lafayette

Purdue University

Steven C Beering, MD PhD, President
Office of the President
Hovde Hall
West Lafayette, IN 47907
317 494-9708
● Athletic Trainer
● Audiologist
● Dietitian/Nutritionist
● Speech Language Pathologist

Iowa

Ames

Iowa State University

Martin C Jischke, President
Ames, IA 50011
515 294-4111
● Dietitian/Nutritionist

Ankeny

Des Moines Area Community College

Joseph A Borgen, PhD, President
2006 S Ankeny Blvd
Ankeny, IA 50021
515 964-6260
● Clin Lab Tech/Med Lab Tech-AD
● Dental Assistant
● Dental Hygienist
● Medical Assistant
● Respiratory Therapist

Bettendorf

Scott Community College

Lenny E Stone, PhD, President
500 Belmont Road
Bettendorf, IA 52722
319 359-7531
● Clin Lab Tech/Med Lab Tech-AD
● Electroneurodiagnostic Tech
● Radiographer

Calmar

Northeast Iowa Community College

Donald Roby, MEd EdS, President
Box 400 Calmar
Calmar, IA 52132
319 562-3263
● Dental Assistant
● Health Information Tech
● Radiographer
● Respiratory Therapist
● Respiratory Therapy Tech

Cedar Falls

University of Northern Iowa

Robert Koob, President
1222 W 27th St
Cedar Falls, IA 50614
319 273-2567
● Audiologist
● Dietitian/Nutritionist
● Speech Language Pathologist
● Therapeutic Recreation Specialist

Cedar Rapids

Kirkwood Community College

Norman R Nielsen, PhD, President
PO Box 2068
6301 Kirkwood Blvd SW
Cedar Rapids, IA 52406-9973
319 398-5500
● Dental Assistant
● Dental Lab Technician
● Electroneurodiagnostic Tech
● Health Information Tech
● Medical Assistant
● Occupational Therapy Asst
● Respiratory Therapist

Mercy/St Luke's Hospitals

Stephen Vanourney, MD, President
1026 A Ave NE
Cedar Rapids, IA 52402
319 369-7204
● Clin Lab Scientist/Med Tech
● Radiographer

Council Bluffs

Iowa Western Community College

Dan Kinney, PhD, President
2700 College Rd Box 4-C
Council Bluffs, IA 51502-3004
712 325-3200
● Dental Assistant
● Medical Assistant

Jennie Edmundson Memorial Hospital

David M Holcomb, MHA, CEO
933 E Pierce St
Council Bluffs, IA 51501
712 328-6239
● Radiographer

Davenport

American Institute of Commerce

John Huston, MBA, President
1801 E Kimberly Rd
Davenport, IA 52807
319 355-3500
● Medical Assistant

Hamilton College

John Huston, MBA, President
American Institute of Commerce
1801 E Kimberly Rd
Davenport, IA 52807
319 355-3500
● Medical Assistant

St Ambrose University

Edward Rogalski, PhD, President
518 W Locust St
Davenport, IA 52803
319 333-6213
● Occupational Therapist

Des Moines

Drake University

Michael R Ferrari, President
25th St and University Ave
Des Moines, IA 50311
515 271-2011
● Rehabilitation Counselor

Iowa Methodist Medical Center

James H Skogsbergh, MS MHA, President
1200 Pleasant St
Des Moines, IA 50309-1453
515 241-6201
- Clin Lab Scientist/Med Tech
- Radiographer

Mercy Hospital Medical Center

Thomas A Reitinger, BA MHA, President/CEO
400 University Ave
Des Moines, IA 50314
515 247-3222
- Clin Lab Scientist/Med Tech
- Cytotechnologist
- Emergency Med Tech-Paramedic
- Radiographer

University of Osteopathic Medicine

Richard Ryan, PhD, President
3440 Grand Ave
Des Moines, IA 50312
515 271-1500
- Physician Assistant

Ft Dodge

Iowa Central Community College

Robert A Paxton, PhD, President
330 Ave M
Ft Dodge, IA 50501
515 576-7201
- Clin Lab Tech/Med Lab Tech-AD
- Medical Assistant
- Radiographer

Iowa City

University of Iowa

Mary Sue Coleman, PhD, President
101 Jessup Hall
Iowa City, IA 52242
319 335-3549
- Athletic Trainer
- Audiologist
- Clin Lab Scientist/Med Tech
- Music Therapist
- Nuclear Medicine Tech
- Physician Assistant
- Rehabilitation Counselor
- Speech Language Pathologist
- Therapeutic Recreation Specialist

University of Iowa Hospitals and Clinics

R Edward Howell, CEO
200 Hawkins Dr 1353 JCP
Iowa City, IA 52242-1059
319 356-3155
- Diagnostic Med Sonographer
- Dietitian/Nutritionist
- Perfusionist
- Radiation Therapist
- Radiographer

Marshalltown

Marshalltown Community College

Paul A Tambrino, EdD, President
3702 S Center St
Marshalltown, IA 50158
515 752-4643
- Dental Assistant
- Surgical Technologist

Mason City

North Iowa Mercy Health Center

David H Vellinga, CEO
84 Beaumont Dr
Mason City, IA 50401
515 424-7722
- Radiographer

Ottumwa

Indian Hills Community College

Lyle Hellyer, PhD, President
525 Grandview
Ottumwa, IA 52501
515 683-5100
- Health Information Tech
- Radiographer

Sioux City

Marian Health Center

Douglas Johnson, MBA, President/CEO
801 Fifth St
Sioux City, IA 51101
712 279-2018
- Clin Lab Scientist/Med Tech
- Radiographer

St Luke's Regional Medical Center

John Daniels, Acting President&CEO
2720 Stone Park Blvd
Sioux City, IA 51104
712 279-3500
- Clin Lab Scientist/Med Tech

Western Iowa Tech Community College

Robert Dunker, PhD, President
4647 Stone Ave PO Box 265
Sioux City, IA 51102-0265
712 274-6400
- Dental Assistant
- Occupational Therapy Asst
- Surgical Technologist

Spencer

Iowa Lakes Community College

James E Billings, President
1900 N Grand Ave
Spencer, IA 51301
712 362-2601
- Medical Assistant

Waterloo

Allen College

Jane Hasek, Chancellor
1825 Logan Ave
Waterloo, IA 50703
319 235-3545
- Radiographer

Covenant Medical Center

Raymond Burfeind, CEO/Administrator
3421 W 9th
Waterloo, IA 50702
319 236-4014
- Radiographer

Hawkeye Community College

William J Hierstein, Presiden
PO Box 8015
Waterloo, IA 50704
319 296-2320
- Clin Lab Tech/Med Lab Tech-AD
- Dental Assistant
- Dental Hygienist
- Respiratory Therapy Tech

Waverly

Wartburg College

Robert L Vogel, President
Waverly, IA 50677-1003
319 352-8200
- Music Therapist

West Burlington

Southeastern Community College

R Gene Gardner, PhD, President
1015 S Gear Ave Drawer F
West Burlington, IA 52655
319 752-2731
- Medical Assistant

Kansas

Dodge City

Dodge City Community College

Richard Drum, PhD, President
2501 N 14th Ave
Dodge City, KS 67801
316 227-9249
- Health Information Tech

Emporia

Emporia State University

Robert E Glennen, President
1200 Commercial St
Emporia, KS 66801
316 343-1200
- Art Therapist
- Rehabilitation Counselor

Flint Hills Technical School

3301 W 18th Ave
Emporia, KS 66801
316 341-2300
- Dental Assistant

Great Bend

Barton County Community College

Veldon L Law, EdD, President
RR 3 Box 136Z
Great Bend, KS 67530-9283
316 792-2701
- Clin Lab Tech/Med Lab Tech-AD
- Occupational Therapy Asst

Hays

Ft Hays State University
Rodolfo Arevalo, PhD, Provost
600 W Park St
Hays, KS 67601
913 628-4231
- Dietitian/Nutritionist
- Radiographer
- Speech Language Pathologist

Hays Pathology Laboratories
Ward M Newcomb, MD, CEO
1300 E 13th St
Hays, KS 67601
913 625-5646
- Clin Lab Scientist/Med Tech

Hutchinson

Hutchinson Community College
Edward E Berger, EdD, President
1300 N Plum St
Hutchinson, KS 67501
316 665-3505
- Health Information Tech
- Radiographer

Kansas City

Bethany Med Ctr/Kansas City Kansas Comm Coll
Patricia Rycken, RRT, Consortial Comm Chair
51 N 12th St
Kansas City, KS 66102
913 281-8750
- Respiratory Therapist
- Respiratory Therapy Tech

Bethany Medical Center
John L Millard, MHA FACHE, President
51 N 12th St
Kansas City, KS 66102
913 281-8703
- Radiographer

University of Kansas Medical Center
Donald F Hagen, MD, Exec Vice Chancellor
3901 Rainbow Blvd
2nd Fl Murphy
Kansas City, KS 66160
913 588-1433
- Clin Lab Scientist/Med Tech
- Cytotechnologist
- Dietitian/Nutritionist
- Health Information Admin
- Nuclear Medicine Tech
- Occupational Therapist
- Radiation Therapist
- Respiratory Therapist

Lawrence

University of Kansas
Robert E Hemenway, Chancellor
3031 Dole Ctr
Lawrence, KS 66045
913 864-0630
- Audiologist
- Music Therapist
- Speech Language Pathologist

Liberal

Seward County Community College
James R Grote, PhD, President
PO Box 1137
Liberal, KS 67901
316 629-2610
- Clin Lab Tech/Med Lab Tech-AD
- Respiratory Therapist
- Respiratory Therapy Tech

Manhattan

Kansas State University
Jon Wefald, President
Anderson Hall
Manhattan, KS 66506-5301
913 532-6221
- Athletic Trainer
- Dietitian/Nutritionist
- Speech Language Pathologist

Overland Park

Johnson County Community College
Charles J Carlsen, EdD, President
12345 College Blvd
Overland Park, KS 66210-1299
913 469-8500
- Dental Hygienist
- Emergency Med Tech-Paramedic
- Respiratory Therapist

Parsons

Labette Community College
Joseph Birmingham, EdD, President
200 S 14th St
Parsons, KS 67357
316 421-6700
- Radiographer
- Respiratory Therapist

Salina

Salina Area Vocational Technical School
2562 Scanlan Ave
Salina, KS 67401
913 827-0134
- Dental Assistant

Topeka

Washburn University of Topeka
Hugh L Thompson, PhD, President
1700 SW College
Topeka, KS 66621
913 231-1010
- Health Information Tech
- Radiation Therapist
- Radiographer
- Respiratory Therapist
- Respiratory Therapy Tech

Wichita

Kansas Newman College
Sr Tarcisia Roths, PhD, President
3100 McCormick Ave
Wichita, KS 67213-2097
316 942-4291
- Occupational Therapist
- Perfusionist
- Radiographer

Wichita Area Technical College
Rosemary A Kirby, PhD, President
324 N Emporia
Wichita, KS 67202
316 833-4664
- Clin Lab Tech/Med Lab Tech-C
- Dental Assistant
- Medical Assistant
- Surgical Technologist

Wichita State University
Eugene Hughes, PhD, President
1845 N Fairmont
Campus Box 1
Wichita, KS 67260-0001
316 978-3001
- Audiologist
- Clin Lab Scientist/Med Tech
- Dental Hygienist
- Histologic Technician-Cert
- Physician Assistant
- Respiratory Therapist
- Speech Language Pathologist

Kentucky

Ashland

Kentucky Tech - Ashland Campus
Richard Kendall, School Director
4818 Roberts Dr
Ashland, KY 41102-9046
606 928-6427
- Surgical Technologist

King's Daughter's Medical Center
Fred Jackson, President
2201 Lexington Ave
Ashland, KY 41101
606 327-4000
- Radiographer

Rowan State Voc Tech School
Howard Moore, MS, Director
Ashland State Voc Tech
4818 Roberts Dr
Ashland, KY 41101
606 928-4256
- Respiratory Therapy Tech

Berea

Berea College
Larry D Shinn, President
Berea, KY 40404
606 986-9341
- Dietitian/Nutritionist

Bowling Green

Bowling Green State Voc Tech School
Donald R Williams, MA, Director
1845 Loop Dr
Bowling Green, KY 42101
502 746-7461
● Dental Assistant
● Radiographer
● Respiratory Therapy Tech
● Surgical Technologist

Western Kentucky University
Thomas Meredith, EdD, President
Office of the President
Wetherby Bldg
Bowling Green, KY 42101
502 745-4346
● Dental Hygienist
● Dietitian/Nutritionist
● Health Information Tech
● Speech Language Pathologist

Covington

Maysville Comm Coll/N Kentucky Univ
James C Shires, President
Hankins Hall
1401 Dixie Hwy
Covington, KY 41011
606 799-7141
● Dental Hygienist

Cumberland

Southeast Community College
W Bruce Ayers, EdD, President
300 College Rd
Cumberland, KY 40823-1099
606 589-2145
● Respiratory Therapist

Edgewood

St Elizabeth Medical Center
Joseph Gross, FACHE, President/CEO
One Medical Village Dr
Edgewood, KY 41017
606 344-2111
● Clin Lab Scientist/Med Tech

Elizabethtown

Hopkinsville Community College
A James Kerley, President
PO Box 2100
Elizabethtown, KY 42701
502 886-3921
● Dental Hygienist

Ky Tech Elizabethtown State Voc Tech School
505 University Dr
Elizabethtown, KY 42701
● Radiographer

Hazard

Hazard Community College
G Edwards Hughes, PhD, President
One Community College Dr
HWY 15 S
Hazard, KY 41701
606 436-5721
● Clin Lab Tech/Med Lab Tech-AD
● Radiographer

Henderson

Henderson Community College
Patrick R Lake, EdD, Director
2660 S Green St
Henderson, KY 42420
502 827-1867
● Clin Lab Tech/Med Lab Tech-AD

Highland

Northern Kentucky University
Jack Moreland, Interim President
Office of the President
Admin Ctr 800B
Highland, KY 41099-2104
606 572-5123
● Radiographer
● Respiratory Therapist

Lexington

Fugazzi College
Frank E Longaker, Chair
406 Lafayette Ave
Lexington, KY 40502
606 266-0401
● Medical Assistant

Kentucky College of Business
Richard G Wood, MA, President
628 E Main St
Lexington, KY 40508
606 253-0621
● Medical Assistant

Kentucky Tech Central Campus
Ron Baugh, MEd, Director
104 Vo-Tech Rd
Lexington, KY 40511-1020
606 246-2400
● Clin Lab Tech/Med Lab Tech-C
● Dental Assistant
● Medical Assistant
● Radiographer
● Respiratory Therapy Tech
● Surgical Technologist

Lexington Community College
Janice N Friedel, PhD, President
Cooper Dr
Oswald Bldg, Rm 209
Lexington, KY 40506-0235
606 257-4831
● Dental Hygienist
● Dental Lab Technician
● Nuclear Medicine Tech
● Radiographer
● Respiratory Therapist

Pathology and Cytology Laboratories, Inc
James L Bauer, MD, President
290 Big Run Rd
Lexington, KY 40503
606 278-9513
● Cytotechnologist

St Joseph Hospital
William Fuchs, President/CEO
One St Joseph Dr
Lexington, KY 40504
606 278-3436
● Radiographer

Univ of Kentucky Chandler Med Ctr
Charles Wethington, PhD, President
103 Administration Plaza Rm A311
Lexington, KY 40536-2231
606 323-5126
● Clin Lab Scientist/Med Tech
● Dietitian/Nutritionist
● Physician Assistant
● Radiation Therapist

University of Kentucky
Charles T Wethington, President
Lexington, KY 40506
606 257-9000
● Dietitian/Nutritionist
● Rehabilitation Counselor
● Speech Language Pathologist

Louisville

Jefferson Community College
Richard Green, EdD, President
109 E Broadway
Louisville, KY 40202
502 584-0181
● Respiratory Therapist

JG Brown Cancer Ctr/U of Louisville Hosp
J Paul Jennings, MBA MHS, Administrator
University of Louisville Hospital
529 S Jackson St
Louisville, KY 40202
502 588-6905
● Radiation Therapist

Kentucky Tech/Jefferson State Campus
Marvin Copes, PhD, Director
727 W Chestnut St
Louisville, KY 40203
502 595-4136
● Clin Lab Tech/Med Lab Tech-C
● Medical Assistant
● Respiratory Therapy Tech

Spalding University
Thomas R Oates, President
851 S Fourth St
Louisville, KY 40203
502 585-9911
● Dietitian/Nutritionist

Spencerian College
Alva R Sullivan, BSC, CEO
4627 Dixie Hwy
Louisville, KY 40216
502 447-1000
● Medical Assistant

University of Louisville
Donald R Kmetz, MD, Interim VP for Hlth Aff
Abell Administration Center
Belknap Campus
Louisville, KY 40292
502 852-5420
- Art Therapist
- Audiologist
- Clin Lab Scientist/Med Tech
- Cytotechnologist
- Dental Hygienist
- Nuclear Medicine Tech
- Radiographer
- Respiratory Therapist
- Speech Language Pathologist

Madisonville

Madisonville Community College
Arthur D Stumpf, PhD, President
College Dr
Madisonville, KY 42431
502 821-2250
- Respiratory Therapist

Madisonville Health Technology Center
Mike Wright, MS, Director Region 2
100 School Ave
KY Tech West Region
Madisonville, KY 42431
502 824-7546
- Clin Lab Tech/Med Lab Tech-C
- Radiographer
- Respiratory Therapy Tech
- Surgical Technologist

Morehead

Morehead State University
Ronald G Eaglin, PhD, President
201 Howell McDowell Admin Bldg
Morehead, KY 40351
606 783-2022
- Dietitian/Nutritionist
- Radiographer

Mt Vernon

KY Tech-Rockcastle County Area Tech Ctr
Donna Hopkins, MA, Principal
PO Box 275
Mt Vernon, KY 40456
606 256-4346
- Respiratory Therapy Tech

Murray

Murray State University
Donald Kurth, PhD, President
Murray, KY 42071
502 762-3763
- Dietitian/Nutritionist
- Speech Language Pathologist

Owensboro

Kentucky Tech - Owensboro Campus
Ray Gillaspie, MS, Director
1501 Frederica St
Owensboro, KY 42301
502 686-3206
- Surgical Technologist

Owensboro Community College
John McGuire, PhD, President
4800 New Hartford Rd
Owensboro, KY 42303-1899
502 686-4400
- Radiographer

Owensboro Mercy Health System
Greg Carlson, CEO
811 E Parrish Ave
PO Box 20007
Owensboro, KY 42303
502 688-2100
- Clin Lab Scientist/Med Tech

Paducah

Lourdes Hospital
Jeff Comer, CEO
1530 Lone Oak Rd
Paducah, KY 42001
502 444-2101
- Clin Lab Scientist/Med Tech

West Kentucky Tech
Lee E Hicklin, MA, Director
PO Box 7408 Blandville Rd
Paducah, KY 42002-7408
502 554-4991
- Dental Assistant
- Diagnostic Med Sonographer
- Medical Assistant
- Radiographer
- Respiratory Therapy Tech
- Surgical Technologist

Paintsville

KY Tech - Mayo Regional Tech Ctr
Gary Coleman, Principal
513 Third St
Paintsville, KY 41240
606 789-5321
- Respiratory Therapy Tech

Pikeville

Pikeville Methodist Hospital
Martha O'Regan Chill, MA, Administrator
911 S Bypass
Pikeville, KY 41501
606 437-3500
- Clin Lab Scientist/Med Tech

Pineville

Cumberland Valley Health Technology Ctr
Denise R Sharpe, Director
PO Box 187 US 25E S
Pineville, KY 40977
606 337-3106
- Clin Lab Tech/Med Lab Tech-C
- Radiographer
- Respiratory Therapy Tech
- Surgical Technologist

Richmond

Eastern Kentucky University
Hanly Funderburk, PhD, President
Coates Admin Bldg Rm 107
Richmond, KY 40475-3101
606 622-2101
- Athletic Trainer
- Clin Lab Scientist/Med Tech
- Clin Lab Tech/Med Lab Tech-AD
- Dietitian/Nutritionist
- Emergency Med Tech-Paramedic
- Health Information Admin
- Health Information Tech
- Medical Assistant
- Occupational Therapist
- Speech Language Pathologist
- Therapeutic Recreation Specialist

Somerset

Somerset Community College
Rollin Watson, PhD, President
808 Monticello Rd
Somerset, KY 42501
606 679-8501
- Clin Lab Tech/Med Lab Tech-AD

Louisiana

Alexandria

Rapides Regional Medical Center
Lynn Truelove, BS MS, President
211 Fourth St
PO Box 30101
Alexandria, LA 71301
318 473-3150
- Clin Lab Scientist/Med Tech
- Dental Hygienist

Baton Rouge

Baton Rouge General Medical Center
James Brexler, President/CEO
3600 Florida St
PO Box 2511-70821
Baton Rouge, LA 70806
504 387-7767
- Radiographer

Louisiana State Univ and A & M College
William E Davis, Chancellor
Baton Rouge, LA 70803
504 388-3202
- Audiologist
- Dietitian/Nutritionist
- Speech Language Pathologist

Our Lady of the Lake Coll
James W Firnberg, EdD, President
5345 Brittany Dr
Baton Rouge, LA 70808
504 768-1710
- Radiographer
- Surgical Technologist

Institutions

Our Lady of the Lake College
James W Firnberg, EdD, President
5345 Brittany Dr
Baton Rouge, LA 70808
504 765-8802
• Clin Lab Scientist/Med Tech

Southern Univ and A & M College
Marvin L Yates, Chancellor
Baton Rouge, LA 70813
504 771-4500
• Dietitian/Nutritionist
• Rehabilitation Counselor
• Speech Language Pathologist

Bossier City

Bossier Parish Community College
Tom Carleton, MA, Chancellor
2719 Airline Dr
Bossier City, LA 71111
318 746-9851
• Respiratory Therapist
• Respiratory Therapy Tech

Eunice

Louisiana State University at Eunice
William J Nunez III, PhD, Interim Chancellor
PO Box 1129
Eunice, LA 70535
318 457-7311
• Radiographer
• Respiratory Therapy Tech

Grambling

Grambling State University
Raymond A Hicks, President
Grambling, LA 71245
318 247-3811
• Therapeutic Recreation Specialist

Hammond

North Oaks Health System
James E Cathey Jr, Administrator
15790 Medical Ctr Dr
Hammond, LA 70403
504 543-6600
• Dietitian/Nutritionist
• Radiographer

Southeastern Louisiana University
Sally Clausen, EdD, President
PO Box 784
Hammond, LA 70402
504 549-2280
• Speech Language Pathologist

Harvey

LA Tech College-West Jefferson Campus
Donna Higgins-Wilson, MEd, Director
475 Manhattan Blvd
Harvey, LA 70058
504 361-6464
• Respiratory Therapy Tech

Lafayette

Lafayette General Medical Center
John J Burdin Jr, MHA, President
1214 Coolidge Ave/PO Box 52009 OCS
Lafayette, LA 70505
318 289-7381
• Radiographer

Louisiana Technical College
Shelton J Cobb, Director
1101 Bertrand Dr PO Box 4909
Lafayett Campus Medical
Lafayette, LA 70502-4909
318 235-5541
• Clin Lab Tech/Med Lab Tech-C

University Medical Center
Lawrence T Dorsey, Hosp Director
2390 W Congress/PO Box 4016-C
Lafayette, LA 70502-4016
318 261-6004
• Radiographer

University of Southwestern Louisiana
Ray Authement, PhD, President
USL Drawer 41008
Lafayette, LA 70504
318 482-6203
• Audiologist
• Dietitian/Nutritionist
• Emergency Med Tech-Paramedic
• Health Information Admin
• Speech Language Pathologist

Lake Charles

Lake Charles Mem Hosp Sch of Med Tech
Elton Williams, CPA, President
1701 Oak Park Blvd
Lake Charles, LA 70601
318 494-3200
• Clin Lab Scientist/Med Tech

McNeese State University
Robert D Hebert, PhD, President
PO Box 93300
Lake Charles, LA 70609
318 475-5556
• Dietitian/Nutritionist
• Radiographer

St Patrick Hospital
J William Hankins, MBA, Administrator
524 S Ryan St
Lake Charles, LA 70601
318 491-7730
• Clin Lab Scientist/Med Tech

Monroe

Northeast Louisiana University
Lawson L Swearingen Jr, JD, President
700 University Ave
NE Station
Monroe, LA 71209-0430
318 342-1010
• Dental Hygienist
• Occupational Therapist
• Occupational Therapy Asst
• Radiographer
• Speech Language Pathologist

St Francis Medical Center
H Gerald Smith, MHA, President/CEO
309 Jackson St
Monroe, LA 71201
318 327-4141
• Clin Lab Scientist/Med Tech

Natchitoches

Northwestern State University
Robert A Alost, PhD, President
Natchitoches, LA 71497
318 357-5701
• Radiographer

New Orleans

Alton Ochsner Medical Foundation
George H Porter III, MD, President
1516 Jefferson Hwy
New Orleans, LA 70121
504 842-3000
• Clin Lab Scientist/Med Tech
• Diagnostic Med Sonographer
• Nuclear Medicine Tech
• Radiation Therapist
• Radiographer
• Respiratory Therapist
• Respiratory Therapy Tech
• Specialist in BB Tech
• Surgical Technologist

Delgado Community College
Ione Elioff, EdD, President
615 City Park Ave
New Orleans, LA 70119-4399
504 483-4400
• Clin Lab Tech/Med Lab Tech-AD
• Dietetic Technician
• Health Information Tech
• Nuclear Medicine Tech
• Radiographer
• Respiratory Therapist
• Respiratory Therapy Tech
• Surgical Technologist

Louisiana State Univ Med Ctr - New Orleans
Mervin L Trail, MD, Chancellor
433 Bolivar St
New Orleans, LA 70112-2223
504 568-4800
• Audiologist
• Clin Lab Scientist/Med Tech
• Occupational Therapist
• Ophthalmic Med Technician
• Rehabilitation Counselor
• Respiratory Therapist
• Speech Language Pathologist

Louisiana State University
Mervin Trail, Chancellor,
1100 Florida Ave
New Orleans, LA 70119
504 948-8530
• Dental Hygienist
• Dental Lab Technician

Loyola University New Orleans
Bernard P Knoth, SJ, President
6363 St Charles Ave
New Orleans, LA 70118
504 865-2011
• Music Therapist

Medical Center of LA - Charity Campus

Jonathan Roberts, DrPH
LHCA-Louisiana Health Care Authority
1532 Tulane Ave
New Orleans, LA 70112-2860
504 568-2311
● Specialist in BB Tech

Ochsner School of Allied Health Sciences

880 Commerce Rd W
New Orleans, LA 70123
504 842-3352
● Dietitian/Nutritionist

Touro Infirmary School of Med Tech

Gary M Stein, MA, President
1401 Foucher St
New Orleans, LA 70115
504 897-8244
● Clin Lab Scientist/Med Tech
● Dietitian/Nutritionist

Tulane University

Eamon M Kelly, President
New Orleans, LA 70118
504 865-5000
● Dietitian/Nutritionist

Ruston

Louisiana Tech University

Daniel D Reneau, PhD, President
PO Box 3168
Ruston, LA 71272
318 257-3785
● Audiologist
● Dietitian/Nutritionist
● Health Information Admin
● Health Information Tech
● Speech Language Pathologist

Shreveport

Louisiana State Univ Med Ctr - Shreveport

Ike Muslow, MD, Vice Chancellor
1501 Kings Hwy
PO Box 33932
Shreveport, LA 71130
318 675-5400
● Physician Assistant

Overton Brooks VA Medical Center

Michael E Hamilton, MHA, Director
510 E Stoner Ave
Shreveport, LA 71101-4295
318 424-6037
● Clin Lab Scientist/Med Tech
● Nuclear Medicine Tech

Southern Univ at Shreveport - Bossier City

Jerome G Green Jr, PhD, Chancellor
3050 Martin Luther King Jr Dr
Shreveport, LA 71107-8032
318 674-3300
● Clin Lab Tech/Med Lab Tech-AD
● Health Information Tech
● Radiographer
● Respiratory Therapist

Thibodaux

Nicholls State University

Donald J Ayo, PhD, President
PO Box 2004 University Station
Thibodaux, LA 70310
504 448-4003
● Dietitian/Nutritionist
● Respiratory Therapist
● Respiratory Therapy Tech

Maine

Augusta

University of Maine - Bangor

Owen Cargol, President
University of Maine-Augusta
46 University Dr.
Augusta, ME 04330
207 621-3000
● Dental Assistant
● Dental Hygienist
● Health Information Tech

University of Maine at Augusta

Owen F Cargol, EdD, President
46 University Dr
Augusta, ME 04330
207 621-3403
● Clin Lab Tech/Med Lab Tech-AD

Bangor

Beal College

Allen Stehle, BS, President
629 Main St
Bangor, ME 04401
207 947-4591
● Medical Assistant

Eastern Maine Medical Center

Norman A Ledwin, President and CEO
489 State St
Bangor, ME 04401
207 973-7051
● Clin Lab Scientist/Med Tech

Eastern Maine Technical College

Joyce E Hedlund, EdD, President
354 Hogan Rd
Bangor, ME 04401
207 941-4691
● Clin Lab Tech/Med Lab Tech-AD
● Radiographer

Husson College

William H Beardsly, PhD, President
One College Circle
Bangor, ME 04401
207 941-7138
● Medical Assistant

Biddeford

University of New England

Sandra Featherman, PhD, President
Hills Beach Rd
Biddeford, ME 04005-9599
207 283-0171
● Dental Hygienist
● Occupational Therapist

Fairfield

Kennebec Valley Technical College

Barbara W Woodlee, EdD, President
92 Western Ave
Fairfield, ME 04937-1367
207 453-5129
● Health Information Tech
● Occupational Therapy Asst
● Respiratory Therapist

Lewiston

Central Maine Medical Center

William W Young Jr, MHA, President
300 Main St
Lewiston, ME 04240
207 795-2700
● Radiographer

Orono

University of Maine - Orono

Frederick E Hutchinson, President
Orono, ME 04469
207 581-1110
● Dietitian/Nutritionist
● Speech Language Pathologist

Portland

Maine Medical Center

Donald McDowell, BS, President
22 Bramhall St
Portland, ME 04102
207 871-2491
● Clin Lab Scientist/Med Tech
● Surgical Technologist

Mercy Hospital

Howard R Buckely, MBA, President
144 State St
Portland, ME 04029
207 879-3000
● Radiographer

University of Southern Maine

Richard L Pattenaude, President
96 Falmouth St
Portland, ME 04103
207 780-4141
● Occupational Therapist
● Rehabilitation Counselor

Presque Isle

University of Maine at Presque Isle

W Michael Easton, PhD, President
181 Main St
22 Preble Hall
Presque Isle, ME 04769
207 768-9525
● Clin Lab Tech/Med Lab Tech-AD

South Portland

Southern Maine Technical College

Wayne H Ross, MPA, President
Fort Rd
South Portland, ME 04106
207 767-9500
- Dietetic Technician
- Radiation Therapist
- Radiographer
- Respiratory Therapist

Waterville

Mid Maine Medical Center Thayer Unit

Scott Bullock, MHA, President
149 North St
Waterville, ME 04901
207 872-4315
- Radiographer

Maryland

Andrews AFB

Malcolm Grow USAF Medical Center

Col. James F. Geiger,
Malcolm Grow USAF Medical Center
Andrews AFB, MD 20762-6600
301 981-3002
- Clin Lab Scientist/Med Tech
- Dietitian/Nutritionist

Arnold

Anne Arundel Community College

Martha R Smith, PhD, President
101 College Pkwy
Arnold, MD 21012-1875
410 541-2222
- Radiographer

Baltimore

Baltimore City Community College

James D Tschechtelin, PhD, President
2901 Liberty Heights Ave
Baltimore, MD 21215-7893
410 333-5800
- Dental Hygienist
- Dietetic Technician
- Health Information Tech

Coppin State College

Calvin W Burnett, President
2500 W North Ave
Baltimore, MD 21216
410 383-5400
- Rehabilitation Counselor

Essex Community College

Donald J Slowinski, EdD, President
7201 Rossville Blvd
Baltimore, MD 21237-3899
410 780-6322
- Clin Lab Tech/Med Lab Tech-AD
- Physician Assistant
- Radiation Therapist
- Radiographer

Greater Baltimore Medical Center

Robert P Kowal, MBA, President
6701 N Charles St
Baltimore, MD 21204
301 828-2121
- Radiographer

Johns Hopkins Hospital

James A Block, MD, President
600 N Wolfe St Admin 126
Baltimore, MD 21287
410 955-0428
- Cytotechnologist
- Diagnostic Med Sonographer
- Nuclear Medicine Tech
- Perfusionist
- Radiographer
- Specialist in BB Tech

Johns Hopkins School of Medicine

Edward D Miller Jr, MD, Intrim Dean
100 Medical Admin Bldg
720 N Rutland Ave
Baltimore, MD 21205
410 955-3180
- Medical Illustrator

Loyola College of Maryland

Harold E Ridley, SJ, President
4501 N Charles St
Baltimore, MD 21210
410 617-2000
- Speech Language Pathologist

Maryland Dept of Hlth & Mental Hygiene

6 St Paul St
Baltimore, MD 21202
410 767-8440
- Dietitian/Nutritionist

Maryland General Hospital

James R Wood, President
827 Linden Ave
Baltimore, MD 21201
301 995-8600
- Radiographer

Mercy Medical Center

Sr Helen Amos, RSM, President
301 St Paul Pl
Baltimore, MD 21202-2165
301 332-9202
- Dietitian/Nutritionist
- Radiographer

Morgan State University

Earl S Richardson, EdD, President
Coldspring Ln and Hillen Rd
Baltimore, MD 21239
410 319-3200
- Clin Lab Scientist/Med Tech
- Dietitian/Nutritionist

University of Maryland

David J Ramsay, DM PhD, President
Office of the Chancellor Davidge Hall
522 W Lombard St
Baltimore, MD 21201-1627
410 706-7002
- Clin Lab Scientist/Med Tech
- Dental Hygienist
- Rehabilitation Counselor

University of Maryland Baltimore County

Freeman A Hrabowski, PhD, President
1000 Hill Top Circle
Admin Rm 1008
Baltimore, MD 21250
410 455-2274
- Diagnostic Med Sonographer
- Emergency Med Tech-Paramedic

University of Maryland Medical System

22 S Greene St
Baltimore, MD 21201-1544
410 328-2561
- Dietitian/Nutritionist

Bel Air

Harford Community College

Claudia E Chiesi, PhD, President
401 Thomas Run Rd
Bel Air, MD 21015
410 836-4200
- Histologic Technician-AD

Bethesda

National Institutes of Health

10 Ctr Dr
Bethesda, MD 20892
301 496-3311
- Dietitian/Nutritionist

Naval School of Health Sciences - MD

Harry C Coffey, Capt MSC USN, Comm Ofcr
8901 Wisconsin Ave
Bethesda, MD 20889-5611
301 295-1204
- Cardiovascular Technologist
- Clin Lab Tech/Med Lab Tech-C
- Cytotechnologist
- Electroneurodiagnostic Tech
- Nuclear Medicine Tech
- Surgical Technologist

NIH Clinical Center Blood Bank

Walter L Jones, Deputy Director
NIH/CC/DTM Bldg 10 Rm IC-711
10 Ctr Dr MSC 1184
Bethesda, MD 20892-1184
301 496-4506
- Specialist in BB Tech

Catonsville

Catonsville Community College

Frederick Walsh, PhD, President
800 S Rolling Rd
Catonsville, MD 21228-9987
410 455-4100
- Occupational Therapy Asst

College Park

Univ of Maryland at College Park

William E Kirwan, President
College Park, MD 20742
301 405-1000
- Audiologist
- Dietitian/Nutritionist
- Speech Language Pathologist

Cumberland

Allegany College of Maryland

Donald L Alexander, EdD, President
12401 Willowbrook Rd SE
Cumberland, MD 21502-2596
301 724-7700
- Clin Lab Tech/Med Lab Tech-AD
- Dental Hygienist
- Occupational Therapy Asst
- Radiographer
- Respiratory Therapist

Frederick

Frederick Community College

Lee J Betts, EdD, President
7932 Opossumtown Pike
Frederick, MD 21702
301 846-2442
- Respiratory Therapist

Hood College

Martha E Church, PhD, President
Rosemont Ave
Frederick, MD 21701
301 663-3131
- Dietitian/Nutritionist

Hagerstown

Hagerstown Business College

Jim Gifford, MEd, President
18618 Crestwood Dr
Hagerstown, MD 21742
301 739-2670
- Health Information Tech

Hagerstown Junior College

Norman P Shea, EdD, President
11400 Robinwood Dr
Hagerstown, MD 21742-6590
301 790-2800
- Radiographer

Largo

Prince George's Community College

Robert I Bickford, PhD, President
301 Largo Rd
Largo, MD 20772
301 322-0400
- Health Information Tech
- Nuclear Medicine Tech
- Radiographer
- Respiratory Therapist

Princess Anne

University of Maryland Eastern Shore

William P Hytche, President
Princess Anne, MD 21853
410 651-2200
- Dietitian/Nutritionist

Rockville

Montgomery College

Robert E Parilla, PhD, President
Central Admin Office
900 Hungerford
Rockville, MD 20850
301 279-5264
- Clin Lab Tech/Med Lab Tech-AD
- Diagnostic Med Sonographer
- Health Information Tech
- Radiographer

Salisbury

Salisbury State University

William C Merwin, EdD, President
Holloway Hall
Salisbury, MD 21801
410 543-6011
- Clin Lab Scientist/Med Tech
- Respiratory Therapist

Wor-Wic Community College

Arnold H Maner, PhD, President
3200 Campus Dr
Salisbury, MD 21801
410 334-2800
- Radiographer

Silver Spring

Holy Cross Hospital

James P Hamill, MHA, President
1500 Forest Glen Rd
Silver Spring, MD 20910
301 905-1216
- Radiographer

Stevenson

Villa Julie College

Carolyn Manuszak, JD, President
Greenspring Valley Rd
Stevenson, MD 21153
410 486-7000
- Clin Lab Tech/Med Lab Tech-AD

Takoma Park

Columbia Union College

Charles Scriven, PhD, President
Office of the President
7600 Flower Ave
Takoma Park, MD 20912
301 891-4119
- Clin Lab Scientist/Med Tech
- Clin Lab Tech/Med Lab Tech-AD
- Respiratory Therapist

Washington Adventist Hospital

Brian Breckenridge, President
7600 Carroll Ave
Takoma Park, MD 20912
301 891-7600
- Radiographer

Towson

Medix School

Bernard E Wilke, Director
1017 York Rd
Towson, MD 21204
410 337-5155
- Dental Assistant
- Medical Assistant

Towson State University

Hoke L Smith, PhD, President
Admin Bldg
Towson, MD 21252-7097
410 830-2356
- Audiologist
- Occupational Therapist
- Speech Language Pathologist

Wye Mills

Chesapeake College

John R Kotula, EdD, President
PO Box 8
Wye Mills, MD 21679
410 822-5400
- Radiographer

Massachusetts

Amherst

University of Massachusetts - Amherst

David K Scott, Chancellor
Amherst, MA 01003
413 545-0111
- Audiologist
- Dietitian/Nutritionist
- Speech Language Pathologist

Bedford

Middlesex Community College - Bedford

Carole A Cowan, EdD, President
Springs Rd
Bedford, MA 01730
617 280-3100
- Clin Lab Tech/Med Lab Tech-AD
- Diagnostic Med Sonographer
- Radiographer

Boston

Bay State College

Frederick K G Afannenstien, BA, President
122 Commonwealth Ave
Boston, MA 02116
617 236-8000
- Occupational Therapy Asst

Berklee College of Music

Lee Eliot Berk, President
1140 Boylston St
Boston, MA 02215
617 266-1400
- Music Therapist

Beth Israel Healthcare

330 Brookline Ave
Boston, MA 02215-5491
617 667-2539
- Dietitian/Nutritionist

Boston University
Jon Westling, President
147 Bay State Rd
Boston, MA 02215
617 353-2209
- Audiologist
- Dietitian/Nutritionist
- Occupational Therapist
- Rehabilitation Counselor
- Speech Language Pathologist

Brigham and Women's Hospital
75 Francis St
Boston, MA 02115-6195
617 732-7493
- Dietitian/Nutritionist

Bunker Hill Community College
Mon O'Shea, Interim President
New Rutherford Ave
Boston, MA 02129
617 228-2000
- Nuclear Medicine Tech
- Radiographer

Children's Hospital
David S Weiner, MBA, President
300 Longwood Ave
Boston, MA 02115
617 355-6433
- Electroneurodiagnostic Tech

Emerson College
Jacqueline W Liebergott, President
100 Beacon St
Boston, MA 02116
617 578-8500
- Speech Language Pathologist

Fisher College
Christian C Fisher, MBA, President
118 Beacon St
Boston, MA 02116
617 236-8800
- Health Information Tech

Forsyth School
Donald I Hay, PhD, Interim Director
140 The Fenway
Boston, MA 02115
617 262-5200
- Dental Hygienist

Laboure College
Sr Clarisse Correia, MS RN, President
2120 Dorchester Ave
Boston, MA 02124-5698
617 296-8300
- Dietetic Technician
- Electroneurodiagnostic Tech
- Health Information Tech
- Radiation Therapist

Mass Coll of Pharmacy & Allied Hlth Sci
Albert Belmont, PhD, Dean/Interim President
179 Longwood Ave
Boston, MA 02115
617 732-2880
- Nuclear Medicine Tech
- Radiation Therapist

Massachusetts General Hospital
J Robert Buchanan, MD, Gen Director
32 Fruit St
Boston, MA 02114
617 726-2101
- Dietitian/Nutritionist

MGH Institute of Health Professions
101 Merrimac St
Boston, MA 02114
617 726-8019
- Speech Language Pathologist

New England Deaconess Hospital
Robert Norton, MHA, President
One Deaconess Rd Farr 1
Boston, MA 02215
617 632-8008
- Clin Lab Scientist/Med Tech
- Specialist in BB Tech

New England Med Ctr/Frances Stern Nutri Ctr
Jerome H Grossman, MD, President
750 Washington St PO Box 451
Boston, MA 02111
617 956-7655
- Dietitian/Nutritionist

Northeastern University
Richard M Freeland, PhD, President
360 Huntington Ave
110 Churchill Hall
Boston, MA 02115
617 373-2101
- Audiologist
- Clin Lab Scientist/Med Tech
- Clin Lab Tech/Med Lab Tech-AD
- Health Information Admin
- Perfusionist
- Physician Assistant
- Radiographer
- Rehabilitation Counselor
- Respiratory Therapist
- Speech Language Pathologist

Simmons College
Barbara Graham, President
300 The Fenway
Boston, MA 02115
617 521-2000
- Dietitian/Nutritionist

University of Massachusetts at Boston
Sherry H Penney, Chancellor
Boston, MA 02125
617 287-5000
- Rehabilitation Counselor

Veterans Administration Medical Center
Elwood Headley, MD, Medical Center Director
150 S Huntington Ave
Boston, MA 02130
617 232-9500
- Clin Lab Scientist/Med Tech

Bridgewater

Bridgewater State College
Adrian Tinsley, PhD, President
Bridgewater, MA 02325
508 697-1210
- Athletic Trainer

Brockton

Massasoit Community College
Louis R Colombo, Interim President
One Massasoit Blvd
Brockton, MA 02402
508 588-9100
- Clin Lab Tech/Med Lab Tech-AD
- Dental Assistant
- Radiographer
- Respiratory Therapist

Brookline

Newbury College
Edward J Tassinari, MEd, President
129 Fisher Ave
Brookline, MA 02146
617 739-0510
- Respiratory Therapist
- Respiratory Therapy Tech

Cambridge

Lesley College
Margarert A McKenna, President
29 Everett St
Cambridge, MA 02138
617 868-9600
- Art Therapist

Mt Auburn Hospital
Francis P Lynch, President
330 Mt Auburn St
Cambridge, MA 02238
617 492-3500
- Dietitian/Nutritionist

Danvers

North Shore Community College
George Traicoff, EdD, President
PO Box 3340
1 Ferncroft Rd
Danvers, MA 01923-0840
508 762-4000
- Occupational Therapy Asst
- Radiographer
- Respiratory Therapist

Fall River

Bristol Community College
Eileen Farley, MA, President
777 Elsbree St
Fall River, MA 02777
508 678-2811
- Clin Lab Tech/Med Lab Tech-AD
- Dental Hygienist
- Occupational Therapy Asst
- Radiographer

Fitchburg

Fitchburg State College
Michael P Riccards, PhD, President
160 Pearl St
Fitchburg, MA 01420
508 665-3112
- Clin Lab Scientist/Med Tech

Framingham

Framingham State College
Paul F Weller, President
100 State St
Framingham, MA 01701
508 620-1220
● Dietitian/Nutritionist

Gardner

Mt Wachusett Community College
Daniel M Asquino, PhD, President
444 Green St
Gardner, MA 01440
508 632-6600
● Clin Lab Tech/Med Lab Tech-AD

Greenfield

Greenfield Community College
Charles Wall, PhD, President
One College Dr
Greenfield, MA 01301
413 774-3131
● Occupational Therapy Asst

Hathorne

Essex Agriculture and Tech Institute
562 Maple St
Hathorne, MA 01937
508 774-0050
● Dietetic Technician

Haverhill

Northern Essex Community College
David F Hartleb, President
Elliott Way
Haverhill, MA 01830
508 374-3900
● Dental Assistant
● Health Information Tech
● Medical Assistant
● Radiographer
● Respiratory Therapist
● Respiratory Therapy Tech

Holyoke

Holyoke Community College
David M Bartley, EdD LLD, President
303 Homestead Ave
Holyoke, MA 01040
413 538-7000
● Health Information Tech
● Radiographer

Lawrence

Lawrence General Hospital
Joseph S McManus, MPH, CEO/President
One General St
Lawrence, MA 01842
508 683-4000
● Clin Lab Scientist/Med Tech

Longmeadow

Bay Path College
Carol A Leary, PhD, President
588 Longmeadow St
Longmeadow, MA 01106
413 567-0621
● Occupational Therapy Asst

Lowell

Middlesex Community College - Lowell
33 Kearney Square
Lowell, MA 01852
508 656-3200
● Dental Assistant
● Dental Hygienist
● Dental Lab Technician

University of Massachusetts - Lowell
William T Hogan, DSc, Chancellor
One University Ave
Lowell, MA 01854
508 934-2201
● Clin Lab Scientist/Med Tech

Medford

Tufts University
John DiBiaggio, PhD, President
Ballou Hall
Medford, MA 02155-7084
617 627-3300
● Occupational Therapist

Milton

Aquinas College at Milton
Mary Huegel, President
303 Adams St
Milton, MA 02186
617 696-3100
● Medical Assistant

New Bedford

St Luke's Hospital/Marriott Corporation
101 Page St
New Bedford, MA 02740-3464
508 997-1525
● Dietitian/Nutritionist

Newton

Newton Wellesley Hospital
John P Bihldorff, MPH, President
2014 Washington St
Newton, MA 02162
617 243-6255
● Clin Lab Scientist/Med Tech

Newton Centre

Mt Ida College
Bryan E Carlson, EdD, President
Sch of Science and Allied Health
777 Dedham St
Newton Centre, MA 02159-3310
617 928-4500
● Dental Assistant
● Occupational Therapy Asst
● Ophthalmic Dispenser

North Adams

Charles H McCann Technical School
Hodges Crossroad
North Adams, MA 01247
413 663-5383
● Dental Assistant

North Dartmouth

University of Massachusetts Dartmouth
Peter H Cressy, PhD, Chancellor
Office of the Chancellor
North Dartmouth, MA 02747
508 999-8000
● Clin Lab Scientist/Med Tech

Paxton

Anna Maria College
Bernard Parker, President
Sunset Ln
Paxton, MA 01612-1198
508 849-3335
● Music Therapist

Pittsfield

Berkshire Community College
Barbara A Viniar, EdD, President
West St
Pittsfield, MA 01201
413 499-4660
● Respiratory Therapist

Berkshire Medical Center
Ruth P Blodgett, COO
725 North St
Pittsfield, MA 01201
413 447-2144
● Clin Lab Scientist/Med Tech
● Cytotechnologist

Quincy

Quincy College
G Jeremiah Ryan, President
34 Coddington St
Quincy, MA 02169
617 984-1776
● Surgical Technologist

Salem

Salem State College
Nancy D Harrington, EdD, President
352 Lafayette St
Salem, MA 01970
508 741-6000
● Nuclear Medicine Tech

South Easton

Southeastern Technical Institute
Paul K O'Leary, MEd, Superintendent
250 Foundry St
South Easton, MA 02375
508 238-4374
● Clin Lab Tech/Med Lab Tech-C
● Dental Assistant
● Medical Assistant

Institutions

Springfield

Life Laboratories

Kenneth Geromini, MT(ASCP)MST, President
299 Carew St
Springfield, MA 01104
413 748-9500
• Clin Lab Scientist/Med Tech

Springfield College

Randolph W Bromery, PhD, President
Marsh Memorial
263 Alden St
Springfield, MA 01109
413 748-3241
• Athletic Trainer
• Occupational Therapist
• Physician Assistant
• Rehabilitation Counselor
• Therapeutic Recreation Specialist

Springfield Technical Community College

Andrew M Scibelli, EdD, President
One Armory Square
PO Box 9000
Springfield, MA 01105
413 781-7822
• Clin Lab Tech/Med Lab Tech-AD
• Dental Assistant
• Dental Hygienist
• Medical Assistant
• Nuclear Medicine Tech
• Occupational Therapy Asst
• Radiation Therapist
• Radiographer
• Respiratory Therapist
• Surgical Technologist

Waltham

Sodexho USA

153 Second Ave
Waltham, MA 02254-3730
800 926-7429
• Dietitian/Nutritionist

Wellesley Hills

Massachusetts Bay Community College

Roger A Van Winkle, MA, President
Wellesley Hills Campus
50 Oakland St
Wellesley Hills, MA 02181-5399
617 239-3100
• Occupational Therapy Asst
• Radiographer

West Barnstable

Cape Cod Community College

Richard A Kraus, President
Rte 132
West Barnstable, MA 02668
508 362-2131
• Dental Hygienist

Worcester

Assumption College

Joseph H Hagan, President
500 Salisbury St
Worcester, MA 01615
508 767-7000
• Rehabilitation Counselor

Becker College

Arnold C Weller Jr, MA MAT, President
61 Sever St Box 15071
Worcester, MA 01615-0071
508 791-9241
• Occupational Therapy Asst

Quinsigamond Community College

Sandra Kurtinitis, PhD, President
670 W Boylston St
Worcester, MA 01606
508 853-2300
• Dental Hygienist
• Occupational Therapy Asst
• Radiographer
• Respiratory Therapist

Univ Mass Med Ctr/Worcester State Coll

Arthur Russo, MD, CEO Clinical Systems
55 Lake Ave N
Worcester, MA 01655
508 856-4114
• Nuclear Medicine Tech
• Radiation Therapist

Worcester State College

Kalyan K Ghosh, PhD, President
486 Chandler St
Worcester, MA 01602-2597
508 793-8020
• Occupational Therapist
• Speech Language Pathologist

Worcester Technical Institute

John C Orrell, Superintendent
Worcester Vocational School System
Wheaton Square
Worcester, MA 01605
508 799-1940
• Dental Assistant
• Medical Assistant
• Ophthalmic Dispenser
• Surgical Technologist

Michigan

Allendale

Grand Valley State University

Arend D Lubbers, MA, President
One Campus Dr
Allendale, MI 49401
616 895-2182
• Athletic Trainer

Ann Arbor

University of Michigan

Homer A Neal, PhD, Interim President
2068 Fleming Adm Bldg
Ann Arbor, MI 48109
313 764-6270
• Dental Hygienist
• Dietitian/Nutritionist

University of Michigan Hospital

1500 E Medical Ctr Dr
Ann Arbor, MI 48109-0056
313 936-5199
• Dietitian/Nutritionist

University of Michigan Medical Center

Gilbert Whitaker, PhD, Provost Academic Affairs
U of Michigan Medical School
3068 Fleming Admin Box 1340
Ann Arbor, MI 48109-0608
313 764-2104
• Medical Illustrator
• Radiation Therapist

Washtenaw Community College

Gunder M Myran, EdD, President
4800 E Huron River Dr
Ann Arbor, MI 48106
313 973-3491
• Dental Assistant
• Radiographer
• Respiratory Therapist

Battle Creek

Kellogg Community College

Paul R Ohm, PhD, President
450 North Ave
Battle Creek, MI 49017
616 965-3931
• Clin Lab Tech/Med Lab Tech-AD
• Dental Hygienist
• Radiographer

Benton Harbor

Lake Michigan College

Richard Pappas, EdD, President
2755 E Napier Ave
Benton Harbor, MI 49022-1899
616 927-8100
• Dental Assistant
• Occupational Therapy Asst
• Radiographer

Berrien Springs

Andrews University

Niels-Erik Andreasen, PhD, President
Berrien Springs, MI 49104
616 471-3100
• Clin Lab Scientist/Med Tech
• Dietitian/Nutritionist

Big Rapids

Ferris State University

William Sederburg, PhD, President
1349 Cramer Circle B-H 421E
Big Rapids, MI 49307-2737
616 592-2500
• Clin Lab Scientist/Med Tech
• Clin Lab Tech/Med Lab Tech-AD
• Dental Hygienist
• Dental Lab Technician
• Health Information Admin
• Health Information Tech
• Nuclear Medicine Tech
• Ophthalmic Dispenser
• Radiographer
• Respiratory Therapist

Bloomfield Hills

Oakland Community College

Richard T Thompson, Chancellor
George A Bee Administrative Ctr
2480 Opdyke Rd
Bloomfield Hills, MI 48304-2266
810 552-2600
- Diagnostic Med Sonographer
- Radiographer
- Respiratory Therapist

Dearborn

Henry Ford Community College

Andrew A Mazzara, PhD, President
5101 Evergreen Rd
Dearborn, MI 48128
313 845-9650
- Health Information Tech
- Medical Assistant
- Respiratory Therapist

Oakwood Hospital and Medical Center

Gerald Fitzgerald, President
18101 Oakwood Blvd PO Box 2500
Dearborn, MI 48170-2500
313 593-7005
- Radiographer

Detroit

Detroit Health Department

1151 Taylor St
Detroit, MI 48202-1732
313 876-4090
- Dietitian/Nutritionist

DMC University Laboratories

Mark McNash, MBA, President
4201 St Antoine Blvd
Detroit, MI 48201
313 745-3053
- Clin Lab Scientist/Med Tech
- Cytotechnologist
- Histologic Technician-Cert

Grace Hospital

Edward S Thomas, Interim Senior vice-Pres.
6071 W Outer Dr
Detroit, MI 48235
313 966-3525
- Radiographer

Harper Hospital

Paul Broughton, President
3990 John R
Detroit, MI 48201-2097
313 745-9375
- Dietitian/Nutritionist

Henry Ford Hospital

Stephen H Velick, MBA, CEO
2799 W Grand Blvd
Detroit, MI 48202
313 876-1257
- Cytotechnologist
- Diagnostic Med Sonographer
- Dietitian/Nutritionist
- Radiation Therapist
- Radiographer

Marygrove College

John E Shay Jr, PhD, President
8425 W McNichols Rd
Detroit, MI 48221-2599
313 862-8000
- Dietitian/Nutritionist
- Radiographer
- Respiratory Therapist

St John Hospital and Medical Center

Timothy Grajewski, MBA, President/CEO
22101 Moross Rd
Detroit, MI 48236
313 343-7531
- Clin Lab Scientist/Med Tech
- Radiographer
- Respiratory Therapy Tech

University of Detroit Mercy

Sr Maureen A Fay, OP PhD, President
PO Box 19900
Detroit, MI 48219-3599
313 993-1455
- Dental Hygienist
- Physician Assistant

Wayne County Community College

Curtis L Ivery, President
801 W Fort St
Detroit, MI 48226-9975
313 496-2510
- Dental Assistant
- Dental Hygienist
- Dietetic Technician
- Occupational Therapy Asst

Wayne State University

David W Adamany, PhD, President
Office of the President
4200 Faculty Admin Bldg
Detroit, MI 48202-3489
313 577-2230
- Art Therapist
- Audiologist
- Clin Lab Scientist/Med Tech
- Dietitian/Nutritionist
- Occupational Therapist
- Radiation Therapist
- Rehabilitation Counselor
- Speech Language Pathologist

East Lansing

Michigan State University

Louanna K Simon, PhD, Provost
438 Admin Bldg
East Lansing, MI 48824
517 355-1524
- Audiologist
- Clin Lab Scientist/Med Tech
- Dietitian/Nutritionist
- Music Therapist
- Rehabilitation Counselor
- Speech Language Pathologist

Flint

Baker College

Julianne T Princinsky, EdD, President
G 1050 W Bristol Rd
Flint, MI 48507-5508
810 766-4036
- Health Information Admin
- Health Information Tech
- Medical Assistant
- Occupational Therapist

Charles Stewart Mott Community College

Allen D Arnold, EdD, President
1401 E Court St
Flint, MI 48503
810 762-0200
- Dental Assistant
- Dental Hygienist
- Occupational Therapy Asst
- Respiratory Therapist

Genesys Regional Medical Center

Young S Suh, President/CEO
302 Kensington Ave
Flint, MI 48503-2000
810 762-8899
- Radiographer

Hurley Medical Center

Glenn A Fosdick, President/CEO
One Hurley Plaza
Flint, MI 48503
810 257-9237
- Clin Lab Scientist/Med Tech
- Dietitian/Nutritionist
- Histologic Technician-Cert
- Radiographer

Garden City

Garden City Hospital, Osteopathic

Gary Ley, MS, President/CEO
6245 N Inkster Rd
Garden City, MI 48135
313 458-4421
- Clin Lab Scientist/Med Tech

Grand Rapids

Butterworth Hospital

Philip H McCorkle, BS MA, CEO
100 Michigan NE
Grand Rapids, MI 49503
616 774-1605
- Clin Lab Scientist/Med Tech

Davenport College

Donald W Maine, MA, President
415 E Fulton St
Grand Rapids, MI 49503
616 451-3511
- Medical Assistant

Grand Rapids Community College

Richard W Calkins, MA, President
143 Bostwick Ave NE
Grand Rapids, MI 49503-3295
616 771-3901
- Dental Assistant
- Dental Hygienist
- Occupational Therapy Asst
- Radiographer

Grosse Pointe Park

Detroit Institute of Ophthalmology

Philip C Hessburg, MD, President
15415 E Jefferson Ave
Grosse Pointe Park, MI 48230
313 824-4800
• Ophthalmic Med Technician

Harrison

Mid Michigan Community College

Ronald Verch, MS, Interim President
1375 S Clare Ave
Harrison, MI 48625
517 386-6642
• Radiographer

Highland Park

Highland Park Community College

Thomas Lloyd Jr, PhD, President
Glendale at Third
Highland Park, MI 48203
313 252-0475
• Surgical Technologist

Ironwood

Gogebic Community College

Donald J Foster, PhD, President
E4946 Jackson Rd
Ironwood, MI 49938
906 932-4231
• Health Information Tech

Jackson

Jackson Community College

E Lee Howser, PhD, President
2111 Emmons Rd
Jackson, MI 49201-8399
517 787-0800
• Diagnostic Med Sonographer
• Medical Assistant
• Radiographer

Kalamazoo

Davenport College - Kalamazoo

Dexter Rohm, BA, VP/Dean
4123 W Main St
Kalamazoo, MI 49006
616 382-2835
• Health Information Tech

Kalamazoo Valley Community College

Marilyn J Schlack, EdD, President
Texas Township Campus
6767 West O Ave PO Box 4070
Kalamazoo, MI 49003-4070
616 372-5000
• Dental Hygienist
• Medical Assistant
• Respiratory Therapist

Western Michigan University

Timothy Light, PhD, Acting Provost & VP
3600 Siebert Admin Bldg
Kalamazoo, MI 49008-5130
616 387-2351
• Audiologist
• Dietitian/Nutritionist
• Music Therapist
• Occupational Therapist
• Physician Assistant
• Speech Language Pathologist

Lansing

Davenport College - Lansing

Don Colizzi, BS, Sr VP and Dean
220 E Kalamazoo St
Lansing, MI 48933
517 484-2600
• Histologic Technician-Cert

Lansing Community College

Abel B Sykes Jr, PhD, President
PO Box 40010
Lansing, MI 48901
517 483-1852
• Dental Assistant
• Dental Hygienist
• Emergency Med Tech-Paramedic
• Radiation Therapist
• Radiographer
• Respiratory Therapist

Livonia

Madonna University

Mary Francilene, President
36600 Schoolcraft Rd
Livonia, MI 48150
313 591-5000
• Dietitian/Nutritionist

Schoolcraft College

Richard W McDowell, PhD, President
18600 Haggerty Rd
Livonia, MI 48152-2696
313 462-4400
• Health Information Tech
• Occupational Therapy Asst

Marquette

Marquette General Hospital

Robert C Neldberg, CEO
420 W Magnetic St
Marquette, MI 49855
906 225-3434
• Radiographer

Northern Michigan University

William E Vandament, PhD, President
602 Cohodas Admin Ctr
Marquette, MI 49855
906 227-2242
• Clin Lab Scientist/Med Tech
• Clin Lab Tech/Med Lab Tech-AD
• Dietitian/Nutritionist
• Speech Language Pathologist

Monroe

Monroe County Community College

Gerald Welch, MA, President
1555 S Raisinville Rd
Monroe, MI 48161
313 242-7300
• Respiratory Therapist
• Respiratory Therapy Tech

Mt Pleasant

Central Michigan University

Leonard E Plachta, PhD, President
165 Warriner Hall
Mt Pleasant, MI 48859
517 774-3131
• Athletic Trainer
• Audiologist
• Dietitian/Nutritionist
• Speech Language Pathologist
• Therapeutic Recreation Specialist

Muskegon

Baker College of Muskegon

Rick E Amidon, President
123 Apple Ave
Muskegon, MI 49442-9982
616 726-4904
• Health Information Tech
• Medical Assistant
• Occupational Therapy Asst
• Surgical Technologist

Muskegon Community College

Frank Marczak, PhD, President
221 S Quarterline Rd
Muskegon, MI 49442
616 777-0303
• Respiratory Therapist
• Respiratory Therapy Tech

Owosso

Baker College of Owosso

Denise Bannan, MA, President and CEO
Owosso Campus
1020 S Washington St
Owosso, MI 48867
517 723-5251
• Clin Lab Tech/Med Lab Tech-AD
• Medical Assistant
• Radiographer

Pontiac

Oakland County Health Division

1200 N Telegraph Rd
Pontiac, MI 48341-0432
810 858-1832
• Dietitian/Nutritionist

Port Huron

Baker College of Port Huron

3403 Lapeer Rd
Port Huron, MI 48060
810 985-7000
• Dental Hygienist

Port Huron Hospital
Donald D Fletcher, MBA, President
1001 Kearney St PO Box 5011
Port Huron, MI 48061-5011
313 987-5000
● Radiographer

Royal Oak

William Beaumont Hospital
Kenneth Myers, MBA, President
3601 W 13 Mile Rd
Royal Oak, MI 48073-6769
810 551-0681
● Clin Lab Scientist/Med Tech
● Histologic Technician-Cert
● Histotechnologist
● Nuclear Medicine Tech
● Radiation Therapist
● Radiographer

Saginaw

Great Lakes Junior College - Bay City
William F Guerriero, MSA, President
320 S Washington Ave
Saginaw, MI 48607
517 755-3457
● Medical Assistant

Great Lakes Junior College - Caro
William F Guerriero, MSA, President
320 S Washington
Saginaw, MI 48607
517 755-3457
● Medical Assistant

Great Lakes Junior College - Midland
William F Guerriero, MSA, President
320 S Washington Ave
Saginaw, MI 48607
517 755-3457
● Medical Assistant

Great Lakes Junior College - Saginaw
William F Guerriero, MSA, President
320 S Washington
Saginaw, MI 48607
517 755-3457
● Medical Assistant

St Mary's Medical Center
Frederic L Fraizer, MS, President/CEO
830 S Jefferson
Saginaw, MI 48601
517 776-8176
● Clin Lab Scientist/Med Tech

Southfield

Providence Hospital and Medical Centers
Michael A Slubowski, CEO Providence Oper Unit
16001 W Nine Mile Rd
Southfield, MI 48037
810 424-3000
● Diagnostic Med Sonographer
● Radiographer

Traverse City

Munson Medical Center
Ralph J Cerny, MA, President
1105 Sixth St
Traverse City, MI 49684
616 935-6501
● Clin Lab Scientist/Med Tech

Northwestern Michigan College
Timothy G Quinn, President
1701 E Front St
Traverse City, MI 49684
616 922-1000
● Dental Assistant

Troy

Carnegie Institute
Gloria J McEachern, CMA, President/CEO
550 Stephenson Hwy Ste 100
Troy, MI 48083
810 589-1078
● Medical Assistant

University Center

Delta College
Peter D Boyse, PhD, President
A-200
University Center, MI 48710
517 686-9201
● Dental Assistant
● Dental Hygienist
● Radiographer
● Respiratory Therapist
● Surgical Technologist

Saginaw Valley State University
Eric R Gilbertson, JD, President
7400 Bay Rd
University Center, MI 48710-0001
517 790-4041
● Occupational Therapist

Warren

Macomb Community College
Albert L Lorenzo, PhD, President
14500 E Twelve Mile Rd
Warren, MI 48093-3896
810 445-7241
● Medical Assistant
● Respiratory Therapist

Waterford

Oakland Community College - Waterford
Preston Pulliams, PhD, President
7350 Cooley Lake Rd
Waterford, MI 48327
313 360-3032
● Dental Hygienist
● Medical Assistant

Wayne

Oakwood-United Hospitals Inc
Charles Bruhn, MHA, Administrator
Annapolis Hospital Unit
33155 Annapolis Ave
Wayne, MI 48184
313 467-4000
● Radiographer

Ypsilanti

Eastern Michigan University
William E Shelton, PhD, President
202 Welch Hall
Ypsilanti, MI 48197-2239
313 487-2211
● Clin Lab Scientist/Med Tech
● Dietitian/Nutritionist
● Music Therapist
● Occupational Therapist
● Speech Language Pathologist

Minnesota

Alexandria

Alexandria Technical College
Larry Shellito, MS, President
1601 Jefferson St
Alexandria, MN 56308
612 762-0221
● Clin Lab Tech/Med Lab Tech-AD
● Clin Lab Tech/Med Lab Tech-C

Anoka

Anoka-Hennepin Technical College
Clifford Korkowski, EdD, President
1355 W Hwy 10
Anoka, MN 55303-1590
612 576-4709
● Health Information Tech
● Medical Assistant
● Occupational Therapy Asst
● Ophthalmic Dispenser
● Surgical Technologist

Austin

Minnesota Riverland Tech College-Austin
John Gedker, President
1600 8th Ave NW
Austin, MN 55912
507 433-0600
● Radiographer

Riverland Community College
John Gedker, President
1900 8th Ave NW
Austin, MN 55912-1407
507 433-0508
● Occupational Therapy Asst

Bemidji

Northwest Technical Coll - Bemidji
Ray Cross, PhD, CEO
Regional Office
1103 Roosevelt SE
Bemidji, MN 56601
218 759-3496
● Dental Assistant

Institutions

Northwest Technical Coll - E Grand Forks

Ray Cross, PhD, President
Regional Office
1103 Roosevelt SE
Bemidji, MN 56601
218 759-3496
- Cardiovascular Technologist
- Clin Lab Tech/Med Lab Tech-AD
- Dietitian/Nutritionist
- Emergency Med Tech-Paramedic
- Medical Assistant
- Occupational Therapy Asst
- Radiographer
- Respiratory Therapist
- Respiratory Therapy Tech
- Surgical Technologist

Northwest Technical Coll - Moorhead

Ray Cross, PhD, CEO/President
Regional Office
1103 Roosevelt SE
Bemidji, MN 56601
218 759-3496
- Dental Assistant
- Dental Hygienist
- Health Information Tech

Bloomington

Medical Institute of Minnesota

Phillip Miller, JD, President
5503 Green Valley Dr
Bloomington, MN 55437
612 844-0064
- Clin Lab Tech/Med Lab Tech-AD
- Histologic Technician-AD
- Medical Assistant
- Radiographer

Normandale Community College

Tom Horak, President
9700 France Ave S
Bloomington, MN 55431
612 832-6301
- Dental Assistant
- Dental Hygienist
- Dietetic Technician

Brainerd

Central Lakes College

Sally J Ihne, President
300 Quince St
Brainerd, MN 56401
218 828-2525
- Dental Assistant

Brooklyn Center

Minnesota School of Business - Brooklyn Ctr

Terry Myhre
Minnesota School of Business
6120 Earle Brown Dr
Brooklyn Center, MN 55430
612 566-7777
- Dental Assistant

Brooklyn Park

Hennepin Technical College

Sharon Grossbach, PhD, President
9000 Brooklyn Blvd
Brooklyn Park, MN 55445
612 550-2118
- Dental Assistant
- Health Information Tech

North Hennepin Community College

Yvette Jackson, PhD, Interim President
7411 85th Ave N
Brooklyn Park, MN 55445
612 424-0820
- Clin Lab Tech/Med Lab Tech-AD

Canby

Minnesota West Comm and Tech College

1011 First St West
Canby, MN 56220
507 223-7252
- Dental Assistant

Crookston

University of Minnesota - Crookston

Donald G Sargeant, Chancellor
Crookston, MN 56716
218 281-6510
- Dietetic Technician

Duluth

College of St Scholastica

Daniel H Pilon, EdD, President
1200 Kenwood Ave
Duluth, MN 55811
218 723-6033
- Clin Lab Scientist/Med Tech
- Dietitian/Nutritionist
- Health Information Admin
- Occupational Therapist

Duluth Business Univ/MN Sch of Business

Bonnie L Kupczynski, Director
412 W Superior St
Duluth, MN 55802
218 722-3361
- Dental Assistant
- Medical Assistant

Lake Superior College

Harold Erickson, PhD, President
2101 Trinity Rd
Duluth, MN 55811-3399
218 722-2801
- Clin Lab Tech/Med Lab Tech-AD
- Dental Hygienist
- Occupational Therapy Asst
- Radiographer
- Respiratory Therapist

University of Minnesota - Duluth

Kathryn A Martin, Chancellor
Duluth, MN 55812
218 726-8000
- Speech Language Pathologist

Faribault

Minnesota Riverland Tech Coll-Faribault

Kenneth H Mills, Vice President
1225 SW Third St
South Central Technical College
Faribault, MN 55021
507 334-3965
- Clin Lab Tech/Med Lab Tech-AD
- Diagnostic Med Sonographer
- Medical Assistant

Fergus Falls

Fergus Falls Community College

Dan True, MSE, President
1414 College Way
Fergus Falls, MN 56537
218 739-7503
- Clin Lab Tech/Med Lab Tech-AD
- Histologic Technician-AD

Hibbing

Hibbing Community College

Tony Kuznik, PhD, President
1515 E 25th St
Hibbing, MN 55746
218 262-7200
- Clin Lab Tech/Med Lab Tech-AD
- Dental Assistant

Mankato

Mankato State University

Richard R Rush, PhD, President
MSU Box 24
PO Box 8400
Mankato, MN 56002-8400
507 389-1111
- Athletic Trainer
- Dental Hygienist
- Dietitian/Nutritionist
- Rehabilitation Counselor
- Speech Language Pathologist

Minneapolis

Abbott Northwestern Hospital

Robert K Spinner, MHA, President
800 E 28th St at Chicago Ave
Minneapolis, MN 55407
612 863-4204
- Radiation Therapist

Augsburg College

Charles S Anderson, PhD, President
2211 Riverside Ave/CB 131
Minneapolis, MN 55454
612 330-1212
- Music Therapist
- Physician Assistant

Hennepin County Medical Center

Charles Richards, Acting Administrator
701 Park Ave S
Minneapolis, MN 55415
612 347-2352
- Clin Lab Scientist/Med Tech

Lakeland Medical Dental Academy
Lorrie Laurin, BA MT(ASCP), President
1402 W Lake St
Minneapolis, MN 55408
612 827-5656
- Clin Lab Tech/Med Lab Tech-AD
- Dental Assistant
- Medical Assistant

Memorial Blood Center of Minneapolis
Jerome Haarmann, MD, Director
2304 Park Ave
Minneapolis, MN 55404
612 871-3300
- Specialist in BB Tech

Minneapolis Technical College
1415 Hennepin Ave S Rm 446
Minneapolis, MN 55403
612 370-9472
- Dental Assistant

Minneapolis Veterans Affairs Medical Ctr
Charles A Milbrandt, FACHE, Director
One Veteran's Dr Mail Rte 114
Minneapolis, MN 55417
612 725-2000
- Dietitian/Nutritionist
- Radiographer

Univ of Minnesota Hosp and Clinic
Frank B Cerra, MD, Provost
Academic Health Ctr/Box 501 Mayo
410 Children's Rehab Center
Minneapolis, MN 55455-0110
612 626-3700
- Clin Lab Scientist/Med Tech
- Dietitian/Nutritionist
- Occupational Therapist
- Perfusionist
- Radiation Therapist
- Radiographer

University of Minnesota - Twin Cities
Nils Hasselmo, President
164 Pillsbury Dr SE
Minneapolis, MN 55455
612 625-5000
- Audiologist
- Dental Hygienist
- Dietitian/Nutritionist
- Music Therapist
- Speech Language Pathologist
- Therapeutic Recreation Specialist

Minnetonka

Rasmussen Colleges
Bob Nemitz, CEO
12450 Wayzata Blvd/Ste 226
Minnetonka, MN 55305
612 545-4058
- Health Information Tech

Moorhead

Concordia College - Moorhead
Paul J Dovre, President
Moorhead, MN 56562
218 299-3947
- Dietitian/Nutritionist

Moorhead State University
Roland E Barden, President
1104 7th Ave S
Moorhead, MN 56563
218 236-2011
- Speech Language Pathologist

North Mankato

South Central Technical College
Kenneth Mills, President
1920 Lee Blvd
North Mankato, MN 56002-1920
507 389-7200
- Dental Assistant

Richfield

Minnesota School of Business - Richfield
Terry Myhre, BS, President
1401 W 76th St/Ste 500
Richfield, MN 55423
612 861-2000
- Medical Assistant

Robbinsdale

North Memorial Medical Center
Scott R Anderson, MHA, CEO President
3300 N Oakdale
Robbinsdale, MN 55422
612 520-5000
- Radiographer

Rochester

Mayo Clinic/Mayo Foundation
Robert R Waller, MD, Chair
200 First St SW
Rochester, MN 55905
507 284-3678
- Clin Lab Tech/Med Lab Tech-C
- Cytotechnologist
- Diagnostic Med Sonographer
- Nuclear Medicine Tech
- Radiation Therapist
- Radiographer

Minnesota Riverland Technical College
Karen Nagle, PhD, Interim Presidnet
University Center of Rochester
851 30th Avenue SE
Rochester, MN 55904-4999
507 285-7216
- Surgical Technologist

Rochester Community and Technical College
Karen E Nagle, PhD, President
851 30th Ave SE
Rochester, MN 55904-4999
507 285-7215
- Dental Assistant
- Dental Hygienist
- Medical Assistant
- Respiratory Therapist

St Marys Hospital/Mayo Medical Center
1216 2nd St SW
Rochester, MN 55902-1906
507 255-5221
- Dietitian/Nutritionist

Rosemount

Dakota County Technical College
David Schroeder, BA, College President
1300 E 145th St
Rosemount, MN 55068-2999
612 423-2281
- Dental Assistant
- Medical Assistant

Roseville

Minneapolis Business College
David Whitman, Director
1711 W County Rd B
Roseville, MN 55113
612 636-7406
- Medical Assistant

St Cloud

St Cloud Hospital
John R Frobenius, President
1406 Sixth Ave N
St Cloud, MN 56303
320 255-5666
- Clin Lab Scientist/Med Tech
- Radiographer

St Cloud State University
Bruce F Grube, President
720 4th Ave S
St Cloud, MN 56301
320 255-2240
- Rehabilitation Counselor
- Speech Language Pathologist

St Cloud Technical College
Larry Barnhardt, MS EdD, President
1540 Northway Dr
St Cloud, MN 56301
320 654-5001
- Dental Assistant
- Dental Hygienist
- Surgical Technologist

St Joseph

College of St Benedict
Colman O'Connell, President
37 S College Ave
St Joseph, MN 56374
612 363-5011
- Dietitian/Nutritionist

St Louis Park

Health System Minnesota/Methodist Hospital
James Reinsrtsen, CEO
6500 Excelsior Blvd
St Louis Park, MN 55426
612 932-5010
- Radiographer

Institutions

St Paul

College of St Catherine
Anita Pampusch, PhD, President
2004 Randolph Ave
St Paul, MN 55105-1794
612 690-6525
- Diagnostic Med Sonographer
- Dietitian/Nutritionist
- Health Information Tech
- Occupational Therapist
- Occupational Therapy Asst
- Radiographer
- Respiratory Therapist

Globe College of Business
Terry L Myrhe, President
175 Fifth St E
Box 60 Ste 201 Galtier Plaza
St Paul, MN 55101-2901
612 224-4378
- Medical Assistant

St Paul Ramsey Medical Center
James B Dixon, MHA, President/CEO
640 Jackson St
St Paul, MN 55101
612 221-2181
- Clin Lab Scientist/Med Tech
- Dietitian/Nutritionist
- Ophthalmic Med Technician

St Paul Technical College
Donovan Schwichtenberg, PhD, President
235 Marshall Ave
St Paul, MN 55102
612 221-1364
- Clin Lab Tech/Med Lab Tech-AD
- Respiratory Therapist

University of Minnesota - St Paul
1334 Eckles Ave
St Paul, MN 55108
612 624-9278
- Dietitian/Nutritionist

St Peter

Gustavus Adolphus College
Axel Steuer, PhD, President
800 W College Ave
St Peter, MN 56082
507 933-7537
- Athletic Trainer

White Bear Lake

Century College
James Mezner, PhD, President
Century Community and Technical College
3300 Century Ave
White Bear Lake, MN 55110
612 779-3342
- Dental Assistant
- Dental Hygienist
- Dental Lab Technician
- Dietetic Technician
- Emergency Med Tech-Paramedic
- Medical Assistant
- Radiographer

Willmar

Rice Memorial Hospital
Lawrence Massa, CEO
301 Becker Ave SW
Willmar, MN 56201
320 235-4543
- Radiographer

Ridgewater College - Willmar Campus
Mary E Retteter, PhD, President
2101 15th Ave NW
PO Box 1097
Willmar, MN 56201
320 231-2901
- Health Information Tech
- Medical Assistant

Winona

St Mary's University of Minnesota
Louis DeThomasis, PhD, President
700 Terrace Heights #30
Winona, MN 55987-1399
507 457-1503
- Nuclear Medicine Tech

Mississippi

Booneville

Northeast Mississippi Community College
Joe M Childers, MEd, President
Cunningham Blvd
Booneville, MS 38829
601 728-7751
- Clin Lab Tech/Med Lab Tech-AD
- Dental Hygienist
- Medical Assistant
- Radiographer
- Respiratory Therapy Tech

Columbus

Mississippi University for Women
Clyda S Rent, President
PO Box W-1340
Columbus, MS 39701
601 329-4750
- Speech Language Pathologist

Ellisville

Jones County Junior College
Terrell Tisdale, EdD, President
900 S Court St
Ellisville, MS 39437
601 477-4100
- Emergency Med Tech-Paramedic
- Radiographer

Fulton

Itawamba Community College
David Cole, EdD, President
602 W Hill St
Fulton, MS 38843
601 862-3101
- Emergency Med Tech-Paramedic
- Radiographer
- Respiratory Therapist
- Respiratory Therapy Tech

Gulfport

Garden Park Community Hospital
William E Peaks, BS MS CPA, CEO
PO Box 1240
Gulfport, MS 39502
601 865-1340
- Perfusionist

Hattiesburg

Forrest General Hospital
Lowery A Woodall, FACHE, Exec Dir
6051 US Hwy 49 S
Hattiesburg, MS 39401
601 288-4201
- Emergency Med Tech-Paramedic

Hattiesburg Radiology Group
Jim Sumrall, Administrator
5000 W Fourth St
Hattiesburg, MS 39402
601 288-4241
- Radiographer

University of Southern Mississippi
Horace Fleming, PhD, President
Box 5001
Hattiesburg, MS 39406-5001
601 266-5001
- Athletic Trainer
- Audiologist
- Clin Lab Scientist/Med Tech
- Dietitian/Nutritionist
- Speech Language Pathologist
- Therapeutic Recreation Specialist

William Carey College
James W Edwards, PhD, President
Tuscan Ave
Hattiesburg, MS 39401-9913
601 582-6223
- Music Therapist

Jackson

Jackson State University
James E Lyons Sr, President
1440 JR Lynch St
Jackson, MS 39217
601 968-2100
- Rehabilitation Counselor

Mississippi Baptist Medical Center
Gerald Cofton, Acting Exec Dir
1225 N State St
Jackson, MS 39202
601 968-5130
- Clin Lab Scientist/Med Tech
- Radiographer

St Dominic-Jackson Memorial Hospital
969 Lakeland Dr
Jackson, MS 39216-4699
601 364-6935
- Dietitian/Nutritionist

University of Mississippi Medical Center

A Wallace Conerly, MD, Vice Chancellor
2500 N State St
Jackson, MS 39216-4505
601 984-1010
- Clin Lab Scientist/Med Tech
- Cytotechnologist
- Dental Hygienist
- Emergency Med Tech-Paramedic
- Health Information Admin
- Nuclear Medicine Tech
- Occupational Therapist
- Radiographer

Lorman

Alcorn State University

Rudolph E Waters, Interim President
Lorman, MS 39096
601 877-6100
- Dietitian/Nutritionist

McComb

Southwest Mississippi Regional Medical Center

Norman M Price, MS, Administrator
PO Box 1307
McComb, MS 39648
601 249-1807
- Emergency Med Tech-Paramedic

Meridian

Meridian Community College

William F Scaggs, PhD, President
910 Hwy 19 N
Meridian, MS 39307
601 483-8241
- Clin Lab Tech/Med Lab Tech-AD
- Dental Hygienist
- Health Information Tech
- Radiographer
- Respiratory Therapy Tech

Mississippi State

Mississippi State University

Donald W Zacharias, President
Mississippi State, MS 39762
601 325-2131
- Dietitian/Nutritionist
- Rehabilitation Counselor

Moorhead

Mississippi Delta Community College

Bobby S Garvin, EdD, President
PO Box 668
Moorhead, MS 38761
601 246-6300
- Clin Lab Tech/Med Lab Tech-AD
- Radiographer

Perkinston

Mississippi Gulf Coast Community College

Barry L Mellinger, PhD, President
PO Box 67
Perkinston, MS 39573
601 928-6335
- Clin Lab Tech/Med Lab Tech-AD
- Emergency Med Tech-Paramedic
- Radiographer
- Respiratory Therapist

Poplarville

Pearl River Community College

Ted J Alexander, BA MEd EdD, President
Station A
Poplarville, MS 39470
601 795-6801
- Clin Lab Tech/Med Lab Tech-AD
- Dental Assistant
- Dental Hygienist
- Respiratory Therapist

Pearl River Jr College - Forest Cty Branch

Ted J Alexander, EdD, President
Station A
Poplarville, MS 39470
601 795-6801
- Respiratory Therapy Tech

Raymond

Hinds Community College District

Clyde H Muse, PhD, President
Raymond Campus
Raymond, MS 39154
601 857-5261
- Clin Lab Tech/Med Lab Tech-AD
- Dental Assistant
- Health Information Tech
- Medical Assistant
- Respiratory Therapist
- Respiratory Therapy Tech
- Surgical Technologist

Senatobia

Northwest Mississippi Community College

David M Haraway, PhD, President
510 N Panola
Senatobia, MS 38668
601 562-3227
- Respiratory Therapist

Tupelo

North Mississippi Medical Center

Jeff Barber, Dr PH, CEO
830 S Gloster
Tupelo, MS 38801
601 841-3136
- Clin Lab Scientist/Med Tech

University

University of Mississippi

Robert C Khayat, Chancellor
University, MS 38677
601 232-7211
- Audiologist
- Dietitian/Nutritionist
- Speech Language Pathologist

Wesson

Copiah - Lincoln Community College

Billy B Thames, EdD, President
PO Box 649
Wesson, MS 39191-0457
601 643-5101
- Clin Lab Tech/Med Lab Tech-AD
- Radiographer
- Respiratory Therapist
- Respiratory Therapy Tech

Missouri

Cape Girardeau

Cape Girardeau Area Voc Tech School

Harold C Tilley, Director
Special School Administrator
301 N Clark
Cape Girardeau, MO 63701
314 334-3358
- Respiratory Therapy Tech

Southeast Missouri State University

Bill L Atchley, Interim President
1 University Plaza
Cape Girardeau, MO 63701
314 651-2000
- Dietitian/Nutritionist
- Speech Language Pathologist

Columbia

Stephens College

Marcia S Kierscht, PhD, President
Campus Box 2001
Columbia, MO 65215
573 876-7210
- Health Information Admin

University of Missouri - Columbia

Charles Kiesler, PhD, Chancellor
105 Jesse Hall
Columbia, MO 65211
573 882-3387
- Dietitian/Nutritionist
- Nuclear Medicine Tech
- Occupational Therapist
- Radiographer
- Rehabilitation Counselor
- Respiratory Therapist
- Speech Language Pathologist
- Therapeutic Recreation Specialist

Farmington

Mineral Area Regional Medical Center

Kenneth C West, Administrator
1212 Weber Rd
Farmington, MO 63640
573 756-4581
- Radiographer

Hannibal

Hannibal Area Voc Tech School

Harold D Ward, Director
4550 McMasters Ave
Hannibal, MO 63401
314 221-4430
- Respiratory Therapy Tech

Independence

Independence Regional Health Center

Joseph E Lammers, President
1509 W Truman Rd
Independence, MO 64050
816 836-8100
• Radiographer

Jefferson City

Missouri Dept of Mental Health

Office of Administration
1706 E Elm St PO Box 687
Jefferson City, MO 65102
314 751-8145
• Dietitian/Nutritionist

Nichols Career Center

Chris Straub, EdD, Superintendent
609 Union
Jefferson City, MO 65101
573 659-3012
• Dental Assistant
• Radiographer

Joplin

Missouri Southern State College

Julio S Leon, President
3950 E Newman Rd
Joplin, MO 64801-1595
417 624-8181
• Dental Hygienist
• Radiographer

St John's Regional Medical Center

Robert Brueckner, President
2727 McClelland Blvd
Joplin, MO 64804
417 781-2727
• Clin Lab Scientist/Med Tech

Kansas City

ARAMARK Healthcare Support Services SW

St Joseph Health System
1000 Carondelet Dr
Kansas City, MO 64114-4802
816 943-2146
• Dietitian/Nutritionist

Avila College

Larry Kramer, EdD, President
11901 Wornall Rd
Kansas City, MO 64145
816 942-8400
• Clin Lab Scientist/Med Tech
• Radiographer

ConCorde Career Institute

Jack F Brozman, Exec Director
1100 Main 10th Fl
Kansas City, MO 66105
816 474-4750
• Medical Assistant

ConCorde Career Institute

Harold Dotson, MS, School Director
3239 Broadway
Kansas City, MO 64111
816 531-5223
• Respiratory Therapy Tech

Penn Valley Community College

E Paul Williams, PhD, President
3201 SW Trafficway
Kansas City, MO 64111-2764
816 759-4201
• Health Information Tech
• Occupational Therapy Asst
• Radiographer

Research Medical Center

Dan H Anderson, BS, President
2316 E Meyer Blvd
Kansas City, MO 64132-1199
816 276-4101
• Nuclear Medicine Tech
• Radiographer

Rockhurst College

Fr Thomas Savage, SJ EdD, President
1100 Rockhurst Rd
Kansas City, MO 64110-2561
816 501-4250
• Occupational Therapist

St Luke's Hospital of Kansas City

G. Richard Hastings, CEO
4400 Wornall Rd
Kansas City, MO 64111
816 932-2101
• Clin Lab Scientist/Med Tech
• Radiation Therapist

Trinity Lutheran Hospital

Ronald A Ommen, President/CEO
3030 Baltimore St
Kansas City, MO 64108
816 751-2000
• Histologic Technician-Cert

Truman Medical Center

E Ratcliffe Anderson Jr, MD, Executive Director
2301 Holmes
Kansas City, MO 64108
816 556-3153
• Cytotechnologist
• Histologic Technician-Cert

University of Missouri - Kansas City

Eleanor B Schwartz, Chancellor
650 E 25th St
Kansas City, MO 64108
816 235-1000
• Dental Hygienist
• Music Therapist

Kirksville

Kirksville Coll of Osteopathic Med-SW Center

Fred C Tinning, PhD, President
800 W Jefferson St
Kirksville, MO 63501
816 626-2391
• Physician Assistant

Truman State University

Jack MacGruder, President
Kirksville, MO 63501
816 785-4000
• Speech Language Pathologist

Maryville

Northwest Missouri State University

Dean L Hubbard, President
Maryville, MO 64468
816 562-1212
• Dietitian/Nutritionist

North Kansas City

North Kansas City Hospital

Michael E Payne, MBA, President
2800 Clay Edwards Dr
North Kansas City, MO 64116
816 691-2000
• Clin Lab Scientist/Med Tech
• Radiographer

Park Hills

Mineral Area College

Dixie A Kohn, President
PO Box 1000
Park Hills, MO 63601
314 431-4593
• Dental Assistant

Point Lookout

College of the Ozarks

Jerry C Davis, President
Point Lookout, MO 65726
417 334-6411
• Dietitian/Nutritionist

Poplar Bluff

Three Rivers Community College

Steven M Poort, EdD, President
Three Rivers Blvd
Poplar Bluff, MO 63901
314 840-9600
• Clin Lab Tech/Med Lab Tech-AD

Rolla

Rolla Technical Institute

Bob Chapman, EdD, School Director
1304 E 10th St
Rolla, MO 65401-3699
573 364-3726
• Radiographer
• Respiratory Therapy Tech

Sedalia

State Fair Community College

Marvin Fielding, PhD, President
3201 W 16th
Sedalia, MO 65301
816 826-7100
• Respiratory Therapy Tech

Springfield

Cox Medical Centers

Larry D Wallis, MHA, Administrator
1423 N Jefferson St
Springfield, MO 65802
417 836-3108
• Clin Lab Scientist/Med Tech
• Radiographer

Ozarks Technical Community College

Norman Meyers, EdD, President
1417 N Jefferson
Springfield, MO 65802
417 895-7000
- Dental Assistant
- Health Information Tech
- Respiratory Therapist
- Respiratory Therapy Tech

Southwest Missouri State University

John Keiser, PhD, President
901 S National Ave
Springfield, MO 65804-0089
417 836-8500
- Athletic Trainer
- Audiologist
- Dietitian/Nutritionist
- Speech Language Pathologist

Springfield College

Barbara Loven, MS, President
1010 W Sunshine
Springfield, MO 65807
417 864-7220
- Medical Assistant

St John's Regional Health Center

Allen Shockley, President
1235 E Cherokee
Springfield, MO 65804
417 885-2845
- Clin Lab Scientist/Med Tech
- Radiographer

St Joseph

Missouri Western State College

Janet G Murphy, EdD, President
4525 Downs Dr
St Joseph, MO 64507
816 271-4237
- Health Information Tech

St Louis

Barnes-Jewish Hospital

John McGuire, Administrator
Barnes-Jewish Hospital
One Barnes Hospital Plaza
St Louis, MO 63110
314 362-5190
- Dietitian/Nutritionist
- Radiation Therapist
- Radiographer

Central Institute for the Deaf

Washington University
818 S Euclid Ave
St Louis, MO 63110-1594
314 652-3200
- Audiologist

Fontbonne College

Dennis Golden, President
6800 Wydown Blvd
St Louis, MO 63105
314 862-3456
- Dietitian/Nutritionist
- Speech Language Pathologist

Jewish Hosp-Coll of Nursing/Allied Hlth

Sharon Pontious, PhD, President
306 S Kingshighway Blvd
St Louis, MO 63110
314 454-7250
- Clin Lab Scientist/Med Tech
- Cytotechnologist

Maryville University

Keith Lovin, President
13550 Conway Rd
St Louis, MO 63141-7299
314 529-9300
- Music Therapist

Sanford Brown College Hazelwood Campus

Brett Combs, MBA, President
1655 Des Peres Rd Ste 150
St Louis, MO 63131
314 965-6606
- Occupational Therapy Asst

St John's Mercy Medical Center

Mark Weber, President
615 S New Ballas Rd
St Louis, MO 63141-8221
314 569-6182
- Clin Lab Scientist/Med Tech
- Radiographer

St Louis Comm Coll at Florissant Valley

Irving P McPhail, President
3400 Pershall Rd
St Louis, MO 63135
314 595-4200
- Dietetic Technician

St Louis Comm College at Forest Park

Henry Shannon, EdD, President
5600 Oakland Ave
St Louis, MO 63110
314 644-9743
- Clin Lab Tech/Med Lab Tech-AD
- Dental Hygienist
- Diagnostic Med Sonographer
- Radiographer
- Respiratory Therapist
- Surgical Technologist

St Louis Community College at Meramec

Richard Black, President
11333 Big Bend Blvd
St Louis, MO 63122
314 984-7762
- Occupational Therapy Asst

St Louis Institute of Art Psychotherapy

308A N Euclid
St Louis, MO 63108
314 367-8550
- Art Therapist

St Louis University Health Sciences Ctr

James R Kimmey, MD, VP of Hlth Sciences Ctr
3556 Caroline St
St Louis, MO 63104-1085
314 577-8101
- Clin Lab Scientist/Med Tech
- Dietitian/Nutritionist
- Health Information Admin
- Nuclear Medicine Tech
- Occupational Therapist
- Physician Assistant
- Speech Language Pathologist

St Louis University Med Ctr/Barnes Hosp

Richard S Kurz, PhD, Chairman
Saint Louis University
3663 Lindell Blvd
St Louis, MO 63108-3342
314 768-1000
- Emergency Med Tech-Paramedic

Veterans Affairs Medical Center

Jefferson Barracks Div
1 Jefferson Barracks Dr
St Louis, MO 63125
314 894-6631
- Dietitian/Nutritionist

Washington University

Mark S Wrighton, PhD, Chancellor
Brookings Dr Campus Box 1192
St Louis, MO 63130-4899
314 935-5100
- Occupational Therapist

St Peters

St Charles County Community College

Donald D Shook, EdD, President
4601 Mid Rivers Mall Dr
St Peters, MO 63376
314 922-8000
- Health Information Tech

Union

East Central College

Dale L Gibson, President
Box 529 Hwy 50 and Prairie Dell
Union, MO 63084
314 583-5193
- Dental Assistant

Warrensburg

Central Missouri State University

Ed M Elliott, President
Warrensburg, MO 64093
816 543-4111
- Audiologist
- Dietitian/Nutritionist
- Speech Language Pathologist

Montana

Billings

Montana State University-Billings

Ronald P Sexton, Chancellor
1500 N 30th St
Billings, MT 59101
406 657-2011
- Rehabilitation Counselor

St Vincent Hospital & Health Center

Jim Paquette, MBA, President
PO Box 35200
Billings, MT 59107
406 657-7102
- Radiographer

Bozeman

Montana State University
Michael Malone, President
Bozeman, MT 59717
406 994-0211
• Dietitian/Nutritionist

Great Falls

Benefits Health Care-West Campus
Lloyd Smith, President
500 15th Ave S PO Box 5013
Benefits Health Care
Great Falls, MT 59403
406 727-3333
• Clin Lab Scientist/Med Tech
• Radiographer

Montana State Univ Coll of Technology
Willard R Weaver, MS, Dean
2100 16th Ave S
Great Falls, MT 59405-4998
406 771-4306
• Dental Assistant
• Health Information Tech
• Occupational Therapy Asst
• Respiratory Therapist
• Respiratory Therapy Tech

Helena

Carroll College
Matthew J Quinn, PhD JD, President
1601 N Benton Ave
Helena, MT 59625
406 447-4402
• Health Information Admin

Missoula

St Patrick Hospital
Lawrence L White Jr, MHA, President
PO Box 4587
Missoula, MT 59806
406 543-7271
• Radiographer

University of Montana-Missoula
George Dennison, PhD, President
University Hall 109
Missoula, MT 59812
• Respiratory Therapy Tech
• Surgical Technologist

Pablo

Salish Kootenai College
Joseph F McDonald, PhD, President
PO Box 117
Pablo, MT 59855
406 675-4800
• Dental Assistant
• Health Information Tech

Nebraska

Grand Island

Central Community College
Joseph W Preusser, PhD, President
PO Box 4903
Grand Island, NE 68802-4903
308 384-5220
• Dental Assistant
• Dental Hygienist
• Medical Assistant

Spencer School of Business
Connie J Collin, BS, Dir
410 W Second St
Grand Island, NE 68801
308 382-8044
• Medical Assistant

Hastings

Central Technical Community College
PO Box 1024
Hastings, NE 68902-1024
402 461-2466
• Dental Lab Technician

Mary Lanning Memorial Hospital
W Michael Kearney, MHA, Administrator
715 N St Joseph
Hastings, NE 68901
402 463-4521
• Radiographer

Kearney

University of Nebraska at Kearney
Gladys S Johnston, Chancellor
25th St and Ninth Ave
Kearney, NE 68849
308 865-8441
• Dietitian/Nutritionist
• Speech Language Pathologist

Lincoln

Southeast Community College
Jeanette Volker, MA, President
8800 O St Lincoln Campus
Lincoln, NE 68520
402 437-2554
• Clin Lab Tech/Med Lab Tech-AD
• Dental Assistant
• Dietetic Technician
• Medical Assistant
• Radiographer
• Respiratory Therapist
• Surgical Technologist

University of Nebraska
L Dennis Smith, President
3835 Holdrege St
Lincoln, NE 68583
402 472-2111
• Dental Hygienist
• Dietitian/Nutritionist

University of Nebraska - Lincoln
Joan R Leitzel, Interim Chancellor
14th and R Sts
Lincoln, NE 68588
402 472-7211
• Audiologist
• Speech Language Pathologist

North Platte

Mid Plains Community College
Greg G Fitch, PhD, Chancellor
416 North Jeffers
North Platte, NE 69101
308 532-8980
• Clin Lab Tech/Med Lab Tech-AD
• Dental Assistant

Omaha

Alegent Health/Immanuel Medical Center
Charles J Marr, FACHE, President/CEO
6901 N 72nd St
Omaha, NE 68122
402 572-2270
• Radiographer
• Respiratory Therapist

Bishop Clarkson Memorial Hospital
Louis W Burgher, MD PhD
4350 Dewey Ave.
Omaha, NE 68105
402 552-3203
• Clin Lab Scientist/Med Tech

Clarkson College
Fay L Bower, DNSc FAAN, President
101 S 42nd St
Omaha, NE 68131-2739
402 552-3394
• Occupational Therapy Asst
• Radiographer

College of St Mary
Maryanne Stevens, RSM PhD, President
1901 S 72nd St
Omaha, NE 68124
402 399-2435
• Health Information Admin
• Health Information Tech

Creighton University
Michael G Morrison, SJ PhD, President
2500 California Plaza
Omaha, NE 68178-0001
402 280-2974
• Emergency Med Tech-Paramedic
• Occupational Therapist

Gateway Electronics Institute
John E Queen, Board Chairman
Gateway College
808 S 74th Plaza Ste 100
Omaha, NE 68114
402 398-0900
• Medical Assistant

Metropolitan Community College
J Richard Gilliland, EdD, President
PO Box 3777
Omaha, NE 68103
402 449-8415
- Dental Assistant
- Respiratory Therapist
- Respiratory Therapy Tech
- Surgical Technologist

NE Methodist Coll Nursing & Allied Hlth
Roger A Koehler, PhD, President
8501 W Dodge Rd
Omaha, NE 68114
402 354-4915
- Diagnostic Med Sonographer
- Radiation Therapist
- Respiratory Therapist

Nebraska Methodist Hospital
Stephen D Long, President/CEO
8303 Dodge St
Omaha, NE 68114
402 354-4436
- Clin Lab Scientist/Med Tech

Omaha College of Health Careers
William J Stuckey, MS, President
10845 Harney St
Omaha, NE 68154-2655
402 333-1400
- Dental Assistant
- Medical Assistant

St Joseph Hospital
Matthew Kurs, MS, President/CEO
601 N 30th St
Omaha, NE 68131-2197
402 449-5021
- Radiographer

University of Nebraska at Omaha
Delbert D Weber, Chancellor
Omaha, NE 68182-0167
402 554-2800
- Speech Language Pathologist

University of Nebraska Medical Center
William O Bernadt, PhD, Chancellor
600 S 42nd St
Omaha, NE 68198-6605
402 559-4200
- Clin Lab Scientist/Med Tech
- Cytotechnologist
- Diagnostic Med Sonographer
- Dietitian/Nutritionist
- Nuclear Medicine Tech
- Perfusionist
- Physician Assistant
- Radiation Therapist
- Radiographer

Scottsbluff

Regional West Medical Center
David Nitschke, CEO
4021 Ave B
Scottsbluff, NE 69361
308 635-3711
- Radiographer

Nevada

Las Vegas

Associated Pathologist Laboratories
John P Schwartz, MBA, President
4230 Burnham Ave
Las Vegas, NV 89119
702 733-7866
- Cytotechnologist

University of Nevada Las Vegas
Carol C Harter, PhD, President
4505 Maryland Pkwy
Las Vegas, NV 89154
702 895-3201
- Clin Lab Scientist/Med Tech
- Nuclear Medicine Tech
- Radiographer

North Las Vegas

Community College of Southern Nevada
Richard Moore, PhD, President
3200 E Cheyenne
North Las Vegas, NV 89030-4296
702 651-4491
- Clin Lab Tech/Med Lab Tech-AD
- Dental Hygienist
- Health Information Tech

Reno

Truckee Meadows Community College
Kenneth Wright, PhD, President
7000 Dandini Blvd
Reno, NV 89512-3999
702 673-7025
- Dental Assistant
- Radiographer

University of Nevada - Reno
Joseph N Crowley, PhD, President
Reno, NV 89557-0046
702 784-4805
- Clin Lab Scientist/Med Tech
- Clin Lab Tech/Med Lab Tech-C
- Dietitian/Nutritionist
- Speech Language Pathologist

New Hampshire

Claremont

New Hampshire Community Technical College
Keith W Bird, PhD, President
One College Dr
Claremont, NH 03743-9707
603 542-7744
- Clin Lab Tech/Med Lab Tech-AD
- Medical Assistant
- Occupational Therapy Asst
- Respiratory Therapist

Concord

New Hampshire Technical Institute
William Siminton, EdD, President
11 Institute Dr
Concord, NH 03301-7412
603 225-1800
- Dental Assistant
- Dental Hygienist
- Emergency Med Tech-Paramedic
- Radiographer

Durham

University of New Hampshire
Joan Leitzel, PhD, President
Thompson Hall
Durham, NH 03824-3547
603 862-2450
- Athletic Trainer
- Clin Lab Scientist/Med Tech
- Dietitian/Nutritionist
- Dietetic Technician
- Occupational Therapist
- Speech Language Pathologist

Keene

Keene State College
Stanley J Yarosewick, President
229 Main
Keene, NH 03431
603 352-1909
- Dietitian/Nutritionist

Manchester

Northeast Career Schools
Chris Liponis, BS, President
749 E Industrial Park Dr
Manchester, NH 03109
603 669-1151
- Medical Assistant

Nashua

New Hampshire Tech College - Nashua
Keith W Bird, President
505 Amherst St
Nashua, NH 03061
603 882-6923
- Ophthalmic Dispenser

New Jersey

Atlantic City

Atlantic City Medical Center
David P Tilton, BS MBA, President/CEO
1925 Pacific Ave
Atlantic City, NJ 08401
609 344-4081
- Radiographer

Institutions

Bayonne

Hudson Area School of Radiologic Tech

Michael R D'Agnes, MBA, President/CEO
29 E 29th St
Bayonne, NJ 07002
201 858-5202
● Radiographer

Blackwood

Camden County College

Phyllis Della Vecchia, PhD, President
PO Box 200
Blackwood, NJ 08012
609 227-7200
● Clin Lab Tech/Med Lab Tech-AD
● Dental Assistant
● Dental Hygienist
● Dietetic Technician
● Ophthalmic Dispenser

Bridgeton

Cumberland County Technical Education Center

601 Bridgeton Ave
Bridgeton, NJ 08302
609 451-9000
● Dental Assistant

S Jersey Hosp System/Bridgeton Hosp Div

Paul S Cooper, BA, President
Irving Ave
Bridgeton, NJ 08302
609 451-6600
● Radiographer

Camden

Cooper Hospital/University Medical Ctr

Kevin G Halpern, MPA FACHE, President
One Cooper Plaza
Camden, NJ 08103
609 342-2010
● Clin Lab Scientist/Med Tech
● Histologic Technician-Cert
● Perfusionist
● Radiation Therapist
● Radiographer

West Jersey Hospital System

Richard Miller, President
1000 Atlantic Ave
Camden, NJ 08104
609 342-4600
● Radiographer

Cape May CourtHouse

Burdette Tomlin Memorial Hospital

Thomas Scott, FACHE, President
Rte 9 and Stone Harbor Blvd
Cape May CourtHouse, NJ 08210
609 463-2180
● Radiographer

Cranford

Union County College

Thomas H Brown, PhD, President
1033 Springfield Ave
Cranford, NJ 07016-1599
908 709-7100
● Occupational Therapy Asst
● Respiratory Therapist

Denville

Northwest NJ Consortium Resp Care Educ

Edward Condit, MBA RRT, Chairman Regl Oper Cncl
C/O NW Covenant Med Ctr Denville Campus
25 Pocono Rd
Denville, NJ 07934
201 625-6720
● Respiratory Therapist

Edison

Middlesex County College

John Bakum, EdD, President
155 Mill Rd PO Box 3050
Edison, NJ 08818-3050
908 906-2517
● Clin Lab Tech/Med Lab Tech-AD
● Dental Hygienist
● Dietetic Technician
● Radiographer

Elizabeth

Elizabeth General Medical Center

David A Fletcher, President
925 E Jersey St
Elizabeth, NJ 07201
908 965-7390
● Diagnostic Med Sonographer
● Radiographer

Englewood

Englewood Hospital and Medical Center

Daniel A Kane, PhD, President/CEO
350 Engle St
Englewood, NJ 07631
201 894-3002
● Radiographer

Glen Ridge/Montclair

Mountainside Hospital

Robert A Silver, MPH, President/CEO
Bay and Highland Aves
Glen Ridge/Montclair, NJ 07042
201 429-6850
● Histologic Technician-Cert

Hackensack

Hackensack Medical Center

John P Ferguson, President
30 Prospect Ave
One Conklin
Hackensack, NJ 07601
201 996-2000
● Radiographer

Jersey City

Hudson County Community College

Glen Gabert, PhD, President
26 Journal Sq.
Jersey City, NJ 07306
201 714-2100
● Health Information Tech
● Medical Assistant

Lincroft

Brookdale Community College

Peter F Burnham, PhD, President
765 Newman Springs Rd
Lincroft, NJ 07738-1522
908 224-2417
● Clin Lab Tech/Med Lab Tech-AD
● Respiratory Therapist

Livingston

St Barnabas Medical Center

Cynthia Sparer, Chief Operating Officer
Old Short Hill Rd
Livingston, NJ 07039
201 533-5628
● Radiation Therapist

Lodi

Felician College

Sr Theresa M Martin, MA, President
262 S Main St
Lodi, NJ 07644
201 778-1190
● Clin Lab Tech/Med Lab Tech-AD

Long Branch

Monmouth Medical Center

Cynthia N Sparer, Executive Director
300 Second Ave
Long Branch, NJ 07740
908 222-5200
● Clin Lab Scientist/Med Tech

Mays Landing

Atlantic Community College

John T May, PhD, President
5100 Black Horse Pike
Mays Landing, NJ 08330-9888
609 343-4901
● Clin Lab Tech/Med Lab Tech-AD
● Occupational Therapy Asst

Atlantic County Vocational Tech School

5080 Atlantic Ave
Mays Landing, NJ 08330
609 625-2249
● Dental Assistant

Morristown

College of St Elizabeth

Jacqueline Burns, President
2 Convent Rd
Morristown, NJ 07960
201 292-6300
● Dietitian/Nutritionist

Morristown Memorial Hospital
Richard P Oths, MBA, President and CEO
100 Madison Ave
Morristown, NJ 07962-1956
201 971-5177
- Cardiovascular Technologist
- Clin Lab Scientist/Med Tech
- Radiographer

Mount Holly

Memorial Hospital of Burlington County
Chester B Kaletkowski, MA BS, President/CEO
175 Madison Ave
Mount Holly, NJ 08060
609 267-0700
- Radiographer

Neptune

Jersey Shore Medical Center
John K Lloyd, MHA, President
1945 Corlies Ave
Neptune, NJ 07753
908 775-5500
- Clin Lab Scientist/Med Tech

New Brunswick

Rutgers SUNJ New Brunswick Campus
Joseph A Potenza, Provost
New Brunswick, NJ 08903
908 932-1766
- Dietitian/Nutritionist

Newark

Essex County College
A Zachery Yamba, President
303 University Ave
Newark, NJ 07102
201 877-3021
- Ophthalmic Dispenser
- Radiographer

Univ of Med & Dent of New Jersey
Stanley S Bergen Jr, MD, President
65 Bergen St Rm 1535
Newark, NJ 07107-3001
201 982-4400
- Clin Lab Scientist/Med Tech
- Clin Lab Tech/Med Lab Tech-AD
- Cytotechnologist
- Dental Assistant
- Dental Hygienist
- Diagnostic Med Sonographer
- Dietitian/Nutritionist
- Nuclear Medicine Tech
- Physician Assistant
- Respiratory Therapist
- Respiratory Therapy Tech
- Surgical Technologist

Univ of Med & Dent of New Jersey
Stanley J Bergen Jr, MD, President
Sch of Hlth Related Professions S
65 Bergen St
Newark, NJ 07107-3000
201 982-4400
- Clin Lab Tech/Med Lab Tech-AD
- Respiratory Therapist

Paramus

Bergen Community College
Judith K Winn, PhD, President/CEO
400 Paramus Rd
Paramus, NJ 07652-1595
201 447-7127
- Clin Lab Tech/Med Lab Tech-AD
- Dental Hygienist
- Diagnostic Med Sonographer
- Medical Assistant
- Radiographer
- Respiratory Therapist
- Surgical Technologist

Passaic

Eastern Heart Inst Gen Hosp Ctr-Passaic
Daniel L Marcantuono, President/CEO
350 Blvd
Passaic, NJ 07053
201 365-4568
- Perfusionist

Paterson

Passaic County Community College
Steven M Rose, EdD, VP for Academic Affairs
One College Blvd
Paterson, NJ 07505-1179
201 684-6300
- Radiographer
- Respiratory Therapist
- Respiratory Therapy Tech

Pemberton

Burlington County College
Robert C Messina Jr, PhD, President
Cnty Rte 530
Pemberton, NJ 08068-1599
609 894-9311
- Health Information Tech

Plainfield

Muhlenberg Regional Medical Center
John R Kopicki, MBA, President
Park Ave and Randolph Rd
Plainfield, NJ 07061
908 668-2250
- Radiographer

Randolph

County College of Morris
Edward J Yaw, EdD, President
Rte 10 and Ctr Grove Rd
Randolph, NJ 07869
201 328-5370
- Clin Lab Tech/Med Lab Tech-AD

Red Bank

Riverview Medical Center
Laurence M Merlis, President/CEO
One Riverview Plaza
Red Bank, NJ 07701
908 530-2232
- Nuclear Medicine Tech
- Radiographer

Ridgewood

The Valley Hospital
Michael W Azzara, MBA, President
223 N Van Dien Ave
Ridgewood, NJ 07450
201 447-8002
- Clin Lab Scientist/Med Tech
- Radiographer

Sewell

Gloucester County College
Richard H Jones, EdD, President
1400 Tanyard Rd
Sewell, NJ 08080
609 468-5000
- Diagnostic Med Sonographer
- Nuclear Medicine Tech
- Respiratory Therapy Tech

Sicklerville

Technical Institute of Camden County
R Sanders Haldeman, MA, Superintendent
Cross Keys Rd PO Box 566
Berlin 343
Sicklerville, NJ 08081-9709
609 767-7000
- Dental Assistant
- Medical Assistant

Somers Point

Shore Memorial Hospital
Richard A Pitman, MBA, President
Shore Rd
Somers Point, NJ 08244
609 653-3545
- Radiographer

Somerville

Raritan Valley Community College
Cary A Israel, President
PO Box 3300
Somerville, NJ 08876
908 526-1200
- Ophthalmic Dispenser

Toms River

Ocean County College
Milton Shaw, MD, President
Ocean County College Dr
CN 2001
Toms River, NJ 08754
908 255-4000
- Clin Lab Tech/Med Lab Tech-C

Totowa

Berdan Institute
Wes Henry, President
265 Rte 46 W
Totowa, NJ 07512
201 256-3444
- Dental Assistant
- Medical Assistant

Trenton

Marriott Health Care/Helene Fuld Med Ctr
Ira G Shimp, CEO
750 Brunswick Ave
Trenton, NJ 08638
609 394-6071
● Dietitian/Nutritionist
● Radiographer

Mercer County Community College
Thomas Sepe, PhD, President
PO Box B
Trenton, NJ 08690
609 586-4800
● Clin Lab Tech/Med Lab Tech-AD
● Radiographer

St Francis Medical Center
Judith Persichilli, President/CEO
601 Hamilton Ave
Trenton, NJ 08629-1986
609 599-5000
● Radiographer

Trenton State College
Harold W Eickhoff, President
Hillwood Lakes CN 4700
Trenton, NJ 08650-4700
609 771-1855
● Audiologist
● Speech Language Pathologist

Union

Kean College of New Jersey
Ronald L Applebaum, PhD, President
1000 Morris Ave
Union, NJ 07083-9982
908 527-2222
● Health Information Admin
● Occupational Therapist
● Speech Language Pathologist

Upper Montclair

Montclair State University
Irvin D Reid, President
Upper Montclair, NJ 07043
201 655-4000
● Dietitian/Nutritionist
● Music Therapist
● Speech Language Pathologist

Vineland

Cumberland County College
Roland J Chapdelaine, EdD, President
College Dr PO Box 517
Vineland, NJ 08360-0517
609 691-8600
● Radiographer

Wayne

William Paterson College
Arnold Speert, PhD, President
300 Pompton Rd
Wayne, NJ 07470
201 595-2222
● Athletic Trainer
● Speech Language Pathologist

Westwood

Pascack Valley Hospital
Louis R Ycre Jr, President
Old Hook Rd
Westwood, NJ 07675
201 358-3010
● Radiographer

New Mexico

Alamogordo

New Mexico State U at Alamogordo
Charles E Reidlinger, PhD, Provost
2400 N Scenic Dr
PO Box 477
Alamogordo, NM 88310
505 439-3640
● Clin Lab Tech/Med Lab Tech-AD

Albuquerque

Albuquerque Tech Voc Institute
Alex Sanchez, EdD, President
525 Buena Vista, SE
Albuquerque, NM 87106
505 224-4411
● Clin Lab Tech/Med Lab Tech-AD

PIMA Medical Institute - Albuquerque
Richard L Luebke Jr, BS, Executive Director
201 San Pedro NE/Bldg 3
Albuquerque, NM 87110
505 881-1234
● Clin Lab Tech/Med Lab Tech-AD
● Radiographer

Southwestern Indian Polytechnic Institute
Carolyn Elgin, President
Box 10146
9169 Coors NW
Albuquerque, NM 87184
505 897-5347
● Ophthalmic Dispenser
● Ophthalmic Laboratory Technologist

Univ of New Mexico School of Medicine
Jane E Henney, MD, Vice President
Health Sciences Center
University of New Mexico
Albuquerque, NM 87131
505 277-5849
● Clin Lab Scientist/Med Tech
● Diagnostic Med Sonographer
● Emergency Med Tech-Paramedic
● Nuclear Medicine Tech
● Radiographer

University of New Mexico
Richard E Peck, PhD, President
Albuquerque, NM 87131-5641
505 277-2626
● Art Therapist
● Audiologist
● Dental Hygienist
● Dietitian/Nutritionist
● Occupational Therapist
● Speech Language Pathologist

Clovis

Clovis Community College
Jay Gurley, EdD, President
417 Schepps Blvd
Clovis, NM 88101
505 769-4000
● Radiographer

Espanola

Northern New Mexico Community College
Connie Valdez, MA, President
1002 N Onate St
Espanola, NM 87532
505 747-2100
● Radiographer

Gallup

University of New Mexico - Gallup/IHS
Robert Carlson, EdD, Campus Director
200 College Rd
Gallup, NM 87301
505 863-7600
● Clin Lab Tech/Med Lab Tech-AD
● Dental Assistant
● Health Information Tech

Hobbs

New Mexico Junior College
Charles D Hays, PhD, President
5317 Lovington Hwy
Hobbs, NM 88240
505 392-4510
● Clin Lab Tech/Med Lab Tech-AD

Las Cruces

Dona Ana Branch Community College
James McLaughlin, EdD, Acting Provost
Box 30001 Dept 3DA
Las Cruces, NM 88003-0001
505 527-7510
● Emergency Med Tech-Paramedic
● Radiographer
● Respiratory Therapist

New Mexico State University
J Michael Ovenduff, President
Box 30001
Dept 3z
Las Cruces, NM 88003-0001
505 646-2035
● Athletic Trainer
● Dietitian/Nutritionist
● Speech Language Pathologist

Portales

Eastern New Mexico University
Everett L Frost, President
Portales, NM 88130
505 562-1011
● Speech Language Pathologist

Roswell

Eastern New Mexico University-Roswell

Joseph Roberts, EdD, Provost
52 University Blvd
PO Box 6000
Roswell, NM 88202-6000
505 624-7112
- Emergency Med Tech-Paramedic
- Occupational Therapy Asst

Silver City

Western New Mexico University

John Counts, PhD, President
PO Box 680
Silver City, NM 88062-0680
505 538-6238
- Occupational Therapy Asst

New York

Albany

Albany Medical Center Hospital

James J Barba, President/CEO
47 New Scotland Ave
Albany, NY 12208
518 262-3830
- Clin Lab Scientist/Med Tech

Albany Medical College

Richard M Ryan Jr, DSc, President/CEO
47 New Scotland Ave A81
Albany, NY 12208
518 262-3830
- Cytotechnologist

Albany Memorial Hospital

Bernard Shapiro, MBA FACHE, CEO
600 Northern Blvd
Albany, NY 12204
518 471-3224
- Radiographer

College of St Rose

Louis C Vaccaro, PhD, President
432 Western Ave
Albany, NY 12203
518 454-5111
- Speech Language Pathologist

Maria College

Sr Laureen Fitzgerald, RSM MA MS, President
700 New Scotland Ave
Albany, NY 12208-1798
518 438-3111
- Occupational Therapy Asst

SUNY at Albany

Karen R Hitchcock, President
1400 Washington Ave
Albany, NY 12222
518 442-3300
- Rehabilitation Counselor

Alfred

SUNY College of Technology at Alfred

William D Rezak, PhD, President
Admin Bldg ASC Rm 229
Alfred, NY 14802
607 587-4211
- Clin Lab Tech/Med Lab Tech-AD
- Health Information Tech

Amherst

Daemen College

Martin J Anisman, PhD, President
4380 Main St
Amherst, NY 14226-3592
716 829-8210
- Clin Lab Scientist/Med Tech

Batavia

Genesee Community College

Stuart Steiner, JD EdD, President
One College Rd
Batavia, NY 14020-9704
716 343-0055
- Occupational Therapy Asst

Binghamton

Broome Community College

Donald A Dellow, EdD, President
Wales Bldg PO Box 1017
Binghamton, NY 13902
607 778-5000
- Clin Lab Tech/Med Lab Tech-AD
- Dental Hygienist
- Health Information Tech
- Medical Assistant
- Radiographer

Ridley-Lowell Business & Technical Institute

Wilfred T Weymouth, MS, President
116 Front St
Binghamton, NY 13905
607 724-2941
- Medical Assistant

Brentwood

Suffolk Community College

Salvatore J LaLima, BBA MS, Provost
Western Campus
Crooked Hill Rd
Brentwood, NY 11717
516 851-6789
- Medical Assistant

Bronx

Bronx Lebanon Hospital Center

Miguel Fuentes, MBA, CEO
1650 Grand Concourse
Bronx, NY 10457
718 518-1800
- Cytotechnologist
- Physician Assistant

CUNY Bronx Community College

Carolyn Williams, President
University Ave and W 181st St
Bronx, NY 10453
718 289-5151
- Nuclear Medicine Tech
- Radiographer

CUNY Herbert H Lehman College

Ricardo R Fernandez, President
Bedford Park Blvd W
Bronx, NY 10468
718 960-8000
- Audiologist
- Dietitian/Nutritionist
- Speech Language Pathologist

Hostos Community College of CUNY

Isaura Santiago, PhD, President
475 Grand Concourse
Bronx, NY 10451
718 518-4300
- Dental Hygienist
- Radiographer

Montefiore Medical Center

Spencer Foreman, MD, President
111 E 210th St
Bronx, NY 10467
718 920-4001
- Radiation Therapist

Veterans Affairs Medical Center

130 W Kingsbridge Rd
Bronx, NY 10468-3904
718 579-1640
- Dietitian/Nutritionist

Brooklyn

ARAMARK Healthcare Support Services

Kingsbrook Jewish Medical Ctr
585 Schenectady Ave
Brooklyn, NY 11203
718 604-5757
- Dietitian/Nutritionist

CUNY Brooklyn College

Vernon E Lattin, President
2900 Bedford Ave
Brooklyn, NY 11210
718 951-5000
- Audiologist
- Dietitian/Nutritionist
- Speech Language Pathologist

CUNY New York City Technical College

Provost Emilie Cozzi, Acting President
300 Jay St N319
Brooklyn, NY 11201
718 260-5400
- Clin Lab Tech/Med Lab Tech-AD
- Dental Hygienist
- Dental Lab Technician
- Ophthalmic Dispenser
- Radiographer

Long Island College Hospital

Harold L Light, President
340 Henry St
Brooklyn, NY 11201
212 780-4651
- Dietitian/Nutritionist
- Radiographer

Institutions

Long Island University - Brooklyn Campus
Gale Stevens-Haynes, Provost
One University Plaza
Brooklyn, NY 11201
718 488-1000
● Respiratory Therapist
● Speech Language Pathologist

New York Methodist Hospital
Mark J Mundy, MSHA, President
506 Sixth St
Brooklyn, NY 11215
718 780-3101
● Clin Lab Scientist/Med Tech
● Radiation Therapist
● Radiographer

Pratt Institute
Thomas F Schutte, President
200 Willoughby Ave
Brooklyn, NY 11205
718 636-3600
● Art Therapist

SUNY Health Science Center - Brooklyn
Russell L Miller, MD, President
450 Clarkson Ave Box 1
Brooklyn, NY 11203-2098
718 270-2611
● Diagnostic Med Sonographer
● Health Information Admin
● Occupational Therapist
● Perfusionist
● Physician Assistant
● Radiographer

The Brooklyn Hosp/Long Island Univ
Frederick Alley, MS FACHE, President
121 DeKalb Ave
Brooklyn, NY 11201
718 250-8005
● Physician Assistant

Buffalo

Byrant & Stratton Business Institute
William B Schatt, Institute Director
1028 Main St
Buffalo, NY 14202
716 884-9120
● Medical Assistant

Canisius College
Vincent M Cooke, SJ PhD, President
2001 Main St
Buffalo, NY 14208-1098
716 888-2100
● Athletic Trainer

D'Youville College
Sr Denise A Roche, GNSH PhD, President
One D'Youville Square
320 Porter Ave
Buffalo, NY 14201-1084
716 881-7624
● Dietitian/Nutritionist
● Occupational Therapist
● Physician Assistant

Erie Community College - City Campus
Louis M Ricci, PhD, President
121 Ellicott St
Buffalo, NY 14203
716 851-1200
● Clin Lab Tech/Med Lab Tech-AD
● Dental Hygienist
● Dental Lab Technician
● Health Information Tech
● Medical Assistant
● Occupational Therapy Asst
● Radiation Therapist
● Respiratory Therapist

Millard Fillmore Health Systems
Charles B Van Vorst, MBA, President/CEO
3 Gates Circle
Buffalo, NY 14209
716 887-4830
● Radiographer

SUNY at Buffalo
William R Greiner, JD LLM, President
501 Capen Hall
Buffalo, NY 14260-0001
716 645-2901
● Audiologist
● Clin Lab Scientist/Med Tech
● Nuclear Medicine Tech
● Occupational Therapist
● Rehabilitation Counselor
● Speech Language Pathologist

SUNY College at Buffalo
F C Richardson, President
1300 Elmwood Ave
Buffalo, NY 14222
716 878-4000
● Dietitian/Nutritionist
● Speech Language Pathologist

SUNY Educational Opportunity Center
465 Washington St
Buffalo, NY 14203
716 849-6725
● Dental Assistant

Trocaire College
Sr Barbara Ciarico, RSM, President
110 Red Jacket Pkwy
Buffalo, NY 14220-2094
716 826-1200
● Clin Lab Tech/Med Lab Tech-AD
● Health Information Tech
● Radiographer
● Surgical Technologist

Canton

SUNY College of Technology at Canton
Joseph L Kennedy, PhD, President
Cornell Dr
Canton, NY 13617
315 386-7204
● Clin Lab Tech/Med Lab Tech-AD

Cobleskill

SUNY Agric & Tech College at Cobleskill
Kenneth Wing, President
Cobleskill, NY 12043
518 234-5111
● Histologic Technician-AD

Cortland

SUNY College at Cortland
Judson H Taylor, PhD, President
Box 2000
Cortland, NY 13045
607 753-2201
● Athletic Trainer
● Therapeutic Recreation Specialist

Dix Hills

Western Suffolk BOCES
Daniel A Domenech, PhD, Dist Super
507 Deer Park Rd
Dix Hills, NY 11746
516 549-4900
● Diagnostic Med Sonographer

Dobbs Ferry

Mercy College
Jay Sexter, PhD, President
555 Broadway
Dobbs Ferry, NY 10522
914 693-4500
● Occupational Therapist

Elmira

Arnot Ogden Medical Center
Anthony J Cooper, CHE, President/CEO
600 Roe Ave
Elmira, NY 14905-1676
607 737-4231
● Radiographer

Far Rockaway

Peninsula Hospital Center
Robert A Levine, MBA,
51-15 Beach Channel Dr
Far Rockaway, NY 11691-1074
718 945-7100
● Radiographer

Farmingdale

SUNY at Farmingdale
Frank A Cipriani, PhD, President
SUNY at Farmingdale
Route 110 Horton Hall
Farmingdale, NY 11735
516 420-2145
● Clin Lab Tech/Med Lab Tech-AD
● Dental Hygienist

Flushing

CUNY Queens College
Allen Lee Sessoms, President
65-30 Kissena Blvd
Flushing, NY 11367
718 997-5000
● Audiologist
● Dietitian/Nutritionist
● Speech Language Pathologist

Fredonia

SUNY College at Fredonia
Donald A MacPhee, President
Fredonia, NY 14063
716 673-3111
- Audiologist
- Music Therapist
- Speech Language Pathologist

Garden City

Adelphi University
Peter Diamandopoulos, President
Garden City, NY 11530
516 877-3000
- Audiologist
- Speech Language Pathologist

Nassau Community College
Sean A Fanelli, PhD, President
Stewart Ave
Garden City, NY 11530
516 572-7205
- Radiation Therapist
- Radiographer
- Respiratory Therapist
- Surgical Technologist

Geneso

SUNY College at Geneseo
Christopher C Dahl, Interim President
1 College Circle
Geneso, NY 14454
716 245-5211
- Speech Language Pathologist

Glens Falls

Glens Falls Hospital
David Kruczlnicki, CEO
100 Park St
Glens Falls, NY 12801
518 792-3151
- Radiographer

Greenvale

Long Island Univ - C W Post Campus
David J Steinberg, PhD, President
University Ctr
Northern Blvd
Greenvale, NY 11548
516 299-0200
- Art Therapist
- Clin Lab Scientist/Med Tech
- Dietitian/Nutritionist
- Health Information Admin
- Radiographer
- Speech Language Pathologist

Hempstead

Hofstra University
James M Shuart, President
Hempstead, NY 11550
516 463-6600
- Art Therapist
- Audiologist
- Rehabilitation Counselor
- Speech Language Pathologist

Herkimer

Herkimer County Community College
Ronald F Williams, EdD, President
100 Reservoir Rd
Herkimer, NY 13350-1598
315 866-0300
- Occupational Therapy Asst

Hornell

St James Mercy Hospital
Paul Shephard, MBA, Administrator
411 Canisteo St
Hornell, NY 14843
607 324-3900
- Radiographer

Ithaca

Cayuga Medical Center at Ithaca
Bonnie H Howell, Administrator
101 Dates Dr
Ithaca, NY 14850
607 274-4443
- Radiographer

Cornell University
Hunter R Rawlings, President
Ithaca, NY 14853
607 255-2000
- Dietitian/Nutritionist

Ithaca College
James J Whalen, PhD LLD, President
953 Danby Rd
Ithaca, NY 14850-7001
607 274-3111
- Audiologist
- Health Information Admin
- Speech Language Pathologist

Jamaica

Catholic Medical Center
William McGuire, President and CEO
Catholic Medical Center
153 Street
Jamaica, NY 11432
718 558-6900
- Clin Lab Scientist/Med Tech
- Physician Assistant
- Radiographer

CUNY York College
Charles C Kidd Sr, President
94-20 Guy R Brewer Blvd
Jamaica, NY 11451-9902
718 262-2350
- Occupational Therapist

St John's University
Donald J Harrington, CM, President
Grand Central and Utopia Pkwys
Jamaica, NY 11439
718 990-6161
- Audiologist
- Speech Language Pathologist

Jamestown

Woman's Christian Association Hospital
Mark E Celmer, President/CEO
207 Foote Ave
Jamestown, NY 14701
716 664-8110
- Clin Lab Scientist/Med Tech
- Radiographer

Johnson City

United Health Services Hospital
Gennaro J Vasile, PhD, President/CEO
PO Box 540
Johnson City, NY 13790
607 770-6140
- Dietitian/Nutritionist

Keuka Park

Keuka College
Arthur F Kirk Jr, EdD, President
Keuka Park, NY 14478-0098
315 536-5201
- Occupational Therapist

Kingston

Ulster Cnty Residential Healthcare Fac
Golden Hill Dr
Kingston, NY 12401
914 339-4540
- Dietitian/Nutritionist

Long Island City

LaGuardia Community College
Raymond C Bowen, PhD, President
31-10 Thomson Ave
Long Island City, NY 11101-3083
718 482-5401
- Dietetic Technician
- Occupational Therapy Asst

Middletown

Orange County Community College
Preston Pulliams, President
115 South St
Middletown, NY 10940-6404
914 341-4700
- Clin Lab Tech/Med Lab Tech-AD
- Dental Hygienist
- Occupational Therapy Asst
- Radiographer

Mineola

Winthrop University Hospital
Ronald L Applbaum, President
259 First St
Mineola, NY 11501
516 663-2201
- Radiographer

Morrisville

SUNY Agric & Tech College at Morrisville
Frederick W Woodward, President
Morrisville, NY 13408
315 684-6000
- Dietetic Technician

New Paltz

SUNY College at New Paltz

Alice Chandler, President
New Paltz, NY 12561
914 257-2121
- Audiologist
- Music Therapist
- Speech Language Pathologist

New Rochelle

College of New Rochelle

Dorothy Ann Kelly, OSU, President
29 Castle Pl
New Rochelle, NY 10805
914 632-5300
- Art Therapist

New York

Bellevue Hospital Center

Pamela Brier, MPH AB, Exec Dir
First Ave and 27th St
New York, NY 10016
212 561-4132
- Radiographer

City of New York Medical School

Yolanda Moses, PhD, President
138 St and Convent Ave A-300
New York, NY 10031
212 650-7285
- Physician Assistant

Columbia University

George Rupp, PhD, President
Ofc of the President 202 Low Library
Morningside Campus
New York, NY 10027
212 280-2825
- Occupational Therapist

Cornell University Medical College

Carl Nathan, MD, Acting Dean
1300 York Ave
New York, NY 10021
212 746-5144
- Physician Assistant

CUNY Borough of Manhattan Community Coll

Antonio Perez, PhD, President
199 Chambers St
New York, NY 10007
212 346-8800
- Emergency Med Tech-Paramedic
- Health Information Tech
- Respiratory Therapist

CUNY Hunter College

David Caputo, President
695 Park Ave
New York, NY 10021
212 772-4000
- Audiologist
- Dietitian/Nutritionist
- Rehabilitation Counselor
- Speech Language Pathologist

Harlem Hospital Center

Bruce Goldman, MPH, Exec Director
506 Lenox Ave
New York, NY 10037
212 939-1340
- Radiographer

Institute of Allied Medical Professions

Thomas Haggerty, ScD, President
405 Park Ave/Ste 501
New York, NY 10022-4405
212 758-1410
- Nuclear Medicine Tech

Interboro Institute

Bruce R Kalisch, President
450 W 56th St
New York, NY 10019
212 399-0091
- Ophthalmic Dispenser

Memorial Sloan - Kettering Cancer Ctr

Paul A Marks, MD, President
1275 York Ave
New York, NY 10021
212 639-6561
- Cytotechnologist
- Radiation Therapist

New York Eye and Ear Infirmary

Joseph P Corcoran, President
310 E 14th St
New York, NY 10003
212 979-4300
- Ophthalmic Med Technician

New York Hospital

David B Skinner, MD, President/CEO
525 E 68th St
New York, NY 10021
212 746-4000
- Cytotechnologist
- Dietitian/Nutritionist

New York University

L Jay Oliva, PhD, President
70 Washington Square S
New York, NY 10003
212 998-2345
- Art Therapist
- Dental Assistant
- Dental Hygienist
- Dietitian/Nutritionist
- Occupational Therapist
- Rehabilitation Counselor
- Speech Language Pathologist

New York University Medical Center

Theresa Bischoff, EVP Deputy Provost
550 First Ave
New York, NY 10016
212 263-5111
- Cytotechnologist
- Diagnostic Med Sonographer
- Nuclear Medicine Tech
- Respiratory Therapist
- Surgical Technologist

St Vincent's Hosp & Med Ctr of New York

Karl P Adler, MD, President/CEO
153 W 11th St
New York, NY 10011
212 604-7500
- Clin Lab Scientist/Med Tech
- Nuclear Medicine Tech

Teachers College Columbia University

Arthur Levine, President
525 W 120th St
New York, NY 10027
212 678-3000
- Dietitian/Nutritionist
- Speech Language Pathologist

Touro College

Bernard Lander, PhD, President
Empire State Bldg
350 Fifth Ave Ste 5122
New York, NY 10118-5198
212 643-0700
- Occupational Therapist
- Physician Assistant

Wood-Tobe Coburn School

Rosemary Duggan, BA, President
8 E 40th St
New York, NY 10016
212 686-9040
- Medical Assistant

Northport

Northport VA Medical Center #632C

Eleanor M Travers, MD, Director
Middleville Rd
Northport, NY 11768
516 261-4400
- Nuclear Medicine Tech
- Radiographer

Oceanside

Hochstim Sch Radiography/S Nassau Hosp

Michael Rodzenko, MA MSHA MSHyg, Exec
Director
2445 Oceanside Rd
Oceanside, NY 11572
516 763-2030
- Radiographer

Marriott/Metro New York AP4 Programs

South Nassau Communities Hospital
2445 Oceanside Rd
Oceanside, NY 11572-1548
516 763-3903
- Dietitian/Nutritionist

Ogdensburg

Mater Dei College

Ronald Mrozinski, President
5428 State Hwy 37
Ogdensburg, NY 13669
315 393-5930
- Ophthalmic Dispenser

Old Westbury

New York Institute of Technology

Mathew Schure, PhD MPH MA, President
Wheatley Rd
Old Westbury, NY 11568
516 686-7650
- Clin Lab Scientist/Med Tech
- Dietitian/Nutritionist

Oneonta

SUNY College at Oneonta
Alan B Donovan, President
Oneonta, NY 13820
607 436-3500
● Dietitian/Nutritionist

Orangeburg

Dominican College
Kathleen Sullivan, OP MA, President
10 Western Hwy
Orangeburg, NY 10962-1299
914 359-7800
● Occupational Therapist

Plattsburgh

Champlain Valley Phys Hospital Med Ctr
Kevin Carroll, JD, President
100 Beekman St
Plattsburgh, NY 12901
518 561-2000
● Radiographer

Clinton Community College
Jay L Fennell, PhD, President
Lake Shore Rd Rte 9 S
136 Clinton Point Dr
Plattsburgh, NY 12901
518 562-4100
● Clin Lab Tech/Med Lab Tech-AD

SUNY College at Plattsburgh
Horace A Judson, President
Plattsburgh, NY 12901
518 564-2000
● Audiologist
● Dietitian/Nutritionist
● Speech Language Pathologist

Port Chester

United Hospital Medical Center
Havva S Idriss, MS, President
406 Boston Post Rd
Port Chester, NY 10573
914 939-7000
● Radiographer

Poughkeepsie

Dutchess Community College
David Conklin, PhD, President
53 Pendell Rd
Poughkeepsie, NY 12601
914 431-8312
● Clin Lab Tech/Med Lab Tech-AD
● Dietetic Technician

Marist College
Dennis J Murray, PhD, President
North Rd
Poughkeepsie, NY 12601
914 575-3000
● Clin Lab Scientist/Med Tech

Queensbury

Adirondack Community College
Roger C Andersen, EdD, President
634 Bay Rd
Queensbury, NY 12804-1498
518 743-2237
● Health Information Tech

Riverdale

Manhattan College
Br Thomas J Scanlan, FSC, CEO
Manhattan College Pkwy
Riverdale, NY 10471
718 862-7301
● Nuclear Medicine Tech

Riverhead

Central Suffolk Hospital
Joseph F Turner, MBA ACHE, President
1300 Roanoke Ave
Riverhead, NY 11901
516 548-6000
● Radiographer

Suffolk County Community College
Elizabeth Blake, Provost
Eastern Campus
Riverhead, NY 11901
516 548-2500
● Dietetic Technician

Rochester

Bryant & Stratton Business Institute
Francis J Felser, BS MBA CPA,
82 St Paul St
Rochester, NY 14604
716 325-6010
● Medical Assistant

Bryant & Stratton Business Institute
Fran J Felser, CPA MBA BS, Campus Dir
Henrietta Campus
1225 Jefferson Rd
Rochester, NY 14623-3136
716 292-5627
● Medical Assistant

Monroe Community College
Peter A Spina, PhD, President
1000 E Henrietta Rd
Rochester, NY 14623
716 292-2100
● Dental Hygienist
● Health Information Tech
● Radiographer

Nat'l Tech Inst for Deaf/Rochester Inst Tech
Robert Davila, PhD, CEO
52 Lomb Memorial Drive
Lyndon Baines Johnson Building
Rochester, NY 14623-5604
716 475-6585
● Ophthalmic Laboratory Technologist

Nazareth College of Rochester
Rose Marie Beston, PhD, President
4245 East Ave
Rochester, NY 14618-2790
716 586-2525
● Art Therapist
● Music Therapist
● Speech Language Pathologist

Rochester General Hospital
Steven I Goldstein, MS, President/CEO
1425 Portland Ave
Rochester, NY 14621
716 338-4430
● Clin Lab Scientist/Med Tech

Rochester Institute of Technology
Albert J Simone, PhD, President
Two Lomb Memorial Dr
Rochester, NY 14623-5604
716 475-2394
● Diagnostic Med Sonographer
● Dietitian/Nutritionist
● Nuclear Medicine Tech
● Physician Assistant

St Mary's Hospital
Stewart Putnam, President/CEO
89 Genesee St
Rochester, NY 14611
716 464-3357
● Clin Lab Scientist/Med Tech

University of Rochester Cancer Center
Thomas Jackson, PhD, President
Admin Bldg
Rochester, NY 14627
716 275-8356
● Radiation Therapist

Rockville Centre

Mercy Medical Center
Vincent DiRubbio, FACHE, President/CEO
1000 N Village Ave
Rockville Centre, NY 11570-1098
516 255-2201
● Radiographer

Molloy College
Martin Snyder, PhD, President
1000 Hempstead Ave
Rockville Centre, NY 11570
516 678-5000
● Health Information Tech
● Nuclear Medicine Tech
● Respiratory Therapist
● Respiratory Therapy Tech

Sanborn

Niagara County Community College
Gerald L Miller, President
3111 Saunders Settlement Rd
Sanborn, NY 14132
716 731-3271
● Electroneurodiagnostic Tech
● Radiographer

Saranac Lake

North Country Community College

Gail Rogers Rice, EdD, President
20 Winona Ave/PO Box 89
Saranac Lake, NY 12983
518 891-2915
● Radiographer

Staten Island

Bayley Seton Hospital

Dominick Stenzione, Exec VP
75 Vanderbilt Ave
Staten Island, NY 10304-3850
718 390-6007
● Physician Assistant

CUNY College of Staten Island

Marlene Springer, PhD, President
2800 Victory Blvd
Staten Island, NY 10314
718 982-2400
● Clin Lab Tech/Med Lab Tech-AD

St Vincent's Medical Center of Richmond

Dominick Stanzione, MPA, Executive VP
355 Bard Ave
Staten Island, NY 10310
718 876-2413
● Nuclear Medicine Tech

Stony Brook

SUNY Health Science Ctr at Stony Brook

Shirley Strum Kenny, PhD, President
Admin Bldg Third Fl
Stony Brook, NY 11794
516 632-6265
● Clin Lab Scientist/Med Tech
● Occupational Therapist
● Physician Assistant
● Radiation Therapist
● Respiratory Therapist

Suffern

Rockland Community College

Neal Raisman, PhD, President
145 College Rd
Suffern, NY 10901-3699
914 574-4214
● Dietetic Technician
● Health Information Tech
● Occupational Therapy Asst
● Respiratory Therapist

Syracuse

Bryant & Stratton Business Institute

Edward J Heinrich, Campus Director
953 James St
Syracuse, NY 13202
315 472-6603
● Medical Assistant

Onondaga Community College

Barrett Jones, Interim President
4941 Onondaga Road
Syracuse, NY 13215
315 469-2211
● Dental Hygienist
● Health Information Tech
● Respiratory Therapist
● Respiratory Therapy Tech
● Surgical Technologist

SUNY Health Science Center at Syracuse

Gregory L Eastwood, MD, President
750 E Adams St
Syracuse, NY 13210
315 464-4513
● Clin Lab Scientist/Med Tech
● Cytotechnologist
● Nuclear Medicine Tech
● Perfusionist
● Radiation Therapist
● Radiographer
● Respiratory Therapist
● Specialist in BB Tech

Syracuse University Main Campus

Kenneth A Shaw, Chancellor & President
Syracuse, NY 13244
315 443-1870
● Audiologist
● Dietitian/Nutritionist
● Rehabilitation Counselor
● Speech Language Pathologist

Tarrytown

Marymount College

Brigid Driscoll, President
Tarrytown, NY 10591
914 631-3200
● Dietitian/Nutritionist

Troy

Hudson Valley Community College

Stephen Curtis, PhD, President
Vandenburgh Ave
Troy, NY 12180
518 270-1530
● Clin Lab Tech/Med Lab Tech-AD
● Dental Hygienist
● Diagnostic Med Sonographer
● Physician Assistant
● Radiographer
● Respiratory Therapist

Russell Sage College

Jeanne H Neff, President
45 Ferry St
Troy, NY 12180
518 270-2000
● Dietitian/Nutritionist

Sage Graduate School

Sage Graduate School
45 Ferry St
Troy, NY 12180-4115
518 270-2075
● Dietitian/Nutritionist

The Sage Colleges

Jeanne H Neff, PhD, President
Office of the President
45 Ferry St
Troy, NY 12180-4115
518 270-2214
● Occupational Therapist

Utica

Mohawk Valley Community College

Michael I Schafer, EdD, President
Payne Hall 305
1105 Sherman Dr
Utica, NY 13501
315 792-5333
● Health Information Tech
● Respiratory Therapy Tech

St Elizabeth Hospital

Sr Rose Vincent, OSF, Administrator
2209 Genesee St
Utica, NY 13501
315 798-8123
● Radiographer

St Luke's Memorial Hospital Center

Andrew E Peterson, MS, Exec Director
Champlin Ave PO Box 479
Utica, NY 13503-0479
315 798-6001
● Radiographer

SUNY Institute of Tech - Utica/Rome

Peter J Cayan, EdD, President
PO Box 3050
Utica, NY 13504-3050
315 792-7400
● Health Information Admin

Utica College of Syracuse University

Michael K Simpson, PhD, President
1600 Burrstone Rd
Utica, NY 13502-4892
315 792-3222
● Occupational Therapist

Valhalla

Westchester Community College

Joseph N Hankin, EdD, President
75 Grasslands Rd
Valhalla, NY 10595
914 785-6706
● Dietetic Technician
● Radiographer
● Respiratory Therapist

Westchester County Medical Center

Grasslands Rd
Valhalla, NY 10595
914 285-7276
● Dietitian/Nutritionist

Watertown

Samaritan Medical Center

Willliam Koughan, President/CEO
830 Washington St
Watertown, NY 13601
315 785-4000
● Clin Lab Tech/Med Lab Tech-C

Williamsville

Erie Community College - North Campus

Dennis D Digiacomo, Dean of Students
6205 Main St
Williamsville, NY 14221
716 851-1002
- Dietetic Technician
- Ophthalmic Dispenser

North Carolina

Albemarle

Stanly Community College

Michael R Taylor, EdD, President
141 College Dr
Albemarle, NC 28001-9402
704 982-0121
- Occupational Therapy Asst
- Respiratory Therapist
- Respiratory Therapy Tech

Asheville

Asheville Buncombe Technical Comm Coll

K Ray Bailey, MEd, President
340 Victoria Rd
Asheville, NC 28801
704 254-1921
- Clin Lab Tech/Med Lab Tech-AD
- Dental Assistant
- Dental Hygienist
- Radiographer

Boone

Appalachian State University

Harvey R Durham, PhD, Provost/Vice Chancellor
Boone, NC 28608
704 262-2070
- Athletic Trainer
- Dietitian/Nutritionist
- Speech Language Pathologist

Burlington

Roche Biomedical Laboratories, Inc

J B Powell, MD, CEO
430 S Spring St
Burlington, NC 27215
910 229-1127
- Cytotechnologist

Chapel Hill

Univ of North Carolina at Chapel Hill

Michael K Hooker, PhD, Chancellor
130 South Bldg CB #9100
Chapel Hill, NC 27599-9100
919 962-1365
- Audiologist
- Clin Lab Scientist/Med Tech
- Cytotechnologist
- Dental Assistant
- Dental Hygienist
- Dietitian/Nutritionist
- Occupational Therapist
- Radiographer
- Rehabilitation Counselor
- Speech Language Pathologist

University of North Carolina Hospitals

Eric B Munson, MBA, Director
101 Manning Dr
Chapel Hill, NC 27514
919 966-5111
- Nuclear Medicine Tech
- Radiation Therapist

Charlotte

Carolinas College of Health Sciences

Clara B Smith, RN BSN MEd, President
PO Box 32861
1200 Blythe Rd
Charlotte, NC 28232-2861
704 355-5043
- Clin Lab Scientist/Med Tech
- Surgical Technologist

Central Piedmont Community College

P Anthony Zeiss, PhD, President
PO Box 35009
Charlotte, NC 28235
704 330-6566
- Cytotechnologist
- Dental Assistant
- Dental Hygienist
- Health Information Tech
- Medical Assistant
- Respiratory Therapist

King's College

Gary L Pritchett, President
322 Lamar Ave
Charlotte, NC 28204
704 372-0266
- Medical Assistant

Presbyterian Hospital

Paul F Betzold, FACHE, President/CEO
200 Hawthorne Ln PO Box 33549
Charlotte, NC 28233-3549
704 384-4942
- Histotechnologist
- Radiographer
- Surgical Technologist

Queens College

Billy O Wireman, President
1900 Selwyn Ave
Charlotte, NC 28274-0001
704 337-2200
- Music Therapist

Clyde

Haywood Community College

Wayne Hawkins, Interim President
Freedlander Dr
Clyde, NC 28721-9454
704 627-2821
- Medical Assistant

Cullowhee

Western Carolina University

John W Bardo, PhD, Chancellor
HF Robinson Admin Bldg
Cullowhee, NC 28723
704 227-7100
- Clin Lab Scientist/Med Tech
- Dietitian/Nutritionist
- Emergency Med Tech-Paramedic
- Health Information Admin
- Speech Language Pathologist

Dallas

Gaston College

Patricia A Skinner, PhD, President
201 Hwy 321 S
Dallas, NC 28034-1499
704 922-6475
- Medical Assistant

Durham

Duke University Medical Center

Ralph Snyderman, MD, Chancellor
Health Affairs
PO Box 3701 M106A Davison Bldg
Durham, NC 27710
919 684-2255
- Clin Lab Scientist/Med Tech
- Ophthalmic Med Technician
- Physician Assistant

Durham Technical Community College

Phail Wynn Jr, EdD MBA, President
1637 Lawson St
Durham, NC 27703-5023
919 598-9374
- Dental Lab Technician
- Occupational Therapy Asst
- Ophthalmic Dispenser
- Respiratory Therapist
- Respiratory Therapy Tech

North Carolina Central University

Julius Chambers, Chancellor
Durham, NC 27707
919 560-6100
- Dietitian/Nutritionist
- Speech Language Pathologist

Fayetteville

Fayetteville Technical Community College

Linwood Powell, EdD, Interim President
PO Box 35236
Fayetteville, NC 28303-0236
910 678-8321
- Dental Assistant
- Dental Hygienist
- Radiographer
- Respiratory Therapist
- Surgical Technologist

Gastonia

Gaston Memorial Hospital

Wayne F Shovelin, MHA, President
2525 Court Dr PO Box 1747
Gastonia, NC 28053-1747
704 834-2121
- Radiographer

Institutions

Goldsboro

Wayne Community College
Edward H Wilson, President
Caller Box 8002
Goldsboro, NC 27530
919 735-5151
- Dental Assistant
- Dental Hygienist

Graham

Alamance Community College
W Ronald McCarter, EdD, President
PO Box 8000
Graham, NC 27253-8000
919 578-2002
- Clin Lab Tech/Med Lab Tech-AD
- Dental Assistant

Greensboro

Bennett College
Gloria R Scott, President
900 E Washington St
Greensboro, NC 27401
910 273-4431
- Dietitian/Nutritionist

Moses H Cone Memorial Hospital
Dennis R Barry, MBA, President
1200 N Elm St
Greensboro, NC 27401-1020
910 574-7881
- Clin Lab Scientist/Med Tech
- Radiographer

North Carolina A & T State University
Edward B Fort, Chancellor
1601 E Market St
Greensboro, NC 27411
910 334-7500
- Dietitian/Nutritionist

Univ of North Carolina at Greensboro
Patricia A Sullivan, Chancellor
1000 Spring Garden St
Greensboro, NC 27412
910 334-5000
- Audiologist
- Dietitian/Nutritionist
- Speech Language Pathologist
- Therapeutic Recreation Specialist

Greenville

East Carolina University
Richard R Eakin, PhD, Chancellor
103 Spilman Bldg
Greenville, NC 27858
919 328-6212
- Athletic Trainer
- Audiologist
- Clin Lab Scientist/Med Tech
- Cytotechnologist
- Dietitian/Nutritionist
- Health Information Admin
- Music Therapist
- Occupational Therapist
- Rehabilitation Counselor
- Speech Language Pathologist

Pitt Community College
Charles E Russell, EdD, President
PO Drawer 7007
Hwy 11 S
Greenville, NC 27835-7007
919 321-4200
- Diagnostic Med Sonographer
- Health Information Tech
- Medical Assistant
- Nuclear Medicine Tech
- Occupational Therapy Asst
- Radiation Therapist
- Radiographer
- Respiratory Therapist

Henderson

Vance Granville Community College
Ben F Currin, EdD, President
PO Box 917
Henderson, NC 27536
919 492-2061
- Radiographer

Hickory

Catawba Valley Community College
Cuyler Dunbar, EdD, President
2550 Hwy 70 SE
Hickory, NC 28602-9699
704 327-7000
- Emergency Med Tech-Paramedic
- Health Information Tech
- Respiratory Therapist
- Respiratory Therapy Tech
- Surgical Technologist

Lenoir-Rhyne College
Ryan LaHurd, PhD, President
Box 7163
Hickory, NC 28601
704 328-7333
- Occupational Therapist

High Point

High Point University
Jacob Martinson, BA MDIV DDIV, President
University Station Montlieu Ave
High Point, NC 27262
919 841-9202
- Athletic Trainer

Hudson

Caldwell Comm College & Tech Institute
Kenneth A Boham, EdD, President
2855 Hickory Blvd
Hudson, NC 28638-1399
704 726-2200
- Diagnostic Med Sonographer
- Nuclear Medicine Tech
- Occupational Therapy Asst
- Radiographer

Jacksonville

Coastal Carolina Community College
Ronald K Lingle, PhD, President
444 Western Blvd
Jacksonville, NC 28546-6877
910 938-6210
- Clin Lab Tech/Med Lab Tech-AD
- Dental Assistant
- Dental Hygienist
- Surgical Technologist

Jamestown

Guilford Technical Community College
Donald C Cameron, EdD, President
PO Box 309
Jamestown, NC 27282
910 334-4822
- Dental Assistant
- Dental Hygienist
- Medical Assistant

Kenansville

James Sprunt Community College
Donald L Reichard, EdD, President
PO Box 398
Kenansville, NC 28349
910 296-2414
- Medical Assistant

Kinston

Lenoir Community College
Lonnie H Blizzard, EdD, President
PO Box 188
Kinston, NC 28501
919 527-6223
- Surgical Technologist

Lenoir Memorial Hospital
Gary Black, President
100 Airport Rd
Kinston, NC 28501
919 522-7797
- Radiographer

Lexington

Davidson County Community College
J Bryan Brooks, EdD, President
PO Box 1287
Lexington, NC 27293-1287
704 249-8189
- Health Information Tech

Lumberton

Robeson Community College
Fred G Williams, President
PO Box 1420
Lumberton, NC 28359
910 738-7101
- Respiratory Therapist

Morehead City

Carteret Community College
Donald W Bryant, EdD, President
3505 Arendell St
Morehead City, NC 28557
919 247-6000
• Medical Assistant
• Radiographer
• Respiratory Therapist
• Respiratory Therapy Tech

Morganton

Western Piedmont Community College
James A Richardson, EdD, President
1001 Burkemont Ave
Morganton, NC 28655
704 438-6010
• Clin Lab Tech/Med Lab Tech-AD
• Dental Assistant
• Medical Assistant

North Wilkesboro

Wilkes Regional Medical Center
David Henson, CEO
PO Box 609
North Wilkesboro, NC 28659
919 651-8100
• Radiographer

Pinehurst

Sandhills Community College
John R Dempsey, PhD, President
2200 Airport Rd
Pinehurst, NC 28374
910 695-3700
• Clin Lab Tech/Med Lab Tech-AD
• Radiographer
• Respiratory Therapist
• Surgical Technologist

Raleigh

Meredith College
John E Weems, President
Raleigh, NC 27607
919 829-8600
• Dietitian/Nutritionist

Wake Technical Community College
Bruce I Howell, EdD, President
9101 Fayetteville Rd
Raleigh, NC 27603
919 662-3301
• Clin Lab Tech/Med Lab Tech-AD
• Dental Assistant
• Medical Assistant
• Radiographer

Salisbury

Rowan-Cabarrus Community College
Richard L Brownell, EdD, President
PO Box 1595
Salisbury, NC 28145-1595
704 637-0760
• Dental Assistant
• Radiographer

Shelby

Cleveland Community College
L Steve Thornburg, EdD, President
137 S Post Rd
Shelby, NC 28150
704 484-4089
• Radiographer

Smithfield

Johnston Community College
John L Tart, EdD, President
PO Box 2350
Smithfield, NC 27577
919 934-3051
• Radiographer

Statesville

Mitchell Community College
Douglas O Eason, PhD, President
West Broad St
Statesville, NC 28677
704 878-3200
• Medical Assistant

Supply

Southeastern Regl Allied Hlth Consortium
W Michael Reaves, EdD, President
PO Box 30
Supply, NC 28462
910 754-6900
• Health Information Tech

Sylva

Southwestern Community College
Barry W Russell, EdD, President
447 College Dr
Sylva, NC 28779
704 586-4091
• Clin Lab Tech/Med Lab Tech-AD
• Occupational Therapy Asst
• Radiographer
• Respiratory Therapist
• Respiratory Therapy Tech

Tarboro

Edgecombe Community College
Hartwell H Fuller, EdD, President
PO Box 550
Tarboro, NC 27886
919 823-5166
• Health Information Tech
• Radiographer
• Respiratory Therapist
• Respiratory Therapy Tech

Washington

Beaufort County Community College
Ron Champion, PhD, President
PO Box 1069
Washington, NC 27889
919 946-6194
• Clin Lab Tech/Med Lab Tech-AD

Weldon

Halifax Community College
Elton Newbern Jr, EdD, President
PO Box 809
Weldon, NC 27890
919 536-2551
• Clin Lab Tech/Med Lab Tech-AD

Wilkesboro

Wilkes Community College
Gordon Burns, Interim President
Collegiate Dr
Wilkesboro, NC 28697-0120
910 838-6100
• Dental Assistant

Wilmington

Cape Fear Community College
Eric B McKeithan, President
411 N Front St
Wilmington, NC 28401-3993
910 251-5100
• Dental Assistant

Miller-Motte Business College
Richard D Craig, MS, President
606 S College Rd
Wilmington, NC 28403
919 392-4660
• Medical Assistant

New Hanover Regional Medical Center
Jim Hobbs, CHE BMA, President
2131 S 17th St PO Box 9000
Wilmington, NC 28402
919 343-7074
• Clin Lab Scientist/Med Tech

Univ of North Carolina - Wilmington
James R Leutze, Chancellor
601 S College Rd
Wilmington, NC 28403
910 395-3000
• Therapeutic Recreation Specialist

Wingate

Wingate College
Jerry McGee, EdD, President
Box 3055
Wingate, NC 28174
704 233-8000
• Medical Assistant

Winston-Salem

Bowman Gray School of Medicine
Richard Janeway, MD, Exec Vice President
Medical Ctr Blvd
Winston-Salem, NC 27157-1003
910 716-4424
• Clin Lab Scientist/Med Tech
• Physician Assistant

Forsyth Memorial Hospital
Paul M Wiles, MHA, President
3333 Silas Creek Pkwy
Winston-Salem, NC 27103
919 718-2023
• Clin Lab Scientist/Med Tech

Institutions

Forsyth Technical Community College
Desna L Wallin, EdD, President
2100 Silas Creek Pky
Winston-Salem, NC 27103
910 723-0371
- Diagnostic Med Sonographer
- Nuclear Medicine Tech
- Radiation Therapist
- Radiographer
- Respiratory Therapist

Winston-Salem State University
Alvin J Schexinder, Chancellor
Office of the Chancellor
Blair Hall 2nd Fl
Winston-Salem, NC 27110
919 750-2041
- Clin Lab Scientist/Med Tech

North Dakota

Bismarck

Bismarck State College
Donna Thigpen, EdD, President
1500 Edwards Ave
Bismarck, ND 58501
701 224-5430
- Clin Lab Tech/Med Lab Tech-AD

Medcenter One Health Systems
Terrance Brosseau, President
222 N Seventh St PO Box 1818
Bismarck, ND 58506-5525
701 222-5413
- Radiographer

St Alexius Medical Center
Richard A Tschider, MA, Administrator
900 E Broadway PO Box 5510
Bismarck, ND 58502-5510
701 224-7600
- Radiographer
- Respiratory Therapist

United Tribes Technical College
David M Gipp, BA, President
3315 University Dr
Bismarck, ND 58504
701 255-3285
- Health Information Tech

University of Mary
Thomas Welder, OSB MM, President
7500 University Dr
Bismarck, ND 58504-9652
701 255-7500
- Athletic Trainer

Fargo

Interstate Business College
Carol A Johnson, Director
2720 32nd Ave SW
Fargo, ND 58103
701 232-2477
- Dental Assistant

MeritCare
Roger Gilbertson, MD, President
720 4th St N
Fargo, ND 58122
701 234-6954
- Clin Lab Scientist/Med Tech
- Radiographer

NDSU/Merit Care Hospital RC Prgm
Larry McGuire, Vice President
720 Fourth St N
Fargo, ND 58122
701 234-5260
- Respiratory Therapist

North Dakota State University
Thomas Plough, President
Fargo, ND 58105
701 231-8011
- Athletic Trainer
- Dietitian/Nutritionist

Grand Forks

Univ of No Dakota Sch of Med and Hlth Sci
Kendall Baker, PhD, President
Box 8193
Grand Forks, ND 58202-8193
701 777-2121
- Athletic Trainer
- Clin Lab Scientist/Med Tech
- Cytotechnologist
- Dietitian/Nutritionist
- Occupational Therapist
- Physician Assistant
- Speech Language Pathologist

Minot

Minot School for Allied Health
C Milton Smith, MD, President/Board of Dir
Trinity Medical Ctr
110 Burdick Expy W
Minot, ND 58701
701 857-5620
- Radiographer

Minot State University
H Erik Shaar, President
500 Ninth Ave NW
Minot, ND 58701
701 857-3030
- Audiologist
- Speech Language Pathologist

Trinity Medical Center
Terry G Hoff, FCHA, President
3 Burdick Expwy at Main St
Minot, ND 58701
701 857-5000
- Clin Lab Scientist/Med Tech

UniMed Medical Center
Gary Kenner, President
Third St SE and Burdick Expwy
Minot, ND 58701
701 857-2300
- Clin Lab Scientist/Med Tech

Wahpeton

North Dakota State College of Science
Jerry C Olson, PhD, President
800 N Sixth St
Wahpeton, ND 58076-0002
701 671-2221
- Dental Assistant
- Dental Hygienist
- Health Information Tech
- Occupational Therapy Asst

Ohio

Akron

Akron General Medical Center
Michael A West, MHA, President
400 Wabash Ave
Akron, OH 44307
330 846-6548
- Cytotechnologist
- Emergency Med Tech-Paramedic

Children's Hospital Medical Ctr of Akron
William H Considine, MHA, President
One Perkins Square
Akron, OH 44308-1062
330 379-8293
- Clin Lab Scientist/Med Tech
- Radiographer

Southern Ohio College - NE
Richard M Thome, MT MSEd, Director
2791 Mogadore Rd
Akron, OH 44312
330 733-8766
- Medical Assistant

Summa Health System
Albert F Gilbert, PhD, President/CEO
525 E Market St
Akron, OH 44309-2090
330 375-3101
- Radiographer

University of Akron
Marion Ruebel, PhD, President
302 E Buchtel Ave
Akron, OH 44325-4702
330 972-7074
- Audiologist
- Dietitian/Nutritionist
- Medical Assistant
- Respiratory Therapist
- Speech Language Pathologist
- Surgical Technologist

Ashland

Ashland County-West Holmes Career Center
David A Kovach, BS MEd, Superintendent
1783 State Rte 60
Ashland, OH 44805
419 289-3313
- Medical Assistant

Athens

Ohio University Main Campus

Robert Glidden, President
Athens, OH 45701
614 593-1000
- Audiologist
- Dietitian/Nutritionist
- Music Therapist
- Rehabilitation Counselor
- Speech Language Pathologist

Berea

Baldwin-Wallace College

Neal Malicky, President
275 Eastland Rd
Berea, OH 44017
216 826-2900
- Music Therapist

Bluffton

Bluffton College

Elmer Neufeld, President
280 W College Ave
Bluffton, OH 45817
419 358-3000
- Dietitian/Nutritionist

Bowling Green

Bowling Green State University

Sidney A Ribeau, PhD, President
220 McFall Ctr
Bowling Green, OH 43403
419 372-2211
- Audiologist
- Clin Lab Scientist/Med Tech
- Dietitian/Nutritionist
- Health Information Tech
- Rehabilitation Counselor
- Respiratory Therapist
- Speech Language Pathologist

Canton

Aultman Hospital

Richard J Pryce, MBA, President
2600 Sixth St SW
Canton, OH 44710
330 438-6241
- Diagnostic Med Sonographer
- Nuclear Medicine Tech
- Radiation Therapist
- Radiographer

Stark State College of Technology

John J McGrath, EdD, President
6200 Frank Ave NW
Canton, OH 44720-7299
330 494-6170
- Clin Lab Tech/Med Lab Tech-AD
- Health Information Tech
- Medical Assistant
- Occupational Therapy Asst
- Respiratory Therapist

Timken Mercy Medical Center

Jack W Topoleski, MHA, President/CEO
1320 Timken Mercy Dr NW
Canton, OH 44708
330 489-1001
- Radiographer

Chesapeake

Collins Career Center

Perry Walls, MS Ed, Superintendent
11627 State Rte 243
Chesapeake, OH 45619
614 867-6641
- Respiratory Therapy Tech

Cincinnati

Christ Hospital

Jack Cook, MHA, President
2139 Auburn Ave
Cincinnati, OH 45219
513 369-2201
- Dietitian/Nutritionist
- Perfusionist

Cincinnati State Tech and Comm College

Jean Patrice Herrington, PhD, Interim President
3520 Central Pkwy
Cincinnati, OH 45223
513 569-1511
- Clin Lab Tech/Med Lab Tech-AD
- Dietetic Technician
- Health Information Tech
- Medical Assistant
- Occupational Therapy Asst
- Respiratory Therapist
- Surgical Technologist

Good Samaritan Hospital

375 Dixmyth Ave
Cincinnati, OH 45220-2489
513 872-1983
- Dietitian/Nutritionist

Southern Ohio College - Woodlawn

G Stephen Coppock, EdD, Director
1011 Glendale-Milford Rd
Cincinnati, OH 45215-1107
513 771-2424
- Medical Assistant

Univ Affl Cincinnati for Devel Disorders

Children's Hospital Medical Ctr
Elland and Bethesda Aves
Cincinnati, OH 45229-2899
513 559-4614
- Dietitian/Nutritionist

Univ of Cincinnati

Joseph A Steger, PhD, President
President's Office
PO Box 210063
Cincinnati, OH 45221-0063
513 556-2201
- Audiologist
- Dental Hygienist
- Dietitian/Nutritionist
- Radiation Therapist
- Radiographer
- Speech Language Pathologist

University of Cincinnati Hospital

Karen Bankston, Admin/Patient Care Serv
University of Cincinnati Hospital
231 Bethesda Ave
Cincinnati, OH 45267-0769
513 558-5319
- Dietitian/Nutritionist
- Emergency Med Tech-Paramedic

University of Cincinnati Medical Center

Joseph A Steger, PhD, President
Admin Bldg
Cincinnati, OH 45221-0063
513 556-2201
- Clin Lab Scientist/Med Tech
- Nuclear Medicine Tech
- Specialist in BB Tech

Xavier University

Rev James E Hoff, SJ PhD, President
3800 Victory Pkwy
Cincinnati, OH 45207-2111
513 745-3501
- Occupational Therapist
- Radiographer

Cleveland

Amer RC Blood Services Northern Ohio Reg

David H Plate, Principal Officer
3747 Euclid Ave
Cleveland, OH 44115
216 431-3152
- Specialist in BB Tech

Case-Western Reserve University

Agnar Pytte, President
University Circle
Cleveland, OH 44106
216 368-2000
- Anesthesiologist Asst
- Dietitian/Nutritionist
- Speech Language Pathologist

Cleveland Clinic Foundation

Floyd D Loop, MD, Chair
(H18)
9500 Euclid Ave
Cleveland, OH 44195-5108
216 444-2300
- Clin Lab Scientist/Med Tech
- Dietitian/Nutritionist
- Perfusionist
- Radiation Therapist

Cleveland State University

Claire Van Ummersen, PhD, President
Euclid Ave at E 24th St
Rhodes Tower 1207
Cleveland, OH 44115-2440
216 687-3544
- Audiologist
- Occupational Therapist
- Speech Language Pathologist

Cleveland Veterans Affairs Med Ctr

10701 E Blvd
Cleveland, OH 44106-1702
216 421-3028
- Dietitian/Nutritionist

Institutions

Cuyahoga Community College

Jerry Sue Thorton, PhD, President
District Administration
700 Carnegie Ave
Cleveland, OH 44115-3196
216 987-4850
- Cardiovascular Technologist
- Clin Lab Tech/Med Lab Tech-AD
- Dental Assistant
- Dental Hygienist
- Dental Lab Technician
- Dietetic Technician
- Health Information Tech
- Medical Assistant
- Occupational Therapy Asst
- Physician Assistant
- Radiographer
- Respiratory Therapist

MetroHealth Medical Center

Terry R White, MBA, President/CEO
2500 Metro Health Dr
Cleveland, OH 44109-1998
216 459-5700
- Diagnostic Med Sonographer
- Dietitian/Nutritionist

MTI Business College

Charles M Kramer, BS, President
1140 Euclid Ave 2nd Flr
Cleveland, OH 44115-1603
216 621-8228
- Medical Assistant

St Luke's Medical Center

Sam Houston, MA, President
11311 Shaker Blvd
Cleveland, OH 44104
216 368-7000
- Cytotechnologist

University Hospitals of Cleveland

Farah M Walters, MS, President/CEO
11100 Euclid Ave
Cleveland, OH 44106
216 844-7565
- Clin Lab Scientist/Med Tech
- Dietitian/Nutritionist
- Radiation Therapist

Columbus

Arthur G James Cancer Hosp & Res Inst

Dennis Smith, BS, Dir of Admin
300 W 10th Ave 519 CHRI
Columbus, OH 43210-1228
614 293-5485
- Radiation Therapist

Bradford School

Gary Pritchett, CEO
6170 Busch Blvd
Columbus, OH 43229
614 846-9410
- Medical Assistant

Capital University

Josiah Blackmore, JD, President
Yochum Hall
2199 E Main St
Columbus, OH 43209
614 236-6908
- Athletic Trainer

Columbus State Community College

Valeriana Moeller, PhD, President
550 E Spring St
PO Box 1609
Columbus, OH 43216-1609
614 227-2400
- Clin Lab Tech/Med Lab Tech-AD
- Dental Lab Technician
- Dietetic Technician
- Emergency Med Tech-Paramedic
- Health Information Tech
- Histologic Technician-Cert
- Respiratory Therapist
- Respiratory Therapy Tech

Mt Carmel College of Nursing

Ann E Schiele, President
127 S Davis Ave
Columbus, OH 43222
614 234-5800
- Dietitian/Nutritionist

Ohio State University

E Gordon Gee, PhD, President
190 N Oval Mall
Columbus, OH 43210-1234
614 292-2424
- Audiologist
- Clin Lab Scientist/Med Tech
- Dental Hygienist
- Dietitian/Nutritionist
- Health Information Admin
- Occupational Therapist
- Perfusionist
- Radiographer
- Rehabilitation Counselor
- Respiratory Therapist
- Speech Language Pathologist

Ohio State University Hospitals

R Reed Fraley, MBA, Assoc VP Health Services
450 W 10th Ave
Columbus, OH 43210
614 293-5555
- Nuclear Medicine Tech
- Specialist in BB Tech

Riverside Methodist Hospitals

Nancy M Schlichting, President/CEO
3535 Olentangy River Rd
Columbus, OH 43214
614 566-5424
- Dietitian/Nutritionist

Cuyahoga Falls

Akron Medical-Dental Institute

Ann C Kindleburg, BBA, School Director
1625 Portage Trail
Cuyahoga Falls, OH 44223
330 928-3400
- Medical Assistant

Dayton

Miami Valley Hospital

Karl R Tague, President/CEO
1 Wyoming St
Dayton, OH 45409
513 223-6192
- Dietitian/Nutritionist

Miami-Jacobs College

Charles Campbell, BA MBA, President
400 E Second St PO Box 1433
Dayton, OH 45401
513 461-5174
- Medical Assistant

Ohio Institute of Photography and Technology

Cecil W Johnston, MSEd, Executive Director
2029 Edgefield Rd
Dayton, OH 45439
513 294-6155
- Medical Assistant

Sinclair Community College

Ned J Sifferlen, EdD, Provost
444 W Third St
Dayton, OH 45402-1460
513 449-5300
- Dental Hygienist
- Dietetic Technician
- Health Information Tech
- Medical Assistant
- Occupational Therapy Asst
- Radiographer
- Respiratory Therapist

University of Dayton

Rev James Heft, PhD SM, Provost
300 College Pk
Dayton, OH 45469-0800
513 229-1000
- Dietitian/Nutritionist
- Music Therapist

Wright State University

Harley E Flack, PhD, President
113 Admin Wing
Dayton, OH 45435
513 873-2312
- Clin Lab Scientist/Med Tech
- Rehabilitation Counselor

East Liverpool

Ohio Valley Business College

Debra A Sanford, BS, President
500 Maryland St PO Box 7000
East Liverpool, OH 43920
330 385-1070
- Medical Assistant

Elyria

Lorain County Community College

Roy A Church, EdD, President
1005 N Abbe Rd
Elyria, OH 44035
216 366-4016
- Clin Lab Tech/Med Lab Tech-AD
- Diagnostic Med Sonographer
- Radiographer

Findlay

The University of Findlay

Kenneth Zirkle, EdD, President
1000 N Main St
Findlay, OH 45840
419 424-4510
- Nuclear Medicine Tech
- Occupational Therapist

Groveport

Fairfield Career Center (EVSD)

Claude Graves, MEd, Superintendent
4465 S Hamilton Rd
Groveport, OH 43125
614 836-5725
• Medical Assistant

Hillsboro

Southern State Community College

Lawrence N Dukes, EdD, President
200 Hobart Dr
Hillsboro, OH 45133
513 393-3431
• Medical Assistant

Kent

Kent State University

Carol A Cartwright, PhD, President
Office of the President
Kent, OH 44242-0001
330 672-2210
• Audiologist
• Dietitian/Nutritionist
• Occupational Therapy Asst
• Radiographer
• Rehabilitation Counselor
• Speech Language Pathologist

Kettering

Kettering College of Medical Arts

Peter D H Bath, DMin, President
3737 Southern Blvd
Kettering, OH 45429
513 296-7218
• Diagnostic Med Sonographer
• Physician Assistant
• Radiographer
• Respiratory Therapist

Kirtland

Lakeland Community College

Ralph R Doty, EdD, President
7700 Clocktower Dr
Kirtland, OH 44094-5198
216 953-7118
• Clin Lab Tech/Med Lab Tech-AD
• Dental Hygienist
• Radiographer
• Respiratory Therapist

Lima

Lima Technical College

James J Countryman, PhD, President
4240 Campus Dr
Lima, OH 45804
419 995-8200
• Dental Hygienist
• Dietetic Technician
• Radiographer
• Respiratory Therapist
• Respiratory Therapy Tech

Mansfield

North Central Technical College

Byron E Kee, EdD, President
2441 Kenwood Circle
PO Box 698
Mansfield, OH 44901
419 755-4800
• Radiographer
• Respiratory Therapist

Marietta

Marietta College

Lauren R Wilson, PhD, President
215 Fifth St
Marietta, OH 45750
614 376-4701
• Athletic Trainer

Marietta Memorial Hospital

Larry J Unroe, MHA, President
401 Matthew St
Marietta, OH 45750
614 374-1412
• Radiographer

Washington State Community College

Carson K Miller, PhD, CEO
710 Colegate Dr
Marietta, OH 45750
614 374-8716
• Clin Lab Tech/Med Lab Tech-AD

Marion

Marion General Hospital

Frank Swinehart, BS, President
McKinley Park Dr
Marion, OH 43302
614 383-8700
• Radiographer

Marion Technical College

J Richard Bryson, PhD, President
1467 Mt Vernon Ave
Marion, OH 43302
614 389-4636
• Clin Lab Tech/Med Lab Tech-AD

Mayfield Village

Meridia Health System

Charles B Miner, CEO & President
6700 Beta Drive, Suite 200
Mayfield Village, OH 44143
216 446-8260
• Radiographer

Medina

Medina County Career Center

Thomas Horwedel, Superintendent
1101 W Liberty St
Medina, OH 44256-9969
216 725-8461
• Medical Assistant

Middleburg Heights

Southwest General Health Center

L Jon Schurmeier, MA, President
18697 Bagley Rd
Middleburg Heights, OH 44130
216 816-6801
• Clin Lab Scientist/Med Tech
• Radiographer

Middletown

Middletown Regional Hospital

Douglas W McNeill, FACHE, President/CEO
105 McKnight Dr
Middletown, OH 45044-8787
513 420-5100
• Clin Lab Tech/Med Lab Tech-C

Mt St Joseph

College of Mount St Joseph

Sr Francis M Thrailkill, PhD OSH, Pres
5701 Delhi Pike
Mt St Joseph, OH 45051
513 244-4232
• Music Therapist

Mt Vernon

Knox County Career Center

Ray Richardson, Superintendent
306 Martinsburg Rd
Mt Vernon, OH 43050
614 397-5820
• Medical Assistant

Nelsonville

Hocking Technical College

John J Light, PhD, President
3301 Hocking Pkwy
Nelsonville, OH 45764
614 753-3591
• Dietetic Technician
• Health Information Tech
• Medical Assistant

Newark

Central Ohio Technical College

Rafael L Cortada, PhD, President
1179 University Dr
Newark, OH 43055-1767
614 366-9211
• Diagnostic Med Sonographer
• Radiographer

Oregon

St Charles Hospital

Kathleen Nelson, CEO
2600 Navarre Ave
Oregon, OH 43616
419 698-7341
• Clin Lab Scientist/Med Tech

Institutions

Oxford

Miami University
Paul G Risser, President
Oxford, OH 45056
513 529-1809
- Audiologist
- Dietitian/Nutritionist
- Speech Language Pathologist

Parma

Parma Community General Hospital
Thomas A Selden Jr, President and CEO
7007 Powers Blvd
Parma, OH 44129-5495
216 888-1800
- Emergency Med Tech-Paramedic

Pepper Pike

Ursuline College
Anne Marie Diederich, President
2550 Lander Rd
Pepper Pike, OH 44124
216 449-4200
- Art Therapist

Portsmouth

Shawnee State University
Clive C Veri, PhD, President
940 Second St
Portsmouth, OH 45662-4303
614 355-2202
- Clin Lab Tech/Med Lab Tech-AD
- Dental Hygienist
- Occupational Therapist
- Occupational Therapy Asst
- Radiographer
- Respiratory Therapist

Rio Grande

University of Rio Grande
Barry M Dorsey, PhD, President
Berry Ctr
Rio Grande, OH 45674
614 245-7204
- Clin Lab Tech/Med Lab Tech-AD

Sandusky

Providence Hospital, Inc
Sr Nancy Linenkugel, OSF, President
1912 Hayes Ave
Sandusky, OH 44870
419 621-7070
- Radiographer

South Euclid

Notre Dame College
Robert E Karsten, Interim President
4545 College Rd
South Euclid, OH 44121
216 381-1680
- Dietitian/Nutritionist

Springfield

Clark State Community College
Albert A Salerno, MA, President
570 E Leffel Ln
Springfield, OH 45505
513 328-6001
- Clin Lab Tech/Med Lab Tech-AD

Comm Hosp of Springfield & Clark County
Neal E Kresheck, MHA, President
2615 E High St
Springfield, OH 45501
513 325-0531
- Radiographer

St Clairsville

Belmont Technical College
W R Channell, PhD, President
120 Fox-Shannon Pl
St Clairsville, OH 43950
614 695-9500
- Medical Assistant

Steubenville

Jefferson Community College
Edward L Florak, EdD, President
4000 Sunset Blvd
Steubenville, OH 43952
614 264-5591
- Clin Lab Tech/Med Lab Tech-AD
- Dental Assistant
- Medical Assistant
- Radiographer
- Respiratory Therapist

Trinity Medical Center East
Fred Brower, MS, President
380 Summit Ave
Steubenville, OH 43952
614 283-7213
- Clin Lab Scientist/Med Tech

Sylvania

Lourdes College
Sr M A Francis Klimkowski, PhD, President
6832 Convent Blvd
Sylvania, OH 43560-2898
419 885-3211
- Occupational Therapy Asst

Toledo

Davis Junior College of Business
Diane Brunner, MEd, President/CEO
4747 Monroe St
Toledo, OH 43623
419 473-2700
- Medical Assistant

Medical College of Ohio
Frank S McCullough, MD, Acting President
3000 Arlington Ave
Toledo, OH 43614
419 381-4260
- Occupational Therapist

Owens Community College
Daniel H Brown, EdD, President
PO 10000 Oregon Rd
Toledo, OH 43699-1947
419 661-7000
- Dental Hygienist
- Diagnostic Med Sonographer
- Dietetic Technician
- Radiation Therapist
- Radiographer
- Surgical Technologist

Riverside Hospital
Scott E Shook, MBA, President/CEO
1600 N Superior St
Toledo, OH 43604
419 729-6059
- Clin Lab Scientist/Med Tech

St Vincent Medical Center
Steven C Mickus, President
2213 Cherry St
Toledo, OH 43608
419 321-4152
- Radiographer

University of Toledo
Frank E Horton, PhD, President
2801 W Bancroft St
Toledo, OH 43606
419 530-2211
- Athletic Trainer
- Cardiovascular Technologist
- Medical Assistant
- Respiratory Therapist
- Respiratory Therapy Tech
- Speech Language Pathologist
- Therapeutic Recreation Specialist

Worthington

Harding Graduate Clinical Art Therapy Prgm
445 E Granville Rd
Worthington, OH 43085
614 785-7443
- Art Therapist

Youngstown

St Elizabeth Health Center
Kevin Nolan, MHA, President/CEO
1044 Belmont Ave
Youngstown, OH 44501-1790
330 746-7211
- Clin Lab Scientist/Med Tech
- Cytotechnologist
- Nuclear Medicine Tech
- Radiographer

Western Reserve Care System
Gary Kaatz, President/CEO
345 Oak Hill Ave Corp Office
Youngstown, OH 44501
330 747-0777
- Clin Lab Scientist/Med Tech
- Radiographer

Youngstown Pub Sch/Choffin Career Center
Joseph Conley, Superintendent
20 W Wood St
Youngstown, OH 44501
330 744-6915
- Dental Assistant
- Surgical Technologist

Youngstown State University
Leslie H Cochran, EdD, President
One University Plaza
Youngstown, OH 44555
330 742-3106
- Clin Lab Tech/Med Lab Tech-AD
- Dental Hygienist
- Dietitian/Nutritionist
- Dietetic Technician
- Emergency Med Tech-Paramedic
- Medical Assistant
- Respiratory Therapist

Zanesville

Muskingum Area Technical College
Lynn H Willett, PhD, President
1555 Newark Rd
Zanesville, OH 43701-2694
614 454-2501
- Clin Lab Tech/Med Lab Tech-AD
- Dietetic Technician
- Medical Assistant
- Occupational Therapy Asst
- Radiographer

Oklahoma

Ada

East Central University
Bill S Cole, EdD, President
Ada, OK 74820
405 332-8000
- Health Information Admin
- Rehabilitation Counselor

Valley View Regional Hospital
Phillip H Fisher, MHA, President
Health Administration
430 N Monta Vista
Ada, OK 74820
405 332-2323
- Clin Lab Scientist/Med Tech

Edmond

University of Central Oklahoma
George Nigh, President
100 N University Dr
Edmond, OK 73034
405 341-2980
- Dietitian/Nutritionist
- Speech Language Pathologist

El Reno

Canadian Valley Area Vocational Tech Sch
Earl Cowan, EdD, Superintendent
6505 E Hwy 66
El Reno, OK 73036
405 262-2629
- Medical Assistant

Enid

O T Autry Area Voc Tech Center
James Strate, EdD, Superintendent
1201 W Willow
Enid, OK 73703
405 242-2750
- Radiographer
- Surgical Technologist

Phillips University
G Curtis Jones Jr, President
100 S University Ave
Enid, OK 73701
405 237-4433
- Music Therapist

ST. Mary's Hospital
Frank Lopez, CEO, Admin
305 S Fifth St PO Box 232
Enid, OK 73702-0232
405 233-6100
- Clin Lab Scientist/Med Tech

Langston

Langston University
Ernest L Holloway, President
Langston, OK 73050
405 466-2231
- Dietitian/Nutritionist

Lawton

Comanche County Memorial Hospital
Randy Curry, MHA, President
3401 W Gore Blvd Box 129
Lawton, OK 73502
405 355-8620
- Clin Lab Scientist/Med Tech

Great Plains Area Voc Tech School
James Nisbett, MSEd, Superintendent
4500 W Lee Blvd
Lawton, OK 73505
405 355-6371
- Radiographer
- Respiratory Therapy Tech
- Surgical Technologist

Miami

Northeastern Oklahoma A & M College
Jerry Carroll, MD, President
Second and I Sts NE
PO Box 1 Station 1
Miami, OK 74354
918 542-8441
- Clin Lab Tech/Med Lab Tech-AD
- Surgical Technologist

Midwest City

Rose State College
Larry Nutter, PhD, President
6420 SE 15th
Midwest City, OK 73110-2797
405 733-7300
- Clin Lab Tech/Med Lab Tech-AD
- Dental Assistant
- Dental Hygienist
- Health Information Tech
- Radiographer
- Respiratory Therapist

Muskogee

Bacone College
Dennis Tanner, PhD, President
Office of the President
Muskogee, OK 74403-1597
918 683-4581
- Radiographer

Muskogee Regional Medical Center
Bill Kennedy, MS, CEO
300 Rockefeller Dr
Muskogee, OK 74401
918 682-5501
- Clin Lab Scientist/Med Tech

Oklahoma City

Francis Tuttle Vocational Technical Ctr
Bruce Gray, MBA, Superintendent
12777 N Rockwell Ave
Oklahoma City, OK 73142
405 722-7799
- Respiratory Therapy Tech

Metro Area Vocational - Technical School
Kara Gae Wilson, EdD, Superintendent
1900 Springlake Dr
Oklahoma City, OK 73111
405 424-8324
- Radiographer
- Surgical Technologist

Oklahoma City Community College
Robert P Todd, EdD, President
7777 S May Ave
Oklahoma City, OK 73159-4444
405 682-7502
- Occupational Therapy Asst

St Anthony Hospital
Steve Hunter, President
1000 N Lee St PO Box 205
Oklahoma City, OK 73101
405 272-7273
- Clin Lab Scientist/Med Tech

Univ of Oklahoma Health Sciences Center
Joseph J Ferretti, PhD, SVP/Provost
University of Oklahoma at Oklahoma City
1000 Stanton L Young Blvd Rm 221
Oklahoma City, OK 73126-1090
405 271-2332
- Audiologist
- Cytotechnologist
- Dental Hygienist
- Diagnostic Med Sonographer
- Dietitian/Nutritionist
- Nuclear Medicine Tech
- Occupational Therapist
- Physician Assistant
- Radiation Therapist
- Radiographer
- Speech Language Pathologist

University Hospitals of Oklahoma City
R Timothy Coussons, MD, CEO
PO Box 26307
Oklahoma City, OK 73126
405 271-4000
- Clin Lab Scientist/Med Tech
- Cytotechnologist

Institutions

Okmulgee

Oklahoma State University - Okmulgee
Robert E Klabenes, Provost & Vice Pres
Okmulgee, OK 74447
918 756-6211
- Dietetic Technician

Seminole

Seminole State College
Jack Medlock, PhD, Interim President
PO Box 351
Seminole, OK 74818-0351
405 382-9950
- Clin Lab Tech/Med Lab Tech-AD

Stillwater

Meridian Technology Center
Fred A Shultz, EdD, Superintendent
1312 S Sangre St
Stillwater, OK 74074
405 377-3333
- Radiographer

Oklahoma State University Main Campus
James E Halligan, President
Stillwater, OK 74078
405 744-5000
- Dietitian/Nutritionist
- Speech Language Pathologist
- Therapeutic Recreation Specialist

Tahlequah

Northeastern State University
W Roger Webb, President
Tahlequah, OK 74464
918 456-5511
- Dietitian/Nutritionist
- Speech Language Pathologist

Tulsa

St Francis Hospital
James R Hardman, FACHE, CEO
6161 S Yale Ave
Tulsa, OK 74136
918 494-1370
- Clin Lab Scientist/Med Tech

Tulsa Community College
Dean P VanTrease, PhD, President
Central Office
6111 E Skelly Dr
Tulsa, OK 74135-6198
918 595-7000
- Clin Lab Tech/Med Lab Tech-AD
- Dental Hygienist
- Health Information Tech
- Medical Assistant
- Occupational Therapy Asst
- Radiographer
- Respiratory Therapist
- Respiratory Therapy Tech

Tulsa Technology Center
Gene Callahan, EdD, Superintendent
3420 S Memorial Dr
Tulsa, OK 74145-1390
918 627-7200
- Radiographer
- Surgical Technologist

University of Tulsa
Robert H Donaldson, President
600 S College Ave
Tulsa, OK 74104
918 631-2000
- Speech Language Pathologist

Weatherford

Southwestern Oklahoma State University
JoeAnna Hibler, EdD, President
100 Campus Dr
Weatherford, OK 73096
405 774-3766
- Health Information Admin
- Music Therapist
- Radiographer

Oregon

Albany

Linn-Benton Community College
Jon Carnahan, President
6500 SW Pacific Blvd
Albany, OR 97321
503 917-4999
- Dental Assistant

Bend

Central Oregon Community College
Robert Barber, EdD, President
NW College Way
Bend, OR 97701
503 382-6112
- Health Information Tech

Corvallis

Oregon State University
Paul Risser, PhD, President
Admin Services Bldg
Corvallis, OR 97331
541 737-2565
- Athletic Trainer
- Dietitian/Nutritionist

Eugene

Lane Community College
Jerry Moskus, PhD, President
4000 E 30th Ave
Eugene, OR 97405
541 747-4501
- Dental Assistant
- Dental Hygienist
- Respiratory Therapist

University of Oregon
David B Frohnmayer, President
Eugene, OR 97403
503 346-3111
- Speech Language Pathologist

Forest Grove

Pacific University
Faith Gabelnick, PhD, President
2043 College Way
Forest Grove, OR 97116-1797
503 357-6151
- Occupational Therapist

Grants Pass

Rogue Community College
Harvey Bennett, PhD, President
3345 Redwood Hwy
Grants Pass, OR 97527
503 471-3500
- Respiratory Therapist
- Respiratory Therapy Tech

Gresham

Mt Hood Community College
Joel Vela, PhD, President
26000 SE Stark St
Gresham, OR 97030-3300
503 667-7211
- Dental Hygienist
- Medical Assistant
- Occupational Therapy Asst
- Respiratory Therapist
- Surgical Technologist

Klamath Falls

Oregon Institute of Technology
Lawrence J Wolf, PhD, President
3201 Campus Dr
Klamath Falls, OR 97601-8801
503 885-1101
- Dental Hygienist
- Radiographer

Marylhurst

Marylhurst College
Nancy Wilgenbusch, President
PO Box 261
Marylhurst, OR 97036
503 636-8141
- Art Therapist

Monmouth

Western Oregon State College
Betty J Youngblood, President
345 N Monmouth Ave
Monmouth, OR 97361
503 838-8000
- Rehabilitation Counselor

Pendleton

Blue Mountain Community College
Ronald L Daniels, President
2411 NW Carden
Pendleton, OR 97801
541 276-1260
- Dental Assistant

Portland

CollegeAmerica
Mardell Lanfranco, Director
921 SW Washington Ste 200
Portland, OR 97205
503 242-9000
- Dental Assistant
- Medical Assistant

ConCorde Career Institute
1827 NE 44th Ave
Portland, OR 97213
503 281-4181
- Dental Assistant

Oregon Health Sciences University
Peter O Kohler, MD, President
3181 SW Sam Jackson Pk Rd/L101
Portland, OR 97201
503 494-8252
- Clin Lab Scientist/Med Tech
- Dental Hygienist
- Dietitian/Nutritionist
- Emergency Med Tech-Paramedic
- Physician Assistant
- Radiation Therapist

Portland Community College
Daniel F Moriarty, EdD, President
PO Box 19000
Portland, OR 97280-0990
503 977-4362
- Clin Lab Tech/Med Lab Tech-AD
- Dental Assistant
- Dental Hygienist
- Dental Lab Technician
- Dietetic Technician
- Health Information Tech
- Medical Assistant
- Ophthalmic Dispenser
- Ophthalmic Med Technician
- Radiographer

Portland State University
Judith A Ramaley, President
Portland, OR 97207-0751
503 725-3000
- Audiologist
- Rehabilitation Counselor
- Speech Language Pathologist

Providence/St. Vincent & Medical Center
Don S Elson, COO,
Administration 9205 SW Barnes Rd
Portland, OR 97225
503 216-3031
- Perfusionist

Veterans Administration Medical Center
Barry L Bell, Director
PO Box 1034
Portland, OR 97207
503 220-8262
- Nuclear Medicine Tech

Salem

Chemeketa Community College
Gerald Berger, EdD, President
4000 Lancaster Dr NE PO Box 14007
Salem, OR 97309
503 399-5121
- Dental Assistant
- Medical Assistant

Mid Willamette Vlly Dietetec Internship
Capital Manor Retirement Community
1955 Dallas Hwy NW Ste 1200
Salem, OR 97304
503 362-4101
- Dietitian/Nutritionist

Willamette University
Jerry E Hudson, President
900 State St
Salem, OR 97301
503 370-6300
- Music Therapist

Pennsylvania

Abington

Abington Memorial Hospital
Felix M Pilla, MS, President
1200 Old York Rd
Abington, PA 19001
215 576-2000
- Clin Lab Scientist/Med Tech
- Radiographer

Aliquippa

Aliquippa Hospital
Charles Van Sluyter, MS, Pres/CEO
2500 Hospital Dr
Aliquippa, PA 15001
412 857-1224
- Radiographer

Allentown

Cedar Crest College
Dorothy G Blaney, PhD, President
100 College Dr
Allentown, PA 18104-6196
610 437-4471
- Dietitian/Nutritionist
- Nuclear Medicine Tech

Lehigh Valley Hospital
Elliot J Sussman, MD MBA, President/CEO
Cedar Crest and I-78
PO Box 689
Allentown, PA 18105-1556
610 402-2204
- Radiographer

Sacred Heart Hospital
Joseph M Cimerola, MHA MBA, Chief Executive Officer
421 Chew St
Allentown, PA 18102-3490
610 776-4900
- Clin Lab Scientist/Med Tech
- Surgical Technologist

The Wood Company
PO Box 3501
6081 Hamilton Blvd
Allentown, PA 18106-0501
610 395-3800
- Dietitian/Nutritionist

Altoona

Altoona Hospital
James W Barner, MBA, President/CEO
620 Howard Ave
Altoona, PA 16601-4899
814 946-2223
- Clin Lab Scientist/Med Tech

Mercy Regional Health System
David J Davies, CEO
2500 Seventh Ave
Altoona, PA 16603-2099
814 944-4101
- Radiation Therapist
- Radiographer

Aston

Neumann College
Rosalie Mirenda, DNSC, President
One Neumann Way
Aston, PA 19014
610 558-5501
- Clin Lab Scientist/Med Tech

Beaver

The Medical Center Beaver PA, Inc
Larry Crowell, President
1000 Dutch Ridge Rd
Beaver, PA 15009
412 728-7000
- Radiographer

Bethlehem

Northampton Community College
Robert J Kopecek, EdD, President
3835 Green Pond Rd
Bethlehem, PA 18017
610 861-5458
- Dental Hygienist
- Radiographer

Bloomsburg

Bloomsburg University
Jessica S Kozloff, President
Bloomsburg, PA 17815
717 389-4000
- Audiologist
- Speech Language Pathologist

Blue Bell

Montgomery County Community College
Edward M Sweitzer, PhD, President
340 DeKalb Pike
218 College Hall
Blue Bell, PA 19422
215 641-6501
- Clin Lab Tech/Med Lab Tech-AD
- Dental Hygienist

Bradford

Bradford Regional Medical Center
George E Leonhardt, President/CEO
116 Interstate Pkwy PO Box 0218
Bradford, PA 16701-0218
814 368-4143
● Radiographer

Bryn Mawr

Harcum College
Patricia Ryan, EdD, President
750 Montgomery Ave
Bryn Mawr, PA 19010
610 525-4100
● Clin Lab Tech/Med Lab Tech-AD
● Dental Assistant
● Dental Hygienist
● Occupational Therapy Asst

Butler

Butler County Community College
Frederick F Bartok, PhD, President
PO Box 1203
Butler, PA 16003-1203
412 287-8711
● Medical Assistant

California

California University of Pennsylvania
Angelo Armenti Jr, President
California, PA 15419
412 938-4000
● Speech Language Pathologist

Camp Hill

Holy Spirit Hospital
Romaine Niemeyer, MHA, President
503 N 21st St
Camp Hill, PA 17011-2288
717 763-2106
● Radiographer

Chambersburg

Chambersburg Hospital
Norman B Epstein, MBA, President
112 N Seventh St
PO Box 187
Chambersburg, PA 17201-0187
717 267-7138
● Clin Lab Tech/Med Lab Tech-C
● Radiographer

Clarion

Clarion University of Pennsylvania
Diane L Reinhard, President
Clarion, PA 16214
814 226-2000
● Audiologist
● Speech Language Pathologist

Clearfield

Clearfield Hospital
Stephen A Wolfe, MS, President/CEO
PO Box 992
Clearfield, PA 16830
814 768-2496
● Radiographer

Coatesville

Brandywine Hospital
James H Thornton, President/CEO
201 Reeceville Rd
Coatesville, PA 19320
610 383-8000
● Radiographer

Coraopolis

Robert Morris Coll/Ohio Valley Gen Hosp
Narrows Run Rd
Coraopolis, PA 15108
412 777-6210
● Radiographer

Cresson

Mt Aloysius College
Edward F Pierce, EdD PD, President
7373 Admiral Peary Hwy
Cresson, PA 16630
814 886-6411
● Clin Lab Tech/Med Lab Tech-AD
● Medical Assistant
● Occupational Therapy Asst
● Surgical Technologist

Dallas

College Misericordia
Albert B Anderson, PhD, President
301 Lake St
Dallas, PA 18612-1098
717 674-6216
● Occupational Therapist
● Radiographer

Danville

Geisinger Medical Center
Stuart Heydt, MD, President
100 N Academy Ave
Danville, PA 17822-2201
717 271-5200
● Cardiovascular Technologist
● Clin Lab Scientist/Med Tech
● Dietitian/Nutritionist
● Histologic Technician-Cert
● Radiographer

East Stroudsburg

East Stroudsburg University
James E Gilbert, PhD, President
200 Prospect St
East Stroudsburg, PA 18301
717 422-3545
● Athletic Trainer

Edinboro

Edinboro University of Pennsylvania
Foster F Diebold, President
Edinboro, PA 16444
814 732-2000
● Dietitian/Nutritionist
● Rehabilitation Counselor
● Speech Language Pathologist

Elizabethtown

Elizabethtown College
Theodore E Long, PhD, President
One Alpha Dr
Elizabethtown, PA 17022-2298
717 361-1193
● Music Therapist
● Occupational Therapist

Elkins Park

Allegheny University Hospitals Elkins Park
Meg McGoldrick, MBA, Exec Director/CEO
60 E Township Line Rd
Elkins Park, PA 19027
215 663-6150
● Clin Lab Scientist/Med Tech
● Radiographer

Erie

Gannon University
Rev Msgr David A Rubino, PhD, President
University Square
Erie, PA 16541-0001
814 871-5800
● Dietitian/Nutritionist
● Occupational Therapist
● Physician Assistant
● Radiographer
● Respiratory Therapist

Mercyhurst College
William P Harvey, President
501 E 38th St
Erie, PA 16546
814 824-2200
● Dietitian/Nutritionist

St Vincent Health Center
Sr Catherine Manning, MBA, President
232 W 25th St
Erie, PA 16544
814 452-5111
● Clin Lab Scientist/Med Tech

Franklin

Northwest Medical Center-Franklin Campus
Michael Reichfield, MHA, President/COO
One Spruce St
Franklin, PA 16323
814 437-7000
● Radiographer

Grantham

Messiah College
Rodney J Sawatsky, PhD, President
Grantham, PA 17027
717 766-2511
● Athletic Trainer
● Dietitian/Nutritionist

Greensburg

Seton Hill College
JoAnne W Boyle, President
Greensburg, PA 15601
412 834-2200
- Dietitian/Nutritionist

Greenville

Thiel College
C Carlyle Haaland, PhD, President
75 College Ave
Greenville, PA 16125
412 589-2100
- Respiratory Therapy Tech

Gwynedd Valley

Gwynedd-Mercy College
Sr Linda Bevilacqua, PhD, President
Sumneytown Pike
Gwynedd Valley, PA 19437
215 641-5560
- Cardiovascular Technologist
- Health Information Admin
- Health Information Tech
- Radiation Therapist
- Respiratory Therapist
- Respiratory Therapy Tech

Harrisburg

Harrisburg Area Community College
Paul B Hurley Jr, PhD, President
One HACC Dr
Harrisburg, PA 17110-2999
717 780-2340
- Clin Lab Tech/Med Lab Tech-AD
- Dental Assistant
- Dental Hygienist
- Emergency Med Tech-Paramedic
- Respiratory Therapist
- Respiratory Therapy Tech

Health Hospitals/Polyclinic Hospital
Stephen F Franklin, MS FACHE, Pres/CEO
P. O. Box 8700
Harrisburg, PA 17105-8700
717 231-8180
- Clin Lab Scientist/Med Tech
- Radiographer

Thompson Learning Corporation
Rita Girondi, EdD, President
5650 Derry St
Harrisburg, PA 17111
717 564-6993
- Medical Assistant

Hazleton

Hazleton-St Joseph Medical Center
Bernard C Rudegeair, FACHA, President/CEO
687 N Church St
Hazleton, PA 18201-3198
717 459-4444
- Radiographer

Penn State University - Hazleton
David Orbid, PhD, Campus Exec Off
Hazleton, PA 18201
717 450-3033
- Clin Lab Tech/Med Lab Tech-AD

Hershey

M S Hershey Med Center/Penn State Univ
Bruce H Hamory, MD, COO of HMC/Exec Dir
PO Box 850
Hershey, PA 17033
717 531-8803
- Perfusionist

Penn State University - Hershey
Bruce Hamary, MD, Chief Operating Officer
500 University Dr
Hershey, PA 17033
610 799-2121
- Radiographer

Immaculata

Immaculata College
Marie Roseanne, President
Immaculata, PA 19345
610 647-4400
- Dietitian/Nutritionist

Jeannette

Monsour Medical Center
Jerry A Joseph, MBA, Administrator
70 Lincoln Way E
Jeannette, PA 15644
412 527-0600
- Radiographer

Jenkintown

Manor Junior College
Sr Mary Cecilia, OSBM, President
700 Fox Chase Rd
Jenkintown, PA 19046
215 885-2360
- Clin Lab Tech/Med Lab Tech-AD
- Dental Assistant
- Dental Hygienist

Johnstown

Conemaugh Valley Memorial Hospital
Timothy J Karnes, MHA, President
1086 Franklin St
Johnstown, PA 15905
814 534-9000
- Clin Lab Scientist/Med Tech
- Clin Lab Tech/Med Lab Tech-C
- Histologic Technician-Cert
- Radiographer
- Surgical Technologist

Greater Johnstown Area Voc - Tech School
Barry Dallara, MA, Administrative Dir
445 Schoolhouse Rd
Johnstown, PA 15904-2998
814 269-3874
- Respiratory Therapy Tech

Lee Hospital
John W Ungar, FACHA, President
320 Main St
Johnstown, PA 15901
814 533-0821
- Dietitian/Nutritionist
- Radiographer

University of Pittsburgh - Johnstown
Albert L Etheridge, PhD, President
153 Biddle Hall
Johnstown, PA 15904
814 269 2090
- Respiratory Therapist

Kittanning

Armstrong County Memorial Hospital
Jack Gary, President/CEO
One Nolte Dr
Kittanning, PA 16201
412 543-8404
- Radiographer

Lancaster

Lancaster Institute for Health Education
Michael A Young, MHA, President/CEO
Lancaster General Hospital
PO Box 3555
Lancaster, PA 17603
717 290-5511
- Cardiovascular Technologist
- Clin Lab Scientist/Med Tech
- Diagnostic Med Sonographer
- Nuclear Medicine Tech
- Radiographer
- Surgical Technologist

St Joseph Hospital
John T Tolmie, MHA, President/CEO
250 College Ave PO Box 3509
Lancaster, PA 17604
717 291-8123
- Emergency Med Tech-Paramedic

Latrobe

Latrobe Area Hospital
Douglas A Clark, FACHE, Exec Director
W Second Ave
Latrobe, PA 15650
412 537-1001
- Clin Lab Scientist/Med Tech

Lincoln University

Lincoln University
Niara Sudarkasa, President
Lincoln University, PA 19352
610 932-8300
- Therapeutic Recreation Specialist

Lock Haven

Lock Haven University
Craig Dean Willis, PhD, President
Sullivan 202
Lock Haven, PA 17745
717 893-2000
- Athletic Trainer

Loretto

St Francis College
Christian R Oravec, TOR, President
PO Box 600
Loretto, PA 15940
814 472-3000
- Physician Assistant

Institutions

Mansfield

Mansfield University
Rodney C Kelchner, MS, President
Mansfield, PA 16933
717 662-4046
- Dietitian/Nutritionist
- Music Therapist
- Radiographer
- Respiratory Therapist

Media

Crozer-Chester Med Ctr/Delaware Co CC
Richard D DeDosmo, President
901 S Media Lane Road
Media, PA 19063-5000
610 359-5000
- Electroneurodiagnostic Tech
- Radiographer
- Respiratory Therapist

Delaware County Community College
Richard D DeCosmo, EdD, President
901 S Media Line Rd
Media, PA 19603-1094
610 359-5100
- Medical Assistant
- Surgical Technologist

Millersville

Millersville University of Pennsylvania
Joseph A Caputo, PhD, President
Biemesderfer Executive Ctr
Millersville, PA 17551
717 872-3592
- Respiratory Therapist

Monaca

Community College of Beaver County
Margaret Williams-Betlyn, PhD, President
College Dr
Monaca, PA 15061
412 775-8561
- Clin Lab Tech/Med Lab Tech-AD

Monroeville

Career Training Academy, Inc
John M Reddy, BS, President
ExpoMart
105 Mall Blvd/Ste 300-W
Monroeville, PA 15146
412 372-3900
- Medical Assistant

Nanticoke

Luzerne County Community College
Thomas Moran, MS, President
Prospect St and Middle Rd
Nanticoke, PA 18634
717 829-7385
- Dental Assistant
- Dental Hygienist
- Respiratory Therapy Tech

Natrona Heights

Allegheny Valley Hospital
John R England, MBA, President/CEO
1301 Carlisle St
Natrona Heights, PA 15065
412 226-7000
- Radiographer

New Castle

St Francis Hospital of New Castle
Sr Donna Zwigart, MA, CEO
1000 S Mercer St
New Castle, PA 16101
412 658-3511
- Radiographer

New Kensington

Penn State Univ - New Kensington Campus
Catherine Gannon, PhD, Campus Exec
3550 Seventh St Rd
New Kensington, PA 15068
412 339-6050
- Clin Lab Tech/Med Lab Tech-AD
- Radiographer

Philadelphia

Albert Einstein Medical Center
Martin G Goldsmith, MBA, President
5501 Old York Rd
Philadelphia, PA 19141-3098
215 456-7010
- Radiographer

Allegheny University of the Health Sciences
Sherif S Abdelhak, President
Broad and Vine Sts
Philadelphia, PA 19102-1192
215 762-8450
- Art Therapist
- Clin Lab Scientist/Med Tech
- Clin Lab Tech/Med Lab Tech-AD
- Music Therapist
- Perfusionist
- Physician Assistant
- Radiographer

Community College of Philadelphia
Frederick W Capshaw, PhD, President
1700 Spring Garden St
Philadelphia, PA 19130
215 751-8028
- Clin Lab Tech/Med Lab Tech-AD
- Dental Assistant
- Dental Hygienist
- Dietetic Technician
- Health Information Tech
- Medical Assistant
- Radiographer
- Respiratory Therapist

Drexel University
Constantine N Papadakis, President
32nd and Chestnut Sts
Philadelphia, PA 19104
215 895-2000
- Dietitian/Nutritionist

Episcopal Hospital
Mark Bateman, President
Front & Lehigh Ave
Philadelphia, PA 19125
215 427-7168
- Perfusionist

Germantown Hospital & Medical Center
David A Ricci, President
One Penn Blvd
Philadelphia, PA 19144
215 951-8000
- Radiographer

Holy Family College
Sr M Francesca Onley, PhD CSFN, Pres
Grant and Frankford Aves
Philadelphia, PA 19114
215 637-7700
- Radiographer

Marriott/Health Care Svcs-Philadelphia
Graduate Hospital
One Graduate Plaza
Philadelphia, PA 19146
215 893-2553
- Dietitian/Nutritionist

Nazareth Hospital
Daniel J Sinnott,
2601 Holme Ave
Philadelphia, PA 19152
215 335-6000
- Clin Lab Scientist/Med Tech

Pennsylvania Hospital
John R Ball, MD JD, President
800 Spruce St
Philadelphia, PA 19107
215 829-3312
- Clin Lab Scientist/Med Tech

Philadelphia College of Textiles and Science
James P Gallagher, PhD, President
School House Ln and Henry Ave
Philadelphia, PA 19144
215 951-2970
- Physician Assistant

Temple University
Peter J Liacouras, LLM, President
Executive Office of the President
Broad St and Montgomery Ave
Philadelphia, PA 19122
215 204-7000
- Athletic Trainer
- Audiologist
- Health Information Admin
- Music Therapist
- Occupational Therapist
- Speech Language Pathologist
- Therapeutic Recreation Specialist

Temple University Hospital
Leon S Malmud, MD, CEO
Broad and Ontario Sts
Philadelphia, PA 19140
215 221-4638
- Radiographer

Thomas Jefferson University

Paul C Brucker, MD, President
1020 Walnut St
641 Scott Bldg
Philadelphia, PA 19107-5587
215 503-6617
● Clin Lab Scientist/Med Tech
● Cytotechnologist
● Diagnostic Med Sonographer
● Occupational Therapist
● Radiographer

Pittsburgh

Allegheny General Hospital

Anthony M Sanzo, MHA, President/CEO
320 E North Ave
Pittsburgh, PA 15212
412 359-5000
● Clin Lab Scientist/Med Tech

Bradford School-Pittsburgh

Vincent Graziano, MBA, President
Gulf Tower
707 Grant St
Pittsburgh, PA 15219
412 391-6710
● Medical Assistant

Chatham College

Esther L Barazzone, PhD, President
Woodland Rd
Pittsburgh, PA 15232-2826
412 365-1100
● Occupational Therapist

Ctr for Emer Med of Western Pennsylvania

Donald Goodman, COO/CFO
230 McKee Pl Ste 500
Pittsburgh, PA 15213
412 578-3200
● Emergency Med Tech-Paramedic

Duffs Business Institute

Mark A Scott, Director
110 Ninth St
Pittsburgh, PA 15222
412 261-4520
● Medical Assistant

Duquesne University

John E Murray Jr, JD, President
600 Forbes Ave
Administration Bldg Rm 510
Pittsburgh, PA 15282
412 396-6060
● Athletic Trainer
● Health Information Admin
● Music Therapist
● Occupational Therapist
● Perfusionist
● Physician Assistant

Family Health Council Inc

625 Stanwix St
Pittsburgh, PA 15222-1417
412 288-9039
● Dietitian/Nutritionist

ICM School of Business and Medical Careers

Gerry Kosentos, Executive Director
10 Wood St
Pittsburgh, PA 15222
412 261-2647
● Medical Assistant

Indiana University of Pennsylvania

Charles M O'Brien Jr, President and CEO
West Penn Hospital
4800 Friendship Ave
Pittsburgh, PA 15224
412 578-5000
● Dietitian/Nutritionist
● Respiratory Therapist
● Speech Language Pathologist

Marriott Corp/St Francis Med Ctr

Thomas Wiles, Acting Chair
45th St off Penn Ave
Pittsburgh, PA 15201
412 622-4212
● Dietitian/Nutritionist

Median School of Allied Health Careers

Frances D Mosle, CEO, President
125 Seventh St
Pittsburgh, PA 15222
412 391-0422
● Dental Assistant
● Medical Assistant

Point Park College/St Francis Med Ctr

Mark O Farrell, PhD, Chair
School of Respiratory Care
201 Wood St
Pittsburgh, PA 15222
412 392-3879
● Respiratory Therapy Tech

Robert Morris College/Allegheny Gen Hosp

Anthony M Sanzo, MHA, President/CEO
320 E North Ave
Pittsburgh, PA 15212
412 359-5000
● Radiographer

Sawyer School

Thomas B Sapienza, MS, President
717 Liberty Ave
Pittsburgh, PA 15222
412 261-5700
● Health Information Tech
● Medical Assistant

Shadyside Hospital

Henry Mordoh, President
5230 Centre Ave
Pittsburgh, PA 15232
412 622-2010
● Dietitian/Nutritionist
● Perfusionist

U Hlth Ctr Pittsburgh/Magee Women's Hosp

Irma Goertzen, MS, CEO
Magee Women's Hospital
300 Halket St
Pittsburgh, PA 15213
412 641-4664
● Cytotechnologist

University of Pittsburgh

Mark A Nordenberg, JD, Chancellor
Rm 107 Cathedral of Learning
Pittsburgh, PA 15260
412 624-4200
● Audiologist
● Clin Lab Scientist/Med Tech
● Dental Hygienist
● Dietitian/Nutritionist
● Health Information Admin
● Occupational Therapist
● Rehabilitation Counselor
● Speech Language Pathologist

University of Pittsburgh Medical Center

Jeff Romoff,
200 Lothrop St
PIttsburgh, PA 15213-2582
412 647-3528
● Radiographer

Western Sch of Hlth & Business Careers

Ross M Perilman, MA CCC, President
Pittsburgh Campus
421 Seventh Ave
Pittsburgh, PA 15219-1907
412 281-2600
● Diagnostic Med Sonographer
● Histologic Technician-AD
● Radiographer
● Respiratory Therapist

Radnor

ARAMARK Healthcare Support Services

Mid-Atlantic Reg/Great Philadelphia Area
Three Radnor Corporate
Radnor, PA 19087
610 687-8600
● Dietitian/Nutritionist

Reading

Community General Hospital

S Michael Francis, MPA, President/CEO
145 N Sixth St PO Box 1728
Reading, PA 19603
215 376-2100
● Radiographer

Reading Area Community College

Gust Zogas, EdD, President
10 S Second St PO Box 1706
Reading, PA 19603
610 372-4721
● Clin Lab Tech/Med Lab Tech-AD
● Respiratory Therapist
● Respiratory Therapy Tech

Reading Hospital and Medical Center

Charles Sullivan, MS, President
PO Box 16052
Reading, PA 19612-6052
610 378-6664
● Clin Lab Scientist/Med Tech
● Radiographer

St Joseph Hospital

Patrick Roche, President/CEO
12th and Walnut Sts
PO Box 316
Reading, PA 19603
610 378-2000
● Radiographer

Institutions

Sayre

Robert Packer Hospital
Russell M Knight, MSHA, President
Guthrie Square
Sayre, PA 18840
717 888-6666
● Clin Lab Scientist/Med Tech

Schnecksville

Lehigh Carbon Community College
James Davis, EdD, President
4525 Education Pk Dr
Schnecksville, PA 18078-2598
610 799-2121
● Health Information Tech
● Medical Assistant
● Occupational Therapy Asst
● Respiratory Therapist
● Respiratory Therapy Tech

Schuylkill Haven

Penn State University - Schuylkill
Wayne D Lammie, PhD, Campus Exec Dir
200 University Dr
Schuylkill Haven, PA 17972-2208
717 385-6000
● Radiographer

Scranton

Community Medical Center
C Richard Hartman, MD, President-CEO
1822 Mulberry St
Scranton, PA 18510
717 969-8241
● Radiographer

Marywood College
Mary Reap, President
Scranton, PA 18509
717 348-6211
● Art Therapist
● Dietitian/Nutritionist
● Music Therapist

Scranton Medical Technology Consortium
Harold E Anderson, President
Moses Taylor Hospital
700 Quincy Ave
Scranton, PA 18510
717 963-2100
● Clin Lab Scientist/Med Tech

University of Scranton
J A Panuska, SJ, President
Scranton, PA 18510
717 941-7400
● Rehabilitation Counselor

Sewickley

Sewickley Valley Hospital
Donald W Spalding, FACHE MFHA, President
Blackburn Rd
Sewickley, PA 15143
412 741-6600
● Radiographer

Sharon

Sharon Regional Health System
Wayne Johnston, MHA, President
740 E State St
Sharon, PA 16146
412 983-3911
● Radiographer

Slippery Rock

Slippery Rock University
Robert Aebersold, PhD, President
300 Old Main
Slippery Rock, PA 16057
412 738-2000
● Athletic Trainer
● Music Therapist

Somerset

Somerset Hospital
Michael J Farrell, Administrator
225 S Ctr Ave
Somerset, PA 15501
814 443-5221
● Radiographer

St Davids

Eastern College
Roberta Hestenes, BA, President
10 Fairview Dr
St Davids, PA 19087-3696
610 341-5890
● Cardiovascular Technologist

State College

South Hills Business School
S Paul Mazza, JD, President
480 Waupelani Dr
State College, PA 16801
814 234-7755
● Health Information Tech

Summerdale

Central Pennsylvania Business School
Todd A Milano, BS, President
Campus on College Hill Rd
Summerdale, PA 17093-0309
717 732-0702
● Medical Assistant

University Park

Penn State University
Graham Spanier, President
201 Old Main
University Park, PA 16802
814 865-7611
● Occupational Therapy Asst

Penn State University - Main Campus
Joab L Thomas, President
201 Old Main
University Park, PA 16802
814 865-4700
● Audiologist
● Dietitian/Nutritionist
● Dietetic Technician
● Rehabilitation Counselor
● Speech Language Pathologist

Washington

Washington Hospital
Telford W Thomas, MHA, President/CEO
155 Wilson Ave
Washington, PA 15301
412 223-3007
● Clin Lab Scientist/Med Tech
● Radiographer

West Chester

West Chester University
Madeleine Wing Adler, PhD, President
102 Phillips Hall
West Chester, PA 19383
610 436-2471
● Athletic Trainer
● Respiratory Therapist
● Speech Language Pathologist

West Mifflin

Comm Coll of Allegheny Cnty-Alleg Campus
James C Holmberg, PhD, VP for Academic Affairs
1750 Clairton Road
West Mifflin, PA 15122-3097
412 469-6300
● Dietetic Technician
● Health Information Tech
● Medical Assistant
● Nuclear Medicine Tech
● Radiation Therapist
● Respiratory Therapist

Comm Coll of Allegheny Cnty-Boyce Campus
James C Holnberg, PhD, VP of Academic Affairs
Community College of Allegheny County
1750 Clairton Rd
West Mifflin, PA 15122-3097
412 469-6300
● Diagnostic Med Sonographer
● Occupational Therapy Asst
● Radiographer
● Surgical Technologist

Comm Coll of Allegheny Cnty-South Campus
James Holmberg, PhD, VP President Exec Dean
1750 Clairton Rd
West Mifflin, PA 15122
412 469-6300
● Clin Lab Tech/Med Lab Tech-AD

Wilkes-Barre

King's College
Rev James Lackenmier, CSC, President
133 N River St
Wilkes-Barre, PA 18711
717 826-5899
● Physician Assistant

Wilkes-Barre General Hospital
Steven C Bjelich, MHA, Executive Director
N River and Auburn Sts
Wilkes-Barre, PA 18764
717 829-8111
● Clin Lab Scientist/Med Tech

Wyoming Valley Health Care System Inc
Ron Stern, President/CEO
N River and Auburn Sts
Wilkes-Barre, PA 18764
717 552-3014
● Nuclear Medicine Tech
● Radiographer

Williamsport

Divine Providence Hospital
Kirby Smith, President
1100 Grampian Blvd
Williamsport, PA 17701
717 326-8101
● Clin Lab Scientist/Med Tech

Pennsylvania College of Technology
Robert L Breuder, PhD, President
One College Ave
Williamsport, PA 17701
717 326-3761
● Dental Hygienist
● Occupational Therapy Asst
● Radiographer

Williamsport Hospital
Steven P Johnson, MBA, President
777 Rural Ave
Williamsport, PA 17701
717 321-2101
● Emergency Med Tech-Paramedic

Wynnewood

Lankenau Hospital
Kenneth Hanover, President/CEO
100 Lancaster Ave
Wynnewood, PA 19096
610 526-3019
● Radiographer

Wyomissing

Berks Technical Institute
Kenneth S Snyder, President
4 Park Plaza
Wyomissing, PA 19610
610 372-1722
● Medical Assistant

York

York College of Pennsylvania
George W Waldner, PhD, President
Country Club Rd
York, PA 17405-7199
717 846-7788
● Health Information Admin
● Respiratory Therapist
● Respiratory Therapy Tech

York Hospital
Bruce M Bartels, MBA, President
1001 S George St
York, PA 17405
717 851-2121
● Clin Lab Scientist/Med Tech
● Radiographer

Youngwood

Westmoreland County Community College
Daniel C Krezenski, President
Armbrust Rd
Youngwood, PA 15697-1895
412 925-4000
● Dental Hygienist
● Dietetic Technician

Puerto Rico

Bayamon

Universidad Central del Caribe
Nilda Candelario, MD, President
Hosp Universitario Ramon Ruiz Arnau
Call Box 60-327
Bayamon, PR 00960-6032
809 798-3001
● Radiographer

Caguas

Huertas Junior College
Felix Rodriguez Matos, PhD, President
PO Box 8429
Caguas, PR 00726
809 743-1242
● Health Information Tech

Carolina

Colegio Universitario Del Este
Alberto Maldonado-Ruiz, Esq, Chancellor
Apartado 2010
Carolina, PR 00984-2010
809 257-7373
● Health Information Tech

Coto Laurel

Ponce Paramedical College
Alberto Aristizabal, President
PO Box 106
Coto Laurel, PR 00780-0106
809 848-1589
● Respiratory Therapy Tech

Humacao

Humacao University College
Roberto Marrero, PhD, Chancellor
University of Puerto Rico
CUH Postal Station
Humacao, PR 00791-9998
787 850-9375
● Occupational Therapy Asst

Mayaguez

Universidad Adventista de las Antillas
Myrna Colon-Contreras, PhD, President
PO Box 118
Mayaguez, PR 00681
787 834-9595
● Health Information Tech
● Respiratory Therapist

Ponce

Catholic University of Puerto Rico
Lorenzo M Albacete, President
2250 Las Americas Ave Ste 564
Ponce, PR 00731-6382
787 841-2000
● Clin Lab Scientist/Med Tech

Rio Piedras

Universidad Metropolitana
Jose F Mendez, CEO
PO Box 21150
Rio Piedras, PR 00928
809 766-1717
● Respiratory Therapist

San German

Interamerican University - San German
Prof Agnes Mojica, MA, Chancellor
Call Box 5100
San German, PR 00683
809 892-4320
● Clin Lab Scientist/Med Tech
● Health Information Tech

San Juan

Interamerican University - Metro Campus
Jose R Gonzalez, PhD, President
GPO Box 3255
San Juan, PR 00936
787 766-1912
● Clin Lab Scientist/Med Tech

Puerto Rico Department of Health
PO Box 70184
San Juan, PR 00936
787 274-6831
● Dietitian/Nutritionist

University of Puerto Rico
Jorge L Sanchez, MD, Chancellor
Medical Sciences Campus
PO Box 365067
San Juan, PR 00936-5067
787 758-2525
● Clin Lab Scientist/Med Tech
● Cytotechnologist
● Dental Assistant
● Dental Hygienist
● Dietitian/Nutritionist
● Health Information Admin
● Nuclear Medicine Tech
● Occupational Therapist
● Radiographer
● Rehabilitation Counselor
● Respiratory Therapist

Veterans Affairs Medical Center
One Veterans Plaza
San Juan, PR 00927-5800
787 758-7575
• Dietitian/Nutritionist

Santurce

University of the Sacred Heart
Jose Jaime Rivera, PhD, President
PO Box 12383 Loiza Station
Santurce, PR 00914
809 728-1515
• Clin Lab Scientist/Med Tech

Rhode Island

Kingston

University of Rhode Island
Robert L Carothers, President
8 Washburn Hall
Kingston, RI 02881-0817
401 792-1000
• Audiologist
• Dietitian/Nutritionist
• Speech Language Pathologist

North Providence

Our Lady of Fatima Hospital
John H Keimig, MHA, President
200 High Service Ave
North Providence, RI 02904
401 456-3000
• Clin Lab Scientist/Med Tech
• Cytotechnologist

Providence

Rhode Island Hospital
Steve Baron, President/CEO
593 Eddy St
Providence, RI 02905
401 444-5123
• Clin Lab Scientist/Med Tech
• Diagnostic Med Sonographer
• Nuclear Medicine Tech
• Radiation Therapist
• Radiographer

Women & Infants' Hospital
Thomas G Parris Jr, President/CEO
101 Dudley St
Providence, RI 02905
401 274-1100
• Cytotechnologist

Warwick

Community College of Rhode Island
Edward J Liston, MBA, President
400 East Ave
Warwick, RI 02886
401 825-1000
• Clin Lab Tech/Med Lab Tech-AD
• Dental Assistant
• Dental Hygienist
• Radiographer
• Respiratory Therapist

New England Institute of Technology
Richard I Gouse, BA, President
2500 Post Rd
Warwick, RI 02886-2266
401 739-5000
• Surgical Technologist

South Carolina

Aiken

Aiken Technical College
Kathleen A obles, President
PO Drawer 696
Aiken, SC 29802
805 593-9231
• Dental Assistant

Anderson

Anderson Area Medical Center
D Kirk Oglesby, MHA, President
800 N Fant St
Anderson, SC 29621
803 261-1109
• Clin Lab Scientist/Med Tech
• Radiographer

Forrest Junior College
Charles Palmer, MEd BA, Exec Director
601 E River St
Anderson, SC 29624
803 225-7653
• Medical Assistant

Charleston

Charleston Southern University
Jairy C Hunter, President
PO Box 118087
Charleston, SC 29423-8087
803 863-7000
• Music Therapist

Medical University of South Carolina
James B Edwards, DMD, President
171 Ashley Ave Rm 225
Charleston, SC 29425-2701
803 792-2211
• Clin Lab Scientist/Med Tech
• Cytotechnologist
• Dietitian/Nutritionist
• Health Information Admin
• Occupational Therapist
• Perfusionist
• Physician Assistant
• Radiation Therapist

Trident Technical College
Mary D Thornley, EdD, President
PO Box 118067
Charleston, SC 29423-8067
803 572-6241
• Clin Lab Tech/Med Lab Tech-AD
• Dental Assistant
• Dental Hygienist
• Medical Assistant
• Occupational Therapy Asst
• Radiographer
• Respiratory Therapist

Clemson

Clemson University
Constantine W Curris, President
201 Sikes Hall
Clemson, SC 29634
803 656-3311
• Dietitian/Nutritionist
• Therapeutic Recreation Specialist

Columbia

Baptist Medical Center at Columbia
Charles D Beaman Jr, President
Taylor at Marion St
Columbia, SC 29220
803 771-5042
• Clin Lab Scientist/Med Tech
• Radiographer

Midlands Technical College
James L Hudgins, PhD, President
PO Box 2408
Columbia, SC 29202
803 738-1400
• Clin Lab Tech/Med Lab Tech-AD
• Dental Assistant
• Dental Hygienist
• Health Information Tech
• Medical Assistant
• Nuclear Medicine Tech
• Radiographer
• Respiratory Therapist
• Respiratory Therapy Tech
• Surgical Technologist

So Carolina Hlth & Environmental Control
Mills Complex
PO Box 101106
Columbia, SC 29211-0106
803 737-3954
• Dietitian/Nutritionist

University of South Carolina
John M Palms, PhD, President
Osborne 203
Columbia, SC 29208
803 777-2001
• Athletic Trainer
• Rehabilitation Counselor
• Speech Language Pathologist

Conway

Horry-Georgetown Technical College
D Kent Sharples, PhD, President
P O Box 26004
Conway, SC 29528-6004
803 347-3786
• Radiographer

Florence

Florence-Darlington Technical College

Charles W Gould, PhD, President
PO Box 100548
Florence, SC 29501-0548
803 661-8000
- Clin Lab Tech/Med Lab Tech-AD
- Dental Assistant
- Dental Hygienist
- Health Information Tech
- Radiographer
- Respiratory Therapist
- Respiratory Therapy Tech
- Surgical Technologist

McLeod Regional Medical Center

J Bruce Barragan, MA, President
555 E Cheves St PO Box 100551
Florence, SC 29501-0551
803 667-2297
- Clin Lab Scientist/Med Tech

Greenville

Greenville Technical College

Thomas E Barton Jr, EdD, CEO
PO Box 5616 Station B
Greenville, SC 29606-5616
864 250-8175
- Clin Lab Tech/Med Lab Tech-AD
- Dental Assistant
- Dental Hygienist
- Dietetic Technician
- Emergency Med Tech-Paramedic
- Radiographer
- Respiratory Therapist
- Respiratory Therapy Tech
- Surgical Technologist

Greenwood

Piedmont Technical College

Lex D Walters, PhD, President
PO Drawer 1467 Emerald Rd
Greenwood, SC 29647
864 941-8536
- Radiographer
- Respiratory Therapist
- Respiratory Therapy Tech

Orangeburg

Orangeburg Calhoun Technical College

Jeffrey R Olson, PhD, President
3250 St Matthews Rd
Orangeburg, SC 29118
803 535-1200
- Clin Lab Tech/Med Lab Tech-AD
- Medical Assistant
- Radiographer
- Respiratory Therapy Tech

South Carolina State University

Leroy Davis, President
Orangeburg, SC 29117
803 536-7014
- Dietitian/Nutritionist
- Rehabilitation Counselor
- Speech Language Pathologist

Pendleton

Tri-County Technical College

Don C Garrison, EdD, President
PO Box 587
Pendleton, SC 29670-0587
864 225-2250
- Clin Lab Tech/Med Lab Tech-AD
- Dental Assistant
- Surgical Technologist

Rock Hill

Winthrop University

Anthony J Digiorgio, President
Oakland Ave
Rock Hill, SC 29733
803 323-2211
- Dietitian/Nutritionist

York Technical College

Dennis Merrell, EdD, President
452 S Anderson Rd
Rock Hill, SC 29730
803 327-8050
- Clin Lab Tech/Med Lab Tech-AD
- Dental Assistant
- Dental Hygienist
- Radiographer

Spartanburg

Spartanburg Technical College

Dan L Terhune, EdD, President
PO Drawer 4386
Spartanburg, SC 29305-4386
803 591-3610
- Clin Lab Tech/Med Lab Tech-AD
- Dental Assistant
- Radiographer
- Respiratory Therapist
- Respiratory Therapy Tech
- Surgical Technologist

South Dakota

Aberdeen

Presentation College

Lorraine Hale, PhD, President
1500 N Main St
Aberdeen, SD 57401-1299
605 229-8404
- Clin Lab Tech/Med Lab Tech-AD
- Surgical Technologist

St Luke's-Midland Regional Medical Ctr

Dale J Stein, MHA, Hosp Administrator
305 S State St
Aberdeen, SD 57401
605 622-5230
- Clin Lab Scientist/Med Tech
- Radiographer

Brookings

South Dakota State University

Robert T Wagner, President
Brookings, SD 57007
605 688-4151
- Dietitian/Nutritionist

Madison

Dakota State University

Jerald A Tunheim, PhD, President
314 Heston Hall
Madison, SD 57042-1799
605 256-5112
- Health Information Admin
- Health Information Tech
- Respiratory Therapist

Mitchell

Mitchell Technical Institute

John Christiansen, EdD, Superintendent
117 E Fourth Ave PO Box 7760
Mitchell, SD 57301
605 995-3000
- Clin Lab Tech/Med Lab Tech-AD

Queen of Peace Hospital

Ronald L Jacobson, MHA, Exec Dir
Fifth and Foster
Mitchell, SD 57301
605 995-2250
- Radiographer

Rapid City

National College

Jerry L Gallentine, PhD, President
321 Kansas City St PO Box 1780
Rapid City, SD 57709
605 394-4900
- Health Information Tech
- Medical Assistant

Rapid City Regional Hospital

Adil M Ameer, MBA, President/CEO
353 Fairmont Blvd
Rapid City, SD 57709
605 341-8100
- Clin Lab Scientist/Med Tech
- Radiographer

Sioux Falls

LCM Pathologists PC

Thomas J Schnabel, MBA, Business Manager
1212 S Euclid Ave
PO Box 5134
Sioux Falls, SD 57117-5134
605 333-1725
- Cytotechnologist

McKennan Hospital

Fred Slunecka, MHA, President/CEO
800 E 21st St
Sioux Falls, SD 57117-5045
605 339-8113
- Radiographer

Sioux Valley Hospital

Lyle E Schroeder, MHA, President
1100 S Euclid Ave PO Box 5039
Sioux Falls, SD 57117-5039
605 333-6424
- Clin Lab Scientist/Med Tech
- Radiographer

Institutions

Southeast Technical Institute
Terrence Sullivan, MS, Director
2301 Career Pl
Sioux Falls, SD 57107
605 331-7624
- Cardiovascular Technologist
- Nuclear Medicine Tech

Vermillion

University of South Dakota
Paul Olscamp, PhD, Interim President
414 E Clark St
Vermillion, SD 57069-2390
605 677-5641
- Audiologist
- Dental Hygienist
- Dietitian/Nutritionist
- Occupational Therapist
- Physician Assistant
- Speech Language Pathologist

Watertown

Lake Area Technical Institute
Rick Melmer, MEd, Superintendent
200 NE 9th
Watertown, SD 57201
605 886-7276
- Clin Lab Tech/Med Lab Tech-AD
- Dental Assistant
- Medical Assistant

Yankton

Mt Marty College
Sr Jacquelyn Ernster, PhD, President
Yankton, SD 57078
605 668-1514
- Dietitian/Nutritionist

Sacred Heart Hospital
Dennis A Sokol, MHA, Exec Director
501 Summit St
Yankton, SD 57078
605 655-9371
- Radiographer

Tennessee

Blountville

Northeast State Technical Comm College
William W. Locke, PhD, President
PO Box 246
Blountville, TN 37617-0246
615 323-3191
- Emergency Med Tech-Paramedic

Chattanooga

Chattanooga State Technical Comm College
James L Catanzaro, PhD, President
4501 Amnicola Hwy
Chattanooga, TN 37406-1097
423 697-4455
- Dental Assistant
- Dental Hygienist
- Diagnostic Med Sonographer
- Health Information Tech
- Nuclear Medicine Tech
- Radiation Therapist
- Radiographer
- Respiratory Therapist

University of Tennessee at Chattanooga
Frederick W Obear, Chancellor
615 McCallie Ave
Chattanooga, TN 37403
615 755-4141
- Dietitian/Nutritionist

Clarksville

Austin Peay State University
Sal D Rinella, PhD, President
Office of the President
Clarksville, TN 37044
615 648-7566
- Clin Lab Scientist/Med Tech

Miller-Motte Business College
Raymond Green, BS, President
1820 Business Park Dr
Clarksville, TN 37040
616 553-0071
- Medical Assistant

Cleveland

Cleveland State Community College
Renee Basham, Interim President
PO Box 3750
Cleveland, TN 37320-3570
615 472-7141
- Clin Lab Tech/Med Lab Tech-AD

Columbia

Columbia State Community College
L Paul Sands, PhD, President
Hwy 412 PO Box 1315
Columbia, TN 38401
615 540-2722
- Clin Lab Tech/Med Lab Tech-AD
- Radiographer
- Respiratory Therapist

Cookeville

Cumberland School of Technology
LaVerne Floyd, MA MT(ASCP), President
1065 E 10th St
Cookeville, TN 38501
615 526-3660
- Clin Lab Tech/Med Lab Tech-AD

Tennessee Technological University
Angelo A Volpe, President
Cookeville, TN 38505
615 372-3101
- Dietitian/Nutritionist
- Music Therapist

Gallatin

Volunteer State Community College
Hal R Ramer, PhD, President
1480 Nashville Pike
Gallatin, TN 37066-3188
615 452-8600
- Dental Assistant
- Emergency Med Tech-Paramedic
- Health Information Tech
- Radiographer
- Respiratory Therapy Tech

Harriman

Roane State Community College
Sherry L Hoppe, EdD, President
276 Patton Ln
Harriman, TN 37748-5011
423 882-4501
- Clin Lab Tech/Med Lab Tech-AD
- Dental Hygienist
- Emergency Med Tech-Paramedic
- Health Information Tech
- Occupational Therapy Asst
- Ophthalmic Dispenser
- Radiographer
- Respiratory Therapist

Harrogate

Lincoln Memorial University
Scott D Miller, PhD, President
Cumberland Gap Pkwy
Harrogate, TN 37752-0901
423 869-6391
- Clin Lab Scientist/Med Tech

Jackson

Jackson State Community College
Walter L Nelms, EdD, President
2046 N Parkway St
Jackson, TN 38301-3797
901 424-3520
- Clin Lab Tech/Med Lab Tech-AD
- Emergency Med Tech-Paramedic
- Radiographer
- Respiratory Therapist

Jefferson City

Carson-Newman College
J Cordell Maddox, President
1646 Russell Ave
Jefferson City, TN 37760
615 471-4000
- Dietitian/Nutritionist

Johnson City

East Tennessee State University
Roy S Nicks, EdD, President
Box 70734
Johnson City, TN 37614
423 439-4211
- Audiologist
- Clin Lab Tech/Med Lab Tech-AD
- Dental Assistant
- Dental Hygienist
- Dental Lab Technician
- Dietitian/Nutritionist
- Medical Assistant
- Radiographer
- Respiratory Therapist
- Respiratory Therapy Tech
- Speech Language Pathologist
- Surgical Technologist

Knoxville

Tennessee Technical Center - Knoxville
1100 Liberty St
Knoxville, TN 37919
615 546-5567
- Dental Assistant

Univ of Tennessee Med Ctr at Knoxville
Charles Mercer, MD, CEO
600 Henley St Ste 100
Knoxville, TN 37902-2911
423 544-6404
- Clin Lab Scientist/Med Tech
- Cytotechnologist
- Nuclear Medicine Tech
- Radiographer

University of Tennessee - Knoxville
William T Snyder, Chancellor
Knoxville, TN 37996
615 974-1000
- Audiologist
- Dietitian/Nutritionist
- Rehabilitation Counselor
- Speech Language Pathologist

Livingston

Tennessee Technology Center - Livingston
Ralph E Robbins, BS, Director
PO Box 219
740 High Tech Dr
Livingston, TN 38570
615 823-5525
- Medical Assistant

Martin

University of Tennessee at Martin
Margaret N Perry, Chancellor
Martin, TN 38238
901 587-7000
- Dietitian/Nutritionist

Memphis

Baptist Memorial Health Care Systems
Stephen C Reynolds, MHA, President
899 Madison Ave
Memphis, TN 38146
901 227-5121
- Diagnostic Med Sonographer
- Nuclear Medicine Tech
- Radiation Therapist
- Radiographer

Methodist Hospitals of Memphis
Gary Shorb, President
1265 Union Ave
Memphis, TN 38104
901 726-8274
- Nuclear Medicine Tech
- Radiation Therapist
- Radiographer

Shelby State Community College
Floyd F. Amann, PhD, President
PO Box 40568
Memphis, TN 38174-0568
901 544-5020
- Clin Lab Tech/Med Lab Tech-AD
- Dietetic Technician
- Emergency Med Tech-Paramedic
- Medical Assistant
- Radiographer

St Joseph Hospital
Joan Carlson, CEO
220 Overton Ave PO Box 178
Memphis, TN 38101-0178
901 529-2830
- Radiographer

Tennessee Technology Center - Memphis
James King, PhD, Director
550 Alabama Ave
Memphis, TN 38105-3799
901 543-6100
- Dental Assistant
- Respiratory Therapy Tech
- Surgical Technologist

University of Memphis
V Lane Rawlins, President
Memphis, TN 38152
901 678-2000
- Audiologist
- Dietitian/Nutritionist
- Rehabilitation Counselor
- Speech Language Pathologist

University of Tennessee Memphis
William R Rice, JD, Chancellor & VP
220 Hyman Admin Bldg
Memphis, TN 38163
901 448-4796
- Clin Lab Scientist/Med Tech
- Cytotechnologist
- Dental Hygienist
- Health Information Admin
- Occupational Therapist

Morristown

Walters State Community College
Jack E Campbell, EdD, President
500 S Davy Crockett Pkwy
Morristown, TN 37813-6899
423 585-2600
- Respiratory Therapy Tech

Murfreesboro

Middle Tennessee State University
James E Walker, President
Murfreesboro, TN 37132
615 898-2300
- Dietitian/Nutritionist

National HealthCare LP
PO Box 1398
Murfreesboro, TN 37133-1398
615 890-2020
- Dietitian/Nutritionist

Nashville

David Lipscomb University
Harold Hazelip, President
Nashville, TN 37204
615 269-1000
- Dietitian/Nutritionist

Metropolitan Nashville General Hospital
John M Stone, MBA, Director
72 Hermitage Ave
Nashville, TN 37210
615 862-4490
- Radiographer

Nashville State Technical Institute
George H Van Allen, EdD, President
120 White Bridge Rd
PO Box 90285
Nashville, TN 37209-4515
615 353-3383
- Occupational Therapy Asst

St Thomas Hospital
John Tighe, President
4220 Harding Rd PO Box 380
Nashville, TN 37202
615 222-2111
- Clin Lab Scientist/Med Tech

Tennessee State University
James A Hefner, PhD, President
3500 John A Merritt Blvd
Nashville, TN 37209-1561
615 963-7401
- Clin Lab Scientist/Med Tech
- Dental Hygienist
- Dietitian/Nutritionist
- Health Information Admin
- Occupational Therapist
- Respiratory Therapist
- Speech Language Pathologist

Trevecca Nazarene University
Millard Reed, DMin, President
333 Murfreesboro Rd
Nashville, TN 37210
615 248-1251
- Physician Assistant

Vanderbilt University Medical Center

Norman B Urmy, MBA, Executive Director
AA 1214 Med Ctr N
Nashville, TN 37232-2101
615 322-2415
- Audiologist
- Clin Lab Scientist/Med Tech
- Dietitian/Nutritionist
- Nuclear Medicine Tech
- Perfusionist
- Radiation Therapist
- Speech Language Pathologist

Texas

Abilene

Abilene Christian University

Royce L Money, President
Box 8363
Abilene, TX 79699
915 674-2000
- Dietitian/Nutritionist

Hendrick Medical Center

Michael C Waters, FACHE, President
1242 N 19th
Abilene, TX 79601-2316
915 670-2201
- Radiographer

Alvin

Alvin Community College

A Rodney Allbright, JD, President
3110 Mustang Rd
Alvin, TX 77511
713 388-4612
- Clin Lab Tech/Med Lab Tech-AD
- Respiratory Therapist
- Respiratory Therapy Tech

Amarillo

Amarillo College

Luther Bud Joyner, EdD, President
2201 S Washington
P. O. Box 447
Amarillo, TX 79178-0001
806 371-5123
- Clin Lab Tech/Med Lab Tech-AD
- Dental Hygienist
- Nuclear Medicine Tech
- Occupational Therapy Asst
- Radiation Therapist
- Radiographer
- Respiratory Therapist
- Surgical Technologist

Northwest Texas Healthcare System

William Webster, MS, Managing Director\CEO
Northwest Texas Healthcare System
PO Box 1110
Amarillo, TX 79175
806 354-1110
- Clin Lab Scientist/Med Tech

Athens

Trinity Valley Community College

Ronald C Baugh, MS, President
Cardinal Dr
Athens, TX 75751
214 675-6211
- Surgical Technologist

Austin

Austin Community College

Hosni Nabi, Interim President
5930 Middle Fiskville Rd
Austin, TX 78752-4390
512 223-7598
- Clin Lab Tech/Med Lab Tech-AD
- Diagnostic Med Sonographer
- Emergency Med Tech-Paramedic
- Occupational Therapy Asst
- Radiographer
- Surgical Technologist

Austin State Hospital

Diane Faucher, Superintendent
4110 Guadalupe St
Austin, TX 78751
512 452-0381
- Clin Lab Scientist/Med Tech

University of Texas at Austin

Robert M Berdahl, President
Austin, TX 78712
512 471-3434
- Audiologist
- Dietitian/Nutritionist
- Rehabilitation Counselor
- Speech Language Pathologist

Baytown

Lee College

Jackson N Sasser, PhD, President
511 S Whiting St
Baytown, TX 77520
713 425-6300
- Emergency Med Tech-Paramedic
- Health Information Tech

Beaumont

Baptist Hospital of Southeast Texas

David Parmer, MS, President
Hospital Admin and Accounting
PO Drawer 1591
Beaumont, TX 77704
409 654-5351
- Radiographer

Lamar Univ Institute of Tech - Beaumont

Robert Krienke, EdD, President
Institute of Technology
Beaumont, TX 77710
409 880-8185
- Audiologist
- Dental Hygienist
- Dietitian/Nutritionist
- Radiographer
- Respiratory Therapist
- Respiratory Therapy Tech
- Speech Language Pathologist

St Elizabeth Hospital

Sr M Fatima McCarthy, MHA RN, Administrator
2830 Calder St/PO Box 5405
Beaumont, TX 77726-5405
409 892-7171
- Clin Lab Scientist/Med Tech

Beeville

Bee County College

Norman E Wallace, President
3800 Charco Rd
Beeville, TX 78102
512 358-3130
- Dental Hygienist

Big Spring

Howard College

Cheryl T Sparks, EdD, President
1001 Birdwell Ln
Big Spring, TX 79720
915 264-5000
- Dental Hygienist
- Health Information Tech
- Respiratory Therapy Tech

Scenic Mountain Medical Center

Ken Randall,
1601 W 11th Pl
Big Spring, TX 79720-9990
915 263-1211
- Radiographer

Brenham

Blinn College

Don E Voelter, PhD, President
902 College Ave
Brenham, TX 77833
409 830-4112
- Radiographer

Brownsville

Univ Tx at Brownsville/TX Southmost Coll

Juliet Garcia, PhD, President
83 Ft Brown
Brownsville, TX 78520
210 541-1241
- Clin Lab Tech/Med Lab Tech-AD
- Radiographer
- Respiratory Therapist
- Respiratory Therapy Tech

Canyon

West Texas A & M University

Russell C Long, President
Canyon, TX 79016
806 656-2000
- Music Therapist

Cisco

Cisco Junior College

Roger Schustereit, PhD, President
Box 3 Rte 3
Cisco, TX 76437
817 442-2567
- Medical Assistant

College Station

Texas A & M University

Ray M Bowen, President
College Station, TX 77843
409 845-3211
• Dietitian/Nutritionist

Corpus Christi

Corpus Christi State University

Robert R Furgason, PhD, President
6300 Ocean Dr
Corpus Christi, TX 78412
512 994-2621
• Clin Lab Scientist/Med Tech

Del Mar College

Terry L Dicianna, PhD, President
Baldwin and Ayers
Corpus Christi, TX 78404
512 886-1203
• Clin Lab Tech/Med Lab Tech-AD
• Dental Assistant
• Dental Hygienist
• Diagnostic Med Sonographer
• Radiographer
• Respiratory Therapist
• Respiratory Therapy Tech
• Surgical Technologist

Corsicana

Navarro College

Gerald Burson, EdD, President
3200 W 7th Ave
Corsicana, TX 75110-4818
903 874-6501
• Occupational Therapy Asst

Dallas

ATI Health Education Centers

Joe Mehlmann, President
ATI Enterprises of Florida Inc
2777 Stemmons Freeway
Dallas, TX 75207
214 630-5651
• Respiratory Therapist
• Respiratory Therapy Tech

Baylor University Medical Center

Boone Powell Jr, FACHA, President
3500 Gaston Ave
Dallas, TX 75246
214 828-0377
• Dental Hygienist
• Dietitian/Nutritionist
• Radiographer

El Centro College

Wright L Lassiter Jr, EdD, President
Main and Lamar Sts
Dallas, TX 75202-3604
214 860-2010
• Cardiovascular Technologist
• Clin Lab Tech/Med Lab Tech-AD
• Diagnostic Med Sonographer
• Radiographer
• Respiratory Therapist
• Surgical Technologist

Presbyterian Hospital of Dallas

8200 Walnut Hill Ln
Dallas, TX 75231-4402
214 345-7558
• Dietitian/Nutritionist

Southern Methodist University

R Gerald Turner, President
6425 Boaz St/PO Box 296
Dallas, TX 75275
214 768-2000
• Music Therapist

Univ of Tx Southwestern Med Ctr - Dallas

Kern Wildenthal, MD PhD, President
5323 Harry Hines Blvd
Dallas, TX 75235-9002
214 648-2508
• Clin Lab Scientist/Med Tech
• Dietitian/Nutritionist
• Emergency Med Tech-Paramedic
• Medical Illustrator
• Physician Assistant
• Rehabilitation Counselor
• Specialist in BB Tech

Denison

Grayson County College

Alan Scheibmeir, PhD, President
6101 Grayson Dr
Denison, TX 75020
903 465-6030
• Clin Lab Tech/Med Lab Tech-AD
• Dental Assistant

Denton

Texas Woman's University

Carol Surles, PhD, President
Box 425587
TWU Station (ACT-15)
Denton, TX 76204-3587
817 898-3201
• Dental Hygienist
• Dietitian/Nutritionist
• Music Therapist
• Occupational Therapist
• Speech Language Pathologist

University of North Texas

Alfred F Hurley, President/CEO
Denton, TX 76203-5008
817 565-2000
• Audiologist
• Rehabilitation Counselor
• Speech Language Pathologist
• Therapeutic Recreation Specialist

Edinburg

Univ of Texas - Pan American

Miguel Nevarez, PhD, President
1201 W University Dr
Edinburg, TX 78539
210 381-2011
• Clin Lab Scientist/Med Tech
• Dietitian/Nutritionist
• Speech Language Pathologist

El Paso

El Paso Community College

Adriana Barrera, PhD, Interim President
PO Box 20500
El Paso, TX 79998
915 594-2112
• Clin Lab Tech/Med Lab Tech-AD
• Dental Assistant
• Dental Hygienist
• Diagnostic Med Sonographer
• Dietetic Technician
• Health Information Tech
• Medical Assistant
• Ophthalmic Dispenser
• Radiographer
• Respiratory Therapist
• Surgical Technologist

University of Texas at El Paso

Diana Natalicio, PhD, President
Admin Bldg 500
El Paso, TX 77902
915 747-5555
• Clin Lab Scientist/Med Tech
• Speech Language Pathologist

Western Technical Institute

Randy L Kuykendall, President
4710 Alabama St
El Paso, TX 79930
915 566-9621
• Medical Assistant

Ft Sam Houston

Army Medical Dept Center and School

James B Peake, MC, Major General
Ft Sam Houston, TX 78234-6100
210 221-6325
• Dental Lab Technician
• Occupational Therapy Asst
• Physician Assistant
• Radiographer
• Respiratory Therapy Tech

Brooke Army Medical Center

Robert G Claypool, BG MC MD, Commdg Gen
Ft Sam Houston, TX 78234-6200
210 916-8125
• Cytotechnologist
• Dietitian/Nutritionist

Ft Worth

Harris Methodist Ft Worth

Barclay Berdan, Sr VP/Managing Dir
1301 Pennsylvania
Ft Worth, TX 76104
817 878-2106
• Clin Lab Scientist/Med Tech

JPS Health Network

Anthony Aleini, CEO
1500 S Main St
Ft Worth, TX 76104
817 927-1230
• Radiographer

Institutions

Tarrant County Junior Coll - South

Jerry Mullen, Dean Instruction
5301 Campus Dr
Ft Worth, TX 76119-5998
817 534-4861
- Dietetic Technician

Texas Christian University

William E Tucker, PhD, Chancellor
PO 32909
Ft Worth, TX 76129
817 921-7783
- Athletic Trainer
- Dietitian/Nutritionist
- Speech Language Pathologist

Gainesville

North Central Texas College

Ronnie Glasscock, PhD, President
1525 W California St
Gainesville, TX 76240
817 668-7731
- Health Information Tech
- Occupational Therapy Asst

Galveston

Galveston College-University of Texas

C B Rathburn III, President
4015 Ave Q
Galveston, TX 77550-2782
409 772-1221
- Nuclear Medicine Tech
- Radiation Therapist
- Radiographer

University of Texas Medical Branch

Thomas N James, MD, President
301 University Blvd
Galveston, TX 77555-1029
409 772-2331
- Clin Lab Scientist/Med Tech
- Health Information Admin
- Occupational Therapist
- Physician Assistant
- Specialist in BB Tech

Harlingen

Texas State Technical College

J Gilbert Leal, PhD MEd, President
2424 Boxwood
Harlingen, TX 78551-3697
210 425-0601
- Dental Assistant
- Health Information Tech

Houston

Baylor College of Medicine

Ralph D Feigin, MD, President/CEO
BCMC 143A/One Baylor Plaza
Houston, TX 77030
713 798-4433
- Audiologist
- Nuclear Medicine Tech
- Perfusionist
- Physician Assistant

Bradford School

Julie H Hayes, President
4669 SW Freeway/Ste 300
Houston, TX 77027
713 629-8940
- Medical Assistant

Gulf Coast Regional Blood Center

Bill T Teague, BS MT(ASCP)SBB, President/CEO
1400 La Concha Ln
Houston, TX 77054-1802
713 790-1200
- Specialist in BB Tech

Harris County Hosp Dist/Ben Taub Hosp

Lois J Moore, MS, CEO/President
2525 Holly Hall
Houston, TX 77266
713 746-6400
- Clin Lab Scientist/Med Tech
- Radiographer

Houston Community College Central

Ruth Burgae-Sasscer, PhD, Chancellor
22 Waugh Dr
Houston, TX 77007
713 718-5059
- Clin Lab Tech/Med Lab Tech-AD
- Dental Assistant
- Dietetic Technician
- Emergency Med Tech-Paramedic
- Health Information Tech
- Nuclear Medicine Tech
- Occupational Therapy Asst
- Radiographer
- Respiratory Therapist
- Respiratory Therapy Tech
- Surgical Technologist

Memorial Hospital System

Dan S Wilford, CEO
7737 SW Freeway
Houston, TX 77074
713 776-5100
- Radiographer

Methodist Hospital

Larry Mathis, CEO/President
6565 Fannin Mail Station D 200
Houston, TX 77030
713 790-2481
- Clin Lab Scientist/Med Tech
- Histologic Technician-Cert

San Jacinto College South

Parker Williams, PhD, President
South Campus
13735 Beamer Rd
Houston, TX 77089
713 484-1900
- Occupational Therapy Asst

Texas Heart Institute

Denton A Cooley, MD, President
PO Box 20345/MC 1-224
Houston, TX 77225
713 791-4026
- Perfusionist

Texas Southern University

James Douglas, ESQ, President
3100 Cleburne St
Houston, TX 77004
713 313-7034
- Clin Lab Scientist/Med Tech
- Dietitian/Nutritionist
- Health Information Admin
- Respiratory Therapist

Texas Woman's University

1130 M D Anderson Blvd
Houston, TX 77030-2804
713 794-2376
- Dietitian/Nutritionist

Univ of Texas Hlth Sci Ctr at Houston

M David Low, MD PhD, President
PO Box 20036
Houston, TX 77225-0708
713 792-4975
- Clin Lab Scientist/Med Tech
- Dental Hygienist
- Dietitian/Nutritionist

Univ of Texas M D Anderson Cancer Ctr

John Mendelsohn, MD, President
1515 Holcombe Blvd Box 213
Houston, TX 77030
713 792-6000
- Clin Lab Scientist/Med Tech
- Cytotechnologist
- Histologic Technician-Cert
- Radiation Therapist

University of Houston

Thomas M Stauffer, PhD, President
2700 Bay Area Blvd
Houston, TX 77058-1098
713 488-9336
- Dietitian/Nutritionist
- Speech Language Pathologist

Veterans Affairs Medical Center

Robert F Stott, MPH, Hosp Director
2002 Holcombe Blvd 00/580
Houston, TX 77030
713 794-7100
- Clin Lab Scientist/Med Tech
- Dietitian/Nutritionist

Huntsville

Sam Houston State University

Martin J Anisman, President
Box 2026
Huntsville, TX 77341
409 294-1111
- Dietitian/Nutritionist
- Music Therapist

Hurst

Tarrant Junior College

Larry Darlage, PhD, President, NE Campus
828 Harwood Rd
Hurst, TX 76054
817 515-6200
- Dental Hygienist
- Health Information Tech
- Radiographer
- Respiratory Therapist
- Surgical Technologist

Kilgore

Kilgore College

William M Holda, EdD, President
1100 Broadway
Kilgore, TX 75662
903 983-8100
- Clin Lab Tech/Med Lab Tech-AD
- Radiographer
- Surgical Technologist

Killeen

Central Texas College

James R Anderson, PhD, Chancellor
US Hwy 190 W
Killeen, TX 76541-9990
817 526-1211
- Clin Lab Tech/Med Lab Tech-AD

Kingsville

Texas A & M University - Kingsville

Manuel L Ibanez, President
Santa Gertrudis
Kingsville, TX 78363
512 595-2111
- Dietitian/Nutritionist

Kingwood

Kingwood College - NHMCCD

Steve Head, PhD, President
20000 Kingwood Dr
Kingwood, TX 77339
713 359-1600
- Respiratory Therapist
- Respiratory Therapy Tech

Laredo

Laredo Community College

Roger Worsley, EdD, President
West End Washington St
Laredo, TX 78040-4395
512 721-5102
- Clin Lab Tech/Med Lab Tech-AD
- Radiographer

Lubbock

Methodist Hospital

Byron Hale Sr, VP/ CFO
3615 19th St PO Box 1201
Lubbock, TX 79408
806 792-1011
- Radiation Therapist
- Radiographer

South Plains College

Richard Walsh, EdD, Provost
1302 Main St
Lubbock, TX 79401
806 747-0576
- Health Information Tech
- Radiographer
- Respiratory Therapist
- Respiratory Therapy Tech
- Surgical Technologist

Texas Tech Univ Hlth Sci Ctr

John T Montford, JD, Chancellor
3601 4th St
Lubbock, TX 79409-2013
806 743-2900
- Audiologist
- Clin Lab Scientist/Med Tech
- Dietitian/Nutritionist
- Emergency Med Tech-Paramedic
- Occupational Therapist
- Speech Language Pathologist

Lufkin

Angelina College

Larry M Phillips, EdD, President
PO Box 1768
Lufkin, TX 75902-1768
409 639-1301
- Radiographer
- Respiratory Therapy Tech

McKinney

Collin County Community Coll District

John H Anthony, EdD, President
2200 W University Dr
McKinney, TX 75070
214 548-6790
- Respiratory Therapist

Midland

Memorial Hospital and Medical Center

Harold Rubin, BS, President
2200 W Illinois St
Midland, TX 79701
915 685-1533
- Clin Lab Scientist/Med Tech

Midland College

David Daniel, EdD, President
3600 N Garfield
Midland, TX 79705
915 685-4500
- Radiographer
- Respiratory Therapist
- Respiratory Therapy Tech

Nacogdoches

Stephen F Austin State University

Daniel D Angel, President
1936 North St
Nacogdoches, TX 75962
409 468-2011
- Dietitian/Nutritionist
- Rehabilitation Counselor
- Speech Language Pathologist

Odessa

Odessa College

Vance W Gipson, EdD, President
201 W University
Odessa, TX 79764-8299
915 335-6410
- Clin Lab Tech/Med Lab Tech-AD
- Radiographer
- Respiratory Therapist
- Respiratory Therapy Tech
- Surgical Technologist

Orange

Baptist Hospital, Orange

Kevin Ioleman, Interim Administrator
608 Strickland
Orange, TX 77630
409 883-9361
- Clin Lab Tech/Med Lab Tech-C

Pasadena

San Jacinto College Central Campus

Monte Blue, EdD, President
8060 Spencer Hwy
PO Box 2007
Pasadena, TX 77501-2007
713 476-1501
- Clin Lab Tech/Med Lab Tech-AD
- Dietetic Technician
- Radiographer
- Respiratory Therapist
- Respiratory Therapy Tech
- Surgical Technologist

Prairie View

Prairie View A & M University

Charles A Hines, President
Prairie View, TX 77446
409 857-3311
- Dietitian/Nutritionist

Richardson

University of Texas at Dallas

Franklyn G Jenifer, President
PO Box 8630688
Richardson, TX 75083
214 883-2111
- Audiologist
- Speech Language Pathologist

San Angelo

Shannon West Texas Memorial Hospital

John Geanes, CEO
120 E Harris PO Box 1879
San Angelo, TX 76902
915 653-6741
- Clin Lab Scientist/Med Tech

San Antonio

Baptist Memorial

Fred R Mills, FACHE, President/CEO
660 N Main St Ste 300
San Antonio, TX 78205-1222
210 302-3000
- Clin Lab Scientist/Med Tech
- Radiographer
- Surgical Technologist

Cancer Therapy & Research Center

Charles A Coltman Jr, MD, Med Admin
4450 Medical Dr
San Antonio, TX 78229
512 616-5580
- Radiation Therapist

Our Lady of the Lake University
Elizabeth A Sueltenfuss, President
411 S W 24th St
San Antonio, TX 78207
210 434-6711
- Speech Language Pathologist

San Antonio College
Robert E Zeigler, PhD, Interim President
1300 San Pedro Ave
San Antonio, TX 78212-4299
210 733-2000
- Dental Assistant
- Medical Assistant

St Philip's College
Charles A Taylor, EdD, President
1801 Martin Luther King St
San Antonio, TX 78203-2098
210 531-3591
- Clin Lab Tech/Med Lab Tech-AD
- Dietetic Technician
- Health Information Tech
- Occupational Therapy Asst
- Radiographer
- Respiratory Therapy Tech
- Surgical Technologist

Univ of Texas Hlth Sci Ctr at San Antonio
John P Howe, MD, President
7703 Floyd Curl Dr
San Antonio, TX 78284-7834
210 567-2000
- Clin Lab Scientist/Med Tech
- Dental Hygienist
- Dental Lab Technician
- Emergency Med Tech-Paramedic
- Occupational Therapist

University Hospital of San Antonio
John A Guest, President/CEO
University Health System
4502 Medical Dr
San Antonio, TX 78229-4493
210 616-2000
- Cytotechnologist
- Histologic Technician-Cert
- Specialist in BB Tech

University of the Incarnate Word
Louis Agnese, PhD, President
4301 Broadway
San Antonio, TX 78209
210 829-6000
- Dietitian/Nutritionist
- Nuclear Medicine Tech

San Marcos

Southwest Texas State University
Jerome H Supple, PhD, President
601 University Dr
San Marcos, TX 78666
512 245-2121
- Clin Lab Scientist/Med Tech
- Dietitian/Nutritionist
- Health Information Admin
- Respiratory Therapist
- Respiratory Therapy Tech
- Speech Language Pathologist

Sheppard AFB

882 Training Group
Robert H Brannon, Col USAF MSC,
939 Missile Rd/CC
Sheppard AFB, TX 76311-2262
817 676-2700
- Clin Lab Tech/Med Lab Tech-C
- Dental Assistant
- Dental Lab Technician
- Physician Assistant
- Radiographer
- Surgical Technologist

Stephenville

Tarleton State University
Dennis P McCabe, PhD, President
Tarleton Station
Stephenville, TX 76402
817 968-9100
- Clin Lab Scientist/Med Tech
- Dietitian/Nutritionist

Temple

Scott & White Memorial Hosp and Clinic
Robert Myers, MD, President
2401 S 31st St
Temple, TX 76508
817 774-2111
- Clin Lab Scientist/Med Tech

Temple College
Marc A Nigliazzo, PhD, President
2600 S First St
Temple, TX 76504
817 773-9961
- Clin Lab Tech/Med Lab Tech-AD
- Respiratory Therapist
- Surgical Technologist

Texarkana

Wadley Regional Medical Center
Hugh Hallgren, MBA, President
1000 Pine St
Texarkana, TX 75501
903 798-8000
- Clin Lab Scientist/Med Tech
- Radiographer

Texas City

College of the Mainland
Larry Stanley, MA, President
1200 Amburn Rd
Texas City, TX 77591
409 938-1211
- Emergency Med Tech-Paramedic

Tyler

Tyler Junior College
William R Crowe, PhD, President
PO Box 9020
Tyler, TX 75711
903 510-2380
- Clin Lab Tech/Med Lab Tech-AD
- Dental Hygienist
- Health Information Tech
- Radiographer
- Respiratory Therapist
- Respiratory Therapy Tech

University of Texas at Tyler
George F Hamm, PhD, President
3900 University Blvd
Tyler, TX 75701
903 566-7100
- Clin Lab Scientist/Med Tech

Victoria

Citizens Medical Center
David Brown, FACHE, Administrator
2701 Hospital Dr
Victoria, TX 77901
512 573-9181
- Radiographer

Victoria College
Jimmy Goodson, EdD, President
2200 E Red River
Victoria, TX 77901
512 573-3291
- Clin Lab Tech/Med Lab Tech-AD
- Respiratory Therapist
- Respiratory Therapy Tech

Waco

Baylor University
Robert B Sloan Jr, President/CEO
Waco, TX 76798
817 755-1011
- Dietitian/Nutritionist
- Speech Language Pathologist

Hillcrest Baptist Medical Center
Richard Scott, President
3000 Herring Ave
Waco, TX 76708
817 756-8551
- Clin Lab Scientist/Med Tech

McLennan Community College
Dennis F Michaelis, PhD, President
1400 College Dr
Waco, TX 76708
817 299-8601
- Clin Lab Tech/Med Lab Tech-AD
- Radiographer
- Respiratory Therapy Tech

Wharton

Wharton County Junior College
Frank R Vivelo, PhD, President
911 Boling Hwy
Wharton, TX 77488
409 532-6400
- Clin Lab Tech/Med Lab Tech-AD
- Dental Hygienist
- Health Information Tech
- Radiographer

Wichita Falls

Midwestern State University
Louis J Rodriguez, PhD, President
3410 Taft Blvd
Wichita Falls, TX 76308-2099
817 689-4211
- Dental Hygienist
- Radiographer
- Respiratory Therapist

Wichita General Hospital
Jeff Hausler, CEO
1600 Eighth St
Wichita Falls, TX 76301
817 723-1461
- Clin Lab Scientist/Med Tech

Utah

Logan

Utah State University
George H Emert, President
Logan, UT 84322
801 797-1000
- Audiologist
- Dietitian/Nutritionist
- Music Therapist
- Rehabilitation Counselor
- Speech Language Pathologist

Ogden

Weber State University
Paul H Thompson, PhD, President
3902 University Circle
Ogden, UT 84408-3904
801 626-7071
- Clin Lab Scientist/Med Tech
- Clin Lab Tech/Med Lab Tech-AD
- Dental Hygienist
- Emergency Med Tech-Paramedic
- Health Information Tech
- Respiratory Therapist
- Respiratory Therapy Tech

Provo

American Inst of Med/Dental Tech
Keith Van Soest, MA, President
1675 N Freedom Blvd Bldg 9A
Provo, UT 84604
801 377-2900
- Dental Assistant
- Medical Assistant

Brigham Young University
Merrill J Bateman, PhD, President
D 346 ASB
Provo, UT 84602
801 378-2521
- Athletic Trainer
- Audiologist
- Clin Lab Scientist/Med Tech
- Dietitian/Nutritionist
- Speech Language Pathologist
- Therapeutic Recreation Specialist

Provo College
1450 W 820 N
Provo, UT 84601
801 375-1861
- Dental Assistant

Utah Valley Regional Medical Center
Larry Dursteler, CEO
1034 N 500 W
Provo, UT 84603
801 373-7850
- Radiographer

Salt Lake City

Bryman School
Edward J Rogan, Director
1144 W 3300 S
Salt Lake City, UT 84119
801 975-7000
- Medical Assistant

Latter Day Saints Business College
Steven K Woodhouse, MBA, President
411 E South Temple
Salt Lake City, UT 84111
801 524-8101
- Medical Assistant

Salt Lake Community College
Frank W Budd, PhD, President
4600 S Redwood Rd
PO Box 30808
Salt Lake City, UT 84130-0808
801 957-4225
- Clin Lab Tech/Med Lab Tech-AD
- Medical Assistant
- Occupational Therapy Asst
- Radiographer
- Surgical Technologist

Univ of Utah Health Sciences Center
Arthur K Smith, PhD, President
203 Park Bldg
Salt Lake City, UT 84112
540 722-8000
- Audiologist
- Clin Lab Scientist/Med Tech
- Cytotechnologist
- Nuclear Medicine Tech
- Physician Assistant
- Speech Language Pathologist
- Therapeutic Recreation Specialist

University of Utah
Arthur K Smith, President
Salt Lake City, UT 84112
801 581-7200
- Dietitian/Nutritionist

Veterans Affairs Medical Center (120D)
500 Foothill Blvd
Salt Lake City, UT 84148-0001
801 582-1565
- Dietitian/Nutritionist

Vermont

Burlington

Champlain College
Rober H Perry, PhD, President
163 S Willard St
Burlington, VT 05402
802 860-2700
- Radiographer
- Respiratory Therapist

Fletcher Allen Health Care
John Frymoyer, MD, CEO
School of Cytotechnology
111 Colchester Ave
Burlington, VT 05401-1429
802 656-2455
- Cytotechnologist
- Dietitian/Nutritionist

University of Vermont
Thomas P Salmon, JD, President
349 Waterman Bldg
Burlington, VT 05405
802 656-3186
- Athletic Trainer
- Clin Lab Scientist/Med Tech
- Dental Hygienist
- Dietitian/Nutritionist
- Nuclear Medicine Tech
- Radiation Therapist
- Speech Language Pathologist

Essex Junction

Essex Technical Center
3 Educational Dr
Essex Junction, VT 05452
- Dental Assistant

Northfield

Vermont College of Norwich University
Richard Schneider, President
Northfield, VT 05764
802 485-2000
- Art Therapist

Rutland

Rutland Regional Medical Center
James T Bowse, President
160 Allen St
Rutland, VT 05701
802 775-7111
- Radiographer

Virginia

Annandale

Northern Virginia Community College
Richard J Ernst, EdD, President
8333 Little River Trnpk
Annandale, VA 22003
703 323-3101
- Clin Lab Tech/Med Lab Tech-AD
- Dental Hygienist
- Dietetic Technician
- Emergency Med Tech-Paramedic
- Health Information Tech
- Radiographer
- Respiratory Therapist
- Respiratory Therapy Tech

Big Stone Gap

Mountain Empire Community College
Robert H Sandel, EdD, President
PO Drawer 700
Big Stone Gap, VA 24219
703 523-2400
- Respiratory Therapy Tech

Blacksburg

Virginia Polytechnic Inst & State Univ
Paul E Torgersen, President
Blacksburg, VA 24061
540 231-6000
- Dietitian/Nutritionist

Charlottesville

Univ of Virginia Health Sciences Center
Michael J Halseth, MS, Exec Director
Box 148 M4
Charlottesville, VA 22908
804 924-2258
- Audiologist
- Clin Lab Scientist/Med Tech
- Dietitian/Nutritionist
- Nuclear Medicine Tech
- Radiation Therapist
- Radiographer
- Speech Language Pathologist

Falls Church

Fairfax Hospital
Jolene Tournabeni, Administrator
3300 Gallows Rd
Falls Church, VA 22046
703 698-3371
- Clin Lab Scientist/Med Tech

Farmville

Longwood College
Patricia Cormier, President
Longwood College
201 High St
Farmville, VA 23909-1899
804 395-2000
- Therapeutic Recreation Specialist

Fishersville

Augusta Medical Center
David Deering, MBA, COO
Augusta Medical Ctr
PO Box 1000
Fishersville, VA 22939
540 332-4500
- Clin Lab Scientist/Med Tech

Fredericksburg

Mary Washington Hospital
Fred M Rankin III, MPH, President/CEO
1001 Sam Perry Blvd
Fredericksburg, VA 22401
703 899-1571
- Radiographer

Hampton

Commonwealth College - Hampton College
Dana Klakeg, Campus Director
1120 W Mercury Blvd
Hampton, VA 23666-3309
804 838-2122
- Medical Assistant

Hampton University
William R Harvey, President
Hampton, VA 23668
804 727-5000
- Dietitian/Nutritionist
- Speech Language Pathologist

Thomas Nelson Community College
Shirley R Pippins, EdD, President
PO Box 9407
Hampton, VA 23670
757 825-2711
- Clin Lab Tech/Med Lab Tech-AD

Harrisonburg

Dominion Business School of Harrisonburg
Dianne Phipps, Director
933 Reservoir St
Harrisonburg, VA 22801
540 433-6977
- Medical Assistant

James Madison University
Ronald E Carrier, President
Harrisonburg, VA 22807
540 568-6211
- Audiologist
- Dietitian/Nutritionist
- Speech Language Pathologist

Rockingham Memorial Hospital
T Carter Melton Jr, MHA, President
235 Cantrell Ave
Harrisonburg, VA 22801
540 433-4101
- Clin Lab Scientist/Med Tech
- Radiographer

Lynchburg

Centra Health Systems of Lynchburg
George W Dawson, MHA, President/CEO
1920 Atherholt Rd
Lynchburg, VA 24501
804 947-4705
- Clin Lab Tech/Med Lab Tech-C

Central Virginia Community College
Belle S Wheelan, PhD, President
3506 Wards Rd
Lynchburg, VA 24502
804 386-4504
- Radiographer
- Respiratory Therapy Tech

Newport News

Riverside Regional Med Ctr - Newport News
Gerald R Brink, MHA, President
500 J Clyde Morris Blvd
Newport News, VA 23601
804 695-4010
- Clin Lab Tech/Med Lab Tech-C

Riverside School of Health Occupations
Gerald R Brink, MHA, Exec Vice President
Newport News Public Schools
12420 Warwick Blvd Ste 6G
Newport News, VA 23606
804 594-2020
- Radiographer
- Surgical Technologist

Norfolk

Commonwealth College - Richmond Campus
Edward A Abrams, Campus Director
300 Boush St
Norfolk, VA 23510-1216
757 625-5892
- Medical Assistant

DePaul Medical Center
Kevin P Conlin, MS, President
150 Kingsley Ln
Norfolk, VA 23505
757 489-5120
- Radiographer

Eastern Virginia Medical School
Edward E Brickell, EdD, President
PO Box 1980
Norfolk, VA 23501
757 446-5600
- Art Therapist

Norfolk State University
Harrison B Wilson, PhD, President
2401 Corprew Ave
Norfolk, VA 23504
757 683-8670
- Clin Lab Scientist/Med Tech
- Dietitian/Nutritionist
- Health Information Admin

Old Dominion University
James V Koch, PhD, President
New Admin Bldg
Norfolk, VA 23529-0001
757 683-3159
- Clin Lab Scientist/Med Tech
- Cytotechnologist
- Dental Assistant
- Dental Hygienist
- Nuclear Medicine Tech
- Ophthalmic Med Technician
- Speech Language Pathologist

Sentara Norfolk General Hospital
Howard P Kern, CEO
600 Gresham Dr
Norfolk, VA 23507
757 668-3361
- Cardiovascular Technologist
- Clin Lab Tech/Med Lab Tech-C
- Electroneurodiagnostic Tech
- Radiation Therapist
- Surgical Technologist

Tidewater Technical
Jerry Yagen
1760 E Little Creek Rd
Norfolk, VA 23518
757 588-2121
- Dental Assistant

Petersburg

Southside Regional Medical Center
David S Dunham, MHA, Exec Director
801 S Adams St
Petersburg, VA 23803
804 862-5903
- Radiographer

Virginia State University
Eddie N Moore Jr, President
Petersburg, VA 23806
804 524-5000
- Dietitian/Nutritionist

Portsmouth

Naval School of Health Sciences
Charles L Anderson, Capt MSC, USN, CO
Portsmouth, VA 23708-5000
804 398-5032
- Surgical Technologist

Radford

Radford University
Douglas Covington, President
Radford, VA 24142
540 831-5000
- Audiologist
- Dietitian/Nutritionist
- Music Therapist
- Speech Language Pathologist
- Therapeutic Recreation Specialist

Richlands

Southwest Virginia Community College
Charles R King, EdD, President
PO Box SVCC
Richlands, VA 24641-1510
703 964-2555
- Radiographer
- Respiratory Therapist
- Respiratory Therapy Tech

Richmond

J Sargeant Reynolds Community College
Simeon A Burnette, PhD, President
PO Box 85622
Richmond, VA 23285-5622
804 371-3200
- Clin Lab Tech/Med Lab Tech-AD
- Dental Assistant
- Dental Lab Technician
- Dietetic Technician
- Occupational Therapy Asst
- Ophthalmic Dispenser
- Respiratory Therapist
- Respiratory Therapy Tech

Med Coll of VA/Virginia Commonwealth U
John E Jones, MD, VP for Hlth Sciences
PO Box 980549
Richmond, VA 23298-0549
804 828-9770
- Clin Lab Scientist/Med Tech
- Dental Hygienist
- Dietitian/Nutritionist
- Nuclear Medicine Tech
- Occupational Therapist
- Radiation Therapist
- Radiographer
- Rehabilitation Counselor
- Therapeutic Recreation Specialist

St Mary's Hospital
Ann Honeycutt, Exec VP\Administrator
5801 Bremo Rd
Richmond, VA 23226
804 285-2011
- Radiographer

Virginia Department of Health
Div of Public Health Nutrition
1500 E Main St Rm 132
Richmond, VA 23219
804 786-5420
- Dietitian/Nutritionist

Roanoke

Carilion Health System/Carilion Roanoke Mem Hosp
Nancy H Agee, RN MN
PO Box 13367
Roanoke, VA 24033-3367
540 981-8385
- Clin Lab Scientist/Med Tech
- Nuclear Medicine Tech
- Radiation Therapist
- Radiographer

College of Health Sciences
Harry C Nickens, EdD, President/CEO
Comm Hospital of Roanoke Valley
PO Box 13186
Roanoke, VA 24031-3186
540 985-8491
- Emergency Med Tech-Paramedic
- Health Information Tech
- Occupational Therapy Asst
- Respiratory Therapist

Dominion Business School of Roanoke
Kathleen Duncan, Director
4142 Melrose Ave NW/Ste 1
Roanoke, VA 24017
540 362-7738
- Medical Assistant

National Business College
Frank Longaker, MA, President
PO Box 6400
Roanoke, VA 24017-0400
540 986-1800
- Medical Assistant

Virginia Western Community College
Charles L Downs, PhD, President
3095 Colonial Ave SW PO Box 14045
Roanoke, VA 24038
540 982-7311
- Dental Hygienist
- Radiographer

Staunton

Dominion Business School of Staunton
Susan Race, BA, School Director
825 Richmond Rd
Staunton, VA 24401
703 886-3596
- Medical Assistant

Virginia Beach

Commonwealth College - Virginia Beach Campus
Kenneth R Sigmon, Director
301 Centre Pointe Dr
Virginia Beach, VA 23462
804 499-7900
- Medical Assistant

Computer Dynamics Institute
400 S Witchduck Rd #10
Virginia Beach, VA 23462
- Dental Assistant

Tidewater Community College
Larry L Whitworth, EdD, President
1700 College Crescent
Virginia Beach, VA 23456
804 484-2121
- Diagnostic Med Sonographer
- Dietetic Technician
- Health Information Tech
- Radiographer
- Respiratory Therapist
- Respiratory Therapy Tech

Winchester

Shenandoah University
James A Davis, President
1460 University Dr
Winchester, VA 22601
540 665-4500
- Music Therapist
- Occupational Therapist
- Respiratory Therapist

Winchester Medical Center
George Caley, FACHE MHA, President
1840 Amherst St
PO Box 3340
Winchester, VA 22601-2540
540 722-8000
- Radiographer
- Surgical Technologist

Wytheville

Wytheville Community College
William F Snyder, EdD, President
1000 E Main St
Wytheville, VA 24382
540 223-4700
- Clin Lab Tech/Med Lab Tech-AD
- Dental Assistant
- Dental Hygienist

Yorktown

Tri-Service Optician Schools (TOPS)
HMC William J Dufort, USN,
Naval Ophthalmic Support & Trng Activity
NWS PO Box 350
Yorktown, VA 23691-0350
804 887-7148
- Ophthalmic Dispenser
- Ophthalmic Laboratory Technologist

Washington

Auburn

Green River Community College
Richard Rutkowski, MBA, President
12401 SE 320th St
Auburn, WA 98002-3699
206 833-9111
- Occupational Therapy Asst

Bellevue

Bellevue Community College
B Jean Floten, MS, President
3000 Landerholm Circle SE
Bellevue, WA 98007-6484
206 641-2301
- Diagnostic Med Sonographer
- Nuclear Medicine Tech
- Radiation Therapist
- Radiographer

Bellingham

Bellingham Technical College
Desmond McArdle, MEd, President
3028 Lindbergh Ave
Bellingham, WA 98225
360 738-3105
- Dental Assistant

Western Washington University
Karen W Morse, President
Bellingham, WA 98225
360 676-3000
- Audiologist
- Speech Language Pathologist

Cheney

Eastern Washington University
Marshall E Drummond, President
Cheney, WA 99004
509 359-6200
- Speech Language Pathologist
- Therapeutic Recreation Specialist

Des Moines

Highline Community College
Edward Command, EdD, President
PO Box 98000
Des Moines, WA 98198-9800
206 878-3710
- Dental Assistant
- Medical Assistant
- Respiratory Therapist

Ellensburg

Central Washington University
Ivory V Nelson, PhD, President
400 E Eighth Ave
Ellensburg, WA 98926-7501
509 963-2111
- Clin Lab Scientist/Med Tech
- Dietitian/Nutritionist
- Emergency Med Tech-Paramedic

Everett

Everett Community College
Susan Carroll, President
801 Wetmore
Everett, WA 98201
206 388-9202
- Medical Assistant

Kirkland

Lake Washington Technical College
Donald W Fowler, President
11605 132nd Ave NE
Kirkland, WA 98034
206 828-5600
- Dental Assistant
- Dental Hygienist

Olympia

South Puget Sound Community College
Kenneth J Minnaert, PhD, President
2011 Mottman Rd SW
Olympia, WA 98502-6218
206 754-7711
- Dental Assistant
- Medical Assistant

Pullman

Washington State University
Samuel H Smith, President
President's Office French 422B
Pullman, WA 99164-1048
509 335-6666
- Athletic Trainer
- Audiologist
- Dietitian/Nutritionist
- Speech Language Pathologist

Renton

Renton Technical College
Robert C Roberts, EdD, President
3000 NE Fourth St
Renton, WA 98056
206 235-2235
- Dental Assistant
- Surgical Technologist

Seattle

Bastyr University
Joseph E Pizzorno Jr, President
144 NE 54th St
Seattle, WA 98105
206 523-9585
- Dietitian/Nutritionist

Harborview Med Ctr - Univ of Washington
David Jaffe, MPA, Admin/Executive Dir
325 Ninth Ave
Seattle, WA 98104
206 731-3036
- Cytotechnologist
- Emergency Med Tech-Paramedic

North Seattle Community College
Constance W Rice, PhD, President
9600 College Way N
Seattle, WA 98103
206 527-3602
- Medical Assistant

Pima Medical Institute - Seattle
Richard Luebke Sr, BS, President
1627 Eastlake Ave E
Seattle, WA 98102
602 326-1600
- Clin Lab Tech/Med Lab Tech-AD
- Radiographer

Sea Mar Community Health Center
8720 14th Ave S
Seattle, WA 98108-4807
206 726-3730
- Dietitian/Nutritionist

Seattle Central Community College

Charles Mitchell, EdD, President
1701 Broadway, 2EB4180
Seattle, WA 98122
206 587-4144
• Ophthalmic Dispenser
• Respiratory Therapist
• Surgical Technologist

Seattle Pacific University

3307 Third Ave W
Seattle, WA 98119
206 281-2050
• Dietitian/Nutritionist

Seattle University

William J Sullivan, PhD SJ, President
Broadway and Madison
Seattle, WA 98122-4460
206 296-1891
• Diagnostic Med Sonographer

Shoreline Community College

Gary Oertli, MEd, President
16101 Greenwood Ave N
Seattle, WA 98133
206 546-4551
• Clin Lab Tech/Med Lab Tech-AD
• Dental Hygienist
• Dietetic Technician
• Health Information Tech
• Histologic Technician-AD

University of Washington

Richard L McCormick, PhD, President
Office of the President
Seattle, WA 98195
206 543-5010
• Audiologist
• Clin Lab Scientist/Med Tech
• Dietitian/Nutritionist
• Health Information Admin
• Occupational Therapist
• Physician Assistant
• Speech Language Pathologist

Spokane

East Washington University

Marshall Drummond, CEO
Paulsen Bldg Rm 252
Spokane, WA 99201
509 623-4319
• Dental Hygienist

Holy Family Hospital

Ronald J Schurra, President
N 5633 Lidgerwood Ave
Spokane, WA 99207
509 482-2450
• Radiographer

Sacred Heart Medical Center

Gerald P Leahy, MHA, President/CEO
W 101 Eighth Ave PO Box 2555
Spokane, WA 99220-2555
509 455-3040
• Clin Lab Scientist/Med Tech

Spokane Community College

James Williams, PhD, President
N 1810 Greene St MS 2150
Spokane, WA 99207
509 533-7042
• Cardiovascular Technologist
• Dental Assistant
• Dietetic Technician
• Emergency Med Tech-Paramedic
• Health Information Tech
• Respiratory Therapist
• Surgical Technologist

Tacoma

Bates Technical College

Bill Mohler, President
1101 S Yakima Ave
Tacoma, WA 98405
206 596-1577
• Dental Assistant
• Dental Lab Technician

Clover Park Technical College

Alson E Green Jr, President
4500 Steilacoom Blvd SW
Tacoma, WA 98499
206 589-5500
• Clin Lab Tech/Med Lab Tech-C
• Dental Assistant

Pierce College

George A Delaney, President
9401 Farwest Dr SW
Tacoma, WA 98498
206 964-6500
• Dental Hygienist

Tacoma Community College

Raymond Needham, PhD, President
6501 S 19th St
Tacoma, WA 98466
206 566-5100
• Emergency Med Tech-Paramedic
• Health Information Tech
• Radiographer
• Respiratory Therapist
• Respiratory Therapy Tech

University of Puget Sound

Susan Resneck Pierce, PhD, President
1500 N Warner St
Tacoma, WA 98416-0510
206 756-3201
• Occupational Therapist

Vancouver

Clark College

Earl P Johnson, President
1800 E McLoughlin Blvd
Vancouver, WA 98663
360 992-2000
• Dental Hygienist

Wenatchee

Wenatchee Valley College

Woody Ahn, EdD, President
1300 Fifth St
Wenatchee, WA 98801
509 662-1651
• Clin Lab Tech/Med Lab Tech-AD
• Radiographer

Yakima

Yakima Valley Community College

Linda J Kaminski, EdD, President
PO Box 1647
Yakima, WA 98907-1647
509 574-4635
• Dental Hygienist
• Occupational Therapy Asst
• Radiographer

West Virginia

Beckley

College of West Virginia

Charles H Polk, EdD, President
PO Box AG
Beckley, WV 25802
304 253-7351
• Diagnostic Med Sonographer
• Physician Assistant
• Respiratory Therapist

Dept of Veterans Affairs Medical Center

Gerard P Husson, Med Ctr Director
200 Veterans Ave
Beckley, WV 25801
304 255-2121
• Clin Lab Tech/Med Lab Tech-C

Bluefield

Bluefield Regional Medical Center

Eugene Pawlowski, MBA, President
500 Cherry St
Bluefield, WV 24701
304 327-1701
• Clin Lab Tech/Med Lab Tech-C

Bluefield State College

Robert E Moore, EdD, President
Rock St
Bluefield, WV 24701
304 327-4030
• Radiographer

Buckhannon

West Virginia Wesleyan College

William R Haden, President
Buckhannon, WV 26201
304 473-8000
• Dietitian/Nutritionist

Charleston

Carver Career & Tech Education Center

Norma Miller, MA, Principal
4799 Midland Dr
Charleston, WV 25306
304 348-1965
• Respiratory Therapy Tech

Charleston Area Medical Center

Phil Goodwin, Exec Vice President
Elmwood Ave
Charleston, WV 25301
304 348-7628
• Cytotechnologist

Institutions

University of Charleston
Edwin H Welch, PhD, President
2300 McCorkle Ave SE
Charleston, WV 25304
304 357-4713
- Radiographer
- Respiratory Therapist

Clarksburg

United Hospital Center
Bruce C Carter, MS, President
#3 Hospital Plaza
Clarksburg, WV 26301
304 624-2332
- Radiographer

Fairmont

Fairmont State College
Janet Dudley-Eshbach, PhD, President
Locust Ave
Fairmont, WV 26554
304 367-4151
- Clin Lab Tech/Med Lab Tech-AD
- Health Information Tech

Huntington

Cabell Huntington Hospital
W Don Smith, BS, President
1340 Hal Greer Blvd
Huntington, WV 25701
304 526-2111
- Cytotechnologist

Marshall University
J Wade Gilley, PhD, President
Community and Technical College
400 Hal Greer Blvd
Huntington, WV 25755
304 696-2300
- Clin Lab Scientist/Med Tech
- Clin Lab Tech/Med Lab Tech-AD
- Dietitian/Nutritionist
- Health Information Tech
- Speech Language Pathologist

St Mary's Hospital
J Thomas Jones, BS MHA, Exec Director/CEO
2900 First Ave
Huntington, WV 25702
304 526-1270
- Radiographer

Institute

West Virginia State College
Hazo W Carter Jr, PhD, President
PO Box 399
Institute, WV 25112
304 766-3111
- Nuclear Medicine Tech

Montgomery

West Virginia Institute of Technology
John P Carrier, President
Montgomery, WV 25136
304 442-3071
- Dental Hygienist

Morgantown

Monongalia County Tech Education Center
Director
1000 Mississippi St
Morgantown, WV 26505
304 291-9240
- Surgical Technologist

West Virginia University
David C Hardesty, JD, President
Stewart Hall
PO Box 6201
Morgantown, WV 26506-6201
304 293-5531
- Athletic Trainer
- Audiologist
- Clin Lab Scientist/Med Tech
- Dental Hygienist
- Dietitian/Nutritionist
- Rehabilitation Counselor
- Speech Language Pathologist

West Virginia University Hospitals, Inc
Bernard G Westfall, MBA, President
PO Box 8150 Medical Ctr Dr
Morgantown, WV 26506-8150
304 598-4000
- Diagnostic Med Sonographer
- Dietitian/Nutritionist
- Nuclear Medicine Tech
- Radiation Therapist
- Radiographer

Mt Gay

Southern West Virginia Community College
Travis Kirkland, PhD, President
PO Box 2900
Mt Gay, WV 25637
304 792-4300
- Clin Lab Tech/Med Lab Tech-AD
- Radiographer

Parkersburg

Camden-Clark Memorial Hospital
Thomas J Corder, President/CEO
800 Garfield Ave
Parkersburg, WV 26101
304 424-2204
- Radiographer

West Liberty

West Liberty State College
Ronald M Zaccari, PhD,
West Liberty, WV 26074
304 336-8000
- Clin Lab Scientist/Med Tech
- Dental Hygienist

Wheeling

Ohio Valley Medical Center
Thomas Galinski, MS, President
2000 Eoff St
Wheeling, WV 26003
304 234-8294
- Radiographer

West Virginia Northern Community College
Linda Dunn, EdD, President
1704 Market St
Wheeling, WV 26003
304 233-5900
- Clin Lab Tech/Med Lab Tech-AD
- Respiratory Therapist
- Surgical Technologist

Wheeling Hospital
Donald H Hofreuter, MD, Administrator
Medical Park
Wheeling, WV 26003
304 243-3000
- Radiographer

Wheeling Jesuit University
Rev Thomas S Acker, SJ PhD, President
316 Washington Ave
Wheeling, WV 26003
304 243-2233
- Nuclear Medicine Tech
- Respiratory Therapist

Wisconsin

Appleton

Fox Valley Technical College
H Victor Baldi, PhD, President
1825 N Bluemound Dr
PO Box 2277
Appleton, WI 54913-2277
414 735-5731
- Dental Assistant
- Occupational Therapy Asst

St Elizabeth Hospital
Otto L Cox, MS, President
1506 S Oneida St
Appleton, WI 54915
414 738-2015
- Clin Lab Scientist/Med Tech

Beloit

Beloit Memorial Hospital
Gregory K Britton, President/CEO
1969 W Hart Rd
Beloit, WI 53511
608 364-5011
- Radiographer

Cleveland

Lakeshore Technical College
Dennis Ladwig, EdD, Director
1290 North Ave
Cleveland, WI 53015
414 458-4183
- Dental Assistant
- Medical Assistant
- Radiographer

Eau Claire

Chippewa Valley Technical College

William A Ihlenfeldt, PhD, President
620 W Clairemont Ave
Eau Claire, WI 54701
715 833-6211
- Clin Lab Tech/Med Lab Tech-AD
- Diagnostic Med Sonographer
- Health Information Tech
- Histologic Technician-AD
- Radiographer

Sacred Heart Hospital

Matthew W Hubler, MHA, Exec Vice President
900 W Clairemont Ave
Eau Claire, WI 54701
715 839-4131
- Clin Lab Scientist/Med Tech

University of Wisconsin - Eau Claire

Larry Schnack, Chancellor
Eau Claire, WI 54702-4004
715 836-2637
- Music Therapist
- Speech Language Pathologist

Fond du Lac

Moraine Park Technical College

John J Shanahan, PhD, President
235 N National Ave/PO Box 1940
Fond du Lac, WI 54936-1940
414 922-8611
- Health Information Tech

Green Bay

Bellin Memorial Hospital

George Kerwin, MBA, Administrator
744 S Webster Ave PO Box 23400
Green Bay, WI 54305-3400
414 433-3899
- Radiographer

Northeast Wisconsin Technical College

Gerald Prindiville, PhD, President
2740 W Mason St PO Box 19042
Green Bay, WI 54307-9042
414 498-5411
- Clin Lab Tech/Med Lab Tech-AD
- Dental Assistant
- Dental Hygienist
- Health Information Tech
- Medical Assistant
- Respiratory Therapist
- Surgical Technologist

St Vincent Hospital

Joseph J Neidenbach, MHA, Administrator
PO Box 13508
Green Bay, WI 54307-3508
414 433-8155
- Clin Lab Scientist/Med Tech

University of Wisconsin - Green Bay

Mark L Perkins, Chancellor
Green Bay, WI 54311
414 465-2000
- Dietitian/Nutritionist

Janesville

Blackhawk Technical College

James Catania, PhD, District Director
6004 Prairie Rd PO Box 5009
Janesville, WI 53547
608 756-4121
- Dental Assistant
- Medical Assistant

Kenosha

Gateway Technical College

Carole Johnson, PhD, President
3520 30th Ave
Kenosha, WI 53141-1690
414 656-6916
- Dental Assistant
- Health Information Tech
- Medical Assistant
- Surgical Technologist

La Crosse

Gundersen Med Found/La Crosse Lutheran

John Katrana, PhD, Clinic Administrator
1836 South Ave
La Crosse, WI 54601
608 782-7300
- Nuclear Medicine Tech

Viterbo College

Robert E Gibbons, PhD, President
818 S 9th St
La Crosse, WI 54601
608 784-0040
- Dietitian/Nutritionist

Western Wisconsin Technical College

J Lee Rasch, EdD, President/District Dir
304 N Sixth St PO BoxC-0908
La Crosse, WI 54601-0908
608 758-9210
- Clin Lab Tech/Med Lab Tech-AD
- Dental Assistant
- Electroneurodiagnostic Tech
- Health Information Tech
- Medical Assistant
- Radiographer
- Respiratory Therapist
- Surgical Technologist

LaCrosse

University of Wisconsin - LaCrosse

Judith L Kuipers, PhD, Chancellor
135a Main Hall
LaCrosse, WI 54601
608 785-8004
- Athletic Trainer
- Therapeutic Recreation Specialist

Madison

Madison Area Technical College

Beverly Simone, EdD, CEO/President
3550 Anderson St
Madison, WI 53704-2599
608 246-6676
- Clin Lab Tech/Med Lab Tech-AD
- Dental Assistant
- Dental Hygienist
- Dietetic Technician
- Medical Assistant
- Occupational Therapy Asst
- Radiographer
- Respiratory Therapist
- Surgical Technologist

State Laboratory of Hygiene

R H Laessig, PhD, Director
Center for Health Studies - UW Madison
465 Henry Hall
Madison, WI 53706
608 262-1293
- Cytotechnologist

University of Wisconsin - Madison

David Ward, PhD, Chancellor
500 Lincoln Dr
158 Bascom Hall
Madison, WI 53706-1380
608 262-9946
- Audiologist
- Clin Lab Scientist/Med Tech
- Dietitian/Nutritionist
- Occupational Therapist
- Physician Assistant
- Rehabilitation Counselor
- Speech Language Pathologist

University of Wisconsin Hosp & Clinics

Gordon M Derzon, MHA, Superintendent
600 Highland Ave
Madison, WI 53792-3252
608 263-8025
- Diagnostic Med Sonographer
- Dietitian/Nutritionist
- Radiation Therapist
- Radiographer

Marshfield

Marshfield Clinic

Robert J DeVita, MBA, Exec Director
1000 N Oak Ave
Marshfield, WI 54449
715 387-5123
- Cytotechnologist

St Joseph's Hospital

Michael A Schmidt, CPA, President/CEO
611 St Joseph Ave
Marshfield, WI 54449-1898
715 387-1713
- Clin Lab Scientist/Med Tech
- Histologic Technician-Cert
- Nuclear Medicine Tech
- Radiographer

Institutions

Menomonie

University of Wisconsin - Stout
Charles W Sorensen, Chancellor
Menomonie, WI 54751
715 232-1123
- Dietitian/Nutritionist
- Rehabilitation Counselor

Mequon

Concordia University Wisconsin
R John Buuck, PhD DMin, President
12800 N Lake Shore Dr
Mequon, WI 53097
414 243-5700
- Medical Assistant
- Occupational Therapist

Milwaukee

Alverno College
Sr Joel Read, President
3401 S 39th St/Box 343922
Milwaukee, WI 53234-3922
414 382-6000
- Music Therapist

Aurora Health Care
G Edwin Howe, MBA, President
3000 W Montana Ave PO Box 343910
Milwaukee, WI 53234-3910
414 647-3000
- Clin Lab Scientist/Med Tech

Blood Center of Southeast Wisconsin
William V. Miller, MD, President
PO Box 2178
Milwaukee, WI 53201-2178
414 937-6338
- Specialist in BB Tech

Clement J Zablocki VA Medical Center
Russell Struble, FACHE, Director
5000 W National Ave
Milwaukee, WI 53295
414 384-2000
- Clin Lab Scientist/Med Tech

Columbia Hospital
Susan Henckel, Executive VP/CEO
Hospital and Health Services
2025 E Newport Ave
Milwaukee, WI 53211
414 961-3800
- Radiographer

Froedtert Memorial Lutheran Hospital
William D Petasnick, MHA, President
9200 W Wisconsin Ave
PO Box 26099
Milwaukee, WI 53226
414 259-2606
- Clin Lab Scientist/Med Tech
- Cytotechnologist
- Nuclear Medicine Tech
- Radiographer

Marquette University
John P Raynor, SJ, Chancellor
619 N 16th St
Milwaukee, WI 53233
414 288-7700
- Dental Hygienist
- Speech Language Pathologist

Milwaukee Area Technical College
John R Birkholz, EdD, President
700 W State St
Milwaukee, WI 53233-1443
414 297-6320
- Clin Lab Tech/Med Lab Tech-AD
- Dental Hygienist
- Dental Lab Technician
- Dietetic Technician
- Medical Assistant
- Occupational Therapy Asst
- Radiographer
- Respiratory Therapist
- Surgical Technologist

Milwaukee School of Engineering
Hermann Viets, PhD, President
1025 N Broadway
Milwaukee, WI 53202-3109
414 277-7100
- Perfusionist

Mt Mary College
Sally Mahoney, Interim President
2900 N Menomonee River Pkwy
Milwaukee, WI 53222-4597
414 258-4810
- Art Therapist
- Dietitian/Nutritionist
- Occupational Therapist

St Francis Hospital
Gregory Banaszynski, BA MBA, President
3237 S 16th St
Milwaukee, WI 53215
414 647-5106
- Diagnostic Med Sonographer

St Joseph's Hospital
Jon Wachs, President & COO
5000 W Chambers St
Milwaukee, WI 53210
414 447-2355
- Radiation Therapist

St Luke's Medical Center
Mark R Ambrosius, MHA, President
2900 W Oklahoma Ave PO Box 2901
Milwaukee, WI 53201-2901
414 649-7500
- Diagnostic Med Sonographer
- Nuclear Medicine Tech
- Radiation Therapist
- Radiographer

St Mary's Hospital
Charles Lobeck, Exec VP/CEO
2323 N Lake Dr
PO Box 503
Milwaukee, WI 53201
414 291-1000
- Diagnostic Med Sonographer
- Radiographer

St Michael Hospital
Jeffery K Jenkins, MHA, President/CEO
2400 W Villard Ave
Milwaukee, WI 53209
414 527-8123
- Radiographer

Stratton College
Robert H Ley, MA, Director/VP
1300 N Jackson St
Milwaukee, WI 53202
414 276-5200
- Medical Assistant

University of Wisconsin - Milwaukee
John H Schroeder, PhD, Chancellor
PO Box 413
Milwaukee, WI 53201
414 229-4331
- Clin Lab Scientist/Med Tech
- Health Information Admin
- Occupational Therapist
- Rehabilitation Counselor
- Speech Language Pathologist

Neenah

Theda Clark Regional Medical Center
Paul E Macek, President
130 Second St PO Box 2021
Neenah, WI 54957-2021
414 729-2004
- Radiographer

New Richmond

Wisconsin Indianhead Technical College
Timothy O Schreiner, AA BS MS, Regl Admin
1019 S Knowles Ave
New Richmond, WI 54017
715 246-6561
- Medical Assistant

Oshkosh

Mercy Medical Center
Otto Cox, President
PO Box 1100
Oshkosh, WI 54902
414 233-5110
- Radiographer

University of Wisconsin - Oshkosh
John E Kerrigan, Chancellor
800 Algoma Blvd
Oshkosh, WI 54901
414 424-1234
- Audiologist
- Music Therapist
- Speech Language Pathologist

Pewaukee

Waukesha County Technical College
Richard T Anderson, EdD, President
800 Main St
Pewaukee, WI 53072
414 691-5201
- Dental Hygienist
- Medical Assistant
- Surgical Technologist

Racine

All Saints Healthcare System Inc
Edward Demeulenaere,
1320 Wisconsin Ave
Racine, WI 53403
414 636-2846
- Radiographer

River Falls

University of Wisconsin - River Falls
Gary A Thibodeau, Chancellor
River Falls, WI 54022
715 425-3911
- Speech Language Pathologist

Stevens Point

University of Wisconsin - Stevens Point
H Howard Thoyre, Acting Chancellor
Stevens Point, WI 54481
715 346-0123
- Audiologist
- Dietitian/Nutritionist
- Speech Language Pathologist

Wausau

Northcentral Technical College
Robert C Ernst, PhD, President
1000 Campus Dr
Wausau, WI 54401-1899
715 675-3331
- Dental Hygienist
- Radiographer
- Surgical Technologist

Wausau Hospital
Paul Spaude, MHA, President
333 Pine Ridge Blvd
Wausau, WI 54401
715 847-2117
- Clin Lab Scientist/Med Tech

Whitewater

University of Wisconsin - Whitewater
H Gaylon Greenhill, Chancellor
800 W Main
Whitewater, WI 53190-1791
414 472-1234
- Speech Language Pathologist

Wisconsin Rapids

Mid-State Technical College
Brian G Oehler, President
500 32nd St N
Wisconsin Rapids, WI 54494
715 423-5650
- Medical Assistant
- Respiratory Therapist
- Surgical Technologist

Wyoming

Casper

Casper College
LeRoy Strausner, PhD, President
125 College Dr
Casper, WY 82601
307 268-2548
- Occupational Therapist
- Radiographer

Cheyenne

Laramie County Community College
Charles Bohlen, PhD, President
1400 E College Dr
Cheyenne, WY 82007
307 778-5222
- Dental Hygienist
- Radiographer

Cody

West Park Hospital
Gary Bishop, MBA, Administrator
707 Sheridan Ave
Cody, WY 82414
307 527-7501
- Radiographer

Laramie

University of Wyoming
Terry P Roark, PhD, President
University Station PO Box 3434
Laramie, WY 82071
307 766-4121
- Audiologist
- Clin Lab Scientist/Med Tech
- Dietitian/Nutritionist
- Speech Language Pathologist

Rock Springs

Western Wyoming Community College
Tex Boggs, PhD, President
2500 College Dr PO Box 428
Rock Springs, WY 82902-0428
307 382-1600
- Respiratory Therapist
- Respiratory Therapy Tech

Sheridan

Sheridan College
Steve Maier, EdD, President
3059 Coffeen Ave
Sheridan, WY 82801
307 674-6446
- Dental Assistant
- Dental Hygienist

Institutions

Section IV

Health Professions Education Data

Section IV—Health Professions Education Data—highlights data collected on the Annual Survey of Accredited Health Professions Education Programs conducted by the American Medical Association, with participation from 10 of the 13 health professions' accrediting agencies:

- Accreditation Council for Occupational Therapy Education
- American Art Therapy Association
- Commission on Accreditation of Allied Health Education Programs
- Commission on Dental Accreditation of the American Dental Association
- Commission on Opticianry Accreditation
- Commission on Standards and Accreditation of the Council on Rehabilitation Education
- Council on Accreditation of the National Recreation and Park Association
- Joint Review Committee on Educational Programs in Nuclear Medicine Technology
- Joint Review Committee on Education in Radiologic Technology
- National Accrediting Agency for Clinical Laboratory Sciences

The population was established from 1996 accreditation data provided by each agency and information submitted by educational programs and sponsoring institutions. Data are provided for educational programs in 35 health professions.

Information about specific accredited programs can be found in Section II: Occupational Descriptions and Educational Programs. Information about institutions that sponsor accredited programs is included in Section III: Institutions Sponsoring Accredited Programs.

1996 Survey of Accredited Health Professions Education Programs

In fall 1996, 3,928 pretested questionnaires were sent to directors of programs accredited as of July 1996. The survey collected data on program enrollments, graduates, and attrition by gender, as well as tuition cost(s), class capacity, availability of evening/weekend classes, program length(s), starting date(s), and credential(s) awarded, along with the name, address, telephone/fax numbers, and e-mail addresses of institution and program officials.

Questionnaires were completed by program directors and verified by principal administrative officers at sponsoring institutions. To ensure a high response rate, non-respondents received reminder mailings after the original surveys were sent. Telephone calls were made to those who did not respond to the reminder mailings. Ninety-six percent (3,768) of the 3,928 surveys sent to directors of accredited programs were returned. Before data entry, questionnaires were individually examined and data were verified by AMA staff; questionnaires that required additional information were returned to respondents for completion.

Enrollment, graduate, and attrition data are reported for the 1995-1996 academic year. Although precise dates vary with institutional calendars, the *1995-1996 academic year* was defined as the period between the beginning of the 1995 fall term/semester and the end of the 1996 summer term/semester. For programs not following an academic calendar, the 1995-1996 academic year reflects September 1, 1995, to August 31, 1996.

Enrollees were defined as students who were enrolled in an accredited program after the institution's cutoff date for adding or dropping courses in fall 1995. *Graduates* were defined as students who successfully completed the program and who were awarded a degree or credential by the end of summer 1996. (Graduates included students in Occupational Therapy Field Work II who had completed baccalaureate requirements by the end of summer 1996.)

Attrition was defined as the number of students who were enrolled but for various reasons ceased to be enrolled in an accredited program during the 1995-1996 academic year. Attrition data reflect the number of students who dropped out, stopped out, or transferred to another program or institution, as well as those who were lost due to academic failure during the 1995-1996 academic year.

Since the early seventies, the AMA has annually collected program enrollment and graduate data. Beginning in 1989, enrollment, attrition, and graduate data have been compiled by gender (collection of data on race/ethnic origin was discontinued after the 1995 survey).

For more information on these or other health professions data, contact:

American Medical Association
Medical Education Products
515 N State St
Chicago, IL 60610
312 464-5333
312 464-5830 Fax

Table 1. Accredited or Approved Programs by Occupation, 1985, 1990, 1995, and 1996*

Occupation	1985	1990	1995	1996
Anesthesiologist Assistant (AA)	0	2	2	2
Art Therapist (ATR)	—	—	—	27
Athletic Trainer (AT)	—	—	29	55
Audiologist (AUD)	149	111	120	120
Cardiovascular Technologist (CVT)	0	2	14	16
Clinical Laboratory Scientist/Medical Technologist (CLS/MT)	584	420	357	339
Clin Lab Tech/Med Lab Tech-Associate Degree (CLT/MLT AD)	225	215	223	24
Clin Lab Tech/Med Lab Tech-Certificate (CLT/MLT C)	56	41	37	38
Cytotechnologist (CYTO)	58	46	67	64
Dental Assistant (DA)	290	244	229	237
Dental Hygienist (DH)	198	202	212	222
Dental Laboratory Technician (DLT)	58	49	37	35
Diagnostic Medical Sonographer (DMS)	24	43	77	75
Dietetic Technician (DT)	80	62	70	72
Dietitian/Nutrionist (DN)	444	439	529	536
Electroneurodiagnostic Technologist (ET)	20	14	14	11
Emergency Medical Technician-Paramedic (EMTP)	20	72	96	98
Health Information Administrator (HIA)	54	55	53	53
Health Information Technician (HIT)	85	108	142	158
Histologic Technician-Associate Degree (HTAD)	+	+	+	9
Histologic Technician-Certificate (HTC)	+	+	+	23
Histotechnologist (HTL)	43++	37++	31++	3
Medical Assistant (MA)	168	185	221	272
Medical Illustrator (MI)	5	6	5	5
Music Therapist (MT)	—	—	—	61
Nuclear Medicine Technologist (NMT)	141	107	120	118
Occupational Therapist (OT)	61	69	98	105
Occupational Therapy Assistant (OTA)	60	69	108	117
Ophthalmic Dispensing Optician (OD)	—	—	—	24
Ophthalmic Laboratory Technician (OLT)	—	—	—	3
Ophthalmic Medical Technician/Technologist (OMT)	9	10	10	11
Orthotist/Prosthetist (OP)	—	—	1	2
Pathologist's Assistant (PTHA)	0	0	0	2
Perfusionist (PERF)	19	26	33	31
Physician Assistant (PA)	52	48	64	87
Radiation Therapist (RADT)	101	104	120	106
Radiographer (RAD)	744	672	677	648
Rehabilitation Counselor (RC)	—	—	—	84
Respiratory Therapist (REST)	232	259	286	293
Respiratory Therapy Technician (RESTT)	182	159	174	162
Specialist in Blood Banking Technology (SBBT)	59	29	24	22
Speech-Language Pathologist (SLP)	**	194	222	223
Surgeon Assistant (SA)	3	3	+	+
Surgical Technologist (ST)	102	113	143	145
Therapeutic Recreation Specialist (TRS)	—	—	—	41
Total	**4,326**	**3,795**	**4,645**	**4,979**

* Table 1 contains the total number of programs for all occupations with accredited programs listed in this *Directory*. Tables 2 through 7 present data only for programs accredited by the 10 agencies listed on p. 447.

— These occupations were not part of the accreditation systems reflected in this *Directory*.

**The number of speech-language pathologist programs for 1985 is included in the number of audiologist programs.

+ Surgeon assistant programs are now listed with physician assistant programs.

++ Before 1996, numbers for HTAD, HTC, and HTL were not broken out.

Health Professions Education Data

Table 2. Number of Programs and Enrollments, Attrition, and Graduates by Occupation, Academic Year 1995–1996*

Occupation	Responding Programs	Enrollments	Attrition	Graduates
Anesthesiologist Assistant	1	12	0	8
Art Therapist	25	1,107	31	376
Athletic Trainer	36	1,455	78	393
Cardiovascular Technologist	14	503	74	226
Clinical Laboratory Scientist/Medical Technologist	346	6,985	536	3,155
Clin Lab Tech/Med Lab Tech-Associate Degree	218	6,439	1,309	2,269
Clin Lab Tech/Med Lab Tech-Certificate	36	957	215	661
Cytotechnologist	62	378	30	315
Dental Assistant	237	6,496	1,341	4,341
Dental Hygienist	219	9,776	554	4,001
Dental Laboratory Technician	34	939	127	398
Diagnostic Medical Sonographer	75	1,342	134	766
Dietetic Technician	0	6,562	NA	732
Dietitian/Nutritionist	0	28,336	NA	5,769
Electroneurodiagnostic Technologist	13	177	39	86
Emergency Medical Technician-Paramedic	91	5,062	942	2,756
Health Information Administrator	53	2,590	128	758
Health Information Technician	144	6,244	735	2,049
Histologic Technician-Associate Degree	8	124	18	34
Histologic Technician-Certificate	20	44	6	38
Histotechnologist	3	9	1	6
Medical Assistant	231	20,512	4,715	8,443
Medical Illustrator	5	78	1	37
Nuclear Medicine Technologist	111	1,537	175	732
Occupational Therapist	92	13,339	397	4,270
Occupational Therapy Assistant	108	6,631	607	2,722
Ophthalmic Dispensing Optician	11	410	56	214
Ophthalmic Laboratory Technician	1	12	9	4
Ophthalmic Medical Technician/Technologist	11	137	11	58
Orthotist/Prosthetist	1	29	3	26
Perfusionist	31	302	28	150
Physician Assistant	64	5,793	213	2,138
Radiation Therapist	109	1,144	154	649
Radiographer	639	19,908	2,468	8,595
Rehabilitation Counselor	66	2,837	141	893
Respiratory Therapist	289	11,081	1,848	4,348
Respiratory Therapy Technician	170	5,587	1,229	2,994
Specialist in Blood Banking Technology	23	51	2	32
Surgical Technologist	140	3,480	831	2,086
Therapeutic Recreation Specialist	29	2,266	194	683
Total	**3,766**	**180,671**	**19,380**	**68,211**

* Data were provided by 3,557 programs (94%) of the responding programs accredited by the 10 agencies listed on page 447.

Table 3. Enrollments, Attrition, and Graduates by Occupation and Gender, Academic Year 1995–1996*

Occupation**	Valid Responses*	Enrollments					Attrition					Graduates				
		Male		Female			Male		Female			Male		Female		
		N	(%)	N	(%)	Total	N	(%)	N	(%)	Total	N	(%)	N	(%)	Total
AA	1	7	58	5	42	12	0	0	0	0	0	5	63	3	38	8
AT	36	723	50	732	50	1,455	40	51	38	49	78	202	51	191	49	393
ATR	25	149	14	958	87	1,107	3	10	28	90	31	30	8	346	92	376
CLS/MT	346	2,083	30	4,902	70	6,985	197	37	339	63	536	863	27	2,292	73	3,155
CLT/MLT AD	218	1,518	24	4,921	76	6,439	340	26	969	74	1,309	490	22	1,779	78	2,269
CLT/MLT C	36	410	43	547	57	957	72	34	143	67	215	313	47	348	53	661
CVT	14	171	34	332	66	503	32	43	42	57	74	72	32	154	68	226
CYTO	62	109	29	269	71	378	11	37	19	64	30	94	30	221	70	315
DA	237	237	4	6,259	96	6,496	50	4	1,291	97	1,341	129	3	4,212	97	4,341
DH	219	317	3	9,459	97	9,776	30	5	524	95	554	81	2	3,920	98	4,001
DLT	34	459	49	480	51	939	77	61	50	39	127	176	44	222	56	398
DMS	75	164	12	1,178	88	1,342	32	24	102	76	134	85	11	681	89	766
DN	0	2,988	11	25,348	89	28,336	NA	NA	NA	NA	NA	635	11	5,134	89	5,769
DT	0	927	14	5,635	86	6,562	NA	NA	NA	NA	NA	102	14	630	86	732
ET	13	59	33	118	67	177	13	33	26	67	39	26	30	60	70	86
EMTP	91	3,768	74	1,294	26	5,062	684	73	258	27	942	2,151	78	605	22	2,756
HIA	53	334	13	2,256	87	2,590	20	16	108	84	128	102	14	656	87	758
HIT	144	472	8	5,772	92	6,244	57	8	678	92	735	125	6	1,924	94	2,049
HTAD	8	42	34	82	66	124	9	50	9	50	18	13	38	21	62	34
HTC	20	10	23	34	77	44	1	17	5	83	6	9	24	29	76	38
HTL	3	1	11	8	89	9	0	0	1	100	1	1	17	5	83	6
MA	231	1,388	7	19,124	93	20,512	431	9	4,284	91	4,715	462	6	7,981	95	8,443
MI	5	33	42	45	58	78	1	10	0	0	1	13	35	24	65	37
NMT	111	694	45	843	55	1,537	83	47	92	53	175	353	48	379	52	732
OD	11	197	48	213	52	410	33	59	23	41	56	122	57	92	43	214
OLT	1	9	75	3	25	12	6	67	3	33	9	3	75	1	25	4
OMT	11	29	21	108	79	137	4	36	7	64	11	15	26	43	74	58
OP	1	16	55	13	45	29	2	67	1	33	3	14	54	12	46	26
OT	92	2,001	15	11,338	85	13,339	74	19	323	81	397	579	14	3,691	86	4,270
OTA	108	986	15	5,645	85	6,631	122	20	485	80	607	407	15	2,315	85	2,722
PA	64	2,311	40	3,482	60	5,793	96	45	117	55	213	841	39	1,297	61	2,138
PERF	31	194	64	108	36	302	18	64	10	36	28	100	67	50	33	150
RAD	639	6,020	30	13,888	70	19,908	761	31	1,707	69	2,468	2,762	32	5,833	68	8,595
RADT	109	432	38	712	62	1,144	65	42	89	58	154	232	36	417	64	649
RC	66	831	29	2,006	71	2,837	28	20	113	80	141	238	27	655	73	893
REST	289	3,862	35	7,219	65	11,081	625	34	1,223	66	1,848	1,574	36	2,774	64	4,348
RESTT	170	1,812	32	3,775	68	5,587	415	34	814	66	1,229	982	33	2,012	67	2,994
SBBT	23	16	31	35	69	51	0	0	2	100	2	10	31	22	69	32
ST	140	752	22	2,728	78	3,480	171	21	660	79	831	492	24	1,594	76	2,086
TRS	29	728	32	1,538	68	2,266	63	33	131	68	194	211	31	472	69	683
Total	**3,766**	**37,259**	**21**	**143,412**	**79**	**180,671**	**4,666**	**24**	**14,714**	**76**	**19,380**	**15,114**	**22**	**53,097**	**78**	**68,211**

* Data were provided by 3,557 (94%) of the 3,766 responding programs accredited by the 10 agencies identified on p. 447.
** See Table 1 for a key to occupational abbreviations.
Percentages are computed on a row basis.

Table 4. Graduates by Occupation and Degree/Award, Academic Year 1995–1996*

Occupation**	1 yr UndGrd Certificate	2 yr UndGrd Certificate	Associate	Bacca-laureate	Post-bacca-laureate	Master's	Total Graduates
AA	0	0	0	0	0	8	8
AT	0	0	0	393	0	0	393
ATR	0	24	0	0	20	332	376
CLS/MT	235	0	1	2,316	579	24	3,155
CLT/MLT AD	0	147	2,122	0	0	0	2,269
CLT/MLT C	599	40	22	0	0	0	661
CVT	27	4	195	0	0	0	226
CYTO	76	0	0	146	84	9	315
DA	4,139	55	147	0	0	0	4,341
DH	37	219	3,121	616	2	6	4,001
DLT	112	90	194	2	0	0	398
DMS	321	45	319	81	0	0	766
DN	0	0	0	3,932	1,837	0	5,769
DT	0	0	732	0	0	0	732
EMTP	2,173	260	290	33	0	0	2,756
ET	21	1	64	0	0	0	86
HIA	0	0	0	701	34	23	758
HIT	78	164	1,799	8	0	0	2,049
HTAD	0	0	29	5	0	0	34
HTC	38	0	0	0	0	0	38
HTL	0	0	0	4	2	0	6
MA	6,136	305	2,002	0	0	0	8,443
MI	0	0	0	0	0	37	37
NMT	266	19	238	173	36	0	732
OD	99	38	77	0	0	0	214
OLT	0	4	0	0	0	0	4
OMT	2	21	32	3	0	0	58
OP	0	0	0	0	26	0	26
OT	0	0	0	3,191	159	920	4,270
OTA	76	132	2,475	39	0	0	2,722
PA	80	342	182	1,096	65	373	2,138
PERF	8	14	2	47	73	6	150
RAD	542	2,683	5,051	319	0	0	8,595
RADT	300	74	192	83	0	0	649
RC	0	0	0	20	0	873	893
REST	156	588	3,184	419	0	1	4,348
RESTT	2,008	209	754	23	0	0	2,994
SBBT	10	0	0	5	10	7	32
ST	1,729	1	356	0	0	0	2,086
TRS	0	0	0	626	0	57	683
Total	**19,268**	**5,479**	**23,580**	**14,281**	**2,927**	**2,676**	**68,211**

* Data on degree/awards were provided by 3,557 programs accredited by the 10 agencies identified in Table 1 that responded to the survey.
** See Table 1 for a key to occupational abbreviations.

Table 5. Accredited Programs by Type of Sponsoring Institution, Academic Year 1995–1996*

	Sponsoring Institution	Institutions		Programs	
		N	%	N	%
AH	Academic Health Ctr/Medical School	87	4.2	428	8.6
DD	Department of Defense	10	0.5	32	0.6
VA	Department of Veterans Affairs	11	0.5	21	0.4
UC	Four-year College or University	544	26.0	1,497	30.1
H1	Hospital or Medical Center: 1-99 Beds	3	0.1	3	0.1
H2	Hospital or Medical Center: 100-299 Beds	130	6.2	147	3.0
H3	Hospital or Medical Center: 300-499 Beds	177	8.5	247	5.0
H4	Hospital or Medical Center: 500 or More Beds	165	7.9	352	7.1
CC	Junior or Community College	533	25.5	1,553	31.2
HC	Nonhospital Health Care Facility, Blood Bank, or Laboratory	28	1.3	31	0.6
VT	Vocational or Technical School	275	13.1	517	10.4
CO	Consortium	9	0.4	16	0.3
OC	Not Known or Other	122	5.8	135	2.7
Total		**2,094**	**100**	**4,979**	**100**

* Includes data for all 13 accrediting agencies with programs in this *Directory*.

Table 6. Accredited Programs by Occupation and Type of Sponsoring Institution, Academic Year 1995–1996

Occupation**	AH* N	AH* %	CC N	CC %	CO N	CO %	DD N	DD %	H1 N	H1 %	H2 N	H2 %	H3 N	H3 %	H4 N	H4 %	HC N	HC %	OC N	OC %	UC N	UC %	VA N	VA %	VT N	VT %	Total	%
AA	2	100.0	0	0.0	0	0.0	0	0.0	0	0.0	0	0.0	0	0.0	0	0.0	0	0.0	0	0.0	0	0.0	0	0.0	0	0.0	2	0.0
AT	3	5.5	1	1.8	0	0.0	0	0.0	0	0.0	0	0.0	0	0.0	0	0.0	0	0.0	0	0.0	51	92.7	0	0.0	0	0.0	55	1.1
ATR	6	22.2	0	0.0	0	0.0	0	0.0	0	0.0	0	0.0	0	0.0	0	0.0	0	0.0	3	11.1	18	66.7	0	0.0	0	0.0	27	0.5
AUD	18	15.0	0	0.0	1	0.8	0	0.0	0	0.0	0	0.0	0	0.0	1	0.8	0	0.0	3	2.5	98	81.7	0	0.0	0	0.0	120	2.4
CLS/MT	47	13.9	2	0.6	1	0.3	2	0.6	0	0.0	34	10.0	70	20.6	85	25.1	5	1.5	0	0.0	86	25.4	7	2.1	0	0.0	339	6.8
CLT/MLT AD	3	1.3	165	73.7	0	0.0	0	0.0	0	0.0	0	0.0	0	0.0	0	0.0	0	0.0	0	0.0	28	12.5	0	0.0	28	12.5	224	4.5
CLT/MLT C	1	2.6	2	5.3	0	0.0	3	7.9	0	0.0	4	10.5	3	7.9	3	7.9	1	2.6	0	0.0	1	2.6	1	2.6	19	50.0	38	0.8
CVT	0	0.0	8	50.0	0	0.0	1	6.3	0	0.0	0	0.0	1	6.3	3	18.8	0	0.0	0	0.0	1	6.3	0	0.0	2	12.5	16	0.3
CYTO	21	32.8	1	1.6	0	0.0	2	3.1	0	0.0	1	1.6	8	12.5	21	32.8	7	10.9	0	0.0	3	4.7	0	0.0	0	0.0	64	1.3
DA	5	2.1	119	50.2	0	0.0	1	0.4	0	0.0	0	0.0	0	0.0	0	0.0	0	0.0	22	9.3	11	4.6	0	0.0	79	33.3	237	4.8
DH	23	10.4	124	55.9	0	0.0	0	0.0	0	0.0	0	0.0	0	0.0	0	0.0	0	0.0	17	7.7	47	21.2	0	0.0	11	5.0	222	4.5
DLT	2	5.7	17	48.6	0	0.0	3	8.6	0	0.0	0	0.0	0	0.0	0	0.0	0	0.0	1	2.9	6	17.1	0	0.0	6	17.1	35	0.7
DMS	11	14.7	33	44.0	0	0.0	0	0.0	0	0.0	1	1.3	4	5.3	13	17.3	0	0.0	0	0.0	7	9.3	0	0.0	6	8.0	75	1.5
DN	45	8.4	0	0.0	1	0.2	3	0.6	0	0.0	4	0.7	14	2.6	22	4.1	0	0.0	68	12.7	374	69.8	4	0.7	1	0.2	536	10.8
DT	0	0.0	57	79.2	0	0.0	0	0.0	0	0.0	0	0.0	0	0.0	0	0.0	0	0.0	0	0.0	10	13.9	0	0.0	5	6.9	72	1.4
EMTP	8	8.2	53	54.1	2	2.0	0	0.0	0	0.0	2	2.0	6	6.1	9	9.2	0	0.0	0	0.0	9	9.2	0	0.0	7	7.1	98	2.0
ET	0	0.0	6	54.5	0	0.0	1	9.1	0	0.0	0	0.0	2	18.2	1	9.1	0	0.0	0	0.0	0	0.0	0	0.0	1	9.1	11	0.2
HIA	12	22.6	0	0.0	0	0.0	0	0.0	0	0.0	0	0.0	0	0.0	1	1.9	0	0.0	0	0.0	40	75.5	0	0.0	0	0.0	53	1.1
HIT	2	1.3	111	70.3	0	0.0	0	0.0	0	0.0	0	0.0	0	0.0	0	0.0	0	0.0	0	0.0	29	18.4	0	0.0	16	10.1	158	3.2
HTAD	0	0.0	5	55.6	0	0.0	0	0.0	0	0.0	0	0.0	0	0.0	0	0.0	0	0.0	0	0.0	0	0.0	0	0.0	4	44.4	9	0.2
HTC	0	0.0	1	4.3	1	4.3	0	0.0	0	0.0	1	4.3	8	34.8	10	43.5	0	0.0	0	0.0	1	4.3	0	0.0	0	0.0	23	0.5
HTL	0	0.0	0	0.0	0	0.0	0	0.0	0	0.0	0	0.0	0	0.0	3	100.0	0	0.0	0	0.0	0	0.0	0	0.0	0	0.0	3	0.1
MA	1	0.4	112	41.2	0	0.0	0	0.0	0	0.0	0	0.0	0	0.0	0	0.0	0	0.0	0	0.0	17	6.3	0	0.0	142	52.2	272	5.5
MI	5	100.0	0	0.0	0	0.0	0	0.0	0	0.0	0	0.0	0	0.0	0	0.0	0	0.0	0	0.0	0	0.0	0	0.0	0	0.0	5	0.1
MT	3	4.9	0	0.0	0	0.0	0	0.0	0	0.0	0	0.0	0	0.0	0	0.0	0	0.0	3	4.9	55	90.2	0	0.0	0	0.0	61	1.2
NMT	24	20.3	28	23.7	0	0.0	1	0.8	0	0.0	0	0.0	8	6.8	23	19.5	0	0.0	4	3.4	22	18.6	5	4.2	3	2.5	118	2.4
OD	0	0.0	17	70.8	0	0.0	1	4.2	0	0.0	0	0.0	0	0.0	0	0.0	0	0.0	0	0.0	3	12.5	0	0.0	3	12.5	24	0.5
OLT	0	0.0	1	33.3	0	0.0	1	33.3	0	0.0	0	0.0	0	0.0	0	0.0	0	0.0	0	0.0	0	0.0	0	0.0	1	33.3	3	0.1
OMT	5	45.5	2	18.2	0	0.0	0	0.0	0	0.0	1	9.1	0	0.0	1	9.1	0	0.0	0	0.0	1	9.1	0	0.0	1	9.1	11	0.2
OP	0	0.0	0	0.0	0	0.0	0	0.0	1	50.0	0	0.0	0	0.0	0	0.0	0	0.0	0	0.0	1	50.0	0	0.0	0	0.0	2	0.0
OT	30	28.6	1	1.0	0	0.0	0	0.0	0	0.0	0	0.0	0	0.0	2	1.9	0	0.0	0	0.0	72	68.6	0	0.0	0	0.0	105	2.1
OTA	1	0.9	85	72.6	0	0.0	1	0.9	0	0.0	0	0.0	0	0.0	0	0.0	0	0.0	0	0.0	15	12.8	0	0.0	15	12.8	117	2.3
PA	37	42.5	8	9.2	0	0.0	3	3.4	0	0.0	1	1.1	0	0.0	4	4.6	0	0.0	4	4.6	30	34.5	0	0.0	0	0.0	87	1.7
PERF	8	25.8	0	0.0	1	3.2	1	3.2	0	0.0	3	9.7	4	12.9	6	19.4	0	0.0	0	0.0	8	25.8	0	0.0	0	0.0	31	0.6
PTHA	1	50.0	0	0.0	0	0.0	0	0.0	0	0.0	0	0.0	0	0.0	0	0.0	0	0.0	0	0.0	1	50.0	0	0.0	0	0.0	2	0.0
RAD	25	3.9	227	35.0	3	0.5	2	0.3	1	0.2	88	13.6	103	15.9	86	13.3	1	0.2	5	0.8	58	9.0	3	0.5	46	7.1	648	13.0
RADT	19	17.9	22	20.8	1	0.9	0	0.0	0	0.0	4	3.8	5	4.7	35	33.0	5	4.7	0	0.0	13	12.3	1	0.9	1	0.9	106	2.1
RC	12	14.3	0	0.0	0	0.0	0	0.0	0	0.0	0	0.0	0	0.0	0	0.0	0	0.0	0	0.0	72	85.7	0	0.0	0	0.0	84	1.7
REST	12	4.1	187	63.8	2	0.7	0	0.0	0	0.0	2	0.7	2	0.7	4	1.4	0	0.0	0	0.0	60	20.5	0	0.0	25	8.5	293	5.9
RESTT	4	2.5	89	54.9	1	0.6	0	0.0	0	0.0	0	0.0	3	1.9	4	2.5	0	0.0	0	0.0	12	7.4	0	0.0	49	30.2	162	3.3
SBBT	4	18.2	1	4.5	0	0.0	0	0.0	0	0.0	0	0.0	3	13.6	6	27.3	8	36.4	0	0.0	0	0.0	0	0.0	0	0.0	22	0.4
SLP	20	9.0	0	0.0	1	0.4	0	0.0	0	0.0	1	0.7	1	0.4	0	0.0	0	0.0	8	3.6	192	86.1	0	0.0	0	0.0	223	4.5
ST	5	3.4	67	46.2	0	0.0	4	2.8	0	0.0	0	0.0	6	4.1	9	6.2	0	0.0	0	0.0	8	5.5	0	0.0	46	31.7	145	2.9
TRS	3	7.3	1	2.4	0	0.0	0	0.0	0	0.0	0	0.0	0	0.0	0	0.0	0	0.0	0	0.0	37	90.2	0	0.0	0	0.0	41	0.8
Total	428	8.6	1,553	31.2	16	0.3	32	0.6	3	0.1	147	3.0	247	5.0	352	7.1	31	0.6	135	2.7	1,497	30.1	21	0.4	517	10.4	4,979	100.0

* See Table 5 for a key to sponsoring institution type abbreviations.
** See Table 1 for a key to occupational abbreviations.
Percentages computed on a row basis.

Health Professions Education Data

Table 7. Enrollments, Graduates, and Number of Programs by State and Occupation, Academic Year 1995–1996*

	AA**	AT	ATR	AUD	CLS/ MT	CLT/ MLTAD	CLT/ MLTC	CVT	CYTO	DA	DH	DLT	DMS	DN	DT	EMTP	ET	HIA	HIT	HTAD	HTC	HTL	MA
AL	0	0	0	0	123	169	0	0	12	114	41	0	17	0	0	491	0	9	111	0	5	0	257
	0	0	0	0	69	54	0	0	10	63	12	0	15	0	0	159	0	8	11	0	3	0	64
	0	1	0	4	8	4	0	0	1	6	1	1	1	11	0	8	0	1	2	0	1	0	4
AK	0	0	0	0	0	0	0	0	0	16	24	0	0	0	0	0	0	0	26	0	0	0	81
	0	0	0	0	0	0	0	0	0	15	12	0	0	0	0	0	0	0	6	0	0	0	26
	0	0	0	0	0	0	0	0	0	1	1	0	0	1	0	0	0	0	1	0	0	0	1
AR	0	0	0	0	71	156	0	0	5	42	0	0	0	0	0	0	0	42	28	0	4	0	29
	0	0	0	0	45	48	0	0	5	34	0	0	0	0	0	0	0	26	10	0	3	0	10
	0	0	0	1	3	7	0	0	1	2	1	0	0	7	1	0	0	1	1	0	1	0	1
AZ	0	0	0	0	237	0	0	0	0	24	145	20	9	0	0	0	16	0	49	0	0	0	419
	0	0	0	0	40	0	0	0	0	13	71	9	7	0	0	0	5	0	19	0	0	0	328
	0	0	0	2	2	1	0	0	0	2	3	1	2	11	1	0	0	0	1	0	0	0	1
BC	0	0	0	0	0	0	0	0	0	0	0	0	0	0	0	0	0	0	0	0	0	0	0
	0	0	0	0	0	0	0	0	0	0	0	0	0	0	0	0	0	0	0	0	0	0	0
	0	0	0	0	0	0	0	0	0	0	0	0	0	0	0	0	0	0	0	0	0	0	0
CA	0	30	119	0	106	0	118	111	18	747	498	79	55	0	0	258	43	19	437	0	0	0	2,830
	0	8	0	0	86	0	90	43	18	497	240	56	28	0	0	79	19	5	97	0	0	0	1,406
	0	2	2	7	23	0	1	1	4	24	14	3	2	42	7	3	1	1	8	0	0	0	21
CO	0	0	0	0	40	40	9	0	0	108	127	0	12	0	0	148	0	54	54	0	2	0	308
	0	0	0	0	38	8	7	0	0	88	55	0	12	0	0	76	0	10	22	0	2	0	75
	0	1	0	2	4	1	1	0	0	6	4	0	2	6	1	3	0	1	2	0	1	0	7
CT	0	23	0	0	74	84	0	0	8	92	124	0	0	0	0	28	0	0	0	0	4	0	1,168
	0	6	0	0	27	19	0	0	3	81	52	0	0	0	0	20	0	0	0	0	3	0	414
	0	1	0	2	8	2	0	0	1	5	3	0	0	9	2	1	0	0	1	0	1	0	11
DC	0	0	50	0	116	0	0	0	0	33	0	0	15	0	0	0	0	0	0	0	0	0	0
	0	0	13	0	27	0	0	0	0	16	0	0	6	0	0	0	0	0	0	0	0	0	0
	0	0	1	0	3	4	0	0	0	1	1	0	1	4	0	0	0	0	0	0	0	0	0
DE	0	0	0	0	108	52	0	0	0	0	45	0	11	0	0	18	0	0	0	8	0	0	0
	0	0	0	0	26	8	0	0	0	0	22	0	5	0	0	18	0	0	0	3	0	0	0
	0	1	0	0	1	1	0	0	0	1	1	0	1	3	0	2	0	0	0	1	0	0	0
FL	0	42	0	0	385	298	42	37	7	573	592	196	118	0	0	1384	16	199	212	10	0	0	910
	0	17	0	0	103	98	22	12	5	305	260	38	43	0	0	820	5	49	100	1	0	0	292
	0	1	0	2	11	7	2	1	2	18	15	4	5	13	4	24	1	3	8	1	1	0	11
GA	0	28	0	0	116	96	178	35	4	456	363	30	20	0	0	0	0	77	35	0	3	0	822
	0	12	0	0	49	32	63	13	3	330	153	9	13	0	0	0	0	24	4	0	3	0	463
	1	1	0	1	7	5	7	1	1	6	9	2	2	12	0	0	0	2	2	0	1	0	10
HI	0	0	0	0	51	32	0	0	0	0	0	0	0	0	0	0	0	0	0	0	0	0	83
	0	0	0	0	15	8	0	0	0	0	0	0	0	0	0	0	0	0	0	0	0	0	18
	0	0	0	1	1	1	0	0	0	0	1	0	0	2	0	0	0	0	0	0	0	0	1
ID	0	0	0	0	12	0	0	0	0	18	59	16	0	0	0	0	0	0	84	0	0	0	12
	0	0	0	0	10	0	0	0	0	16	28	6	0	0	0	0	0	0	34	0	0	0	12
	0	1	0	1	2	0	0	0	0	1	1	1	0	3	1	0	0	0	2	0	0	0	1
IL	0	126	74	0	345	240	3	0	0	155	403	19	46	0	0	46	6	200	327	0	0	0	271
	0	34	33	0	145	103	3	0	0	98	168	11	20	0	0	35	6	58	119	0	0	0	133
	0	3	3	6	15	11	1	0	1	8	8	2	2	21	3	2	1	3	8	0	2	1	8
IN	0	82	0	0	88	145	4	0	8	114	290	16	0	0	0	0	0	25	121	0	0	0	2,196
	0	27	0	0	82	46	4	0	6	87	120	9	0	0	0	0	0	20	58	0	0	0	717
	0	3	0	3	12	6	1	0	1	7	5	1	0	10	2	2	0	2	3	0	0	0	19
IA	0	46	0	0	49	85	0	0	4	161	62	17	7	0	0	21	30	0	130	0	0	0	310
	0	14	0	0	44	36	0	0	4	113	38	7	6	0	0	14	15	0	48	0	0	0	112
	0	1	0	2	6	4	0	0	1	7	2	1	1	5	0	1	2	0	3	0	0	0	8
KS	0	19	37	0	72	35	21	0	4	30	105	0	0	0	0	20	0	22	73	0	0	0	17
	0	7	0	0	49	5	11	0	4	28	50	0	0	0	0	17	0	21	22	0	0	0	14
	0	1	1	2	3	1	1	0	1	3	2	0	0	4	0	1	0	1	3	0	0	0	1
KY	0	28	37	0	158	114	57	0	25	50	121	25	5	0	0	120	0	62	86	0	0	0	347
	0	7	14	0	75	37	21	0	16	32	58	9	5	0	0	28	0	7	21	0	0	0	132
	0	1	1	1	7	4	4	0	2	3	5	1	1	12	0	1	0	1	2	0	0	0	8
LA	0	0	0	0	124	22	46	0	0	0	120	26	3	0	0	136	0	375	151	0	0	0	0
	0	0	0	0	92	12	15	0	0	0	66	12	3	0	0	17	0	45	39	0	0	0	0
	0	0	0	4	9	2	1	0	0	0	2	1	1	15	1	1	0	2	3	0	0	0	0
ME	0	0	0	0	9	62	0	0	0	9	137	0	0	0	0	0	0	0	45	0	0	0	117
	0	0	0	0	8	25	0	0	0	5	40	0	0	0	0	0	0	0	15	0	0	0	38
	0	0	0	0	2	3	0	0	0	1	2	0	0	2	1	0	0	0	2	0	0	0	2

* Data were provided by 3,557 (94%) of the responding programs accredited by the 10 agencies listed on p. 447.

** See Table 1 for a key to occupational abbreviations.

MI	MT	NMT	OD	OLT	OMT	OP	OT	OTA	PA	PERF	PTHA	RAD	RADT	RC	REST	RESTT	SBBT	SLP	ST	TRS		Total	State
0	0	21	0	0	0	0	225	112	39	0	0	403	13	23	169	0	2	0	0	0	Enrollments	2,356	Alabama
0	0	11	0	0	0	0	80	71	18	0	0	141	7	6	56	0	1	0	0	0	Graduates	859	
0	1	1	0	0	0	0	3	2	2	0	0	11	2	3	4	0	1	5	0	0	Programs	89	
0	0	0	0	0	0	0	0	0	0	0	0	0	0	0	0	0	0	0	0	0	Enrollments	147	Alaska
0	0	0	0	0	0	0	0	0	0	0	0	0	0	0	0	0	0	0	0	0	Graduates	59	
0	0	0	0	0	0	0	0	0	0	0	0	0	0	0	0	0	0	0	0	0	Programs	5	
0	0	13	0	0	0	0	0	354	0	8	0	218	0	108	231	323	0	0	0	0	Enrollments	2174	Arizona
0	0	0	0	0	0	0	0	109	0	1	0	72	0	0	106	107	0	0	0	0	Graduates	887	
0	1	1	0	0	0	0	0	1	1	1	0	4	0	1	6	4	0	3	0	0	Programs	50	
0	0	16	0	0	0	0	94	0	0	0	0	292	6	111	54	152	0	0	36	0	Enrollments	1138	Arkansas
0	0	15	0	0	0	0	46	0	0	0	0	134	4	17	18	87	0	0	31	0	Graduates	533	
0	0	4	0	0	0	0	1	0	0	0	0	12	2	2	2	6	0	4	2	0	Programs	62	
0	0	0	0	0	0	0	0	0	0	0	0	0	0	0	0	0	0	0	0	0	Enrollments	0	British
0	0	0	0	0	0	0	0	0	0	0	0	0	0	0	0	0	0	0	0	0	Graduates	0	Columbia
0	0	1	0	0	0	0	0	0	0	0	0	0	0	0	0	0	0	0	0	0	Programs	1	
0	0	12	0	0	0	0	691	267	586	0	0	1,378	106	283	1,640	1,283	2	0	293	63	Enrollments	12,072	California
0	0	12	0	0	0	0	298	112	219	0	0	599	45	58	755	707	2	0	159	20	Graduates	5658	
0	3	8	0	0	0	1	4	5	6	0	0	37	8	6	22	9	1	14	7	5	Programs	302	
0	0	10	0	0	0	0	179	166	65	0	0	225	5	0	113	96	0	0	64	14	Enrollments	1,839	Colorado
0	0	7	0	0	0	0	77	64	19	0	0	94	5	0	51	26	0	0	16	7	Graduates	759	
0	1	1	0	0	0	0	1	4	1	0	0	8	0	1	3	2	0	2	3	1	Programs	70	
0	0	14	0	0	0	29	585	0	138	10	0	269	24	0	181	12	0	0	37	92	Enrollments	2,996	Connecticut
0	0	4	0	0	0	26	131	0	51	4	0	101	6	0	42	7	0	0	19	70	Graduates	1,086	
0	0	3	1	0	0	1	2	1	2	1	0	12	3	0	5	1	0	2	2	1	Programs	84	
0	0	22	0	0	0	0	0	37	0	0	0	69	0	0	40	0	0	0	0	0	Enrollments	410	Delaware
0	0	6	0	0	0	0	0	14	0	0	0	27	0	0	18	0	0	0	0	0	Graduates	147	
0	0	1	0	0	0	0	0	1	0	0	0	3	0	0	2	0	0	0	0	0	Programs	18	
0	0	5	0	0	17	0	127	0	232	8	0	148	18	20	48	0	11	0	0	23	Enrollments	871	District of
0	0	3	0	0	8	0	31	0	6	6	0	127	2	10	16	0	6	0	0	3	Graduates	280	Columbia
0	1	1	0	0	1	0	1	0	2	1	0	3	2	2	1	0	1	4	0	1	Programs	36	
0	0	102	0	0	11	0	595	167	248	26	0	871	96	10	757	194	4	0	127	0	Enrollments	8,229	Florida
0	0	37	0	0	6	0	95	79	114	10	0	383	63	5	211	131	3	0	90	0	Graduates	3,397	
0	2	7	2	0	1	0	5	4	2	1	0	26	7	3	19	11	2	6	6	2	Programs	240	
20	0	15	40	0	0	0	87	13	218	0	0	654	21	101	272	142	5	0	147	545	Enrollments	4,543	Georgia
10	0	12	14	0	0	0	43	13	77	0	0	264	17	35	93	46	5	0	71	108	Graduates	1,979	
1	2	1	1	0	0	0	1	2	2	0	0	22	4	3	8	5	1	3	7	1	Programs	134	
0	0	0	0	0	0	0	0	0	0	0	0	37	0	24	27	0	0	0	0	0	Enrollments	254	Hawaii
0	0	0	0	0	0	0	0	0	0	0	0	14	0	4	13	0	0	0	0	0	Graduates	72	
0	0	0	0	0	0	0	0	1	0	1	1	0	0	0	0	0	0	1	0	0	Programs	11	
0	0	0	0	0	0	0	0	37	0	0	0	52	0	21	29	15	0	0	15	0	Enrollments	370	Idaho
0	0	0	0	0	0	0	0	22	0	0	0	31	0	2	12	12	0	0	15	0	Graduates	200	
0	0	0	0	0	0	0	0	1	0	0	0	1	0	1	1	1	0	1	1	0	Programs	21	
25	0	56	0	0	42	0	265	232	324	10	0	1,205	64	149	303	232	2	0	147	182	Enrollments	5,499	Illinois
11	0	31	0	0	14	0	112	132	127	4	0	489	32	28	133	135	0	0	101	51	Graduates	2,366	
1	2	4	0	0	1	0	3	6	3	2	0	31	5	4	11	10	1	11	7	4	Programs	215	
0	0	22	0	0	0	0	429	39	23	0	0	428	39	0	209	71	0	0	210	92	Enrollments	4,651	Indiana
0	0	10	0	0	0	0	185	19	8	0	0	203	18	0	103	54	0	0	74	42	Graduates	1,892	
0	2	2	0	0	0	0	3	1	1	0	0	19	4	0	7	3	0	4	7	1	Programs	131	
0	0	8	0	0	0	0	108	90	106	7	0	354	5	88	129	39	0	0	42	0	Enrollments	1,898	Iowa
0	0	8	0	0	0	0	54	23	53	4	0	124	5	43	45	19	0	0	29	0	Graduates	858	
0	2	1	0	0	0	0	1	2	2	1	0	13	1	2	3	2	0	2	2	2	Programs	80	
0	0	4	0	0	0	0	186	66	89	2	0	258	23	44	175	67	0	0	20	0	Enrollments	1,389	Kansas
0	0	3	0	0	0	0	82	28	33	0	0	90	23	16	99	34	0	0	15	0	Graduates	651	
0	1	1	0	0	0	0	2	1	1	1	0	6	2	1	8	3	0	4	1	0	Programs	57	
0	0	11	0	0	0	0	374	0	91	0	0	481	5	55	146	229	0	0	97	160	Enrollments	2,884	Kentucky
0	0	5	0	0	0	0	125	0	0	0	0	225	4	26	65	101	0	0	77	160	Graduates	1,250	
0	0	2	0	0	0	0	1	0	1	0	0	14	2	1	6	9	0	5	7	1	Programs	103	
0	0	22	0	0	9	0	210	72	0	4	0	480	8	85	170	278	3	0	57	0	Enrollments	2,401	Louisiana
0	0	19	0	0	0	0	87	39	0	4	0	193	7	25	77	53	0	0	44	0	Graduates	849	
0	1	3	0	0	1	0	2	1	1	0	0	12	1	2	6	6	2	7	3	1	Programs	91	
0	0	0	0	0	0	0	207	48	0	0	0	102	11	25	38	0	0	0	35	0	Enrollments	845	Maine
0	0	0	0	0	0	0	49	22	0	0	0	55	5	6	22	0	0	0	26	0	Graduates	316	
0	0	0	0	0	0	0	2	1	1	0	0	5	1	1	2	0	0	1	1	0	Programs	30	

Table 7. Enrollments, Graduates, and Number of Programs by State and Occupation, Academic Year 1995–1996* (cont.)

	AA**	AT	ATR	AUD	CLS/ MT	CLT/ MLTAD	CLT/ MLTC	CVT	CYTO	DA	DH	DLT	DMS	DN	DT	EMTP	ET	HIA	HIT	HTAD	HTC	HTL	MA
MD	0	0	0	0	248	81	76	18	16	61	105	0	68	0	0	30	7	0	179	16	0	0	398
	0	0	0	0	68	28	64	12	10	47	44	0	33	0	0	14	6	0	48	1	0	0	249
	0	0	0	2	5	5	1	1	2	1	3	0	3	10	1	1	1	0	4	1	0	0	1
MA	0	26	121	0	367	180	10	0	4	111	273	29	27	0	0	0	9	55	97	0	0	0	174
	0	3	121	0	81	55	6	0	4	75	99	14	13	0	0	0	5	16	46	0	0	0	103
	0	2	1	3	10	6	1	0	1	8	6	1	1	15	2	0	2	1	5	0	0	0	6
MI	0	109	13	0	392	111	0	0	12	94	546	24	52	0	0	44	0	58	370	0	6	5	680
	0	34	13	0	164	53	0	0	12	44	243	19	41	0	0	27	0	23	161	0	5	4	259
	0	2	1	4	14	4	0	0	2	8	12	1	4	20	1	1	0	2	7	0	4	1	14
MN	0	16	0	0	111	303	20	0	5	799	243	0	24	0	0	83	0	81	193	24	0	0	770
	0	7	0	0	53	130	8	0	5	397	97	0	17	0	0	53	0	15	39	7	0	0	349
	0	2	0	1	5	10	2	1	1	16	8	1	2	12	3	2	0	1	5	2	0	0	12
MS	0	0	0	0	214	191	0	0	18	12	89	0	0	0	0	82	0	37	46	0	0	0	40
	0	0	0	0	57	79	0	0	9	12	40	0	0	0	0	65	0	18	13	0	0	0	18
	0	1	0	2	4	7	0	0	1	2	4	0	0	8	0	6	0	1	2	0	0	0	2
MO	0	57	25	0	109	92	0	0	12	72	151	0	12	0	0	62	0	198	164	0	0	0	107
	0	9	20	0	53	33	0	0	11	57	76	0	12	0	0	27	0	34	87	0	0	0	13
	0	1	1	3	9	2	0	0	2	4	3	0	1	12	1	1	0	2	4	0	2	0	1
MT	0	0	0	0	3	0	0	0	0	70	0	0	0	0	0	0	0	21	62	0	0	0	0
	0	0	0	0	3	0	0	0	0	35	0	0	0	0	0	0	0	7	18	0	0	0	0
	0	0	0	0	1	0	0	0	0	2	0	0	0	1	0	0	0	1	2	0	0	0	0
NE	0	0	0	0	36	57	0	0	4	104	30	14	14	0	0	80	0	26	16	0	0	0	221
	0	0	0	0	36	18	0	0	4	50	15	5	10	0	0	41	0	7	3	0	0	0	122
	0	0	0	1	3	2	0	0	1	5	2	1	2	4	1	1	0	1	1	0	0	0	5
NV	0	0	0	0	94	20	0	0	10	25	33	0	0	0	0	0	0	0	60	0	0	0	0
	0	0	0	0	5	7	0	0	9	16	13	0	0	0	0	0	0	0	5	0	0	0	0
	0	0	0	0	2	1	1	0	1	1	1	0	0	0	2	0	0	0	1	0	0	0	0
NH	0	0	0	0	92	20	0	0	0	24	0	0	0	0	0	38	0	0	0	0	0	0	194
	0	0	0	0	17	8	0	0	0	19	0	0	0	0	0	14	0	0	0	0	0	0	146
	0	1	0	0	1	1	0	0	1	1	0	0	0	3	1	1	0	0	0	0	0	0	2
NJ	0	0	0	0	61	282	8	9	7	244	202	0	72	0	0	0	0	65	89	0	0	0	449
	0	0	0	0	47	81	7	8	5	115	68	0	44	0	0	0	0	13	22	0	0	0	268
	0	1	0	1	6	10	1	1	1	6	4	0	4	7	2	0	0	1	2	0	2	0	4
NM	0	0	10	0	29	62	0	0	0	0	69	0	7	0	0	60	0	0	0	0	0	0	0
	0	0	0	0	12	21	0	0	0	0	43	0	7	0	0	54	0	0	0	0	0	0	0
	0	1	1	1	1	5	0	0	0	1	1	0	1	3	0	3	0	0	1	0	0	0	0
NY	0	62	346	0	408	591	4	0	43	87	728	112	186	0	0	65	13	170	656	34	0	0	987
	0	23	76	0	165	157	3	0	34	74	288	43	76	0	0	20	8	53	189	13	0	0	188
	0	2	6	13	14	12	1	0	6	2	10	2	5	38	7	1	1	4	11	1	0	0	9
NC	0	66	0	0	193	248	0	0	17	229	214	18	38	0	0	86	0	70	134	0	0	0	830
	0	20	0	0	120	99	0	0	12	165	80	6	20	0	0	26	0	34	56	0	0	0	335
	0	3	0	3	10	9	0	0	4	13	7	1	3	16	0	2	0	2	6	0	0	1	13
ND	0	22	0	0	121	21	0	0	6	37	55	0	0	0	0	0	0	0	50	0	0	0	0
	0	4	0	0	29	7	0	0	6	34	27	0	0	0	0	0	0	0	21	0	0	0	0
	0	3	0	1	4	1	0	0	1	2	1	0	0	4	0	0	0	0	2	0	0	0	0
OH	12	81	79	0	191	479	4	56	8	52	484	66	87	0	0	235	0	34	357	0	0	0	1,484
	8	23	26	0	111	185	4	31	8	31	199	10	44	0	0	151	0	19	117	0	0	0	507
	1	3	2	8	13	14	1	2	3	3	9	2	6	30	9	5	0	1	7	0	1	0	25
OK	0	0	0	0	37	81	0	0	0	12	99	0	36	0	0	0	0	105	58	0	0	0	88
	0	0	0	0	37	33	0	0	0	12	48	0	16	0	0	0	0	28	19	0	0	0	43
	0	0	0	1	7	4	0	0	1	1	3	0	1	9	1	0	0	2	2	0	0	0	2
OR	0	130	26	0	19	42	0	0	0	159	226	38	0	0	0	111	0	0	94	0	0	0	64
	0	15	0	0	18	16	0	0	0	123	126	20	0	0	0	48	0	0	39	0	0	0	51
	0	1	1	1	1	1	0	0	0	7	5	1	0	3	1	1	0	0	2	0	0	0	3
PA	0	196	73	0	234	328	5	55	24	126	418	0	64	0	0	205	10	213	227	0	8	0	1,490
	0	36	17	0	185	112	5	30	21	100	172	0	42	0	0	142	4	83	81	0	8	0	746
	0	7	2	5	24	12	2	4	2	6	10	0	4	26	4	4	1	5	6	1	2	0	16
PR	0	0	0	0	284	0	0	0	0	0	0	0	0	0	0	0	0	24	159	0	0	0	0
	0	0	0	0	171	0	0	0	0	0	0	0	0	0	0	0	0	8	48	0	0	0	0
	0	0	0	0	5	0	0	0	1	1	1	0	0	4	0	0	0	1	4	0	0	0	0
QU	0	0	0	0	0	0	0	0	0	0	0	0	0	0	0	0	0	0	0	0	0	0	0
	0	0	0	0	0	0	0	0	0	0	0	0	0	0	0	0	0	0	0	0	0	0	0
	0	0	1	0	0	0	0	0	0	0	0	0	0	0	0	0	0	0	0	0	0	0	0

* Data were provided by 3,557 (94%) of the responding programs accredited by the 10 agencies listed on p. 447.

** See Table 1 for a key to occupational abbreviations.

MI	MT	NMT	OD	OLT	OMT	OP	OT	OTA	PA	PERF	PTHA	RAD	RADT	RC	REST	RESTT	SBBT	SLP	ST	TRS		Total	State
11	0	48	0	0	0	0	208	150	75	11	0	327	11	16	207	0	5	0	97	0	Enrollments	2,469	Maryland
5	0	33	0	0	0	0	61	81	44	9	0	147	6	5	83	0	5	0	92	0	Graduates	1,195	
1	0	3	0	0	0	0	1	2	2	1	0	14	1	2	5	0	2	3	1	0	Programs	80	
0	0	86	41	0	0	0	801	425	163	8	0	294	73	239	236	58	1	0	94	0	Enrollments	4,002	Massa-
0	0	25	18	0	0	0	234	174	43	3	0	143	24	107	97	33	0	0	68	0	Graduates	1,610	chusetts
0	2	5	2	0	1	0	4	10	2	1	0	10	4	5	8	2	1	6	3	1	Programs	138	
15	0	69	23	0	0	0	663	244	101	0	0	654	11	44	460	36	0	0	55	106	Enrollments	4,997	Michigan
8	0	32	12	0	0	0	223	119	37	0	0	249	11	19	178	29	0	0	30	99	Graduates	2,148	
1	3	2	1	0	1	0	5	6	4	0	1	23	5	2	12	3	0	6	3	1	Programs	181	
0	0	14	0	0	11	0	376	375	0	5	0	295	13	69	153	56	0	0	143	0	Enrollments	4,182	Minnesota
0	0	10	0	0	5	0	121	117	0	5	0	126	11	23	50	18	0	0	74	0	Graduates	1,737	
0	2	2	1	0	1	0	3	5	1	1	0	13	3	2	5	1	1	5	4	1	Programs	137	
0	0	0	6	0	0	0	53	0	0	0	0	280	0	31	200	203	0	0	26	55	Enrollments	1,583	Mississippi
0	0	0	6	0	0	0	25	0	0	0	0	121	0	7	101	121	0	0	16	14	Graduates	722	
0	1	1	0	0	0	0	1	0	0	1	0	10	0	2	6	6	0	3	1	1	Programs	73	
0	0	41	0	0	0	0	550	229	66	0	0	452	12	16	89	67	1	0	22	0	Enrollments	2,606	Missouri
0	0	12	0	0	0	0	225	83	28	0	0	194	8	0	51	57	1	0	16	0	Graduates	1,107	
0	2	3	0	0	0	0	4	3	1	0	0	16	2	1	3	6	0	7	1	1	Programs	99	
0	0	0	0	0	0	0	0	46	0	0	0	36	0	34	33	43	0	0	15	0	Enrollments	363	Montana
0	0	0	0	0	0	0	0	17	0	0	0	18	0	22	14	22	0	0	0	0	Graduates	156	
0	0	0	0	0	0	0	0	1	1	0	0	3	0	1	1	2	0	0	1	0	Programs	17	
0	0	6	0	0	0	0	154	0	120	10	0	154	4	0	86	18	0	0	58	0	Enrollments	1,212	Nebraska
0	0	4	0	0	0	0	19	0	40	0	0	75	4	0	55	17	0	0	42	0	Graduates	567	
0	0	1	0	0	0	0	1	1	1	1	0	7	2	0	4	1	0	3	2	0	Programs	54	
0	0	19	0	0	0	0	0	0	0	0	0	31	0	0	0	0	0	0	0	0	Enrollments	292	Nevada
0	0	17	0	0	0	0	0	0	0	0	0	16	0	0	0	0	0	0	0	0	Graduates	88	
0	0	1	0	0	0	0	0	0	0	0	0	2	0	0	0	0	0	0	1	0	Programs	14	
0	0	0	0	0	0	0	285	54	0	0	0	45	0	0	19	0	0	0	0	0	Enrollments	771	New
0	0	0	0	0	0	0	70	21	0	0	0	14	0	0	8	0	0	0	0	0	Graduates	317	Hampshire
0	0	0	1	0	0	0	1	1	0	0	0	1	0	0	1	0	0	0	1	0	Programs	18	
0	0	27	84	0	0	0	101	77	123	19	0	640	11	0	205	69	0	0	37	0	Enrollments	2,881	New Jersey
0	0	17	27	0	0	0	28	37	33	4	0	281	10	0	97	55	0	0	29	0	Graduates	1,296	
0	1	3	3	0	0	0	1	2	1	2	0	24	2	0	7	3	0	4	3	0	Programs	109	
0	0	4	0	0	0	0	48	118	0	0	0	122	0	0	41	24	0	0	0	0	Enrollments	594	New
0	0	4	0	0	0	0	20	44	0	0	0	57	0	0	22	6	0	0	0	0	Graduates	290	Mexico
0	0	1	1	1	0	0	1	2	0	0	0	5	0	0	1	0	0	3	0	0	Programs	34	
0	0	254	34	12	2	0	1,688	648	923	7	0	908	123	228	928	84	0	0	144	90	Enrollments	10,565	New York
0	0	114	8	4	2	0	499	200	379	2	0	405	66	88	260	54	0	0	74	32	Graduates	3,597	
0	3	11	4	1	1	0	13	7	14	2	0	37	8	6	12	3	1	21	4	1	Programs	294	
0	0	52	42	0	6	0	112	227	180	0	0	615	31	63	298	112	0	0	100	60	Enrollments	4,041	North
0	0	26	23	0	2	0	37	87	86	0	0	257	20	0	147	67	0	0	70	14	Graduates	1,809	Carolina
0	2	4	1	0	1	0	3	5	4	0	1	20	3	2	12	6	0	6	7	2	Programs	171	
0	0	0	0	0	0	0	0	96	81	0	0	35	0	0	27	0	0	0	0	0	Enrollments	551	North
0	0	0	0	0	0	0	0	40	80	0	0	18	0	0	19	0	0	0	0	0	Graduates	285	Dakota
0	0	0	0	0	0	0	1	1	1	0	0	4	0	0	2	0	0	2	0	0	Programs	30	
0	0	158	0	0	0	0	522	442	176	39	0	1,005	85	135	655	65	2	0	131	0	Enrollments	7,214	Ohio
0	0	70	0	0	0	0	179	167	75	22	0	402	37	41	246	39	2	0	66	0	Graduates	2,820	
0	4	5	0	0	0	0	6	8	4	3	0	29	6	5	16	4	3	10	4	1	Programs	253	
0	0	16	0	0	0	0	71	36	100	0	0	258	22	25	64	81	0	0	52	0	Enrollments	1,241	Oklahoma
0	0	6	0	0	0	0	34	35	45	0	0	115	10	10	28	45	0	0	42	0	Graduates	606	
0	2	1	0	0	0	0	1	2	1	0	0	10	1	1	2	3	0	5	5	1	Programs	69	
0	0	0	0	0	33	0	46	38	0	4	0	365	12	64	118	13	0	0	38	0	Enrollments	1,640	Oregon
0	0	0	0	0	18	0	21	18	0	4	0	75	7	22	44	11	0	0	11	0	Graduates	687	
0	1	1	1	0	1	0	1	1	1	1	0	2	1	2	4	2	0	2	1	0	Programs	50	
0	0	87	0	0	0	0	1,141	632	704	83	0	1,211	87	87	578	171	0	0	148	162	Enrollments	8,767	Penn-
0	0	47	0	0	0	0	249	259	212	37	0	508	56	43	180	74	0	0	70	30	Graduates	3,549	sylvania
0	7	4	0	0	0	0	8	6	8	5	0	54	3	4	15	9	0	9	6	2	Programs	283	
0	0	8	0	0	0	0	105	67	0	0	0	106	0	115	140	140	0	0	0	0	Enrollments	1,148	Puerto Rico
0	0	6	0	0	0	0	27	18	0	0	0	37	0	0	55	98	0	0	0	0	Graduates	468	
0	0	1	0	0	0	0	1	1	0	0	0	2	0	1	3	1	0	0	0	0	Programs	27	
0	0	0	0	0	0	0	0	0	0	0	0	0	0	0	0	0	0	0	0	0	Enrollments	0	Quebec
0	0	0	0	0	0	0	0	0	0	0	0	0	0	0	0	0	0	0	0	0	Graduates	0	
0	0	0	0	0	0	0	0	0	0	0	0	0	0	0	0	0	0	0	0	0	Programs	1	

Table 7. Enrollments, Graduates, and Number of Programs by State and Occupation, Academic Year 1995–1996* (cont.)

	AA**	AT	ATR	AUD	CLS/ MT	CLT/ MLTAD	CLT/ MLTC	CVT	CYTO	DA	DH	DLT	DMS	DN	DT	EMTP	ET	HIA	HIT	HTAD	HTC	HTL	MA
RI	0	0	0	0	14	32	0	0	14	23	0	0	4	0	0	0	0	0	0	0	0	0	0
	0	0	0	0	14	11	0	0	14	16	0	0	4	0	0	0	0	0	0	0	0	0	0
	0	0	0	1	2	1	0	0	2	1	1	0	1	2	0	0	0	0	0	0	0	0	0
SC	0	0	0	0	40	239	0	0	11	133	309	0	0	0	0	34	0	19	22	0	0	0	134
	0	0	0	0	34	74	0	0	9	103	105	0	0	0	0	15	0	15	6	0	0	0	50
	0	1	0	0	4	8	0	0	1	8	5	0	0	6	1	1	0	1	2	0	0	0	4
SD	0	0	0	0	18	71	0	90	3	36	59	0	0	0	0	0	0	36	52	0	0	0	55
	0	0	0	0	17	30	0	45	3	25	27	0	0	0	0	0	0	6	20	0	0	0	11
	0	0	0	1	3	3	0	1	1	1	1	0	0	3	0	0	0	1	2	0	0	0	2
TN	0	0	0	0	147	210	0	0	12	82	222	0	24	0	0	192	0	68	141	0	0	0	334
	0	0	0	0	67	98	0	0	10	55	72	0	23	0	0	109	0	25	61	0	0	0	72
	0	0	0	4	7	7	0	0	2	5	5	1	2	16	1	5	0	2	3	0	0	0	4
TX	0	22	0	0	487	506	321	23	10	434	661	116	33	0	0	594	0	103	532	0	8	0	389
	0	5	0	0	241	180	301	6	10	386	210	89	30	0	0	433	0	64	149	0	7	0	30
	0	1	0	6	27	20	2	1	3	7	14	3	4	37	5	7	0	3	11	0	3	0	5
UT	0	127	0	0	129	87	0	0	4	115	61	0	0	0	0	44	0	0	29	0	0	0	334
	0	45	0	0	52	25	0	0	4	88	29	0	0	0	0	43	0	0	13	0	0	0	133
	0	1	0	3	3	2	0	0	1	2	1	0	0	5	0	1	0	0	1	0	0	0	4
VT	0	32	33	0	82	0	0	0	6	28	47	0	0	0	0	0	0	0	0	0	0	0	0
	0	10	12	0	13	0	0	0	6	28	18	0	0	0	0	0	0	0	0	0	0	0	0
	0	1	1	0	1	0	0	0	1	1	1	0	0	2	0	0	0	0	0	0	0	0	0
VA	0	0	30	0	137	131	11	14	7	214	243	0	76	0	0	280	0	68	81	0	0	0	138
	0	0	13	0	71	49	9	4	7	162	116	0	60	0	0	133	0	8	22	0	0	0	64
	0	0	1	3	8	4	3	1	1	5	5	1	1	13	3	2	0	1	3	0	0	0	7
WA	0	27	0	0	65	61	11	55	0	232	286	55	77	0	0	67	0	14	158	8	0	0	110
	0	10	0	0	36	18	10	22	0	152	88	12	36	0	0	58	0	9	45	2	0	0	68
	0	1	0	3	3	3	1	1	1	8	6	1	2	11	2	4	0	1	3	1	0	0	4
WV	0	31	0	0	65	96	9	0	10	0	215	0	25	0	0	0	0	0	60	0	0	0	0
	0	7	0	0	27	50	8	0	8	0	77	0	25	0	0	0	0	0	36	0	0	0	0
	0	1	0	1	3	4	2	0	2	0	3	0	2	6	0	0	0	0	2	0	0	0	0
WI	0	27	34	0	199	217	0	0	20	124	387	23	98	0	0	0	27	41	189	24	4	0	865
	0	10	18	0	107	73	0	0	20	85	110	14	50	0	0	0	13	0	60	7	4	0	364
	0	1	1	3	10	5	0	0	3	7	6	1	5	14	2	0	1	1	5	1	1	0	12
WY	0	0	0	0	75	0	0	0	0	15	65	0	0	0	0	0	0	0	0	0	0	0	0
	0	0	0	0	14	0	0	0	0	14	26	0	0	0	0	0	0	0	0	0	0	0	0
	0	0	0	1	1	0	0	0	0	1	2	0	0	0	0	0	0	0	0	0	0	0	0
Totals	12	1,455	1,107	0	6,985	6,439	957	503	378	6,496	9,776	939	1,377	28,336+	6,562+	5,062	177	2,590	6,244	124	44	9	20,512
	8	393	376	0	3,155	2,269	661	226	315	4,341	4,001	398	782	5,769+	732+	2,756	86	758	2,049	34	38	6	8,443
	2	55	27	120	339	224	38	16	64	237	222	35	75	536	72	98	11	53	158	9	23	3	272

* Data were provided by 3,557 (94%) of the responding programs accredited by the 10 agencies listed on p. 447.

** See Table 1 for a key to occupational abbreviations.

+ These data were provided on an aggregate rather than state-by-state basis.

MI	MT	NMT	OD	OLT	OMT	OP	OT	OTA	PA	PERF	PTHA	RAD	RADT	RC	REST	RESTT	SBBT	SLP	ST	TRS		Total	State
0	0	4	0	0	0	0	0	0	0	0	0	86	4	0	36	0	0	0	0	0	Enrollments	217	Rhode
0	0	4	0	0	0	0	0	0	0	0	0	37	4	0	17	0	0	0	0	0	Graduates	121	Island
0	0	1	0	0	0	0	0	0	0	0	0	2	1	0	1	0	0	1	1	0	Programs	18	
0	0	7	0	0	0	0	69	22	57	0	0	274	17	88	101	138	0	0	109	83	Enrollments	1,906	South
0	0	6	0	0	0	0	28	21	22	0	0	119	8	43	70	53	0	0	77	22	Graduates	880	Carolina
0	1	1	0	0	0	0	1	1	1	1	0	11	1	2	6	6	0	2	5	1	Programs	82	
0	0	32	0	0	0	0	75	0	29	0	0	70	0	0	47	0	0	0	11	0	Enrollments	684	South
0	0	14	0	0	0	0	21	0	12	0	0	35	0	0	12	0	0	0	4	0	Graduates	282	Dakota
0	0	1	0	0	0	0	1	0	1	0	0	6	0	0	1	0	0	1	1	0	Programs	31	
0	0	35	30	0	0	0	137	84	59	3	0	421	32	53	184	75	0	0	30	0	Enrollments	2,575	Tennessee
0	0	33	14	0	0	0	48	41	50	0	0	175	27	22	77	55	0	0	24	0	Graduates	1,158	
0	1	5	1	0	0	0	2	2	1	1	0	12	4	2	6	4	0	5	2	0	Programs	112	
7	0	120	13	0	0	0	1,066	420	430	32	0	1,830	72	61	780	644	9	0	353	0	Enrollments	10,076	Texas
3	0	27	5	0	0	0	329	246	123	29	0	949	44	20	231	404	5	0	208	0	Graduates	4,764	
1	4	5	1	0	0	0	4	8	5	2	0	36	5	4	21	18	4	14	16	1	Programs	308	
0	0	2	0	0	0	0	0	40	64	0	0	61	1	72	22	33	0	0	25	140	Enrollments	1,390	Utah
0	0	1	0	0	0	0	0	29	32	0	0	32	1	16	18	17	0	0	18	9	Graduates	605	
0	1	1	0	0	0	0	0	1	1	0	0	2	0	1	1	1	0	3	1	2	Programs	39	
0	0	11	0	0	0	0	0	0	0	0	0	49	12	0	22	0	0	0	0	0	Enrollments	322	Vermont
0	0	3	0	0	0	0	0	0	0	0	0	23	6	0	7	0	0	0	0	0	Graduates	126	
0	0	1	0	0	0	0	0	0	0	0	0	2	1	0	1	0	0	1	0	0	Programs	14	
0	0	46	103	0	6	0	248	118	0	0	0	392	25	113	189	214	0	0	111	140	Enrollments	3,135	Virginia
0	0	11	93	0	3	0	81	44	0	0	0	186	18	50	76	112	0	0	91	57	Graduates	1,540	
0	2	4	2	1	1	0	2	2	0	0	0	15	4	1	6	6	0	5	4	3	Programs	120	
0	0	2	0	0	0	0	161	124	126	0	0	244	26	0	104	19	0	0	97	44	Enrollments	2,173	Washington
0	0	2	0	0	0	0	91	19	57	0	0	88	12	0	52	14	0	0	58	25	Graduates	984	
0	0	1	1	0	0	0	2	2	1	0	0	6	1	0	4	1	0	4	3	1	Programs	83	
0	0	12	0	0	0	0	0	0	57	0	0	258	4	52	119	26	0	0	33	0	Enrollments	1,072	West
0	0	11	0	0	0	0	0	0	15	0	0	121	4	39	47	20	0	0	25	0	Graduates	520	Virginia
0	0	3	0	0	0	0	0	0	2	0	0	9	1	1	4	1	0	2	2	0	Programs	51	
0	0	18	0	0	0	0	297	219	0	6	0	418	12	85	202	35	4	0	224	215	Enrollments	4,014	Wisconsin
0	0	18	0	0	0	0	105	58	0	2	0	188	12	35	65	24	2	0	114	60	Graduates	1,618	
0	3	4	0	0	0	0	4	3	1	1	0	18	3	3	5	0	1	8	8	1	Programs	142	
0	0	0	0	0	0	0	0	0	0	0	0	48	0	0	7	30	0	0	0	0	Enrollments	240	Wyoming
0	0	0	0	0	0	0	0	0	0	0	0	18	0	0	6	30	0	0	0	0	Graduates	108	
0	0	0	0	0	0	0	1	0	0	0	0	3	0	0	1	1	0	1	0	0	Programs	13	
78	0	1,532	410	12	137	29	13,339	6,631	5,793	302	0	19,908	1,144	2,837	11,081	5,587	51	0	3,480	2,266	Total Enrollments		145,773
37	0	732	214	4	58	26	4,270	2,722	2,138	150	0	8,595	649	893	4,348	2,994	32	0	2,086	683	Total Graduates		61,710
5	61	118	24	3	11	2	105	117	87	31	2	648	106	84	293	162	22	223	145	41	Total Programs		4,979